Essentials of
Psychiatric Mental Health Nursing

3RD EDITION

Mary C. Townsend, RN, MN, CS
Clinical Nurse Specialist
Psychiatric/Mental Health Nursing
Private Practice

Formerly Assistant Professor and Coordinator,
Mental Health Nursing
Kramer School of Nursing
Oklahoma City University
Oklahoma City, Oklahoma

F.A. Davis Company • Philadelphia

F. A. Davis Company
1915 Arch Street
Philadelphia, PA 19103
www.fadavis.com

Printed in the United States of America

Last digit indicates print number: 10 9 8 7 6 5 4 3 2 1

Publisher, Nursing: Robert G. Martone
Design Manager: Joan Wendt

As new scientific information becomes available through basic and clinical research, recommended treatments and drug therapies undergo changes. The author(s) and publisher have done everything possible to make this book accurate, up to date, and in accord with accepted standards at the time of publication. The author(s), editors, and publisher are not responsible for errors or omissions or for consequences from application of the book, and make no warranty, expressed or implied, in regard to the contents of the book. Any practice described in this book should be applied by the reader in accordance with professional standards of care used in regard to the unique circumstances that may apply in each situation. The reader is advised always to check product information (package inserts) for changes and new information regarding dose and contraindications before administering any drug. Caution is especially urged when using new or infrequently ordered drugs.

Library of Congress Cataloging-in-Publication Data

Townsend, Mary C., 1941-
Essentials of psychiatric mental health nursing / Mary C. Townsend.— 3rd ed.
p. ; cm.
Includes bibliographical references and index.
ISBN 0-8036-1267-2 (hardcover : alk. paper)
1. Psychiatric nursing.
[DNLM: 1. Psychiatric Nursing—methods. 2. Mental Disorders—nursing. WY 160 T749e 2005] I. Title.
RC440.T689 2005
616.89′0231—dc22

2004006560

- New research studies with **Implications of Research for Evidence-Based Practice** throughout each of the major diagnostic chapters, describing studies that provide research-based evidence for specific nursing interventions
- **New and updated psychotropic medication** information
- **Test Your Critical Thinking Skills** boxes—with case studies and exercises
- **Care Plans** for clients with DSM-IV-TR diagnoses, with interventions and rationales for commonly observed nursing diagnoses
- **Critical Pathways of Care**
- **Case Studies**
- Twenty-one sample **Client Teaching Guides** containing information related to psychotropic medications and psychiatric illnesses—that can be reproduced as handouts for client education
- Appendices providing all the DSM-IV-TR classifications, NANDA diagnoses and behaviors, critical pathways, and guidelines for mental health assessment, as well as a glossary to the entire textbook

CHAPTER 22 ● VICTIMS OF ABUSE OR NEGLECT 523

INTERNET REFERENCES

- Additional information related to child abuse may be located at the following Web sites:
  a http://www.childabuse.org/
  b http://www.fvpf.org
  c http://www.child-abuse.com
- Additional information related to sexual assault may be located at the following Web sites:
  a http://www.vaw.umn.edu/Vawnet/mrape.htm
  b http://www.ncweb.com/org/rapecrisis
- Additional information related to domestic violence may be located at the following Web sites:
  a http://www.ndvh.org/
  b http://www.cpsdv.org/
  c http://home.cybergrrl.com/dv/book/toc.html
  d http://crisis-support.org/
  e http://www.ama-assn.org/ama/pub/category/3242.html

TEST YOUR CRITICAL THINKING SKILLS

Sandy is a psychiatric nurse who works at the safe house for battered women. Lisa has just been admitted with her two small children after she was treated in the emergency department. She had been beaten severely by her husband when he was intoxicated last night. She escaped with her children after he passed out in their bedroom.

In her initial assessment, Sandy learns from Lisa that she has been battered by her husband for 5 years, beginning shortly after their marriage. She explained that she "knew he drank quite a lot before we were married, but thought he would stop after we had kids." Instead, the drinking has increased. Sometimes he doesn't even get home from work until 11:00 or midnight, after stopping to drink at the bar with his buddies.

IMPLICATIONS OF RESEARCH FOR EVIDENCE BASED PRACTICE

Sachs, B., Hall, L.A., Lutenbacher, M., and Rayens, M.K.: **Potential for abusive parenting by rural mothers with low-birth-weight children.** Image: Journal of Nursing Scholarship (1999); 31(1):21–25.

Description of the Study: The purpose of this study was to describe factors influencing the potential for abusive parenting by rural mothers of low birth weight (LBW) children. The convenience sample in this study included 48 mothers of LBW children, ranging in age from 18 to 39 years, all living in a rural area of the state, and all living with their LBW infant at the time of the study. Average length of the children's hospitalization after birth was 6 weeks, and the average age at time of the study was 9 months. In-home interviews were conducted using structured questionnaires to assess the mothers' everyday stressors, depressive symptoms, functional social support, quality of family relationships, and child abuse potential.

Results of the Study: According to the questionnaires used for measurement, 54 percent of the mothers indicated a high level of depressive symptoms, and 63 percent indicated a high potential for physical child abuse. No significant differences were noted in depressive symptoms and potential for child abuse by birth weight, health status of the child, or time since hospital discharge. Mothers with high child abuse potential reported more everyday stressors and depressive symptoms, less functional social support, and poorer family functioning. Because in this study everyday stressors and the two social support systems (functional social support and quality of family relationships) were examined as predictors of depressive symptoms, it is suggested that everyday stressors exert both a direct and an indirect effect on mothers' potential for child abuse. The strongest predictor of child abuse potential was mothers' depressive symptoms.

Implications for Nursing Practice: The researchers conclude that rural mothers of LBW children are at risk for abusive parenting. This study demonstrated the ad-

148 UNIT II ● PSYCHIATRIC/MENTAL HEALTH NURSING INTERVENTIONS

TABLE 9–2 Care Plan for the Client Who Has Experienced a Traumatic Event[1]

Nursing Diagnosis: ANXIETY (PANIC)/FEAR
Related to: Real or perceived threat to physical well-being; threat of death; situational crisis; exposure to toxins; unmet needs
Evidenced by: Persistent feelings of apprehension and uneasiness; sense of impending doom; impaired functioning; verbal expressions of having no control or influence over situation, outcome, or self-care; sympathetic stimulation; extraneous physical movements

Outcome Criteria	Nursing Interventions	Rationale
Client will maintain anxiety at manageable level.	1. Determine degree of anxiety/fear present, associated behaviors (e.g., laughter, crying, calm or agitation, excited/hysterical behavior, expressions of disbelief and/or self-blame), and reality of perceived threat.	1. Clearly understanding client's perception is pivotal to providing appropriate assistance in overcoming the fear. Individual may be agitated or totally overwhelmed. Panic state increases risk for client's own safety as well as the safety of others in the environment.
	2. Note degree of disorganization.	2. Client may be unable to handle ADLs or work requirements and need more intensive intervention.
	3. Create as quiet an area as possible. Maintain a calm confident manner. Speak in even tones, using short simple sentences.	3. Decreases sense of confusion or overstimulation; enhances sense of safety. Helps client focus on what is said and reduces transmission of anxiety.
	4. Develop trusting relationship with the client.	4. Trust is the basis of a therapeutic nurse/client relationship and enables them to work effectively together.
	5. Identify whether incident has reactivated preexisting or coexisting situations (physical or psychological).	5. Concerns and psychological issues will be recycled every time trauma is reexperienced and affect how the client views the current situation.
	6. Determine presence of physical symptoms (e.g., numbness, headache, tightness in chest, nausea, and pounding heart).	6. Physical problems need to be differentiated from anxiety symptoms so appropriate treatment can be given.
	7. Identify psychological responses (e.g., anger, shock, acute anxiety, panic, confusion, denial). Record emotional changes.	7. Although these are normal responses at the time of the trauma, they will recycle again and again until they are dealt with adequately.
	8. Discuss with client the perception of what is causing the anxiety.	8. Increases the ability to connect symptoms to subjective feeling of anxiety, providing opportunity to gain insight/control and make desired changes.
	9. Assist client to correct any distortions being experienced. Share perceptions with client.	9. Perceptions based on reality will help to decrease fearfulness. How the nurse views the situation may ... it differently.

CHAPTER 16 ● ANXIETY DISORDERS 359

CASE STUDY

John was afraid to ride on elevators. He had been known to climb 24 flights of stairs in an office building to avoid riding the elevator. John's own insurance office had plans for moving the company to a high-rise building soon, with offices on the 32nd floor. John sought assistance from a therapist who employed systematic desensitization for this problem. He was taught to achieve a sense of calmness and well-being by using a combination of mental imagery and progressive relaxation techniques. In the relaxed state, John was initially instructed to imagine the entry level of his office building, with a clear image of the bank of elevators. In subsequent sessions, and always in the relaxed state, John progressed to images of walking onto an elevator, having the elevator door close after he had entered, riding the elevator to the 32nd floor, and emerging from the elevator once the doors were

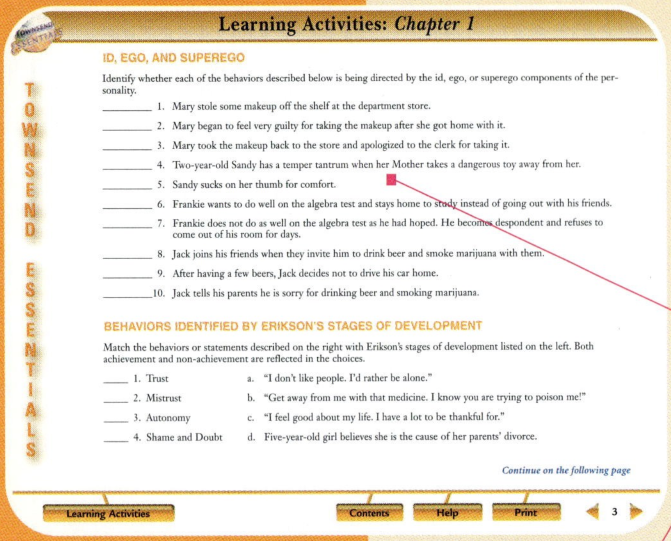

Learning Activities: *Chapter 1*

ID, EGO, AND SUPEREGO

Identify whether each of the behaviors described below is being directed by the id, ego, or superego components of the personality.

_________ 1. Mary stole some makeup off the shelf at the department store.
_________ 2. Mary began to feel very guilty for taking the makeup after she got home with it.
_________ 3. Mary took the makeup back to the store and apologized to the clerk for taking it.
_________ 4. Two-year-old Sandy has a temper tantrum when her Mother takes a dangerous toy away from her.
_________ 5. Sandy sucks on her thumb for comfort.
_________ 6. Frankie wants to do well on the algebra test and stays home to study instead of going out with his friends.
_________ 7. Frankie does not do as well on the algebra test as he had hoped. He becomes despondent and refuses to come out of his room for days.
_________ 8. Jack joins his friends when they invite him to drink beer and smoke marijuana with them.
_________ 9. After having a few beers, Jack decides not to drive his car home.
_________10. Jack tells his parents he is sorry for drinking beer and smoking marijuana.

BEHAVIORS IDENTIFIED BY ERIKSON'S STAGES OF DEVELOPMENT

Match the behaviors or statements described on the right with Erikson's stages of development listed on the left. Both achievement and non-achievement are reflected in the choices.

____ 1. Trust	a. "I don't like people. I'd rather be alone."
____ 2. Mistrust	b. "Get away from me with that medicine. I know you are trying to poison me!"
____ 3. Autonomy	c. "I feel good about my life. I have a lot to be thankful for."
____ 4. Shame and Doubt	d. Five-year-old girl believes she is the cause of her parents' divorce.

Continue on the following page

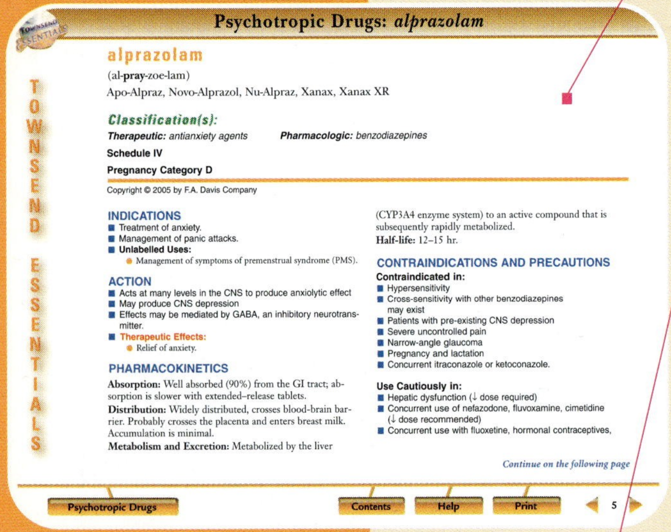

Psychotropic Drugs: *alprazolam*

alprazolam

(al-pray-zoe-lam)

Apo-Alpraz, Novo-Alprazol, Nu-Alpraz, Xanax, Xanax XR

Classification(s):

Therapeutic: *antianxiety agents* ***Pharmacologic:*** *benzodiazepines*

Schedule IV

Pregnancy Category D

INDICATIONS

- Treatment of anxiety.
- Management of panic attacks.
- **Unlabelled Uses:**
  - Management of symptoms of premenstrual syndrome (PMS).

ACTION

- Acts at many levels in the CNS to produce anxiolytic effect
- May produce CNS depression
- Effects may be mediated by GABA, an inhibitory neurotransmitter.
- **Therapeutic Effects:**
  - Relief of anxiety.

PHARMACOKINETICS

Absorption: Well absorbed (90%) from the GI tract; absorption is slower with extended-release tablets.
Distribution: Widely distributed, crosses blood-brain barrier. Probably crosses the placenta and enters breast milk. Accumulation is minimal.
Metabolism and Excretion: Metabolized by the liver (CYP3A4 enzyme system) to an active compound that is subsequently rapidly metabolized.
Half-life: 12–15 hr.

CONTRAINDICATIONS AND PRECAUTIONS

Contraindicated in:

- Hypersensitivity
- Cross-sensitivity with other benzodiazepines may exist
- Patients with pre-existing CNS depression
- Severe uncontrolled pain
- Narrow-angle glaucoma
- Pregnancy and lactation
- Concurrent itraconazole or ketoconazole.

Use Cautiously in:

- Hepatic dysfunction (↓ dose required)
- Concurrent use of nefazodone, fluvoxamine, cimetidine (↓ dose recommended)
- Concurrent use with fluoxetine, hormonal contraceptives,

Continue on the following page

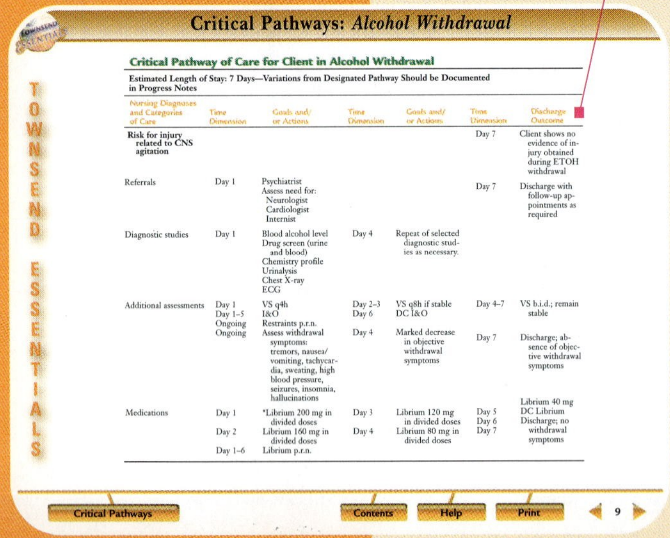

Critical Pathways: *Alcohol Withdrawal*

Critical Pathway of Care for Client in Alcohol Withdrawal

Estimated Length of Stay: 7 Days—Variations from Designated Pathway Should be Documented in Progress Notes

Nursing Diagnoses and Categories of Care	Time Dimension	Goals and/or Actions	Time Dimension	Goals and/or Actions	Time Dimension	Discharge Outcome
Risk for injury related to CNS agitation					Day 7	Client shows no evidence of injury obtained during ETOH withdrawal
Referrals	Day 1	Psychiatrist Assess need for: Neurologist Cardiologist Internist			Day 7	Discharge with follow-up appointments as required
Diagnostic studies	Day 1	Blood alcohol level Drug screen (urine and blood) Chemistry profile Urinalysis Chest X-ray ECG	Day 4	Repeat of selected diagnostic studies as necessary.		
Additional assessments	Day 1 Day 1–5 Ongoing Ongoing	VS q4h I&O Restraints p.r.n. Assess withdrawal symptoms: tremors, nausea/vomiting, tachycardia, sweating, high blood pressure, seizures, insomnia, hallucinations	Day 2–3 Day 6 Day 4	VS q8h if stable DC I&O Marked decrease in objective withdrawal symptoms	Day 4–7 Day 7	VS b.i.d.; remain stable Discharge; absence of objective withdrawal symptoms
Medications	Day 1 Day 2 Day 1–6	*Librium 200 mg in divided doses Librium 160 mg in divided doses Librium p.r.n.	Day 3 Day 4	Librium 120 mg in divided doses Librium 80 mg in divided doses	Day 5 Day 6 Day 7	Librium 40 mg DC Librium Discharge; no withdrawal symptoms

On the attached Student CD-ROM, you will find helpful learning and teaching aids

- **Electronic Test Bank**
  - **220 NCLEX-style questions,** including the new alternate formats
- **Electronic Student Workbook**
  - Hundreds of **Learning Activities**
  - 55 **Psychotropic Drug Monographs**
  - 21 Sample **Client Education Teaching Guides** that can be reproduced as client handouts
  - **Care Plans** and **Critical Pathways** that you can customize
  - Psychotropic **Drug Classifications** with dosage information
  - Helpful Assessments, Tools and Tables
    - Levels of Anxiety
    - Global Assessment Functioning Scale
    - Medication Assessment Tool
    - Mental Status Assessment
    - Cultural Assessment Tool
    - Glossary

An Instructor's Resource Disk is available for educators with teaching aids to assist you with your lessons

- **Updated and Expanded Electronic Test Bank**
  - 400 NCLEX-style questions ***with page and chapter references***
- **Instructor's Guide**
  - **Chapter Focus, Key Terms** and **Chapter Outline/Lecture Notes**
  - Answers to the Critical Thinking Exercises from the text
  - Clinical Exercises
  - Case Studies for Use with Student Learning
- **PowerPoint presentation covering *all* 25 chapters**

Written by only one author,
Essentials of Psychiatric Mental Health Nursing
is straightforward, consistent, easy-to-read, and user-friendly.
And now it's in full color.

Townsend Essentials

The concise format of Townsend *Essentials* provides the fundamental psychiatric nursing information you need.

AS OUR HEALTH CARE SYSTEM continues to evolve, the amount of information that nursing students need to know is growing, too. For the third edition of *Essentials of Psychiatric Mental Health Nursing*, Mary C. Townsend, RN, MN, CS, presents an evidence-based, holistic approach to psychiatric nursing that addresses this expanding knowledge base and incorporates years of experience as a clinical nurse specialist and educator. Regardless of how many or how few weeks are devoted to the topic, Townsend's easy-to-follow approach and singular voice will provide students with the understanding of how to care for their clients.

Time and again, students and educators talk about how much they appreciate that Mary Townsend's books are so user-friendly. The author has often shared stories from students and instructors who say ***Essentials of Psychiatric Mental Health Nursing*** is easier to follow than other textbooks covering comparable material.

MARY C. TOWNSEND has loved psychiatric nursing since the first day of her psychiatric nursing course in college and knew right away that would be her specialty. This full-color, third edition of Townsend *Essentials* conveys the author's enthusiasm for the nursing profession and helps students in their commitment to psychiatric nursing.

Because client education is a vital nursing function, Townsend *Essentials of Psychiatric Mental Health Nursing* contains an appendix with 21 sample client teaching guides.

TOWNSEND *ESSENTIALS* ANSWERS THE QUESTION
"WHAT DO PSYCHIATRIC NURSES DO?"
IN A LANGUAGE THAT CAN BE UNDERSTOOD BY ALL

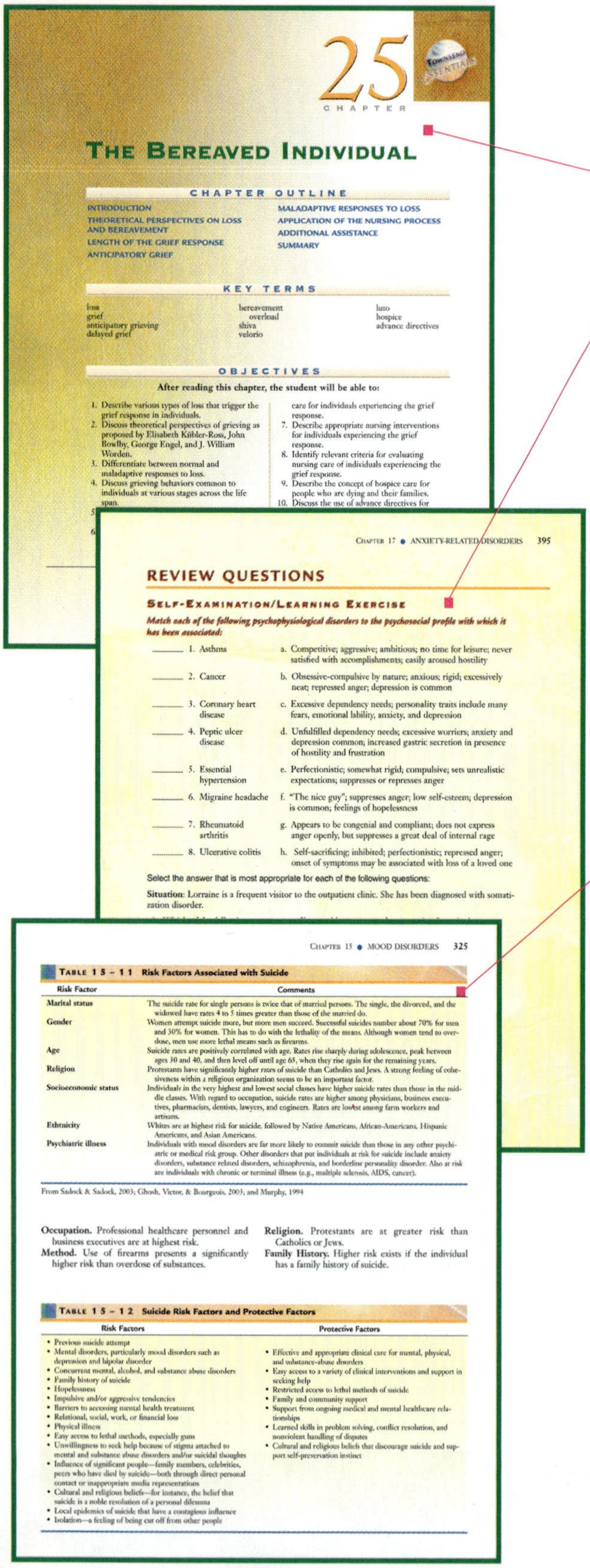

25

CHAPTER

THE BEREAVED INDIVIDUAL

CHAPTER OUTLINE

INTRODUCTION
THEORETICAL PERSPECTIVES ON LOSS AND BEREAVEMENT
LENGTH OF THE GRIEF RESPONSE
ANTICIPATORY GRIEF
MALADAPTIVE RESPONSES TO LOSS
APPLICATION OF THE NURSING PROCESS
ADDITIONAL ASSISTANCE
SUMMARY

KEY TERMS

loss
grief
anticipatory grieving
delayed grief
bereavement overload
shiva
velorio
luto
hospice
advance directives

OBJECTIVES

After reading this chapter, the student will be able to:

1. Describe various types of loss that trigger the grief response in individuals.
2. Discuss theoretical perspectives of grieving as proposed by Elisabeth Kübler-Ross, John Bowlby, George Engel, and J. William Worden.
3. Differentiate between normal and maladaptive responses to loss.
4. Discuss grieving behaviors common to individuals at various stages across the life span.

care for individuals experiencing the grief response.

7. Describe appropriate nursing interventions for individuals experiencing the grief response.
8. Identify relevant criteria for evaluating nursing care of individuals experiencing the grief response.
9. Describe the concept of hospice care for people who are dying and their families.
10. Discuss the use of advance directives for

CHAPTER 17 • ANXIETY-RELATED DISORDERS 395

REVIEW QUESTIONS

SELF-EXAMINATION/LEARNING EXERCISE

Match each of the following psychophysiological disorders to the psychosocial profile with which it has been associated:

______ 1. Asthma	a. Competitive; aggressive; ambitious; no time for leisure; never satisfied with accomplishments; easily aroused hostility
______ 2. Cancer	b. Obsessive-compulsive by nature; anxious; rigid; excessively neat; repressed anger; depression is common
______ 3. Coronary heart disease	c. Excessive dependency needs; personality traits include many fears, emotional lability, anxiety, and depression
______ 4. Peptic ulcer disease	d. Unfulfilled dependency needs; excessive worriers; anxiety and depression common; increased gastric secretion in presence of hostility and frustration
______ 5. Essential hypertension	e. Perfectionistic; somewhat rigid; compulsive; sets unrealistic expectations; suppresses or represses anger
______ 6. Migraine headache	f. "The nice guy"; suppresses anger; low self-esteem; depression is common; feelings of hopelessness
______ 7. Rheumatoid arthritis	g. Appears to be congenial and compliant; does not express anger openly, but suppresses a great deal of internal rage
______ 8. Ulcerative colitis	h. Self-sacrificing; inhibited; perfectionistic; repressed anger; onset of symptoms may be associated with loss of a loved one

Select the answer that is most appropriate for each of the following questions:

Situation: Lorraine is a frequent visitor to the outpatient clinic. She has been diagnosed with somatization disorder.

CHAPTER 15 • MOOD DISORDERS 325

TABLE 15-11 Risk Factors Associated with Suicide

Risk Factor	Comments
Marital status	The suicide rate for single persons is twice that of married persons. The single, the divorced, and the widowed have rates 4 to 5 times greater than those of the married do.
Gender	Women attempt suicide more, but more men succeed. Successful suicides number about 70% for men and 30% for women. This has to do with the lethality of the means. Although women tend to overdose, men use more lethal means such as firearms.
Age	Suicide rates are positively correlated with age. Rates rise sharply during adolescence, peak between ages 30 and 40, and then level off until age 65, when they rise again for the remaining years.
Religion	Protestants have significantly higher rates of suicide than Catholics and Jews. A strong feeling of cohesiveness within a religious organization seems to be an important factor.
Socioeconomic status	Individuals in the very highest and lowest social classes have higher suicide rates than those in the middle classes. With regard to occupation, suicide rates are higher among physicians, business executives, pharmacists, dentists, lawyers, and engineers. Rates are lowest among farm workers and artisans.
Ethtnicity	Whites are at highest risk for suicide, followed by Native Americans, African-Americans, Hispanic Americans, and Asian Americans.
Psychiatric illness	Individuals with mood disorders are far more likely to commit suicide than those in any other psychiatric or medical risk group. Other disorders that put individuals at risk for suicide include anxiety disorders, substance related disorders, schizophrenia, and borderline personality disorder. Also at risk are individuals with chronic or terminal illness (e.g., multiple sclerosis, AIDS, cancer).

From Sadock & Sadock, 2003; Ghosh, Victor, & Bourgeois, 2003; and Murphy, 1994

Occupation. Professional healthcare personnel and business executives are at highest risk.
Method. Use of firearms presents a significantly higher risk than overdose of substances.
Religion. Protestants are at greater risk than Catholics or Jews.
Family History. Higher risk exists if the individual has a family history of suicide.

TABLE 15-12 Suicide Risk Factors and Protective Factors

Risk Factors	Protective Factors
• Previous suicide attempt • Mental disorders, particularly mood disorders such as depression and bipolar disorder • Concurrent mental, alcohol, and substance abuse disorders • Family history of suicide • Hopelessness • Impulsive and/or aggressive tendencies • Barriers to accessing mental health treatment • Relational, social, work, or financial loss • Physical illness • Easy access to lethal methods, especially guns • Unwillingness to seek help because of stigma attached to mental and substance abuse disorders and/or suicidal thoughts • Influence of significant people—family members, celebrities, peers who have died by suicide—both through direct personal contact or inappropriate media representations • Cultural and religious beliefs—for instance, the belief that suicide is a noble resolution of a personal dilemma • Local epidemics of suicide that have a contagious influence • Isolation—a feeling of being cut off from other people	• Effective and appropriate clinical care for mental, physical, and substance-abuse disorders • Easy access to a variety of clinical interventions and support in seeking help • Restricted access to lethal methods of suicide • Family and community support • Support from ongoing medical and mental healthcare relationships • Learned skills in problem solving, conflict resolution, and nonviolent handling of disputes • Cultural and religious beliefs that discourage suicide and support self-preservation instinct

MARY TOWNSEND'S SIMPLE AND STRAIGHTFORWARD STYLE MAKES IT EASY TO LEARN

Each chapter includes **Chapter Outline, Key Terms,** and **Objectives,** as well as

- Chapter Review Questions
- Up-to-date topics with **Classical, Contemporary,** and **Internet References**
- **NANDA Taxonomy II** (2003-2004) used throughout the text
- Terminology and diagnostic criteria from the latest DSM-IV-TR

Throughout the text, you'll find new chapters, insets, and other special features

- New or expanded content on **disaster nursing** (Chapter 9) and **suicide** (Chapter 15)
- New section covering **psychosocial therapies** (Chapter 11), including psychoanalysis, interpersonal psychotherapy, reality therapy, relaxation therapy, assertiveness training, and cognitive therapy
- New chapter, **The Bereaved Individual** (Chapter 25), identifying theoretical perspectives, grieving behaviors from life stage and cultural points of view (normal and maladaptive), discussing the concepts of hospice care and advanced directives, and applying the nursing process—including a nursing care plan—to bereaved individuals

DEDICATION

To my best friend,

Jimmy

ACKNOWLEDGMENTS

My special thanks to:

Robert Martone and the editorial and production staffs of the F.A. Davis Company, who are always willing to provide assistance when requested.

Nursing faculty, colleagues, and students who have provided me with valuable feedback so that I can strive to achieve excellence in my publications.

Nursing administrators and staff from area facilities who provide input and help keep me informed about current clinical and state-of-the-discipline issues.

TO THE INSTRUCTOR

The 21st century continues to bring about a great deal of change in the healthcare system in general, and to nursing in particular. The psychiatric nurse/nurse practitioner now may provide services in a variety of settings—hospitals, community mental health centers, rape crisis centers, hospices, correctional facilities, drug and alcohol rehabilitation centers, and in private practice, to name a few.

The body of knowledge in nursing continues to grow and expand as rapidly as nursing undergoes change. Nurses must draw upon this research base to support the care that they provide for their clients. The third edition of *Essentials of Psychiatric Mental Health Nursing* strives to present an evidence-based, holistic approach to psychiatric nursing practice.

Psychiatric nurses continue to face numerous complex challenges. The biological shift in psychiatry, which had its roots in the 1990s "decade of the brain," made it necessary for psychiatric nurses to be familiar with the concepts of psychoimmunology, neuroendocrinology, and genetics, and the role they may play in mental illness.

Now, well into the first decade of the new century, new challenges must be faced. On September 25, 2000, in a ceremony on Capitol Hill, the American Psychological Association launched the initiative declaring the decade of 2000 to 2010 as the "decade of behavior." This initiative has been endorsed by the American Psychiatric Nurses Association (APNA).

The "decade of behavior" involves more than 50 professional societies (including APNA), representing the behavioral and social sciences, which have joined to focus their talents, energy, and creativity on meeting many of society's most significant challenges. These include ensuring and improving education; improving health and access to healthcare; ensuring safety in homes and communities; curbing drug use and abuse, poverty, racism, cynicism toward institutions of government, crime, and high risk behaviors; and actively addressing an aging population. At the heart of meeting these and many other national challenges lies behavior.

In 2020, the ten leading causes of mortality throughout the world are projected to include heart disease; cerebrovascular disease; pulmonary disease; lower respiratory infections; tracheal, bronchial and lung cancers; traffic accidents; tuberculosis; stomach cancer; HIV/AIDS; and suicide. Behavior is an important element in prevention of these causes of mortality and in their treatment. In 2020, the three leading causes of disability throughout the world are projected to include heart disease, major depression, and traffic accidents. Behavior is once again an important underpinning of these three contributors of disability, and behavioral and social science research can lower the impact of these causes of morbidity and mortality. Many of these issues are addressed in this new edition.

Content and Features New to This Edition

New content on Disaster Nursing (Chapter 9)

New content on Psychosocial Therapies (Chapter 11). An explanation of various psychosocial therapies includes the following: Psychoanalysis, Interpersonal Psychotherapy, Reality Therapy, Relaxation Therapy, Assertiveness Training, and Cognitive Therapy.

Expanded content on Suicide (Chapter 15)

New chapter on The Bereaved Individual (Chapter 25). This chapter identifies various theoretical perspectives of grieving. Normal and maladaptive responses to loss are described. Grieving behaviors common to individuals of various ages and cultures are discussed. The nursing process, including a nursing care plan, is applied to bereaved individuals. The concepts of hospice care and advanced directives are presented.

Client Teaching Guides (Appendix H). A set of 21 sample teaching guides that may be reproduced and given to clients. These handouts contain information related to psychotropic medications and psychiatric illnesses that nurses can use when implementing client teaching.

NANDA Taxonomy II (2003–2004). Used throughout the text

New and updated psychotropic medication information (Chapter 10 and in relevant clinical chapters)

New Mental Status Examination for Dementia (Chapter 12)

New research studies with implications for evidence-based practice. (In all relevant clinical chapters.)

A new Student CD-ROM.

Features that Have Been Retained

The concept of **holistic nursing** is retained in the third edition. An attempt has been made to ensure that the physical aspects of psychiatric/mental health nursing are not overlooked. Both physical and psychosocial nursing diagnoses are included for physiological disorders (such as asthma, migraine headache, and hypertension) and for psychological disorders (such as somatoform and eating disorders). In all relevant situations, the mind/body connection is addressed.

Nursing process is retained in the second edition as the tool for delivery of care to the individual with a psychiatric disorder or to assist in the primary prevention or exacerbation of mental illness symptoms. The six steps of the nursing process, as described in the American Nurses Association Standards of Clinical Nursing Practice are used to provide guidelines for the nurse. These standards of care are included for the DSM-IV-TR diagnoses, as well as the aging individual, the bereaved individual, victims of abuse and neglect, and as examples in several of the therapeutic approaches. The six steps include:

Assessment: Background assessment data, including a description of symptomatology, provides an extensive knowledge base from which the nurse may draw when performing an assessment. Several assessment tools are also included.

Diagnosis: Analysis of the data is included, from which nursing diagnoses common to specific psychiatric disorders are derived.

Outcome Identification: Outcomes are derived from the nursing diagnoses and stated as measurable goals.

Planning: A plan of care is presented with selected nursing diagnoses for the DSM-IV-TR diagnoses, as well as for the elderly client, the bereaved individual, victims of abuse and neglect, the elderly homebound client, and the primary caregiver of the client with a chronic mental illness. Critical Pathways of Care are included for clients in alcohol withdrawal, schizophrenic psychosis, depression, manic episode, PTSD, and anorexia nervosa. (Appendix E). The planning standard also includes tables that list topics for educating clients and families about mental illness.

Implementation: The interventions that have been identified in the plan of care are included along with rationale for each. Case studies at the end of each DSM-IV-TR chapter assist the student in the practical application of theoretical material. Also included as a part of this particular standard is Unit II of the textbook: Psychiatric/Mental Health Nursing Interventions. This section of the textbook addresses psychiatric nursing intervention in depth, and frequently speaks to the differentiation in scope of practice between the basic level psychiatric nurse and the advanced practice level psychiatric nurse. Advanced practice nurses with prescriptive authority will find the extensive chapter on psychopharmacology particularly helpful.

Evaluation: The evaluation standard includes a set of questions that the nurse may use to assess whether the nursing actions have been successful in achieving the objectives of care.

Internet references for each DSM-IV-TR diagnosis, with Web site listings for information related to the disorder

Tables that list topics for client education (Clinical chapters)

Assigning nursing diagnoses to client behaviors (Appendix C)

Additional Educational Resources

Faculty may also find the following teaching aids that accompany this textbook helpful:

- Five psychotropic Appendices that provide all the *DSM-IV-TR* classifications, NANDA diagnoses and behaviors, and guidelines for mental health assessment as well as a glossary to the entire textbook.

- **Instructor's Guide (IG).** Contains chapter outlines with lecture notes, case studies, and answers to the Critical Thinking Exercises from the textbook.
- A computerized bank of NCLEX-style test questions that reference the information in the textbook
- A Student CD-ROM with hundreds of test questions and learning activities to help students in the profession.
- PowerPoint Presentation. An extensive collection of slides to accompany lectures for all chapters.

All chapters throughout the text have been updated and revised to reflect today's healthcare reformation and to provide information based on the latest, current state of the discipline of nursing. It is hoped that the revisions and additions to this 3rd edition continue to satisfy a need within psychiatric/mental health nursing practice. Many of the changes reflect feedback that I have received from users of the previous editions. To those individuals I express heartfelt thanks. I welcome comments in an effort to retain what some have called the "user friendliness" of the text. I hope that this third edition continues to promote and advance the commitment to psychiatric/mental health nursing.

MARY C. TOWNSEND

CONTENTS

Sample Client Teaching Guides

Unit One

Introduction to Psychiatric/ Mental Health Concepts

CHAPTER 1

Mental Health and Mental Illness

CHAPTER OUTLINE

KEY TERMS

fight-or-flight syndrome
bereavement overload
ego defense mechanisms
anxiety
grief
neurosis
psychosis
anticipatory grief
Diagnostic and Statistical Manual of Mental Disorders, Fourth Edition, Text Revision (DSM-IV-TR)

OBJECTIVES

After reading this chapter, the student will be able to:

1. Define *mental health* and *mental illness.*
2. Discuss cultural elements that influence attitudes toward mental health and mental illness.
3. Identify physiological responses to stress.
4. Discuss the concepts of anxiety and grief as psychological responses to stress.
5. Describe the DSM-IV-TR multiaxial evaluation system for classification of mental disorders.

INTRODUCTION

The concepts of mental health and mental illness are culturally defined. Some cultures are quite liberal in the range of behaviors that are considered acceptable, whereas others have very little tolerance for behaviors that deviate from the cultural norms. A study of the history of psychiatric care reveals some shocking truths about past treatment of mentally ill individuals. Many were kept in control by means that could be considered less than humane.

This chapter defines mental health and mental illness and describes physical and psychological responses to stress. ***The Diagnostic and Statistical Manual of Mental Disorders, 4th Edition, Text Revision (DSM-IV-TR)***, multiaxial evaluation system is also presented.

MENTAL HEALTH

A number of theorists have attempted to define the concept of mental health. Many of these concepts deal with various aspects of individual functioning. Maslow (1970) emphasized an individual's motivation in the continuous quest for self-actualization. He identified a "hierarchy of needs," the lower ones requiring fulfillment before those at higher levels can be achieved, with self-actualization being fulfillment of one's highest potential. This hierarchy of needs is presented in Figure 1–1. An individual's position in the hierarchy may change from a higher level to a lower level based on life circumstances. For example, an individual facing major surgery who has been working on tasks to achieve self-actualization may become preoccupied, if only temporarily, with the need for physiological safety.

Maslow described self-actualization as being "psychologically healthy, fully human, highly evolved, and fully mature." He believed that healthy, or self-actualized, individuals possessed the following characteristics:

- An appropriate perception of reality
- The ability to accept oneself, others, and human nature
- The ability to manifest spontaneity
- The capacity for focusing concentration on problem solving
- A need for detachment and desire for privacy
- Independence, autonomy, and a resistance to enculturation
- An intensity of emotional reaction
- A frequency of "peak" experiences that validate the worthwhileness, richness, and beauty of life
- An identification with humankind
- The ability to achieve satisfactory interpersonal relationships
- A democratic character structure and strong sense of ethics
- Creativeness
- A degree of nonconformance

The American Psychiatric Association (APA) (1980) defines mental health as:

> Simultaneous success at working, loving, and creating with the capacity for mature and flexible resolution of conflicts between instincts, conscience, important other people, and reality.

Townsend (2003) defines mental health as:

> The successful adaptation to stressors from the internal or external environment, evidenced by thoughts, feelings, and behaviors that are age-appropriate and congruent with local and cultural norms.

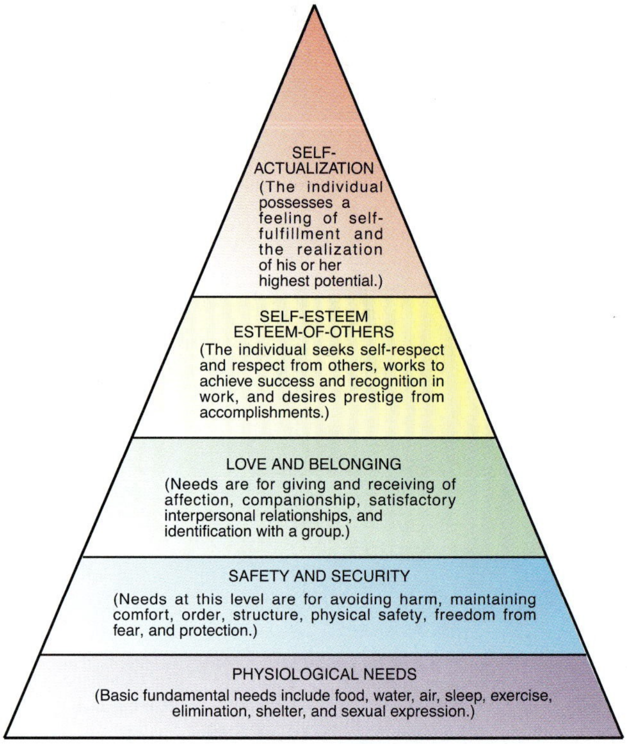

FIGURE 1–1 Maslow's hierarchy of needs.

This definition of mental health will be used for purposes of this text.

MENTAL ILLNESS

A universal concept of mental illness is difficult to define, because of the cultural factors that influence such a concept. However, certain elements are associated with individuals' perceptions of mental illness, regardless of cultural origin. Horwitz (1982) identifies two of these elements as *incomprehensibility* and *cultural relativity*.

Incomprehensibility relates to the inability of the general population to understand the motivation behind the behavior. When observers are unable to find meaning or comprehensibility in behavior, they are likely to label that behavior as mental illness. Horwitz states:

> Observers attribute labels of mental illness when the rules, conventions, and understandings they use to interpret behavior fail to find any intelligible motivation behind an action.

TABLE 1 – 1 Cultural Aspects of Mental Illness

1. The initial recognition that an individual's behavior deviates from the social norms usually is by members of the lay community rather than by a psychiatric professional.
2. People who are related to an individual, or who are of the same cultural or social group, are less likely to label an individual's behavior as mentally ill, than someone who is relationally or culturally distant. Family members (or people of the same cultural or social group) try to "normalize" the behavior and try to find an explanation for the behavior.
3. Psychiatrists see a mentally ill person most often when the family members can no longer deny the illness, often when the behavior is at its worst. The local or cultural norms define pathological behavior.
4. The lowest social class usually displays the highest amount of mental illness symptoms. However, they tend to tolerate a wider range of behaviors that deviate from societal norms and are less likely to consider these behaviors as indicative of mental illness. Mental illness labels are most often applied by psychiatric professionals.
5. The higher the social class, the greater the recognition of mental illness behaviors (as defined by societal norms). Members of the higher social classes are likely to be self-labeled or labeled by family members or friends. Psychiatric assistance is sought soon after the first signs of emotional disturbance.
6. The more highly educated a person is, the greater the recognition of mental illness behaviors. However, even more relevant than amount of education is type of education. Individuals in the more humanistic types of professions (e.g., lawyers, social workers, artists, teachers, nurses) are more likely to seek psychiatric assistance than are other types of professionals (e.g., business executives, computer specialists, accountants, engineers).
7. In terms of religion, people who are Jewish are more likely to seek psychiatric assistance than are people who are Catholic or Protestant.
8. Women are more likely than men are to recognize the symptoms of mental illness and seek assistance.
9. The greater the cultural distance from the mainstream of society (i.e., the fewer the ties with conventional society), the greater the likelihood of negative response by society to their illness. For example, immigrants have a greater distance from the mainstream than the native-born, blacks more than whites, and "bohemians" more than bourgeoisie. They are more likely to be subjected to coercive treatment, and involuntary psychiatric commitments are more common.

Source: Adapted from Horwitz (1982).

The element of *cultural relativity* considers that these rules, conventions, and understandings are conceived within an individual's own particular culture. Behavior is categorized as "normal" or "abnormal" according to one's cultural or societal norms. Therefore, a behavior that is recognized as evidence of mental illness in one society may be viewed as normal in another society, and vice versa. Horwitz identified a number of cultural aspects of mental illness, which are presented in Table 1–1.

In the DSM-IV-TR (APA, 2000), the APA defines mental illness or a mental disorder as:

> A clinically significant behavioral or psychological syndrome or pattern that occurs in an individual and that is associated with present distress (e.g., a painful symptom) or disability (i.e., impairment in one or more important areas of functioning), or with a significantly increased risk of suffering death, pain, disability, or an important loss of freedom … and is not merely an expectable … response to a particular event.

Townsend (2003) defines mental illness as:

> Maladaptive responses to stressors from the internal or external environment, evidenced by thoughts, feelings, and behaviors that are incongruent with the local and cultural norms, and interfere with the individual's social, occupational, and/or physical functioning. This definition of mental illness will be used for purposes of this text.

PHYSICAL AND PSYCHOLOGICAL RESPONSES TO STRESS

Physical Responses

In 1956, Hans Selye published the results of his research concerning the physiological response of a biological system to a change imposed on it. Since the initial publication of his findings, he has revised his definition of stress to "the state manifested by a specific syndrome which consists of all the nonspecifically-induced changes within a biologic system" (Selye, 1976). This syndrome of symptoms has come to be known as the **fight-or-flight syndrome.** Selye called this general reaction of the body to stress the *general adaptation syndrome*. He described the reaction in three distinct stages:

1. Alarm Reaction Stage. During this stage, the physiological responses of the fight-or-flight syndrome are initiated.

2. Stage of Resistance. The individual uses the physiological responses of the first stage as a defense in the attempt to adapt to the stressor. If adaptation occurs, the third stage is prevented or delayed. Physiological symptoms may disappear.
3. Stage of Exhaustion. This stage occurs when there is a prolonged exposure to the stressor to which the body has become adjusted. The adaptive energy is depleted, and the individual can no longer draw from the resources for adaptation described in the first two stages. Diseases of adaptation (e.g., headaches, mental disorders, coronary artery disease, ulcers, colitis) may occur. Without intervention for reversal, exhaustion and even death ensues (Selye, 1956, 1974).

Biological responses associated with the fight-or-flight syndrome include the following:

1. The Immediate Response. The hypothalamus stimulates the sympathetic nervous system, which results in the following physical effects:
    - The adrenal medulla releases norepinephrine and epinephrine into the bloodstream.
    - The pupils of the eye dilate.
    - Secretion from the lacrimal (tear) glands is increased.
    - In the lungs, the bronchioles dilate and the respiration rate is increased.
    - The force of cardiac contraction increases, as does cardiac output, heart rate, and blood pressure.
    - Gastrointestinal motility and secretions decrease, and sphincters contract.
    - In the liver, there is increased glycogenolysis and gluconeogenesis and decreased glycogen synthesis.
    - The bladder muscle contracts and the sphincter relaxes; there is increased ureter motility.
    - Secretion from the sweat glands is increased.
    - Lipolysis occurs in the fat cells.
2. The Sustained Response. When an individual experiences stress over a long time, the hypothalamus stimulates the pituitary gland to release hormones that produce the following effects:
    - Adrenocorticotropic hormone (ACTH) stimulates the adrenal cortex to release glucocorticoids and mineralocorticoids, resulting in increased gluconeogenesis and retention of sodium and water and decreased immune and inflammatory responses.
    - Vasopressin (antidiuretic hormone) increases fluid retention and increases blood pressure through constriction of blood vessels.
    - Growth hormone has a direct effect on protein, carbohydrate, and lipid metabolism, resulting in increased serum glucose and free fatty acids.
    - Thyrotropic hormone stimulates the thyroid gland to increase the basal metabolic rate.
    - Gonadotropins cause a decrease in secretion of sex hormones, resulting in decreased libido and impotence.

This "fight-or-flight" response undoubtedly served our ancestors well. Those *Homo sapiens* who had to face the giant grizzly bear or the saber-toothed tiger as a facet of their struggle for survival must have used these adaptive resources to their advantage. The response was elicited in emergencies, used in the preservation of life, and followed by restoration of the compensatory mechanisms to the pre-emergent condition (homeostasis).

Selye performed his extensive research in a controlled setting with laboratory animals as subjects. He elicited the physiological responses with physical stimuli, such as exposure to hot or cold temperatures, electric shock, injection of toxic agents, restraint, and surgical injury. Since the publication of Selye's original research, it has become apparent that the fight-or-flight syndrome occurs in response to psychological or emotional stimuli, just as it does to physical stimuli. The psychological or emotional stressors are often not resolved as rapidly as some physical stressors; therefore, the body may be depleted of its adaptive energy more readily than it is from physical stressors. The fight-or-flight response may be inappropriate or even dangerous to the lifestyle of today, in which stress has been described as "a pervasive, chronic, and relentless psychosocial situation" (Wallis, 1983). This chronic response maintains the body in the aroused condition for extended periods, which promotes susceptibility to diseases of adaptation.

Psychological Responses

Anxiety and **grief** have been described as two major, primary psychological response patterns to stress. A variety of thoughts, feelings, and behaviors are associated with each of these response patterns. Adaptation is determined by the degree to which the thoughts, feelings, and behaviors interfere with an individual's functioning.

Anxiety

Anxiety has been defined as a diffuse apprehension that is vague in nature and is associated with feelings of uncertainty and helplessness. Feelings of anxiety are so common as to be considered almost universal in our society. Low levels of anxiety are adaptive and can provide the motivation required for survival. Anxiety becomes problematic when the individual is unable to prevent the anxiety from escalating to a level that interferes with the ability to meet basic needs.

Peplau (1963) described four levels of anxiety: mild, moderate, severe, and panic. Nurses must be able to recognize the symptoms associated with each level to plan for appropriate intervention with anxious individuals.

1. Mild Anxiety. This level of anxiety is seldom a problem for the individual. It is associated with the tension experienced in response to the events of day-to-day living. Mild anxiety prepares people for action. It sharpens the senses, increases motivation for productivity, increases the perceptual field, and results in a heightened awareness of the environment. Learning is enhanced and the individual is able to function at his or her optimal level.
2. Moderate Anxiety. As the level of anxiety increases, the extent of the perceptual field diminishes. The moderately anxious individual is less alert to events occurring within the environment. The individual's attention span and ability to concentrate decrease, although, with direction, he or she may still attend to needs. Assistance with problem solving may be required. Increased muscular tension and restlessness are evident.
3. Severe Anxiety. The perceptual field of the severely anxious individual is so greatly diminished that concentration centers on one particular detail only or on many extraneous details. Attention span is extremely limited, and the individual has much difficulty completing even the simplest task. Physical symptoms (e.g., headaches, palpitations, insomnia) and emotional symptoms (e.g., confusion, dread, horror) may be evident. Discomfort is experienced to the degree that virtually all overt behavior is aimed at relieving the anxiety.
4. Panic Anxiety. In this most intense state of anxiety, the individual is unable to focus on even one detail within the environment. Misperceptions are common, and a loss of contact with reality may occur. The individual may experience hallucinations or delusions. Behavior may be characterized by wild and desperate actions or extreme withdrawal. Human functioning and communication with others are ineffective. Panic anxiety is associated with a feeling of terror, and individuals may be convinced that they have a life-threatening illness or fear that they are "going crazy," are losing control, or are emotionally weak (APA, 2000). Prolonged panic anxiety can lead to physical and emotional exhaustion and can be life threatening.

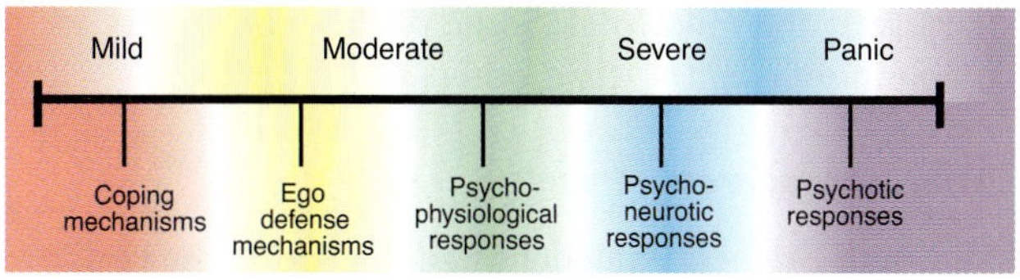

FIGURE 1–2 Adaptation responses on a continuum of anxiety.

A variety of behavioral adaptation responses occurs at each level of anxiety. Figure 1–2 depicts these behavioral responses on a continuum of anxiety ranging from mild to panic.

Mild Anxiety

At the mild level, individuals use any of a number of coping behaviors that satisfy their needs for comfort. Menninger (1963) described the following types of coping mechanisms that individuals use to relieve anxiety in stressful situations:

- Sleeping
- Eating
- Physical exercise
- Smoking
- Crying
- Yawning
- Drinking
- Daydreaming
- Laughing
- Cursing
- Pacing
- Foot swinging
- Fidgeting
- Nail biting
- Finger tapping
- Talking to someone with whom one feels comfortable

Undoubtedly there are many more responses too numerous to mention here, considering that each individual develops his or her own unique ways to relieve anxiety at the mild level. Some of these behaviors are much more adaptive than others.

Mild to Moderate Anxiety

Sigmund Freud (1961) identified the ego as the reality component of the personality that governs problem solving and rational thinking. As the level of anxiety increases, the strength of the ego is tested, and energy is mobilized to confront the threat. Anna Freud (1953) identified a number of defense mechanisms employed by the ego in the face of threat to biological or psychological integrity (Table 1–2). Some of these **ego defense mechanisms** are more adaptive than others, but all are used (either consciously or unconsciously) as protective devices for the ego in an effort to relieve mild to moderate anxiety. They become maladaptive when used by an individual to such a degree that there is interference with the ability to deal with reality, with interpersonal relations, or with occupational performance.

Moderate to Severe Anxiety

Anxiety at the moderate to severe level that remains unresolved over an extended period can contribute to a number of physiological disorders. The DSM-IV-TR (APA, 2000) describes these disorders as "the presence of one or more specific psychological or behavioral factors that adversely affect a general medical condition." The psychological factors may exacerbate symptoms of, delay recovery from, or interfere with treatment of the medical condition. The condition may be initiated or exacerbated by an environmental situation that the individual perceives as stressful. Measurable pathophysiology can be demonstrated. The DSM-IV-TR states:

> Psychological and behavioral factors may affect the course of almost every major category of disease, including cardiovascular conditions, dermatological conditions, endocrinological conditions, gastrointestinal conditions, neoplastic conditions, neurological conditions, pulmonary conditions, renal conditions, and rheumatological conditions. (p. 732)

Severe Anxiety

Extended periods of repressed severe anxiety can result in psychoneurotic patterns of behaving. **Neurosis** is no longer a separate category of disorders in the DSM-IV-TR (APA, 2000). However, the term is still used in the literature to further describe the symptomatology of certain disorders. Neuroses are psychiatric disturbances, characterized by excessive anxiety that is expressed directly or altered through defense mechanisms. It appears as a symptom, such as an obsession, a compulsion, a phobia, or a sexual dysfunction (Sadock & Sadock, 2003). The following are common characteristics of people with neuroses:

1. They are aware that they are experiencing distress.
2. They are aware that their behaviors are maladaptive.
3. They are unaware of any possible psychological causes of the distress.
4. They feel helpless to change their situation.
5. They experience no loss of contact with reality.

The following disorders are examples of psychoneurotic responses to severe anxiety as they appear in the DSM-IV-TR:

1. Anxiety Disorders. Disorders in which the characteristic features are symptoms of anxiety and avoidance behavior (e.g., phobias, obsessive-compulsive disorder, panic disorder, generalized anxiety disorder, post-traumatic stress disorder).
2. Somatoform Disorders. Disorders in which the characteristic features are physical symptoms for which there is no demonstrable organic pathology. Psychological factors are judged to play a significant role in the onset, severity, exacerbation, or maintenance of the symptoms (e.g., hypochondriasis, conversion disorder, somatization disorder, pain disorder).
3. Dissociative Disorders. Disorders in which the characteristic feature is a disruption in the usually integrated functions of consciousness, memory, identity, or perception of the environment (e.g., dissociative amnesia, dissociative fugue, dissociative identity disorder, depersonalization disorder).

Panic Anxiety

At this extreme level of anxiety, an individual is not capable of processing what is happening in the environment and may lose contact with reality. **Psychosis** is defined as a loss of ego boundaries or a gross impairment in reality testing (APA, 2000). Psychoses are serious psychiatric disturbances characterized by the presence of delusions or hallucinations and the impairment of interpersonal functioning and relationship to the external world. The following are common characteristics of people with psychoses:

TABLE 1 – 2 Ego Defense Mechanisms

Defense Mechanism	Example	Defense Mechanism	Example
Compensation Covering up a real or perceived weakness by emphasizing a trait one considers more desirable	A physically handicapped boy is unable to participate in football, so he compensates by becoming a great scholar.	**Projection** Attributing feelings or impulses unacceptable to one's self to another person.	Sue feels a strong sexual attraction to her track coach and tells her friend, "He's coming on to me!"
Denial Refusing to acknowledge the existence of a real situation or the feelings associated with it	A woman drinks alcohol every day and cannot stop, failing to acknowledge that she has a problem.	**Rationalization** Attempting to make excuses or formulate logical reasons to justify unacceptable feelings or behaviors	John tells the rehab nurse, "I drink because it's the only way I can deal with my bad marriage and my worse job."
Displacement The transfer of feelings from one target to another that is considered less threatening or that is neutral	A client is angry at his doctor, does not express it, but becomes verbally abusive with the nurse.	**Reaction Formation** Preventing unacceptable or undesirable thoughts or behaviors from being expressed by exaggerating opposite thoughts or types of behaviors	Jane hates nursing. She attended nursing school to please her parents. During career day, she speaks to prospective students about the excellence of nursing as a career.
Identification An attempt to increase self-worth by acquiring certain attributes and characteristics of an individual one admires	A teenaged boy who required lengthy rehabilitation after an accident decides to become a physical therapist as a result of his experiences.	**Regression** Responding to stress by retreating to an earlier level of development and the comfort measures associated with that level of functioning	When 2-year-old Jay is hospitalized for tonsillitis he will drink only from a bottle, although his mother states he has been drinking from a cup for 6 months.
Intellectualization An attempt to avoid expressing actual emotions associated with a stressful situation by using the intellectual processes of logic, reasoning, and analysis	Susan's husband is being transferred with his job to a city far away from her parents. She hides anxiety by explaining to her parents the advantages associated with the move.	**Repression** Involuntarily blocking unpleasant feelings and experiences from one's awareness	An accident victim can remember nothing about the accident.
Introjection Integrating the beliefs and values of another individual into one's own ego structure	Children integrate their parents' value system into the process of conscience formation. A child says to a friend, "Don't cheat. It's wrong."	**Sublimation** Rechanneling of drives or impulses that are personally or socially unacceptable into activities that are constructive	A mother whose son was killed by a drunk driver channels her anger and energy into being the president of the local chapter of Mothers Against Drunk Drivers.
Isolation Separating a thought or memory from the feeling tone or emotion associated with it	Without showing any emotion, a young woman describes being attacked and raped.	**Suppression** The voluntary blocking of unpleasant feelings and experiences from one's awareness	Scarlett O'Hara says, "I don't want to think about that now. I'll think about that tomorrow."
		Undoing Symbolically negating or canceling out an experience that one finds intolerable	Joe is nervous about his new job and yells at his wife. On his way home he stops and buys her some flowers.

1. They exhibit minimal distress (emotional tone is flat, bland, or inappropriate).
2. They are unaware that their behavior is maladaptive.
3. They are unaware of any psychological problems.
4. They are exhibiting a flight from reality into a less stressful world or into one in which they are attempting to adapt.

Examples of psychotic responses to anxiety include the schizophrenic, schizoaffective, and delusional disorders.

Grief

Grief is a subjective state of emotional, physical, and social responses to the loss of a valued entity. The loss may be *real,* in which case it can be substantiated by others (e.g., death of a loved one, loss of personal possessions), or it may be *perceived* by the individual alone and cannot be shared or identified by others (e.g., loss of the feeling of femininity following a mastectomy). Any situation that creates *change* for an individual can be identified as a loss. *Failure* (either real or perceived) can be viewed as a loss.

The loss, or anticipated loss, of anything of value to an individual can trigger the grief response. This period of characteristic emotions and behaviors is called *mourning.* The "normal" mourning process is adaptive and is characterized by feelings of sadness, guilt, anger, helplessness, hopelessness, and despair. Indeed, an absence of mourning may be considered maladaptive.

Stages of Grief

Kübler-Ross (1969), in extensive research with terminally ill patients, identified five stages of feelings and behaviors that individuals experience in response to a real, perceived, or anticipated loss:

Stage 1—Denial: This is a stage of shock and disbelief. The response may be one of "No, it can't be true!" The reality of the loss is not acknowledged. Denial is a protective mechanism that allows the individual to cope within an immediate time period while organizing more effective defense strategies.

Stage 2—Anger: "Why me?" and "It's not fair!" are comments often expressed during the anger stage. Envy and resentment toward individuals not affected by the loss are common. Anger may be directed at the self or displaced on loved ones, caregivers, and even God. There may be a preoccupation with an idealized image of the lost entity.

Stage 3—Bargaining: "If God will help me through this, I promise I will go to church every Sunday and volunteer my time to help others." During this stage, which is usually not visible or evident to others, a "bargain" is made with God in an attempt to reverse or postpone the loss. Sometimes the promise is associated with feelings of guilt for not having performed satisfactorily, appropriately, or sufficiently.

Stage 4—Depression: During this stage, the full impact of the loss is experienced. The sense of loss is intense, and feelings of sadness and depression prevail. This is a time of quiet desperation and disengagement from all association with the lost entity. This stage differs from pathological depression in that this is a stage of advancement toward resolution rather than the fixation in an earlier stage of the grief process.

Stage 5—Acceptance: The final stage brings a feeling of peace regarding the loss. It is a time of quiet expectation and resignation. The focus is on the reality of the loss and its meaning for the individuals affected by it.

Not all individuals experience each of these stages in response to a loss, nor do they necessarily experience them in this order. Some individuals' grieving behaviors may fluctuate, and even overlap, among the stages.

Anticipatory Grief

When a loss is anticipated, individuals often begin the work of grieving before the actual loss occurs. This is called **anticipatory grief.** Most people re-experience the grieving behaviors once the loss occurs, but having this time to prepare for the loss can facilitate the process of mourning and actually decreasing the length and intensity of the response. Problems arise, particularly in anticipating the death of a loved one, when family members experience anticipatory grieving and the mourning process is completed prematurely. They disengage emotionally from the dying person, who then may feel rejected by loved ones at a time when this psychological support is so vital.

Resolution

The grief response can last from weeks to years. It cannot be hurried, and individuals must be allowed to progress at their own pace. In the loss of a loved one, grief work usually lasts for at least a year, during which the grieving person experiences each significant "anniversary" date for the first time without the loved one present.

Length of the grief process may be prolonged by a number of factors. If the relationship with the lost entity had been marked by ambivalence or if there had been an enduring "love-hate" association, reaction to the loss may be burdened with guilt. Guilt lengthens the grief reaction by promoting feelings of anger toward the self for having committed a wrongdoing or behaved in an unacceptable manner toward that which is now lost. It may even lead to feeling that one's behavior has contributed to the loss.

Anticipatory grieving is thought to shorten the grief response in some individuals who are able to work through some of the feelings before the loss occurs. If the loss is sudden and unexpected, mourning may take longer than it would if individuals were able to grieve in anticipation of the loss.

Length of the grieving process is also affected by the number of recent losses experienced by an individual and whether he or she is able to complete one grieving process before another loss occurs. This is particularly true for elderly individuals who may be experiencing numerous losses—such as spouse, friends, other relatives, independent functioning, home, personal possessions, and pets—in a relatively short time. As grief accumulates, a type of **bereavement overload** occurs, which for some individuals presents an impossible task of grief work.

Resolution of the process of mourning is thought to have occurred when an individual can look back on the relationship with the lost entity and accept both the pleasures and the disappointments (both the positive and the negative aspects) of the association (Bowlby and Parkes, 1970). Disorganization and emotional pain have been experienced and tolerated. Preoccupation with the lost entity has been replaced with energy and the desire to pursue new situations and relationships.

Maladaptive Grief Responses

Maladaptive responses to loss occur when an individual is not able to satisfactorily progress through the stages of grieving to achieve resolution. Maladaptive responses generally occur when an individual becomes fixed in the denial or anger stage of the grief process. Several types of grief responses have been identified as pathological. They include responses that are prolonged, delayed or inhibited, or distorted. The *prolonged* response is characterized by an intense preoccupation with memories of the lost entity for many years after the loss has occurred. Behaviors associated with the stages of denial or anger are manifested, and disorganization of functioning and intense emotional pain related to the lost entity are evidenced.

In the *delayed or inhibited* response, the individual becomes fixed in the denial stage of the grieving process. The emotional pain associated with the loss is not experienced, but anxiety disorders (e.g., phobias, hypochondriasis) or sleeping and eating disorders (e.g., insomnia, anorexia) may be evident. The individual may remain in denial for many years, until the grief response is triggered by a reminder of the loss, or even by another, unrelated loss.

The individual who experiences a *distorted* response is fixed in the anger stage of grieving. In the distorted response, all the normal behaviors associated with grieving, such as helplessness, hopelessness, sadness, anger, and guilt, are exaggerated out of proportion to the situation. The individual turns the anger inward on the self, is consumed with overwhelming despair, and is unable to function in normal activities of daily living. Pathological depression is a distorted grief response.

THE DSM-IV-TR MULTIAXIAL EVALUATION SYSTEM

The APA (2000) endorses case evaluation on a multiaxial system, "to facilitate comprehensive and systematic evaluation with attention to the various mental disorders and general medical conditions, psychosocial and environmental problems, and level of functioning that might be overlooked if the focus were on assessing a single presenting problem." Each individual is evaluated on five axes. They are defined by the DSM-IV-TR in the following manner:

Axis I—Clinical Disorders and Other Conditions That may be a Focus of Clinical Attention: This includes all mental disorders (except personality disorders and mental retardation.

Axis II—Personality Disorders and Mental Retardation: These disorders usually begin in childhood or adolescence and persist in a stable form into adult life.

Axis III—General Medical Conditions: These include any current general medical condition that is potentially relevant to the understanding or management of the individual's mental disorder.

Axis IV—Psychosocial and Environmental Problems:

These are problems that may affect the diagnosis, treatment, and prognosis of mental disorders named on axes I and II. These include problems related to primary support group, social environment, education, occupation, housing, economics, access to health care services, interaction with the legal system or crime, and other types of psychosocial and environmental problems.

Axis V—Global Assessment of Functioning: This allows the clinician to rate the individual's overall functioning on the Global Assessment of Functioning (GAF) scale. This scale represents in global terms a single measure of the individual's psychological, social, and occupational functioning.

The DSM-IV-TR outline of axis I and axis II categories and codes is presented in Appendix A.

SUMMARY

A number of definitions of mental health and mental illness can be found in the literature. For purposes of this text, *mental health* is defined as "the successful adaptation to stressors from the internal or external environment, evidenced by thoughts, feelings, and behaviors that are age-appropriate and congruent with local and cultural norms" (Townsend, 2003). *Mental illness* is defined as "maladaptive responses to stressors from the internal or external environment, evidenced by thoughts, feelings, and behaviors that are incongruent with the local and cultural norms, and interfere with the individual's social, occupational, and/or physical functioning" (Townsend, 2003).

Most cultures label behavior as mental illness based on *incomprehensibility* and *cultural relativity*. When observers are unable to find meaning or comprehensibility in behavior, they are likely to label that behavior as mental illness. The meaning of behaviors is determined within individual cultures.

Selye, who has become known as the founding father of stress research, defined stress as "the state manifested by a specific syndrome which consists of all the non-specifically-induced changes within a biological system" (Selye, 1976). He determined that physical beings respond to stressful stimuli with a predictable set of physiological changes. He described the response in three distinct stages: (1) the alarm reaction stage, (2) the stage of resistance, and (3) the stage of exhaustion. Many illnesses, or diseases of adaptation, have their origin in this aroused state, which is the preparation for the fight-or-flight response.

Anxiety and *grief* have been identified as the two major, primary responses to stress. Peplau (1963) defined anxiety by levels of symptom severity: mild, moderate, severe, and panic. Behaviors associated with levels of anxiety include coping mechanisms, ego defense mechanisms, psychophysiological responses, psychoneurotic responses, and psychotic responses.

Grief is described as a response to loss of a valued entity. Stages of normal mourning as identified by Kübler-Ross (1969) are denial, anger, bargaining, depression, and acceptance. Anticipatory grief is grief work that is begun, and sometimes completed, before the loss occurs. Resolution is thought to occur when an individual is able to remember and accept both the positive and negative aspects associated with the lost entity. Grieving is thought to be maladaptive when the mourning process is prolonged, delayed or inhibited, or becomes distorted and exaggerated out of proportion to the situation. Pathological depression is considered a distorted reaction. The DSM-IV-TR multiaxial system of diagnostic classification, which defines five axes in which each individual case is evaluated, was described.

REVIEW QUESTIONS

SELF-EXAMINATION

Please answer the questions based on the following case study:

Anna is 72 years old. She has been a widow for 20 years. When Anna's husband had been dead for a year, Anna's daughter gave her a puppy, which she named Lucky. Lucky was a happy, lively mutt of unknown origin, and he and Anna soon became inseparable. Lucky lived to a ripe old age of 16 and died in Anna's arms 3 years ago. Anna's daughter has consulted the community mental health nurse practitioner about her mother, stating, "She doesn't do a thing for herself anymore, and all she wants to talk about is Lucky. She visits his grave every day! She still cries when she talks about him. I don't know what to do!"

1. Anna's behavior would be considered maladaptive because:
   a. It has been over 3 years since Lucky died.
   b. Her grief is too intense to be over just the loss of a dog.
   c. She continues to be preoccupied with Lucky's loss after a prolonged period.
   d. People in this culture would not comprehend such behavior over loss of a pet.
2. Anna's grieving behavior would most likely be considered to be:
   a. Delayed
   b. Inhibited
   c. Prolonged
   d. Distorted
3. Anna is most likely fixed in which stage of the grief process?
   a. Denial
   b. Anger
   c. Depression
   d. Acceptance
4. Anna is of the age when she may have experienced many losses coming close together. What is this called?
   a. Bereavement overload
   b. Normal mourning
   c. Isolation
   d. Cultural relativity
5. Anna's daughter has likely put off seeking help for Anna because:
   a. Women are less likely to seek help for emotional problems than men.
   b. Relatives often try to "normalize" the behavior, rather than label it mental illness.
   c. She knows that all old people are expected to be a little depressed.
   d. She is afraid that the neighbors "will think her mother is crazy."
6. Lucky got away from Anna while they were taking a walk. He ran into the street and was hit by a car. Anna cannot remember any of these circumstances of his death. This is an example of what defense mechanism?
   a. Rationalization
   b. Suppression
   c. Denial
   d. Repression

7. Lucky sometimes refused to obey Anna, and indeed did not come back to her when she called to him on the day he was killed. However, Anna continues to insist, "He was the very best dog. He always minded me. He always did everything I told him to do." This represents the defense mechanism of:
   a. Sublimation
   b. Compensation
   c. Reaction formation
   d. Undoing
8. Anna's maladaptive grief response may be attributed to:
   a. Unresolved grief over loss of her husband.
   b. Loss of several relatives and friends over the last few years.
   c. Repressed feelings of guilt over the way in which Lucky died.
   d. Any or all of the above.
9. For what reason would Anna's illness be considered a neurosis rather than a psychosis?
   a. She is unaware that her behavior is maladaptive.
   b. She exhibits inappropriate affect (emotional tone).
   c. She experiences no loss of contact with reality.
   d. She tells the nurse, "There is nothing wrong with me!"
10. Which of the following statements by Anna might suggest that she is achieving resolution of her grief over Lucky's death?
   a. "I don't cry anymore when I think about Lucky."
   b. "It's true. Lucky didn't always mind me. Sometimes he ignored my commands."
   c. "I remember how it happened now. I should have held tighter to his leash!"
   d. "I won't ever have another dog. It's just too painful to lose them."

REFERENCES

American Psychiatric Association. (2000). Diagnostic and statistical manual of mental disorders—text revision (4th ed.). Washington, DC: American Psychiatric Association.

American Psychiatric Association. (1980). A psychiatric glossary (5th ed.) Washington, DC: American Psychiatric Press.

Sadock, B.J., and Sadock, V.A. (2003). Synopsis of psychiatry: Behavioral sciences/clinical psychiatry (9th ed.). Baltimore: Lippincott Williams & Wilkins.

Townsend, M.C. (2003). Psychiatric/mental health nursing: Concepts of care (4th ed.). Philadelphia: F.A. Davis.

Wallis, C. (1983, June 6). Stress: Can we cope? Time, pp. 48–54.

CLASSICAL REFERENCES

Bowlby, J., and Parkes, C.M. (1970). Separation and loss. In E.J. Anthony & C. Koupernik (Eds.), International yearbook for child psychiatry and allied disciplines: The child and his family, (Vol. 1). New York: John Wiley & Sons.

Freud, A. (1953). The ego and mechanisms of defense. New York: International Universities Press.

Freud, S. (1961). The ego and the id. In Standard edition of the complete psychological works of Freud, Vol. XIX. London: Hogarth Press.

Horwitz, A.V. (1982). The social control of mental illness. New York: Academic Press.

Kübler-Ross, E. (1969). On death and dying. New York: Macmillan.

Maslow, A. (1970). Motivation and personality (2nd ed.). New York: Harper & Row.

Menninger, K. (1963). The vital balance. New York: Viking Press.

Peplau, H. (1963). A working definition of anxiety. In S. Burd & M. Marshall (Eds.), Some clinical approaches to psychiatric nursing. New York: Macmillan.

Selye, H. (1956). The stress of life. New York: McGraw-Hill.

Selye, H. (1974). Stress without distress. New York: Signet Books.

Selye, H. (1976). The stress of life (rev. ed.). New York: McGraw-Hill.

Townsend Essentials

CHAPTER 2

Concepts of Personality Development

CHAPTER OUTLINE

KEY TERMS

ego
id
superego
libido
personality
surrogate
temperament
psychodynamic nursing
counselor
technical expert

OBJECTIVES

After reading this chapter, the student will be able to:

1. Define *personality*.
2. Identify the ways in which knowledge of personality development is relevant to nursing in the psychiatric/mental health setting.
3. Discuss the major components of the following developmental theories: (a) Psychoanalytic theory—Freud; (b) Interpersonal theory—Sullivan; (c) Theory of psychosocial development—Erikson; (d) Theory of object relations development—Mahler; and (e) A nursing model of interpersonal development—Peplau

INTRODUCTION

The DSM-IV-TR (American Psychiatric Association [APA], 2000) defines **personality** as "enduring patterns of perceiving, relating to, and thinking about the environment and oneself that are exhibited in a wide range of social and personal contexts" (p. 686). Nurses must have a basic knowledge of human personality development to understand maladaptive behavioral responses commonly seen in psychiatric clients. Developmental theories identify behaviors associated with various *stages* through which individuals pass, thereby specifying what is appropriate or inappropriate at each developmental level.

Specialists in child development believe that infancy and early childhood are the major life periods during which developmental change originates and occurs. Specialists in life cycle development believe that people continue to develop and change throughout life, thereby suggesting the possibility for renewal and growth in adults.

Developmental stages are identified by age. Behaviors can then be evaluated for age-appropriateness. Ideally, an individual successfully fulfills all the tasks associated with one stage before moving on to the next stage (at the appropriate age). Realistically, however, this seldom happens. One reason is related to **temperament,** the inborn personality characteristics that influence an individual's manner of reacting to the environment, and ultimately his or her developmental progression (Chess & Thomas, 1986). The environment may also influence one's developmental pattern. Individuals who are reared in a dysfunctional family system often have retarded ego development. According to specialists in life-cycle development, behaviors from an unsuccessfully completed stage can be modified and corrected in a later stage.

Stages overlap, and an individual may be working on tasks associated with several stages at one time. When an individual becomes fixed in a lower level of development, with age-inappropriate behaviors focused on fulfillment of those tasks, psychopathology may become evident. Only when personality traits are inflexible and maladaptive and cause either significant functional impairment or subjective distress do they constitute *personality disorders* (APA, 2000).

PSYCHOANALYTIC THEORY

Sigmund Freud (1961), who has been called the father of psychiatry, is credited as the first to identify development by stages. He considered the first 5 years of a child's life to be the most important, because he believed that an individual's basic character had been formed by the age of 5.

Freud's personality theory can be conceptualized according to structure and dynamics of the personality, topography of the mind, and stages of personality development.

Structure of the Personality

Freud organized the structure of the personality into three major components: the **id, ego**, and **superego**. They are distinguished by their unique functions and different characteristics.

Id

The *id* is the locus of instinctual drives—the "pleasure principle." Present at birth, it endows the infant with instinctual drives that seek to satisfy needs and achieve immediate gratification. Id-driven behaviors are impulsive and may be irrational.

Ego

The *ego*, also called the *rational self* or the "reality principle," begins to develop between the ages of 4 and 6 months. The ego experiences the reality of the external world, adapts to it, and responds to it. As the ego develops and gains strength, it seeks to bring the influences of the external world to bear upon the id, to substitute the reality principle for the pleasure principle (Marmer, 1999). A primary function of the ego is one of mediator, that is, to maintain harmony among the external world, the id, and the superego.

Superego

If the id is identified as the pleasure principle, and the ego the reality principle, the *superego* might be referred to as the "perfection principle." The superego, which develops between ages 3 and 6 years, internalizes the values and morals set forth by primary caregivers. Derived from a system of rewards and punishments, the superego is composed of two major components: the *ego-ideal* and the *conscience.* When a child is consistently rewarded for "good" behavior, the self-esteem is enhanced, and the behavior becomes part of the ego-ideal; that is, it is internalized as part of his or her value system. The conscience is formed when the child is consistently punished for "bad" behavior. The child learns what is considered morally right or wrong from feedback received from parental figures and from society or culture. When moral and ethical principles or even internalized ideals and values are disregarded, the conscience generates a feeling of guilt within the individual. The superego is important in the socialization of the individual because it assists the ego in the control of id impulses. When the superego becomes rigid and punitive, problems with low self-confidence and low self-esteem arise.

Topography of the Mind

Freud classified all mental contents and operations into three categories: the conscious, the preconscious, and the unconscious.

- The *conscious* includes all memories that remain within an individual's awareness. It is the smallest of the three categories. Events and experiences that are easily remembered or retrieved are considered to be within one's conscious awareness. Examples include telephone numbers, birthdays of self and significant others, dates of special holidays, and what one consumed for lunch that day. The conscious mind is thought to be under the control of the ego, the rational and logical structure of the personality.
- The *preconscious* includes all memories that may have been forgotten or are not in present awareness but, with attention, can readily be recalled into consciousness. Examples include telephone numbers or addresses once known but little used and feelings associated with significant life events that may have occurred at some time in the past. The preconscious enhances awareness by helping to *suppress* unpleasant or nonessential memories from consciousness. It is thought to be partially under the control of the superego, which helps to suppress unacceptable thoughts and behaviors.
- The *unconscious* includes all memories that one is unable to bring to conscious awareness. It is the largest of the three topographical levels. Unconscious material consists of unpleasant or nonessential memories that have been *repressed* and can be retrieved only through therapy, hypnosis, and with certain substances that alter the awareness and have the capacity to restructure repressed memories. Unconscious material may also emerge in dreams and in seemingly incomprehensible behavior.

Dynamics of the Personality

Freud believed that *psychic energy* is the force or impetus required for mental functioning. Originating in the id, it instinctually fulfills basic physiological needs. Freud called this psychic energy (or the drive to fulfill basic physiological needs such as hunger, thirst, and sex) the **libido.** As the child matures, psychic energy is diverted from the id to form the ego and then from the ego to form the superego. Psychic energy is distributed within these three components, with the ego retaining the largest share to maintain a balance between the impulsive behaviors of the id and the idealistic behaviors of the superego. If an excessive amount of psychic energy is stored in one of these personality components, behavior reflects that part of the personality. For instance, impulsive behavior prevails when excessive psychic energy is stored in the id. Overinvestment in the ego reflects self-absorbed, or narcissistic, behaviors; an excess within the superego results in rigid, self-deprecating behaviors.

Freud used the terms *cathexis* and *anticathexis* to describe the forces within the id, ego, and superego that are used to invest psychic energy in external sources to satisfy needs. Cathexis is the process by which the id invests energy into an object in an attempt to achieve gratification. An example is the individual who instinctively turns to alcohol to relieve stress. Anticathexis is the use of psychic energy by the ego and the superego to control id impulses. In the example cited, the ego would attempt to control the use of alcohol with rational thinking, such as, "I already have ulcers from drinking too much. I will call my Alcoholics Anonymous sponsor for support. I will not drink." The superego would exert control with such thinking as, "I shouldn't drink. If I drink, my family will be hurt and angry. I should think of how it affects them. I'm such a weak person." Freud believed that an imbalance between cathexis and anticathexis resulted in internal conflicts, producing tension and anxiety within the individual. Freud's daughter Anna devised a comprehensive list of defense mechanisms, believed to be used by the ego as a protective device against anxiety, in mediating between the excessive demands of the id, and the excessive restrictions of the superego (see Chapter 1).

Freud's Stages of Personality Development

Freud described formation of the personality through five stages of *psychosexual* development. He placed

TABLE 2 – 1 Freud's Stages of Psychosexual Development

Age	Stage	Major Developmental Tasks
Birth–18 months	Oral	Relief from anxiety through oral gratification of needs
18 months–3 years	Anal	Learning independence and control, with focus on the excretory function
3–6 years	Phallic	Identification with parent of same sex; development of sexual identity; focus on genital organs
6–12 years	Latency	Sexuality repressed; focus on relationships with same-sex peers
13–20 years	Genital	Libido reawakened as genital organs mature; focus on relationships with members of the opposite sex

much emphasis on the first five years of life, and believed that characteristics developed during these early years bore heavily on one's adaptation patterns and personality traits in adulthood. Fixation in an early stage of development almost certainly results in psychopathology. An outline of these five stages is presented in Table 2–1.

Oral Stage: Birth to 18 Months

During the oral stage, behavior is directed by the id, and the goal is immediate gratification of needs. The focus of energy is the mouth, and behaviors include sucking, chewing, and biting. The infant feels a sense of attachment and is unable to differentiate the self from the person who is providing the mothering. This includes feelings such as anxiety. Because of this lack of differentiation, a pervasive feeling of anxiety on the part of the mother may be passed on to her infant, leaving the child vulnerable to similar feelings of insecurity. With the beginning of development of the ego at age 4 to 6 months, the infant starts to view the self as separate from the mothering figure. A sense of security and the ability to trust others are derived out of gratification from fulfillment of basic needs during this stage.

Anal Stage: 18 Months to 3 Years

The major task in the anal stage is gaining independence and control, with particular focus on the excretory function. Freud believed that the manner in which the parents and other primary caregivers approach the task of toilet training may have far-reaching effects on the child in terms of values and personality characteristics. When toilet training is strict and rigid, the child may choose to retain the feces, becoming constipated. Adult retentive personality traits influenced by this type of training include stubbornness, stinginess, and miserliness. An alternate reaction to strict toilet training is for the child to expel feces in an unacceptable manner or at inappropriate times. Far-reaching effects of this behavior pattern include malevolence, cruelty to others, destructiveness, disorganization, and untidiness.

Toilet training that is more permissive and accepting attaches the feeling of importance and desirability to feces production. The child becomes extroverted, productive, and altruistic.

Phallic Stage: 3 to 6 Years

In this stage, the focus of energy shifts to the genital area. Discovery of differences between genders results in a heightened interest in the sexuality of self and others. This interest may be manifested in sexual self-exploratory or group-exploratory play. Freud proposed that the development of the *Oedipus complex* occurred during this stage of development. He described this as the child's unconscious desire to eliminate the parent of the same sex and to possess the parent of the opposite sex for himself or herself. Guilt feelings result with the emergence of the superego during these years. Resolution of this internal conflict occurs when the child develops a strong identification with the parent of the same sex and internalizes that parent's attitudes, beliefs, and value system.

Latency Stage: 6 to 12 Years

During the elementary school years, the focus changes from egocentrism to one of more interest in group activities, learning, and socialization with peers. Sexuality is not absent during this period but remains obscure and imperceptible to others. The preference is homosexual; children of this age show a distinct preference for same-sex relationships, even rejecting members of the opposite sex.

Genital Stage: 13 to 20 Years

In the genital stage, the maturing of the genital organs results in a reawakening of the libidinal drive. The focus is on relationships with members of the opposite sex and preparations for selecting a mate. The development of sexual maturity evolves from self-gratification to behaviors deemed acceptable by societal norms. Interpersonal relationships are based on genuine pleasure derived from the interaction rather than from the more self-serving implications of childhood associations.

Relevance of Psychoanalytic Theory to Nursing Practice

Knowledge of the structure of the personality can assist nurses who work in the mental health setting. The ability to recognize behaviors associated with the id, the ego, and the superego assists in the assessment of developmental level. Understanding the use of ego defense mechanisms is important in making determinations about maladaptive behaviors, in planning care for clients to assist in creating change (if desired), or in helping clients accept themselves as unique individuals.

INTERPERSONAL THEORY

Sullivan (1953) believed that individual behavior and personality development are the direct result of interpersonal relationships. Before the development of his own theoretical framework, Sullivan embraced the concepts of Freud. Later, he changed the focus of his work from the *intrapersonal* view of Freud to one with a more *interpersonal* flavor in which human behavior could be observed in social interactions with others. His ideas, which were not universally accepted at the time, have been integrated into the practice of psychiatry through publication only since his death in 1949. Sullivan's major concepts include the following:

Anxiety is a feeling of emotional discomfort, toward the relief or prevention of which all behavior is aimed. Sullivan believed that anxiety is the "chief disruptive force in interpersonal relations and the main factor in the development of serious difficulties in living." It arises out of one's inability to satisfy needs or achieve interpersonal security.

Satisfaction of needs is the fulfillment of all requirements associated with an individual's physiochemical environment. Sullivan identified examples of these requirements as oxygen, food, water, warmth, tenderness, rest, activity, sexual expression—virtually anything that, when absent, produces discomfort in the individual.

Interpersonal security is the feeling associated with relief from anxiety. When all needs have been met, one experiences a sense of total well-being, which Sullivan termed *interpersonal security*. He believed individuals have an innate need for interpersonal security.

Self-system is a collection of experiences, or security measures, adopted by the individual to protect against anxiety. Sullivan identified three components of the self-system, which are based on interpersonal experiences early in life.

- The *"good me"* is the part of the personality that develops in response to positive feedback from the primary caregiver. Feelings of pleasure, contentment, and gratification are experienced. The child learns which behaviors elicit this positive response as it becomes incorporated into the self-system.
- The *"bad me"* is the part of the personality that develops in response to negative feedback from the primary caregiver. Anxiety is experienced, eliciting feelings of discomfort, displeasure, and distress. The child learns to avoid negative feelings by altering certain behaviors.
- The *"not me"* is the part of the personality that develops in response to situations that produce intense anxiety in the child. Feelings of horror, awe, dread, and loathing are experienced in response to these situations, leading the child to deny these feelings in an effort to relieve anxiety. These feelings, having then been denied, become "not me," but someone else. This withdrawal from emotions has serious implications for mental disorders in adult life.

Sullivan's Stages of Personality Development

Sullivan describes six stages of personality development. An outline of the stages of personality development according to Sullivan's interpersonal theory is presented in Table 2–2.

Infancy: Birth to 18 Months

During this beginning stage, the major developmental task for the child is the gratification of needs. This is

TABLE 2 – 2 Stages of Development in Sullivan's Interpersonal Theory

Age	Stage	Major Developmental Tasks
Birth–18 months	Infancy	Relief from anxiety through oral gratification of needs
18 months–6 years	Childhood	Learning to experience a delay in personal gratification without undue anxiety
6–9 years	Juvenile	Learning to form satisfactory peer relationships
9–12 years	Preadolescence	Learning to form satisfactory relationships with persons of same sex; initiating feelings of affection for another person
12–14 years	Early adolescence	Learning to form satisfactory relationships with persons of the opposite sex; developing a sense of identity
14–21 years	Late adolescence	Establishing self-identity; experiencing satisfying relationships; working to develop a lasting, intimate, opposite-sex relationship

accomplished through activity associated with the mouth, such as crying, nursing, and thumb sucking.

Childhood: 18 Months to 6 Years

At ages 18 months to 6 years, the child learns that interference with fulfillment of personal wishes and desires may result in delayed gratification. He or she learns to accept this and feel comfortable with it, recognizing that delayed gratification often results in parental approval, a more lasting type of reward. Tools of this stage include the mouth, the anus, language, experimentation, manipulation, and identification.

Juvenile: 6 to 9 Years

The major task of the juvenile stage is formation of satisfactory relationships within the peer group. This is accomplished using competition, cooperation, and compromise.

Preadolescence: 9 to 12 Years

The tasks of the preadolescence stage focus on developing relationships with persons of the same sex. One's ability to collaborate with and show love and affection for another person begins at this stage.

Early Adolescence: 12 to 14 Years

During early adolescence, the child is struggling with developing a sense of identity, separate and independent from the parents. The major task is formation of satisfactory relationships with members of the opposite sex. Sullivan saw the emergence of lust in response to biological changes as a major force occurring during this period.

Late Adolescence: 14 to 21 Years

The late adolescent period is characterized by tasks associated with the attempt to achieve interdependence within the society and the formation of a lasting, intimate relationship with a selected member of the opposite sex. The genital organs are the major developmental focus of this stage.

Relevance of Interpersonal Theory to Nursing Practice

The interpersonal theory has significant relevance to nursing practice. Relationship development, which is a major concept of this theory, is a major psychiatric nursing intervention. Nurses develop therapeutic relationships with clients in an effort to help them generalize this ability to interact successfully with others.

With knowledge about the behaviors associated with all levels of anxiety and methods for alleviating anxiety, nurses can help clients achieve interpersonal security and a sense of well-being. Nurses use the concepts of Sullivan's theory to help clients achieve a higher degree of independent and interpersonal functioning.

THEORY OF PSYCHOSOCIAL DEVELOPMENT

Erikson (1963) studied the influence of social processes on the development of the personality. He described eight stages of the life cycle during which individuals struggle with developmental "crises." Specific tasks associated with each stage must be com-

TABLE 2 – 3 Stages of Development in Erikson's Psychosocial Theory

Age	Stage	Major Developmental Tasks
Infancy (Birth–18 months)	Trust vs. mistrust	To develop a basic trust in the mothering figure and be able to generalize it to others
Early childhood (18 months–3 years)	Autonomy vs. shame and doubt	To gain some self-control and independence within the environment
Late childhood (3–6 years)	Initiative vs. guilt	To develop a sense of purpose and the ability to initiate and direct own activities
School age (6–12 years)	Industry vs. inferiority	To achieve a sense of self-confidence by learning, competing, performing successfully, and receiving recognition from significant others, peers, and acquaintances
Adolescence (12–20 years)	Identity vs. role confusion	To integrate the tasks mastered in the previous stages into a secure sense of self
Young adulthood (20–30 years)	Intimacy vs. isolation	To form an intense, lasting relationship or a commitment to another person, cause, institution, or creative effort
Adulthood (30–65 years)	Generativity vs. stagnation	To achieve the life goals established for oneself, while also considering the welfare of future generations
Old age (65 years–death)	Ego integrity vs. despair	To review one's life and derive meaning from both positive and negative events, while achieving a positive sense of self-worth

pleted for resolution of the crisis and for emotional growth to occur. An outline of Erikson's stages of psychosocial development is presented in Table 2–3.

Erikson's Stages of Personality Development

Trust versus Mistrust: Birth to 18 Months

MAJOR DEVELOPMENTAL TASK. In this stage, the major task is to develop a basic trust in the mothering figure and be able to generalize it to others.

- Achievement of the task results in self-confidence, optimism, faith in the gratification of needs and desires, and hope for the future. The infant learns to trust when basic needs are met consistently.
- Nonachievement results in emotional dissatisfaction with the self and others, suspiciousness, and difficulty with interpersonal relationships. The task remains unresolved when primary caregivers fail to respond to the infant's distress signal promptly and consistently.

Autonomy versus Shame and Doubt: 18 Months to 3 Years

MAJOR DEVELOPMENTAL TASK. The major task in this stage is to gain some self-control and independence within the environment.

- Achievement of the task results in a sense of self-control and the ability to delay gratification, and a feeling of self-confidence in one's ability to perform. Autonomy is achieved when parents encourage and provide opportunities for independent activities.
- Nonachievement results in a lack of self-confidence, a lack of pride in the ability to perform, a sense of being controlled by others, and a rage against the self. The task remains unresolved when primary caregivers restrict independent behaviors, both physically and verbally, or set the child up for failure with unrealistic expectations.

Initiative versus Guilt: 3 to 6 Years

MAJOR DEVELOPMENTAL TASK. During this stage, the goal is to develop a sense of purpose and the ability to initiate and direct one's own activities.

- Achievement of the task results in the ability to exercise restraint and self-control of inappropriate social behaviors. Assertiveness and dependability increase, and the child enjoys learning and personal achievement. The conscience develops, thereby controlling the impulsive behaviors of the id. Initiative is achieved when creativity is encouraged and performance is recognized and positively reinforced.
- Nonachievement results in feelings of inadequacy

and a sense of defeat. Guilt is experienced to an excessive degree, even to the point of accepting liability in situations for which one is not responsible. The child may view himself or herself as evil and deserving of punishment. The task remains unresolved when creativity is stifled and parents continually expect a higher level of achievement than the child produces.

Industry versus Inferiority: 6 to 12 Years

MAJOR DEVELOPMENTAL TASK. The major task of this stage is to achieve a sense of self-confidence by learning, competing, performing successfully, and receiving recognition from significant others, peers, and acquaintances.

- Achievement of the task results in a sense of satisfaction and pleasure in the interaction and involvement with others. The individual masters reliable work habits and develops attitudes of trustworthiness. He or she is conscientious, feels pride in achievement and enjoys play, but desires a balance between fantasy and "real world" activities. Industry is achieved when encouragement is given to activities and responsibilities in the school and community, as well as those within the home, and recognition is given for accomplishments.
- Nonachievement results in difficulty in interpersonal relationships because of feelings of personal inadequacy. The individual can neither cooperate and compromise with others in group activities, nor problem solve or complete tasks successfully. He or she may become either passive and meek or overly aggressive to cover up for feelings of inadequacy. If this occurs, the individual may manipulate or violate the rights of others to satisfy his or her own needs or desires; he or she may become a workaholic with unrealistic expectations for personal achievement. This task remains unresolved when parents set unrealistic expectations for the child, when discipline is harsh and tends to impair self-esteem, and when accomplishments are consistently met with negative feedback.

Identity versus Role Confusion: 12 to 20 Years

MAJOR DEVELOPMENTAL TASK. At this stage, the goal is to integrate the tasks mastered in the previous stages into a secure sense of self.

- Achievement of the task results in a sense of confidence, emotional stability, and a view of the self as a unique individual. Commitments are made to a value system, to the choice for a career, and to relationships with members of both genders. Identity is achieved when adolescents are allowed to experience independence by making decisions that influence their lives. Parents should be available to offer support when needed but should gradually relinquish control to the maturing individual in an effort to encourage the development of an independent sense of self.
- Nonachievement results in a sense of self-consciousness, doubt, and confusion about one's role in life. Personal values or goals for one's life are absent. Commitments to relationships with others are nonexistent or superficial and brief. A lack of self-confidence is often expressed by delinquent and rebellious behavior. Entering adulthood, with its accompanying responsibilities, may be an underlying fear. This task can remain unresolved for many reasons (e.g., when independence is discouraged by the parents and the adolescent is nurtured in the dependent position; when discipline within the home has been overly harsh, inconsistent, or absent; and when parental rejection or frequent shifting of parental figures has occurred).

Intimacy versus Isolation: 20 to 30 Years

MAJOR DEVELOPMENTAL TASK. The objective during this stage is to form an intense, lasting relationship, or a commitment to another person, a cause, an institution, or a creative effort (Murray & Zentner, 2001).

- Achievement of the task results in the capacity for mutual love and respect between two people and the ability of an individual to pledge a total commitment to another. The intimacy goes far beyond the sexual contact between two people. It describes a commitment in which personal sacrifices are made for another, whether it be another person, or if one chooses, a career or other type of cause or endeavor to which an individual elects to devote his or her life. Intimacy is achieved when an individual has developed the capacity for giving of oneself to another. This is learned when one has been the recipient of this type of giving within the family unit.
- Nonachievement results in withdrawal, social isolation, and aloneness. The individual is unable to form lasting, intimate relationships, often seeking intimacy through numerous superficial sexual contacts. No career is established; he or she may have a history of occupational changes (or may fear change

and thus remain in an undesirable job situation). The task remains unresolved when love in the home has been deprived or distorted through the younger years (Murray & Zentner, 2001). One fails to achieve the ability to give of the self without having been the recipient early on from primary caregivers.

Generativity versus Stagnation or Self-Absorption: 30 to 65 Years

MAJOR DEVELOPMENTAL TASK. The major task of this stage is to achieve the life goals established for oneself, while also considering the welfare of future generations.

- Achievement of the task results in a sense of gratification from personal and professional achievements and from meaningful contributions to others. The individual is active in the service of and to society. Generativity is achieved when the individual expresses satisfaction with this stage in life and demonstrates responsibility for leaving the world a better place in which to live.
- Nonachievement results in lack of concern for the welfare of others and total preoccupation with the self. He or she becomes withdrawn, isolated, and highly self-indulgent, with no capacity for giving of the self to others. The task remains unresolved when earlier developmental tasks are not fulfilled and the individual does not achieve the degree of maturity required to derive gratification out of a personal concern for the welfare of others.

Ego Integrity versus Despair: 65 Years to Death

MAJOR DEVELOPMENTAL TASK. During this stage, the goal is to review one's life and derive meaning from both positive and negative events, while achieving a positive sense of self.

- Achievement of the task results in a sense of self-worth and self-acceptance as one reviews life goals, accepting that some were achieved and some were not. The individual derives a sense of dignity from his or her life experiences and does not fear death, rather viewing it as another stage of development. Ego integrity is achieved when individuals have successfully completed the developmental tasks of the other stages and have little desire to make major changes in the ways their lives have progressed.
- Nonachievement results in a sense of self-contempt and disgust with how life has progressed. The individual would like to start over and have a second chance at life. He or she feels worthless and helpless to change. Anger, depression, and loneliness are evident. The focus may be on past failures or perceived failures. Impending death is feared or denied, or ideas of suicide may prevail. The task remains unresolved when earlier tasks are not fulfilled: self-confidence, a concern for others, and a strong sense of self-identity were never achieved.

Relevance of Psychosocial Development Theory to Nursing Practice

Erikson's theory is particularly relevant to nursing practice in that it incorporates sociocultural concepts into the development of personality. Erikson provides a systematic, stepwise approach and outlines specific tasks that should be completed during each stage. This information can be used quite readily in psychiatric/mental health nursing. Many individuals with mental health problems are still struggling to achieve tasks from a number of developmental stages. Nurses can plan care to assist these individuals in fulfilling these tasks and in moving on to a higher developmental level.

THEORY OF OBJECT RELATIONS

Mahler (Mahler, Pine, & Bergman, 1975) formulated a theory that describes the separation-individuation process of the infant from the maternal figure (primary caregiver). She describes this process as progressing through three major phases, and she further delineates phase III, the separation-individuation phase, into four subphases. Mahler's developmental theory is outlined in Table 2–4.

Phase I: The Autistic Phase (Birth to 1 Month). In this phase, also called *normal autism*, the infant exists in a half-sleeping, half-waking state and does not perceive the existence of other people or an external environment. The fulfillment of basic needs for survival and comfort is the focus and is merely accepted as it occurs. This theory suggests that fixation in this phase may predispose the child to autistic disorder.

Phase II: The Symbiotic Phase (1 to 5 Months). *Symbiosis* is a type of "psychic fusion" of mother and child. The child views the self as an extension of the mother, but with a developing awareness that she

TABLE 2 – 4 Stages of Development in Mahler's Theory of Object Relations

Age	Phase/Subphase	Major Developmental Tasks
Birth–1 month	I. Normal autism	Fulfillment of basic needs for survival and comfort
1–5 months	II. Symbiosis	Development of awareness of external source of need fulfillment
	III. Separation-Individuation	
5–10 months	a. Differentiation	Commencement of a primary recognition of separateness from the mothering figure
10–16 months	b. Practicing	Increased independence through locomotor functioning; increased sense of separateness of self
16–24 months	c. Rapprochement	Acute awareness of separateness of self; learning to seek "emotional refueling" from mothering figure to maintain feeling of security
24–36 months	d. Consolidation	Sense of separateness established; on the way to object constancy (i.e., able to internalize a sustained image of loved object/person when it is out of sight); resolution of separation anxiety

fulfills the child's every need. Mahler suggests that absence of, or rejection by, the maternal figure at this phase can lead to symbiotic psychosis. This theory suggests that fixation in the symbiotic phase of development may predispose the child to adolescent- or adult-onset psychotic disorder.

Phase III: Separation-Individuation (5 to 36 Months). This third phase represents what Mahler calls the "psychological birth" of the child. *Separation* is defined as the physical and psychological attainment of a sense of personal distinction from the mothering figure. *Individuation* occurs with a strengthening of the ego and an acceptance of a sense of "self," with independent ego boundaries. Four subphases are described through which the child evolves in his or her progression from a symbiotic extension of the mothering figure to a distinct and separate being.

Subphase 1—Differentiation (5 to 10 Months). The differentiation phase begins with the child's initial physical movements away from the mothering figure. A primary recognition of separateness commences.

Subphase 2—Practicing (10 to 16 Months). With advanced locomotor functioning, the child experiences feelings of exhilaration from increased independence. He or she is now able to move away from and return to the mothering figure. A sense of omnipotence is manifested.

Subphase 3—Rapprochement (16 to 24 Months). This third subphase is critical to the child's healthy ego development. During this time the child becomes increasingly aware of his or her separateness from the mothering figure, while the sense of fearlessness and omnipotence diminishes. The child, now recognizing the mother as a separate individual, wishes to reestablish closeness with her but shuns the total reengulfment of the symbiotic stage. The child needs the mothering figure to be available to provide "emotional refueling" on demand. Critical to this subphase is the mothering figure's response to the child. If the mothering figure is available to fulfill emotional needs as they are required, the child develops a sense of security in the knowledge that he or she is loved and will not be abandoned. However, if emotional needs are inconsistently met or if the mother rewards clinging, dependent behaviors and withholds nurturing when the child demonstrates independence, feelings of rage and fear of abandonment develop and often persist into adulthood.

Subphase 4—Consolidation (24 to 36 Months). With achievement of consolidation, a definite individuality and sense of separateness of self are established. Objects are represented as whole, with the ability to integrate both "good" and "bad." A degree of object constancy is established, as the child is able to internalize a sustained image of the mothering figure as enduring and loving, while maintaining the perception of her as a separate person in the outside world.

Relevance of Object Relations Theory to Nursing Practice

Understanding of the concepts of Mahler's theory of object relations helps the nurse assess the client's level of individuation from primary caregivers. The emotional problems of many individuals can be traced to lack of fulfillment of the tasks of separation/individuation. Examples include problems related to dependency and excessive anxiety. The individual with borderline personality disorder is thought to be fixed in the rapprochement phase of development, harboring fears of abandonment and underlying rage. This knowledge is important in providing nursing care to these individuals.

A NURSING MODEL—HILDEGARD E. PEPLAU

Peplau (1991) applied interpersonal theory to nursing practice and, most specifically, to nurse-client relationship development. She established a framework for **psychodynamic nursing**, the interpersonal involvement of the nurse with a client in a given nursing situation. Peplau stated, "Nursing is helpful when both the patient and the nurse grow as a result of the learning that occurs in the nursing situation."

Peplau correlated the stages of personality development in childhood to stages through which clients advance during the progression of an illness. She also viewed these interpersonal experiences as learning situations for nurses to facilitate forward movement in the development of personality. She believed that when there is fulfillment of psychological tasks associated with the nurse-client relationship, the personalities of both could be strengthened. Key concepts include the following:

- *Nursing* is a human relationship between an individual who is sick, or in need of health services, and a nurse especially educated to recognize and to respond to the need for help.
- *Psychodynamic nursing* is being able to understand one's own behavior, to help others identify felt difficulties, and to apply principles of human relations to the problems that arise at all levels of experience.
- *Roles* are sets of values and behaviors that are specific to functional positions within social structures. Peplau identified the following *nursing roles:*
    - *Resource person* is one who provides specific, needed information that helps the client understand his or her problem and the new situation.
    - **Counselor** is one who listens as the client reviews feelings related to difficulties he or she is experiencing in any aspect of life. "Interpersonal techniques" have been identified to facilitate the nurse's interaction in the process of helping the client solve problems and make decisions concerning these difficulties.
    - *Teacher* is one who identifies learning needs and provides information to the client or family that may aid in improvement of the life situation.
    - *Leader* is one who directs the nurse-client interaction and ensures that appropriate actions are undertaken to facilitate achievement of the designated goals.
    - **Technical expert** is one who understands various professional devices and possesses the clinical skills necessary to perform the interventions that are in the best interest of the client.
    - **Surrogate** is one who serves as a substitute figure for another.
- *Phases of nurse-client relationship* are stages of overlapping roles or functions in relation to health problems, during which the nurse and client learn to work cooperatively to resolve difficulties. Peplau identified four phases:
    - *Orientation* is the phase during which the client, nurse, and family work together to recognize, clarify, and define the existing problem.
    - *Identification* is the phase after which the client's initial impression has been clarified and during which he or she begins to respond selectively to persons who seem to offer the help that is needed. Clients may respond in one of three ways: (1) on the basis of participation or interdependent relations with the nurse, (2) on the basis of independence or isolation from the nurse, or (3) on the basis of helplessness or dependence on the nurse (Peplau, 1991).
    - *Exploitation* is the phase during which the client proceeds to take full advantage of the services offered to him or her. Having learned which services are available, feeling comfortable within the setting, and serving as an active participant in his or her own health care, the client exploits the services available and explores all possibilities of the changing situation.
    - *Resolution* occurs when the client is freed from

TABLE 2 – 5 Stages of Development in Peplau's Interpersonal Theory

Age	Stage	Major Developmental Tasks
Infancy	Learning to count on others	Learning to communicate in various ways with the primary caregiver to have comfort needs fulfilled
Toddlerhood	Learning to delay satisfaction	Learning the satisfaction of pleasing others by delaying self-gratification in small ways
Early childhood	Identifying oneself	Learning appropriate roles and behaviors by acquiring the ability to perceive the expectations of others
Late childhood	Developing skills in participation	Learning the skills of compromise, competition, and cooperation with others; establishing a more realistic view of the world and a feeling of one's place in it

identification with helping persons and gathers strength to assume independence. Resolution is the direct result of successful completion of the other three phases.

- *Psychological tasks* are developmental lessons that must be on the way to achieving maturity of the personality.

Peplau's Stages of Personality Development

Peplau (1991) identified four psychological tasks that she associated with the stages of infancy and childhood described by Freud and Sullivan. She stated:

> When psychological tasks are successfully learned at each era of development, biological capacities are used productively and relations with people lead to productive living. When they are not successfully learned they carry over into adulthood and attempts at learning continue in devious ways, more or less impeded by conventional adaptations that provide a superstructure over the baseline of actual learning. (p. 166)

In the context of nursing, Peplau (1991) related these four psychological tasks to the demands made on nurses in their relations with clients. She maintained that:

> nursing can function as a maturing force in society. Since illness is an event that is experienced along with feelings that derive from older experiences, but are re-enacted in the relationship of nurse-to-patient, the nurse-patient relationship is seen as an opportunity for nurses to help patients complete the unfinished psychological tasks of childhood in some degree. (p. 159)

Peplau's psychological tasks of personality development include the following four stages. An outline of the stages of personality development according to Peplau's theory is presented in Table 2–5.

Learning to Count on Others

Nurses and clients first come together as strangers. Both bring to the relationship certain "raw materials," such as inherited biological components, personality characteristics (*temperament*), individual intellectual capacity, and specific cultural or environmental influences. Peplau related these to the same "raw materials" with which an infant comes into this world. The newborn is capable of experiencing *comfort* and *discomfort*. He or she soon learns to communicate feelings in a way that results in the fulfillment of comfort needs by the mothering figure who provides love and care unconditionally. However, fulfillment of these dependency needs is inhibited when goals of the mothering figure become the focus, and love and care are contingent upon meeting the needs of the caregiver rather than the infant.

Clients with unmet dependency needs regress during illness and demonstrate behaviors that relate to this stage of development. Other clients regress to this level because of physical disabilities associated with their illness. Peplau believed that, when nurses provide unconditional care, they help these clients progress toward more mature levels of functioning. This may involve the role of "surrogate mother," in which the nurse fulfills needs for the client with the intent of helping him or her grow, mature, and become more independent.

Learning to Delay Satisfaction

Pepleu related this stage to that of toddlerhood, or the first step in the development of interdependent social relations. Psychosexually, it is compared to the anal stage of development, when a child learns that, because of cultural mores, he or she cannot empty the bowels for relief of discomfort at will, but must delay to use the toilet, which is considered more culturally acceptable. Toilet training that occurs too early, is very rigid and renders the child powerless, is presented as a dirty and disgusting behavior, or is set forth as a condition for love and caring results in a child's unfulfillment of the tasks associated with this stage. The child fails to learn the satisfaction of pleasing others by delaying self-gratification in small ways. He or she may also exhibit rebellious behavior by failing to comply with demands of the mothering figure in an effort to counter feelings of powerlessness. The child may accomplish this by withholding the fecal product or failing to deposit it in the culturally acceptable manner.

Peplau cites Fromm (1949) in describing the following potential behaviors of individuals who have failed to complete the tasks of the second stage of development:

- Exploitation and manipulation of others to satisfy their own desires because they are unable to do so independently
- Suspiciousness and envy of others, directing hostility toward others in an effort to enhance their own self-image
- Hoarding and withholding possessions from others; miserliness
- Inordinate neatness and punctuality
- Inability to relate to others through sharing of feelings, ideas, or experiences
- Ability to vary the personality characteristics to those required to satisfy personal desires at any given time

When nurses observe these types of behaviors in clients, it is important to encourage full expression and to convey unconditional acceptance. When the client learns to feel safe and unconditionally accepted, he or she is more likely to let go of the oppositional behavior and advance in the developmental progression. Peplau (1991) stated:

> Nurses who aid patients to feel safe and secure, so that wants can be expressed and satisfaction eventually achieved, also help them to strengthen personal power that is needed for productive social activities. (p. 207)

Identifying Oneself

"A concept of self develops as a product of interaction with adults" (Peplau, 1991, p. 211). A child learns to structure self-concept by observing how others interact with him or her as a person. Roles and behaviors are established out of the child's perception of the expectations of others. When children perceive that adults expect them to maintain more or less permanent roles as infants, they perceive themselves as helpless and dependent. When the perceived expectation is that the child must behave in a manner beyond his or her maturational level, the child is deprived of the fulfillment of emotional and growth needs at the lower levels of development. Children who are given freedom to respond to situations and experiences unconditionally (i.e., with behaviors that are appropriate to their feelings) learn to improve on and reconstruct behavioral responses at their own pace. Peplau (1991) stated:

> The ways in which adults appraise the child, and the way he functions in relation to his experiences and perceptions, are taken in or introjected and become the child's view of himself. (p. 213)

In nursing, it is important for the nurse to recognize cues that communicate how the client feels about himself or herself, and about the presenting medical problem. In the initial interaction, it is difficult for the nurse to perceive the "wholeness" of the client, for the focus is on the condition that has caused him or her to seek help. Likewise, it is difficult for the client to perceive the nurse as a "mother (or father)" or "somebody's wife (or husband)" or as having a life aside from being there to offer assistance with the immediate presenting problem. As the relationship develops, nurses must be able to recognize client behaviors that indicate unfulfilled needs and provide experiences that promote growth. For example, the client who very proudly announces that he or she has completed activities of daily living independently and wants the nurse to come and inspect her room may still be craving the positive reinforcement that is so necessary at lower levels of development.

Nurses must also be aware of the predisposing factors that they bring to the relationship. Attitudes and beliefs about certain issues can have a deleterious effect on the client and interfere not only with the therapeutic relationship but also with the client's ability for growth and development. For example, a nurse who has strong beliefs against abortion may treat a client who has just undergone an abortion with disapproval and disrespect. The nurse may respond in this manner without even realizing he or she is doing so. Attitudes and values are introjected during early development and can be integrated so completely as to become a part of the self-system. Nurses must have knowledge and appreciation of their own concept of self to develop the flexibility required to accept all clients as they are, unconditionally. Effective resolution of problems that arise in the interdependent relationship can be the means for both client and nurse to reinforce positive personality traits and modify those more negative views of self.

Developing Skills in Participation

Peplau cites Sullivan's (1953) description of the "juvenile" stage of personality development (ages 6 through 9). During this stage, the child develops the capacity to "compromise, compete, and cooperate" with others. These skills are considered basic to one's ability to participate collaboratively with others. If a child tries to use the skills of an earlier level of development (e.g., crying, whining, or demanding), he or she may be rejected by peers of this juvenile stage. As this stage progresses, children begin to view themselves through the eyes of their peers. Sullivan (1953) called this "consensual validation." Preadolescents take on a more realistic view of the world and a feeling of their place in it. The capacity to love others (besides the mother figure) develops at this time, and is expressed in relation to one's self-acceptance.

Failure to develop appropriate skills at any point along the developmental progression results in an individual's difficulty with participation in confronting the recurring problems of life. It is not the responsibility of the nurse to teach solutions to problems, but rather to help clients improve their problem-solving skills so that they may achieve their own resolution. This is accomplished through development of the skills of competition, compromise, cooperation, consensual validation, and love of self and others. Nurses can assist clients to develop or refine these skills by helping them to identify the problem, define a goal, and take the responsibility for performing the actions necessary to reach that goal. Peplau (1991) stated:

> Participation is required by a democratic society. When it has not been learned in earlier experiences, nurses have an opportunity to facilitate learning in the present and thus to aid in the promotion of a democratic society. (p. 259)

Relevance of Peplau's Model to Nursing Practice

Peplau's model provides nurses with a framework to interact with clients, many of whom are fixed in—or, because of illness, have regressed to—an earlier level of development. She suggests roles that nurses may assume to assist clients to progress, thereby achieving or resuming their appropriate developmental level. Appropriate developmental progression arms the individual with the ability to confront the recurring problems of life. Nurses serve to facilitate learning of that which has not been learned in earlier experiences.

SUMMARY

Growth and development are unique to each individual and continue throughout the life span. With each stage, there evolves an increasing complexity in the growth of the personality. This chapter has provided a description of the theories of Freud, Sullivan, Erikson, and Mahler. In addition, the theoretical concepts of Peplau, and their application to interpersonal relations in nursing, were presented. These theorists together provide a multifaceted approach to personality development.

Nurses must have a basic knowledge of human personality development to understand maladaptive behavioral responses commonly seen in psychiatric clients. Knowledge of the appropriateness of behaviors at each developmental level is vital to the planning and implementation of quality nursing care.

REVIEW QUESTIONS

SELF-EXAMINATION

Please answer the questions based on the following case study:

Mr. J. is 35 years old. He has been admitted to the psychiatric unit for observation and evaluation following his arrest on charges that he robbed a convenience store and sexually assaulted the store clerk. Mr. J. was the illegitimate child of a teenage mother who deserted him when he was 6 months old. He was shuffled from one relative to another until it was clear that no one wanted him. Social Services placed him in foster homes, from which he continuously ran away. During his teenage years he was arrested a number of times for stealing, vandalism, arson, and other infractions of the law. He was shunned by his peers and to this day has little interaction with others. On the unit, he appears very anxious, paces back and forth, and darts his head from side to side in a continuous scanning of the area. He is unkempt and unclean. He has refused to eat, making some barely audible comment related to "being poisoned." He has shown no remorse for his misdeeds.

1. Theoretically, in which level of psychosocial development (according to Erikson) would you place Mr. J.?
   a. Intimacy vs. isolation
   b. Generativity vs. self-absorption
   c. Trust vs. mistrust
   d. Autonomy vs. shame and doubt
2. According to Erikson's theory, where would you place Mr. J. based on his behavior?
   a. Intimacy vs. isolation
   b. Generativity vs. self-absorption
   c. Trust vs. mistrust
   d. Autonomy vs. shame and doubt
3. According to Mahler's theory, Mr. J. did not receive the critical "emotional refueling" required during the rapprochement phase of development. What are the consequences of this deficiency?
   a. He has not yet learned to delay gratification.
   b. He does not feel guilt about wrongdoings to others.
   c. He is unable to trust others.
   d. He has internalized rage and fears of abandonment.
4. In what stage of development is Mr. J. fixed according to Sullivan's interpersonal theory?
   a. Infancy. He relieves anxiety through oral gratification.
   b. Childhood. He has not learned to delay gratification.
   c. Early adolescence. He is struggling to form an identity.
   d. Late adolescence. He is working to develop a lasting relationship.
5. Which of the following describes the psychoanalytical structure of Mr. J.'s personality?
   a. Weak id, strong ego, weak superego
   b. Strong id, weak ego, weak superego
   c. Weak id, weak ego, punitive superego
   d. Strong id, weak ego, punitive superego
6. In which of Peplau's stages of development would you assess Mr. J.?
   a. Learning to count on others
   b. Learning to delay gratification
   c. Identifying oneself
   d. Developing skills in participation

7. In planning care for Mr. J., on which of the following would be the primary focus for nursing?
   a. To decrease anxiety and develop trust
   b. To set limits on his behavior
   c. To ensure that he gets to group therapy
   d. To attend to his hygiene needs

Match the nursing role as described by Peplau with the nursing care behaviors listed on the right:

_____	8. Surrogate	a. "Mr. J., please tell me what it was like when you were growing up."
_____	9. Counselor	b. "What questions do you have about being here on this unit?"
_____	10. Resource person	c. "Some changes will have to be made in your behavior. I care about what happens to you."

REFERENCES

American Psychiatric Association (2000). Diagnostic and statistical manual of mental disorders—text revision (4th ed.). Washington, DC: APA.

Marmer, S.S. (1999). Theories of the mind and psychopathology. In R.E. Hales & S.C. Yudofsky (Eds.), Essentials of clinical psychiatry. Washington, DC: American Psychiatric Press.

Murray, R.B., & Zentner, J.P. (2001). Health promotion strategies through the life span (7th ed.). Upper Saddle River, NJ: Prentice Hall.

Peplau, H.E. (1991). Interpersonal relations in nursing. New York: Springer.

CLASSICAL REFERENCES

Chess, S., & Thomas, A. (1986). Temperament in clinical practice. New York: The Guilford Press.

Erikson, E. (1963). Childhood and society (2nd ed.). New York: WW Norton.

Freud, S. (1961). The ego and the id. Standard edition of the complete psychological works of Freud (Vol XIX). London: Hogarth Press.

Fromm, E. (1949). Man for himself. New York: Farrar & Rinehart.

Mahler, M., Pine, F., & Bergman, A. (1975). The psychological birth of the human infant. New York: Basic Books.

Sullivan, H.S. (1953). The interpersonal theory of psychiatry. New York: W.W. Norton.

3

CHAPTER

Biological Implications

CHAPTER OUTLINE

KEY TERMS

limbic system
neurons
dendrites
neurotransmitters
receptor sites
neuroendocrine system
synapse
axon
cell body

OBJECTIVES

After reading this chapter, the student will be able to:

1. Identify gross anatomical structures of the brain and describe their functions.
2. Discuss the physiology of neurotransmission within the central nervous system.
3. Describe the role of neurotransmitters in human behavior.
4. Discuss the association of endocrine functioning to the development of psychiatric disorders.
5. Discuss the correlation of alteration in brain function to various psychiatric disorders.
6. Identify various diagnostic procedures used to detect alteration in biological functioning that may be contributing to psychiatric disorders.
7. Discuss the implications of psychobiological concepts to the practice of psychiatric/mental health nursing.

INTRODUCTION

In recent years, a greater emphasis has been placed on the study of the organic basis for psychiatric illness. This "neuroscientific revolution" began in earnest when the 101st legislature of the United States designated the 1990s as the "decade of the brain." With this legislation came the challenge for studying the biological basis of behavior. Several mental illnesses are now being considered as physical disorders that are the result of malfunctions and/or malformations of the brain.

This is not to imply that psychosocial and sociocultural influences are totally discounted. The systems of biology, psychology, and sociology are not mutually exclusive—they are interacting systems. This is clearly indicated by the fact that individuals experience biological changes in response to various environmental events. Indeed, each of these disciplines may be, at various times, most appropriate for explaining behavioral phenomena.

This chapter presents an overview of neurophysiological, neurochemical, and endocrine influences on psychiatric illness. Various diagnostic procedures used to detect alterations in biological function that may contribute to psychiatric illness are identified. A discussion of the implications for nursing is included.

NEUROPHYSIOLOGICAL INFLUENCES

The Nervous System

The nervous system is composed of two major divisions: the central nervous system (CNS) and the peripheral nervous system (PNS). An outline of the components of these two divisions is presented in Table 3–1. A discussion of the primary functions of these components follows.

TABLE 3 – 1 Components of the Nervous System

- I. Central Nervous System
  - A. Brain
    - 1. Forebrain
      - a. Cerebrum
        - i. Frontal lobes
        - ii. Parietal lobes
        - iii. Temporal lobes
        - iv. Occipital lobes
      - b. Diencephalon
        - i. Thalamus
        - ii. Hypothalamus
        - iii. Limbic system
    - 2. Midbrain
      - a. Mesencephalon
    - 3. Hindbrain
      - a. Pons
      - b. Medulla
      - c. Cerebellum
  - B. Nerve Tissue
    - 1. Neurons
    - 2. Synapses
    - 3. Neurotransmitters
  - C. Spinal Cord
    - 1. Fiber tracts
    - 2. Spinal nerves
- II. Peripheral Nervous System
  - A. Afferent System
    - 1. Sensory neurons
      - a. Somatic
      - b. Visceral
  - B. Efferent System
    - 1. Somatic nervous system
      - a. Somatic motor neurons
    - 2. Autonomic nervous system
      - a. Sympathetic nervous system
        - i. Visceral motor neurons
      - b. Parasympathetic nervous system
        - i. Visceral motor neurons

The Central Nervous System

The Brain

The brain has three main divisions, which are subdivided into six major parts. The forebrain is made up of the cerebrum and diencephalon. The midbrain is the mesencephalon. The pons, medulla, and cerebellum make up the hindbrain. These six structures will be discussed individually. Diagrams of these structures are presented in Figures 3–1, 3–2, and 3–3.

CEREBRUM. The cerebrum is composed of two hemispheres separated by a deep groove that houses a band of 200 million **neurons** (nerve cells) called the corpus callosum. The outer shell is called the cortex. It is extensively folded and consists of billions of neurons. The left hemisphere appears to be dominant in most people. It controls speech, comprehension, rationality, and logic. The right hemisphere is nondominant in most people. Sometimes called the "creative" brain, the right hemisphere is associated with affect, behavior, and spatial perceptual functions. Each hemisphere is divided into four lobes.

- Frontal Lobes. The frontal lobes control voluntary body movement, including movements that permit speaking, thinking, and judgment formation. The frontal lobe may also play a role in the emotional experience, as evidenced by changes in mood and character after damage to this area. The alterations include fear, aggressiveness, depression, rage, euphoria, irritability, and apathy and are likely related to a frontal lobe connection to the **limbic system**.
- Parietal Lobes. The parietal lobes control perception and interpretation of most sensory information (including touch, pain, taste, and body position). Language interpretation is associated with the left hemisphere of the parietal lobe.
- Temporal Lobes. The upper anterior temporal lobe is concerned with auditory functions, and the lower part is dedicated to short-term memory. The sense

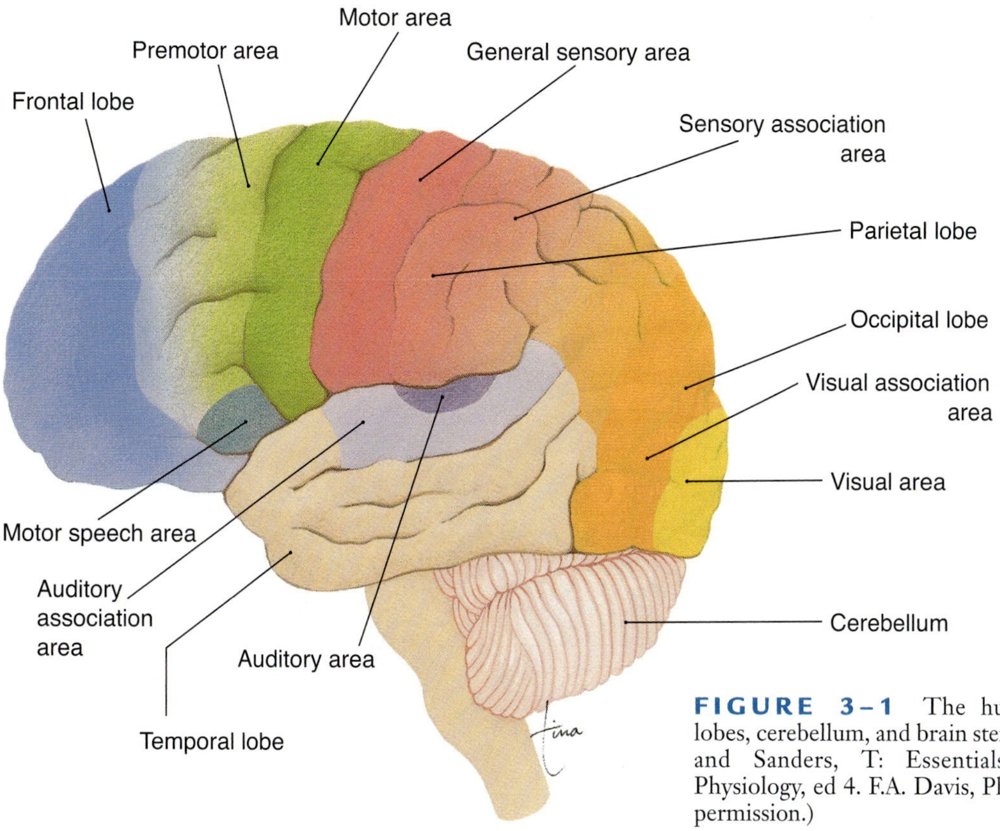

FIGURE 3–1 The human brain: cerebral lobes, cerebellum, and brain stem. (From Scanlon, VC and Sanders, T: Essentials of Anatomy and Physiology, ed 4. F.A. Davis, Philadelphia, 2003, with permission.)

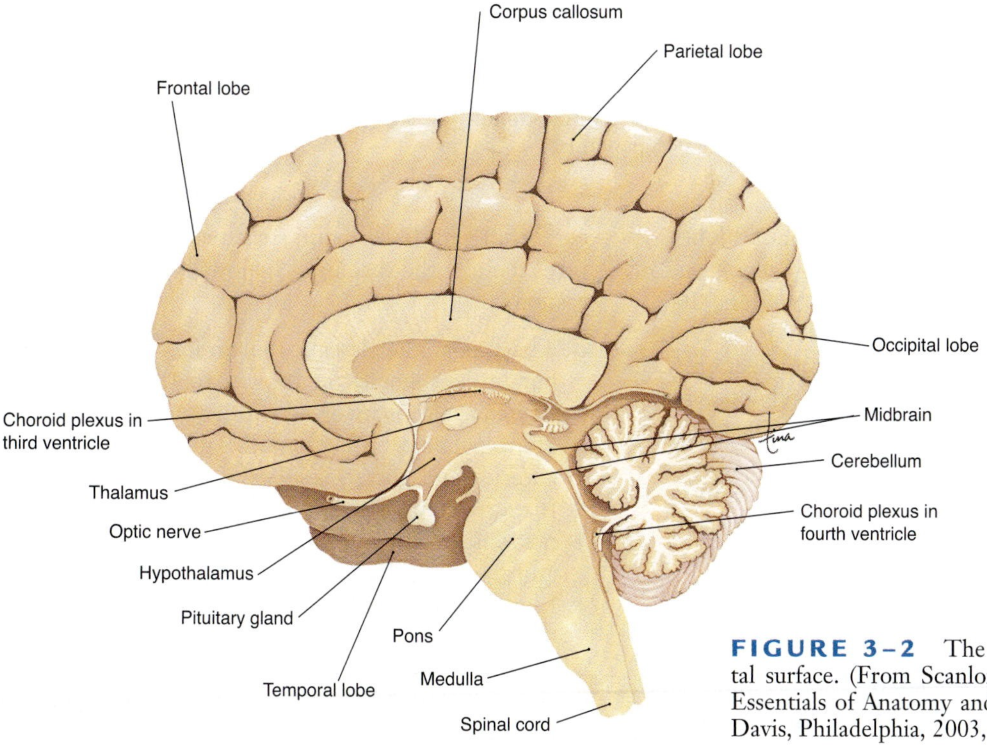

FIGURE 3–2 The human brain: midsagittal surface. (From Scanlon, VC and Sanders, T: Essentials of Anatomy and Physiology, ed 4. F.A. Davis, Philadelphia, 2003, with permission.)

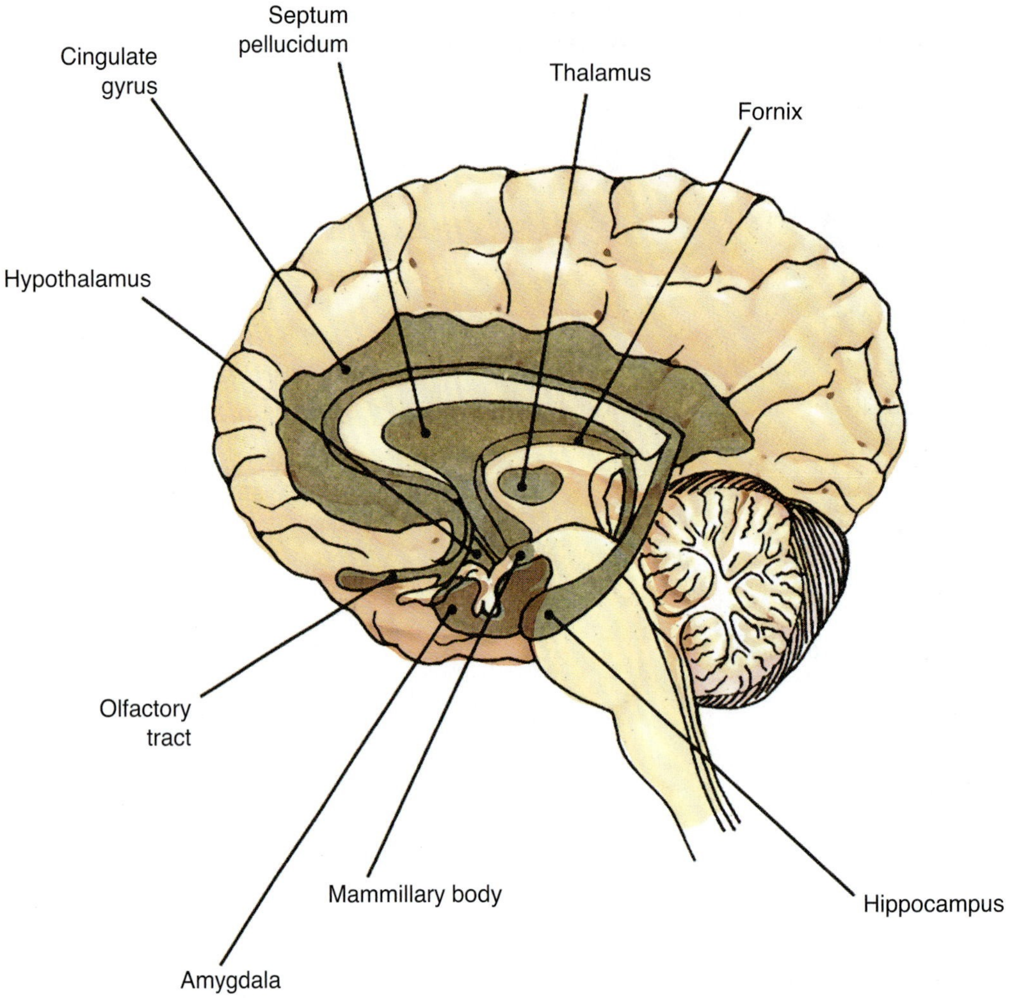

FIGURE 3–3 Structures of the limbic system. (Adapted from Scanlon, VC and Sanders, T: Essentials of Anatomy and Physiology, ed 4. F.A. Davis, Philadelphia, 2003, with permission.)

of smell has a connection to the temporal lobes, as the impulses carried by the olfactory nerves end in this area of the brain (Scanlon & Sanders, 2003). The temporal lobes also play a role in the expression of emotions through an interconnection with the limbic system. The left temporal lobe, along with the left parietal lobe, is involved in language interpretation.

- Occipital Lobes. The occipital lobes are the primary area of visual reception and interpretation. Visual perception, which gives individuals the ability to judge spatial relationships such as distance and to see in three dimensions, is also processed in this area (Scanlon & Sanders, 2003). Language interpretation is influenced by the occipital lobes through an association with the visual experience.

DIENCEPHALON. The diencephalon connects the cerebrum with lower brain structures. Its major structures include the thalamus, hypothalamus, and limbic system.

- Thalamus. The thalamus integrates all sensory input (except smell) on its way to the cortex. The thalamus also is involved with emotions and mood.
- Hypothalamus. The hypothalamus regulates the anterior and posterior lobes of the pituitary gland. It exerts control over the actions of the autonomic nervous system and regulates appetite and temperature.
- Limbic System. The limbic system consists of medially placed cortical and subcortical structures and the fiber tracts connecting them with one another and with the hypothalamus. These structures include the hippocampus, mammillary body, amygdala, olfactory tract, hypothalamus, cingulate gyrus,

septum pellucidum, thalamus, and fornix. The limbic system, which is sometimes called the "emotional brain," is associated with fear and anxiety; anger and aggression; love, joy, and hope; and sexuality and social behavior.

MESENCEPHALON. Structures of major importance in the mesencephalon, or midbrain, include nuclei and fiber tracts. They extend from the pons to the hypothalamus and are responsible for the integration of various reflexes, including visual reflexes (e.g., automatically turning away from a dangerous object when it comes into view), auditory reflexes (e.g., automatically turning toward a sound that is heard), and righting reflexes (e.g., automatically keeping the head upright and maintaining balance) (Scanlon & Sanders, 2003).

PONS. The pons is the bulbous structure that lies between the midbrain and the medulla (see Fig. 3–2). It is composed of large bundles of fibers and forms a major connection between the cerebellum and the brainstem. It also contains the central connections of cranial nerves V through VIII and centers for respiration and skeletal muscle tone.

MEDULLA. The medulla provides a pathway for all ascending and descending fiber tracts. It contains vital centers that regulate heart rate, blood pressure, respiration, and reflex centers for swallowing, sneezing, coughing, and vomiting (Scanlon & Sanders, 2003). It also contains nuclei for cranial nerves IX through XII. The medulla, pons, and midbrain form the structure known as the brainstem. These structures are identified in Figure 3–2.

CEREBELLUM. The cerebellum is separated from the brainstem by the fourth ventricle, but it has connections to the brainstem through bundles of fiber tracts. It is situated just below the occipital lobes of the cerebrum (see Figs. 3–1 and 3–2). The functions of the cerebellum are concerned with involuntary movement, such as muscular tone and coordination and the maintenance of posture and equilibrium.

Nerve Tissue

NEURONS. The tissue of the CNS consists of nerve cells called neurons that generate and transmit electrochemical impulses. The structure of a neuron is composed of a **cell body**, an **axon**, and **dendrites**. The cell body contains the nucleus and is essential for the continued life of the neuron. The dendrites are processes that transmit impulses toward the cell body, and the axon transmits impulses away from the cell body. Cells called *afferent* (or *sensory*) *neurons* carry impulses from the periphery to the CNS, where they are interpreted into various sensations. The *efferent* or *motor neurons* carry impulses from the CNS to the muscles and glands of the periphery. Cells of a third type, called *interneurons*, exist entirely within the CNS and comprise 99 percent of all nerve cells. They may carry only sensory or motor impulses, or they may serve as integrators in the pathways between afferent and efferent neurons. They account in large part for thinking, feelings, learning, language, and memory.

SYNAPSES. Some messages may be processed through only a few neurons, while others may require thousands of neuronal connections. The neurons that transmit the impulses do not actually touch each other. The junction between two neurons is called a **synapse**. The small space between the axon terminals of one neuron and the cell body or dendrites of another is called the *synaptic cleft*. Neurons conducting impulses toward the synapse are called *presynaptic neurons*, and those conducting impulses away are called *postsynaptic neurons* (Fig. 3–4).

NEUROTRANSMITTERS. Chemicals called **neurotransmitters** are stored in the axon terminals of presynaptic neurons. Electrical impulses cause the release of these chemicals into the synaptic cleft. The neurotransmitter combines with **receptor sites** on the postsynaptic neuron, resulting in a determination of whether another electrical impulse is generated (see Fig. 3–4).

Neurotransmitters are responsible for essential functions in the role of human emotion and behavior. They are also the targets for the mechanism of action of many of the psychotropic medications. After a neurotransmitter has performed its function in the synaptic cleft, either it returns to the vesicles in the axon terminals to be stored and used again or it is inactivated and dissolved by enzymes. The process of being stored for reuse is called *reuptake*, a function that holds significance for understanding the mechanism of action of certain psychotropic medications.

Many neurotransmitters exist within the central and peripheral nervous systems, but only a limited number have implications for psychiatry. Major categories include the cholinergics, monoamines, amino acids, and neuropeptides.

Cholinergics

ACETYLCHOLINE. Acetylcholine was the first chemical to be identified and proven as a neurotransmitter.

- Location: It is a major effector chemical within the autonomic nervous system (ANS), producing activity at all sympathetic and parasympathetic presy-

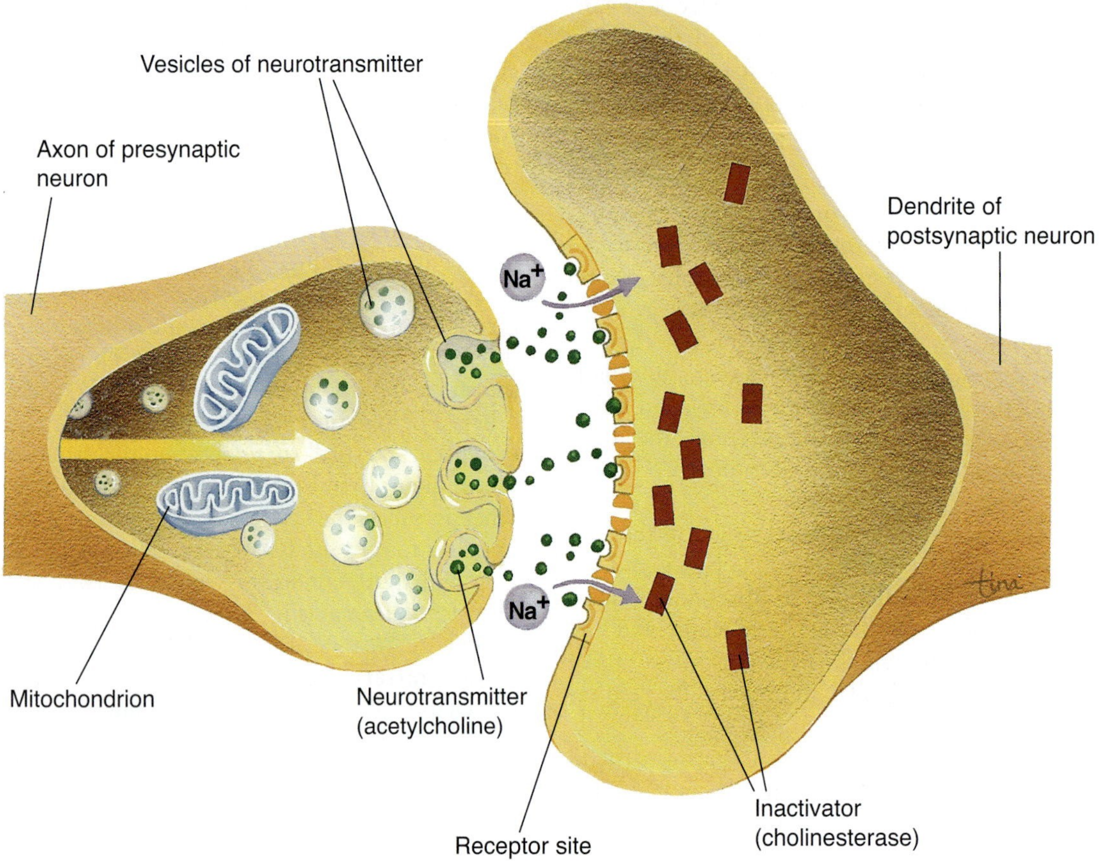

FIGURE 3–4 Impulse transmission at a synapse. The *arrow* indicates the direction of the electrical impulse. (From Scanlon, VC and Sanders, T: Essentials of Anatomy and Physiology, ed 4. F.A. Davis, Philadelphia, 2003, with permission.)

naptic nerve terminals and all parasympathetic postsynaptic nerve terminals. It is highly significant in the neurotransmission that occurs at the junctions of nerve and muscles. In the CNS, acetylcholine neurons innervate the cerebral cortex, hippocampus, and limbic structures. The pathways are especially dense through the area of the basal ganglia in the brain.

- Functions: Acetylcholine is implicated in sleep, arousal, pain perception, the modulation and coordination of movement, and memory acquisition and retention.
- Possible Implications for Mental Illness: Cholinergic mechanisms may have some role in certain disorders of motor behavior and memory, such as Parkinson's disease, Huntington's chorea, and Alzheimer's disease. Increased levels have been associated with depression.

Monoamines

NOREPINEPHRINE. Norepinephrine is the neurotransmitter associated with the "fight or flight" syndrome of symptoms that occurs in response to stress.

- Location: Norepinephrine is found in the ANS at the sympathetic postsynaptic nerve terminals. In the CNS, norepinephrine pathways originate in the pons and medulla and innervate the thalamus, dorsal hypothalamus, limbic system, hippocampus, cerebellum, and cerebral cortex.
- Functions: Norepinephrine may have a role in the regulation of mood, in cognition and perception, in cardiovascular functioning, and in sleep and arousal.
- Possible Implications for Mental Illness: The mechanism of norepinephrine transmission has

been implicated in certain mood disorders such as depression and mania, in anxiety states, and in schizophrenia (Sadock & Sadock, 2003). Levels of the neurotransmitter are thought to be decreased in depression and increased in mania, anxiety states, and schizophrenia.

DOPAMINE. Dopamine is derived from the amino acid tyrosine and may play a role in physical activation of the body.

- Location: Dopamine pathways arise from the midbrain and hypothalamus and terminate in the frontal cortex, limbic system, basal ganglia, and thalamus. Dopamine neurons in the hypothalamus innervate the posterior pituitary, and those from the posterior hypothalamus project to the spinal cord.
- Functions: Dopamine is involved in the regulation of movements and coordination, emotions, and voluntary decision-making ability, and because of its influence on the pituitary gland, it inhibits the release of prolactin (Sadock & Sadock, 2003).
- Possible Implications for Mental Illness: Decreased levels of dopamine have been implicated in the etiology of Parkinson's disease and depression (Sadock & Sadock, 2003). Increased levels of dopamine are associated with mania (Dubovsky, Davies, & Dubovsky, 2003) and schizophrenia (Ho, Black, & Andreasen, 2003).

SEROTONIN. Serotonin is derived from the dietary amino acid tryptophan. The antidepressants called selective serotonin reuptake inhibitors (SSRIs) block the reuptake of this neurotransmitter to increase levels in the brain.

- Location: Serotonin pathways originate from cell bodies located in the pons and medulla and project to areas including the hypothalamus, thalamus, limbic system, cerebral cortex, cerebellum, and spinal cord. Serotonin that is not returned to be stored in the axon terminal vesicles is catabolized by the enzyme monoamine oxidase.
- Functions: Serotonin may play a role in sleep and arousal, libido, appetite, mood, aggression, and pain perception.
- Possible Implications for Mental Illness: Increased levels of serotonin have been implicated in schizophrenia and anxiety states (Sadock & Sadock, 2003). Decreased levels of the neurotransmitter have been associated with depression (Dubovsky, Davies, & Dubovsky, 2003).

HISTAMINE. The role of histamine in mediating allergic and inflammatory reactions has been well documented. Its role in the CNS as a neurotransmitter has only recently been confirmed, and the availability of information is limited.

- Location: The highest concentrations of histamine are found within various regions of the hypothalamus.
- Function: The exact processes mediated by histamine within the CNS are unclear.
- Possible Implications for Mental Illness: Some data suggest that histamine may play a role in depressive illness.

Amino Acids

GAMMA-AMINOBUTYRIC ACID (GABA). GABA is associated with short inhibitory interneurons, although some long-axon pathways within the brain have been identified.

- Location: Widespread distribution in the CNS, with high concentrations in the hypothalamus, hippocampus, cortex, cerebellum, and basal ganglia of the brain, in the gray matter of the dorsal horn of the spinal cord, and in the retina.
- Functions: GABA interrupts the progression of the electrical impulse at the synaptic junction, producing a significant slowdown of body activity.
- Possible Implications for Mental Illness: Decreased levels of GABA have been implicated in the etiology of anxiety disorders, movement disorders such as Huntington's chorea, and various forms of epilepsy.

GLYCINE. Glycine is also considered an inhibitory amino acid.

- Location: Highest concentrations of glycine in the CNS are found in the spinal cord and brainstem.
- Functions: Glycine appears to be involved in recurrent inhibition of motor neurons within the spinal cord and is possibly involved in the regulation of spinal and brainstem reflexes.
- Possible Implications for Mental Illness: Decreased levels of glycine have been implicated in the pathogenesis of certain types of spastic disorders. Toxic accumulation of the neurotransmitter in the brain and cerebrospinal fluid can result in "glycine encephalopathy" (Murphy & Deutsch, 1991).

GLUTAMATE. This neurotransmitter appears to be primarily excitatory in nature.

- Location: Glutamate is found in the pyramidal cells of the cortex, the cerebellum, and the primary sensory afferent systems. It is also found in the hippocampus, thalamus, hypothalamus, and spinal cord.
- Functions: Glutamate functions in the relay of sensory information and in the regulation of various motor and spinal reflexes.
- Possible Implications for Mental Illness: Increased receptor activity has been implicated in the etiology of certain neurodegenerative disorders, such as Parkinson's disease. Decreased receptor activity can induce psychotic behavior.

Neuropeptides

ENDORPHINS AND ENKEPHALINS. These neurotransmitters are sometimes called opioid peptides.

- Location: They have been found in various concentrations in the hypothalamus, thalamus, limbic structures, midbrain, and brainstem. Enkephalins are also found in the gastrointestinal (GI) tract.
- Function: With their natural morphine-like properties, they are thought to have a role in pain modulation.
- Possible Implications for Mental Illness: Modulation of dopamine activity by opioid peptides may indicate some link to the symptoms of schizophrenia.

SUBSTANCE P. Substance P was the first neuropeptide to be discovered.

- Location: Substance P is present in high concentrations in the hypothalamus, limbic structures, midbrain, and brainstem and is found in the thalamus, basal ganglia, and spinal cord.
- Functions: Substance P is thought to play a role in sensory transmission, particularly in the regulation of pain.
- Possible Implications for Mental Illness: Decreased concentrations have been found in the substantia nigra of the basal ganglia of clients with Huntington's chorea.

SOMATOSTATIN. Somatostatin is also called the growth hormone-inhibiting hormone.

- Location: Somatostatin is found in the cerebral cortex, hippocampus, thalamus, basal ganglia, brainstem, and spinal cord.
- Functions: Somatostatin exerts inhibitory effects on the release of norepinephrine and stimulatory effects on serotonin. It stimulates the turnover and release of dopamine in the basal ganglia and acetylcholine in the brainstem and hippocampus.
- Possible Implications for Mental Illness: High concentrations of somatostatin have been reported in brain specimens of clients with Huntington's chorea; low concentrations have been reported in clients with Alzheimer's disease.

Spinal Cord

The second major component of the CNS is the spinal cord. It transmits impulses to and from the brain and is the integrating center for the spinal cord reflexes (Scanlon & Sanders, 2003).

FIBER TRACTS. A cross section of the spinal cord reveals an area of gray matter in the central part that is made up of the cell bodies of motor neurons and interneurons. Around the external part of the cord is an area of white matter, so called because the fibers that make up the area are sheathed in a white, lipid substance called myelin. Ascending spinal tracts carry sensory impulses to the brain, and descending tracts carry motor impulses from the brain to the periphery. The center of the spinal cord contains cerebrospinal fluid and is continuous with the ventricles in the brain.

SPINAL NERVES. Thirty-one pairs of nerves emerge from the spinal cord. They do not have names; they are identified by the level of the vertebrae from which they arise. In general, the cervical nerves supply the upper portion of the body, including the diaphragm. Most of the thoracic nerves supply the trunk of the body, and the lumbar and sacral nerves supply the hips, pelvic cavity, and legs (Scanlon & Sanders, 2003). Damage to the spinal cord results in loss of, or alteration in, function to the part of the body innervated by the spinal nerves that arise from the injured area of the cord. Regeneration of damaged neurons depends on extent and severity of the injury and expedience in receiving treatment.

The Peripheral Nervous System

The PNS is composed of the nerve processes that connect the CNS (brain and spinal cord) with the receptors, muscles, and glands in the periphery of the body.

The Afferent System

Afferent, or sensory, neurons convey information from receptors in the periphery to the CNS (Scanlon & Sanders, 2003). Various receptors respond to specific stimuli that generate neuronal impulses to the CNS. For example, receptors in the eye respond to light stimuli; receptors in the skin respond to touch or pain stimuli; and receptors in the ear respond to sound stimuli. Once activated, receptors generate an impulse to the CNS for interpretation of the sensation. Sensory neurons from external areas of the body, such as skin, skeletal muscles, and joints, are called *somatic;* those from receptors in internal organs are called *visceral* (Scanlon & Sanders, 2003).

The Efferent System

Efferent, or motor, neurons carry information from the CNS to peripheral areas of the body. This includes skeletal muscles, smooth and cardiac muscles, and glands.

SOMATIC NERVOUS SYSTEM. The somatic nervous system consists of fibers that go from the CNS (either brain or spinal cord) to skeletal muscle cells. The excitation of these neurons, sometimes called *somatic motor neurons*, always leads to contraction of a skeletal muscle.

AUTONOMIC NERVOUS SYSTEM. Efferent neurons of the ANS innervate smooth muscles, cardiac muscles, and glands. These neurons are sometimes called *visceral motor neurons.* The ANS is further divided into *sympathetic* and *parasympathetic* components, which often function in opposition to each other. Many glands and muscles have dual innervation; that is, they are stimulated by both sympathetic and parasympathetic fibers. In these instances, when the activity of one system is enhanced, the activity of the other is suppressed (Fig. 3–5).

- The Sympathetic Nervous System. The sympathetic nervous system becomes the dominant component during stressful situations. Activation of the sympathetic nervous system results in the fight or flight response that was described in Chapter 1. Examples of this response include increased cardiac and respiratory activity and a decrease in GI functioning. Neurotransmitters involved in impulse transmission within the sympathetic nervous system include acetylcholine and norepinephrine.
- The Parasympathetic Nervous System. The parasympathetic nervous system is dominant in the non-stressful or relaxed state. Parasympathetic dominance promotes efficient GI functioning and maintains heart and respirations at resting rates. The neurotransmitter found in the parasympathetic nervous system is acetylcholine.

The Neuroendocrine System

The **neuroendocrine system** deals with the interaction between the nervous and endocrine systems and the hormones that react to stimulation from the nerve cells.

The Pituitary Gland

The pituitary gland is only about the size of a pea, but despite its size and because of the powerful control it exerts over endocrine functioning in humans, it is sometimes called the "master gland." Many of the hormones subject to hypothalamus-pituitary regulation may have implications for behavioral functioning. Discussion of these hormones is summarized in Table 3–2.

The pituitary gland has two major lobes—the anterior lobe (called the *adenohypophysis*) and the posterior lobe (called the *neurohypophysis*). The pituitary gland is under the direct control of the hypothalamus.

Neurohypophysis

The hypothalamus has direct control over the posterior pituitary through efferent neural pathways. Two hormones are found in the posterior pituitary: vasopressin or antidiuretic hormone (ADH) and oxytocin. They are actually produced by the hypothalamus and stored in the posterior pituitary. Their release is mediated by neural impulses from the hypothalamus (Fig. 3–6).

ANTIDIURETIC HORMONE. The main function of ADH is to conserve body water and maintain normal blood pressure. The release of ADH is stimulated by pain, emotional stress, dehydration, increased plasma concentration, or decreased blood volume. An alteration in the secretion of this hormone may be a factor in the polydipsia observed in about 10 to 15 percent of hospitalized psychiatric patients. Other factors correlated with this behavior include adverse effects of psychotropic medications and features of the behavioral disorder itself. ADH also may play a role in learning and memory, in alteration of the pain response, and in the modification of sleep patterns.

OXYTOCIN. Oxytocin stimulates contraction of the uterus at the end of pregnancy and stimulates release of milk from the mammary glands (Scanlon & Sanders, 2003). It is also released in response to stress and during sexual arousal. Its role in behavioral functioning is unclear, although it is possible that oxytocin may act in certain situations to stimulate the release of adrenocorticotropic hormone (ACTH),

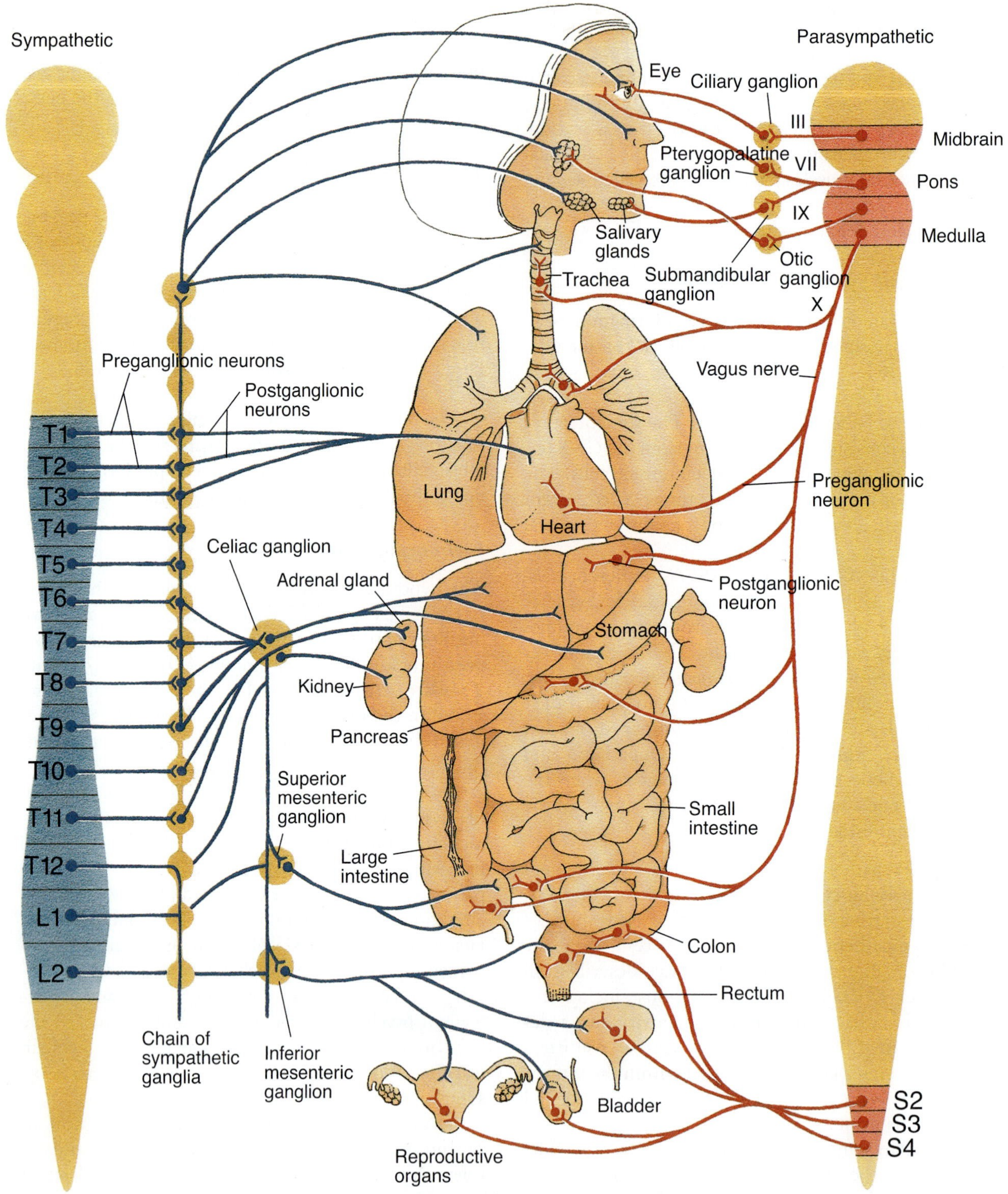

FIGURE 3–5 The autonomic nervous system. (From Scanlon, VC and Sanders, T: Essentials of Anatomy and Physiology, ed 4. F.A. Davis, Philadelphia, 2003, with permission.)

TABLE 3 – 2 Hormones of the Neuroendocrine System

Hormone	Location and Stimulation of Release	Target Organ	Function	Possible Behavioral Correlation to Altered Secretion
Antidiuretic hormone	Posterior pituitary; release stimulated by dehydration, pain, stress	Kidney (causes increased reabsorption)	Conservation of body water and maintenance of blood pressure	Polydipsia; altered pain response; modified sleep pattern
Oxytocin	Posterior pituitary; release stimulated by end of pregnancy, stress, sexual arousal	Uterus; breasts	Contraction of the uterus for labor; release of breast milk	May play role in stress response by stimulation of ACTH
Growth hormone	Anterior pituitary; release stimulated by growth hormone-releasing hormone from hypothalamus	Bones and tissues	Growth in children; protein synthesis in adults	Anorexia nervosa
Thyroid-stimulating hormone	Anterior pituitary; release stimulated by thyrotropin-releasing hormone from hypothalamus	Thyroid gland	Stimulation of secretion of thyroid hormones needed for metabolism of food and regulation of temperature	Increased levels: insomnia, anxiety, emotional lability; Decreased levels: depression, fatigue
Adrenocorticotropic hormone	Anterior pituitary; release stimulated by corticotropin-releasing hormone from hypothalamus	Adrenal cortex	Stimulation of secretion of cortisol, which plays a role in response to stress	Increased levels: mood disorders, psychosis Decreased levels: depression, apathy, fatigue
Prolactin	Anterior pituitary; release stimulated by prolactin-releasing hormone from hypothalamus	Breasts	Stimulation of milk production	Increased levels: depression, anxiety, decreased libido, irritability
Gonadotropic hormone	Anterior pituitary; release stimulated by gonadotropin-releasing hormone from hypothalamus	Ovaries and testes	Stimulation of secretion of estrogen, progesterone, and testosterone; role in ovulation and sperm production	Decreased levels: depression and anorexia nervosa; Increased testosterone, increased sexual behavior and aggressiveness
Melanocyte-stimulating hormone	Anterior pituitary; release stimulated by onset of darkness	Pineal gland	Stimulation of secretion of melatonin	Increased levels: depression

thereby playing a key role in the overall hormonal response to stress.

Adenohypophysis

The hypothalamus produces *releasing hormones* that pass through capillaries and veins of the hypophyseal portal system to capillaries in the anterior pituitary, where they stimulate secretion of specialized hormones. This pathway is presented in Figure 3–6. The hormones of the anterior pituitary gland regulate multiple body functions and include growth hormone (GH), thyroid-stimulating hormone (TSH), ACTH, prolactin, gonadotropin-stimulating hormone, and melanocyte-stimulating hormone (MSH). Most of these hormones are regulated by a *negative feedback* mechanism. Once the hormone has exerted its effects, the information is "fed back" to the anterior pituitary, which inhibits the release, and ultimately decreases the effects, of the stimulating hormones.

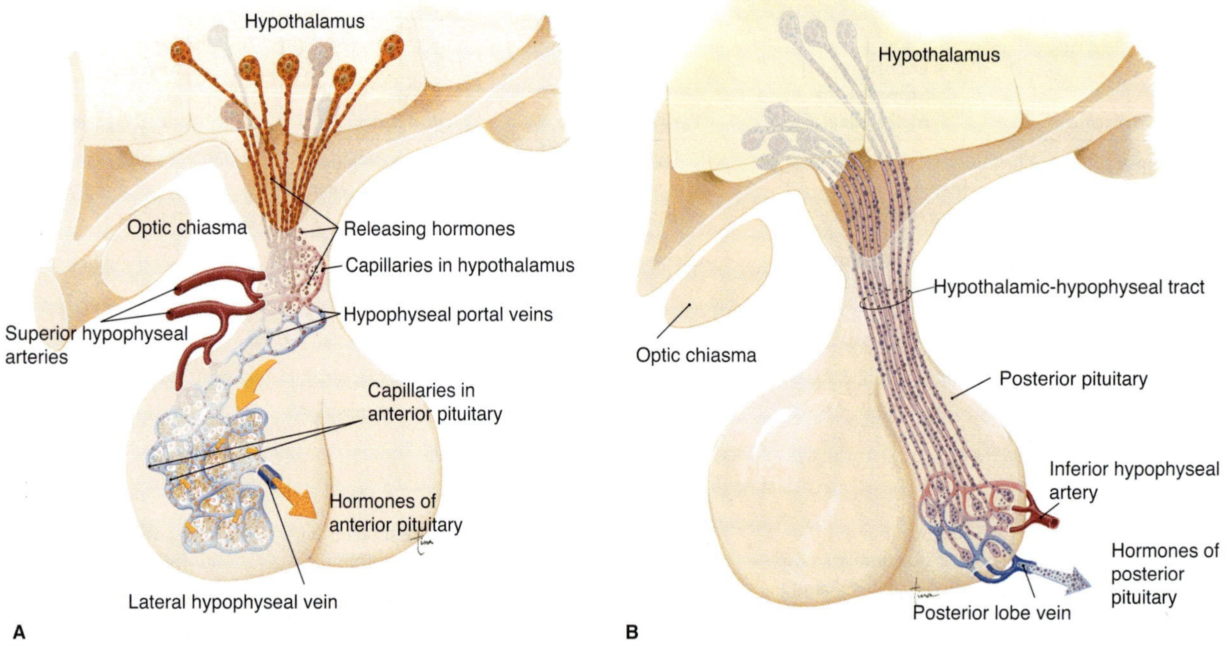

FIGURE 3–6 Hypothalamic regulation of pituitary hormones. (A) Releasing hormones of the hypothalamus circulate directly to the anterior pituitary and influence its secretions. (B) Posterior pituitary stores hormones produced in the hypothalamus. (From Scanlon, VC and Sanders, T: Essentials of Anatomy and Physiology, ed 4. F.A. Davis, Philadelphia, 2003, with permission.)

GROWTH HORMONE. The release of GH, also called somatotropin, is stimulated by growth hormone-releasing hormone (GHRH) from the hypothalamus. Its release is inhibited by growth hormone-inhibiting hormone (GHIH), or somatostatin, also from the hypothalamus. It is responsible for growth in children and continued protein synthesis throughout life. During periods of fasting, it stimulates the release of fat from the adipose tissue to be used for increased energy. The release of GHIH is stimulated in response to periods of hyperglycemia. GHRH is stimulated in response to hypoglycemia and to stressful situations. During prolonged stress, GH has a direct effect on protein, carbohydrate, and lipid metabolism, resulting in increased serum glucose and free fatty acids to be used for increased energy. There has been some indication of a possible correlation between abnormal secretion of growth hormone and anorexia nervosa.

THYROID-STIMULATING HORMONE. Thyrotropin-releasing hormone from the hypothalamus stimulates the release of TSH, or thyrotropin, from the anterior pituitary. TSH stimulates the thyroid gland to secrete triiodothyronine (T_3) and thyroxine (T_4). Thyroid hormones are integral to the metabolism of food and the regulation of temperature.

A correlation between thyroid dysfunction and altered behavioral functioning has been noted. Hyperthyroidism is characterized by irritability, insomnia, anxiety, restlessness, weight loss, and emotional lability. In some instances, serious psychiatric symptoms, such as impairments in memory and orientation, manic excitement, delusions, and hallucinations, are evident (Sadock & Sadock, 2003). Fatigue, weight gain, cold intolerance, depression, hypomania, slowed thinking, and delirium have been associated with hypothyroidism. Studies have correlated various forms of thyroid dysfunction with mood disorders, anxiety, eating disorders, schizophrenia, and dementia.

ADRENOCORTICOTROPIC HORMONE. Corticotropin-releasing hormone (CRH) from the hypothalamus stimulates the release of ACTH from the anterior pituitary. ACTH stimulates the adrenal cortex to secrete cortisol. The role of cortisol in human behavior is not well understood, although it seems to be secreted under stressful situations. Disorders of the adrenal cortex can result in hyposecretion or hypersecretion of cortisol.

Addison's disease is the result of hyposecretion of the hormones of the adrenal cortex. Behavioral symptoms of hyposecretion include mood changes with apathy, social withdrawal, impaired sleep, decreased concentration, and fatigue. Hypersecretion of cortisol results in Cushing's disease and is associated with behaviors that include depression, mania, psychosis, and suicidal ideation. Cognitive impairments also have been commonly observed.

PROLACTIN. Serum prolactin levels are regulated by prolactin-releasing hormone and prolactin-inhibiting hormone from the hypothalamus. Prolactin stimulates milk production by the mammary glands in the presence of high levels of estrogen and progesterone during pregnancy. Behavioral symptoms associated with hypersecretion of prolactin include depression, decreased libido, stress intolerance, anxiety, and increased irritability.

GONADOTROPIC HORMONES. The gonadotropic hormones are so called because they produce an effect on the gonads—the ovaries and the testes. The gonadotropins include follicle-stimulating hormone (FSH) and luteinizing hormone (LH), and their release from the anterior pituitary is stimulated by gonadotropin-releasing hormone (GnRH) from the hypothalamus. In women, FSH initiates maturation of ovarian follicles into the ova and stimulates their secretion of estrogen. LH is responsible for ovulation and the secretion of progesterone from the corpus luteum. In men, FSH initiates sperm production in the testes, and LH increases secretion of testosterone by the interstitial cells of the testes (Scanlon & Sanders, 2003). The gonadotropins are regulated by a negative feedback of gonadal hormones at the hypothalamic or pituitary level.

Limited evidence exists to correlate gonadotropins to behavioral functioning, although some observations warrant hypothetical consideration. Studies have indicated decreased levels of testosterone, LH, and FSH in depressed men. Increased sexual behavior and aggressiveness have been linked to elevated testosterone levels in both men and women. Decreased plasma levels of LH and FSH commonly occur in patients with anorexia nervosa. Supplemental estrogen therapy has resulted in improved mentation and mood in some depressed women.

MELANOCYTE-STIMULATING HORMONE. MSH from the hypothalamus stimulates the pineal gland to secrete melatonin. The release of melatonin appears to depend on the onset of darkness and is suppressed by light. Studies of this hormone have indicated that environmental light can affect neuronal activity and influence circadian rhythms. Correlation between abnormal secretion of melatonin and symptoms of depression has led to the implication of melatonin in the etiology of mood disorders with a seasonal pattern, in which individuals become depressed only during the fall and winter months when the amount of daylight decreases.

IMPLICATIONS FOR PSYCHIATRIC ILLNESS

It is thought that a number of mental disorders have biological bases. As previously stated, this does not imply that psychosocial and sociocultural influences are totally discounted but that the systems of biology, psychology, and sociology are interacting systems. This has been clearly indicated by the fact that individuals experience biological changes in response to various environmental events. Indeed, biological implications present but one etiological explanation for psychiatric illness.

Schizophrenia

Anomalies of the Brain

Some studies have shown a significant enlargement in cerebral ventricular size in the brains of individuals with schizophrenia. Dilation of cortical sulci and fissures were also observed. Several studies have indicated that temporal lobe size may be decreased in schizophrenia (Ho, Black, & Andreasen, 2003).

Functional cerebral asymmetries of the brain occur normally as they relate to language comprehension and speech production. Computerized studies with schizophrenic populations have suggested that some individuals with the disorder exhibit abnormal cerebral asymmetry, reduced cerebellar volume, and brain density changes (Sadock & Sadock, 2003).

A number of studies have reported neuropathology as identified by histological changes in the brains of individuals with schizophrenia (Ho, Black, & Andreasen, 2003). Regions where changes have been noted include the limbic system, thalamus, basal ganglia, hippocampus, and frontal cortex.

Neurotransmitter Hypothesis

The neurotransmitter hypothesis suggests that schizophrenia, (or schizophrenia-like symptoms) may be caused by an excess of dopamine-dependent neuronal activity in the brain (Sadock & Sadock, 2003). This excess activity may be related to increased production or release of the substance at nerve terminals, increased receptor sensitivity, or reduced activity of dopamine antagonists.

Various other biochemicals have been implicated in the predisposition to schizophrenia. Abnormalities in the neurotransmitters norepinephrine, serotonin, acetylcholine, and GABA and the neuroregulators, such as prostaglandins and endorphins, have been suggested.

Possible Endocrine Correlation

Although the exact mechanism is unknown, there may be some correlation between decreased levels of the hormone prolactin and schizophrenia. The neurotransmitter dopamine, which is elevated in schizophrenia, acts as the prolactin-inhibiting factor. By decreasing dopamine, antipsychotic medications increase prolactin synthesis and release. Negative symptoms in schizophrenia may be associated with decreased prolactin levels (Sadock & Sadock, 2003).

Mood Disorders

Neuroanatomical Considerations

The symptoms of mood disorders, as well as biological research findings, support the hypothesis that mood disorders involve pathology of the limbic system, the basal ganglia, and the hypothalamus (Dubovsky, Davies, & Dubovsky, 2003). The limbic system plays a major role in the discharge of emotions. Stooped posture, motor slowness, and the minor cognitive impairment of depression indicate involvement of the basal ganglia. Dysfunction of the hypothalamus is suggested by alterations in sleep, appetite, and sexual behavior.

Neurotransmitter Hypothesis

Early studies have associated symptoms of depression with a functional deficiency of norepinephrine and dopamine, and mania with a functional excess of these amines. The neurotransmitter serotonin appears to remain low in both states (Goodwin & Jamison, 1990). Norepinephrine has been identified as a key component in the mobilization of the body to deal with stressful situations. Neurons that contain serotonin are critically involved in the regulation of such diverse functions as sleep, temperature, pain sensitivity, appetite, locomotor activity, neuroendocrine secretions, and mood. The level of dopamine in the mesolimbic system of the brain is thought to exert a strong influence over human mood and behavior. A diminished supply of these biogenic amines inhibits the transmission of impulses from one neuronal fiber to another, causing a failure of the cells to fire or become charged.

Possible Endocrine Correlation

In clients who are depressed, the normal system of hormonal inhibition fails, resulting in a hypersecretion of cortisol. This elevated serum cortisol is the basis for the dexamethasone suppression test that is sometimes used to determine if an individual has somatically treatable depression.

Hypothyroidism has also been associated with depression. Diminished TSH from the anterior pituitary gland in response to administered thyrotropin-releasing factor is observed in approximately 25 percent of depressed persons. Hyperthyroidism has been associated with symptoms of acute mania.

A correlation may exist between abnormal secretion of melatonin from the pineal gland and mood disorder with seasonal pattern, in which individuals become depressed only during the fall and winter months when the secretion of melatonin increases in response to decreased amounts of daylight.

Anxiety Disorders

Neuroanatomical Considerations

The limbic system has been the focus of study in the correlation of brain pathology to anxiety disorders. Stimulation of this area has produced anxiety and fear responses in nonhuman primates (Sadock & Sadock, 2003). The cingulate gyrus of the limbic system has been implicated in the pathophysiology of obsessive-compulsive disorder. The temporal cortex has also been implicated as a pathophysiological site in anxiety disorders, particularly with obsessive-compulsive disorder (Sadock & Sadock, 2003).

Neurotransmitter Hypothesis

The neurotransmitters most closely associated with anxiety disorders include norepinephrine, serotonin, and GABA. Norepinephrine causes hyperarousal and anxiety, and elevated levels are implicated in the etiology of panic disorder. Serotonin may play a role in the behaviors associated with obsessive-compulsive disorder. This hypothesis has been supported by the positive effects seen when the disorder is treated with

SSRIs, such as fluoxetine and clomipramine. GABA is a neurotransmitter that inhibits postsynaptic excitation, thus interrupting the progression of the electrical impulse at the synaptic junction. Enhancement of the GABA system is the mechanism of action by which the benzodiazepines produce their calming effect in the treatment of anxiety disorders.

Possible Endocrine Correlation

Increased levels of TSH and prolactin have been observed in individuals with anxiety disorders. Some individuals with obsessive-compulsive disorder exhibit increased cortisol levels (similar to those seen in depressive disorder). The role of neuroendocrine dysregulation in the etiology of anxiety disorders has not yet been determined.

Anorexia Nervosa

Neuroanatomical Considerations

Some computed tomographic (CT) studies have revealed enlarged cerebrospinal fluid (CSF) spaces (enlarged sulci and ventricles) during the starvation period in individuals with anorexia nervosa (Sadock & Sadock, 2003). This finding appears to reverse itself by weight gain.

Neurotransmitter Hypothesis

Preliminary studies have indicated that there is probably a dysregulation of dopamine, serotonin, and norepinephrine in individuals with anorexia nervosa (Halmi, 2003). A decrease in serotonin turnover has been found in clients with both bulimia and anorexia, and low CSF norepinephrine levels were discovered in clients with long-term anorexia who have obtained a weight within at least 15 percent of their normal weight range.

Possible Endocrine Correlation

Some speculation has occurred regarding a primary hypothalamic dysfunction in anorexia nervosa. Studies consistent with this theory have revealed elevated CSF cortisol levels and a possible impairment of dopaminergic regulation in people with anorexia (Halmi, 2003). Additional evidence in the etiological implication of hypothalamic dysfunction is gathered from the fact that many individuals with anorexia experience amenorrhea before the onset of starvation and significant weight loss.

Alzheimer's Disease

Neuroanatomical Considerations

Observation of a brain from an individual with Alzheimer's disease reveals diffuse atrophy with flattened cortical sulci and enlarged cerebral ventricles (Sadock & Sadock, 2003). Microscopic findings include senile plaques, neurofibrillary tangles, and neuronal loss.

Neurotransmitter Hypothesis

Research has indicated that in the brains of clients with Alzheimer's disease, the enzyme required to produce acetylcholine is dramatically reduced, leading to a reduction in the amount of neurotransmitter that is released to cells in the cortex and hippocampus. Other neurotransmitters thought to be diminished in Alzheimer's disease are norepinephrine and somatostatin. Diminished concentrations of these neurochemicals have been implicated in the pathophysiology of the disease.

Possible Endocrine Correlation

The hormone corticotropin has been reported to be decreased in Alzheimer's disease (Sadock & Sadock, 2003).

DIAGNOSTIC PROCEDURES USED TO DETECT ALTERED BRAIN FUNCTION

Several diagnostic procedures are used to detect alteration in biological function that may contribute to psychiatric disorders. Following is an explanation of various examinations, the technique used, the purpose of the examination, and possible findings.

Electroencephalography

Technique

For an electroencephalogram (EEG), electrodes are placed on the scalp in a standardized position. Amplitude and frequency of beta, alpha, theta, and delta brain waves are graphically recorded on paper by ink markers for multiple areas of the brain surface.

Purpose/Possible Findings

The EEG measures brain electrical activity and identifies dysrhythmias, asymmetries, or suppression of brain rhythms. It is used in the diagnosis of epilepsy, neoplasm, stroke, metabolic, or degenerative disease.

Computerized EEG Mapping

Technique

EEG tracings are summarized by computer-assisted systems, in which various regions of the brain are identified, and functioning is interpreted by color coding or gray shading.

Purpose/Possible Findings

Computerized EEG mapping measures brain electrical activity. It is used largely in research to represent statistical relationships between individuals and groups or between two populations of subjects (e.g., clients with schizophrenia versus control subjects).

Computed Tomographic Scan

Technique

Computed tomographic scan (CT) may be used with or without contrast medium. X-rays are taken of various transverse planes of the brain while a computerized analysis produces a precise reconstructed image of each segment.

Purpose/Possible Findings

The CT scan measures the accuracy of brain structure to detect possible lesions, abscesses, areas of infarction, or aneurysm. This technology has also been used to identify various anatomical differences in clients with schizophrenia, organic mental disorders, and bipolar disorder.

Magnetic Resonance Imaging

Technique

In magnetic resonance imaging (MRI), within a strong magnetic field, the nuclei of hydrogen atoms absorb and re-emit electromagnetic energy that is computerized and transformed into image information. No radiation or contrast medium is used.

Purpose/Possible Findings

MRI measures the anatomical and biochemical status of various segments of the brain. It also detects brain edema, ischemia, infection, neoplasm, trauma, and other changes such as demyelination. Morphological differences between the brains of clients with schizophrenia and those of control subjects have been noted.

Positron Emission Tomography

Technique

With positron emission tomography (PET), the client receives an intravenous injection of a radioactive substance (the type depends on the brain activity to be visualized). Detectors surround the head and relay data to a computer, which interprets the signals and produces the image.

Purpose/Possible Findings

PET measures specific brain functioning, such as glucose metabolism, oxygen utilization, blood flow, and, of particular interest in psychiatry, neurotransmitter/receptor interaction.

Single Photon Emission Computed Tomography

Technique

The single photon emission computed tomography (SPECT) technique is similar to PET, but a longer-acting radioactive substance must be used to allow time for a gamma camera to rotate about the head and gather the data, which then are computer assembled into a brain image.

Purpose/Possible Findings

SPECT measures various aspects of brain functioning, as with PET; it also has been used to take images of activity or CSF circulation.

IMPLICATIONS FOR NURSING

The discipline of psychiatric/mental health nursing has always spoken of its role in holistic healthcare, but historical review reveals that emphasis has been placed on treatment approaches that focus on psychological and social factors (Abraham, Fox, & Cohen, 1992). Psychiatric nurses must integrate knowledge of the biological sciences into their practices if they are to ensure safe and effective care to people with mental illness. Lowery (1992) states:

> The "medicalization" of psychiatry seems to be well underway. It is psychiatry's turn to reap the benefits of technology and science. Perhaps more than any other specialty, psychiatric nursing will change as the result of these developments that are revolutionizing the way in which we think about our patients and ourselves. (p. 13)

To ensure a smooth transition from a psychosocial focus to one of biopsychosocial emphasis, nurses must have a clear understanding of the following:

- Neuroanatomy and neurophysiology: the structure and functioning of the various parts of the brain and their correlation to human behavior and psychopathology.
- Neuronal processes: the various functions of the nerve cells, including the role of neurotransmitters, receptors, synaptic activity, and informational pathways.
- Neuroendocrinology: the interaction of the endocrine and nervous systems, and the role that the endocrine glands and their respective hormones play in behavioral functioning.
- Circadian rhythms: regulation of biochemical functioning over periods of rhythmic cycles and their influence in predicting certain behaviors.
- Genetic influences: hereditary factors that predispose individuals to certain psychiatric disorders.
- Psychoimmunology: the influence of stress on the immune system and the role of stress in susceptibility to illness.
- Psychopharmacology: the increasing use of psychotropics in the treatment of mental illness, demanding greater knowledge of psychopharmacological principles, and nursing interventions necessary for safe and effective management.
- Diagnostic technology: the importance of keeping informed about the latest in technological procedures for diagnosing alterations in brain structure and function.

Why are these concepts important to the practice of psychiatric/mental health nursing? The interrelationship between psychosocial adaptation and physical functioning has been established. The *bio* must remain an integral part of biopsychosocial nursing. As Lowery (1992) has stated:

> Nursing's near future is full of challenges: we have a major advocacy task to reduce the continuing stigma of mental illness and the implications for delivery of care; we must begin to rationalize the evolving specialty system and our roles in it; and we must begin to incorporate new science and technology into our practice, education, and research. (pp. 9–10)

SUMMARY

The "medicalization of psychiatry" necessitates that nurses be cognizant of the interaction between physical and mental factors in the development and management of psychiatric illness. These current trends have made it essential for nurses to increase their knowledge about the structure and functioning of the brain. This includes the processes of neurotransmission and the function of various neurotransmitters. This is especially important in light of the increasing role of psychotropic medication in the treatment of psychiatric illness. Because the mechanism of action of many of these drugs occurs at synaptic transmission, nurses must understand this process so that they may predict outcomes and safely manage the administration of psychotropic medications.

The endocrine system plays an important role in human behavior through the hypothalamic-pituitary axis. Hormones and their circadian rhythm of regulation significantly influence a number of physiological and psychological life-cycle phenomena, such as moods, sleep-arousal, stress response, appetite, libido, and fertility.

It is important for nurses to keep abreast of the expanding diagnostic technologies available for detecting alterations in physical functioning. These technologies are facilitating the growth of knowledge linking mental illness to disorders of the brain. The expanding biological focus within psychiatry must be integrated into nursing practice as part of the continuing effort to fulfill clients' needs.

REVIEW QUESTIONS

SELF-EXAMINATION/LEARNING EXERCISE

Match the following parts of the brain to their functions described in the right-hand column:

_______ 1. Frontal lobe	a. Sometimes called the “emotional brain”; associated with multiple feelings and behaviors.
_______ 2. Parietal lobe	b. Concerned with visual reception and interpretation.
_______ 3. Temporal lobe	c. Voluntary body movement; thinking and judgment; expression of feeling.
_______ 4. Occipital lobe	d. Integrates all sensory input (except smell) on way to cortex.
_______ 5. Thalamus	e. Part of the cortex that deals with sensory perception and interpretation.
_______ 6. Hypothalamus	f. Hearing, short-term memory, and sense of smell.
_______ 7. Limbic system	g. Control over pituitary gland autonomic nervous system. Regulates appetite and temperature.

Select the answer that is most appropriate for each of the following questions:

8. At a synapse, the determination of further impulse transmission is accomplished by means of
   a. Potassium ions
   b. Interneurons
   c. Neurotransmitters
   d. The myelin sheath
9. A decrease in which of the following neurotransmitters has been implicated in depression?
   a. GABA, acetylcholine, and aspartate
   b. Norepinephrine, serotonin, and dopamine
   c. Somatostatin, substance P, and glycine
   d. Glutamate, histamine, and opioid peptides
10. Which of the following hormones has been implicated in the etiology of mood disorder with seasonal pattern?
    a. Increased levels of melatonin
    b. Decreased levels of oxytocin
    c. Decreased levels of prolactin
    d. Increased levels of thyrotropin

REFERENCES

Abraham, I.L., Fox, J.C., & Cohen, B. T. (1992). Integrating the bio into the biopsychosocial: Understanding and treating biological phenomena in psychiatric-mental health nursing. Archives of Psychiatric Nursing, 6(5), 296–305.

Dubovsky, S.L., Davies, R., & Dubovsky, A.N. (2003). Mood disorders. In R.E. Hales & S.C. Yudofsky (Eds.). Textbook of clinical psychiatry (4th ed.). Washington, DC: American Psychiatric Publishing.

Goodwin, F.K., & Jamison, K.R. (1990). Manic-depressive illness. New York: Oxford University Press.

Halmi, K.A. (2003). Eating disorders: Anorexia nervosa, bulimia nervosa, and obesity. In R.E. Hales & S.C.Yudofsky (Eds.). Textbook of clinical psychiatry (4th ed.). Washington, DC: American Psychiatric Publishing.

Ho, B.C., Black, D.W., & Andreasen, N.C. (2003). Schizophrenia and other psychotic disorders. In R.E. Hales & S.C.Yudofsky (Eds.). Textbook of clinical psychiatry (4th ed.). Washington, DC: American Psychiatric Publishing.

Lowery, B.J. (1992). Psychiatric nursing in the 1990's and beyond. Journal of Psychosocial Nursing, 30(1), 7–13.

Murphy, M., & Deutsch, S.I. (1991). Neurophysiological and neurochemical basis of behavior. In K. Davis, H. Klar, & J.T. Coyle (Eds.). Foundations of psychiatry. Philadelphia: W.B. Saunders.

Sadock, B.J., & Sadock, V.A. (2003). Kaplan & Sadock's synopsis of psychiatry: Behavioral sciences/clinical psychiatry (9th ed.). Philadelphia: Lippincott Williams & Wilkins.

Scanlon, V.C., & Sanders, T. (2003). Essentials of anatomy and physiology (4th ed.). Philadelphia: F.A. Davis.

4

CHAPTER

Ethical and Legal Issues

CHAPTER OUTLINE

KEY TERMS

assault
autonomy
battery
criminal law
beneficence
bioethics
Christian ethics
civil law
common law
defamation of character
ethical dilemma
ethical egoism
ethics
false imprisonment
informed consent
privileged communication
justice
libel
Kantianism
malpractice
moral behavior
natural law theory
negligence
nonmaleficence
right
slander
statutory laws
torts
utilitarianism
values
values clarification
veracity

OBJECTIVES

After reading this chapter, the student will be able to:

1. Differentiate among ethics, morals, values, and rights.
2. Discuss ethical theories including utilitarianism, Kantianism, Christian ethics, natural law theories, and ethical egoism.
3. Define *ethical dilemma.*
4. Discuss the ethical principles of autonomy, beneficence, nonmaleficence, justice, and veracity.
5. Use an ethical decision-making model to make an ethical decision.
6. Describe ethical issues relevant to psychiatric/mental health nursing.
7. Define *statutory law* and *common law.*
8. Differentiate between civil and criminal law.
9. Discuss legal issues relevant to psychiatric/mental health nursing.
10. Differentiate between *malpractice* and *negligence.*
11. Identify behaviors relevant to the psychiatric/mental health setting for which specific malpractice action could be taken.

INTRODUCTION

Nurses are constantly faced with the challenge of making difficult decisions regarding good and evil or life and death. This chapter presents a discussion of ethical theory as a foundation upon which ethical decisions may be made. The American Nurses Association (ANA) (2001) has established a code of ethics for nurses to use as a framework within which to make ethical choices and decisions (Table 4–1).

Because legislation determines what is *right* or *good* within a society, legal issues pertaining to psychiatric/mental health nursing are also discussed. Definitions are presented, along with rights of psychiatric clients of which nurses must be aware. Nursing competency and client care accountability are compromised when the nurse has inadequate knowledge about the laws that regulate the practice of nursing.

Knowledge of the legal and ethical concepts presented in this chapter will enhance the quality of care the nurse provides in his or her psychiatric/mental health nursing practice and also protect the nurse within the parameters of legal accountability. Indeed, the very right to practice nursing carries with it the responsibility to maintain a specific level of competency and to practice in accordance with certain ethical and legal standards of care.

DEFINITIONS

- **Ethics** is the science that deals with the rightness and wrongness of actions (Aiken, 1994).
- **Bioethics** is the term applied to these principles when they refer to concepts within the scope of medicine, nursing, and allied health.
- **Moral behavior** is defined as conduct that results from serious critical thinking about how individuals ought to treat others. Moral behavior reflects the way a person interprets basic respect for other persons, such as the respect for autonomy, freedom, justice, honesty, and confidentiality (Pappas, 1994).
- **Values** are ideals or concepts that give meaning to the individual's life (Aiken, 1994).
- **Value clarification** is a process of self-exploration through which individuals identify and rank their own personal values. This process increases awareness about why individuals behave in certain ways. Values clarification is important in nursing to increase understanding about why certain choices and decisions are made over others and how values affect nursing outcomes.
- **Right** is defined as "a valid, legally recognized claim or entitlement, encompassing both freedom from government interference or discriminatory treatment and an entitlement to a benefit or service" (Levy & Rubenstein, 1996). A right is *absolute* when there is no restriction whatsoever on the individual's entitlement. A *legal right* is one on which the society has agreed and formalized into law. Both the National League for Nursing (NLN) and the American Hospital Association (AHA) have established guidelines of patients' rights. Although these are not considered legal documents, nurses and hospitals are considered responsible for upholding these rights of patients. The AHA Patient's Bill of Rights is presented in Table 4–2.

TABLE 4 – 1 American Nurses Association Code of Ethics for Nurses

1. The nurse, in all professional relationships, practices with compassion and respect for the inherent dignity, worth and uniqueness of every individual, unrestricted by consideration of social or economic status, personal attributes, or the nature of health problems.
2. The nurse's primary commitment is to the patient whether an individual, family, group or community.
3. The nurse promotes, advocates for, and strives to protect the health, safety, and rights of the patient.
4. The nurse is responsible and accountable for individual nursing practice and determines the appropriate delegation of tasks consistent with the nurse's obligation to provide optimum patient care.
5. The nurse owes the same duties to self as to others, including the responsibility to preserve integrity and safety, to maintain competence, and to continue personal and professional growth.
6. The nurse participates in establishing, maintaining, and improving healthcare environments and conditions of employment conducive to the provision of quality healthcare and consistent with the values of the profession through individual and collective action.
7. The nurse participates in the advancement of the profession through contributions to practice, education, administration, and knowledge development.
8. The nurse collaborates with other health professionals and the public in promoting community, national, and international efforts to meet health needs.
9. The profession of nursing, as represented by associations and their members, is responsible for articulating nursing values, for maintaining the integrity of the profession and its practice, and for shaping social policy.

Source: Reprinted with permission from American Nurses Association, Code of Ethics for Nurses with Interpretive Statements, © 2001 American Nurses Publishing, American Nurses Foundation/American Nurses Association, Washington, D.C.

TABLE 4 – 2 American Hospital Association Patient's Bill of Rights

1. The patient has the right to considerate and respectful care.
2. The patient has the right to obtain from his physician complete current information concerning his diagnosis, treatment, and prognosis in terms the patient can be reasonably expected to understand. When it is not medically advisable to give such information to the patient, the information should be made available to an appropriate person in his behalf. He has the right to know by name the physician responsible for coordinating his care.
3. The patient has the right to receive from his physician information necessary to give informed consent prior to the start of any procedure and/or treatment. Except in emergencies, such information for informed consent should include but not necessarily be limited to the specific procedure and/or treatment, the medically significant risks involved, and the probable duration of incapacitation. Where medically significant alternatives for care or treatment exist, or when the patient requests information concerning medical alternatives, the patient has the right to such information. The patient also has the right to know the name of the person responsible for the procedures and/or treatment.
4. The patient has the right to refuse treatment to the extent permitted by law and to be informed of the medical consequences of his action.
5. The patient has the right to every consideration of his privacy concerning his own medical care program. Case discussion, consultation, examination, and treatment are confidential and should be conducted discreetly. Those not directly involved in his care must have the permission of the patient to be present.
6. The patient has the right to expect that all communications and records pertaining to his care should be treated as confidential.
7. The patient has the right to expect that within its capacity a hospital must make reasonable response to the request of a patient for services. The hospital must provide evaluation, service, and/or referral as indicated by the urgency of the case. When medically permissible, a patient may be transferred to another facility only after he has received complete information and explanation concerning the needs for and alternatives to such a transfer. The institution to which the patient is to be transferred must first have accepted the patient for transfer.
8. The patient has the right to obtain information as to any relationship of his hospital to other healthcare and educational institutions insofar as his care is concerned. The patient has the right to obtain information as to the existence of any professional relationships among individuals, by name, who are treating him.
9. The patient has the right to be advised if the hospital proposes to engage in or perform human experimentation affecting his care or treatment. The patient has the right to refuse to participate in such research projects.
10. The patient has the right to expect reasonable continuity of care. He has the right to know in advance what appointment times and physicians are available and where. The patient has the right to expect that the hospital will provide a mechanism whereby he is informed by his physician or a delegate of the physician of the patient's continuing healthcare requirements following discharge.
11. The patient has the right to examine and receive an explanation of his bill regardless of source of payment.
12. The patient has the right to know what hospital rules and regulations apply to his conduct as a patient.

Source: AHA (1992), with permission.

ETHICAL CONSIDERATIONS

Theoretical Perspectives

An *ethical theory* is a moral principle or a set of moral principles that can be used in assessing what is morally right or morally wrong (Ellis & Hartley, 2004). These principles provide guidelines for ethical decision-making.

Utilitarianism

The basis of **utilitarianism** is "the greatest-happiness principle." This principle holds that actions are right in proportion, as they tend to promote happiness, and wrong as they tend to produce the reverse of happiness. Thus, the good is happiness, and the right is that which promotes the good. Conversely, the wrongness of an action is determined by its tendency to bring about unhappiness.

A second principle of utilitarianism is "the end justifies the means." An ethical decision based on the utilitarian view would look at the results of the decision. Action would be taken based on the results that produced the most good (happiness) for the most people.

Kantianism

Named for philosopher Immanuel Kant, **Kantianism** is directly opposed to utilitarianism. Kant argued that it is not the consequences or end results that make an action right or wrong; rather it is the principle or motivation on which the action is based that is the morally decisive factor. Kantianism suggests that our actions are bound by a sense of duty. This theory is often called *deontology* (from the Greek *deon*, which means "that which is binding; duty"). Kantian-directed ethical decisions are made out of respect for moral law. For example, "I make this choice because it is morally right and my duty to do so" (not because of consideration for a possible outcome).

Christian Ethics

A basic principle that might be called a Christian philosophy is that which is also known as the golden rule: "Do unto others as you would have them do unto you" and, alternatively, "Do not do unto others what you would not have them do unto you." The imperative demand of **Christian ethics** is to treat others as moral equals and to recognize the equality of other persons by permitting them to act as we do when they occupy a position similar to ours.

Natural Law Theories

The most general moral precept of the **natural law theory** is "do good and avoid evil." Natural law theorists contend, then, that ethics must be grounded in a concern for the human good. Although the nature of this "human good" is not explained, Catholic theologians view natural law as the law inscribed by God into the nature of things—as a species of divine law. According to this conception, the Creator endows all things with certain potentialities or tendencies that serve to define their natural end. The fulfillment of a thing's natural tendencies constitutes the specific good of that thing. For example, the natural tendency of an acorn is to become an oak. What, then, is the natural potential, or tendency, of human beings? Natural law theorists focus on an attribute that is regarded as distinctively human, as separating human beings from the rest of the worldly creatures; that is, the ability to live according to the dictates of reason. It is with this ability to reason that humans are able to choose "good" over "evil." In natural law, evil acts are never condoned, even if they are intended to advance the noblest of ends.

Ethical Egoism

Ethical egoism espouses that what is right and good is what is best for the individual making the decision. An individual's actions are determined by what is to his or her own advantage. The action may not be best for anyone else involved, but consideration is only for the individual making the decision.

Ethical Dilemmas

An **ethical dilemma** is a situation that requires an individual to make a choice between two equally unfavorable alternatives (Catalano, 1996). Evidence exists to support both moral "rightness" and moral "wrongness" related to a certain action. The individual who must make the choice experiences conscious conflict regarding the decision.

Ethical dilemmas arise when no explicit reasons exist that govern an action. Ethical dilemmas generally create a great deal of emotion. Often the reasons supporting each side of the argument for action are logical and appropriate. The actions associated with both sides are desirable in some respects and undesirable in others. In most situations, taking no action is considered an action taken.

Ethical Principles

Ethical principles are fundamental guidelines that influence decision-making. The ethical principles of autonomy, beneficence, nonmaleficence, veracity, and justice are helpful and used frequently by healthcare workers to assist with ethical decision-making. These principles apply largely to the deontological (Kantianism) ethical theory, in which decisions are made out of a sense of duty.

Autonomy

The principle of **autonomy** arises from the Kantian duty of respect for persons as rational agents. This viewpoint emphasizes the status of persons as autonomous moral agents whose right to determine their destinies should always be respected. This presumes that individuals are always capable of making independent choices for themselves. Healthcare workers know this is not always the case. Children, individuals who are comatose, and the seriously mentally ill are examples of clients who are incapable of making informed choices. In these instances, a representative of the individual is usually asked to intervene and give consent. However, healthcare workers must ensure that respect for an individual's autonomy is not disregarded in favor of what another person may view as best for the client.

Beneficence

Beneficence refers to one's duty to benefit or promote the good of others. Healthcare workers who act in their clients' interests are beneficent, provided their actions really do serve the client's best interest. In fact, some duties do seem to take preference over other duties. For example, the duty to respect the autonomy of an individual may be overridden when that individual has been deemed harmful to self or others. Aiken (1994) states, "The difficulty that sometimes arises in implementing the principle of beneficence lies in determining what exactly is good for another and who can best make the decision about this good."

Nonmaleficence

Nonmaleficence is the requirement that healthcare providers do no harm to their clients, either intentionally or unintentionally (Aiken, 1994). Some philosophers suggest that this principle is more important than beneficence; that is, they support the notion that it is more important to avoid doing harm than it is to do good. In any event, ethical dilemmas often arise when a conflict exists between an individual's rights (the duty to promote good) and what is thought to best represent the welfare of the individual (the duty to do no harm). An example of this conflict might occur when administering chemotherapy to a cancer patient, knowing it will prolong his or her life but creating "harm" (side effects) in the short term.

Justice

The principle of **justice** has been referred to as the "justice as fairness" principle. It is sometimes referred to as *distributive justice*, and its basic premise lies with the right of individuals to be treated equally regardless of race, gender, marital status, medical diagnosis, social standing, economic level, or religious belief (Aiken, 1994). The concept of justice reflects a duty to treat all individuals equally and fairly. When applied to healthcare, this principle suggests that all resources within the society (including healthcare services) ought to be distributed evenly without respect to socioeconomic status. Thus, according to this principle, the vast disparity in the quality of care dispensed to the various classes within our society is considered unjust. A more equitable distribution of care for all individuals would be favored.

Veracity

The principle of **veracity** refers to one's duty always to be truthful. Aiken (1994) states, "Veracity requires that the healthcare provider tell the truth and not intentionally deceive or mislead clients." There are times when limitations must be placed on this principle, such as when the truth would knowingly produce harm or interfere with the recovery process. Being honest is not always easy, but lying is rarely justified. Clients have the right to know about their diagnosis, treatment, and prognosis.

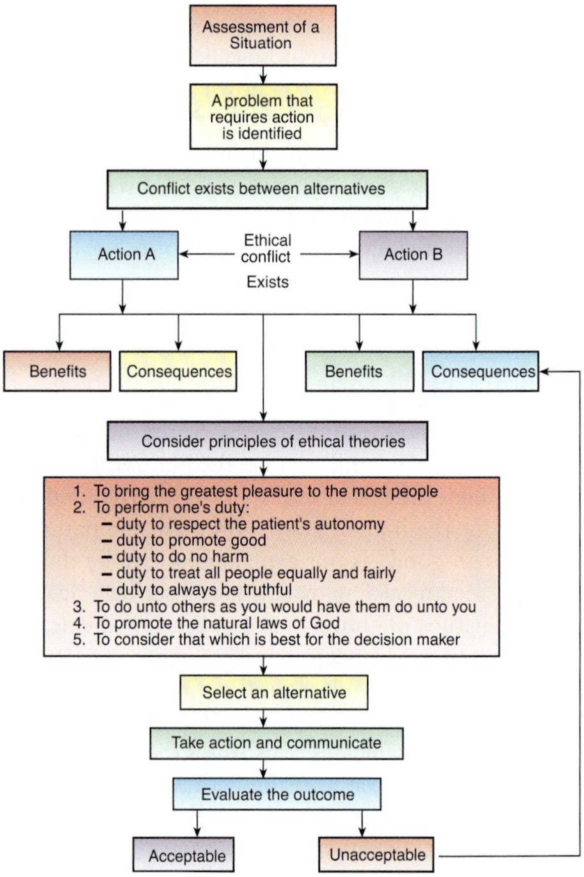

FIGURE 4–1 Ethical decision-making model.

A Model for Making Ethical Decisions

The following is a set of steps that may be used in making an ethical decision. These steps closely resemble the steps of the nursing process.

1. *Assessment.* Gather the subjective and objective data about a situation.
2. *Problem Identification.* Identify the conflict between two or more alternative actions.
3. *Plan.* (a) Explore the benefits and consequences of each alternative; (b) Consider principles of ethical theories; (c) Select an alternative.
4. *Implementation.* Act on the decision made and communicate the decision to others.
5. *Evaluation.* Evaluate outcomes.

A schematic of this model is presented in Figure 4–1. A case study using this decision-making model is presented in Table 4–3. If the outcome is acceptable, action continues in the manner selected. If the outcome is unacceptable, benefits and consequences of the remaining alternatives are reexamined, and Steps three through seven in Table 4–3 are repeated.

TABLE 4 – 3 Ethical Decision-Making—A Case Study

Step 1. Assessment

Tonja is a 17-year-old girl who is currently on the psychiatric unit with a diagnosis of conduct disorder. Tonja reports that she has been sexually active since she was 14. She had an abortion when she was 15, and a second one just 6 weeks ago. She states that her mother told her she has "had her last abortion," and that she has to start taking birth control pills. She asks her nurse, Kimberly, to give her some information about the pills and tell her how to go about getting some. Kimberly believes Tonja desperately needs information about birth control pills, as well as other types of contraceptives, but the psychiatric unit is part of a Catholic hospital, and hospital policy prohibits distributing this type of information.

Step 2. Problem Identification

A conflict exists between the client's need for information, the nurse's desire to provide that information, and the institution's policy prohibiting the provision of that information.

Step 3. Alternatives—Benefits and Consequences

1. Alternative 1. Give the client information and risk losing job.
2. Alternative 2. Do not give client information and compromise own values of holistic nursing.
3. Alternative 3. Refer client to another source outside the hospital and risk reprimand from supervisor.

Step 4. Consider Principles of Ethical Theories

1. Alternative 1. Giving the client information would certainly respect the client's autonomy and would benefit the client by decreasing her chances of becoming pregnant again. It would not be to the best advantage of Kimberly because she would likely lose her job. And according to the beliefs of the Catholic hospital, the natural laws of God would be violated.
2. Alternative 2. Withholding information restricts the client's autonomy. It has the potential for doing harm, in that without the use of contraceptives, the client may become pregnant again (and she implies that this is not what she wants). Kimberly's Christian ethic is violated in that this action is not what she would want "done unto her."
3. Alternative 3. A referral would respect the client's autonomy, would promote good, and would do no harm (except perhaps to Kimberly's ego from the possible reprimand). Also, this decision would comply with Kimberly's Christian ethic.

Step 5. Select an Alternative

Alternative 3 is selected based on the ethical theories of utilitarianism (does the most good for the greatest number), Christian ethics (Kimberly's belief of "Do unto others as you would have others do unto you"), and Kantianism (to perform one's duty) and the ethical principles of autonomy, beneficence, and nonmaleficence. The success of this decision depends upon the client's follow-through with the referral and compliance with use of the contraceptives.

Step 6. Take Action and Communicate

Taking action involves providing information in writing for Tonja, perhaps making a phone call and setting up an appointment for her with Planned Parenthood. Communicating suggests sharing the information with Tonja's mother. Communication also includes documentation of the referral in the client's chart.

Step 7. Evaluate the Outcome

An acceptable outcome might indicate that Tonja did indeed keep her appointment at Planned Parenthood and is complying with the prescribed contraceptive regimen. It might also include Kimberly's input into the change process in her institution to implement these types of referrals to other client's who request them.

An unacceptable outcome might be indicated by Tonja's lack of follow-through with the appointment at Planned Parenthood or lack of compliance in using the contraceptives, resulting in another pregnancy. Kimberly may also view a reprimand from her supervisor as an unacceptable outcome, particularly if she is told that she must select other alternatives should this situation arise in the future. This may motivate Kimberly to make another decision—that of seeking employment in an institution that supports a philosophy more consistent with her own.

Ethical Issues in Psychiatric/Mental Health Nursing

The Right to Refuse Medication

The AHA's (1992) Patient's Bill of Rights states: "The patient has the right to refuse treatment to the extent permitted by law, and to be informed of the medical consequences of his action." In psychiatry, refusal of treatment primarily concerns the administration of psychotropic medications. "To the extent permitted by law" may be defined within the U.S. Constitution and several of its amendments (e.g., the First Amendment, which addresses the rights of speech, thought, and expression; the Eighth Amendment, which grants the right to freedom from cruel and unusual punishment;

and the Fifth and Fourteenth Amendments, which grant due process of law and equal protection for all). In psychiatry, "the medical consequences of his action" may include such steps as involuntary commitment, legal competency hearing, or client discharge from the hospital.

Although many courts are supporting a client's right to refuse medications in the psychiatric area, some limitations do exist. Weiss-Kaffie and Purtell (2001) state:

> The treatment team must determine that three criteria be met to force medication without client consent. The client must exhibit behavior that is dangerous to self or others; the medication ordered by the physician must have a reasonable chance of providing help to the client; and clients who refuse medication must be judged incompetent to evaluate the benefits of the treatment in question. (p. 361)

The Right to the Least-Restrictive Treatment Alternative

Healthcare personnel must attempt to provide treatment in a manner that least restricts the freedom of clients. The "restrictiveness" of psychiatric therapy can be described in the context of a continuum, based on severity of illness. Clients may be treated on an outpatient basis, in day hospitals, or in voluntary or involuntary hospitalization. Symptoms may be treated with verbal rehabilitative techniques and move successively to behavioral techniques, chemical interventions, seclusion, mechanical restraints, or electroconvulsive therapy. The problem appears to arise in selecting the least restrictive means among involuntary chemical intervention, seclusion, and mechanical restraints. Sadock and Sadock (2003) state:

> Distinguishing among these interventions on the basis of restrictiveness proves to be a purely subjective exercise fraught with personal bias. Moreover, each of these three interventions is both more and less restrictive than each of the other two. Nevertheless, the effort should be made to think in terms of restrictiveness when deciding how to treat patients. (p. 1358)

LEGAL CONSIDERATIONS

In 1980, the 96th Congress of the United States passed the Mental Health Systems Act, which includes a Patient's Bill of Rights, for recommendation to the states. An adaptation of these rights is presented in Table 4–4.

Nurse Practice Acts

The legal parameters of professional and practical nursing are defined within each state by the state's nurse practice act. These documents are passed by the state legislature and in general are concerned with such provisions as the following:

- The definition of important terms including the definition of nursing and the various types of nurses recognized

TABLE 4 – 4 Bill of Rights for Psychiatric Patients

1. The right to appropriate treatment and related services in the setting that is most supportive and least restrictive to personal freedom.
2. The right to an individualized, written treatment or service plan; the right to treatment based on such plan; and the right to periodic review and revision of the plan based on treatment needs.
3. The right, consistent with one's capabilities, to participate in and receive a reasonable explanation of the care and treatment process.
4. The right to refuse treatment except in an emergency situation or as permitted by law.
5. The right not to participate in experimentation in the absence of informed, voluntary, written consent.
6. The right to freedom from restraint or seclusion except in an emergency situation.
7. The right to a humane treatment environment that affords reasonable protection from harm and appropriate privacy.
8. The right to confidentiality of medical records (also applicable following patient's discharge).
9. The right of access to medical records except information received from third parties under promise of confidentiality, and when access would be detrimental to the patient's health (also applicable following patient's discharge).
10. The right of access to use of the telephone, personal mail, and visitors, unless deemed inappropriate for treatment purposes.
11. The right to be informed of these rights in comprehensible language.
12. The right to assert grievances if rights are infringed.
13. The right to referral as appropriate to other providers of mental health services upon discharge.

Source: Adapted from Mental Health Systems Act (1980).

- A statement of the education and other training or requirements for licensure and reciprocity
- Broad statements that describe the scope of practice for various levels of nursing (APN, RN, LPN)
- Conditions under which a nurse's license may be suspended or revoked and instructions for appeal
- The general authority and powers of the state board of nursing (Fedorka & Resnick, 2001)

Most nurse practice acts are very general in their terminology, and do not provide specific guidelines for practice. Nurses must understand the scope of practice protected by their license, and should seek assistance from legal counsel if unsure about the proper interpretation of a nurse practice act.

Types of Law

There are two general categories or types of law that are of most concern to nurses: statutory law and common law. These laws are identified by their source or origin.

Statutory Law

A statutory law is a law enacted by a legislative body, such as a county or city council, the state legislature, or the Congress of the United States. An example of statutory law would be the nurse practice acts.

Common Law

Common laws derive from decisions made in previous cases. These laws apply to a body of principles that evolve from court decisions resolving various controversies. Because common law in the United States has been developed on a state basis, the law on specific subjects may differ from state to state. An example of a common law might be how different states deal with a nurse's refusal to provide care for a specific client.

Classifications Within Statutory and Common Law

Broadly speaking, there are two kinds of unlawful acts: civil and criminal. Both statutory law and common law have civil and criminal components.

Civil Law

Civil law protects the private and property rights of individuals and businesses. Private individuals or groups may bring a legal action to court for breach of civil law. These legal actions are of two basic types: torts and contracts.

TORTS. A **tort** is a violation of a civil law in which an individual has been wronged. In a tort action, one party asserts that wrongful conduct on the part of the other has caused harm and seeks compensation for harm suffered. A tort may be *intentional* or *unintentional*. Examples of unintentional torts are malpractice and negligence actions. An example of an intentional tort is the touching of another person without that person's consent. Intentional touching (e.g., a medical treatment) without the client's consent can result in a charge of battery, an intentional tort.

CONTRACTS. In a contract action, one party asserts that the other party, in failing to fulfill an obligation, has breached the contract, and either compensation or performance of the obligation is sought as remedy. An example might be an action by a mental health professional whose clinical privileges have been reduced or terminated in violation of an implied contract between the professional and a hospital.

Criminal Law

Criminal law provides protection from conduct deemed injurious to the public welfare. It provides for punishment of those found to have engaged in such conduct. This commonly includes imprisonment, parole conditions, a loss of privilege (such as a license), a fine, or any combination of these (Ellis & Hartley, 2004). An example of a violation of criminal law is the theft by a hospital employee of supplies or drugs.

Legal Issues in Psychiatric/Mental Health Nursing

Confidentiality and Right to Privacy

An individual's privacy is protected by the Fourth, Fifth, and Fourteenth Amendments to the U.S. Constitution. Most states have statutes protecting the confidentiality of client records and communications. The only individuals who have a right to observe a client or have access to medical information are those involved in his or her medical care.

Pertinent medical information may be released without consent in a life-threatening situation. If information is released in an emergency, the following information must be recorded in the client's record: date of disclosure, person to whom information was disclosed, reason for disclosure, reason written consent could not be obtained, and the specific information disclosed.

Most states have statutes that pertain to the doctrine of **privileged communication**. Although the codes differ markedly from state to state, most grant certain professionals privileges under which they may refuse to reveal information about, and communications with, clients. In most states, the doctrine of privileged communication applies to psychiatrists and attorneys; in some instances, psychologists, clergy, and nurses are included.

In certain instances, nurses may be called on to testify in cases in which the medical record is used as evidence. In most states, the right to privacy pertaining to these records is exempted in civil or criminal proceedings. Therefore, it is important that nurses document with these possibilities in mind. Strict record keeping using statements that are objective and nonjudgmental, having care plans that are specific in their prescriptive interventions, and maintaining documentation that describes those interventions and their subsequent evaluation all serve the best interests of the client, the nurse, and the institution should questions regarding care arise. Documentation very often weighs heavily in malpractice case decisions.

The right to confidentiality is a basic one, and especially so in psychiatry. Although societal attitudes are improving, individuals have been discriminated against in the past for no other reason than for having a history of emotional illness. Nurses working in psychiatry must guard the privacy of their clients with great diligence.

Informed Consent

According to law, all persons have the right to decide whether to accept or reject treatment (Guido, 1997). A healthcare provider can be charged with assault and battery for providing life-sustaining treatment to a client when the client has not agreed to it. The rationale for the doctrine of **informed consent** is the preservation and protection of individual autonomy in determining what will and will not happen to the person's body (Guido, 1997).

Informed consent is a client's permission granted to a physician to perform a therapeutic procedure, before which information about the procedure has been presented to the client with adequate time given for consideration about the pros and cons. The client should receive information such as what treatment alternatives are available; why the physician believes this treatment is most appropriate; the possible outcomes, risks, and adverse effects; the possible outcome should the client select another treatment alternative; and the possible outcome should the client choose to have no treatment. An example of a treatment in the psychiatric area that requires informed consent is electroconvulsive therapy.

There are some conditions under which treatment may be performed without obtaining informed consent. A client's refusal to accept treatment may be challenged under the following circumstances (Cournos & Petrila, 1992; Goldstein, Perdew, & Pruitt, 1989; Guido, 1997; Levy & Rubenstein, 1996):

1. When a client is mentally incompetent to make a decision and treatment is necessary to preserve life or avoid serious harm.
2. When refusing treatment endangers the life or health of another.
3. During an emergency in which a client is in no condition to exercise judgment.
4. When the client is a child (consent is obtained from parent or surrogate).
5. In the case of therapeutic privilege. In therapeutic privilege, information about a treatment may be withheld if the physician can show that full disclosure would hinder or complicate necessary treatment, cause severe psychological harm, or be so upsetting as to render a rational decision by the client impossible.

Although most clients in psychiatric/mental health facilities are competent and capable of giving informed consent, those with severe psychiatric illness do not possess the cognitive ability to do so. If an individual has been determined legally to be mentally incompetent, consent is obtained from the legal guardian. Difficulty arises when there has been no legal determination made, but the individual's current mental state prohibits informed decision-making (e.g., the person who is psychotic, unconscious, or inebriated). In these instances, informed consent is usually obtained from the individual's nearest relative. If none exist and time permits, the physician may ask the court to appoint a conservator or guardian. When time does not permit court intervention, permission may even be sought from the hospital administrator.

A client or guardian always has the right to withdraw consent after it has been given. When this occurs, the physician should inform (or reinform) the client or guardian about the consequences of refusing treatment. If treatment has already been initiated, the physician should terminate treatment in a way least likely to cause injury to the client and inform the client or guardian of the risks associated with interrupted treatment (Guido, 1997).

The nurse's role in obtaining informed consent is usually defined by agency policy. A nurse may sign the consent form as witness for the client's signature. However, legal liability for informed consent lies with the physician. The nurse acts as client advocate to ensure that the following three major elements of informed consent have been addressed:

1. Knowledge—that the client has received adequate information on which to base his or her decision.
2. Competency—that the individual's cognition is not impaired to an extent that would interfere with decision-making or, if so, that the individual has a legal representative.
3. Free Will—that the individual has given consent voluntarily without pressure or coercion from others.

Restraints and Seclusion

An individual's privacy and personal security are protected by the U.S. Constitution and supported by the Mental Health Systems Act of 1980, out of which was conceived a bill of rights for psychiatric patients. These include "the right to freedom from restraint or seclusion except in an emergency situation."

In psychiatry, the term *restraints* generally refers to a set of leather straps that are used to restrain the extremities of an individual whose behavior is out of control and who poses an inherent risk to the physical safety and psychological well-being of the individual and staff (Joint Commission on Accreditation of Healthcare Organizations [JCAHO], 2000). Restraints are never to be used as punishment or for the convenience of staff. Less restrictive measures to decrease agitation, such as "talking down" (verbal intervention) and chemical restraints (tranquilizing medication) are usually tried first. If these interventions are ineffective, mechanical restraints may be instituted. *Seclusion* is another type of physical restraint in which the client is confined alone in a room from which he or she is unable to leave. The room is usually furnished minimally, with items to promote the client's comfort and safety.

The Joint Commission on Accreditation of Healthcare Organizations has released a set of revisions to its previous restraint and seclusion standards. The intent of these revisions is to reduce the use of this intervention, as well as to provide greater assurance of safety and protection to individuals placed in restraint or seclusion for reasons related to psychiatric disorders or substance abuse (Medscape, 2000). In addition to others, these revisions provide the following guidelines:

1. In the event of an emergency, restraints or seclusion may be initiated without a physician's order.
2. As soon as possible, but no longer than 1 hour after the initiation of restraint or seclusion, a qualified staff member must notify the physician about the individual's physical and psychological condition and obtain a verbal or written order for the restraints or seclusion.
3. Orders for restraints or seclusion must be reissued by a physician every 4 hours for adults aged 18 and older, every 2 hours for children and adolescents aged 9 to 17, and every hour for children younger than 9 years.
4. An in-person evaluation of the individual must be made by the physician within 4 hours of the initiation of restraints or seclusion of an adult aged 18 or older, and within 2 hours for children and adolescents aged 17 and younger.
5. Minimum times for in-person re-evaluations by a physician include 8 hours for individuals aged 18 years and older, and 4 hours for individuals aged 17 and younger.
6. If an individual is no longer in restraints or seclusion when an original verbal order expires, the physician must conduct an in-person evaluation within 24 hours of initiation of the intervention.

Clients in restraints or seclusion must be observed and assessed every 10 to 15 minutes with regard to circulation, respiration, nutrition, hydration, and elimination. Such attention should be documented in the client's record.

False imprisonment is the deliberate and unauthorized confinement of a person within fixed limits by the use of verbal or physical means (Ellis & Hartley, 2004). Healthcare workers may be charged with false imprisonment for restraining or secluding—against the wishes of the client—anyone having been admitted to the hospital voluntarily. Should a voluntarily admitted client decompensate to a point that restraint or seclusion for protection of self or others is necessary, court intervention to determine competency and involuntary commitment is required to preserve the client's rights to privacy and freedom.

Commitment Issues

Voluntary Admissions

Each year, more than 1 million persons are admitted to hospitals for psychiatric treatment, of which approximately two thirds are considered voluntary. To be admitted voluntarily, an individual makes direct application to the institution for services and may stay as long as treatment is deemed necessary. He or she may sign out of the hospital at any time, unless the healthcare professional determines, following a mental status examination, that the client may be harmful to self or others and recommends that the admission status be changed from voluntary to involuntary. Durham (1996) states:

> Even though these hospital admissions are considered "voluntary," they are regulated by statute to ensure that (1) persons with mental disorders are sufficiently competent to make decisions of this kind, (2) inappropriate pressure or outright coercion has not been exerted on a person already in custody to admit themselves, and (3) the person is truly "willing" to seek treatment, thereby improving the prospects for success." (p. 17)

Involuntary Commitment

Because involuntary hospitalization results in substantial restrictions of the rights of an individual, the admission process is subject to the guarantee of the Fourteenth Amendment to the U.S. Constitution that provides citizens protection against loss of liberty and ensures due process rights (Weiss-Kaffie & Purtell, 2001). Involuntary commitments are made for various reasons. Most states commonly cite the following criteria:

1. In an emergency situation (for the client who is dangerous to self or others)
2. For observation and treatment of mentally ill persons
3. When an individual is unable to take care of basic personal needs (the "gravely disabled")

Under the Fourth Amendment, individuals are protected from unlawful searches and seizures without probable cause. Therefore, the individual seeking the involuntary commitment must show probable cause why the client should be hospitalized against his or her wishes; that is, that person must show that there is cause to believe that the person would be dangerous to self or others, is mentally ill and in need of treatment, or is gravely disabled.

EMERGENCY COMMITMENTS. Emergency commitments are sought when an individual manifests behavior that is clearly and imminently dangerous to self or others. These admissions are usually instigated by relatives or friends of the individual, police officers, the court, or healthcare professionals. Emergency commitments are time-limited, and a court hearing for the individual is scheduled, usually within 72 hours. At that time, the court may decide that the client may be discharged; or, if deemed necessary, and voluntary admission is refused by the client, an additional period of involuntary commitment may be ordered. In most instances, another hearing is scheduled for a specified time (usually in 7 to 21 days).

THE MENTALLY ILL PERSON IN NEED OF TREATMENT. A second type of involuntary commitment is for the observation and treatment of mentally ill persons in need of treatment. Most states have established definitions of what constitutes "mentally ill" for purposes of state involuntary admission statutes. Some examples include individuals who, because of severe mental illness, are:

- Unable to make informed decisions concerning treatment
- Likely to cause harm to self or others
- Unable to fulfill basic personal needs necessary for health and safety

In determining whether commitment is required, the court looks for substantial evidence of abnormal conduct—evidence that cannot be explained as the result of a physical cause. There must be "clear and convincing evidence" as well as "probable cause" to substantiate the need for involuntary commitment to ensure that an individual's rights under the Constitution are protected. The U.S. Supreme Court in *O'Connor v Donaldson* held that the existence of mental illness alone does not justify involuntary hospitalization. State standards require a specific impact or consequence to flow from the mental illness that involves danger or an inability to care for one's own needs. These clients are entitled to court hearings with representation, at which time determination of commitment and length of stay are considered. Legislative statutes governing involuntary commitments vary from state to state.

INVOLUNTARY OUTPATIENT COMMITMENT. Involuntary outpatient commitment (IOC) is a court-ordered mechanism used to compel a person with mental illness to submit to treatment on an outpatient basis. Maloy (1996) cites three determinants for commitment to outpatient treatment. These include:

1. Conditional release from inpatient hospitalization
2. Commitment to an outpatient program as a less re-

strictive alternative to hospitalization, for persons who meet the inpatient commitment standard, but would benefit from community treatment
3. Commitment to outpatient treatment (sometimes called *preventive commitment*) based on less stringent criteria than are required for inpatient commitment

Most states have already enacted IOC legislation or currently have resolutions that speak to this topic on their agendas. Most commonly, clients who are committed into the IOC programs have severe and persistent mental illness, such as schizophrenia. The rationale behind the legislation is to reduce the numbers of readmissions and lengths of hospital stays of these clients. Concern lies in the possibility of violating the individual rights of psychiatric clients without significant improvement in treatment outcomes. Maloy (1996) states,

> IOC laws do not necessarily lead to improvements in services or enhancements of community mental health programs. Nonetheless, the ongoing attention given to outpatient commitment laws by state legislators suggests that state policymakers view IOC as a useful and appropriate response to the challenges and crises posed by severe and persistent mental illness. (p. 44)

Ongoing research shows that IOC may indeed reduce hospital readmissions and lengths of stays. Continuing research is required to determine if IOC will improve treatment compliance and enhance quality of life in the community for individuals with severe and persistent mental illness.

THE GRAVELY DISABLED CLIENT. A number of states have statutes that specifically define the "gravely disabled" client. For those that do not use this label, the description of the individual who, because of mental illness, is unable to take care of basic personal needs is very similar.

Gravely disabled is generally defined as a condition in which an individual, because of mental illness, is in danger of serious physical harm resulting from inability to provide for basic needs such as food, clothing, shelter, medical care, and personal safety. Inability to care for oneself cannot be established by showing that an individual lacks the resources to provide the necessities of life. Rather, it is the inability to make use of available resources.

Should it be determined that an individual is gravely disabled, a guardian, conservator, or committee will be appointed by the court to ensure the management of the person and his or her estate. To legally restore competency then requires another court hearing to reverse the previous ruling. The individual whose competency is being determined has the right to be represented by an attorney.

Nursing Liability

Mental health practitioners—psychiatrists, psychologists, psychiatric nurses, and social workers—have a duty to provide appropriate care based on the standards of their professions and the standards set by law. The standards of care for psychiatric/mental health nursing are presented in Chapter 6.

Malpractice and Negligence

The terms **malpractice** and **negligence** are often used interchangeably. *Negligence* has been defined as:

> The failure to exercise the standard of care that a reasonably prudent person would have exercised in a similar situation; any conduct that falls below the legal standard established to protect others against unreasonable risk of harm, except for conduct that is intentionally, wantonly, or willfully disregardful of others' rights (Garner, 1999).

Any person may be negligent. In contrast, malpractice is a specialized form of negligence applicable only to professionals.

Black's Law Dictionary defines malpractice as:

> An instance of negligence or incompetence on the part of a professional. To succeed in a malpractice claim, a plaintiff must also prove proximate cause and damages (Garner, 1999).

In the absence of any state statutes, common law is the basis of liability for injuries to clients caused by acts of malpractice and negligence of individual practitioners. In other words, most decisions of negligence in the professional setting are based on legal precedent (decisions that have previously been made about similar cases) rather than any specific action taken by the legislature.

To summarize, when the breach of duty is characterized as malpractice, the action is weighed against the professional standard. When it is brought forth as negligence, action is contrasted with what a reasonably prudent professional would have done in the same or similar circumstances.

Marchand (2001) cites the following basic elements of a nursing malpractice lawsuit:

1. The existence of a duty, owed by the nurse to a patient, to conform to a recognized standard of care

2. A failure to conform to the required nursing standard of care
3. Actual injury
4. A reasonably close causal connection between the nurse's conduct and the patient's injury

For the client to prevail in a malpractice claim, each of these elements must be proved. Juries' decisions are generally based on the testimony of expert witnesses, because members of the jury are laypeople and cannot be expected to know what nursing interventions should have been carried out. Without the testimony of expert witnesses, a favorable verdict usually goes to the defendant nurse.

Types of Lawsuits that Occur in Psychiatric Nursing

Most malpractice suits against nurses are civil actions; that is, they are considered breach of conduct actions on the part of the professional, for which compensation is being sought. The nurse in the psychiatric setting should be aware of the types of behaviors that may result in charges of malpractice.

Basic to the psychiatric client's hospitalization is his or her right to confidentiality and privacy. A nurse may be charged with *breach of confidentiality* for revealing aspects about a client's case, or even for revealing that an individual has been hospitalized, if that person can show that making this information known resulted in harm.

When shared information is detrimental to the client's reputation, the person sharing the information may be liable for **defamation of character**. When the information is in writing, the action is called **libel**. Oral defamation is called **slander**. Defamation of character involves communication that is malicious and false (Ellis & Hartley, 2004). Occasionally, libel arises out of critical, judgmental statements written in the client's medical record. Nurses need to be very objective in their charting, backing up all statements with factual evidence.

Invasion of privacy is a charge that may result when a client is searched without probable cause. Many institutions conduct body searches on mental clients as a routine intervention. In these cases, there should be a physician's order and written rationale should show probable cause for the intervention. Many institutions are re-examining their policies regarding this procedure.

Assault is an act that results in a person's genuine fear and apprehension that he or she will be touched without consent. **Battery** is the touching of another person without consent. These charges can result when a treatment is administered to a client against his or her wishes and outside of an emergency. Harm or injury need not have occurred for these charges to be legitimate.

For confining a client against his or her wishes, and outside of an emergency, the nurse may be charged with false imprisonment. Examples of actions that may invoke these charges include locking an individual in a room; taking a client's clothes for purposes of detainment against his or her will; and mechanically restraining a competent, voluntary client who demands to be released.

Avoiding Liability

Hall and Hall (2001) suggest the following proactive nursing actions in an effort to avoid nursing malpractice:

1. Responding to the patient
2. Educating the patient
3. Complying with the standard of care
4. Supervising care
5. Adhering to the nursing process
6. Documentation
7. Follow up

In addition, it is a positive practice to develop and maintain a good interpersonal relationship with the client and his or her family. Some clients appear to be more "suit-prone" than others are. Suit-prone clients are often very critical, complaining, uncooperative, and even hostile. A natural response by the staff to these clients is to become defensive or withdrawn. Either of these behaviors increases the likelihood of a lawsuit should an unfavorable event occur (Ellis & Hartley, 2004). No matter how high the degree of technical competence and skill of the nurse, his or her insensitivity to a client's complaints and failure to meet the client's emotional needs often influence whether or not a lawsuit is generated. A great deal depends on the psychosocial skills of the healthcare professional.

SUMMARY

This chapter examined some of the ethical and legal issues relevant to psychiatric/mental health nursing in an effort to promote enhancement of quality of client care, as well as provide protection to the nurse within the parameters of legal accountability. Ethics is a branch of philosophy that deals with values related to human conduct, to the rightness and wrongness of certain actions, and to the goodness and badness of the motives and ends of such actions.

Clients have certain rights that are afforded them under the Constitution of the United States. Clients' rights have also been set forth by the AHA, the NLN, the American Civil Liberties Union (ACLU), and the Mental Health Systems Act. Nurse practice acts and standards of professional practice guide the scope within which a nurse may legally practice. The ANA has established a code for nurses under which guidelines the professional nurse is expected to practice ethical nursing.

Ethical theories and principles are foundational guidelines that influence decision-making. Ethical theories include utilitarianism, Kantianism, Christian ethics, natural-law theories, and ethical egoism. Ethical principles include autonomy, beneficence, nonmaleficence, veracity, and justice. An individual's ethical philosophy affects his or her decision-making and ultimately the outcomes of those decisions.

Ethical issues in psychiatric/mental health nursing include the right to refuse medication and the right to the least-restrictive treatment alternative. An ethical decision-making model was presented along with a case study for application of the process.

Statutory laws are those that have been enacted by legislative bodies, and common laws are derived from decisions made in previous cases. Civil law protects the private and property rights of individuals and businesses, and criminal law provides protection from conduct deemed injurious to the public welfare. Both statutory law and common law have civil and criminal components.

Legal issues in psychiatric/mental health nursing center around confidentiality and the right to privacy, informed consent, restraints, seclusion, and commitment issues. Nurses are accountable for their own actions in relation to these issues, and violation can result in malpractice lawsuits against the physician, the hospital, and the nurse. Nurses must be aware of the kinds of behaviors that place them at risk for malpractice action. Developing and maintaining a good interpersonal relationship with the client and his or her family appears to be a positive factor when the question of malpractice is being considered.

REVIEW QUESTIONS

SELF-EXAMINATION/LEARNING EXERCISE

Match the following decision-making examples with the appropriate ethical theory:

_____	1. Carol (a nurse) decides to go against family wishes and tell the client of his terminal status because that is what she would want if she were the client.	a. Utilitarianism
_____	2. Carol decides to respect family wishes and not tell the client of his terminal status because that would bring the most happiness to the most people.	b. Kantianism
_____	3. Carol decides not to tell the client about his terminal status because it would be too uncomfortable for her to do so.	c. Christian ethics
_____	4. Carol decides to tell the client of his terminal status because her reasoning tells her that to do otherwise would be an evil act.	d. Natural law theories
_____	5. Carol decides to tell the client of his terminal status because she believes it is her duty to do so.	e. Ethical egoism

Match the following nursing actions with the possible legal action with which the nurse may be charged:

_____	6. The nurse assists the physician with electroconvulsive therapy on his client who has refused to give consent.	a. Breach of confidentiality
_____	7. When the local newspaper calls to inquire why the mayor has been admitted to the hospital, the nurse replies, "He's here because he is an alcoholic."	b. Defamation of character
_____	8. A competent, voluntary client has stated he wants to leave the hospital. The nurse hides his clothes in an effort to keep him from leaving.	c. Assault
_____	9. Jack recently lost his wife and is very depressed. He is running for re-election to the Senate and asks the staff to keep his hospitalization confidential. The nurse is excited about having a Senator on the unit and tells her boyfriend about the admission, which soon becomes common knowledge. Jack loses the election.	d. Battery
_____	10. Joe is very restless and is pacing a lot. The nurse says to Joe, "If you don't sit down in the chair and be still, I'm going to put you in restraints!"	e. False imprisonment

REFERENCES

Aiken, T.D. (1994). Legal, ethical, and political issues in nursing. Philadelphia: F.A. Davis.

American Hospital Association (AHA). (1992). A patient's bill of rights. Chicago: American Hospital Association.

American Nurses Association. (2001). Code of ethics for nurses with interpretive statements. Washington, D.C.: American Nurses Association.

Catalano, J.T. (1996). Contemporary professional nursing. Philadelphia: FA Davis.

Cournos, F., & Petrila, J. (1992). Legal and ethical issues. In F.I. Kass, J.M. Oldham, & H. Pardes (Eds.), The Columbia University College of Physicians and Surgeons complete guide to mental health. New York: Henry Holt.

Durham, M.L. (1996). Civil commitment of the mentally ill: Research, policy and practice. In B.D Sales & S.A. Shaw (Eds.), Mental health and law: Research, policy and services. Durham, NC: Carolina Academic Press.

Ellis, J.R., & Hartley, C.L. (2004). Nursing in today's world: Trends, issues, and management (8th ed.). Philadelphia: Lippincott Williams & Wilkins.

Fedorka, P., & Resnick, L.K. (2001). Defining nursing practice. In M.E. O'Keefe (Ed.), Nursing practice and the law: Avoiding malpractice and other legal rights. Philadelphia: F.A. Davis.

Garner, B.A. (Ed.). (1999). Black's law dictionary. St. Paul, MN: West Group.

Goldstein, A.S., Perdew, S., & Pruitt, S.S. (1989). The nurse's legal advisor: Your guide to legally safe practice. Philadelphia: J.B. Lippincott.

Guido, G.W. (1997). Legal issues in nursing (2nd ed.). Stamford, CT: Appleton & Lange.

Hall, J.K., & Hall, D. (2001). Negligence specific to nursing. In M.E. O'Keefe (Ed.), Nursing practice and the law: Avoiding malpractice and other legal risks. Philadelphia: F.A. Davis.

Joint Commission on Accreditation of Healthcare Organizations. (2000). Restraint and seclusion standards for behavioral health. Retrieved May 2000 from http://www.jcaho.org/standard/restraint/restraint_stds.html/

Levy, R.M., & Rubenstein, L.S. (1996). The rights of people with mental disabilities. Carbondale, IL: Southern Illinois University Press.

Maloy, K.A. (1996). Does involuntary outpatient commitment work? In B. D. Sales & S. A. Shah (Eds.), Mental health and law: Research, policy and services. Durham, NC: Carolina Academic Press.

Marchand, L. (2001). Legal terminology. In M.E. O'Keefe (Ed.), Nursing practice and the law: Avoiding malpractice and other legal risks. Philadelphia: F.A. Davis.

McGovern, T.F. (1991). Foreword. In P.J. Parker, & S. Baldwin (Eds.), Ethical issues in mental health. London: Chapman & Hall.

Medscape Wire (2000). Joint Commission Releases Revised Restraints Standards for Behavioral Healthcare. Retrieved May 2000 from http://psychiatry.medscape.com/MedscapeWire/2000/0500/medwire.0509.Joint.html

Mental Health Systems Act. P.L. 96–398, Title V, Sect. 501.94 Stat. 1598, Oct 7, 1980.

Pappas A. (1994). Ethical issues. In J. Zerwekl & J.C. Claborn (Eds.), Nursing today: Transition and trends. Philadelphia: W.B. Saunders.

Sadock, B.J. & Sadock, V.A. (2003). Synopsis of psychiatry: Behavioral sciences/clinical psychiatry (9th ed.). Philadelphia: Lippincott Williams & Wilkins.

Weiss-Kaffie, C.J., & Purtell, N.E. (2001). Psychiatric nursing. In M.E. O'Keefe (Ed.), Nursing practice and the law: Avoiding malpractice and other legal risks. Philadelphia: F.A. Davis.

UNIT TWO

PSYCHIATRIC/ MENTAL HEALTH NURSING INTERVENTIONS

5

CHAPTER

Relationship Development and Therapeutic Communication

CHAPTER OUTLINE

KEY TERMS

rapport
concrete thinking
confidentiality
unconditional positive regard
genuineness
empathy
sympathy
territoriality
density
intimate distance
personal distance
social distance
public distance
paralanguage
transference
countertransference

OBJECTIVES

After reading this chapter, the student will be able to:

1. Describe the relevance and dynamics of a therapeutic nurse-client relationship.
2. Identify goals of the nurse-client relationship.
3. Identify and discuss essential conditions for a therapeutic relationship to occur.
4. Describe the phases of relationship development and the tasks associated with each phase.
5. Identify types of preexisting conditions that influence the outcome of the communication process.
6. Define *territoriality*, *density*, and *distance* as components of the environment.
7. Identify components of nonverbal expression.
8. Describe therapeutic and nontherapeutic verbal communication techniques.
9. Describe active listening.
10. Discuss therapeutic feedback.

INTRODUCTION

The nurse-client relationship is the foundation on which psychiatric nursing is established. It is a relationship in which both participants must recognize each other as unique and important human beings. It is also a relationship where mutual learning occurs. Peplau (1991) has stated:

> Shall a nurse do things *for* a patient or can participant relationships be emphasized so that a nurse comes to do things *with* a patient as her share of an agenda of work to be accomplished in reaching a goal—health. It is likely that the nursing process is educative and therapeutic when nurse and patient can come to know and to respect each other, as persons who are alike, and yet different, as persons who share in the solution of problems. (p. 9.)

Hays and Larson (1963) have described the role of the nurse as providing the client with the opportunity to:

1. Identify and explore problems in relating to others.
2. Discover healthy ways of meeting emotional needs.
3. Experience a satisfying interpersonal relationship.

The *therapeutic interpersonal relationship* is the process by which nurses provide care for clients in need of psychosocial intervention. *Therapeutic use of self* is the instrument for delivery of that care. *Interpersonal communication techniques* (both verbal and nonverbal) are the "tools" of psychosocial intervention.

This chapter describes the phases of development of a therapeutic nurse-client relationship. Therapeutic use of self and techniques of interpersonal communication are discussed.

THE THERAPEUTIC NURSE-CLIENT RELATIONSHIP

Travelbee (1971), who expanded on Peplau's theory of interpersonal relations in nursing, has stated that it is only when each individual in the interaction perceives the other as a human being that a relationship is possible. She refers not to a nurse-client relationship, but rather to a human-to-human relationship, which she describes as a "mutually significant experience." That is, both the nurse and the recipient of care have needs met when each views the other as a unique human being, not as "an illness," as "a room number," or as "all nurses" in general.

Therapeutic relationships are goal oriented. Ideally, the nurse and client decide together what the goal of the relationship will be. Most often, the goal is directed at learning and growth promotion in an effort to bring about some type of change in the client's life. In general, the goal of a therapeutic relationship may be based on a problem-solving model.

EXAMPLE:

GOAL

The client will demonstrate more adaptive coping strategies for dealing with (specific life situation).

INTERVENTIONS

1. Identify what is troubling the client at this time.
2. Encourage the client to discuss changes he or she would like to make.
3. Discuss with the client which changes are possible and which are not possible.
4. Have the client explore feelings about aspects that cannot be changed and alternative ways of coping more adaptively.
5. Discuss alternative strategies for creating changes the client desires to make.
6. Weigh the benefits and consequences of each alternative.
7. Assist the client to select an alternative.
8. Encourage the client to implement the change.
9. Provide positive feedback for the client's attempts to create change.
10. Assist the client to evaluate outcomes of the change and make modifications as required.

Therapeutic Use of Self

Travelbee (1971) described the instrument for delivery of the process of interpersonal nursing as the *therapeutic use of self,* which she defined as "the ability to use one's personality consciously and in full awareness in an attempt to establish relatedness and to structure nursing interventions."

Use of the self in a therapeutic manner requires that the nurse have a great deal of self-awareness and self-understanding, having arrived at a philosophical belief about life, death, and the overall human condition. The nurse must understand that the ability and extent to which one can effectively help others in time of need is strongly influenced by this internal value system—a combination of intellect and emotions.

CONDITIONS ESSENTIAL TO DEVELOPMENT OF A THERAPEUTIC RELATIONSHIP

Several characteristics that enhance the achievement of a therapeutic relationship have been identified. These concepts are highly significant to the use of self as the therapeutic tool in interpersonal relationship development.

Rapport

Getting acquainted and establishing rapport is the primary task in relationship development. **Rapport** implies special feelings on the part of both the client and the nurse based on acceptance, warmth, friendliness, common interest, a sense of trust, and a nonjudgmental attitude. Establishing rapport may be accomplished by discussing non–health-related topics. Travelbee (1971) states:

> [To establish rapport] is to create a sense of harmony based on knowledge and appreciation of each individual's uniqueness. It is the ability to be still and experience the other as a human being—to appreciate the unfolding of each personality one to the other. The ability to truly care for and about others is the core of rapport.

Trust

To trust another, one must feel confidence in that person's presence, reliability, integrity, veracity, and sincere desire to provide assistance when requested. As identified in Chapter 2, trust is the initial developmental task described by Erikson. When this task has not been achieved, this component of relationship development becomes more difficult. That is not to say that trust cannot be established, but only that additional time and patience may be required on the part of the nurse.

It is imperative for the nurse to convey an aura of trustworthiness, which requires that he or she possess a sense of self-confidence. Confidence in the self is derived from knowledge gained through achievement of personal and professional goals and the ability to integrate these roles and to function as a unified whole.

Trust cannot be presumed; it must be earned. Trustworthiness is demonstrated through nursing interventions that convey a sense of warmth and caring to the client. These interventions are initiated simply and concretely, and directed toward activities that address the client's basic needs for physiological and psychological safety and security. Many psychiatric clients experience **concrete thinking,** which focuses their thought processes on specifics rather than generalities and immediate issues rather than eventual outcomes. Examples of nursing interventions that would promote trust in an individual who is thinking concretely include the following:

- Providing a blanket when the client is cold
- Providing food when the client is hungry
- Keeping promises
- Being honest (e.g., saying,"I don't know the answer to your question, but I'll try to find out") and then following through.
- Simply and clearly providing reasons for certain policies, procedures, and rules
- Providing a written, structured schedule of activities
- Attending activities with the client if he or she is reluctant to go alone
- Being consistent in adhering to unit guidelines
- Taking the client's preferences, requests, and opinions into consideration when possible in decisions concerning his or her care
- Ensuring **confidentiality**; providing reassurance that what is discussed will not be repeated outside the boundaries of the healthcare team

Trust is the basis of a therapeutic relationship. The nurse working in psychiatry must perfect the skills that foster the development of trust. Trust must be established in order for the nurse-client relationship to progress beyond the superficial level of tending to the client's immediate needs.

Respect

To show respect is to believe in the dignity and worth of an individual regardless of his or her unacceptable behavior. Rogers (1951) called this **unconditional positive regard**. The attitude is nonjudgmental, and the respect is unconditional in that it does not depend on the behavior of the client to meet certain standards. The nurse, in fact, may not approve of the client's lifestyle or pattern of behaving. However, with unconditional positive regard, the client is accepted and respected for no other reason than that he or she is considered a worthwhile and unique human being.

Many psychiatric clients have very little self-respect owing to the fact that, because of their behavior, they have been rejected by others in the past. Recognition gree of rapport has been established. Interactions may remain on a superficial level until anxiety subsides. Several interactions may be required to fulfill the tasks associated with this phase.

The Working Phase

The therapeutic work of the relationship is accomplished during this phase. Tasks include:

1. Maintaining the trust and rapport that was established during the orientation phase.
2. Promoting the client's insight and perception of reality.
3. Problem solving using the model presented earlier in this chapter.
4. Overcoming resistance behaviors on the part of the client, as the level of anxiety rises in response to discussion of painful issues.
5. Continuously evaluating progress toward goal attainment.

Transference and Countertransference

Transference and countertransference are common phenomena that often arise during the course of a therapeutic relationship. **Transference** occurs when the client unconsciously attributes (or "transfers") feelings and behavioral predispositions, formed toward a significant other earlier in life, to the nurse (Campbell & Barringer, 1998). These feelings toward the nurse may be triggered by something about the nurse's appearance or personality characteristics that the client views as similar to the significant other from his or her past. Transference can interfere with the therapeutic interaction when the feelings being expressed include anger and hostility. Anger toward the nurse can be manifested by uncooperativeness and resistance to the therapy.

Transference can also take the form of overwhelming affection for the nurse or excessive dependency on the nurse. The nurse is overvalued, and the client forms unrealistic expectations of the nurse. When the nurse is unable to fulfill those expectations or meet the excessive dependency needs, the client may become angry and hostile.

INTERVENTIONS FOR TRANSFERENCE. Hilz (2001) states,

> In cases of transference, the relationship does not usually need to be terminated, except when the transference poses a serious barrier to therapy or safety. The nurse should work with the patient in sorting out the past from the present, and assist the patient into identifying the transference and reassign a new and more appropriate meaning to the current nurse-patient relationship. The goal is to guide the patient to independence by teaching them to assume responsibility for their own behaviors, feelings, and thoughts, and to assign the correct meanings to the relationships based on present circumstances instead of the past.

Countertransference refers to the nurse's behavioral and emotional response to the client. These responses may be related to unresolved feelings toward significant others from the nurse's past, or they may be generated in response to transference feelings on the part of the client. It is not easy to refrain from becoming angry when the client is consistently antagonistic, to feel flattered when showered with affection and attention by the client, or even to feel quite powerful when the client exhibits excessive dependency on the nurse. These feelings can interfere with the therapeutic relationship when they initiate the following types of behaviors:

- The nurse overidentifies with the client's feelings because they remind him or her of problems from the nurse's past or present.
- The nurse and client develop a social or personal relationship.
- The nurse begins to give advice or attempts to "rescue" the client.
- The nurse encourages and promotes the client's dependence.
- The nurse's anger engenders feelings of disgust toward the client.
- The nurse feels anxious and uneasy in the presence of the client.
- The nurse is bored and apathetic in sessions with the client.
- The nurse has difficulty setting limits on the client's behavior.
- The nurse defends the client's behavior to other staff members.

The nurse may be completely unaware or only minimally aware of the counter-transference as it is occurring (Hilz, 2001).

INTERVENTIONS FOR COUNTERTRANSFERENCE. Hilz (2001) states:

> The relationship usually should not be terminated in the presence of countertransference. Rather, the nurse or staff member experiencing the countertransference should be supportively assisted by other staff members to identify his or her feelings and behaviors and recognize

Sympathetic response: Nurse: "I can certainly identify with what you are feeling. I've been overweight most of my life, too. I just get so angry when people act like that. They are so insensitive! It's just so typical of skinny people to act that way. You have a right to want to stay away from them. We'll just see how loud they laugh when you get to choose what movie is shown on the unit after dinner tonight."

Empathetic response: Nurse: "You feel angry and embarrassed by what happened at lunch today." As tears fill BJ's eyes, the nurse encourages her to cry if she feels like it, and to express her anger at the situation. She stays with BJ, but does not dwell on her own feelings about what happened. Instead she focuses on BJ and what the client perceives are her immediate needs.

PHASES OF A THERAPEUTIC NURSE-CLIENT RELATIONSHIP

Psychiatric nurses use interpersonal relationship development as the primary intervention with clients in various psychiatric/mental health settings. This is congruent with Peplau's (1962) identification of counseling as the major subrole of nursing in psychiatry. If what Sullivan (1953) believed is true (i.e., that all emotional problems stem from difficulties with interpersonal relationships), then this role of the nurse in psychiatry becomes especially meaningful and purposeful. It becomes an integral part of the total therapeutic regimen.

The therapeutic interpersonal relationship is the means by which the nursing process is implemented. Through the relationship, problems are identified, and resolution is sought. Tasks of the relationship have been categorized into four phases:

1. Preinteraction phase
2. Orientation (introductory) phase
3. Working phase
4. Termination phase

Although each phase is presented as specific and distinct from the others, there may be some overlapping of tasks, particularly when the interaction is limited. The major goals during each phase of the nurse-client relationship are listed in Table 5–1.

TABLE 5 – 1 Phases of Relationship Development and Major Nursing Goals

Phase	Goals
Preinteraction	Explore self-perceptions
Orientation (introductory)	Establish trust and formulate contract for intervention
Working	Promote client change
Termination	Evaluate goal attainment and ensure therapeutic closure

The Preinteraction Phase

The preinteraction phase involves preparation for the first encounter with the client. Tasks include:

1. Obtaining available information about the client from his or her chart, significant others, or other health-team members. From this information, the initial assessment is begun. This initial information may also allow the nurse to become aware of personal responses to knowledge about the client.
2. Examining one's feelings, fears, and anxieties about working with a particular client. For example, the nurse may have been reared in an alcoholic family and have ambivalent feelings about caring for a client who is alcohol dependent. All individuals bring attitudes and feelings from prior experiences to the clinical setting. The nurse needs to be aware of how these preconceptions may affect his or her ability to care for individual clients.

The Orientation (Introductory) Phase

During the orientation phase, the nurse and client become acquainted. Tasks include:

1. Creating an environment for the establishment of trust and rapport.
2. Establishing a contract for intervention that details the expectations and responsibilities of both the nurse and client.
3. Gathering assessment information to build a strong client database.
4. Identifying the client's strengths and limitations.
5. Formulating nursing diagnoses.
6. Setting goals that are mutually agreeable to the nurse and client.
7. Developing a plan of action that is realistic for meeting the established goals.
8. Exploring feelings of both the client and nurse in terms of the introductory phase.

Introductions often are uncomfortable, and the participants may experience some anxiety until a degree of rapport has been established. Interactions may remain on a superficial level until anxiety subsides. Several interactions may be required to fulfill the tasks associated with this phase.

The Working Phase

The therapeutic work of the relationship is accomplished during this phase. Tasks include:

1. Maintaining the trust and rapport that was established during the orientation phase.
2. Promoting the client's insight and perception of reality.
3. Problem solving using the model presented earlier in this chapter.
4. Overcoming resistance behaviors on the part of the client, as the level of anxiety rises in response to discussion of painful issues.
5. Continuously evaluating progress toward goal attainment.

Transference and Countertransference

Transference and countertransference are common phenomena that often arise during the course of a therapeutic relationship. **Transference** occurs when the client unconsciously attributes (or "transfers") feelings and behavioral predispositions, formed toward a significant other earlier in life, to the nurse (Campbell & Barringer, 1998). These feelings toward the nurse may be triggered by something about the nurse's appearance or personality characteristics that the client views as similar to the significant other from his or her past. Transference can interfere with the therapeutic interaction when the feelings being expressed include anger and hostility. Anger toward the nurse can be manifested by uncooperativeness and resistance to the therapy.

Transference can also take the form of overwhelming affection for the nurse or excessive dependency on the nurse. The nurse is overvalued, and the client forms unrealistic expectations of the nurse. When the nurse is unable to fulfill those expectations or meet the excessive dependency needs, the client may become angry and hostile.

INTERVENTIONS FOR TRANSFERENCE. Hilz (2001) states,

> In cases of transference, the relationship does not usually need to be terminated, except when the transference poses a serious barrier to therapy or safety. The nurse should work with the patient in sorting out the past from the present, and assist the patient into identifying the transference and reassign a new and more appropriate meaning to the current nurse-patient relationship. The goal is to guide the patient to independence by teaching them to assume responsibility for their own behaviors, feelings, and thoughts, and to assign the correct meanings to the relationships based on present circumstances instead of the past.

Countertransference refers to the nurse's behavioral and emotional response to the client. These responses may be related to unresolved feelings toward significant others from the nurse's past, or they may be generated in response to transference feelings on the part of the client. It is not easy to refrain from becoming angry when the client is consistently antagonistic, to feel flattered when showered with affection and attention by the client, or even to feel quite powerful when the client exhibits excessive dependency on the nurse. These feelings can interfere with the therapeutic relationship when they initiate the following types of behaviors:

- The nurse overidentifies with the client's feelings because they remind him or her of problems from the nurse's past or present.
- The nurse and client develop a social or personal relationship.
- The nurse begins to give advice or attempts to "rescue" the client.
- The nurse encourages and promotes the client's dependence.
- The nurse's anger engenders feelings of disgust toward the client.
- The nurse feels anxious and uneasy in the presence of the client.
- The nurse is bored and apathetic in sessions with the client.
- The nurse has difficulty setting limits on the client's behavior.
- The nurse defends the client's behavior to other staff members.

The nurse may be completely unaware or only minimally aware of the counter-transference as it is occurring (Hilz, 2001).

INTERVENTIONS FOR COUNTERTRANSFERENCE. Hilz (2001) states:

> The relationship usually should not be terminated in the presence of countertransference. Rather, the nurse or staff member experiencing the countertransference should be supportively assisted by other staff members to identify his or her feelings and behaviors and recognize

CONDITIONS ESSENTIAL TO DEVELOPMENT OF A THERAPEUTIC RELATIONSHIP

Several characteristics that enhance the achievement of a therapeutic relationship have been identified. These concepts are highly significant to the use of self as the therapeutic tool in interpersonal relationship development.

Rapport

Getting acquainted and establishing rapport is the primary task in relationship development. **Rapport** implies special feelings on the part of both the client and the nurse based on acceptance, warmth, friendliness, common interest, a sense of trust, and a nonjudgmental attitude. Establishing rapport may be accomplished by discussing non–health-related topics. Travelbee (1971) states:

> [To establish rapport] is to create a sense of harmony based on knowledge and appreciation of each individual's uniqueness. It is the ability to be still and experience the other as a human being—to appreciate the unfolding of each personality one to the other. The ability to truly care for and about others is the core of rapport.

Trust

To trust another, one must feel confidence in that person's presence, reliability, integrity, veracity, and sincere desire to provide assistance when requested. As identified in Chapter 2, trust is the initial developmental task described by Erikson. When this task has not been achieved, this component of relationship development becomes more difficult. That is not to say that trust cannot be established, but only that additional time and patience may be required on the part of the nurse.

It is imperative for the nurse to convey an aura of trustworthiness, which requires that he or she possess a sense of self-confidence. Confidence in the self is derived from knowledge gained through achievement of personal and professional goals and the ability to integrate these roles and to function as a unified whole.

Trust cannot be presumed; it must be earned. Trustworthiness is demonstrated through nursing interventions that convey a sense of warmth and caring to the client. These interventions are initiated simply and concretely, and directed toward activities that address the client's basic needs for physiological and psychological safety and security. Many psychiatric clients experience **concrete thinking,** which focuses their thought processes on specifics rather than generalities and immediate issues rather than eventual outcomes. Examples of nursing interventions that would promote trust in an individual who is thinking concretely include the following:

- Providing a blanket when the client is cold
- Providing food when the client is hungry
- Keeping promises
- Being honest (e.g., saying,"I don't know the answer to your question, but I'll try to find out") and then following through.
- Simply and clearly providing reasons for certain policies, procedures, and rules
- Providing a written, structured schedule of activities
- Attending activities with the client if he or she is reluctant to go alone
- Being consistent in adhering to unit guidelines
- Taking the client's preferences, requests, and opinions into consideration when possible in decisions concerning his or her care
- Ensuring **confidentiality**; providing reassurance that what is discussed will not be repeated outside the boundaries of the healthcare team

Trust is the basis of a therapeutic relationship. The nurse working in psychiatry must perfect the skills that foster the development of trust. Trust must be established in order for the nurse-client relationship to progress beyond the superficial level of tending to the client's immediate needs.

Respect

To show respect is to believe in the dignity and worth of an individual regardless of his or her unacceptable behavior. Rogers (1951) called this **unconditional positive regard**. The attitude is nonjudgmental, and the respect is unconditional in that it does not depend on the behavior of the client to meet certain standards. The nurse, in fact, may not approve of the client's lifestyle or pattern of behaving. However, with unconditional positive regard, the client is accepted and respected for no other reason than that he or she is considered a worthwhile and unique human being.

Many psychiatric clients have very little self-respect owing to the fact that, because of their behavior, they have been rejected by others in the past. Recognition that they are being accepted and respected as unique individuals on an unconditional basis can serve to elevate feelings of self-worth and self-respect. The nurse can convey an attitude of respect by:

- Calling the client by name (and title, if the client prefers)
- Spending time with the client
- Allowing sufficient time to answer the client's questions and concerns
- Promoting an atmosphere of privacy during therapeutic interactions with the client, or when the client may be undergoing physical examination or therapy
- Always being open and honest with the client, even when the truth may be difficult to discuss
- Taking the client's ideas, preferences, and opinions into consideration when planning care
- Striving to understand the motivation behind the client's behavior, regardless how unacceptable it may seem

Genuineness

The concept of **genuineness** refers to the nurse's ability to be open, honest, and "real" in interactions with the client. To be "real" is to be aware of what one is experiencing internally and to allow the quality of this inner experiencing to be apparent in the therapeutic relationship (Raskin & Rogers, 1995). When one is genuine, there is congruence between what is felt and what is being expressed. The nurse who possesses the quality of genuineness responds to the client with truth and honesty, rather than with responses he or she may consider more "professional" or ones that merely reflect the "nursing role."

Genuineness may call for a degree of self-disclosure on the part of the nurse. This is not to say that the nurse must disclose to the client everything he or she is feeling, or *all* personal experiences that may relate to what the client is going through. Indeed, care must be taken when using self-disclosure, to avoid transposing the roles of nurse and client. When the nurse uses self-disclosure, a quality of "humanness" is revealed to the client, creating a role for the client to model in similar situations. The client may then feel more comfortable revealing personal information to the nurse.

Most individuals have an uncanny ability to detect other peoples' artificiality. When the nurse does not bring the quality of genuineness to the relationship, a reality base for trust cannot be established. These qualities are essential if the actualizing potential of the client is to be released and for change and growth to occur (Raskin & Rogers, 1995).

Empathy

Empathy is a process wherein an individual is able to see beyond outward behavior and sense accurately another's inner experience at a given point in time (Travelbee, 1971). With empathy, the nurse can accurately perceive and understand the meaning and relevance of the client's thoughts and feelings. The nurse must also be able to communicate this perception to the client. This is done by attempting to translate words and behaviors into feelings.

It is not uncommon for the concept of empathy to be confused with that of **sympathy**. The major difference is that with empathy the nurse "accurately perceives or understands" what the client is feeling and encourages the client to explore these feelings. With sympathy the nurse actually "shares" what the client is feeling, and experiences a need to alleviate distress.

Empathy is considered one of the most important characteristics of a therapeutic relationship. Accurate empathetic perceptions on the part of the nurse assist the client to identify feelings that may have been suppressed or denied. Positive emotions are generated as the client realizes that he or she is truly understood by another. As the feelings surface and are explored, the client learns aspects about self of which he or she may have been unaware. This contributes to the process of personal identification and the promotion of positive self-concept.

With empathy, while understanding the client's thoughts and feelings, the nurse is able to maintain sufficient objectivity to allow the client to achieve problem resolution with minimal assistance. With sympathy, the nurse actually feels what the client is feeling, objectivity is lost, and the nurse may become focused on relief of personal distress rather than on helping the client resolve the problem at hand. The following is an example of an empathetic and sympathetic response to the same situation.

Situation: BJ is a client on the psychiatric unit with a diagnosis of dysthymic disorder. She is 5 feet 5 inches tall, and weighs 295 pounds. BJ has been overweight all her life. She is single, has no close friends, and has never had an intimate relationship with another person. It is her first day on the unit, and she is refusing to come out of her room. When she appeared for lunch in the dining room following admission, she was embarrassed when several of the other clients laughed aloud and called her "fatso."

the occurrence of the phenomenon. It may be helpful to have evaluative sessions with the nurse after his or her encounter with the patient, in which both the nurse and other staff members (who are observing the interactions) discuss and compare the exhibited behaviors in the relationship.

The Termination Phase

Termination of the relationship may occur for a variety of reasons: the mutually agreed-on goals may have been reached; the client may be discharged from the hospital; or, in the case of a student nurse, it may be the end of a clinical rotation. Termination can be a difficult phase for both the client and nurse. The main task involves bringing a therapeutic conclusion to the relationship. This occurs when:

1. Progress has been made toward attainment of mutually set goals.
2. A plan for continuing care or for assistance during stressful life experiences is mutually established by the nurse and client.
3. Feelings about termination of the relationship are recognized and explored. Both the nurse and client may experience feelings of sadness and loss. The nurse should share his or her feelings with the client. Through these interactions, the client learns that it is acceptable to have these feelings at a time of separation. Through this knowledge, the client experiences growth during the process of termination.

NOTE: When the client feels sadness and loss, behaviors to delay termination may become evident. If the nurse experiences the same feelings, he or she may allow the client's behaviors to delay termination. For therapeutic closure, the nurse must establish the reality of the separation, and resist being manipulated into repeated delays by the client.

INTERPERSONAL COMMUNICATION

It has been said, "You cannot not communicate." Every word that is spoken and every movement that is made gives a message to someone. Interpersonal communication is a transaction between the sender and the receiver. In the transactional model of communication, both participants are simultaneously perceiving each other, listening to each other, and mutually involved in creating meaning in a relationship.

The Impact of Preexisting Conditions

In all interpersonal transactions, both the sender and receiver bring certain preexisting conditions to the exchange that influence both the intended message and the way in which it is interpreted. Examples of these conditions include one's value system, internalized attitudes and beliefs, culture or religion, social status, gender, background knowledge and experience, and age or developmental level. The type of environment in which the communication takes place also may influence the outcome of the transaction.

Values, Attitudes, and Beliefs

Values, attitudes, and beliefs are learned ways of thinking. Children generally adopt the value systems and internalize the attitudes and beliefs of their parents. Children may retain this way of thinking into adulthood or develop a different set of attitudes and values as they mature.

Values, attitudes, and beliefs can influence communication in numerous ways. For example, prejudice can be expressed verbally through negative stereotyping.

One's value system may be communicated with behaviors that are more symbolic in nature. For example, an individual who values youth may dress and behave in a manner that is characteristic of one who is much younger. A person who values freedom and the American way of life may fly the U.S. flag in front of his or her home each day. In each of these situations, a message is being communicated.

Culture or Religion

Communication has its roots in culture. Cultural mores, norms, ideas, and customs provide the basis for our way of thinking. Cultural values are learned, and differ from society to society. For example, in some European countries (e.g., Italy, Spain, and France), men may greet each other with hugs and kisses. These behaviors are appropriate in those cultures, but they would communicate a different message in the United States or England.

Religion also can influence communication. Priests and ministers who wear clerical collars publicly communicate their mission in life. The collar also may influence the way in which others relate to them, either positively or negatively. Other symbolic gestures, such as wearing a cross around the neck or hanging a crucifix on the wall, also communicate an individual's religious beliefs.

Social Status

Studies of nonverbal indicators of social status or power have suggested that high-status persons are associated with gestures that communicate their higher-power position. For example, they use less eye contact, a more relaxed posture, louder voice pitch, more frequent use of hands on hips, "power dressing," greater height, and more distance when communicating with individuals considered to be of lower social status.

Gender

Gender influences the manner in which individuals communicate. Each culture has *signals* that are recognized as either masculine or feminine, and provide a basis for distinguishing between members of each gender. An example is differences in posture, both standing and sitting, between American men and women. Men stand with thighs 10 to 15 degrees apart, the pelvis rolled back, and the arms slightly away from the body. Women stand with legs close together, the pelvis tipped forward, and the arms close to the body. When sitting, men may lean back in the chair with legs apart or may rest the ankle of one leg over the knee of the other. Women tend to sit more upright in the chair with legs together, perhaps crossed at the ankles, or one leg crossed over the other at thigh level.

Roles have traditionally been identified as either male or female. For example, in America, masculinity has been traditionally communicated through such roles as husband, father, breadwinner, doctor, lawyer, or engineer. Traditional female roles have included wife, mother, homemaker, nurse, teacher, or secretary.

Gender signals are changing in American society as gender roles become less distinct. Behaviors that have been considered typically masculine or feminine in the past may now be generally acceptable in both genders. Words such as "unisex" communicate a desire by some individuals to diminish the distinction between the genders and minimize the discrimination of either. Roles are changing as both women and men enter professions that were once dominated by members of the opposite gender.

Age or Developmental Level

Age influences communication, and it is never more evident than during adolescence. In their struggle to separate from parental confines and establish their own identity, adolescents generate a unique pattern of communication that changes from generation to generation. Words such as "awesome," "groovy," and "cool" have had special meaning for different generations of adolescents.

Developmental influences on communication may relate to physiological alterations. One example is American Sign Language, the system of unique gestures used by many people who are deaf or hearing impaired. Individuals who are blind at birth never learn the subtle nonverbal gesticulations that accompany language and can totally change the meaning of the spoken word.

Environment in Which the Transaction Takes Place

The place where the communication occurs influences the outcome of the interaction. Some individuals might feel uncomfortable and refuse to speak during a group therapy session, but may be open and willing to discuss problems on a one-to-one basis with the nurse.

Territoriality, density, and distance are aspects of environment that communicate messages. *Territoriality* is the innate tendency to own space. Individuals lay claim to areas around them as their own. This influences communication when an interaction takes place in the territory "owned" by one or the other. Interpersonal communication can be more successful if the interaction takes place in a "neutral" area. For example, with the concept of territoriality in mind, the nurse may choose to conduct the psychosocial assessment in an interview room rather than in his or her office or in the client's room.

Density refers to the number of people within a given environmental space. It has been shown to influence interpersonal interaction. Some studies indicate that a correlation exists between prolonged high-density situations and certain behaviors, such as aggression, stress, criminal activity, hostility toward others, and a deterioration of mental and physical health.

Distance is the means by which various cultures use space to communicate. Hall (1966) identified four kinds of spatial interaction, or distances, that people maintain from each other in their interpersonal interactions and the kinds of activities in which people engage at these various distances. **Intimate distance** is the closest distance that individuals will allow between themselves and others. In America, this distance, which is restricted to interactions of an intimate nature, is 0 to 18 inches. **Personal distance** is approximately 18 to 40 inches and is reserved for interactions that are personal in nature, such as close conversations with friends or colleagues. **Social distance** is about 4 to 12 feet away from the body. Interactions at this distance include conversations with strangers or acquaintances, such as at a cocktail party or in a public building. A **public distance** is one that exceeds 12 feet. Examples include speaking in public or yelling to someone some distance away. This distance is considered public space, and communicants are free to move about in it during the interaction.

Nonverbal Communication

Some aspects of nonverbal expression have been discussed in the previous section on preexisting conditions that influence communication. Other components of nonverbal communication include physical appearance and dress, body movement and posture, touch, facial expressions, eye behavior, and vocal cues or **paralanguage**. These nonverbal messages vary from culture to culture.

Physical Appearance and Dress

Physical appearance and dress are part of the total nonverbal stimuli that influence interpersonal responses and, under some conditions, they are the primary determinants of such responses. Body coverings—both dress and hair—are manipulated by the wearer in a manner that conveys a distinct message to the receiver. Dress can be formal or casual, stylish or sloppy. Hair can be long or short, and even the presence or absence of hair conveys a message about the person. Other body adornments that are also considered potential communicative stimuli include tattoos, masks, cosmetics, badges, jewelry, and eyeglasses. Some jewelry worn in specific ways can give special messages (e.g., a gold band or diamond ring worn on the fourth finger of the left hand, a boy's class ring worn on a chain around a girl's neck, or a pin bearing Greek letters worn on the lapel). Some individuals convey a specific message with the total absence of any type of body adornment.

Body Movement and Posture

The way in which an individual positions his or her body communicates messages regarding self-esteem, gender identity, status, and interpersonal warmth or coldness. The individual whose posture is slumped, with head and eyes pointed downward, conveys a message of low self-esteem. Specific ways of standing or sitting are considered either feminine or masculine within a defined culture. To stand straight and tall with head high and hands on hips indicates a superior status over the person being addressed.

Reece and Whitman (1962) identified response behaviors that were used to designate individuals as either "warm" or "cold" persons. Individuals who were perceived as warm responded to others with a shift of posture toward the other person, a smile, direct eye contact, and hands that remained still. Individuals who responded to others with a slumped posture, by looking around the room, drumming fingers on the desk, and not smiling were perceived as cold.

Touch

Touch is a powerful communication tool. It can elicit both negative and positive reactions, depending on the people involved and the circumstances of the interaction. It is a very basic and primitive form of communication, and the appropriateness of its use is culturally determined.

Touch can be categorized according to the message communicated (Knapp and Hall, 2001):

1. **Functional-Professional.** This type of touch is impersonal and businesslike. It is used to accomplish a task.
   EXAMPLE: A tailor measuring a customer for a suit or a physician examining a client.
2. **Social-Polite.** This type of touch is still rather impersonal, but it conveys affirmation or acceptance of the other person.
   EXAMPLE: A handshake.
3. **Friendship-Warmth.** Touch at this level indicates a strong liking for the other person—a feeling that he or she is a friend.
   EXAMPLE: Laying one's hand on the shoulder of another.
4. **Love-Intimacy.** This type of touch conveys an emotional attachment or attraction for another person.
   EXAMPLE: Engaging in a strong, mutual embrace.
5. **Sexual Arousal.** Touch at this level is an expression of physical attraction only.
   EXAMPLE: Touching another in the genital region.

Some cultures encourage more touching of various types than others. The nurse should understand the cultural meaning of touch before using this method of communication in specific situations.

Facial Expressions

Next to human speech, facial expression is the primary source of communication. Facial expressions primarily reveal an individual's emotional state, such as happiness, sadness, anger, surprise, or fear. The face is a complex, multimessage system. Facial expressions serve to complement and qualify other communication behaviors, and at times even take the place of verbal messages.

Eye Behavior

Eyes have been called the "windows of the soul." It is through eye contact that individuals view and are viewed by others in a revealing way. An interpersonal connectedness occurs through eye contact. In American culture, eye contact conveys a personal interest in the other person. Eye contact indicates that the communication channel is open, and it is often the initiating factor in verbal interaction between two people.

Patterns of gazing or staring are regulated by social rules. These rules dictate where, when, for how long, and at whom we can look. Staring is often used to register disapproval of the behavior of another. People are extremely sensitive to being looked at, and if the gazing or staring behavior violates social rules, they often assign meaning to it (e.g., "He kept staring at me, and I began to wonder if I was dressed inappropriately or had mustard on my face!").

Vocal Cues or Paralanguage

Paralanguage, or vocal cues, is the gestural component of the spoken word. It consists of pitch, tone, and loudness of spoken messages, the rate of speaking, expressively placed pauses, and emphasis assigned to certain words. These vocal cues greatly influence the way individuals interpret verbal messages. A normally soft-spoken individual whose pitch and rate of speaking increases may be perceived as being anxious or tense.

Different vocal emphases can alter interpretation of the message. For example:

1. "I felt SURE you would notice the change."
   Interpretation: I was SURE you would, but you didn't.
2. "I felt sure YOU would notice the change."
   Interpretation: I thought YOU would, even if nobody else did.
3. "I felt sure you would notice the CHANGE."
   Interpretation: Even if you didn't notice anything else, I thought you would notice the CHANGE.

Verbal cues play a major role in determining responses in human communication situations. *How* a message is verbalized can be as important as *what* is verbalized.

Therapeutic Communication Techniques

Hays and Larson (1963) identified a number of techniques to assist the nurse in interacting more therapeutically with clients. These are the "technical procedures" carried out by the nurse working in psychiatry, and they should serve to enhance development of a therapeutic nurse-client relationship. Table 5–2 includes a list of these techniques, a short explanation of their usefulness, and examples of each.

Nontherapeutic Communication Techniques

Several approaches are considered barriers to open communication between the nurse and client. Hays and Larson (1963) identified a number of these techniques, which are presented in Table 5–3. The nurse should recognize and eliminate the use of these patterns in his or her relationships with clients. Avoiding these communication barriers will maximize the effectiveness of communication and enhance the nurse-client relationship.

Process Recordings

Process recordings are written reports of verbal interactions with clients. They are verbatim (to the extent that this is possible) accounts, written by the nurse or student as a tool for improving interpersonal communication techniques. The process recording can take many forms, but usually includes the verbal and nonverbal communication of both nurse and client. The interaction provides a means for the nurse to analyze both the content and pattern of the interaction. The process recording is not documentation in and of itself, but should be used as a learning tool for professional development. An example of one type of process recording is presented in Table 5–4.

Active Listening

To listen actively is to be attentive to what the client is saying, both verbally and nonverbally. Attentive listening creates a climate in which the client can

TABLE 5 – 2 Therapeutic Communication Techniques

Technique	Explanation/Rationale	Examples
Using silence	Gives the client the opportunity to collect and organize thoughts, to think through a point, or to consider introducing a topic of greater concern than the one being discussed.	
Accepting	Conveys an attitude of reception and regard.	"Yes, I understand what you said." Eye contact; nodding.
Giving recognition	Acknowledging; indicating awareness; better than complimenting, which reflects the nurse's judgment.	"Hello, Mr. J. I notice that you made a ceramic ash tray in OT." "I see you made your bed."
Offering self	Making oneself available on an unconditional basis, increasing client's feelings of self-worth.	"I'll stay with you awhile." "We can eat our lunch together." "I'm interested in you."
Giving broad openings	Allows the client to take the initiative in introducing the topic; emphasizes the importance of the client's role in the interaction.	"What would you like to talk about today?" "Tell me what you are thinking."
Offering general leads	Offers the client encouragement to continue.	"Yes, I see." "Go on." "And after that?"
Placing the event in time or sequence	Clarifies the relationship of events in time so that the nurse and client can view them in perspective.	"What seemed to lead up to…?" "Was this before or after…?" "When did this happen?"
Making observations	Verbalizing what is observed or perceived. This encourages the client to recognize specific behaviors and compare perceptions with the nurse.	"You seem tense." "I notice you are pacing a lot." "You seem uncomfortable when you…"
Encouraging description of perceptions	Asking the client to verbalize what is being perceived; often used with clients experiencing hallucinations.	"Tell me what is happening now." "Are you hearing the voices again?" "What do the voices seem to be saying?"
Encouraging comparison	Asking the client to compare similarities and differences in ideas, experiences, or interpersonal relationships. This helps the client recognize life experiences that tend to recur as well as those aspects of life that are changeable.	"Was this something like…?" "How does this compare with the time when…?" "What was your response the last time this situation occurred?"
Restating	Repeating the main idea of what the client has said. This lets the client know whether an expressed statement has been understood and gives him or her the chance to continue, or to clarify if necessary.	Cl: "I can't study. My mind keeps wandering." Ns: "You have trouble concentrating." Cl: "I can't take that new job. What if I can't do it?" Ns: "You're afraid you will fail in this new position."
Reflecting	Referring questions and feelings back to the client so that they may be recognized and accepted and so that the client may recognize that his or her point of view has value—a good technique to use when the client asks the nurse for advice.	Cl: "What do you think I should do about my wife's drinking problem?" Ns: "What do *you* think you should do?" Cl: "My sister won't help a bit toward my mother's care. I have to do it all!" Ns: "You feel angry when she doesn't help."
Focusing	Taking notice of a single idea or even a single word; works especially well with a client who is moving rapidly from one thought to another. This technique is *not* therapeutic, however, with the client who is very anxious. Focusing should not be pursued until the anxiety level has subsided.	"This point seems worth looking at more closely. Perhaps you and I can discuss it together."

(Continued)

TABLE 5 – 2 Therapeutic Communication Techniques *(Continued)*

Technique	Explanation/Rationale	Examples
Exploring	Delving further into a subject, idea, experience, or relationship; especially helpful with clients who tend to remain on a superficial level of communication. However, if the client chooses not to disclose further information, the nurse should refrain from pushing or probing in an area that obviously creates discomfort.	"Please explain that situation in more detail." "Tell me more about that particular situation."
Seeking clarification and validation	Striving to explain that which is vague or incomprehensible and searching for mutual understanding; clarifying the meaning of what has been said facilitates and increases understanding for both client and nurse.	"I'm not sure that I understand. Would you please explain?" "Tell me if my understanding agrees with yours." "Do I understand correctly that you said…?"
Presenting reality	When the client has a misperception of the environment, the nurse defines reality or indicates his or her perception of the situation for the client.	"I understand that the voices seem real to you, but I do not hear any voices." "There is no one else in the room but you and me."
Voicing doubt	Expressing uncertainty as to the reality of the client's perceptions; often used with clients experiencing delusional thinking.	"I find that hard to believe." "That seems rather doubtful to me."
Verbalizing the implied	Putting into words what the client has only implied or said indirectly; can also be used with the client who is mute or is otherwise experiencing impaired verbal communication. This clarifies that which is *implicit* rather than *explicit*.	Cl: "It's a waste of time to be here. I can't talk to you or anyone." Ns: "Are you feeling that no one understands?" Cl: (Mute) Ns: "It must have been very difficult for you when your husband died in the fire."
Attempting to translate words into feelings	"Desymbolizing" what the client has said and finding clues to the underlying true feelings that have been expressed indirectly.	Cl: "I'm way out in the ocean." Ns: "You must be feeling very lonely right now."
Formulating a plan of action	Having a plan in mind for dealing with what is considered to be a stressful situation may help the client prevent anger or anxiety from escalating to an unmanageable level.	"What could you do to let your anger out harmlessly?" "Next time this comes up, what might you do to handle it more appropriately?"

Adapted from Hays & Larson (1963).

communicate. With active listening, the nurse communicates acceptance and respect for the client, and trust is enhanced. A climate is established within the relationship that promotes openness and honest expression.

Several nonverbal behaviors have been designated as facilitative skills for attentive listening. Those listed here can be identified by the acronym SOLER:

S—Sit squarely facing the client. This gives the message that the nurse is there to listen, and is interested in what the client has to say.

O—Observe an open posture. Posture is considered "open" when arms and legs remain uncrossed. This suggests that the nurse is "open" to what the client has to say. With a "closed" position, the nurse can convey a somewhat defensive stance, possibly invoking a similar response in the client.

L—Lean forward toward the client. This conveys to the client that you are involved in the interaction, interested in what is being said, and making a sincere effort to be attentive.

E—Establish eye contact. Direct eye contact is another behavior that conveys the nurse's involvement and willingness to listen to what the client has to say. The absence of eye contact, or the constant shifting of eye contact, gives the message that the nurse is not really interested in what is being said.

TABLE 5 – 3 Nontherapeutic Communication Techniques

Technique	Explanation/Rationale	Examples
Giving reassurance	Indicating to the client that there is no cause for anxiety, thereby devaluing the client's feelings; may discourage the client from further expression of feelings if he or she believes they will only be downplayed or ridiculed.	"I wouldn't worry about that If I were you" "Everything will be all right." **Better to say:** "We will work on that together."
Rejecting	Refusing to consider or showing contempt for the client's ideas or behavior. This may cause the client to discontinue interaction with the nurse for fear of further rejection.	"Let's not discuss..." "I don't want to hear about..." **Better to say:** "Let's look at that a little closer."
Approving or disapproving	Sanctioning or denouncing the client's ideas or behavior; implies that the nurse has the right to pass judgment on whether the client's ideas or behaviors are "good" or "bad," and that the client is expected to please the nurse. The nurse's acceptance of the client is then seen as conditional depending on the client's behavior.	"That's good. I'm glad that you..." "That's bad. I'd rather you wouldn't..." **Better to say:** "Let's talk about how your behavior invoked anger in the other clients at dinner."
Agreeing or disagreeing	Indicating accord with or opposition to the client's ideas or opinions; implies that the nurse has the right to pass judgment on whether the client's ideas or opinions are "right" or "wrong." Agreement prevents the client from later modifying his or her point of view without admitting error. Disagreement implies inaccuracy, provoking the need for defensiveness on the part of the client.	"That's right. I agree." "That's wrong. I disagree." "I don't believe that." **Better to say:** "Let's discuss what you feel is unfair about the new community rules."
Giving advice	Telling the client what to do or how to behave implies that the nurse knows what is best and that the client is incapable of any self-direction. It nurtures the client in the dependent role by discouraging independent thinking.	"I think you should..." "Why don't you..." **Better to say:** "What do you think you should do?"
Probing	Persistent questioning of the client; pushing for answers to issues the client does not wish to discuss. This causes the client to feel used and valued only for what is shared with the nurse, and places the client on the defensive.	"Tell me how your mother abused you when you were a child." "Tell me how you feel toward your mother now that she is dead." "Now tell me about..." **Better technique:** The nurse should be aware of the client's response and discontinue the interaction at the first sign of discomfort.
Defending	Attempting to protect someone or something from verbal attack. To defend what the client has criticized is to imply that he or she has no right to express ideas, opinions, or feelings. Defending does not change the client's feelings and may cause the client to think the nurse is taking sides with those being criticized and against the client.	"No one here would lie to you." "You have a very capable physician. I'm sure he only has your best interests in mind." **Better to say:** "I will try to answer your questions and clarify some issues regarding your treatment.
Requesting an explanation	Asking the client to provide the reasons for thoughts, feelings, behavior, and events. Asking "why" a client did something or feels a certain way can be very intimidating, and implies that the client must defend his or her behavior or feelings.	"Why do you think that?" "Why do you feel this way?" "Why did you do that?" **Better to say:** "Describe what you were feeling just before that happened."

(Continued)

TABLE 5 – 3 Nontherapeutic Communication Techniques *(Continued)*

Technique	Explanation/Rationale	Examples
Indicating the existence of an external source of power	Attributing the source of thoughts, feelings, and behavior to others or to outside influences. This encourages the client to project blame for his or her thoughts or behaviors on others rather than accepting the responsibility personally.	"What makes you say that?" "What made you do that?" "What made you so angry last night?" **Better to say:** "You became angry when your brother insulted your wife.
Belittling feelings expressed	Misjudging the degree of the client's discomfort, which may convey a lack of empathy and understanding. The nurse may tell the client to "perk up" or "snap out of it." This causes the client to feel insignificant or unimportant. When one is experiencing discomfort, it is no relief to hear that others are or have been in similar situations.	Cl: "I have nothing to live for. I wish I were dead." Ns: "Everybody gets down in the dumps at times. I feel that way myself sometimes." **Better to say:** "You must be very upset. Tell me what you are feeling right now."
Making stereotyped comments	Making empty conversation encourages a similar response from the client. Clichés and trite expressions are meaningless in a nurse-client relationship.	"I'm fine, and how are you?" "Hang in there. It's for your own good." "Keep your chin up." **Better to say:** "The therapy must be difficult for you at times. How do you feel about your progress at this point?"
Using denial	Denying that a problem exists blocks discussion with the client, and avoids helping the client identify and explore areas of difficulty.	Cl: "I'm nothing." Ns: "Of course you're something. Everybody is somebody. **Better to say:** "You're feeling like no one cares about you right now."
Interpreting	Making conscious that which is unconscious, to tell the client the meaning of his or her experience.	"What you really mean is..." "Unconsciously you're saying..." **Better technique:** The nurse must leave interpretation of the client's behavior to the psychiatrist. The nurse has not been prepared to perform this technique, and in attempting to do so, may endanger other nursing roles with the client."
Introducing an unrelated topic	Changing the subject causes the nurse to take over the direction of the discussion. This may occur to get to something that the nurse wants to discuss with the client or to get away from a topic that he or she would prefer not to discuss.	Cl: "I don't have anything to live for." Ns: "Did you have visitors this weekend?" **Better technique:** The nurse must remain open and free to hear the client and to take in all that is being conveyed, both verbally and nonverbally.

Adapted from Hays & Larson (1963).

NOTE: Ensure that eye contact conveys warmth and is accompanied by smiling and intermittent nodding of the head and that it does not come across as staring or glaring, which can create intense discomfort in the client.

R—Relax. Whether sitting or standing during the interaction, the nurse should communicate a sense of being relaxed and comfortable with the client. Restlessness and fidgetiness communicate a lack of interest and a feeling of discomfort that is likely to be transferred to the client.

Feedback

Feedback is a method of communication for helping the client consider a modification of behavior. Feedback gives information to clients about how they are being perceived by others. It should be presented in a manner that discourages defensiveness on the part

TABLE 5 – 4 Sample Process Recording

Nurse (Nonverbal)	Client Verbal (Nonverbal)	Nurse's Thoughts & Feelings About Interaction	Analysis of the Interaction
Do you still have thoughts about harming yourself? (Sitting facing the client; looking directly at client)	Not really. I still feel sad, but I don't want to die. (Looking at hands in lap.)	Feeling a little uncomfortable. Always a hard question to ask.	**Therapeutic.** Asking a direct question about suicidal intent.
Tell me what you were feeling before you took all the pills the other night. (Still using SOLAR techniques of active listening.)	I was just so angry! To think that my husband wants a divorce now that he has a good job. I worked hard to put him through college. (Fists clenched. Face and neck reddened.)	Beginning to feel more comfortable. Client seems willing to talk and I think she trusts me.	**Therapeutic.** Exploring. Delving further into the experience.
You wanted to hurt him because you felt betrayed. (SOLAR)	Yes! If I died, maybe he'd realize that he loved me more than that other woman. (Tears starting to well up in her eyes.)	Starting to feel sorry for her.	**Therapeutic.** Attempting to translate words into feelings.
Seems like a pretty drastic way to get your point across. (Small frown.)	I know. It was a stupid thing to do. (Wiping eyes.)	Trying hard to remain objective.	**Nontherapeutic.** Sounds disapproving. Better to have pursued her feelings.
How are you feeling about the situation now? (SOLAR)	I don't know. I still love him. I want him to come home. I don't want him to marry her. (Starting to cry again.)	Wishing there was an easy way to help relieve some of her pain.	**Therapeutic.** Focusing on her feelings.
Yes, I can understand that you would like things to be the way they were before. (Offer client a tissue.)	(Silence. Continues to cry softly.)	I'm starting to feel some anger toward her husband. Sometimes it's so hard to remain objective!	**Therapeutic.** Conveying empathy.
What do you think are the chances of your getting back together? (SOLAR)	None. He's refused marriage counseling. He's already moved in with her. He says it's over. (Wipes tears. Looks directly at nurse.)	Relieved to know that she isn't using denial about the reality of the situation.	**Therapeutic.** Reflecting. Seeking client's perception of the situation.
So how are you preparing to deal with this inevitable outcome? (SOLAR)	I'm going to do the things we talked about: join a divorced women's support group; increase my job hours to full time; do some volunteer work; and call you or the suicide hot line if I feel like taking pills again. (Looks directly at nurse. Smiles.)	Positive feeling to know that she remembers what we discussed earlier and plans to follow through.	**Therapeutic.** Formulating a plan of action.
It won't be easy. But you have come a long way, and I feel you have gained strength in your ability to cope. (Standing. Looking at client. Smiling.)	Yes, I know I will have hard times. But I also know I have support, and I want to go on with my life and be happy again. (Standing, smiling at nurse)	Feeling confident that the session has gone well; hopeful that the client will succeed in what she wants to do with her life.	**Therapeutic.** Presenting reality.

of the client. Feedback can be useful to the client if presented with objectivity by a trusted individual.

Some criteria about useful feedback include:

1. Feedback should be descriptive rather than evaluative, and focused on the behavior rather than on the client. Avoiding evaluative language reduces the need for the client to react defensively. An objective description allows the client to take the information and use it in whatever way he or she chooses. When the focus is on the client, the nurse makes judgments about the client.

EXAMPLE:

Descriptive and focused on behavior	"Jane was very upset in group today when you called her 'fatty' and laughed at her in front of the others."
Evaluative	"You were very rude and inconsiderate to Jane in group today."
Focus on client	"You are a very insensitive person."

2. Feedback should be specific rather than general. Information that gives details about the client's behavior can be used more easily than a generalized description for modifying the behavior.

EXAMPLE:

General	"You just don't pay attention."
Specific	"You were talking to Joe when we were deciding on the issue. Now you want to argue about the outcome."

3. Feedback should be directed toward behavior that the client has the capacity to modify. To provide feedback about a characteristic or situation that the client cannot change will only provoke frustration.

EXAMPLE:

Can modify	"I noticed that you did not want to hold your baby when the nurse brought her to you."
Cannot modify	"Your baby daughter is mentally retarded because you took drugs when you were pregnant."

4. Feedback should impart information rather than offer advice. Giving advice fosters dependence and may convey the message to the client that he or she is not capable of making decisions and solving problems independently. It is the client's right and privilege to be as self-sufficient as possible.

EXAMPLE:

Imparting information	"There are various methods of assistance for people who want to lose weight, such as Overeaters Anonymous, Weight Watchers, regular visits to a dietitian, the Physician's Weight Loss Program. You can decide what is best for you."
Giving advice	"You obviously need to lose a great deal of weight. I think the Physician's Weight Loss Program would be best for you."

5. Feedback should be well timed. Feedback is most useful when given at the earliest appropriate opportunity following the specific behavior.

EXAMPLE:

Prompt response	"I saw you hit the wall with your fist just now when you hung up the phone from talking to your mother."
Delayed response	"You need to learn some more appropriate ways of dealing with your anger. Last week after group, I saw you pounding your fist against the wall."

SUMMARY

Nurses who work in the psychiatric/mental health field use special skills, or "interpersonal techniques," to assist clients in adapting to difficulties or changes in life experiences. A therapeutic or "helping" relationship is established through use of these interpersonal techniques and is based on knowledge of theories of personality development and human behavior.

Therapeutic nurse-client relationships are goal oriented. Ideally, the goal is mutually agreed on by the nurse and client and is directed at learning and growth promotion. The problem-solving model is used in an attempt to bring about some type of change in the client's life. The instrument for delivery of the process of interpersonal nursing is the therapeutic use of self, which requires that the nurse possess a strong sense of self-awareness and self-understanding.

Several characteristics that enhance the achievement of a therapeutic relationship have been identified. They include rapport, trust, respect, genuineness, and empathy.

The tasks associated with the development of a therapeutic interpersonal relationship have been categorized into four phases: the preinteraction phase, the orientation (introductory) phase, the working phase, and the termination phase.

Interpersonal communication is a transaction between the sender and the receiver. In all interpersonal transactions, both the sender and receiver bring certain preexisting conditions to the exchange that influence both the intended message and the way in which it is interpreted. Examples of these conditions include one's value system, internalized attitudes and beliefs, culture or religion, social status, gender, background knowledge and experience, age or developmental level, and the type of environment in which the communication takes place.

Nonverbal expression is a primary communication system in which meaning is assigned to various gestures and patterns of behavior. Some components of nonverbal communication include physical appearance and dress, body movement and posture, touch, facial expressions, eye behavior, and vocal cues or paralanguage. The meaning of each of these nonverbal components is culturally determined.

Various techniques of communication that can facilitate interaction between nurse and client, as well as a number of barriers to effective communication, were presented in this chapter. Techniques of active listening and examples of feedback as a method of communication for helping the client modify behavior also were presented. The nurse must be aware of the therapeutic or nontherapeutic value of the communication techniques used with the client, as they are the "tools" of psychosocial intervention.

REVIEW QUESTIONS

Self-Examination/Learning Exercise

Match the actions listed on the right to the appropriate phase of nurse-client relationship development on the left:

_______ 1. Preinteraction Phase	a. Kim tells Nurse Jones she wants to learn more adaptive ways to handle her anger. Together, they set some goals.
_______ 2. Orientation (Introductory) Phase	b. The goals of therapy have been met, but Kim cries and says she has to keep coming to therapy in order to be able to handle her anger appropriately.
_______ 3. Working Phase	c. Nurse Jones reads Kim's previous medical records. She explores her feelings about working with a woman who has abused her child.
_______ 4. Termination Phase	d. Nurse Jones helps Kim practice various techniques to control her angry outbursts. She gives Kim positive feedback for attempting to improve maladaptive behaviors.

Identify the correct answer in each of the following questions. Provide explanation where requested. Identify the technique used (both therapeutic and nontherapeutic) in all choices given.

5. A client states: "I refuse to shower in this room. I must be very cautious. The FBI has placed a camera in here to monitor my every move." Which of the following is the therapeutic response? What is this technique called?
   a. "That's not true."
   b. "I have a hard time believing that is true."
6. Nancy, a depressed client who has been unkempt and untidy for weeks, today comes to group therapy wearing makeup and a clean dress, and having washed and combed her hair. Which of the following responses by the nurse is most appropriate? Give your rationale.
   a. "Nancy, I see you have put on a clean dress and combed your hair."
   b. "Nancy, you look wonderful today!"
7. Dorothy was involved in an automobile accident while under the influence of alcohol. She swerved her car into a tree and narrowly missed hitting a child on a bicycle. She is in the hospital with multiple abrasions and contusions. She is talking about the accident with the nurse. Which of the following statements by the nurse is most appropriate? Identify the therapeutic or nontherapeutic technique in each.
   a. "Now that you know what can happen when you drink and drive, I'm sure you won't let it happen again. I'm sure everything will be okay."
   b. "That was a terrible thing you did. You could have killed that child!"
   c. "Now I guess you'll have to buy a new car. Can you afford that?"
   d. "What made you do such a thing?"
   e. "Tell me how you are feeling about what happened."

8. Judy has been in the hospital for 3 weeks. She has used Valium "to settle my nerves" for the past 15 years. She was admitted by her psychiatrist for safe withdrawal from the drug. She has passed the physical symptoms of withdrawal at this time, but states to the nurse, "I don't know if I will make it without Valium after I go home. I'm already starting to feel nervous. I have so many personal problems." Which is the most appropriate response by the nurse? Identify the technique in each.
   a. "Why do you think you have to have drugs to deal with your problems?"
   b. "You'll just have to pull yourself together. Everybody has problems, but not everybody uses drugs to deal with them. They just do the best that they can."
   c. "I don't want to talk about that now. Look at that sunshine. It's beautiful outside. You and I are going to take a walk!"
   d. "Starting today you and I are going to think about some alternative ways for you to deal with those problems—things that you can do to decrease your anxiety without resorting to drugs."
9. Mrs. S. asks the nurse, "Do you think I should tell my husband about my affair with my boss?" Give one therapeutic response and one nontherapeutic response. Give your rationale, and identify the technique used in each response.
10. Carol, an adolescent, just returned from group therapy and is crying. She says to the nurse, "All the other kids laughed at me! I try to fit in, but I always seem to say the wrong thing. I've never had a close friend. I guess I never will." Which is the most appropriate response by the nurse? Identify each technique used.
    a. "You're feeling pretty down on yourself right now."
    b. "Why do you feel this way about yourself?"
    c. "What makes you think you will never have any friends?"
    d. "The next time they laugh at you, you should just get up and leave the room!"
    e. "I'm sure they didn't mean to hurt your feelings."
    f. "Keep your chin up and hang in there. Your time will come."

REFERENCES

Campbell, P., & Barringer. (1998). The nursing process in psychiatric-mental health nursing. In C.A. Glod (Ed.), Contemporary psychiatric-mental health nursing: The brain-behavior connection. Philadelphia: F.A. Davis.

Hilz, L.M. (2001). Transference and countertransference. Kathi's Mental Health Review. Retrieved November 10, 2001, at http://www.toddlertime.com/trans-countertrans-2.htm

Knapp, M.L., & Hall, J.A. (2001). Nonverbal communication in human interaction (5th ed.). Belmont, CA: Wadsworth.

Peplau, H.E. (1991). Interpersonal relations in nursing. New York: Springer.

Raskin, N.J., & Rogers, C.R. (1995). Person-centered therapy. In R.J. Corsini & D. Wedding (Eds.), Current psychotherapies (5th ed.). Itasca, IL: J.E. Peacock.

CLASSICAL REFERENCES:

Hall, E.T. (1966). The hidden dimension. Garden City, NY: Doubleday.

Hays, J.S., & Larson, K.H. (1963). Interacting with patients. New York: Macmillan.

Peplau, H.E. (1962). Interpersonal techniques: The crux of psychiatric nursing. American Journal of Nursing, 62:50–54.

Reece, M., & Whitman, R. (1962). Expressive movements, warmth, and verbal reinforcement. Journal of Abnormal and Social Psychology, 64:234–236.

Rogers, C.R. (1951). Client-centered therapy. Boston: Houghton Mifflin.

Sullivan, H.S. (1953). The interpersonal theory of psychiatry. New York: W.W. Norton.

Travelbee, J. (1971). Interpersonal aspects of nursing (2nd ed.). Philadelphia: F.A. Davis.

TOWNSEND ESSENTIALS

6

CHAPTER

The Nursing Process in Psychiatric/Mental Health Nursing

CHAPTER OUTLINE

KEY TERMS

nursing process
nursing diagnosis
interdisciplinary
problem-oriented recording (POR)
Focus charting®
PIE charting
acculturation
stereotyping
ethnicity
culture
nursing interventions classification (NIC)
nursing outcomes classification (NOC)

OBJECTIVES

After reading this chapter, the student will be able to:

1. Define nursing process.
2. Identify six steps of the nursing process and describe nursing actions associated with each.
3. Describe the benefits of using nursing diagnosis.
4. Discuss the list of nursing diagnoses approved by NANDA International for clinical use and testing.
5. Define and differentiate between *culture* and *ethnicity*.
6. Describe six phenomena with which to identify cultural differences.
7. Apply the six steps of the nursing process in the care of a client within the psychiatric setting.
8. Document client care that validates use of the nursing process.

INTRODUCTION

For many years, the **nursing process** has provided a systematic framework for the delivery of nursing care. It is nursing's means of fulfilling the *scientific methodology* requirement to be considered a profession. This chapter examines the steps of the nursing process as set forth by the American Nurses Association (ANA) in the *Standards of Clinical Nursing Practice* (ANA, 1998). Tools for conducting a biopsychosocial assessment, a mental status examination, and a cultural assessment are included. Nursing diagnoses approved for clinical use and testing by NANDA International are discussed. Documentation that validates the use of the nursing process is presented.

THE NURSING PROCESS

Definition

The nursing process consists of six steps and uses a problem-solving approach that has come to be accepted as nursing's scientific methodology. It is goal-directed, with the objective being delivery of quality client care.

Nursing process is dynamic, not static. It is an ongoing process that continues for as long as the nurse and client have interactions directed toward change in the client's physical or behavioral responses. Figure 6–1 presents a schematic of the ongoing nursing process.

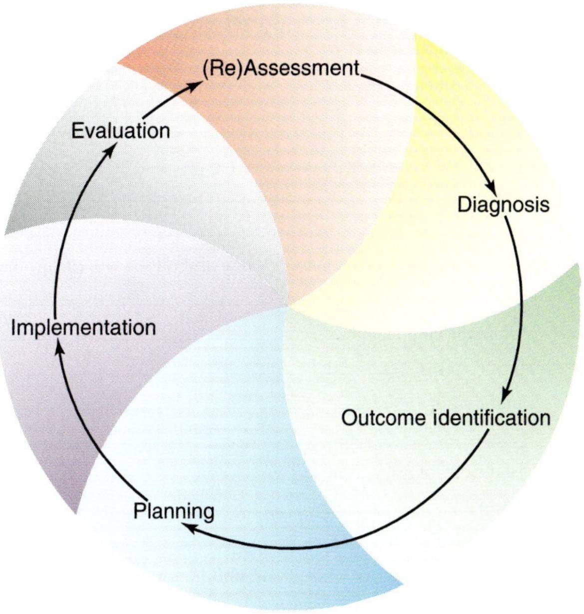

FIGURE 6–1 The ongoing nursing process.

STANDARDS OF CARE

The ANA, in collaboration with the American Psychiatric Nurses Association and the International Society of Psychiatric-Mental Health Nurses, has created a set of standards that psychiatric nurses are expected to follow as they provide care for their clients. The ANA (2000) states:

> Standards of care pertain to professional nursing activities that are demonstrated by the nurse through the nursing process. These involve assessment, diagnosis, outcome identification, planning, implementation, and evaluation. The nursing process is the foundation of clinical decision-making, and encompasses all significant action taken by nurses in providing developmentally and culturally relevant psychiatric-mental health care to all patients. (p. 28)

The standards with rationales as set forth by the ANA (2000) are presented as follows.

Standard I. Assessment

The psychiatric/mental health nurse collects client health data.

Rationale

The assessment interview—which requires linguistically and culturally effective communications skills, interviewing, behavioral observation, record review, and comprehensive assessment of the client and relevant systems—enables the psychiatric-mental health nurse to make sound clinical judgments and plan appropriate interventions with the client (ANA, 2000, p. 28).

In this first step, information is gathered from which to establish a database for determining the best possible care for the client. Information for this database is gathered from a variety of sources, including interviewing the client or family, observing the client and his or her environment, consulting other health team members, reviewing the client's records, and conducting a nursing physical examination. A biopsychosocial assessment tool based on the stress-adaptation framework is included in Table 6–1.

TABLE 6 – 1 Nursing History and Assessment Tool

I. General Information

Client name: ____________________ Allergies: ____________________

Room number: ____________________ Diet: ____________________

Doctor: ____________________ Height/weight: ____________________

Age: ____________________ Vital signs: TPR/BP ____________________

Sex: __________ Name and phone no. of significant other: ____________________

Race: __________ ____________________

Dominant language: ____________________ City of residence: ____________________

Marital status: ____________________ Diagnosis (admitting & current): ____________________

Chief complaint: ____________________ ____________________

____________________ ____________________

Conditions of admission:

Date: ____________________ Time: ____________________

Accompanied by: ____________________ ____________________

Route of admission (wheelchair; ambulatory; cart): ____________________

Admitted from: ____________________

II. Predisposing Factors

A. *Genetic Influences*

1. Family configuration (use genograms):

Family of origin: Present family:

Family dynamics (describe significant relationships between family members): ____________________

____

____

____

____

2. Medical/psychiatric history:

a. Client: ____________________

____

____

b. Family members: ____________________

____

____

3. Other genetic influences affecting present adaptation. This might include effects specific to gender, race, appearance, such as genetic physical defects, or any other factor related to genetics that is affecting the client's adaptation that has not been mentioned elsewhere in this assessment.

____

____

B. *Past Experiences*

1. Cultural and social history:
   a. Environmental factors (family living arrangements, type of neighborhood, special working conditions): ______
   b. Health beliefs and practices (personal responsibility for health; special self-care practices); ______
   c. Religious beliefs and practices: ______
   d. Educational background: ______
   e. Significant losses/changes (include dates): ______
   f. Peer/friendship relationships: ______
   g. Occupational history: ______
   h. Previous pattern of coping with stress: ______
   i. Other lifestyle factors contributing to present adaptation: ______

C. *Existing Conditions*

1. Stage of development (Erikson):
   a. Theoretically: ______
   b. Behaviorally: ______
   c. Rationale: ______
2. Support systems: ______
3. Economic security: ______

(Continued)

TABLE 6 – 1 Nursing History and Assessment Tool *(Continued)*

4. Avenues of productivity/contribution:
   a. Current job status: ______________________________
   ____
   b. Role contributions and responsibility for others: ______________________________
   ____

III. Precipitating Event

Describe the situation or events that precipitated this illness/hospitalization: ______________________________
____
____

IV. Client's Perception of the Stressor

Client's or family member's understanding or description of stressor/illness and expectations of hospitalization: ______________
____
____
____

V. Adaptation Responses

A. ***Psychosocial***

1. Anxiety level (circle level, and check the behaviors that apply): mild moderate severe panic
   calm ________ friendly ________ passive ________ alert ________ perceives environment correctly ________
   cooperative ________ impaired attention ________ "jittery" ________ unable to concentrate ________
   hypervigilant ________ tremors ________ rapid speech ________ withdrawn ________ confused ________
   disoriented ________ fearful ________ hyperventilating ________ misinterpreting the environment (hallucinations or delusions) ________ depersonalization ________ obsessions ________ compulsions ________
   somatic complaints ________ excessive hyperactivity ________ other ______________________________
   ____
2. Mood/affect (circle as many as apply): happiness sadness dejection despair elation
   euphoria suspiciousness apathy (little emotional tone) anger/hostility
3. Ego defense mechanisms (describe how used by client):
   Projection ______________________________
   Suppression ______________________________
   Undoing ______________________________
   Displacement ______________________________
   Intellectualization ______________________________
   Rationalization ______________________________
   Denial ______________________________
   Repression ______________________________
   Isolation ______________________________
   Regression ______________________________
   Reaction Formation ______________________________
   Splitting ______________________________
   Religiosity ______________________________
   Sublimation ______________________________
   Compensation ______________________________

4. Level of self-esteem (circle one): low moderate high

   Things client likes about self ______________________________

   ____

   Things client would like to change about self ______________________________

   ____

   Objective assessment of self-esteem:

   Eye contact ______________________________

   General appearance ______________________________

   ____

   Personal hygiene ______________________________

   Participation in group activities and interactions with others ______________________________

   ____

5. Stage and manifestations of grief (circle one):

   denial anger bargaining depression acceptance

   Describe the client's behaviors that are associated with this stage of grieving in response to loss or change. __________

   ____

   ____

6. Thought processes (circle as many as apply): clear logical easy to follow relevant confused blocking delusional rapid flow of thoughts slowness in thought association suspicious

   Recent memory (circle one): loss intact Remote memory (circle one): loss intact

   Other: ______________________________

   ____

7. Communication patterns (circle as many as apply): clear coherent slurred speech incoherent neologisms loose associations flight of ideas aphasic perseveration rumination tangential speech loquaciousness slow, impoverished speech

   speech impediment (describe) ______________________________

   other ______________________________

   ____

8. Interaction patterns (describe client's pattern of interpersonal interactions with staff and peers on the unit, e.g., manipulative, withdrawn, isolated, verbally or physically hostile, argumentative, passive, assertive, aggressive, passive-aggressive, other): ______________________________

   ____

   ____

   ____

9. Reality orientation (check those that apply):

   Oriented to: time __________ person __________

   place __________ situation __________

10. Ideas of destruction to self/others? Yes No

    If yes, consider plan; available means ______________________________

    ____

    ____

    ____

(Continued)

TABLE 6 – 1 Nursing History and Assessment Tool *(Continued)*

B. *Physiological*

1. Psychosomatic manifestations (describe any somatic complaints that may be stress-related): ______

2. Drug history and assessment:

Use of prescribed drugs:

NAME	DOSAGE	PRESCRIBED FOR	RESULTS

Use of over-the-counter drugs or herbal supplements:

NAME	DOSAGE	USED FOR	RESULTS

Use of street drugs or alcohol:

NAME	AMOUNT USED	HOW OFTEN USED	WHEN LAST USED	EFFECTS PRODUCED

3. Pertinent physical assessments:

a. Respirations: normal ______ labored ______

Rate ______ Rhythm ______

b. Skin: warm ______ dry ______ moist ______ cool ______ clammy ______ pink ______

cyanotic ______ poor turgor ______ edematous ______

Evidence of: rash ______ bruising ______ needle tracts ______ hirsutism ______

loss of hair ______ other ______

c. Musculoskeletal status: weakness ______ tremors ______

Degree of range of motion (describe limitations) ______

Pain (describe) ______

Skeletal deformities (describe) ______

Coordination (describe limitations) ______

d. Neurological status:
History of (check all that apply): seizures ________ (describe method of control) ________
____
headaches (describe location and frequency) ________
fainting spells ________ dizziness ________
tingling/numbness (describe location) ________

e. Cardiovascular: B/P ________ Pulse ________
History of (check all that apply):
hypertension ________ palpitations ________
heart murmur ________ chest pain ________
shortness of breath ________ pain in legs ________
phlebitis ________ ankle/leg edema ________
numbness/tingling in extremities ________
varicose veins ________

f. Gastrointestinal:
Usual diet pattern: ________
Food allergies: ________
Dentures? Upper ________ Lower ________
Any problems with chewing or swallowing? ________
Any recent change in weight? ________
Any problems with:
indigestion/heartburn? ________
relieved by ________
nausea/vomiting? ________
relieved by ________
History of ulcers? ________
Usual bowel pattern ________
Constipation? ________ Diarrhea? ________
Type of self-care assistance provided for either of the above problems ________
____

g. Genitourinary/Reproductive:
Usual voiding pattern ________
Urinary hesitancy? ________ Frequency? ________
Nocturia? ________ Pain/burning? ________
Incontinence? ________
Any genital lesions? ________
Discharge? ________ Odor? ________
History of sexually transmitted disease? ________
If yes, please explain ________
____

(Continued)

TABLE 6 – 1 Nursing History and Assessment Tool *(Continued)*

Any concerns about sexuality/sexual activity? ____________________

____

Method of birth control used ____________________

Females:

Date of last menstrual cycle ____________________

Length of cycle ____________________

Problems associated with menstruation? ____________________

____

Breasts: Pain/tenderness? ____________________

Swelling? __________ Discharge? __________

Lumps? __________ Dimpling? __________

Practice breast self-examination? ____________________

Frequency? ____________________

Males:

Penile discharge? ____________________

Prostate problems? ____________________

h. Eyes:

	YES	NO	EXPLAIN
Glasses?			
Contacts?			
Swelling?			
Discharge?			
Itching?			
Blurring?			
Double vision?			

i. Ears

	YES	NO	EXPLAIN
Pain?			
Drainage?			
Difficulty hearing?			
Hearing aid?			
Tinnitus?			

j. Medication side effects:

What symptoms is the client experiencing that may be attributed to current medication usage?

____

____

k. Altered lab values and possible significance: ____________________

____

____

l. Activity/rest patterns:

Exercise (amount, type, frequency) ____________________

____

Leisure time activities: ____________________

____

Patterns of sleep: Number of hours per night ______

Use of sleep aids? ______

Pattern of awakening during the night? ______

______

Feel rested upon awakening? ______

m. Personal hygiene/activities of daily living:

Patterns of self-care: independent ______

Requires assistance with: mobility ______

hygiene ______

toileting ______

feeding ______

dressing ______

other ______

Statement describing personal hygiene and general appearance ______

______

______

n. Other pertinent physical assessments: ______

______

______

______

VI. Summary of Initial Psychosocial/Physical Assessment:

Knowledge Deficits Identified:

Nursing Diagnoses Indicated:

SOURCE: From Townsend (2003)

Components of the mental status assessment are presented in Table 6–2.

Sociocultural Concepts

What is **culture**? How does it differ from **ethnicity**? Why are these questions important? The answers lie in the changing face of America. Immigration is not new in the United States. Indeed, most U.S. citizens are either immigrants or descendants of immigrants. This pattern continues because of the many individuals who want to take advantage of the technological growth and upward mobility that exists in this country. Gordon (1995) states:

> Although immigration is not new in the United States, its complexion has changed. The fact that the new immigrants are people of color has had a decided impact on many industries, healthcare included. The Bureau of Labor Statistics estimates that by the year 2005, there will be a total of 151 million people, either in the work force or looking for work, an increase of 26 million from 1990. The Bureau predicts a 32 percent increase in African-Americans, a 75 percent increase in Hispanics, and a 74 percent increase in Asians, Native Americans, Pacific Islanders, Native Alaskans, and others. (p. 14)

Culture describes a particular society's entire way of living, encompassing shared patterns of belief, feeling, and knowledge, that guides people's conduct and is

TABLE 6 – 2 Mental Status Assessment

Gathering the correct information about the client's mental status is essential to the development of an appropriate plan of care. The mental status examination describes all areas of the client's mental functioning. Components that are considered critical in the assessment of a client's mental status include the following:

IDENTIFYING DATA

1. Name
2. Sex
3. Age
4. Race/culture
5. Occupational/financial status
6. Educational level
7. Significant other
8. Living arrangements
9. Religious preference
10. Allergies
11. Special diet considerations
12. Chief complaint
13. Medical diagnosis

GENERAL DESCRIPTION

Appearance

1. Grooming and dress
2. Hygiene
3. Posture
4. Height and weight
5. Level of eye contact
6. Hair color and texture
7. Evidence of scars, tattoos, or other distinguishing skin marks
8. Evaluation of client's appearance compared with chronological age

Motor Activity

1. Tremors
2. Tics or other stereotypical movements
3. Mannerisms and gestures
4. Hyperactivity
5. Restlessness or agitation
6. Aggressiveness
7. Rigidity
8. Gait patterns
9. Echopraxia
10. Psychomotor retardation
11. Freedom of movement (range of motion)

Speech Patterns

1. Slowness or rapidity of speech
2. Pressure of speech
3. Intonation
4. Volume
5. Stuttering or other speech impairments
6 Aphasia

General Attitude

1. Cooperative/uncooperative
2. Friendly/hostile/defensive
3. Uninterested/apathetic
4. Attentive/interested
5. Guarded/suspicious

EMOTIONS

Mood

1. Sad
2. Depressed
3. Despairing
4. Irritable
5. Anxious
6. Elated
7. Euphoric
8. Fearful
9. Guilty
10. Labile

Affect

1. Congruence with mood
2. Constricted or blunted (diminished amount/range and intensity of emotional expression)
3. Flat (absence of emotional expression)
4. Appropriate or inappropriate (defines congruence of affect with the situation or with the client's behavior)

THOUGHT PROCESSES

Form of Thought

1. Flight of ideas
2. Associative looseness
3. Circumstantiality
4. Tangentiality
5. Neologisms
6. Concrete thinking
7. Clang associations
8. Word salad
9. Perseveration
10. Echolalia
11. Mutism
12. Poverty of speech (restriction in the amount of speech)
13. Ability to concentrate
14. Attention span

Content of Thought

1. Delusions
   a. Persecutory
   b. Grandiose
   c. Reference
   d. Control or influence
   e. Somatic
   f. Nihilistic
2. Suicidal or homicidal ideas
3. Obsessions
4. Paranoia/suspiciousness
5. Magical thinking
6. Religiosity
7. Phobias
8. Poverty of content (vague, meaningless responses)

PERCEPTUAL DISTURBANCES

1. Hallucinations
   a. Auditory
   b. Visual
   c. Tactile
   d. Olfactory
   e. Gustatory

2. Illusions
3. Depersonalization (altered perception of the self)
4. Derealization (altered perception of the environment)

SENSORIUM AND COGNITIVE ABILITY

1. Level of alertness/consciousness
2. Orientation
   a. Time
   b. Place
   c. Person
   d. Circumstances
3. Memory
   a. Recent
   b. Remote
   c. Confabulation
4. Capacity for abstract thought

IMPULSE CONTROL

1. Ability to control impulses related to the following:
   a. Aggression
   b. Hostility
   c. Fear
   d. Guilt
   e. Affection
   f. Sexual feelings

JUDGMENT AND INSIGHT

1. Ability to solve problems
2. Ability to make decisions
3. Knowledge about self
   a. Awareness of limitations
   b. Awareness of consequences of actions
   c. Awareness of illness
4. Adaptive/maladaptive use of coping strategies and ego defense mechanisms

passed down from generation to generation. *Ethnicity* is a somewhat narrower term and relates to people who identify with each other because of a shared heritage (Griffith, Gonzalez, & Blue, 2003).

Why is this important? Cultural influences affect human behavior, the interpretation of human behavior, and the response to human behavior. It is therefore essential for nurses to understand the effects of these cultural influences if they are to work effectively with this diverse population. However, caution must be taken not to assume that all individuals who share a culture or ethnic group are clones. This constitutes **stereotyping** and must be avoided. Geissler (1994) states, "The different values found within one culture may be as numerous as the variations found when comparing two different cultures." Every individual must be appreciated for his or her uniqueness.

This section explores the concepts in which various cultural differences may occur. These possible differences must be taken into consideration when conducting a nursing assessment. A cultural assessment tool is presented in Table 6–3.

How Do Cultures Differ?

Giger and Davidhizar (1999) suggest six cultural phenomena that vary with application and use but are evidenced among all cultural groups:

TABLE 6–3 Cultural Assessment Tool

Client's name ______________________ Ethnic origin ______________________

Address ______________________________________ Birthdate ______________

Name of significant other ______________________ Relationship ______________________

Primary language spoken ______________________ Second language spoken ______________________

How does client usually communicate with people who speak a different language? ______________________

Is an interpreter required? ______________________ Available? ______________________

Highest level of education achieved: ______________________ Occupation: ______________

Presenting problem: ______________________________________

Has this problem ever occurred before? ______________________________________

If so, in what manner was it handled previously? ______________________________________

What is the client's usual manner of coping with stress? ______________________________________

(Continued)

TABLE 6 – 3 Cultural Assessment Tool *(Continued)*

Who is (are) the client's main support system(s)? ______

Describe the family living arrangements: ______

Who is the major decision maker in the family? ______

Describe client's/family members' roles within the family. ______

______

Describe religious beliefs and practices: ______

Are there any religious requirements or restrictions that place limitations on the client's care? ______

If so, describe: ______

Who in the family takes responsibility for health concerns? ______

Describe any special health beliefs and practices: ______

______

From whom does family usually seek medical assistance in time of need? ______

Describe client's usual emotional/behavioral response to:

Anxiety: ______

Anger: ______

Loss/change/failure: ______

Pain: ______

Fear: ______

Describe any topics that are particularly sensitive or that the client is unwilling to discuss (because of cultural taboos):

______

What are the client's personal feelings regarding touch? ______

What are the client's personal feelings regarding eye contact? ______

What is the client's personal orientation to time? (past, present, future) ______

Describe any particular illnesses to which the client may be bioculturally susceptible (e.g., hypertension and sickle cell anemia in African Americans): ______

Describe any nutritional deficiencies to which the client may be bioculturally susceptible (e.g., lactose intolerance in Native and Asian Americans): ______

Describe client's favorite foods: ______

Are there any foods the client requests or refuses because of cultural beliefs related to this illness (e.g., "hot" and "cold" foods for Latino Americans and Asian Americans)? If so, please describe: ______

______

Describe client's perception of the problem and expectations of health care: ______

______

Townsend (2003).

1. Communication
2. Space
3. Social organization
4. Time
5. Environmental control
6. Biological variations

Communication

All verbal and nonverbal behavior in the presence of another individual is communication. Therapeutic communication has always been considered an essential part of the nursing process and represents a critical element in the curricula of most schools of nursing. Communication has its roots in culture. Cultural mores, norms, ideas, and customs provide the basis for our way of thinking. Cultural values are learned and differ from society to society. Communication is expressed through language (the spoken vocabulary), paralanguage (the voice quality, intonation, rhythm, speed of the spoken word), and gestures (touch, facial expression, eye movements, body posture, physical appearance). The nurse who is planning care must have an understanding of the client's needs and expectations as they are being communicated.

Being a third party, an interpreter often complicates matters, but one may be necessary when the client does not speak the same language as the nurse. However, interpreting is a very complex process that requires a keen sensitivity to cultural nuances, not just translating words into another language.

Space

Spatial determinants relate to the place where the communication occurs and encompass the concepts of territoriality, density, and distance. *Territoriality* refers to the innate tendency to own space. The need for territoriality is met only if the individual has control of a space, can establish rules for that space, and is able to defend the space against invasion or misuse by others (Giger & Davidhizar, 1999). *Density* refers to the number of people within a given environmental space and has been shown to influence interpersonal interaction. *Distance* is the means by which various cultures use space to communicate. Hall (1966) identified three primary dimensions of space in interpersonal interactions in the Western culture: the intimate zone (0 to 18 inches), the personal zone (18 inches to 3 feet), and the social zone (3 to 6 feet). These dimensions of space differ from culture to culture. For example, the personal space of Latino-Americans and African-Americans is smaller than that of Native Americans and Asian-Americans. Caution must be taken with touch in cultures that respect a large personal space.

Social Organization

Cultural behavior is socially acquired through a process called **acculturation**, which involves acquiring knowledge and internalizing values (Giger & Davidhizar, 1999). Children are acculturated by observing adults within their social organizations. Social organizations include families, religious groups, and ethnic groups. It is important for the nurse to understand the importance of these social organizations to certain cultures. African-Americans, Latino-Americans, Asian-Americans, Native Americans, and Western European Americans all have strong ties to these social organizations, which commonly have a great deal of influence on healthcare practices.

Time

An awareness of the concept of time is a gradual learning process. Some cultures place great importance on values measured by clock time. Punctuality and efficiency are highly valued in the United States. Other cultures are actually scornful of clock time. For example, peasants in Algeria live with a total indifference to the passage of clock time and despise haste in human affairs (Giger & Davidhizar, 1999).

Other cultural implications regarding time have to do with perception of time orientation. Whether individuals are present-oriented or future-oriented in their perception of time influences many aspects of their lives. Ethnic Americans who have become highly acculturated within the society are likely to be future-oriented as is the dominant culture. Many less acculturated individuals may be more present-oriented or past-oriented. It is important for the nurse to understand how these differences in perspective of time influence individuals' lives. A present-oriented person may arrive very late for an appointment because of a situation that may have arisen in the family—a situation that is regarded by that person as a personal priority. A future-oriented nurse must take care not to label this person as irresponsible because of the tardiness.

Environmental Control

This variable has to do with the extent to which individuals perceive that they have control over their environment. Cultural beliefs and practices influence how individuals respond to their environment during periods of wellness and illness. To provide culturally appropriate care, the nurse should not only respect the individual's unique beliefs but also should also have an understanding of how these beliefs can be used to promote optimal health in the client's environment (Giger & Davidhizar, 1999). Townsend (2003) provides the following example:

> Religion and health practices are intertwined in the Native American culture. The medicine man (or woman) is called the shaman, and may use a variety of methods in his or her practice. Some depend on "crystal gazing" to diagnose illness, some sing and perform elaborate healing ceremonies, and some use herbs and other plants or roots to concoct remedies with healing properties. The Native American healers and U.S. Indian Health Service have worked together with mutual respect for many years. Research studies have continued to show the importance of each of these healthcare systems in the overall wellness of Native American people. (p. 96)

Biological Variations

Biological differences exist among people in various racial groups (Giger & Davidhizar, 1999). These differences include body structure (both size and shape), skin color, physiological responses to medication, electrocardiographic patterns, susceptibility to disease, and nutritional preferences and deficiencies.

It is difficult to generalize about any one specific group in a country known for its heterogeneity. Within the American "melting pot," any or all of the characteristics described could apply to individuals within any or all of the cultural groups represented. As these stated differences continue to be integrated, one American culture will eventually emerge. This is already in evidence in certain regions of the country today. However, some differences still do exist, and it is important for nurses to be aware of certain cultural influences that may affect individuals' behaviors and beliefs, particularly as they apply to healthcare. A common example is the individual who is accustomed to eating certain foods and insists on having those particular foods to eat while in the hospital. It may be important for the nurse to find a way for this individual to have the food he or she desires if having it is within safe medical practice. It may even be the only means of ensuring that the client receives adequate sustenance during the hospital stay.

Standard II. Diagnosis

The psychiatric/mental health nurse analyzes the assessment data in determining diagnoses.

Rationale

The basis for providing psychiatric-mental health nursing care is the recognition and identification of patterns of response to actual or potential psychiatric illnesses, mental health problems, and potential co-morbid physical illnesses (ANA, 2000, p. 30).

In the second step, data gathered during the assessment are analyzed. Diagnoses and potential problem statements are formulated and prioritized. Diagnoses conform to accepted classification systems, such as the NANDA Nursing Diagnosis Taxonomy II (Appendix B); *International Classification of Diseases* (WHO, 1993); and *DSM-IV-TR* (APA, 2000) (Appendix A).

Why Nursing Diagnosis?

The concept of **nursing diagnosis** is not new. For a very long time, nurses have identified specific client responses for which nursing interventions were used to help improve quality of life. Therefore, it is not surprising for some nurses, who have been in practice for many years, to question the need for change to the specific terminology espoused by NANDA International. However, the autonomy of practice to which nurses were entitled by virtue of their licensure historically was lacking in the provision of nursing care. Nurses were considered "handmaidens" for physicians, and nursing consisted of a traditional set of tasks.

The term *diagnosis* in relation to nursing first began to appear in the literature in the early 1950s. The formalized organization of the concept, however, was initiated only in 1973 with the convening of the First National Conference on Nursing Diagnosis. The National Task Force for Classification of Nursing Diagnoses was developed during this conference. These individuals were charged with the task of identifying and classifying nursing diagnoses.

Additionally, in the 1970s, the ANA began to write standards of practice around the steps of the nursing process, of which nursing diagnosis is an inherent part. This format encompassed both the general and specialty standards outlined by the ANA. The standards of psychiatric/mental health nursing practice are summarized in Table 6–4.

Decisions regarding professional negligence are made based on the standards of practice defined by the ANA and the individual state nursing practice acts. A number of states have incorporated the steps of the nursing process, including nursing diagnosis, into the scope of nursing practice described in their nursing practice acts. When this is the case, it is the legal duty

TABLE 6 – 4 Standards of Psychiatric/Mental Health Clinical Nursing Practice

Standard I. Assessment
The psychiatric-mental health nurse collects client health data.

Standard II. Diagnosis
The psychiatric-mental health nurse analyzes the assessment data in determining diagnoses.

Standard III. Outcome Identification
The psychiatric-mental health nurse identifies expected outcomes individualized to the client.

Standard IV. Planning
The psychiatric-mental health nurse develops a plan of care that is negotiated among the client, nurse, family, and health care team and prescribes evidence-based interventions to attain expected outcomes.

Standard V. Implementation
The psychiatric-mental health nurse implements the interventions identified in the plan of care.

Standard Va. Counseling
The psychiatric-mental health nurse uses counseling interventions to assist clients in improving or regaining their previous coping abilities, fostering mental health, and preventing mental illness and disability.

Standard Vb. Milieu Therapy
The psychiatric-mental health nurse provides, structures, and maintains a therapeutic environment in collaboration with the client and other health care clinicians.

Standard Vc. Promotion of Self-Care Activities
The psychiatric-mental health nurse structures interventions around the client's activities of daily living to foster self-care and mental and physical well-being.

Standard Vd. Psychobiological Interventions
The psychiatric-mental health nurse uses knowledge of psychobiological interventions and applies clinical skills to restore the client's health and prevent further disability.

Standard Ve. Health Teaching
The psychiatric-mental health nurse, through health teaching, assists clients in achieving satisfying, productive, and healthy patterns of living.

Standard Vf. Case Management
The psychiatric-mental health nurse provides case management to coordinate comprehensive health services and ensure continuity of care.

Standard Vg. Health Promotion and Health Maintenance
The psychiatric-mental health nurse employs strategies and interventions to promote and maintain mental health and prevent mental illness.

Advanced Practice Interventions (Vh, Vi, & Vj)

Standard Vh. Psychotherapy
The advanced practice nurse in psychiatric-mental health uses individual, group, and family psychotherapy, and other therapeutic treatments to assist clients in preventing mental illness and disability, treating mental health disorders, and improving mental health status and functional abilities.

Standard Vi. Prescriptive Authority and Treatment
The advanced practice nurse in psychiatric-mental health uses prescriptive authority, procedures, and treatments in accordance with state and federal laws and regulations to treat symptoms of psychiatric illness and improve functional health status.

Standard Vj. Consultation
The advanced practice nurse in psychiatric-mental health provides consultation to enhance the abilities of other clinicians to provide services for clients and effect change in the system.

Standard VI. Evaluation
The psychiatric-mental health nurse evaluates the client's progress in attaining expected outcomes.

Adapted from ANA, 2000 (with permission).

of the nurse to show that nursing process and nursing diagnosis were accurately implemented in the delivery of nursing care.

Nursing diagnosis is included in the definition of professional nursing as set forth by the ANA. The ANA (2003) defines professional nursing as follows:

> Nursing is the protection, promotion, and optimization of health and abilities, prevention of illness and injury, alleviation of suffering through the diagnosis and treatment of human response, and advocacy in the care of individuals, families, communities, and populations. (p. 6)

NANDA International evolved from the National Task Force for Classification of Nursing Diagnoses. The major purpose of NANDA is to provide a forum for discussion about the development, refinement, and promotion of taxonomy of nursing diagnostic terminology (Lancour, 1990). A list of nursing diagnoses approved by NANDA is in Appendix B. This list is by no means exhaustive or all-inclusive. For purposes of this text, however, the existing list will be used to try to maintain a common language within nursing, and to encourage clinical testing of what is available.

An official definition of nursing diagnosis has been formulated through the work of NANDA and was presented to the membership in 1990. The definition is as follows:

> Nursing diagnosis is a clinical judgment about individual, family, or community responses to actual or potential health problems/life processes. A nursing diagnosis provides the basis for selection of nursing interventions to achieve outcomes for which the nurse is accountable. (NANDA International, 2003)

The use of nursing diagnosis affords some autonomy that historically has been lacking in the practice of nursing. Nursing diagnosis describes the client's condition, facilitating the prescription of interventions and establishment of parameters for outcome criteria based upon what is uniquely nursing. The ultimate benefit is to the client, who receives effective and consistent nursing care based on knowledge of the problems that he or she is experiencing and of the most beneficial nursing interventions to resolve them.

Standard III. Outcome Identification

The psychiatric/mental health nurse identifies expected outcomes individualized to the client.

Rationale

Within the context of providing nursing care, the ultimate goal is to influence health outcomes and improve the client's health status (ANA, 2000, p. 31).

Expected outcomes are derived from the nursing diagnosis. They must be measurable and estimate a time for attainment. They must be realistic for the client's capabilities and are most effective when formulated by the **interdisciplinary** team members, the client, and significant others together.

Nursing Outcomes Classification (NOC)

NOC is a comprehensive, standardized classification of patient/client outcomes developed to evaluate the effects of nursing interventions (Johnson, Maas, & Moorhead, 2001). The outcomes have been linked to NANDA diagnoses and to the **Nursing Interventions Classification (NIC).** NANDA, NIC, and NOC represent all domains of nursing and can be used together or separately (Johnson et al., 2001).

Each NOC outcome has a label name, a definition, a list of indicators to evaluate client status in relation to the outcome, and a five-point Likert scale to measure client status (Johnson, Maas, & Moorhead, 2001). The 260 NOC outcomes include 247 individual-level outcomes, 7 family-level outcomes, and 6 community-level outcomes.

Standard IV. Planning

The psychiatric/mental health nurse develops a plan of care that is negotiated among the client, nurse, family, and healthcare team and prescribes evidence-based interventions to attain expected outcomes.

Rationale

A plan of care is used to guide therapeutic interventions systematically, document progress, and achieve the expected client outcomes (ANA, 2000, p. 32).

The care plan is individualized to the client's mental health problems, condition, or needs and is developed in collaboration with the client, significant others, and interdisciplinary care team members, if possible. For each diagnosis identified, the most appropriate interventions, based on current psychiatric/mental health nursing practice and research, are selected. Client education and necessary referrals are included. Priorities for delivery of nursing care are determined.

Nursing Interventions Classification

NIC is a comprehensive, standardized language describing treatments that nurses perform in all settings and in all specialties. NIC includes both physiological and psychosocial interventions as well as those for illness treatment, illness prevention, and health promotion (Dochterman & Bulechek, 2001). NIC interventions are comprehensive, based on research, and reflect current clinical practice. They were developed inductively, based on existing practice.

NIC contains 486 interventions, each with a definition and a detailed set of activities that describes what a nurse does to implement the intervention. Dochterman and Bulechek (2001) state: "The use of standardized language provides for the continuity of care and enhances communication among nurses and between nurses and other providers."

Standard V. Implementation

The psychiatric/mental health nurse implements the interventions identified in the plan of care.

Rationale

In implementing the plan of care, the psychiatric-mental health nurses use a wide range of interventions designed to prevent mental and physical illness and to promote, maintain, and restore mental and physical health. Psychiatric-mental health nurses select interventions according to their level of practice. At the basic level, the nurse may select counseling, milieu therapy, promotion of self-care activities, intake screening and evaluation, psychobiological interventions, health teaching, case management, health promotion and health maintenance, and a variety of other approaches to meet the mental health needs of clients. In addition to the intervention options available to the basic-level psychiatric-mental health nurse, the advanced practice psychiatric-mental health nurse may provide consultation, engage in psychotherapy, and prescribe pharmacological agents in accordance with state statutes or regulations (ANA, 2000).

Interventions selected during the planning stage are executed, taking into consideration the nurse's level of practice, education, and certification. The care plan serves as a blueprint for delivery of safe, ethical, and appropriate interventions. Documentation of interventions also occurs at this step in the nursing process.

Several specific interventions are included among the standards of psychiatric-mental health clinical nursing practice (ANA, 2000):

Standard Va. Counseling. The psychiatric-mental health nurse uses counseling interventions to assist clients in improving or regaining their previous coping abilities, fostering mental health, and preventing mental illness and disability.

Standard Vb. Milieu Therapy. The psychiatric-mental health nurse provides, structures, and maintains a therapeutic environment in collaboration with the client and other healthcare clinicians.

Standard Vc. Self-Care Activities. The psychiatric-mental health nurse structures interventions around the client's activities of daily living to foster self-care and mental and physical well-being.

Standard Vd. Psychobiological Interventions. The psychiatric-mental health nurse uses knowledge of psychobiological interventions and applies clinical skills to restore the client's health and prevent further disability.

Standard Ve. Health Teaching. The psychiatric-mental health nurse, through health teaching, assists clients in achieving satisfying, productive, and healthy patterns of living.

Standard Vf. Case Management. The psychiatric-mental health nurse provides case management to coordinate comprehensive health services and ensure continuity of care.

Standard Vg. Health Promotion and Health Maintenance. The psychiatric-mental health nurse employs strategies and interventions to promote and maintain mental health and prevent mental illness.

Standards specific to the advanced practice psychiatric-mental health nurse include:

Standard Vh. Psychotherapy. The advanced practice psychiatric-mental health nurse uses individual, group, and family psychotherapy and other therapeutic treatments to assist clients in preventing mental illness and disability, treating mental health disorders, and improving mental health status and functional abilities.

Standard Vi. Prescriptive Authority and Treatment. The advanced practice psychiatric-mental health nurse uses prescriptive authority, procedures, and treatments in accordance with state and federal laws and regulations to treat symptoms of psychiatric illness and improve functional health status.

Standard Vj. Consultation. The advanced practice psychiatric-mental health nurse provides consultation to enhance the abilities of other clinicians to provide services for clients and effect change in the system.

Standard VI. Evaluation

The psychiatric-mental health nurse evaluates the client's progress in attaining expected outcomes.

Rationale

Nursing care is a dynamic process involving change in the client's health status over time, giving rise to the need for data, different diagnoses, and modifications in the plan of care. Therefore, evaluation is a continuous process of appraising the effect of nursing and the treatment regimen on the client's health status and expected outcomes (ANA, 2000).

During the evaluation step, the nurse measures the success of the interventions in meeting the outcome criteria. The client's response to treatment is documented, validating use of the nursing process in the delivery of care. The diagnoses, outcomes, and plan of care are reviewed and revised as need is determined by the evaluation.

APPLYING THE NURSING PROCESS IN THE PSYCHIATRIC SETTING

Based on the definition of mental health set forth in Chapter 1, the role of the nurse in psychiatry focuses on assisting the client to successfully adapt to stressors within the environment. Goals are directed toward change in thoughts, feelings, and behaviors that are age-appropriate and congruent with local and cultural norms.

Therapy within the psychiatric setting is very often team-oriented, or **interdisciplinary.** Therefore, it is important to delineate nursing's involvement in the treatment regimen. Nurses are indeed valuable members of the team. Having progressed beyond the role of custodial caregiver in the psychiatric setting, nurses now provide services that are defined within the scope of nursing practice. Nursing diagnosis is helping to define these nursing boundaries, and thereby providing a measure of autonomy and professionalism that has for so long been unrealized.

For example, a newly admitted client with the medical diagnosis of schizophrenia may be demonstrating the following behaviors:

- Verbalizing hearing voices
- Inability to trust others
- Refusing to interact with staff and peers
- Expressing a fear of failure
- Poor personal hygiene

From these assessments, the treatment team may determine that the client has the following problems:

- Auditory hallucinations
- Paranoid delusions
- Social withdrawal
- Developmental regression

Team goals would be directed toward:

- Terminating hallucinations (or in the case of a chronically ill person, at least helping him or her understand that the voices are not real)
- Reducing suspiciousness
- Increasing feelings of self-worth

From this team treatment plan, nursing may identify the following nursing diagnoses:

1. Disturbed sensory perception, auditory (evidenced by hearing voices)
2. Disturbed thought processes (evidenced by delusions)
3. Low self-esteem (evidenced by fear of failure and social withdrawal)
4. Self-care deficit (evidenced by poor personal hygiene)

Nursing diagnoses are prioritized according to life-threatening potential. Maslow's hierarchy of needs is a good model to follow in prioritizing nursing diagnoses. In this instance, disturbed sensory perception (auditory) is identified as the priority nursing diagnosis, because the client may be hearing voices that command him or her to harm self or others. Nursing in psychiatry, regardless of the setting—hospital (inpatient or outpatient), office, home, community—is goal-directed care. The goals (or expected outcomes) are client-oriented, are measurable, and focus on resolution of the problem if this is realistic or on a more short-term outcome if resolution is unrealistic. For example, in the previous situation, expected outcomes for the identified nursing diagnoses might be as follows:

1. The client will demonstrate trust in one staff member within 5 days.
2. The client will verbalize understanding that the voices are not real (not heard by others) within 10 days.
3. The client will complete one simple craft project within 7 days.
4. The client will take responsibility for own self-care and perform activities of daily living independently by discharge.

Nursing's contribution to the interdisciplinary treatment regimen will focus on establishing trust on a one-to-one basis, reducing the level of anxiety that is promoting hallucinations, giving positive feedback for small day-to-day accomplishments in an effort to build self-esteem, and assisting with and encouraging independent self-care. These interventions describe *independent nursing* actions and goals that are evaluated apart from, while also being directed toward achievement of, the *team's* treatment goals.

In this manner of collaboration with other team members, nursing provides a service that is unique and based on sound knowledge of psychopathology, scope of practice, and legal implications of the role. Although there is no dispute that "following doctor's orders" continues to be accepted in the priority of care, nursing intervention that enhances achievement of the overall goals of treatment is being recognized for its important contribution. The nurse who administers a medication prescribed by the physician to decrease anxiety may also choose to stay with the anxious client and offer reassurance of safety and security, thereby providing an independent nursing action that is distinct from, yet complementary to, the medical treatment.

DOCUMENTATION TO THE NURSING PROCESS

Equally important as using the nursing process in the delivery of care is the written documentation that it has been used. Some contemporary nursing leaders advocate that with solid standards of practice and procedures in place within the institution, nurses need only chart when there has been a deviation in the care as outlined by that standard. However, many legal decisions are still based on the precept that "if it was not charted, it was not done."

Because nursing process and nursing diagnosis are mandated by some nursing practice acts, documentation of their use is considered, in those states, as evidence in determining certain cases of negligence by nurses. Some healthcare organization accrediting agencies also require that nursing process be reflected in the delivery of care. In these instances, documentation must bear written testament to the use of the nursing process.

A variety of documentation methods can be used to reflect use of the nursing process in the delivery of nursing care. Three examples are presented here: **problem-oriented recording (POR), Focus charting®**, and the problem, intervention, evaluation (PIE) system of documentation.

Problem-Oriented Recording (POR)

POR follows the *s*ubjective, *o*bjective, *a*ssessment, *p*lan, *i*mplementation, and *e*valuation (SOAPIE) format. It has as its basis a list of problems. When used in nursing, the problems (nursing diagnoses) are identified on a written plan of care with appropriate nursing interventions described for each. Documentation written in the SOAPIE format includes:

S = Subjective data: Information gathered from what the client, family, or other source has said or reported.

O = Objective data: Information gathered by direct observation of the person performing the assessment; may include a physiological measurement such as blood pressure or a behavioral response such as affect.

A = Assessment: The nurse's interpretation of the subjective and objective data.

P = Plan: The actions or treatments to be carried out (may be omitted in daily charting if the plan is clearly explained in the written nursing care plan and no changes are expected).

I = Intervention: Those nursing actions that were actually carried out.

E = Evaluation of the problem following nursing intervention (some nursing interventions cannot be evaluated immediately, so this section may be optional).

Table 6–5 shows how POR corresponds to the steps of the nursing process. Following is an example of a three-column documentation in the POR format.

EXAMPLE:

Date/ Time	*Problem*	*Progress Notes*
6-22-03 1000	Social isolation	**S:** States he does not want to sit with or talk to others; "they frighten me"

TABLE 6 – 5 Validation of the Nursing Process with Problem-Oriented Recording

Problem-Oriented Recording	What is Recorded	Nursing Process
S and O (Subjective and Objective data)	Verbal reports to, and direct observation and examination by, the nurse	Assessment
A (Assessment)	Nurse's interpretation of S and O	Diagnosis and outcome identification
P (Plan) Omitted in charting if written plan describes care to be given	Description of appropriate nursing actions to resolve the identified problem	Planning
I (Intervention)	Description of nursing actions actually carried out	Implementation
E (Evaluation)	Reassessment of the situation to determine results of nursing actions implemented	Evaluation

O: Stays in room alone unless strongly encouraged to come out; no group involvement; at times listens to group conversations from a distance but does not interact; some hypervigilance and scanning noted
A: Inability to trust; panic level of anxiety; delusional thinking
I: Initiated trusting relationship by spending time alone with the client; discussed his feelings regarding interactions with others; accompanied client to group activities; provided positive feedback for voluntarily participating in assertiveness training

Focus Charting®

Another type of documentation that reflects use of the nursing process is **Focus charting®**. Focus charting differs from POR in that the main perspective has been changed from "problem" to "focus," and data, action, and response (DAR) have replaced SOAPIE.

Lampe (1985) suggests that a focus for documentation can be any of the following:

1. Nursing diagnosis
2. Current client concern or behavior
3. Significant change in the client status or behavior
4. Significant event in the client's therapy

The focus cannot be a medical diagnosis. The documentation is organized in the format of DAR. These categories are defined as follows:

D = Data: Information that supports the stated focus or describes pertinent observations about the client
A = Action: Immediate or future nursing actions that address the focus and evaluation of the present care plan along with any changes required
R = Response: Description of client's responses to any part of the medical or nursing care

Table 6–6 shows how focus charting corresponds to the steps of the nursing process. Following is an example of a three-column documentation in the DAR format.

EXAMPLE:

Date/ Time	*Focus*	*Progress Notes*
6-22-03 1000	Social isolation related to mistrust, panic anxiety, delusions	**D:** States he does not want to sit with or talk to others; they "frighten" him; stays in room alone unless strongly encouraged to come out; no group involvement; at times listens to group conversations from a distance, but does not interact; some hypervigilance and scanning noted **A:** Initiated trusting relationship by spending time alone with client; discussed his feelings regarding interactions with others; accompa-

TABLE 6–6 Validation of the Nursing Process with Focus Charting

Focus Charting	What is Recorded	Nursing Process
D (Data)	Information that supports the stated focus or describes pertinent observations about the client.	Assessment
Focus	A nursing diagnosis; current client concern or behavior; significant change in client status; significant event in the client's therapy. **NOTE:** If outcome appears on written care plan, it need not be repeated in daily documentation unless a change occurs.	Diagnosis and outcome identification
A (Action)	Immediate or future nursing actions that address the focus; appraisal of the care plan along with any changes required.	Plan and implementation
R (Response)	Description of client responses to any part of the medical or nursing care.	Evaluation

TABLE 6 – 7 Validation of the Nursing Process with APIE Method

APIE Charting	What is Recorded	Nursing Process
A (Assessment)	Subjective and objective data about the client that is gathered at the beginning of each shift	Assessment
P (Problem)	Name (or number) of nursing diagnosis being addressed from written problem list, and identified outcome for that problem. **NOTE:** If outcome appears on written care plan, it need not be repeated in daily documentation unless a change occurs	Diagnosis and outcome identification
I (Intervention)	Nursing actions performed, directed at problem resolution	Plan and implementation
E (Evaluation)	Appraisal of client responses to determine effectiveness of nursing interventions	Evaluation

nied client to group activities; provided positive feedback for voluntarily participating in assertiveness training
R: Cooperative with therapy; still acts uncomfortable in the presence of a group of people; accepted positive feedback from nurse

The PIE Method

PIE or, more specifically, APIE (*a*ssessment, *p*roblem, *i*ntervention, *e*valuation), is a systematic method of documenting to nursing process and nursing diagnosis. A problem-oriented system, **PIE charting,** uses accompanying flow sheets that are individualized by each institution. Criteria for documentation are organized in the following manner:

A = Assessment: A complete client assessment is conducted at the beginning of each shift. Results are documented under this section in the progress notes. Some institutions elect instead to use a daily client assessment sheet designed to meet specific needs of the unit. Explanation of any deviation from the norm is included in the progress notes.

P = Problem: A problem list, or list of nursing diagnoses, is an important part of the APIE method of charting. The name or number of the problem being addressed is documented in this section.

I = Intervention: Nursing actions are performed, directed at resolution of the problem.

E = Evaluation: Outcomes of the implemented interventions are documented, including an evaluation of client responses to determine the effectiveness of nursing interventions and the presence or absence of progress toward resolution of a problem.

Table 6–7 shows how APIE charting corresponds to the steps of the nursing process. Following is an example of a three-column documentation in the APIE format.

EXAMPLE:

Date/ Time	*Problem*	*Progress Notes*
6-22-03 1000	Social Isolation	**A:** States he does not want to sit with or talk to others; they "frighten" him; stays in room alone unless strongly encouraged to come out; no group involvement; at times listens to group conversations from a distance but does not interact; some hypervigilance and scanning noted **P:** Social isolation related to inability to trust, panic level of anxiety, and delusional thinking **I:** Initiated trusting relationship by spending time alone with client; discussed his feelings regarding interactions with others; accompanied client to group activities; provided positive feedback for voluntarily participating in assertiveness training **E:** Cooperative with therapy; still uncomfortable in the presence of a group of people; accepted positive feedback from nurse

SUMMARY

The nursing process provides a methodology by which nurses may deliver care using a systematic, scientific approach. The focus is goal directed and based on a decision-making or problem-solving model, consisting of six steps: assessment, diagnosis, outcome identification, planning, implementation, and evaluation.

Sociocultural influences affect human behavior, the interpretation of human behavior, and the response to human behavior. Therefore, it is essential for nurses to understand the effects of these cultural influences if they are to work effectively with diverse populations. This chapter explored the concepts in which various cultural differences may occur and which must be taken into consideration when conducting a nursing assessment. A cultural assessment tool was included.

Nursing diagnosis is inherent within the nursing process. The concept of nursing diagnosis is not new, but has only become formalized with the organization of NANDA in the 1970s. Nursing diagnosis defines the scope and boundaries for nursing, thereby offering a degree of autonomy and independence so long restricted within the practice of nursing. Nursing diagnosis also provides a common language for nursing and helps nurses provide consistent, quality care for their clients based on an increase in the body of nursing knowledge through research. The current list of nursing diagnoses approved by NANDA is in Appendix B.

The psychiatric nurse uses the nursing process to help clients successfully adapt to stressors within the environment. Goals are directed toward change in thoughts, feelings, and behaviors that are age-appropriate and congruent with local and cultural norms. The nurse serves as a valuable member of the interdisciplinary treatment team, working both independently and cooperatively with other team members. Nursing diagnosis, in its ability to define the scope of nursing practice, is facilitating nursing's role in the psychiatric setting by differentiating that which is specifically nursing from interventions associated with other disciplines. Nursing in psychiatry is goal-directed care. These goals are evaluated apart from, while also being directed toward achievement of, the team's treatment goals.

Nurses must document that the nursing process has been used in the delivery of care. Its use is mandated in some states by the nurse practice act and is also required by some healthcare organization accrediting agencies. Three methods of documentation—POR, focus charting, and the PIE system—were presented with examples to demonstrate how they reflect use of the nursing process.

REVIEW QUESTIONS

SELF-EXAMINATION/LEARNING EXERCISE

Select the answer that is most appropriate for each of the following questions.

Situation: Annie is 69 years old. She has been admitted to the psychiatric unit with a diagnosis of major depression. Annie's daughter took her to her family physician because she was concerned about her mother's condition. The family physician performed a complete physical examination, ruled out any physical illness, and referred her to a psychiatrist.

Annie's psychosocial history reveals that her husband died 3 years ago. They had been married for 46 years. Annie has lived alone since her husband's death. Her daughter describes Annie's behaviors in the following way:

"Annie visits her husband's grave site at least twice a week. She has become increasingly isolated and withdrawn and has given up most of the activities in which she previously participated. She still attends her church services regularly. She has quit cooking for herself and eats very little. She has lost about 20 pounds in the last year."

Admission data includes: height 5′ 2″; weight 82 pounds; VS: T 97.6, P 96, R 18, BP 102/67. Annie is a very thin, gray-haired, Asian-American woman who appears to be her stated age. Her mood is depressed, and her affect is flat. She answers some questions, but relies on her daughter to do most of the talking. She has little direct eye contact, and keeps her eyes focused mostly on her hands in her lap, which are fidgeting with a wadded-up tissue. She becomes tearful when she talks about her husband.

1. In assessing Annie, the nurse may want to do a cultural assessment because:
   a. Some Asian-Americans may have needs that differ from the dominant culture.
   b. Asian-Americans have very different ideas about psychiatric care.
   c. Annie's religious beliefs will affect the kind of care she expects to receive.
   d. It is rare for an Asian-American to grieve for such a long period of time.

2. What might the nurse consider in assessing Annie's lack of eye contact?
   a. She is shy.
   b. Eye contact will return when the depression is resolved.
   c. Lack of eye contact may be a cultural influence.
   d. She has chronic low self-esteem.

3. After analyzing the assessment data, which would be the priority nursing diagnosis for Annie?
   a. Chronic low self-esteem related to learned helplessness
   b. Imbalanced nutrition, less than body requirements related to inadequate food intake
   c. Social isolation related to unresolved grief
   d. Fear related to living alone

4. A realistic outcome intervention for working with Annie would be:
   a. Annie will have increased self-esteem within 7 days.
   b. Annie will gain 1 to 2 pounds per week while in the hospital.
   c. Annie will participate in all activities on the unit within 48 hours of admission.
   d. Annie will agree to move to a nursing home so that she will no longer have to fear living alone.

5. Based on information gathered in the cultural assessment, which of the following might be an appropriate nursing intervention for Annie?
   a. Give strong positive feedback every time she makes eye contact.
   b. Help her understand that visiting her husband's grave so often is prolonging resolution of her grief.

c. Ask her family to bring in some of her favorite foods for her to eat while she is in the hospital.
d. Give positive feedback every time she talks about her husband without crying.

The nurse has difficulty getting Annie to attend activities. She tries to stay in her room most of the time and comes out only with strong encouragement. Annie says to the nurse, "I just don't feel like doing anything or seeing anyone since my husband died. I just want to be alone and think about him." Annie's care plan has a nursing diagnosis of social isolation and includes the following interventions: spend one-to-one time with client until trust has been established; attend group activities with client until she is comfortable attending alone; give positive feedback for interactions with others.

Match each part of the progress note on the right with its identifying part of problem-oriented documentation on the left:

_______ 6. S = Subjective	a. Attended group therapy and assertiveness training with Annie. Provided positive feedback for attendance.
_______ 7. O = Objective	b. "I just don't feel like doing anything or seeing anyone since my husband died. I just want to be alone and think about him."
_______ 8. A = Assessment	c. Is beginning to feel more comfortable in groups. Took more active role than previously taken.
_______ 9. I = Intervention	d. Social isolation related to unresolved grief from loss of husband.
_______ 10. E = Evaluation	e. Stays in room alone unless strongly encouraged to come out; activities of daily living completed without assistance; appears relieved to have nurse attend groups with her.

REFERENCES

American Nurses Association. (2000). Scope and standards of psychiatric-mental health nursing practice. Washington, DC: Author.

American Nurses Association. (1998). Standards of clinical nursing practice (2nd ed.). Washington, DC: Author.

American Nurses Association. (2003). Nursing's social policy statement (2nd ed.). Washington, DC: Author.

American Psychiatric Association. (2000). Diagnosis and statistical manual of mental disorders—text revision (4th ed.). Washington, DC: Author.

Dochterman, J.M., & Bulechek, G. (2001). Nursing interventions classification overview. Retrieved November 11, 2001 from http://coninfo.nursing.uiowa.edu/nic/overview.htm

Geissler, E.M. (1994). Pocket guide to cultural assessment. St. Louis: Mosby Year Book.

Giger, J.N., & Davidhizar, R.E. (1999). Transcultural nursing: Assessment and intervention (3rd ed.). St. Louis: Elsevier.

Gordon, B.N. (1995). Cultural diversity: You make a difference. The Oklahoma Nurse, 40:14–15.

Griffith, E.E.H., Gonzalez, C.A., & Blue, H.C. (2003). Introduction to cultural psychiatry. In R.E. Hales & S.C. Yodofsky (Eds.), Textbook of psychiatry (4th ed.). Washington, DC: American Psychiatric Publishing.

Johnson, M., Maas, M., & Moorhead, S. (2001). Nursing outcomes classification: Overview. Retrieved November 20, 2001, from http://coninfo.nursing.uiowa.edu/noc/overview.htm

Johnson, M., et al. (2001). Nursing diagnoses, outcomes, and interventions: NANDA, NOC, and NIC linkages. St. Louis: Mosby.

Lampe, S.S. (1985). Focus charting: Streamlining documentation. Nursing Management, 16:43–46.

Lancour, J. (1990). President's message. Nursing Diagnosis, 1:4.

NANDA International. (2003). Nursing diagnoses: Definitions and classification, 2003–2004. Philadelphia: NANDA International.

Townsend, M.C. (2003). Psychiatric-mental health nursing: Concepts of care (4th ed.). Philadelphia: F.A. Davis.

World Health Organization. (1993). International classification of diseases (10th ed.). Geneva: Author.

CLASSICAL REFERENCES

Hall, E.T. (1966). The hidden dimension. Garden City, N.Y.: Doubleday.

7

CHAPTER

Milieu—The Therapeutic Environment

CHAPTER OUTLINE

KEY TERMS

milieu
milieu therapy
therapeutic community

OBJECTIVES

After reading this chapter, the student will be able to:

1. Define *milieu therapy.*
2. Explain the goal of therapeutic community/ milieu therapy.
3. Identify seven basic assumptions of a therapeutic community.
4. Discuss conditions that characterize a therapeutic community.
5. Identify the various therapies that may be included within the program of the therapeutic community and the healthcare workers that make up the interdisciplinary treatment team.
6. Describe the role of the nurse on the interdisciplinary treatment team.

INTRODUCTION

Standard Vb of the Scope and Standards of Psychiatric-Mental Health Nursing Practice (ANA, 2000) states that, "The psychiatric-mental health nurse provides, structures, and maintains a therapeutic environment in collaboration with the patient and other healthcare clinicians."

This chapter defines and explains the goal of milieu therapy. The conditions necessary for a therapeutic environment are discussed, and the roles of the various healthcare workers within the interdisciplinary team are delineated. An interpretation of the nurse's role in milieu therapy is included.

MILIEU DEFINED

The word **milieu** is French for "middle." The English translation of the word is "surroundings, or environment." In psychiatry, therapy involving the milieu, or environment, may be called **milieu therapy**, therapeutic community, or therapeutic environment. In this context, it is defined as "a scientific structuring of the environment in order to effect behavioral changes and to improve the psychological health and functioning of the individual" (Skinner, 1979). Thus, the goal of milieu therapy is to manipulate the environment so that all aspects of the client's hospital experience are considered therapeutic. Within this therapeutic community setting, the client is expected to learn adaptive coping, interaction, and relationship skills that can be generalized to other aspects of his or her life.

CURRENT STATUS OF THE THERAPEUTIC COMMUNITY

Milieu therapy came into its own during the 1960s, 1970s, and early 1980s. During this period, psychiatric inpatient treatment provided sufficient time to implement programs of therapy that were aimed at social rehabilitation. Nursing's focus of establishing interpersonal relationships with clients fit well within this concept of therapy. Patients were encouraged to be active participants in their therapy, and individual autonomy was emphasized.

The current focus of inpatient psychiatric care has changed. Hall (1995) states:

> Care in inpatient psychiatric facilities can now be characterized as short and biologically based. By the time patients have stabilized enough to benefit from the socialization that would take place in a milieu as treatment program, they [often] have been discharged. (p. 51)

Although strategies for milieu therapy are still used, they have been modified to conform to the short-term approach to care or to outpatient treatment programs. Some programs (e.g., those for children and adolescents, clients with substance addictions, and geriatric clients) have successfully adapted the concepts of milieu treatment to their specialty needs (DeSocio, Bowllan, & Staschak, 1997; Whall, 1991; Bowler, 1991).

Many of the original concepts of milieu therapy are presented in this chapter. It is important to remember that a number of modifications to these concepts have been applied in practice for use in a variety of settings.

BASIC ASSUMPTIONS

Skinner (1979) outlined seven basic assumptions on which a therapeutic community is based:

1. *The health in each individual is to be realized and encouraged to grow.* All individuals are considered to have strengths as well as limitations. These healthy aspects of the individual are identified and serve as a foundation for growth in the personality and in the ability to function more adaptively and productively in all aspects of life.
2. *Every interaction is an opportunity for therapeutic intervention.* Within this structured setting, it is virtually impossible to avoid interpersonal interaction. The ideal situation exists for clients to improve communication and relationship development skills. Learning occurs from immediate feedback of personal perceptions.
3. *The client owns his or her own environment.* Clients make decisions and solve problems related to government of the unit. In this way, personal needs for autonomy as well as needs that pertain to the group as a whole are fulfilled.
4. *Each client owns his or her behavior.* Each individual within the therapeutic community is expected to take responsibility for his or her own behavior.
5. *Peer pressure is a useful and a powerful tool.* Behavioral group norms are established through peer pressure. Feedback is direct and frequent, so that behaving in a manner acceptable to the other members of the community becomes essential.
6. *Inappropriate behaviors are dealt with as they occur.* Individuals examine the significance of their behavior, look at how it affects other people, and discuss appropriate ways of behaving in certain situations.
7. *Restrictions and punishment are to be avoided.* Destructive behaviors can usually be controlled with group discussion. However, if an individual requires external controls, temporary isolation is preferred over lengthy restriction or other harsh punishment.

CONDITIONS THAT PROMOTE A THERAPEUTIC COMMUNITY

In a therapeutic community setting, everything that happens to the client, or within the client's environment, is considered part of the treatment program. The community setting is the foundation for the program of treatment. Community factors—such as social interactions, the physical structure of the unit, and schedule of activities—may generate negative responses from some clients. These stressful experiences are used as examples to help the client learn how to manage stress more adaptively in real-life situations.

Under what conditions, then, is a healthcare environment considered therapeutic? A number of criteria have been identified:

1. *Basic physiological needs are fulfilled.* As Maslow (1968) has suggested, individuals do not move to higher levels of functioning until the basic biological needs for food, water, air, sleep, exercise, elimination, shelter, and sexual expression have been met.
2. *The physical facilities are conducive to achievement of the goals of therapy.* Space is provided so that each client has sufficient privacy, as well as physical space, for therapeutic interaction with others. Furnishings are arranged to present an atmosphere that accommodates communal living, dining, activity areas, and for facilitation of interpersonal interaction and communication.
3. *A democratic form of self-government exists.* In the therapeutic community, clients participate in the decision-making and problem-solving that affect the management of the treatment setting. This is accomplished through regularly scheduled community meetings. These meetings are attended by staff and clients, and all individuals have equal input into the discussions. At these meetings, client norms, rules, and behavioral limits are set forth. This reinforces the democratic posture of the treatment setting because these are expectations that affect all clients on an equal basis. Consequences of violating the rules are explained and enforced.

Other issues that may be discussed at the community meetings include those with which certain clients have some disagreements. A decision is then made by the entire group in a democratic manner. For example, clients in an inpatient unit may disagree with the hours that have been designated for watching television on a weekend night. They may elect to bring up this issue at a community meeting and suggest an extension in television viewing time. After discussion by the group, a vote will be taken, and clients and staff agree to abide by the expressed preference of the majority. Some therapeutic communities elect officers (usually a president and a secretary) who serve for a specified period. The president calls the meeting to order, conducts the business of discussing old and new issues, and asks for volunteers (or makes appointments, alternately, so that all clients have a turn) to accomplish the daily tasks associated with community living; for example, cleaning the tables after each meal and watering plants in the treatment facility. New assignments are made at each meeting. The secretary reads the minutes of the previous meeting and takes minutes of the current meeting. Minutes are important in the event that clients have a disagreement about issues that were discussed at various meetings. Minutes provide written evidence of decisions made by the group.

In treatment settings where clients have short attention spans or disorganized thinking, meetings are brief. Business is generally limited to introductions and expectations of the here and now. Discussions also may include comments about a recent occurrence in the group or something that has been bothering a member and about which he or she has some questions. These meetings are usually conducted by staff, although all clients have equal input into the discussions.

All clients are expected to attend the meetings. Exceptions are made for times when aspects of therapy interfere (e.g., scheduled testing, x-ray examinations, electroencephalograms). An explanation is made to clients present so that false perceptions of danger are not generated by another person's absence.

All staff members are also expected to attend the meetings, unless client care precludes their attendance.

4. *Responsibilities are assigned according to client capabilities.* Increasing self-esteem is an ultimate goal of the therapeutic community. Therefore, a client should not be set up for failure by being assigned a responsibility that is beyond his or her level of ability. By assigning clients responsibilities that promote achievement, self-esteem is enhanced. Consideration must also be given to times during which the client will show some regression in the treatment regimen. Adjustments in assignments

should be made in a way that preserves self-esteem and provides for progression to greater amounts of responsibility as the client returns to previous level of functioning.

5. *A structured program of social and work-related activities is scheduled as part of the treatment program.* Each client's therapeutic program consists of group activities in which interpersonal interaction and communication with other individuals are emphasized. Time is also devoted to personal problems. Various group activities may be selected for clients with specific needs (e.g., an exercise group for a person who expresses anger inappropriately, an assertiveness group for a person who is passive-aggressive, or a stress management group for a person who is anxious). A structured schedule of activities is the major focus of a therapeutic community. Through these activities, change in the client's personality and behavior can be achieved. New coping strategies are learned, and social skills are developed. In the group situation, the client is able to practice what he or she has learned to prepare for transition to the general community.
6. *Community and family are included in the program of therapy in an effort to facilitate discharge from treatment.* An attempt is made to include family members, as well as certain aspects of the community that affect the client, in the treatment program. It is important to keep as many links to the client's life outside of therapy as possible. Family members are invited to participate in specific therapy groups and, in some instances, to share meals with the client in the communal dining room. Connection with community life may be maintained through client group activities, such as shopping, picnicking, attending movies, bowling, and visiting the zoo. Inpatient clients may be awarded passes to visit family or may participate in work-related activities, the length of time being determined by the activity and the client's condition. These connections with family and community facilitate the discharge process and may help to prevent the client from becoming too dependent on the therapy.

THE PROGRAM OF THERAPEUTIC COMMUNITY

Care for clients in the therapeutic community is directed by an interdisciplinary treatment (IDT) team. An initial assessment is made by the admitting psychiatrist, nurse, or other designated admitting agent, who establishes a priority of care. The IDT team determines a comprehensive treatment plan and goals of therapy and assigns intervention responsibilities. All members sign the treatment plan and meet regularly to update the plan as needed. Depending on the size of the treatment facility and scope of the therapy program, members representing a variety of disciplines may participate in the promotion of a therapeutic community. For example, an IDT team may include a psychiatrist, clinical psychologist, psychiatric clinical nurse specialist, psychiatric nurse, mental health technician, psychiatric social worker, occupational therapist, recreational therapist, art therapist, music therapist, psychodramatist, dietitian, and chaplain. Table 7–1 provides an explanation of responsibilities and educational preparation required for these members of the IDT team.

THE ROLE OF THE NURSE

Milieu therapy can take place in a variety of inpatient and outpatient settings. In the hospital, nurses are generally the only members of the IDT team who spend time with the clients on a 24-hour basis, and they assume responsibility for management of the therapeutic milieu. In all settings, the nursing process is used for the delivery of nursing care. Ongoing assessment, diagnosis, outcome identification, planning, implementation, and evaluation of the environment are necessary for the successful management of a therapeutic milieu. Nurses are involved in all day-to-day activities that pertain to client care. Suggestions and opinions of nursing staff are given serious consideration in the planning of care for individual clients. Information from the initial nursing assessment is used to create the IDT plan. Nurses have input into therapy goals and participate in the weekly updates and modification of treatment plans.

In some treatment facilities, a separate nursing care plan is required in addition to the IDT plan. When this is the case, the nursing care plan must reflect diagnoses that are specific to nursing and include problems and interventions from the IDT plan that have been assigned specifically to the discipline of nursing.

In the therapeutic milieu, nurses are responsible for ensuring that clients' physiological needs are met. Clients must be encouraged to perform as independently as possible in fulfilling activities of daily living.

TABLE 7 – 1 The Interdisciplinary Treatment Team in Psychiatry

Team Member	Responsibilities	Education Required
Psychiatrist	Serves as the leader of the team. Responsible for diagnosis and treatment of mental disorders. Performs psychotherapy; prescribes medication and other somatic therapies.	Medical degree with residency in psychiatry and license to practice medicine.
Clinical psychologist	Conducts individual, group, and family therapy. Administers, interprets, and evaluates psychological tests that assist in the diagnostic process.	Doctorate in clinical psychology with 2–3 year internship supervised by a licensed clinical psychologist. State license is required to practice.
Psychiatric clinical nurse specialist	Conducts individual, group, and family therapy. Presents educational programs for nursing staff. Provides consultation services to nurses who require assistance in the planning and implementation of care for individual clients.	Registered nurse with minimum of a master's degree in psychiatric nursing. Some institutions require certification by national credentialing association.
Psychiatric nurse	Provides ongoing assessment of client condition, both mentally and physically. Manages the therapeutic milieu on a 24-hour basis. Administers medications. Assists clients with all therapeutic activities as required. Focus is on one-to-one relationship development.	Registered nurse with hospital diploma, associate degree, or baccalaureate degree. Some psychiatric nurses have national certification.
Mental health technician (also called psychiatric aide or assistant or psychiatric technician)	Functions under the supervision of the psychiatric nurse. Provides assistance to clients in the fulfillment of their activities of daily living. Assists activity therapists as required in conducting their groups. May also participate in one-to-one relationship development.	Varies from state to state. Requirements include high school education, with additional vocational education or on-the-job training. Some hospitals hire individuals with baccalaureate degree in psychology in this capacity. Some states require a licensure examination to practice.
Psychiatric social worker	Conducts individual, group, and family therapy. Is concerned with client's social needs, such as placement, financial support, and community requirements. Conducts in-depth psychosocial history on which the needs assessment is based. Works with client and family to ensure that requirements for discharge are fulfilled and needs can be met by appropriate community resources.	Minimum of a master's degree in social work. Some states require additional supervision and subsequent licensure by examination.
Occupational therapist	Works with clients to help develop (or redevelop) independence in performance of activities of daily living. Focus is on rehabilitation and vocational training in which clients learn to be productive, thereby enhancing self-esteem. Creative activities and therapeutic relationship skills are used.	Baccalaureate or master's degree in occupational therapy.
Recreational therapist	Uses recreational activities to promote clients to redirect their thinking or to rechannel destructive energy in an appropriate manner. Clients learn skills that can be used during leisure time and during times of stress following discharge from treatment. Examples include bowling, volleyball, exercises, and jogging. Some programs include activities such as picnics, swimming, and even group attendance at the state fair when it is in session.	Baccalaureate or master's degree in recreational therapy.

(Continued)

TABLE 7 – 1 The Interdisciplinary Treatment Team in Psychiatry *(Continued)*

Team Member	Responsibilities	Education Required
Music therapist	Encourages clients in self-expression through music. Clients listen to music, play instruments, sing, dance, and compose songs that help them get in touch with feelings and emotions that they may not be able to experience in any other way.	Graduate degree with specialty in music therapy.
Art therapist	Uses the client's creative abilities to encourage expression of emotions and feelings through artwork. Helps clients to analyze their own work in an effort to recognize and resolve underlying conflict.	Graduate degree with specialty in art therapy.
Psychodramatist	Directs clients in the creation of a "drama" that portrays real-life situations. Individuals select problems they wish to enact, and other clients play the roles of significant others in the situations. Some clients are able to "act out" problems that they are unable to work through in a more traditional manner. All members benefit through intensive discussion that follows.	Graduate degree in psychology, social work, nursing, or medicine with additional training in group therapy and specialty preparation to become a psychodramatist.
Dietitian	Plans nutritious meals for all clients. Works on consulting basis for clients with specific eating disorders, such as anorexia nervosa, bulimia nervosa, obesity, and pica.	Baccalaureate or master's degree with specialty in dietetics.
Chaplain	Assesses, identifies, and attends to the spiritual needs of clients and their family members. Provides spiritual support and comfort as requested by client or family. May provide counseling if educational background includes this type of preparation.	College degree with advanced education in theology, seminary, or rabbinical studies.

However, the nurse must make ongoing assessments to provide assistance for those who require it. Assessing physical status is an important nursing responsibility that must not be overlooked in a psychiatric setting that emphasizes holistic care.

Reality orientation for clients who have disorganized thinking or who are disoriented or confused is important in the therapeutic milieu. Clocks with large hands and numbers, calendars that give the day and date in large print, and orientation boards that discuss daily activities and news happenings can help keep clients oriented to reality. Nurses should ensure that clients have written schedules of activities to which they are assigned and that they arrive at those activities on schedule. Some inpatient clients may require an identification sign on their door to remind them which room is theirs. All of these determinations are made from ongoing nursing assessments.

Nurses are responsible for the management of medication administration on inpatient psychiatric units. In some treatment programs, clients are expected to accept the responsibility and request their medication at the appropriate time. Although ultimate responsibility lies with the nurse, he or she must encourage clients to be self-reliant. Nurses must work with the clients to determine methods that result in achievement and provide positive feedback for successes.

A major focus of nursing in the therapeutic milieu is the one-to-one relationship, which grows out of a developing trust between client and nurse. Many clients with psychiatric disorders have never achieved the ability to trust. If this can be accomplished in a relationship with the nurse, the trust may be generalized to other relationships in the client's life. Developing trust means keeping promises that have been made. It means total acceptance of the individual as a person—separate from behavior that is unacceptable. It means responding to the client with concrete behaviors that are understandable to him or her (e.g., "If you are frightened, I will stay with you"; "If you are cold, I will bring you a blanket"; "If you are thirsty, I will bring you a drink of water"). Within an atmosphere of trust, the client is encouraged to express feelings and emotions and to discuss unresolved issues that are creating problems in his or her life.

The nurse is responsible for setting limits on unacceptable behavior in the therapeutic milieu. This requires stating to the client in understandable terminology what behaviors are not acceptable and what the consequences will be should the limits be violated. These limits must be established, written, and carried out by all staff. Consistency in carrying out the consequences of violation of the established limits is essential if the learning is to be reinforced.

The role of client teacher is important in the psychiatric area, as it is in all areas of nursing. Nurses must be able to assess learning readiness in individual clients. Do they want to learn? What is their level of anxiety? What is their level of ability to understand the information being presented? Topics for client education in psychiatry include information about medical diagnoses, side effects of medications, the importance of continuing to take medications, and stress management, among others. Some topics must be individualized for specific clients, whereas others may be taught in group situations. Table 7–2 outlines various topics of nursing concern for client education in psychiatry. Echternacht (2001) states:

> Milieu therapy interventions are recognized as one of the basic-level functions of psychiatric-mental health nurses as addressed [in the American Nurses Association *Scope and Standards of Psychiatric-Mental Health Nursing Practice*, 2000]. Milieu therapy has been described as an excellent framework for operationalizing Peplau's interpretation and extension of Harry Stack Sullivan's Interpersonal Theory for use in nursing practice. (p. 39) ... Now is the time to rekindle interest in the therapeutic milieu concept and to reclaim nursing's traditional milieu intervention functions. Nurses need to identify the number of registered nurses necessary to carry out structured and unstructured milieu functions consistent with their standards of practice. (p. 43)

TABLE 7 – 2 The Therapeutic Milieu—Topics for Client Education

1. Ways to increase self-esteem
2. Ways to deal with anger appropriately
3. Stress-management techniques
4. How to recognize signs of increasing anxiety and intervene to stop progression
5. Normal stages of grieving and behaviors associated with each stage
6. Assertiveness techniques
7. Relaxation techniques:
   a. Progressive relaxation
   b. Tense and relax
   c. Deep breathing
   d. Autogenics
8. Medications (specify)
   a. Reason for taking
   b. Harmless side effects
   c. Side effects to report to physician
   d. Importance of taking regularly
   e. Importance of not stopping abruptly
9. Effects of (substance) on the body
   a. Alcohol
   b. Other depressants
   d. Stimulants
   e. Hallucinogens
   f. Narcotics
   f. Cannabinols
10. Problem-solving skills
11. Thought-stopping/thought-switching techniques
12. Sex education
    a. Structure and function of reproductive system
    b. Contraceptives
    c. Sexually transmitted diseases
13. The essentials of good nutrition
14. (For parents/guardians)
    a. Signs and symptoms of substance abuse
    b. Effective parenting techniques

SUMMARY

In psychiatry, milieu therapy (or a therapeutic community) constitutes a manipulation of the environment in an effort to create behavioral changes and to improve the psychological health and functioning of the individual. The goal of therapeutic community is for the client to learn adaptive coping, interaction, and relationship skills that can be generalized to other aspects of his or her life. The community environment itself serves as the primary tool of therapy.

According to Skinner (1979), a therapeutic community is based on seven basic assumptions:

1. The health in each individual is to be realized and encouraged to grow.
2. Every interaction is an opportunity for therapeutic intervention.
3. The client owns his or her own environment.
4. Each client owns his or her behavior.
5. Peer pressure is a useful and a powerful tool.
6. Inappropriate behaviors are dealt with as they occur.
7. Restrictions and punishment are to be avoided.

Because the goals of milieu therapy relate to helping the client learn to generalize that which is learned to other aspects of his or her life, the conditions that promote a therapeutic community in a treatment setting are similar to the types of conditions that exist in real-life situations. They include the following:

1. The fulfillment of basic physiological needs.
2. Physical facilities that are conducive to achievement of the goals of therapy.
3. The existence of a democratic form of self-government.
4. The assignment of responsibilities according to client capabilities.
5. A structured program of social and work-related activities.
6. The inclusion of community and family in the program of therapy in an effort to facilitate discharge from treatment.

The program of therapy on the milieu unit is conducted by the IDT team. The team includes some, or all, of the following disciplines and may include others that are not specified here: psychiatrist, clinical psychologist, psychiatric clinical nurse specialist, psychiatric nurse, mental health technician, psychiatric social worker, occupational therapist, recreational therapist, art therapist, music therapist, psychodramatist, dietitian, and chaplain.

Nurses play a crucial role in the management of a therapeutic milieu. They are involved in the assessment, diagnosis, outcome identification, planning, implementation, and evaluation of all treatment programs. They have significant input into the IDT plans, which are developed for all clients. They are responsible for ensuring that clients' basic needs are fulfilled; assessing physical and psychosocial status continually; administering medication; helping the client develop trusting relationships; setting limits on unacceptable behaviors; educating clients; and, ultimately, helping clients, within the limits of their capability, to become productive members of society.

REVIEW QUESTIONS

SELF-EXAMINATION/LEARNING EXERCISE

Test your knowledge of milieu therapy by supplying the information requested.

1. Define milieu therapy.
2. What is the goal of milieu therapy/therapeutic community?

Select the best response in each of the following questions:

3. In prioritizing care within the therapeutic environment, which of the following nursing interventions would receive the highest priority?
   a. Ensuring that the physical facilities are conducive to achievement of the goals of therapy.
   b. Scheduling a community meeting for 8:30 each morning.
   c. Attending to the nutritional and comfort needs of all clients.
   d. Establishing contacts with community resources.
4. In the community meeting, which of the following actions is most important for reinforcing the democratic posture of the therapy setting?
   a. Allowing each person specific and equal amount of time to talk.
   b. Reviewing group rules and behavioral limits that apply to all clients.
   c. Reading the minutes from yesterday's meeting.
   d. Waiting until all clients are present before initiating the meeting.
5. One of the goals of therapeutic community is for clients to become more independent and accept self-responsibility. Which of the following approaches by staff best encourages fulfillment of this goal?
   a. Including client input and decisions into the treatment plan.
   b. Insisting that each client take a turn as "president" of the community meeting.
   c. Making decisions for the client regarding plans for treatment.
   d. Requiring that the client be bathed, dressed, and attends breakfast on time each morning.
6. Client teaching is an important nursing function in milieu therapy. Which of the following statements by the client indicates the need for knowledge and a readiness to learn?
   a. "Get away from me with that medicine! I'm not sick!"
   b. "I don't belong on the psych unit. It's my migraine headaches that I need help with."
   c. "I've taken Valium every day of my life for the last 20 years. I'll stop when I'm good and ready!"
   d. "The doctor says I have bipolar disorder. What does that really mean?"

Match the following activities with the responsible therapist from the IDT team:

______	7. Psychiatrist	a. Helps clients plan, shop for, and cook a meal.
______	8. Clinical psychologist	b. Locates halfway house and arranges living conditions for client being discharged from the hospital.
______	9. Psychiatric social worker	c. Helps clients get to know themselves better by having them describe what they feel when they hear a certain song.

______ 10. Psychiatric clinical nurse specialist	d. Helps clients to recognize their own beliefs so that they may draw comfort from those beliefs in time of spiritual need.
______ 11. Psychiatric nurse	e. Accompanies clients on community trip to the zoo.
______ 12. Mental health technician	f. Diagnoses mental disorders, conducts psychotherapy, and prescribes somatic therapies.
______ 13. Occupational therapist	g. Manages the therapeutic milieu on a 24-hour basis.
______ 14. Recreational therapist	h. Conducts group and family therapies and administers and evaluates psychological tests that assist in the diagnostic process.
______ 15. Music therapist	i. Conducts group therapies and provides consultation and education to staff nurses.
______ 16. Art therapist	j. Assists staff nurses in the management of the milieu.
______ 17. Psychodramatist	k. Encourages clients to express painful emotions by drawing pictures on paper.
______ 18. Dietitian	l. Assesses needs, establishes, monitors, and evaluates a nutritional program for a client with anorexia nervosa.
______ 19. Chaplain	m. Directs a group of clients in acting out a situation that is otherwise too painful for a client to discuss openly.

REFERENCES

American Nurses Association (2000). Scope and standards of psychiatric-mental health nursing practice. Washington DC: Author.

Bowler, J.B. (1991). Transformation into a healing healthcare environment: Recovering the possibilities of psychiatric/mental health nursing. Perspectives in Psychiatric Care, 27:21–25.

DeSocio, J., Bowllan, N., & Staschak, S. (1997). Lessons learned in creating a safe and therapeutic milieu for children, adolescents, and families: Developmental considerations. Journal of Child and Adolescent Psychiatric Nursing, 10:18–26.

Echternacht, M.R. (2001). Fluid group: Concept and clinical application in the therapeutic milieu. Journal of the American Psychiatric Nurses Association, 7:39–44.

Hall, B.A. (1995). Use of milieu therapy: The context and environment as therapeutic practice for psychiatric-mental health nurses. In C.A. Anderson (Ed.), Psychiatric nursing 1974 to 1994: A report on the state of the art. St. Louis: Mosby Year Book.

Whall, A.L. (1991). Using the environment to improve the mental health of the elderly. Journal of Gerontological Nursing, 17:39.

CLASSICAL REFERENCES

Maslow, A. (1968). Towards a psychology of being (2nd ed.). New York: Van Nostrand.

Skinner, K. (1979, August). The therapeutic milieu: Making it work. Journal of Psychiatric Nursing and Mental Health Services, 38–44.

8

CHAPTER

TOWNSEND ESSENTIALS

INTERVENTION IN GROUPS

CHAPTER OUTLINE

KEY TERMS

altruism
autocratic
catharsis
democratic
group therapy
laissez-faire
psychodrama
family therapy
universality
genogram
therapeutic group

OBJECTIVES

After reading this chapter, the student will be able to:

1. Define a *group*.
2. Discuss eight functions of a group.
3. Identify various types of groups.
4. Describe physical conditions that influence groups.
5. Discuss "curative factors" that occur in groups.
6. Describe the phases of group development.
7. Identify various leadership styles in groups.
8. Identify various roles that members assume within a group.
9. Discuss psychodrama and family therapy as specialized forms of group therapy.
10. Describe the role of the nurse in group therapy.

INTRODUCTION

Human beings are complex creatures who share their activities of daily living with various *groups* of people. Sampson and Marthas (1990) state:

> We are *biological* organisms possessing qualities shared with all living systems and with others of our species. We are *psychological* beings with distinctly human capabilities for thought, feeling, and action. We are also *social* beings, who function as part of the complex webs that link us with other people. (p. 3)

Healthcare professionals not only share their personal lives with groups of people but also encounter multiple group situations in their professional operations. Some examples include team conferences, committee meetings, grand rounds, and in-service sessions, to name a few. In psychiatry, work with clients and families often takes the form of groups. With group work, not only does the nurse have the opportunity to reach out to a greater number of people at one time but those individuals also assist each other by bringing to the group and sharing their feelings, opinions, ideas, and behaviors. Clients learn from each other in a group setting.

This chapter explores various types and methods of therapeutic groups that can be used with psychiatric clients and the role of the nurse in group intervention. A discussion of the family as a specialized type of group is also presented.

GROUP DEFINED

A *group* is a collection of individuals whose association is founded on shared commonalities of interest, values, norms, or purpose. Membership in a group is generally by chance (born into the group), by choice (voluntary affiliation), or by circumstance (the result of life-cycle events over which an individual may or may not have control).

FUNCTIONS OF A GROUP

Sampson and Marthas (1990) have outlined eight functions that groups serve for their members. They contend that groups may serve more than one function and usually serve different functions for different members of the group. The eight functions are:

1. **Socialization.** The cultural group into which we are born begins the process of teaching social norms. This is continued throughout our lives by members of other groups with which we become affiliated.
2. **Support.** One's fellow group members are available in time of need. Individuals derive a feeling of security from group involvement.
3. **Task completion.** Group members provide assistance in endeavors that are beyond the capacity of one individual alone or when results can be achieved more effectively as a team.
4. **Camaraderie.** Members of a group provide the joy and pleasure that individuals seek from interactions with significant others.
5. **Informational.** Learning takes place within groups. Explanations regarding world events occur in groups. Knowledge is gained when individual members learn how others in the group have resolved situations similar to those with which they are currently struggling.
6. **Normative.** This function relates to the ways in which groups enforce the established norms.
7. **Empowerment.** Groups help to bring about improvement in existing conditions by providing support to individual members who seek to bring about change. Groups have power that individuals alone do not.
8. **Governance.** An example of the governing function is that of rules being made by committees within a larger organization.

TYPES OF GROUPS

The functions of a group vary depending on the reason the group was formed. Clark (2000) identifies three types of groups in which nurses most often participate: task groups, teaching groups, and supportive/therapeutic groups.

Task Groups

The function of a task group is to accomplish a specific outcome or task. The focus is on solving problems and making decisions to achieve this outcome. Often, a deadline is placed on completion of the task, and such importance is placed on a satisfactory outcome that conflict within the group may be smoothed over or ignored in order to focus on the priority at hand.

Teaching Groups

Teaching, or educational, groups exist to convey knowledge and information to a number of individuals. Nurses can be involved in teaching groups of many varieties, such as medication education, childbirth education, breast self-examination, and effective parenting classes. These groups usually have a set time or a set number of meetings. Members learn from each other as well as from the designated instructor. The objective of teaching groups is verbalization or demonstration by the learner of the material presented by the end of the designated period.

Supportive/Therapeutic Groups

The primary concern of support groups is to prevent future upsets by teaching participants effective ways of dealing with emotional stress arising from situational or developmental crises. For the purposes of this text, it is important to differentiate between **therapeutic group** and **group therapy**. Leaders of group therapy generally have advanced degrees in psychology, social work, nursing, or medicine. They often have additional training or experience under the supervision of an accomplished professional in conducting group psychotherapy based on various theoretical frameworks, such as psychoanalytic, psychodynamic, interpersonal, or family dynamics. Approaches based on these theories are used by the group therapy leaders to encourage improvement in the ability of group members to function on an interpersonal level.

Therapeutic groups, on the other hand, are based to a lesser extent in theory. Focus is more on group relations, interactions among group members, and the consideration of a selected issue. Like group therapists, individuals who lead therapeutic groups must be knowledgeable in *group process*; that is, the *ways* in which group members interact with each other. Interruptions, silences, judgments, glares, and scapegoating are examples of group processes (Clark, 2000). They must also have thorough knowledge of *group content*, the topic or issue being discussed within the group, and the ability to present the topic in language that can be understood by all group members. Many nurses who work in psychiatry lead supportive/therapeutic groups.

Self-Help Groups

An additional type of group, in which nurses may or may not be involved, is the self-help group. Self-help groups have grown in numbers and in credibility in recent years. They allow clients to talk about their fears and relieve feelings of isolation while receiving comfort and advice from others undergoing similar experiences (Harvard Medical School, 1998). Examples of self-help groups are Alzheimer's Disease and Related Disorders, Anorexia Nervosa and Associated Disorders, Weight Watchers, Alcoholics Anonymous, Reach to Recovery, Parents Without Partners, Overeaters Anonymous, Adult Children of Alcoholics, and many others related to specific needs or illnesses. These groups may or may not have a professional leader or consultant. They are run by members, and leadership often rotates from member to member.

Nurses may become involved with self-help groups either voluntarily or because their advice or participation has been requested by the members. The nurse may function as a referral agent, resource person, member of an advisory board, or leader of the group. Self-help groups are a valuable source of referral for clients with specific problems. However, nurses must be knowledgeable about the purposes of the group, membership, leadership, benefits, and problems that might threaten the success of the group before making referrals to their clients for a specific self-help group. The nurse may find it necessary to attend several meetings of a particular group, if possible, to assess its effectiveness of purpose and appropriateness for client referral.

PHYSICAL CONDITIONS THAT INFLUENCE GROUP DYNAMICS

Seating

The physical conditions for the group should be set up so that there is no barrier between the members. For example, a circle of chairs is better than chairs set around a table. Members should be encouraged to sit in different chairs each meeting. This openness and change creates an uncomfortableness that encourages anxious and unsettled behaviors that can then be explored within the group.

Size

Various authors have suggested different ranges of size as ideal for group interaction: 4 to 7 (Huber, 1996), 2 to 15 (Sampson & Marthas, 1990), and 4 to 12 (Clark, 2000). Group size does make a difference in the interaction among members. The larger the group, the less time there is available to devote to each member. In fact, in larger groups, those more aggressive individuals are most likely to be heard, whereas quieter members may be left out of the discussions altogether. On the other hand, larger groups provide more opportunities for individuals to learn from other members. The wider range of life experiences and knowledge provides a greater potential for effective group problem-solving. Studies have indicated that a composition of seven or eight members provides a favorable climate for optimal group interaction and relationship development.

Membership

Whether the group is open- or closed-ended is another condition that influences the dynamics of group process. Open-ended groups are those in which members leave and others join at any time during the existence of the group. The continuous movement of members in and out of the group creates the type of uncomfortableness described previously that encourages unsettled behaviors in individual members and fosters the exploration of feelings. These are the most common types of groups held on short-term inpatient units, and they are also used in outpatient and long-term care facilities. Closed-ended groups usually have a predetermined, fixed period. All members join at the time the group is organized, and terminate their membership at the end of the designated period. Closed-ended groups are often composed of individuals with common issues or problems they wish to address.

CURATIVE FACTORS

Why are therapeutic groups helpful? Yalom (1985) identified 11 curative factors that individuals can achieve through interpersonal interactions within the group. Some of the factors are present in most groups in varying degrees. These curative factors identified by Yalom include:

1. **The instillation of hope.** By observing the progress of others in the group with similar problems, a group member garners hope that his or her problems can also be resolved.
2. **Universality.** Individuals come to realize that they are not alone in the problems, thoughts, and feelings they are experiencing. Anxiety is relieved by the support and understanding of others in the group who share similar (universal) experiences.
3. **The imparting of information.** Knowledge is gained through formal instruction and the sharing of advice and suggestions among group members.
4. **Altruism. Altruism** is assimilated by group members through mutual sharing and concern for each other. Providing assistance and support to others creates a positive self-image and promotes self-growth.
5. **The corrective recapitulation of the primary family group.** Group members are able to reexperience early family conflicts that remain unresolved. Attempts at resolution are promoted through feedback and exploration.
6. **The development of socializing techniques.** Through interaction with and feedback from other members in the group, individuals are able to correct maladaptive social behaviors and learn and develop new social skills.
7. **Imitative behavior.** In this setting, one who has mastered a particular psychosocial skill or developmental task can be a valuable role model for others. Individuals may imitate selected behaviors that they wish to develop in themselves.
8. **Interpersonal learning.** The group offers many and varied opportunities for interacting with other people. Insight is gained regarding how one perceives and is perceived by others.
9. **Group cohesiveness.** Members develop a sense of belonging that separates the individual ("I am") from the group ("we are"). Out of this alliance emerges a common feeling that both individual members and the total group are of value to each other.
10. **Catharsis.** Within the group, members are able to express both positive and negative feelings—perhaps feelings that have never been expressed before—in a nonthreatening atmosphere. This **catharsis**, or open expression of feelings, is beneficial for the individual in the group.
11. **Existential factors.** The group is able to help individual members take direction of their own lives and to accept responsibility for the quality of their existence.

It may be helpful for a group leader to explain these curative factors to members of the group. Positive responses are experienced by individuals who understand and are able to recognize curative factors as they occur within the group.

PHASES OF GROUP DEVELOPMENT

Groups, like individuals, move through phases of life-cycle development. Ideally, groups progress from the phase of infancy to advanced maturity in an effort to fulfill the objectives set forth by the membership. Unfortunately, as with individuals, some groups become fixed in early developmental levels and never progress, or they experience periods of regression in the developmental process. Three phases of group development are discussed here.

Phase I. Initial or Orientation Phase

Group Activities

The leader and members work together to establish the rules that will govern the group (e.g., when and where meetings will occur, the importance of confidentiality, how meetings will be structured). Goals of the group are established. Members are introduced to each other.

Leader Expectations

The leader is expected to orient members to specific group processes, encourage members to participate without disclosing too much too soon, promote an environment of trust, and ensure that rules established by the group do not interfere with fulfillment of the goals.

Member Behaviors

In phase I, members have not yet established trust and will respond to this lack of trust by being overly polite. There is a fear of not being accepted by the group. They may try to "get on the good side" of the leader with compliments and conforming behaviors. A power struggle may ensue as members compete for their position in the "pecking order" of the group.

Phase II. Middle or Working Phase

Group Activities

Ideally, during the working phase, cohesiveness has been established within the group. This is when the productive work toward completion of the task is undertaken. Problem-solving and decision-making occur within the group. In the mature group, cooperation prevails, and differences and disagreements are confronted and resolved.

Leader Expectations

The role of leader diminishes and becomes one of facilitator during the working phase. Some leadership functions are shared by certain members of the group as they progress toward resolution. The leader helps to resolve conflict and continues to foster cohesiveness among the members while ensuring that they do not deviate from the intended task or purpose for which the group was organized.

Member Behaviors

At this point, trust has been established among the members. They turn more often to each other and less often to the leader for guidance. They accept criticism from each other, using it in a constructive manner to create change. Occasionally, subgroups will form in which two or more members conspire with each other to the exclusion of the rest of the group. To maintain group cohesion, these subgroups must be confronted and discussed by the entire membership. Conflict is managed by the group with minimal assistance from the leader.

Phase III. Final or Termination Phase

Group Activities

The longer a group has been in existence, the more difficult termination is likely to be for the members. Termination should be mentioned from the outset of group formation. It should be discussed in depth for several meetings before the final session. A sense of loss that precipitates the grief process may be evident, particularly in groups that have been successful in their stated purpose.

Leader Expectations

In the termination phase, the leader encourages the group members to reminisce about what has occurred within the group, to review the goals and discuss the actual outcomes, and to encourage members to provide feedback to each other about individual progress within the group. The leader encourages members to discuss feelings of loss associated with termination of the group.

Member Behaviors

Members may express surprise over the actual materialization of the end. This represents the grief response of denial, which may then progress to anger. Anger toward other group members or toward the leader may reflect feelings of abandonment (Sampson & Marthas, 1990). These feelings may lead to individual members' discussions of previous losses for which similar emotions were experienced. Successful termination of the group may help members develop the skills needed when losses occur in other dimensions of their lives.

LEADERSHIP STYLES

Three of the most common group leadership styles have been described by Lippitt and White (1958). They include **autocratic, democratic**, and **laissez-faire.** Table 8–1 outlines a comparison of the three leadership styles.

Autocratic

Autocratic leaders have personal goals for the group. They withhold information from group members, particularly issues that may interfere with achievement of their own objectives. The message that is conveyed to the group is: "We will do it my way. My way is best." The focus in this style of leadership is on the leader. Members are dependent on the leader for problem-solving, decision-making, and obtaining permission to perform. The approach of the autocratic leader is one of persuasion, striving to persuade others in the group that his or her ideas and methods are superior. Productivity is high with this type of leadership, but often morale within the group is low owing to lack of member input and creativity.

Democratic

The democratic leadership style focuses on the members of the group. Information is shared with members in an effort to allow them to make decisions regarding achieving the goals for the group. Members are encouraged to participate fully in problem-solving of issues that relate to the group, including taking action to effect change. The message conveyed to the group is: "Decide what must be done, consider the alternatives, make a selection, and proceed with the actions required to complete the task." The leader provides guidance and expertise as needed. Productivity is lower than it is with autocratic leadership, but morale is much higher because of the extent of input allowed all members of the group and the potential for individual creativity.

Laissez-Faire

This leadership style allows people to do as they please. There is no direction from the leader. In fact, the laissez-faire leader's approach is noninvolvement. Goals for the group are undefined. No decisions are made, no problems are solved, and no action is taken. Members become frustrated and confused, and productivity and morale are low.

MEMBER ROLES

Benne and Sheats (1948) identified three major types of roles that individuals play within the membership of the group. These are roles that serve to:

1. Complete the task of the group.
2. Maintain or enhance group processes.
3. Fulfill personal or individual needs.

Task roles and maintenance roles contribute to the success or effectiveness of the group. Personal roles satisfy needs of the individual members, sometimes to the extent of interfering with the effectiveness of the group.

TABLE 8 – 1 Leadership Styles—Similarities and Differences

Characteristics	Autocratic	Democratic	Laissez-Faire
1. Focus	Leader	Members	Undetermined
2. Task strategy	Members are persuaded to adopt leader's ideas	Members engage in group problem-solving	No defined strategy
3. Member participation	Limited	Unlimited	Inconsistent
4. Individual creativity	Stifled	Encouraged	Not addressed
5. Member enthusiasm and morale	Low	High	Low
6. Group cohesiveness	Low	High	Low
7. Productivity	High	High (may not be as high as in autocratic)	Low
8. Individual motivation and commitment	Low (tend to work only when leader is present to urge them to do so)	High (satisfaction derived from personal input and participation)	Low (feelings of frustration from lack of direction or guidance)

Table 8–2 presents an outline of specific roles within these three major types and the behaviors associated with each.

PSYCHODRAMA

A specialized type of therapeutic group, called **psychodrama**, was introduced by J. L. Moreno, a Viennese psychiatrist. Moreno's method employs a dramatic approach in which clients become "actors" in life-situation scenarios.

The group leader is called the *director*, group members are the *audience*, and the *set* or *stage* may be specially designed or may just be any room or part of a room selected for this purpose. Actors are members from the audience who agree to take part in the "drama" by role-playing a situation about which they have been informed by the director. Usually the situation is an issue with which an individual client has been struggling. The client plays the role of himself or herself and is called the *protagonist*. In this role, the client is able to express true feelings toward individuals (represented by group members) with whom he or she has unresolved conflicts.

In some instances, the group leader may ask a client to volunteer to be the protagonist for that session. The client may choose a situation he or she wishes to enact and select the audience members to portray the roles of others in the life situation.

The psychodrama setting provides the client with a safer and less-threatening atmosphere than the real situation in which to express true feelings. Resolution of interpersonal conflicts is facilitated.

When the drama has been completed, group members from the audience discuss the situation they have observed, offer feedback, express their feelings, and relate their own similar experiences. In this way, all group members benefit from the session, either directly or indirectly.

TABLE 8 – 2 Member Roles Within Groups

Role	Behaviors
Task Roles	
Coordinator	Clarifies ideas and suggestions that have been made within the group; brings relationships together to pursue common goals
Evaluator	Examines group plans and performance, measuring against group standards and goals
Elaborator	Explains and expands upon group plans and ideas
Energizer	Encourages and motivates group to perform at its maximum potential
Initiator	Outlines the task at hand for the group and proposes methods for solution
Orienter	Maintains direction within the group
Maintenance Roles	
Compromiser	Relieves conflict within the group by assisting members to reach a compromise agreeable to all
Encourager	Offers recognition and acceptance of others' ideas and contributions
Follower	Listens attentively to group interaction; is passive participant
Gatekeeper	Encourages acceptance of, and participation by, all members of the group
Harmonizer	Minimizes tension within the group by intervening when disagreements produce conflict
Individual (Personal) Roles	
Aggressor	Expresses negativism and hostility toward other members; may use sarcasm in effort to degrade the status of others
Blocker	Resists group efforts; demonstrates rigid and sometimes irrational behaviors that impede group progress
Dominator	Manipulates others to gain control; behaves in authoritarian manner
Help-seeker	Uses the group to gain sympathy from others; seeks to increase self-confidence from group feedback; lacks concern for others or for the group as a whole
Monopolizer	Maintains control of the group by dominating the conversation
Mute or silent member	Does not participate verbally; remains silent for a variety of reasons—may feel uncomfortable with self-disclosure or may be seeking attention through silence
Recognition seeker	Talks about personal accomplishments in an effort to gain attention for self
Seducer	Shares intimate details about self with group; is the least reluctant of the group to do so; may frighten others in the group and inhibit group progress with excessive premature self-disclosure

Adapted from Benne and Sheats, 1948.

Nurses often serve as actors, or role players, in psychodrama sessions. Leaders of psychodrama have graduate degrees in psychology, social work, nursing, or medicine, with additional training in group therapy and specialty preparation to become a psychodramatist.

THE FAMILY AS A GROUP

Family therapy is a type of therapeutic modality in which the focus of treatment is on the family as a unit. It represents a form of intervention in which members of a family are assisted to identify and change problematic, maladaptive, self-defeating, repetitive relationship patterns (Goldenberg & Goldenberg, 1995). In family therapy, the family is viewed as a *system* in which the members are interdependent; a change in one part (member) within the system affects or creates change in all the other parts (members). The focus is not on an individual, identified client; it is on the family as a whole. The basic concept of this form of treatment is that it is faster, more logical, more satisfactory, and more economical to treat all members of a system of relationships than to concentrate on the person who is supposed to be in need of treatment (Goldenberg & Goldenberg, 1995).

Because the major goal of family therapy is to bring about positive change in relationships, the therapist ideally conducts the initial assessment with the entire family. If this is not possible, information is gathered from the client who has sought treatment, and an appointment is scheduled to meet with the family later. The initial assessment is not complete until the therapist has had the opportunity to observe the interactions among all family members.

Some family therapists favor the use of a **genogram** in the study of multiple generations within families. Genograms offer the convenience of a great deal of information in a small amount of space. They can also be used as teaching tools with the family itself. An overall picture of the life of the family over several generations can be conveyed, including roles that various family members play, and emotional distance between specific individuals. Areas for change can be easily identified. A sample genogram is presented in Figure 8–1.

Once the assessment has been completed and problems identified, family members establish goals for change with guidance from the therapist. Change occurs through open, honest communication among all family members. The family therapist's role is to facilitate this type of interaction. As goals are achieved and change occurs, family members will demonstrate the ability to communicate effectively, the ability to resolve conflicts adaptively, and the ability for each to

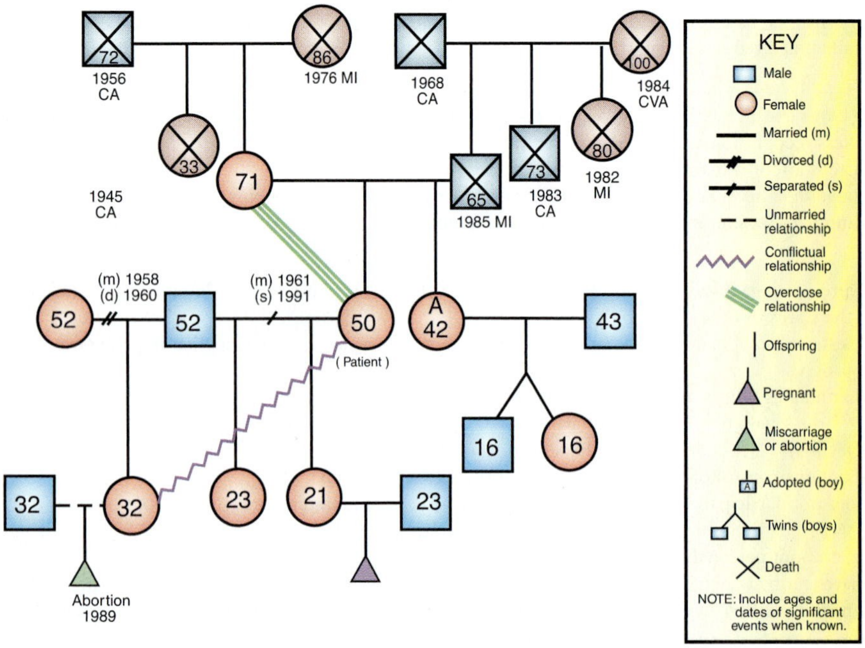

FIGURE 8–1 Sample genogram.

function both independently and interdependently in a healthy manner.

Nurses who conduct family therapy are expected to possess a graduate degree and have considerable knowledge of family theory. However, it is within the realm of the generalist nurse in psychiatry to contribute to the assessment and planning phases of family therapy and to ongoing observation and evaluation. Family consideration in individual client care is also essential. Nurses should have a basic understanding of family dynamics and the ability to distinguish between functional and dysfunctional behaviors within a family system.

THE ROLE OF THE NURSE IN GROUP INTERVENTIONS

Nurses participate in group situations on a daily basis. Within healthcare settings, nurses serve on or lead task groups that create policy, describe procedures, and plan client care. They also participate in a variety of other groups aimed at the institutional effort of serving the consumer. Nurses are encouraged to use the steps of the nursing process as a framework for task group leadership.

In psychiatry, nurses may lead various types of therapeutic groups, such as client education, assertiveness training, support, parenting, and transition to discharge groups, among others. To function effectively in the leadership capacity for these groups, nurses need to be able to recognize various processes that occur in groups (e.g., the phases of group development, the various roles that people play within group situations, and the motivation behind the behavior) and be able to select the most appropriate leadership style for the type of group being led. Generalist nurses may develop these skills as part of their undergraduate education, or they may pursue additional study while serving and learning as the coleader of a group with a more experienced nurse leader.

Generalist nurses in psychiatry rarely serve as leaders of psychotherapy groups. The *Scope and Standards of Psychiatric-Mental Health Nursing Practice* (American Nurses Association, 2000) specifies that nurses who serve as family and group psychotherapists should have a minimum of a master's degree in psychiatric nursing. Other criteria that have been suggested are educational preparation in group theory, extended practice as a group coleader or leader under the supervision of an experienced psychotherapist, and participation in group therapy on an experiential level. Additional specialist training is required beyond the master's level to prepare nurses to become family therapists or psychodramatists.

Leading therapeutic groups is within the realm of nursing practice. Because group work is such a common therapeutic approach in the discipline of psychiatry, nurses working in this field must continually strive to expand their knowledge and use group process as a significant psychiatric nursing intervention.

SUMMARY

A *group* has been defined as "a collection of individuals whose association is founded upon shared commonalities of interest, values, norms, or purpose." Groups serve various functions for their members. Eight group functions were defined by Sampson and Marthas (1990). They include socialization, support, task completion, camaraderie, informational, normative, empowerment, and governance.

Three types of groups were identified: (1) task groups, whose function it is to solve problems, make decisions, and achieve a specific outcome; (2) teaching groups, in which knowledge and information are conveyed to a number of individuals; and (3) supportive/therapeutic groups, whose function it is to educate people to deal effectively with emotional stress in their lives.

Self-help groups also can be beneficial to clients with specific problems. In self-help groups, members share the same type of problem and help each other to prevent decompensation because of that problem. Professionals may or may not be a part of self-help groups.

Group therapy is differentiated from *therapeutic groups* by amount of educational preparation of the leader. Group psychotherapists have advanced degrees in psychology, social work, medicine, or nursing. The focus of group psychotherapy is more theoretically based than it is in therapeutic groups.

Certain physical conditions, such as placement of the seating and size of the group, influence group interaction. Whether the group is open-ended or closed-ended also can affect group performance. In an *open-ended* group, members leave and others join at any time during the existence of the group. *Closed-ended* groups have a predetermined, fixed time frame. All members join the group at the same time and leave at the end of the designated period.

Yalom (1985) identified a number of benefits that individuals derive from participation in therapeutic groups. He called these benefits *curative factors*. They include the instillation of hope, universality, the imparting of information, altruism, the corrective recapitulation of the primary family group, the development of socializing techniques, imitative behavior, interpersonal learning, group cohesiveness, catharsis, and existential factors.

Groups progress through three major phases of development. In the initial (orientation) phase, members are introduced to each other, rules and goals of the group are established, and a trusting relationship is initiated. In the second phase, called the middle or working phase, the actual work of the group takes place. As the group matures, trust is established, and members cooperate in decision-making and problem-solving, with the leader then serving more as a facilitator. The final or termination phase can be difficult, particularly if the group has been together for a long time. A sense of loss can trigger the grief response, and it is essential that members confront these feelings and work through them before the final session.

Group leadership styles may vary. The *autocratic* leader concentrates on fulfillment of his or her own objectives for the group. This is achieved through persuasive selling of personal ideas to the group. Productivity is high with this type of leader, but morale and motivation are low. With a *democratic* leader, group members are encouraged to participate fully in the decision-making process. The leader provides guidance and expertise as needed. Productivity is lower than with autocratic leadership, but morale and motivation are much higher. In a group with *laissez-faire* leadership, the members essentially receive no direction at all. Goals are not established, decisions are not made, everyone does as he or she pleases, and confusion prevails. Productivity, morale, and motivation are low.

Members play various roles within groups. These roles are categorized according to *task roles*, *maintenance roles*, and *personal roles*. Task roles and maintenance roles contribute to the success or effectiveness of the group. Personal roles satisfy needs of the individual members, sometimes to the extent of interfering with the effectiveness of the group.

Psychodrama is a specialized type of group therapy that uses a dramatic approach in which clients become "actors" in life-situation scenarios. The psychodrama setting provides the client with a safer and less threatening atmosphere than the real situation in which to express and work through unresolved conflicts. Specialized training, in addition to a master's degree, is required for nurses to serve as psychodramatists.

Family therapy brings together some or all members of the family in a group situation. The major goal is to bring about positive change in relationships. The therapist helps family members to identify problems, establish goals for change, and work toward achievement of those goals through open, honest communication.

Nurses lead various types of therapeutic groups in the psychiatric setting. Knowledge of human behavior in general and the group process in particular is essential to effective group leadership. Specialized training, in addition to a master's degree, is required for nurses to serve as group psychotherapists, psychodramatists, or family therapists.

REVIEW QUESTIONS

SELF-EXAMINATION/LEARNING EXERCISE

Test your knowledge of group process by supplying the information requested.

1. Define a *group*.
2. Identify the type of group and leadership style in each of the following situations:
   a. NJ is the nurse leader of a childbirth preparation group. Each week she shows various films and sets out various reading materials. She expects the participants to utilize their time on a topic of their choice or practice skills they have observed on the films. Two couples have dropped out of the group, stating, "This is a big waste of time."
   Type of group______________________________________
   Style of leadership___________________________________
   b. MK is a psychiatric nurse who has been selected to lead a group for women who desire to lose weight. The criteria for membership is that they must be at least 20 pounds overweight. All have tried to lose weight on their own many times in the past without success. At their first meeting, MK provided suggestions as the members determine what their goals will be and how they plan to go about achieving those goals. They decided how often they wanted to meet and what they planned to do at each meeting.
   Type of group______________________________________
   Style of leadership___________________________________
   c. JJ is a staff nurse on a surgical unit. He has been selected as leader of a newly established group of staff nurses organized to determine ways to decrease the number of medication errors occurring on the unit. JJ has definite ideas about how to do this. He has also applied for the position of head nurse on the unit and believes that if he is successful in leading the group toward achievement of its goals, he can increase his chances for promotion. At each meeting, he addresses the group in an effort to convince the members to adopt his ideas.
   Type of group______________________________________
   Style of leadership___________________________________

Match the situation on the right to the curative factor or benefit it describes on the left:

______ 3. Instillation of hope	a. Sam admires the way Jack stands up for what he believes. He decides to practice this himself.
______ 4. Universality	b. Nancy sees that Jane has been a widow for 5 years now and has adjusted well. She thinks that maybe she can too.
______ 5. Imparting of information	c. Susan has come to realize that she has the power to shape the direction of her life.
______ 6. Altruism	d. John is able to have a discussion with another person for the first time in his life.
______ 7. Corrective recapitulation of the primary family group	e. Linda now understands that her mother really did love her, although she was not able to show it.
______ 8. Development of socializing techniques	f. Alice has come to feel as though the other group members are like a family to her. She looks forward to the meetings each week.

_______ 9. Imitative behavior	g. Tony talks in the group about the abuse he experienced as a child. He has never told anyone about this before.
_______ 10. Interpersonal learning	h. Sandra felt so good about herself when she left the group tonight. She had provided both physical and emotional support to Judy who shared for the first time about being raped.
_______ 11. Group cohesiveness	i. Judy appreciated Sandra's support as she expressed her feelings related to the rape. She had come to believe that no one else felt as she did.
_______ 12. Catharsis	j. Paul knew that people did not want to be his friend because of his violent temper. In the group he has learned to control his temper and form satisfactory interpersonal relationships with others.
_______ 13. Existential factors	k. Henry learned about the effects of alcohol on the body when a nurse from the chemical dependency unit spoke to the group.

Match the individual on the right to the role he or she is playing within the group:

_______ 14. Aggressor	a. Nancy talks incessantly in the group. When someone else tries to make a comment, she refuses to allow him or her to speak.
_______ 15. Blocker	b. On the first day the group meets, Valerie shares the intimate details of her incestuous relationship with her father.
_______ 16. Dominator	c. Colleen listens with interest to everything the other members say, but she does not say anything herself in the group.
_______ 17. Help seeker	d. Violet is obsessed with her physical appearance. Although she is beautiful, she has little self-confidence and needs continuous positive feedback. She states, "Maybe if I became a blond my boyfriend would love me more."
_______ 18. Monopolizer	e. Larry states to Violet, "Listen, dummy, you need more than blond hair to keep the guy around. A bit more in the brains department would help!"
_______ 19. Mute or silent member	f. At the beginning of the group meeting, Dan says, "All right now, I have a date tonight. I want this meeting over on time! I'll keep track of the time and let everyone know when his or her time is up. When I say you're done, you're done, understand?"

_______ 20. Recognition seeker

_______ 21. Seducer

g. Joyce says, "I won my first beauty contest when I was 6 months old. Can you imagine? And I've been winning them ever since. I was prom queen when I was 16, Miss Rose Petal when I was 19, Miss Silver City at 21. Next, I go to the state contest. It's just all so exciting!"

h. Joe, an RN on the care-planning committee says, "What a stupid suggestion. Nursing diagnosis! I won't even discuss the matter.We have been doing our care plans this way for 20 years. I refuse to even consider changing."

REFERENCES

American Nurses Association (ANA). (2000). Scope and standards of psychiatric-mental health nursing practice. Washington, DC: Author.

Clark, C.C. (2000). The nurse as group leader (3rd ed.). New York: Springer.

Goldenberg, I., & Goldenberg, H. (1995). Family therapy. In R.J. Corsini & D. Wedding (Eds.). Current psychotherapies (5th ed.). Itasca, IL: F.E. Peacock

Harvard Medical School. (1998, March). Cancer in the mind. Harvard Mental Health Letter, 14:1–5.

Huber, D. (1996). Leadership and nursing care management. Philadelphia: W.B. Saunders.

Sampson, E.E., & Marthas, M. (1990). Group process for the health professions (3rd ed.). Albany, NY: Delmar Publishers.

CLASSICAL REFERENCES

Benne, K.B., & Sheats, P. (1948, Spring). Functional roles of group members. Journal of Social Issues, 4:42–49.

Lippitt, R., & White, R.K. (1958). An experimental study of leadership and group life. In E.E., Maccoby, T.M. Newcomb, & E.L. Hartley (Eds.), Readings in social psychology (3rd ed.). New York: Holt, Rinehart, & Winston.

Yalom, I. (1985). The theory and practice of group psychotherapy (3rd ed.). New York: Basic Books.

TOWNSEND ESSENTIALS

9

CHAPTER

INTERVENING IN CRISES

CHAPTER OUTLINE

KEY TERMS

crisis
crisis intervention
prodromal syndrome

OBJECTIVES

After reading this chapter, the student will be able to:

1. Define *crisis*.
2. Describe four phases in the development of a crisis.
3. Identify types of crises that occur in people's lives.
4. Discuss the goal of crisis intervention.
5. Describe the steps in crisis intervention.
6. Identify the role of the nurse in crisis intervention.
7. Apply the nursing process to clients experiencing crises.
8. Apply the nursing process to clients expressing anger or aggression.
9. Apply the nursing process to care of victims of disaster.

INTRODUCTION

Stressful situations are a part of everyday life. Any stressful situation can precipitate a **crisis**. Crises result in a disequilibrium from which many individuals require assistance to recover. **Crisis intervention** requires problem-solving skills that are often diminished by the level of anxiety accompanying disequilibrium. Assistance with problem-solving during the crisis period preserves self-esteem and promotes growth with resolution.

In recent years, individuals in the United States have been faced with a number of catastrophic events, including natural disasters such as tornados, earthquakes, hurricanes, and floods. Also, man-made disasters, such as the Oklahoma City bombing and the attacks on the World Trade Center and the Pentagon, have created psychological stress of astronomical proportions in populations around the world.

This chapter examines the phases in the development of a crisis and the types of crises that occur in people's lives. The methodology of crisis intervention, including the role of the nurse, is explored. A discussion of disaster nursing is also presented.

CRISIS DEFINED

The term *crisis* is defined by Lagerquist (2001) as follows:

> A sudden event in one's life that disturbs homeostasis, during which usual coping mechanisms cannot resolve the problem. (p. 340)

A number of characteristics have been identified that can be viewed as assumptions on which the concept of crisis is based (Caplan, 1964; Kaplan & Sadock, 1998; Aguilera, 1998). They include the following:

1. Crisis occurs in all individuals at one time or another and is not necessarily equated with psychopathology.
2. Crises are precipitated by specific identifiable events.
3. Crises are personal by nature. What may be considered a crisis by one individual may not be so for another.
4. Crises are acute, not chronic, and will be resolved in one way or another within a brief period.
5. A crisis contains the potential for psychological growth or deterioration.

Individuals who are in crisis feel helpless to change. They do not believe they have the resources to deal with the precipitating stressor. Levels of anxiety rise to the point that the individual becomes nonfunctional, thoughts become obsessional, and all behavior is aimed at relief of the anxiety being experienced. The feeling is overwhelming and may affect the individual physically as well as psychologically.

Bateman & Peternelj-Taylor (1998) state:

> Outside Western culture, a crisis is often viewed as a time for movement and growth. The Chinese symbol for crisis consists of the characters for *danger* and *opportunity* [Fig. 9–1]. When a crisis is viewed as an opportunity for growth, those involved are much more capable of resolving related issues and more able to move toward positive changes. When the crisis experience is overwhelming because of its scope and nature or when there has not been adequate preparation for the necessary changes, the dangers seem paramount and overshadow any potential growth. The results are maladaptive coping and dysfunctional behavior. (pp. 144–145)

PHASES IN THE DEVELOPMENT OF A CRISIS

The development of a crisis follows a relatively predictable course. Caplan (1964) outlined four specific phases through which individuals progress in response to a precipitating stressor and which culminate in the state of acute crisis.

PHASE 1. *The individual is exposed to a precipitating stressor.* Anxiety increases; previous problem-solving techniques are used.

PHASE 2. *When previous problem-solving techniques do not relieve the stressor, anxiety increases further.* The individual begins to feel a great deal of discomfort at this point. Coping techniques that have worked in the past are attempted, only to create feelings of helplessness when they are not successful. Feelings of confusion and disorganization prevail.

PHASE 3. *All possible resources, both internal and external, are called on to resolve the problem and relieve the discomfort.* The individual may try to view the problem from a different perspective or even to overlook certain aspects of it. New problem-solving

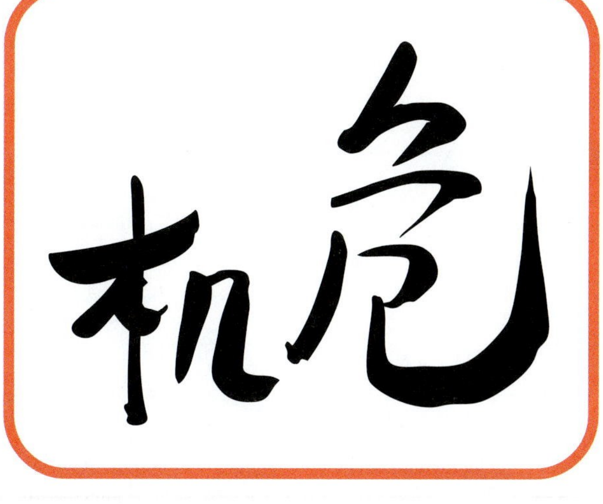

FIGURE 9–1 Chinese symbol for "crisis."

techniques may be used and, if effectual, resolution may occur at this phase, with the individual returning to a higher, a lower, or the previous level of premorbid functioning.

PHASE 4. *If resolution does not occur in previous phases, Caplan states that "the tension mounts beyond a further threshold or its burden increases over time to a breaking point. Major disorganization of the individual with drastic results often occurs."* Anxiety may reach panic levels. Cognitive functions are disordered, emotions are labile, and behavior may reflect the presence of psychotic thinking.

These phases are congruent with the concept of "balancing factors" as described by Aguilera (1998). These factors affect the way in which an individual perceives and responds to a precipitating stressor. A schematic of these balancing factors is illustrated in Figure 9–2.

The paradigm set forth by Aguilera suggests that whether or not an individual experiences a crisis in response to a stressful situation depends on the following three factors:

1. **The individual's perception of the event.** If the event is perceived realistically, the individual is more likely to draw on adequate resources to restore equilibrium. If the perception of the event is distorted, attempts at problem-solving are likely to be ineffective, and restoration of equilibrium goes unresolved.
2. **The availability of situational supports.** Aguilera states, "Situational supports are those persons who are available in the environment and who can be depended on to help solve the problem" (p. 37). Without adequate situational supports during a stressful situation, an individual is most likely to feel overwhelmed and alone.
3. **The availability of adequate coping mechanisms.** When a stressful situation occurs, individuals draw on behavioral strategies that have previously been successful for them. If these coping strategies work, a crisis may be diverted. If not, disequilibrium may continue, and tension and anxiety may increase.

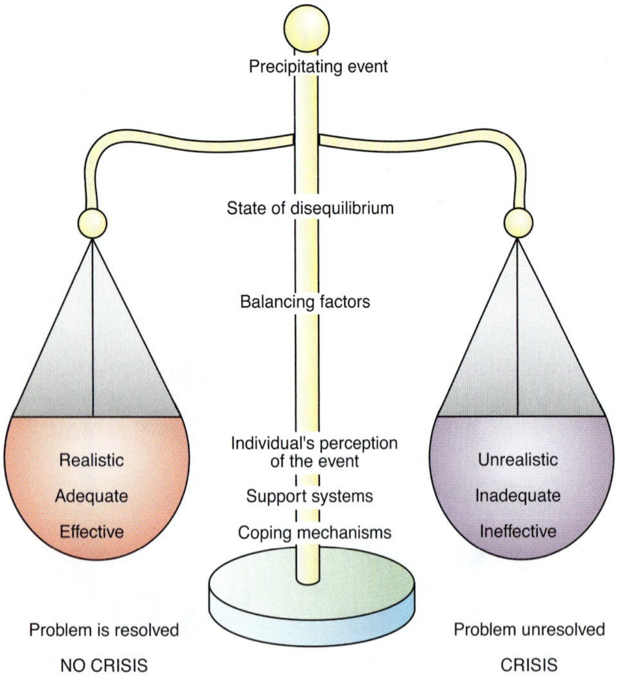

FIGURE 9–2 The effects of balancing factors in a stressful event.

As previously set forth, it is assumed that crises are acute, not chronic, situations that will be resolved in one way or another within a brief period. Kaplan and Sadock (1998) state, "A crisis is self-limited and can last from a few hours to weeks. It is characterized by an initial phase in which anxiety and tension rise, followed by a phase in which problem-solving mechanisms are set in motion." Crises can become growth opportunities when individuals learn new methods of coping that can be preserved and used when similar stressors recur.

TYPES OF CRISES

Baldwin (1978) identified six classes of emotional crises, which progress by degree of severity. As the measure of psychopathology increases, the source of the stressor changes from external to internal. The type of crisis determines the method of intervention selected.

Class 1: Dispositional Crises

Definition: An acute response to an external situational stressor.

EXAMPLE:

Nancy and Ted have been married for 3 years and have a 1-year-old daughter. Ted has been having difficulty with his boss at work. Twice during the past 6 months, he has exploded in anger at home and become abusive with Nancy. Last night he became angry that dinner was not ready when he expected. He grabbed the baby from Nancy and tossed her, screaming, into her crib. He hit and punched Nancy until she feared for her life. This morning when he left for work, she took the baby and went to the emergency department of the city hospital, not having anywhere else to go.

Intervention: Nancy's physical wounds were cared for in the emergency department. The mental health counselor provided support and guidance in terms of presenting alternatives to her. Needs and issues were clarified, and referrals for agency assistance were made.

Class 2: Crises of Anticipated Life Transitions

Definition: Normal life-cycle transitions that may be anticipated but over which the individual may feel a lack of control.

EXAMPLE:

College student JT is placed on probationary status because of low grades this semester. His wife had a baby and had to quit her job. He increased his working hours from part-time to full-time to compensate and therefore had little time for studies. He presents himself to the student-health nurse clinician, complaining of numerous vague physical complaints.

Intervention: Physical examination should be performed (physical symptoms could be caused by depression) and ventilation of feelings encouraged. Reassurance and support should be provided as needed. The client should be referred to services that can provide financial and other types of needed assistance. Problematic areas should be identified and approaches to change discussed.

Class 3: Crises Resulting from Traumatic Stress

Definition: Crises precipitated by unexpected external stresses over which the individual has little or no control and from which he or she feels emotionally overwhelmed and defeated.

EXAMPLE:

Sally was a waitperson whose shift ended at midnight. Two weeks ago, while walking to her car in the deserted parking lot, she was abducted by two men with guns, taken to an abandoned building, raped, and beaten. Since that time, her physical wounds have nearly healed. However, Sally cannot be alone; she is constantly fearful; she relives the experience in flashbacks and dreams; and she is unable to eat, sleep, or work at the restaurant. Her friend offers to accompany her to the mental health clinic.

Intervention: The nurse should encourage Sally to talk about the experience and to ventilate feelings associated with it. The nurse should offer reassurance and support; discuss stages of grief and how rape causes a loss of self-worth, triggering the grief response; identify support systems that can help Sally to resume her normal activities; and explore new methods of coping with emotions arising from a situation with which she has had no previous experience.

Class 4: Maturational/ Developmental Crises

Definition: Crises that occur in response to situations that trigger emotions related to unresolved conflicts in one's life. These crises are of internal origin and reflect underlying developmental issues that involve dependency, value conflicts, sexual identity, control, and capacity for emotional intimacy.

EXAMPLE:

Bob is 40 years old. He has just been passed over for a job promotion for the third time. He has moved many times within the large company for which he works, usually after angering and alienating himself from the supervisor. His father was domineering and became abusive when Bob did not comply with his every command. Over the years, Bob's behavioral response became one of passive-aggressiveness—first with his father, then with his supervisors. This third rejection has created feelings of depression and intense anxiety in Bob. At his wife's insistence, he has sought help at the mental health clinic.

Intervention: The primary intervention is to help Bob identify the unresolved developmental issue that is creating the conflict. Support and guidance are offered during the initial crisis period, and then assistance is given to help him work through the underlying conflict in an effort to change response patterns that are creating problems in his current life situation.

Class 5: Crises Reflecting Psychopathology

Definition: Emotional crises in which preexisting psychopathology has been instrumental in precipitating the crisis or in which psychopathology significantly impairs or complicates adaptive resolution. Examples of psychopathology that may precipitate crises include borderline personality, severe neuroses, characterological disorders, or schizophrenia.

EXAMPLE:

Sonja, aged 29, was diagnosed with borderline personality disorder at age 18. She has been in therapy on a weekly basis for 10 years, with several hospitalizations for suicide attempts during that time. She has had the same therapist for the past 6 years. The therapist told Sonja today that she is to be married in 1 month, and will be moving across the country with her new husband. Sonja is distraught and experiencing intense feelings of abandonment. She is found wandering in and out of traffic on a busy expressway, oblivious to her surroundings. Police bring her to the emergency department of the hospital.
Intervention: The initial intervention is to help bring down the level of anxiety in Sonja that has created feelings of unreality in her. She requires that someone stay with her and reassure her of her safety and security. After the feelings of panic have subsided, she should be encouraged to verbalize her feelings of abandonment. Regressive behaviors should be discouraged. Positive reinforcement should be given for independent activities and accomplishments. The primary therapist will need to pursue this issue of termination with Sonja at length. Referral to a long-term care facility may be required.

Class 6: Psychiatric Emergencies

Definition: Crises in which general functioning has been severely impaired and the individual rendered incompetent or unable to assume personal responsibility. Examples include acutely suicidal individuals, drug overdoses, reactions to hallucinogenic drugs, acute psychoses, uncontrollable anger, and alcohol intoxication.

EXAMPLE:

Jennifer, aged 16, had been dating Joe, the star high school football player, for 6 months. After the game on Friday night, Jennifer and Joe went to Jackie's house, where a number of high school students had gathered for an after-game party. No adults were present. About midnight, Joe told Jennifer that he did not want to date her anymore. Jennifer became hysterical, and Jackie was frightened by her behavior. She took Jennifer to her parents' bedroom and gave her a Valium from a bottle in her mother's medicine cabinet. She left Jennifer lying on her parents' bed and returned to the party downstairs. About an hour later, she returned to her parents' bedroom and found that Jennifer had removed the bottle of Valium from the cabinet and swallowed all of them. Jennifer was unconscious, and Jackie could not awaken her. An ambulance was called, and Jennifer was transported to the local hospital.
Intervention: The crisis team monitored vital signs, ensured maintenance of adequate airway, initiated gastric lavage, and administered activated charcoal to minimize absorption. Jennifer's parents were notified and rushed to the hospital. The situation was explained to them, and they were encouraged to stay by her side. When the physical crisis was resolved, Jennifer was transferred to the psychiatric unit. In therapy, she was encouraged to ventilate her feelings regarding the rejection and subsequent overdose. Family therapy sessions were conducted in an effort to clarify interpersonal issues and to identify areas for change. On an individual level, Jennifer's therapist worked with her to establish more adaptive methods of coping with stressful situations.

CRISIS INTERVENTION

Individuals experiencing crises have an urgent need for assistance. In crisis intervention the therapist, or other intervener, becomes a part of the individual's life situation. Because of the individual's emotional state, he or she is unable to solve problems and therefore requires guidance and support to help mobilize the resources needed to resolve the crisis.

Lengthy psychological interpretations are not appropriate for crisis intervention. It is a time for doing what is needed to help the individual get relief and for calling into action all the people and other resources required to do so. Aguilera (1998) states:

> The goal of crisis intervention is the resolution of an immediate crisis. Its focus is on the supportive, with the restoration of the individual to his pre-crisis level of functioning or possibly to a higher level of functioning. The therapist's role is direct, supportive, and that of an active participant. (p. 24)

Crisis intervention takes place in both inpatient and outpatient settings. The basic methodology relies heavily on orderly problem-solving techniques and structured activities that are focused on change. Through adaptive change, crises are resolved, and growth occurs. Because of the time limitation of crisis intervention, the individual must experience some relief almost from the first interaction. Crisis intervention, then, is not aimed at major personality change or reconstruction (as may be the case in long-term psychotherapy); its goal is using a given crisis situation to, at the very least, restore functioning and, at most, to enhance personal growth.

PHASES OF CRISIS INTERVENTION: THE ROLE OF THE NURSE

Nurses respond to crises on a daily basis. Crises can occur in every unit in the general hospital, the home setting, the community healthcare setting, schools, offices, and private practice. Indeed, nurses may be called on to function as crisis helpers in virtually any setting committed to the practice of nursing.

Aguilera (1998) describes four specific phases in the technique of crisis intervention. These phases are clearly comparable to the steps of the nursing process.

Phase 1. Assessment

In this phase, the crisis helper gathers information regarding the precipitating stressor and the resulting crisis that prompted the individual to seek professional help. A nurse in crisis intervention might perform some of the following assessments:

1. Ask the individual to describe the event that precipitated this crisis.
2. Determine when it occurred.
3. Assess the individual's physical and mental status.
4. Determine if the individual has experienced this stressor before. If so, what methods of coping were used? Have these methods been tried this time?
5. If previous coping methods were tried, what was the result?
6. If new coping methods were tried, what was the result?
7. Assess suicide or homicide potential, plan, and means.
8. Assess the adequacy of support systems.
9. Determine level of pre-crisis functioning. Assess the usual coping methods, available support systems, and ability to solve problems.
10. Assess the individual's perception of personal strengths and limitations.
11. Assess the individual's use of substances.

Information from the comprehensive assessment is then analyzed, and appropriate nursing diagnoses reflecting the immediacy of the crisis are identified. Some nursing diagnoses that may be relevant include:

1. Ineffective coping
2. Anxiety (severe to panic)
3. Disturbed thought processes
4. Risk for self- or other-directed violence
5. Rape-trauma syndrome
6. Post-trauma response
7. Fear

Phase 2. Planning of Therapeutic Intervention

In the planning phase of the nursing process, the nurse selects the appropriate nursing actions for the identified nursing diagnoses. In planning the interventions, the type of crisis (as well as the individual's strengths and available resources for support) is taken into consideration. Goals are established for crisis resolution and a return to or increase in the pre-crisis level of functioning.

Phase 3. Intervention

During Phase 3, the actions that were identified in Phase 2 are implemented. The following interventions are the focus of nursing in crisis intervention:

- Use a reality-oriented approach. The focus of the problem is on the here and now.
- Remain with the individual who is experiencing panic anxiety.
- Establish a rapid working relationship by showing unconditional acceptance, by active listening, and by attending to immediate needs.
- Discourage lengthy explanations or rationalizations of the situation; promote an atmosphere for verbalization of true feelings.
- Set firm limits on aggressive, destructive behaviors. At high levels of anxiety, behavior is likely to be impulsive and regressive. Establish at the outset what is acceptable and what is not, and maintain consistency.

- Clarify the problem the individual is facing. The nurse does this by describing his or her perception of the problem and comparing it with the individual's perception of the problem.
- Help the individual determine what he or she believes precipitated the crisis.
- Acknowledge feelings of anger, guilt, helplessness, and powerlessness, taking care to avoid providing positive feedback for these feelings.
- Guide the individual through a problem-solving process by which he or she may move in the direction of positive life change:
    - Help the individual confront the source of the problem that is creating the crisis response.
    - Encourage the individual to discuss changes he or she would like to make. Jointly determine whether desired changes are realistic.
    - Encourage exploration of feelings about aspects that cannot be changed, and explore alternative ways of coping more adaptively in these situations.
    - Discuss alternative strategies for creating changes that are realistically possible.
    - Weigh benefits and consequences of each alternative.
    - Assist the individual to select alternative coping strategies that will help alleviate future crises.
- Identify external support systems and new social networks from which the individual may seek assistance in times of stress.

Phase 4. Evaluation of Crisis Resolution and Anticipatory Planning

To evaluate the outcome of crisis intervention, a reassessment is made to determine if the stated objective was achieved:

1. Have positive behavioral changes occurred?
2. Has the individual developed more adaptive coping strategies? Have they been effective?
3. Has the individual grown from the experience by gaining insight into his or her responses to crises?
4. Does the individual believe that he or she could respond with healthy adaptation in future stressful situations to prevent crisis development?
5. Can the individual describe a plan of action for dealing with stressors similar to the one that precipitated this crisis?

During the evaluation period, the nurse and client summarize what has occurred during the intervention. They review what the individual has learned and "anticipate" how he or she will respond in the future. A determination is made regarding follow-up therapy; if needed, the nurse provides referral information.

CRISIS ON THE INPATIENT UNIT: ANGER/AGGRESSION MANAGEMENT

Assessment

Nurses must be aware of the symptoms associated with anger and aggression to make an accurate assessment. Because the best intervention is prevention, risk factors for assessing violence potential are also presented.

Anger

Alexander (1991a) identifies a cluster of characteristics that describe anger:

- Intense distress
- Frowning
- Gritting of the teeth
- Pacing
- Eyebrow displacement (raised, lowered, knitted)
- Clenched fists
- Increased energy
- Fatigue
- Withdrawal
- Flushed face
- Emotional overcontrol
- Change in tone of voice (either lowered, with words spoken between clenched teeth, or yelling and shouting)

Anger has been identified as a stage in the grieving process. Individuals who become fixed in this stage may become depressed. In this instance, the anger is turned inward as a way for the individual to maintain control over the pent-up anger. Because of the negative connotation of the word *anger*, some clients will not acknowledge that what they are feeling is anger. These individuals will need assistance to recognize their true feelings and to understand that anger is a perfectly acceptable emotion when it is expressed appropriately.

Aggression

Alexander (1991b) states that aggression can arise from such feeling states as anger, anxiety, tension, guilt, frustration, and hostility. Aggressive behaviors can be classified as mild (e.g., sarcasm), moderate (e.g., slamming doors), severe (e.g., threats of physical violence against others), or extreme (e.g., physical acts of violence against others). Alexander (1991b) identifies aggression by the following defining characteristics:

- Sarcasm
- Verbal or physical threats
- Change in voice tone (raised or quavering voice tone and pitch; rapid or hesitant speech)
- Degrading comments
- Pacing
- Throwing or striking objects or people
- Suspiciousness
- Suicidal ideation
- Homicidal ideation
- Self-mutilation
- Invasion of personal space
- Increase in agitation or irritability
- Disturbed thought process and perception
- Misinterpretation of stimuli
- Anger disproportionate to an event

Warren (1990) states, "Aggression has long-term negative consequences almost all of the time. Even the short-term gains it occasionally produces are usually canceled out over the long term."

Assessing Risk Factors

Prevention is the key issue in the management of aggressive or violent behavior. The individual who becomes violent usually feels an underlying helplessness. Three factors that have been identified as important considerations in assessing for potential violence include:

1. Past history of violence
2. Client diagnosis
3. Current behavior

Blair and New (1991) report the results of several studies that clearly implicate a history of assault as the most widely recognized risk factor for violence in a treatment setting. The second most frequently correlated factor with assaultive behavior is diagnosis. The diagnoses that have a high association with violent behavior are substance abuse/intoxication (either as a primary or secondary diagnosis), schizophrenia, posttraumatic stress disorder, organic brain disorders, personality disorders, and bipolar mania.

Dubin (2003) states:

> The successful management of aggression is predicated on the ability to predict which patients are most likely to become violent. Once such a prediction is made, rapid intervention can defuse the risk of violence. Violence usually does not occur without warning.

He describes a "**prodromal syndrome,**" which is characterized by anxiety and tension, verbal abuse and profanity, and increasing hyperactivity. These escalating behaviors usually do not occur in stages but most often overlap and sometimes occur simultaneously. Behaviors associated with this prodromal stage include rigid posture; clenched fists and jaws; grim, defiant affect; talking in a rapid, raised voice; arguing and demanding; using profanity and threatening verbalizations; agitation and pacing; and pounding and slamming.

Most assaultive behavior is preceded by a period of increasing hyperactivity. Behaviors associated with the prodromal syndrome should be considered emergent and demand immediate attention. Keen observation skills and background knowledge for accurate assessment are critical factors in predicting potential for violent behavior.

Diagnosis/Outcome Identification

NANDA International does not include a separate nursing diagnosis for anger. The nursing diagnosis of dysfunctional grieving may be used when anger is expressed inappropriately and the etiology is related to a loss.

The following nursing diagnoses may be considered for clients demonstrating inappropriate expression of anger or aggression:

Ineffective coping
Risk for self-directed or other-directed violence

Outcome Criteria

The following criteria may be used for measurement of outcomes in the care of the client needing assistance with management of anger and aggression. The client:

1. Is able to recognize when he or she is angry, and seeks out staff to talk about his or her feelings.
2. Is able to take responsibility for own feelings of anger.
3. Demonstrates the ability to exert internal control over feelings of anger.
4. Is able to diffuse anger before losing control.

5. Uses the tension generated by the anger in a constructive manner.
6. Does not cause harm to self or others.
7. Is able to use steps of the problem-solving process rather than becoming violent as a means of seeking solutions.

Planning/Implementation

In Table 9–1, a plan of care is presented for the client who expresses anger inappropriately. Goals of care and appropriate nursing interventions with rationale are included for each diagnosis.

Evaluation

Evaluation consists of reassessment to determine if the nursing interventions have been successful in achieving the objectives of care. The following questions may provide information to determine the success of working with a client exhibiting inappropriate expression of anger.

- Is the client able to recognize when he or she is angry now?
- Can the client take responsibility for these feelings and keep them in check without losing control?
- Does the client seek out staff to talk about feelings when they occur?
- Is the client able to transfer tension generated by the anger into constructive activities?
- Has harm to the client and others been avoided?
- Is the client able to solve problems adaptively without undue frustration and without becoming violent?

DISASTER NURSING

Although there are many definitions of disaster, a common feature is that the event overwhelms local resources and threatens the function and safety of the community (Norwood, Ursano, & Fullerton, 2001). A violent disaster, whether natural or man-made, may leave devastation of property or life. Such tragedies also leave victims with a damaged sense of safety and well-being as well as varying degrees of emotional trauma (Oklahoma State Department of Health, 2001). Children, who lack life experiences and coping skills, are particularly vulnerable. Their sense of order and security has been seriously disrupted, and they are unable to understand that the disruption is time limited and that their world will eventually return to normal.

APPLICATION OF THE NURSING PROCESS

Background Assessment Data

Individuals respond to traumatic events in many ways. Grieving is a natural response following any loss, and it may be more extreme if the disaster is directly experienced or witnessed (Oklahoma State Department of Health, 2001). The emotional effects of loss and disruption may show up immediately or may appear weeks or months later.

Psychological and behavioral responses common in adults following trauma and disaster include anger; disbelief; sadness; anxiety; fear; irritability; arousal; numbing; sleep disturbance; and increases in alcohol, caffeine, and tobacco use (Norwood, Ursano, & Fullerton, 2001). Preschool children commonly experience separation anxiety, regressive behaviors, nightmares, and hyperactive or withdrawn behaviors. Older children may have difficulty concentrating, somatic complaints, sleep disturbances, and concerns about safety. Adolescents' responses are often similar to those of adults.

Norwood, Ursano, and Fullerton (2001) state:

> Traumatic bereavement is recognized as posing special challenges to survivors. While the death of loved ones is always painful, an unexpected and violent death can be more difficult to assimilate. Family members may develop intrusive images of the death based on information gleaned from authorities or the media. Witnessing or learning of violence to a loved one also increases vulnerability to psychiatric disorders. The knowledge that one has been exposed to toxins is a potent traumatic stressor…and the focus of much concern in the medical community preparing for responses to terrorist attacks using biological, chemical, or nuclear agents. (pp. 4, 5)

Nursing Diagnoses/Outcome Identification

Information from the assessment is analyzed, and appropriate nursing diagnoses reflecting the immediacy of the situation are identified. Some nursing diagnoses that may be relevant include:

TABLE 9 – 1 Care Plan for the Individual Who Expresses Anger Inappropriately

Nursing Diagnosis: INEFFECTIVE COPING
Related to: (Possible) negative role modeling; dysfunctional family system
Evidenced by: Yelling, name-calling, hitting others, and temper tantrums as expressions of anger

Outcome Criteria	Nursing Interventions	Rationale
Client will be able to recognize anger in self and take responsibility before losing control.	1. Remain calm when dealing with an angry client.	1. Anger expressed by the nurse will most likely incite increased anger in the client.
	2. Set verbal limits on behavior. Clearly delineate the consequences of inappropriate expression of anger and always follow through.	2. Consistency in enforcing the consequences is essential if positive outcomes are to be achieved. Inconsistency creates confusion and encourages testing of limits.
	3. Have the client keep a diary of angry feelings, what triggered them, and how they were handled.	3. This provides a more objective measure of the problem.
	4. Avoid touching the client when he or she becomes angry.	4. The client may view touch as threatening and could become violent.
	5. Help the client determine the true source of the anger.	5. Many times anger is being displaced onto a safer object or person. If resolution is to occur, the first step is to identify the source of the problem.
	6. It may be constructive to ignore initial derogatory remarks by the client.	6. Lack of feedback often extinguishes an undesirable behavior.
	7. Help the client find alternate ways of releasing tension, such as physical outlets, and more appropriate ways of expressing anger, such as seeking out staff when feelings emerge.	7. Client will likely need assistance to problem-solve more appropriate ways of behaving.
	8. Role model appropriate ways of expressing anger assertively, such as, "I dislike being called names. I get angry when I hear you saying those things about me."	8. Role modeling is one of the strongest methods of learning.

Nursing Diagnosis: RISK FOR SELF-DIRECTED OR OTHER-DIRECTED VIOLENCE
Related to: (Possibly) having been nurtured in an atmosphere of violence.

Outcome Criteria	Nursing Interventions	Rationale
The client will not harm self or others. The client will verbalize anger rather than hit others	1. Observe client for escalation of anger (called the prodromal syndrome): increased motor activity, pounding, slamming, tense posture, defiant affect, clenched teeth and fists, arguing, demanding, and challenging or threatening staff.	1. Violence may be prevented if risks are identified in time.
	2. When these behaviors are observed, first ensure that sufficient staff are available to help with a potentially violent situation. Attempt to defuse the anger beginning with the least restrictive means.	2. The initial consideration must be having enough help to diffuse a potentially violent situation. Client rights must be honored, while preventing harm to client and others on the unit.
	3. Techniques for dealing with aggression include:	3. Aggression control techniques promote safety and reduce risk of harm to client and others:
	a. Talking down. Say, "John, you seem very angry. Let's go to your room and talk about it." (Ensure that client does not position self between door and nurse.)	a. Promotes a trusting relationship and may prevent the client's anxiety from escalating.
	b. Physical Outlets. "Maybe it would help if you punched your pillow or the punching bag for a while" or "I'll stay here with you if you want."	b. Provides effective way for client to release tension associated with high levels of anger.

(Continued)

TABLE 9–1 Care Plan for the Individual Who Expresses Anger Inappropriately *(Continued)*

Nursing Diagnosis: RISK FOR SELF-DIRECTED OR OTHER-DIRECTED VIOLENCE

Related to: (Possibly) having been nurtured in an atmosphere of violence

Outcome Criteria

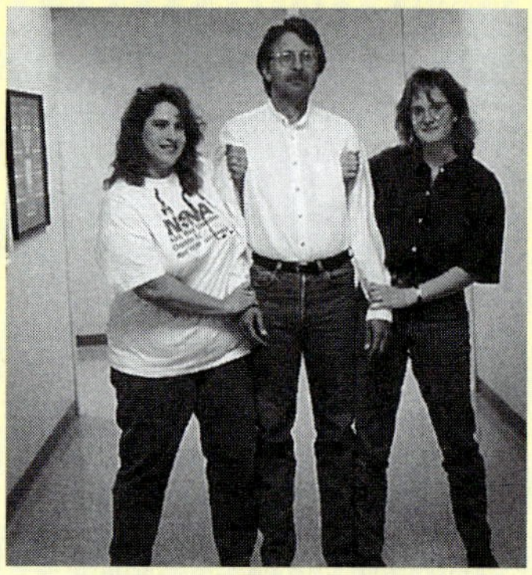

Walking a client to the seclusion room (From Townsend, M.C.: Essentials of Psychiatric Mental Health Nursing, ed. 2. F.A. Davis Company, Philadelphia, 2002, p. 152, with permission.)

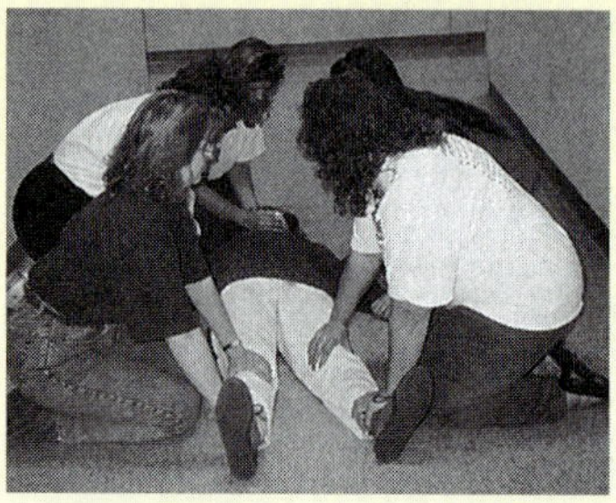

Staff restraint of a client in supine position. The client's head is controlled to prevent biting. (From Townsend, M.C.: Essentials of Psychiatric Mental Health Nursing, ed 2. F.A. Davis Company, Philadelphia, 2002, p. 152, with permission.)

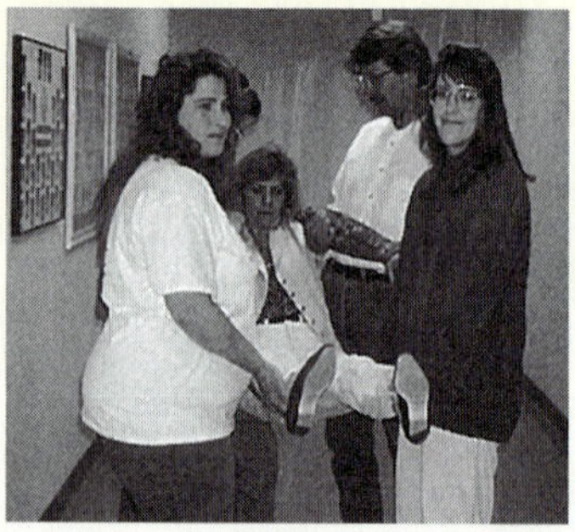

Transporting a client to the seclusion room. (From Townsend, M.C.: Essentials of Psychiatric Mental Health Nursing, ed 2. F.A. Davis Company, Philadelphia, 2002, p. 152, with permission.)

Nursing Interventions	Rationale
c. Medication. If agitation continues to escalate, offer client choice of taking medication voluntarily. If he or she refuses, reassess the situation to determine if harm to self or others is imminent.	c. Provides the least restrictive method of controlling client behavior.
d. Call for assistance. Remove self and other clients from the immediate area. Call violence code, push "panic" button, call for assault team, or institute measures established by institution. Sufficient staff to indicate a show of strength may be enough to deescalate the situation, and client may agree to take the medication.	d. Client and staff safety are of primary concern.
e. Restraints. If client is not calmed by "talking down" or by medication, use of mechanical restraints and/or seclusion may be necessary. Be sure to have sufficient staff available to assist. These three figures illustrate ways in which staff can safely and appropriately deal with an out-of-control client. Follow protocol for restraints/seclusion established by the institution. JCAHO (2000) requires that the physician reissue a new order for restraints every 4 hours for adults and every 1–2 hours for children and adolescents. If the client has previously refused medication, administer after restraints have been applied. Most states consider this intervention appropriate in emergency situations or if a client would likely harm self or others.	e. Clients who do not have internal control over their own behavior may require external controls, such as mechanical restraints, in order to prevent harm to self or others.
f. Observation and documentation. Observe the client in restraints every 15 minutes (or according to institutional policy). Ensure that circulation to extremities is not compromised (check temperature, color, pulses). Assist client with needs related to nutrition, hydration, and elimination. Position client so that comfort is facilitated and aspiration can be prevented. Document all observations.	f. Client well-being is a nursing priority.
g. Ongoing assessment. As agitation decreases, assess client's readiness for restraint removal or reduction. With assistance from other staff members, remove one restraint at a time, while assessing client's response. This minimizes the risk of injury to client and staff.	g. Gradual removal of the restraints allows for testing of the client's self-control. Client and staff safety are of primary concern.
h. Staff debriefing. It is important when a client loses control for staff to follow-up with a discussion about the situation. Tardiff (1994) states, "The violent episode should be discussed in terms of what happened, what would have prevented it, why seclusion or restraint was used (if it was), and how the client or the staff felt in terms of the use of seclusion and restraint." It is also important to discuss the situation with other clients who witnessed the episode. It is important that they understand what happened. Some clients may fear that they could be secluded or restrained at some time for no apparent reason.	h. Debriefing diminishes the emotional impact of the intervention and provides an opportunity to clarify the need for the intervention, offer mutual feedback, and promote client's self-esteem (Norris & Kennedy, 1992).

- Risk for injury (trauma, suffocation, poisoning)
- Risk for infection
- Anxiety (panic)
- Fear
- Spiritual distress
- Risk for post-trauma syndrome
- Ineffective community coping

The following criteria may be used for measurement of outcomes in the care of the client having experienced a traumatic event. The client:

1. Experiences minimal/no injury to self.
2. Demonstrates behaviors necessary to protect self from further injury.
3. Identifies interventions to prevent/reduce risk of infection.
4. Is free of infection.
5. Maintains anxiety at manageable level.
6. Expresses beliefs and values about spiritual issues.
7. Demonstrates ability to deal with emotional reactions in an individually appropriate manner.
8. Demonstrates an increase in activities to improve community functioning.

Planning/Implementation

Table 9–2 provides a plan of care for the client who has experienced a traumatic event. Selected nursing diagnoses are presented, along with outcome criteria, appropriate nursing interventions, and rationales for each.

Evaluation

In the final step of the nursing process, a reassessment is conducted to determine if the nursing actions have been successful in achieving the objectives of care. Evaluation of the nursing actions for the client who has experienced a traumatic event may be facilitated by gathering information utilizing the following types of questions.

1. Has the client escaped serious injury, or have injuries been resolved?
2. Have infections been prevented or resolved?
3. Is the client able to maintain anxiety at a manageable level?
4. Does he or she demonstrate appropriate problem-solving skills?
5. Is the client able to discuss his or her beliefs about spiritual issues?
6. Does the client demonstrate the ability to deal with emotional reactions in an individually appropriate manner?
7. Does he or she verbalize a subsiding of the physical manifestations (e.g., pain, nightmares, flashbacks, fatigue) associated with the traumatic event?
8. Has there been recognition of factors affecting the community's ability to meet its own demands or needs?
9. Has there been a demonstration of increased activities to improve community functioning?
10. Has a plan been established and put in place to deal with future contingencies?

SUMMARY

A *crisis* is defined as "a sudden event in one's life that disturbs homeostasis, during which usual coping mechanisms cannot resolve the problem" (Lagerquist, 2001). All individuals experience crises at one time or another. This does not necessarily indicate psychopathology.

Crises are precipitated by specific identifiable events and are determined by an individual's personal perception of the situation. They are acute rather than chronic and generally last no more than a few hours to a few weeks.

Crises occur when an individual is exposed to a stressor and previous problem-solving techniques are ineffective. This causes the level of anxiety to rise. Panic may ensue when new techniques are used and resolution fails to occur.

Baldwin (1978) identified six types of crises. They include dispositional crises, crises of anticipated life transitions, crises resulting from traumatic stress, maturational/developmental crises, crises reflecting psychopathology, and psychiatric emergencies. The type of crisis determines the method of intervention selected.

Crisis intervention is designed to provide rapid assistance for individuals who have an urgent need. Aguilera (1998) identifies the minimum therapeutic goal of crisis intervention as psychological resolution of the individual's immediate crisis and restoration to at least the level of functioning that existed before the crisis period. A maximum goal is improvement in functioning above the pre-crisis level.

Nurses regularly respond to individuals in crisis in all types of settings. Nursing process is the vehicle by which nurses assist individuals in crisis with a short-term problem-solving approach to change. A

TABLE 9–2 Care Plan for the Client Who Has Experienced a Traumatic Event[1]

Nursing Diagnosis: ANXIETY (PANIC)/FEAR
Related to: Real or perceived threat to physical well-being; threat of death; situational crisis; exposure to toxins; unmet needs
Evidenced by: Persistent feelings of apprehension and uneasiness; sense of impending doom; impaired functioning; verbal expressions of having no control or influence over situation, outcome, or self-care; sympathetic stimulation; extraneous physical movements

Outcome Criteria	Nursing Interventions	Rationale
Client will maintain anxiety at manageable level.	1. Determine degree of anxiety/fear present, associated behaviors (e.g., laughter, crying, calm or agitation, excited/hysterical behavior, expressions of disbelief and/or self-blame), and reality of perceived threat.	1. Clearly understanding client's perception is pivotal to providing appropriate assistance in overcoming the fear. Individual may be agitated or totally overwhelmed. Panic state increases risk for client's own safety as well as the safety of others in the environment.
	2. Note degree of disorganization.	2. Client may be unable to handle ADLs or work requirements and need more intensive intervention.
	3. Create as quiet an area as possible. Maintain a calm confident manner. Speak in even tones, using short simple sentences.	3. Decreases sense of confusion or overstimulation; enhances sense of safety. Helps client focus on what is said and reduces transmission of anxiety.
	4. Develop trusting relationship with the client.	4. Trust is the basis of a therapeutic nurse/client relationship and enables them to work effectively together.
	5. Identify whether incident has reactivated preexisting or coexisting situations (physical or psychological).	5. Concerns and psychological issues will be recycled every time trauma is reexperienced and affect how the client views the current situation.
	6. Determine presence of physical symptoms (e.g., numbness, headache, tightness in chest, nausea, and pounding heart).	6. Physical problems need to be differentiated from anxiety symptoms so appropriate treatment can be given.
	7. Identify psychological responses (e.g., anger, shock, acute anxiety, panic, confusion, denial). Record emotional changes.	7. Although these are normal responses at the time of the trauma, they will recycle again and again until they are dealt with adequately.
	8. Discuss with client the perception of what is causing the anxiety.	8. Increases the ability to connect symptoms to subjective feeling of anxiety, providing opportunity to gain insight/control and make desired changes.
	9. Assist client to correct any distortions being experienced. Share perceptions with client.	9. Perceptions based on reality will help to decrease fearfulness. How the nurse views the situation may help client to see it differently.
	10. Explore with client or significant other the manner in which client has previously coped with anxiety-producing events.	10. May help client regain sense of control and recognize significance of trauma.
	11. Engage client in learning new coping behaviors (e.g., progressive muscle relaxation, thought-stopping).	11. Replacing maladaptive behaviors can enhance ability to manage and deal with stress. Interrupting obsessive thinking allows client to use energy to address underlying anxiety, while continued rumination about the incident can retard recovery.
	12. Encourage use of techniques to manage stress and vent emotions such as anger and hostility.	12. Reduces the likelihood of eruptions that can result in abusive behavior.
	13. Give positive feedback when client demonstrates better ways to manage anxiety and is able to calmly and realistically appraise the situation.	13. Provides acknowledgement and reinforcement, encouraging use of new coping strategies. Enhances ability to deal with fearful feelings and gain control over situation, promoting future successes.
	14. Administer medications as indicated: Antianxiety: diazepam, alprazolam, oxazepam; or Antidepressants: fluoxetine, paroxetine, bupropion.	14. Provides temporary relief of anxiety symptoms, enhancing ability to cope with situation. To lift mood and help suppress intrusive thoughts and explosive anger.

[1]Doenges, Moorhouse, and Geissler, 2002, with permission.

Nursing Diagnosis: Spiritual Distress

Related to: Physical or psychological stress; energy-consuming anxiety; loss(es), intense suffering; separation from religious or cultural ties; challenged belief and value system

Evidenced by: Expressions of concern about disaster and the meaning of life and death or belief systems; inner conflict about current loss of normality and effects of the disaster; anger directed at deity; engaging in self-blame; seeking spiritual assistance

Outcome Criteria	Nursing Interventions	Rationale
Client expresses beliefs and values about spiritual issues.	1. Determine client's religious/spiritual orientation, current involvement, and presence of conflicts.	1. Provides baseline for planning care and accessing appropriate resources.
	2. Establish environment that promotes free expression of feelings and concerns. Provide calm, peaceful setting when possible.	2. Promotes awareness and identification of feelings so they can be dealt with.
	3. Listen to client's and significant others' expressions of anger, concern, alienation from God, belief that situation is a punishment for wrongdoing, etc.	3. It is helpful to understand the client's and significant others' points of view and how they are questioning their faith in the face of tragedy.
	4. Note sense of futility, feelings of hopelessness and helplessness, lack of motivation to help self.	4. These thoughts and feelings can result in the client feeling paralyzed and unable to move forward to resolve the situation.
	5. Listen to expressions of inability to find meaning in life and reason for living. Evaluate for suicidal ideation.	5. May indicate need for further intervention to prevent suicide attempt.
	6. Determine support systems available to client.	6. Presence or lack of support systems can affect client's recovery.
	7. Ask how you can be most helpful. Convey acceptance of client's spiritual beliefs and concerns.	7. Promotes trust and comfort, encouraging client to be open about sensitive matters.
	8. Make time for nonjudgmental discussion of philosophic issues and questions about spiritual impact of current situation.	8. Helps client to begin to look at basis for spiritual confusion. *Note:* There is a potential for care provider's belief system to interfere with client finding own way. Therefore, it is most beneficial to remain neutral and not espouse own beliefs.
	9. Discuss difference between grief and guilt and help client to identify and deal with each, assuming responsibility for own actions, expressing awareness of the consequences of acting out of false guilt.	9. Blaming self for what has happened impedes dealing with the grief process and needs to be discussed and dealt with.
	10. Use therapeutic communication skills of reflection and active listening.	10. Helps client find own solutions to concerns.
	11. Encourage client to experience meditation, prayer, and forgiveness. Provide information that anger with God is a normal part of the grieving process.	11. This can help to heal past and present pain.
	12. Assist client to develop goals for dealing with life situation.	12. Enhances commitment to goal, optimizing outcomes and promoting sense of hope.
	13. Identify and refer to resources that can be helpful, e.g., pastoral/parish nurse or religious counselor, crisis counselor, psychotherapy, Alcoholics/Narcotics Anonymous.	13. Specific assistance may be helpful to recovery, e.g., relationship problems, substance abuse, suicidal ideation.
	14. Encourage participation in support groups.	14. Discussing concerns and questions with others can help client resolve feelings.

Nursing Diagnosis: Risk for Post-Trauma Syndrome

Related to: Events outside the range of usual human experience; serious threat or injury to self or loved ones; witnessing horrors or tragic events; exaggerated sense of responsibility; survivor's guilt or role in the event, inadequate social support

Outcome Criteria	Nursing Interventions	Rationale
Client demonstrates ability to deal with emotional reactions in an individually appropriate manner.	1. Determine involvement in event (e.g., survivor, significant other, rescue/aid worker, healthcare provider, family member).	1. All those concerned with a traumatic event are at risk for emotional trauma and have needs related to their involvement in the event. *Note:* Close involvement with victims affects individual responses and may prolong emotional suffering.
	2. Evaluate current factors associated with the event, such as displacement from home due to illness/injury, natural disaster, or terrorist attack. Identify how client's past experiences may affect current situation.	2. Affects client's reaction to current event and is basis for planning care and identifying appropriate support systems and resources.
	3. Listen for comments of taking on responsibility (e.g., "I should have been more careful or gone back to get her.")	3. Statements such as these are indicators of "survivor's guilt" and blaming self for actions.
	4. Identify client's current coping mechanisms.	4. Noting positive or negative coping skills provides direction for care.
	5. Determine availability and usefulness of client's support systems, family, social contacts, and community resources.	5. Family and others close to the client may also be at risk and require assistance to cope with the trauma.
	6. Provide information about signs and symptoms of post-trauma response, especially if individual is involved in a high-risk occupation.	6. Awareness of these factors helps individual identify need for assistance when signs and symptoms occur.
	7. Identify and discuss client's strengths as well as vulnerabilities.	7. Provides information to build on for coping with traumatic experience.
	8. Evaluate individual's perceptions of events and personal significance (e.g., rescue worker trained to provide lifesaving assistance but recovering only dead bodies).	8. Events that trigger feelings of despair and hopelessness may be more difficult to deal with, and require long-term interventions.
	9. Provide emotional and physical presence by sitting with client/significant other and offering solace.	9. Strengthens coping abilities
	10. Encourage expression of feelings. Note whether feelings expressed appear congruent with events experienced.	10. It is important to talk about the incident repeatedly. Incongruencies may indicate deeper conflict and can impede resolution.
	11. Note presence of nightmares, reliving the incident, loss of appetite, irritability, numbness and crying, and family or relationship disruption.	11. These responses are normal in the early post-incident time frame. If prolonged and persistent, they may indicate need for more intensive therapy.
	12. Provide a calm, safe environment.	12. Helps client deal with the disruption in his or her life.
	13. Encourage and assist client in learning stress-management techniques.	13. Promotes relaxation and helps individual exercise control over self and what has happened.
	14. Recommend participation in debriefing sessions that may be provided following major disaster events.	14. Dealing with the stresses promptly may facilitate recovery from the event or prevent exacerbation.
	15. Identify employment, community resource groups.	15. Provides opportunity for ongoing support to deal with recurrent feelings related to the trauma.
	16. Administer medications as indicated, such as antipsychotics (e.g., chlorpromazine or haloperidol) or carbamazepine (Tegretol).	16. Low doses may be used for reduction of psychotic symptoms when loss of contact with reality occurs, usually for clients with especially disturbing flashbacks. Tegretol may be used to alleviate intrusive recollections/flashbacks, impulsivity, and violent behavior.

Nursing Diagnosis: Ineffective Community Coping

Related to: Natural or man-made disasters (earthquakes, tornados, floods, reemerging infectious agents, terrorist activity); ineffective or nonexistent community systems (e.g., lack of or inadequate emergency medical system, transportation system, or disaster planning systems)

Evidenced by: Deficits of community participation; community does not meet its own expectations; expressed vulnerability; community powerlessness; stressors perceived as excessive; excessive community conflicts; high illness rates

Outcome Criteria	Nursing Interventions	Rationale
Client demonstrates an increase in activities to improve community functioning.	1. Evaluate how community activities are related to meeting collective needs within the community itself and between the community and the larger society. Note immediate needs, such as healthcare, food, shelter, funds.	1. Provides a baseline to determine community needs in relation to current concerns or threats.
	2. Note community reports of functioning including areas of weakness or conflict.	2. Provides a view of how the community itself sees these areas.
	3. Identify effects of related factors on community activities.	3. In the face of a current threat, local or national, community resources need to be evaluated, updated and given priority to meet the identified need.
	4. Determine availability and use of resources. Identify unmet demands or needs of the community.	4. Information necessary to identify what else is needed to meet the current situation.
	5. Determine community strengths.	5. Promotes understanding of the ways in which the community is already meeting the identified needs.
	6. Encourage community members/groups to engage in problem-solving activities.	6. Promotes a sense of working together to meet the needs.
	7. Develop a plan jointly with the members of the community to address immediate needs.	7. Deals with deficits in support of identified goals.
	8. Create plans managing interactions within the community itself and between the community and the larger society.	8. Meets collective needs when the concerns/threats are shared beyond a local community.
	9. Make information accessible to the public. Provide channels for dissemination of information to the community as a whole (e.g., print media, radio/television reports and community bulletin boards, internet sites, speaker's bureau, reports to committees/councils/advisory boards).	9. Readily available accurate information can help citizens deal with the situation.
	10. Make information available in different modalities and geared to differing educational levels/cultures of the community.	10. Using languages other than English and making written materials accessible to all members of the community will promote understanding.
	11. Seek out and evaluate needs of underserved populations.	11. Homeless and those residing in lower income areas may have special requirements that need to be addressed with additional resources.

four-phase technique was outlined: assessment/analysis, planning of therapeutic intervention, intervention, and evaluation of crisis resolution and anticipatory planning. Through this structured method of assistance, nurses help individuals in crisis to develop more adaptive coping strategies for dealing with stressful situations in the future.

Intervention in crises that involve anger and aggression by a client requires special knowledge and skills on the part of the nursing staff. Nurses must be aware of the symptoms associated with anger and aggression to make an accurate assessment. Prevention is the key issue in the management of aggressive or violent behavior. Three elements have been identified as key risk factors in the potential for violence: (1) past history of violence, (2) client diagnosis, and (3) current behaviors. Nursing diagnoses and outcome criteria for working with clients expressing anger or aggression were discussed, and a care plan outlining appropriate interventions was presented.

Nurses have many important skills that can assist individuals and communities in the wake of traumatic events. This chapter presented an example of disaster nursing as it is implemented through the six steps of the nursing process. A care plan for the client who has experienced a traumatic event was included.

REVIEW QUESTIONS

SELF-EXAMINATION/LEARNING EXERCISE

Select the best response to each of the following questions:

1. Which of the following is a correct assumption regarding the concept of crisis?
   a. Crises occur only in individuals with psychopathology.
   b. The stressful event that precipitates crisis is seldom identifiable.
   c. A crisis contains the potential for psychological growth or deterioration.
   d. Crises are chronic situations that recur many times during an individual's life.

2. Crises occur when an individual:
   a. Is exposed to a precipitating stressor
   b. Perceives a stressor to be threatening
   c. Has no support systems
   d. Experiences a stressor and perceives coping strategies to be ineffective

3. Amanda's mobile home was destroyed by a tornado. Amanda received only minor injuries, but she is experiencing disabling anxiety in the aftermath of the event. This type of crisis is called:
   a. Crisis resulting from traumatic stress
   b. Maturational/developmental crisis
   c. Dispositional crisis
   d. Crisis of anticipated life transitions

4. The most appropriate crisis intervention with Amanda would be to:
   a. Encourage her to recognize how lucky she is to be alive
   b. Discuss stages of grief and feelings associated with each
   c. Identify community resources that can help Amanda
   d. Suggest that she find a place to live that provides a storm shelter

5. Jenny reported to the high school nurse that her mother drinks too much. She is drunk every afternoon when Jenny gets home from school. Jenny is afraid to invite friends over because of her mother's behavior. This type of crisis is called:
   a. Crisis resulting from traumatic stress
   b. Maturational/developmental crisis
   c. Dispositional crisis
   d. Crisis reflecting psychopathology

6. The most appropriate nursing intervention with Jenny would be to:
   a. Make arrangements for her to start attending Alateen meetings
   b. Help her identify the positive things in her life and recognize that her situation could be a lot worse than it is
   c. Teach her about the effects of alcohol on the body and that it can be hereditary
   d. Refer her to a psychiatrist for private therapy to learn to deal with her home situation

7. Ginger, age 19 and an only child, left 3 months ago to attend a college of her choice 500 miles away from her parents. It is Ginger's first time away from home. She has difficulty making decisions and will not undertake anything new without first consulting her mother. They talk on the phone almost every day. Ginger has recently started having anxiety attacks. She consults the nurse practitioner in the student health center. This type of crisis is called:

a. Crisis resulting from traumatic stress
b. Dispositional crisis
c. Psychiatric emergency
d. Maturational/developmental crisis

8. The most appropriate nursing intervention with Ginger would be to:
   a. Suggest she move to a college closer to home
   b. Work with Ginger on unresolved dependency issues
   c. Help her find someone in the college town from whom she could seek assistance rather than calling her mother regularly
   d. Recommend that the college physician prescribe an antianxiety medication for Ginger

9. Marie, aged 56, is the mother of five children. Her youngest child, who had been living at home and attending the local college, recently graduated and accepted a job in another state. Marie has never worked outside the home and has devoted her life to satisfying the needs of her husband and children. Since the departure of her last child from home, Marie has become increasingly despondent. Her husband becomes very concerned and takes her to the local mental health center. This type of crisis is called:
   a. Dispositional crisis
   b. Crisis of anticipated life transitions
   c. Psychiatric emergency
   d. Crisis resulting from traumatic stress

10. The most appropriate nursing intervention with Marie would be to:
    a. Refer her to her family physician for a complete physical examination
    b. Suggest she seek outside employment now that her children have left home
    c. Identify convenient support systems for times when she is feeling particularly despondent
    d. Begin grief work and assist her to recognize areas of self-worth separate and apart from her children

Situation: John, age 27, was brought to the emergency department by two police officers. He smelled strongly of alcohol, was loud, verbally abused the staff, slurred his words, and had difficulty standing and walking without assistance. His blood alcohol level was measured at 293 mg/dL. John's girlfriend reported that they were at a party and he became violent, hitting her and threatening to kill others who tried to protect her. She reported that he gets drunk almost every day and has beaten her a number of times. When told that he would be admitted to detox, he started cursing and hitting the staff who were trying to help him. He was admitted to the Detox Center of the Alcohol Treatment Unit with a diagnosis of Alcohol Intoxication. He was restrained for the protection of self and others. His diagnosis was later changed to Alcohol Dependence, following conclusion of the withdrawal syndrome.

11. The nurses give John the nursing diagnosis of Risk for other-directed violence. What is the priority objective for this diagnosis?
    a. The client will not verbalize anger or hit anyone.
    b. The client will verbalize anger rather than hit others.
    c. The client will not harm self or others.
    d. The client will be restrained if he becomes verbally or physically abusive.

12. One evening, the nurse hears John yelling in the dayroom. The nurse observes his increased agitation, clenched fists, and loud demanding voice. He is challenging and threatening staff and the other clients. The nurse's priority intervention would be:
    a. Call for assistance.
    b. Draw up a syringe of PRN haloperidol.
    c. Ask John if he would like to talk about his anger.
    d. Tell John that if he does not calm down, he will have to be restrained.

13. John and his girlfriend had an argument during her visit. Which behavior by John would indicate he is learning to problem-solve his frustrations adaptively?
    a. John says to the nurse, "Give me some of that medication before I end up in restraints!"
    b. When his girlfriend leaves, John goes to the exercise room and punches on the punching bag.
    c. John says to the nurse, "I guess I'm going to have to dump that broad!"
    d. John says to his girlfriend, "You'd better leave before I do something I'm sorry for."

14. Andrew, a New York City firefighter, and his entire unit responded to the terrorist attacks at the World Trade Center. Working as a team, he and his best friend, Carlo, entered the area together. Carlo was killed when the building collapsed. Andrew was injured, but he survived. Since that time, Andrew has had frequent nightmares and anxiety attacks. He says to the mental health worker, "I don't know why Carlo had to die and I didn't!" This statement by Andrew suggests that he is experiencing:
    a. Spiritual distress
    b. Night terrors
    c. Survivor's guilt
    d. Suicidal ideation

15. Intervention with Andrew would include:
    a. Encouraging expression of feelings
    b. Antianxiety medications
    c. Participation in a support group
    d. a and c
    e. All of the above

REFERENCES

Aguilera, D.C. (1998). Crisis intervention: Theory and methodology (8th ed.). St. Louis: C.V. Mosby.

Alexander, D.I. (1991a). Anger. In G.K. McFarland & M.D. Thomas (Eds.), Psychiatric mental health nursing: Application of the nursing process. Philadelphia: J.B. Lippincott.

Alexander, D.I. (1991b). Aggression. In G.K. McFarland & M.D. Thomas (Eds.), Psychiatric mental health nursing: Application of the nursing process. Philadelphia: J.B. Lippincott.

Bateman, A., & Peternelj-Taylor, C. (1998). Crisis intervention. In C.A. Glod (Ed.), Contemporary psychiatric-mental health nursing: The brain-behavior connection. Philadelphia: F.A. Davis.

Blair, D.T., & New, S.A. (1991). Assaultive behavior: Know the risks. Journal of Psychosocial Nursing, 29:25–30.

Doenges, M.E., Moorhouse, M.F., & Geissler, A.C. (2002). Nursing care plans: Guidelines for individualizing patient care (6th ed.). Philadelphia: F.A. Davis.

Dubin, W.R. (2003), Violent patients. In G. Bosker (Ed.), The emergency medicine reports textbook of adult and pediatric emergency medicine. Atlanta, GA: Thomson American Health Consultants.

Joint Commission on Accreditation of Healthcare Organizations. (2000). Restraint and Seclusion Standards for Behavioral Health. Available at: http://www.jcaho.org/standard/restraint/restraint_stds.html/

Kaplan, H.I., & Sadock, B.J. (1998). Synopsis of psychiatry: Behavioral sciences/clinical psychiatry (8th ed.). Baltimore: Williams & Wilkins.

Lagerquist, S.L. (2001). Davis's NCLEX-RN success. Philadelphia: F.A. Davis.

Norris, M.K. & Kennedy, C.W. (1992). How patients perceive the seclusion process. Journal of Psychosocial Nursing and Mental Health Services, 30:7–13.

Norwood, A.E., Ursano, R.J., & Fullerton, C.S. (2001). Disaster psychiatry: Principles and practice. American Psychiatric Association. Retrieved on 11-09-01 from http://www.psych.org/pract_of_psych/principles_and_practice3201.cfm

Oklahoma State Department of Health. (2001). After the storm: Helping families cope with disaster. Oklahoma City: State Department of Health.

Tardiff, K. (1994). Violence. In R.E. Hales, S.C. Yvdofsky, & J.A. Talbott (Eds.), The American psychiatric press textbook of psychiatry (2nd ed.). Washington, D.C.: American Psychiatric Press.

Warren, N.C. (1990). Make anger your ally. Colorado Springs, CO: Focus on the Family.

CLASSICAL REFERENCES

Baldwin, B.A. (1978, July). A paradigm for the classification of emotional crises: Implications for crisis intervention. American Journal of Orthopsychiatry, 48:538–551.

Caplan, G. (1964). Principles of preventive psychiatry. New York: Basic Books.

10

CHAPTER

TOWNSEND ESSENTIALS

PSYCHOPHARMACOLOGY

CHAPTER OUTLINE

KEY TERMS

hypertensive crisis
oculogyric crisis
priapism
tardive dyskinesia
neuroleptic malignant syndrome (NMS)
retrograde ejaculation
gynecomastia
amenorrhea
agranulocytosis
extrapyramidal symptoms (EPS)
akinesia
akathisia
dystonia
serotonin syndrome

OBJECTIVES

After reading this chapter, the student will be able to:

1. Discuss historical perspectives related to psychopharmacology.
2. Describe indications, actions, contraindications, precautions, side effects, and nursing implications for the following classifications of drugs: antianxiety agents, antidepressants, mood stabilizers, antipsychotics, antiparkinsonian agents, sedative-hypnotics, and agents for attention deficit hyperactivity disorder
3. Apply the steps of the nursing process to the administration of psychotropic medications.

INTRODUCTION

The middle of the 20th century identifies a pivotal period in the treatment of the mentally ill. It was during this time that the phenothiazines were introduced into the United States. Before that time they had been used in France as preoperative medications. As Dr. Henri Laborit of the Hospital Boucicaut in Paris stated:

> It was our aim to decrease the anxiety of the patients to prepare them in advance for their postoperative recovery. With these new drugs, the phenothiazines, we were seeing a profound psychic and physical relaxation … a real indifference to the environment and to the upcoming operation. It seemed to me these drugs *must* have an application in psychiatry. (Sage, 1984)

Indeed, they have had a significant application in psychiatry. Not only have they given many individuals a chance, without which they would have been unable to function, but they have also provided researchers and clinicians with information to study the origins and etiologies of mental illness. Knowledge gained from learning how these drugs work has promoted advancement in understanding how behavioral disorders develop. Dr. Arnold Scheibel, Director of the University of California Brain Research Institute, stated:

> [When these drugs came out] there was a sense of disbelief that we could actually do something substantive for the patients ... see them for the first time as sick individuals and not as something bizarre that we could literally not talk to. (Sage, 1984)

This chapter explores historical perspectives in the use of psychotropic medications in the treatment of mental illness. Seven classifications of medications are discussed, and their implications for psychiatric nursing are presented in the context of the steps of the nursing process.

HISTORICAL PERSPECTIVES*

Historically, reaction to and treatment of persons with mental illness ranged from benign involvement to intervention some would consider inhumane. Individuals with mental illness were feared because of common beliefs associating them with demons or the supernatural. They were looked upon as loathsome and often were mistreated.

Beginning in the late 18th century, a type of "moral reform" in the treatment of persons with mental illness began to occur. This resulted in the establishment of community and state hospitals concerned with the needs of persons with mental illness. Considered a breakthrough in the humanization of care, these institutions, however well intentioned, fostered the concept of custodial care. Clients were ensured the provision of food and shelter but received little or no hope of change for the future. As they became increasingly dependent on the institution to fill their needs, the likelihood of their return to the family or community diminished.

The early part of the 20th century saw the advent of the somatic therapies in psychiatry. Individuals with mental illness were treated with insulin shock therapy, wet sheet packs, ice baths, electroconvulsive therapy, and psychosurgery. Before 1950, sedatives and amphetamines were the only significant psychotropic medications available. Even these had limited use because of their toxicity and addicting effects. Since the 1950s, the development of psychopharmacology has expanded to include widespread use of antipsychotic, antidepressant, and antianxiety medications. Research into how these drugs work has provided an understanding of the etiology of many psychiatric disorders.

Psychotropic medications are not intended to "cure" the mental illness. Most physicians who prescribe these medications for their clients use them as an adjunct to individual or group psychotherapy. Although their contribution to psychiatric care cannot be minimized, it must be emphasized that psychotropic medications relieve physical and behavioral symptoms. They do not resolve emotional problems.

Nurses must understand the legal implications associated with administration of psychotropic medications. Laws differ from state to state, but most adhere to the client's right to refuse treatment. Exceptions exist in emergencies when it has been determined that clients are likely to harm themselves or others.

APPLYING THE NURSING PROCESS IN PSYCHOPHARMACOLOGICAL THERAPY

Antianxiey Agents

Background Assessment Data

Indications

Antianxiety drugs are also called *anxiolytics* and *minor tranquilizers.* They are used in the treatment of anxiety disorders, anxiety symptoms, acute alcohol withdrawal, skeletal muscle spasms, convulsive disorders, status epilepticus, and preoperative sedation. Their use and efficacy for periods greater than 4 months have not been evaluated. Examples of commonly used antianxiety agents are presented in Table 10–1.

Action

Antianxiety drugs depress subcortical levels of the central nervous system (CNS), particularly the limbic system and reticular formation. They may potentiate the effects of the powerful inhibitory neurotransmitter gamma-aminobutyric acid in the brain, thereby producing a calmative effect. All levels of CNS depression can be affected, from mild sedation to hypnosis to coma. *Exception:* Buspirone (BuSpar) does not depress the CNS. Although its action is unknown, the drug is believed to produce the desired effects through interactions with serotonin, dopamine, and other neurotransmitter receptors.

*From Townsend, M.C. (2003), p. 291.

TABLE 10–1 Antianxiety Agents

Chemical Class	Generic (Trade) Name	Daily Dosage Range
Antihistamines	Hydroxyzine (Vistaril; Atarax)	50–400 mg
Benzodiazepines	Alprazolam (Xanax)	0.75–4 mg
	Chlordiazepoxide (Librium)	15–100 mg
	Clonazepam (Klonopin)	1.5–20 mg
	Clorazepate (Tranxene)	15–60 mg
	Diazepam (Valium)	4–40 mg
	Lorazepam (Ativan)	2–4 mg
	Oxazepam (Serax)	30–120 mg
Propanediols	Meprobamate (Miltown)	1.2–2.4 g
Azaspirodecanediones	Buspirone (BuSpar)	15–60 mg

Contraindications/Precautions

Antianxiety drugs are contraindicated in individuals with known hypersensitivity to any of the drugs within the classification (i.e., anxiolytics) or group (e.g., benzodiazepines). They should not be taken in combination with other CNS depressants and are contraindicated in pregnancy and lactation, narrow-angle glaucoma, shock, and coma.

Caution should be taken in administering these drugs to elderly or debilitated clients and clients with hepatic or renal dysfunction. (The dosage usually has to be decreased.) Caution is also required with individuals who have a history of drug abuse or addiction and with those who are depressed or suicidal. In depressed clients, CNS depressants can exacerbate symptoms.

Interactions

Increased effects of antianxiety agents can occur when taken concomitantly with alcohol, barbiturates, narcotics, antipsychotics, antidepressants, antihistamines, neuromuscular blocking agents, cimetidine or disulfiram, and with herbal depressants (e.g., kava and valerian). Decreased effects can be noted with cigarette smoking and caffeine consumption.

Diagnosis

The following nursing diagnoses may be considered for clients receiving therapy with antianxiety agents:

1. Risk for injury related to seizures; panic anxiety; abrupt withdrawal after long-term use; effects of medication intoxication or overdose
2. Risk for activity intolerance related to side effects of sedation and lethargy
3. Risk for acute confusion related to action of the medication on the CNS

Planning/Implementation

The plan of care should include monitoring for the following side effects of antianxiety agents. Nursing implications related to each side effect follow the asterisk (*).

1. Drowsiness, confusion, lethargy (most common side effects). *Instruct the client not to drive or operate dangerous machinery when taking the medication.
2. Tolerance; physical and psychological dependence (does not apply to buspirone). *Instruct the client on long-term therapy not to quit taking the drug abruptly. Abrupt withdrawal can be life threatening. Symptoms include depression, insomnia, increased anxiety, abdominal and muscle cramps, tremors, vomiting, sweating, convulsions, and delirium.
3. Ability to potentiate the effects of other CNS depressants. *Instruct the client not to drink alcohol or take other medications that depress the CNS when taking this medication.
4. Possibility of aggravating symptoms in depressed person. *Assess the client's mood daily. Take necessary precautions for potential suicide.
5. Orthostatic hypotension. *Monitor lying and standing blood pressure and pulse every shift. Instruct the client to arise slowly from a lying or sitting position.
6. Paradoxical excitement (client develops symptoms opposite of the medication's desired effect). *Withhold drug, and notify the physician.
7. Dry mouth. *Have the client take frequent sips of water, suck on ice chips or hard candy, or chew sugarless gum.
8. Nausea and vomiting. *Have the client take the drug with food or milk.
9. Blood dyscrasias. *Symptoms of sore throat, fever, malaise, easy bruising, or unusual bleeding should be reported to the physician immediately.
10. Delayed onset (buspirone only). *Ensure that the client understands there is a lag time of 10 days to 2 weeks between onset of therapy with buspirone and subsiding of anxiety symptoms. Client should

continue to take the medication during this time. *Note:* This medication is not recommended for p.r.n. administration because of this delayed therapeutic onset. There is no evidence that buspirone creates tolerance or physical dependence as do the CNS-depressant anxiolytics.

Client/Family Education

The client should:

- Not drive or operate dangerous machinery. Drowsiness and dizziness can occur.
- Not stop taking the drug abruptly because this can produce serious withdrawal symptoms, such as depression, insomnia, anxiety, abdominal and muscle cramps, tremors, vomiting, sweating, convulsions, and delirium.
- (With buspirone only): Be aware of lag time between start of therapy and subsiding of symptoms. Relief is usually evident within 10 to 14 days. The client must take the medication regularly, as ordered, so that it has sufficient time to take effect.
- Not consume other CNS depressants (including alcohol).
- Not take nonprescription medication without approval from physician.
- Rise slowly from sitting or lying position to prevent sudden drop in blood pressure.
- Report symptoms of sore throat, fever, malaise, easy bruising, unusual bleeding, or motor restlessness to physician immediately.
- Be aware of risks of taking this drug during pregnancy. (Congenital malformations have been associated with use during the first trimester.) The client should notify the physician of the desirability to discontinue the drug if pregnancy is suspected or planned.
- Be aware of possible side effects. The client should refer to written materials furnished by healthcare providers regarding the correct method of self-administration.
- Carry a card or piece of paper at all times stating the names of medications being taken.

Outcome Criteria/Evaluation

The following criteria may be used for evaluating the effectiveness of therapy with antianxiety agents. The client:

1. Demonstrates a reduction in anxiety, tension, and restless activity
2. Experiences no seizure activity
3. Experiences no physical injury
4. Is able to tolerate usual activities without excessive sedation
5. Exhibits no evidence of confusion
6. Tolerates the medication without gastrointestinal (GI) distress
7. Verbalizes understanding of the need for, side effects of, and regimen for self-administration
8. Verbalizes possible consequences of abrupt withdrawal from the medication

Antidepressants

Background Assessment Data

Indications

Antidepressant medications are used in the treatment of dysthymic disorder; major depression with melancholia or psychotic symptoms; depression associated with organic disease, alcoholism, schizophrenia, or mental retardation; depressive phase of bipolar disorder; and depression accompanied by anxiety. These drugs elevate mood and alleviate other symptoms associated with moderate to severe depression. Specific groups are also used to treat chronic pain, premenstrual dysphoric disorder, panic disorder, social phobia, generalized anxiety disorder, and obsessive-compulsive disorder. Examples of commonly used antidepressant medications are presented in Table 10–2.

Action

These drugs ultimately work to increase the concentration of norepinephrine, serotonin, and/or dopamine in the body. This is accomplished in the brain by blocking the reuptake of these neurotransmitters by the neurons (tricyclics, tetracyclics, selective serotonin reuptake inhibitors, and others). It also occurs when an enzyme, monoamine oxidase (MAO), that is known to inactivate norepinephrine, serotonin, and dopamine, is inhibited at various sites in the nervous system (MAO inhibitors [MAOIs]).

Contraindications/Precautions

Antidepressant drugs are contraindicated in individuals with hypersensitivity. They are also contraindicated in the acute recovery phase following myocardial infarction and in individuals with angle-closure glaucoma.

Caution should be used in administering these

TABLE 10–2 Antidepressant Medications

Chemical Class	Generic (Trade) Name	Daily Adult Dosage Range*
Tricyclics	Amitriptyline (Elavil)	50–300 mg
	Amoxapine (Asendin)	50–600 mg
	Clomipramine (Anafranil)	25–250 mg
	Desipramine (Norpramin)	25–300 mg
	Doxepin (Sinequan)	25–300 mg
	Imipramine (Tofranil)	30–300 mg
	Nortriptyline (Aventyl; Pamelor)	30–150 mg
	Protriptyline (Vivactil)	15–60 mg
	Trimipramine (Surmontil)	50–300 mg
Heterocyclics	Bupropion (Wellbutrin; Zyban)	200–450 mg
	Maprotiline (Ludiomil)	50–225 mg
	Mirtazapine (Remeron)	15–45 mg
	Trazodone (Desyrel)	150–600 mg
Selective serotonin reuptake inhibitors	Citalopram (Celexa)	20–40 mg
	Escitalopram (Lexapro)	10–20 mg
	Fluoxetine (Prozac)	20–80 mg
	Fluvoxamine (Luvox)	50–300 mg
	Paroxetine (Paxil)	10–50 mg
	Sertraline (Zoloft)	50–200 mg
Nonselective reuptake inhibitors	Venlafaxine (Effexor)	75–375 mg
Monoamine oxidase inhibitors	Isocarboxazid (Marplan)	20–60 mg
	Phenelzine (Nardil)	45–90 mg
	Tranylcypromine (Parnate)	30–60 mg

*Dosage requires slow titration; onset of therapeutic response may be 1 to 4 weeks.

drugs to elderly or debilitated clients and those with hepatic, renal, or cardiac insufficiency. (The dosage usually must be decreased.) Caution is also required with psychotic clients, with clients who have benign prostatic hypertrophy, and with individuals who have a history of seizures (may decrease seizure threshold). *Note:* As these drugs take effect and mood begins to lift, the individual may have increased energy with which to implement a suicide plan. Suicide potential often increases as level of depression decreases. The nurse should be particularly alert to sudden lifts in mood.

Interactions

TRICYCLIC ANTIDEPRESSANTS. Hyperpyretic crisis, **hypertensive crisis**, severe seizures, and tachycardia may occur when used with MAOIs. Use of these drugs may decrease therapeutic response to some antihypertensives (clonidine, guanethidine). Additive CNS depression occurs with concurrent use of CNS depressants. Additive sympathomimetic and anticholinergic effects occur with use of other drugs possessing these same properties. Increased effects of tricyclic antidepressants may occur with bupropion, cimetidine, haloperidol, selective serotonin reuptake inhibitors (SSRIs), and valproic acid.

MAO INHIBITORS. Hypertensive crisis may occur with concurrent use of amphetamines, methyldopa, levodopa, dopamine, epinephrine, norepinephrine, reserpine, vasoconstrictors, or ingestion of tyramine-containing foods (Table 10–3). Hypertension or hypotension, coma, convulsions, and death may occur with meperidine or other narcotic analgesics when used with MAOIs. Additive hypotension may result with concurrent use of antihypertensives or spinal anesthesia and MAOIs. Additive hypoglycemia may result with concurrent use of insulin or oral hypoglycemic agents and MAOIs. Serious, potentially fatal adverse reactions may occur with concurrent use of other antidepressants, carbamazepine, cyclobenzaprine, maprotiline, furazolidone, procarbazine, or selegiline. Avoid using within 2 weeks of each other (5 weeks after therapy with fluoxetine).

SSRIs. Concurrent use with cimetidine may result in increased concentrations of SSRIs. Hypertensive crisis can occur if used within 14 days of MAOIs. Impairment of mental and motor skills may be potentiated with use of alcohol. **Serotonin syndrome** may occur with concurrent use of MAOIs and other drugs that increase serotonin, such as tryptophan, amphetamines, or other psychostimulants; other antidepressants that increase 5-hydroxytryptamine levels; or buspirone, lithium, or dopamine agonists (e.g., amantadine, bromocriptine). Concomitant use of SSRIs may increase effects of hydantoins, tricyclic antidepressants, benzodiazepines, beta-blockers, carbamazepine, clozapine, haloperidol, phenothiazines, St. John's wort, sumatriptan, sympathomimetics, tacrine, theophylline, and warfarin.

Diagnosis

The following nursing diagnoses may be considered for clients receiving therapy with antidepressant medications:

1. Risk for suicide related to depressed mood
2. Risk for injury related to side effects of sedation, lowered seizure threshold, orthostatic hypotension, **priapism**, photosensitivity, arrhythmias, hypertensive crisis, or serotonin syndrome

TABLE 10 – 3 Diet and Drug Restrictions for Clients on MAOI Therapy

Foods Containing Tyramine		
High Tyramine Content (Avoid while on MAOI Therapy)	**Moderate Tyramine Content (May eat occasionally while on MAOI Therapy)**	**Low Tyramine Content (Limited quantities permissible while on MAOI Therapy)**
Aged cheeses (cheddar, Swiss, Camembert, blue cheese, Parmesan, provolone, Romano, brie)	Gouda cheese, processed American cheese, mozzarella	Pasteurized cheeses (cream cheese, cottage cheese, ricotta)
Raisins, fava beans, flat Italian beans, Chinese pea pods	Yogurt, sour cream Avocados, bananas	Figs
Red wines (Chianti, burgundy, cabernet sauvignon)	Beer, white wine, coffee, colas, tea, hot chocolate	Distilled spirits (in moderation)
Smoked and processed meats (salami, bologna, pepperoni, summer sausage)	Meat extracts, such as bouillon	
Caviar, pickled herring, corned beef, chicken or beef liver		
Soy sauce, brewer's yeast, meat tenderizer (MSG)	Chocolate	

Drug Restrictions
Ingestion of the following substances while on MAOI Therapy could result in life-threatening hypertensive crisis. A 14-day interval is recommended between use of these drugs and an MAOI.
Other antidepressants (tricyclic; SSRIs)
Sympathomimetics: (epinephrine, dopamine, norepinephrine, ephedrine, pseudoephedrine, phenylephrine, phenylpropanolamine, over-the-counter cough and cold preparations)
Stimulants (amphetamines, cocaine, methyldopa, diet drugs)
Antihypertensives (methyldopa, guanethidine, reserpine)
Meperidine and (possibly) other opioid narcotics (morphine, codeine)
Antiparkinsonian agents (levodopa)

Adapted from Sadock & Sadock (2003) and Marangell, et al. (2003).

3. Social isolation related to depressed mood
4. Constipation related to side effects of the medication

Planning/Implementation

The plan of care should include monitoring for the following side effects from antidepressant medications. Nursing implications related to each side effect follow the asterisk (*). A general profile of the side effects of antidepressant medications is presented in Table 10–4.

1. May occur with all chemical classes:

   - Dry mouth. *Offer the client sugarless candy, ice, frequent sips of water. Strict oral hygiene is very important.
   - Sedation. *Request an order from the physician for the drug to be given at bedtime. Request that the physician decrease the dosage or perhaps order a less sedating drug. Instruct the client not to drive or use dangerous equipment when experiencing sedation.
   - Nausea. Medication may be taken with food to minimize GI distress.
   - Discontinuation syndrome. *All classes of antidepressants have varying potentials to cause discontinuation syndromes. Abrupt withdrawal following long-term therapy with SSRIs and venlafaxine may result in dizziness, lethargy, headache, and nausea. Fluoxetine is less likely to result in withdrawal symptoms because of its long half-life. Abrupt withdrawal from tricyclics may produce hypomania, akathisia, cardiac arrhythmias, and panic attacks. The discontinuation syndrome associated with MAOIs includes confusion, hypomania, and worsening of depressive symptoms. All antidepressant medication should be tapered gradually to prevent withdrawal symptoms (Haddad, 2001).

TABLE 10–4 Side Effect Profiles of Antidepressant Medications

	CNS Side Effects		Cardiovascular Side Effects		Other Side Effects		
	Sedation	*Insomnia/ Agitation*	*Orthostatic Hypotension*	*Cardiac Arrhythmia*	*Gastrointestinal Distress*	*Weight Gain (>6 kg)*	*Anticholinergic**
Amitriptyline	4+	0	4+	3+	0	4+	4+
Desipramine	1+	1+	2+	2+	0	1+	1+
Doxepin	4+	0	2+	2+	0	3+	3+
Imipramine	3+	1+	4+	3+	1+	3+	3+
Nortriptyline	1+	0	2+	2+	0	1+	1+
Protriptyline	1+	1+	2+	2+	0	0	2+
Trimipramine	4+	0	2+	2+	0	3+	1+
Amoxapine	2+	2+	2+	3+	0	1+	2+
Maprotiline	4+	0	0	1+	0	2+	2+
Mirtazapine	4+	0	0	1+	0	2+	2+
Trazodone	4+	0	1+	1+	1+	1+	0
Bupropion	0	2+	0	1+	1+	0	0
Fluoxetine	0	2+	0	0	3+	0	0
Fluvoxamine	0	2+	0	0	3+	0	0
Paroxetine	0	2+	0	0	3+	0	0
Sertraline	0	2+	0	0	3+	0	0
Monoamine oxidase inhibitors (MAOIs)	1+	2+	2+	0	1+	2+	1+

KEY: 0 = Absent or rare
1+ = Infrequent
2+, 3+ = Relatively common
4+ = Frequent
* Dry mouth, blurred vision, urinary hesitancy, constipation.
Adapted from Depression Guideline Panel (1993); *Drug Facts & Comparisons* (2003); and Schatzberg, Cole, & DeBattista (2003).

2. Most commonly occur with tricyclics or heterocyclics:

- Blurred vision. *Offer reassurance that this symptom should subside after a few weeks. Instruct the client not to drive until vision is clear. Clear small items from routine pathway to prevent falls.
- Constipation. *Order foods high in fiber; increase fluid intake if not contraindicated; and encourage the client to increase physical exercise, if possible.
- Urinary retention. *Instruct the client to report hesitancy or inability to urinate. Monitor intake and output. Try various methods to stimulate urination, such as running water in the bathroom or pouring water over the perineal area.
- Orthostatic hypotension. *Instruct the client to rise slowly from a lying or sitting position. Monitor blood pressure (lying and standing) frequently, and document and report significant changes. Avoid long hot showers or tub baths.
- Reduction of seizure threshold. *Observe clients with history of seizures closely. Institute seizure precautions as specified in hospital procedure manual. Bupropion (Wellbutrin) should be administered in doses of no more than 150 mg and should be given 8 hours apart. Bupropion has been associated with a relatively high incidence of seizure activity in anorexic and cachectic clients.
- Tachycardia; arrhythmias. *Carefully monitor blood pressure and pulse rate and rhythm, and report any significant change to the physician.
- Photosensitivity. *Ensure that client wears protective sunscreens, clothing, and sunglasses when outdoors.
- Weight gain. *Provide instructions for reduced calorie diet. Encourage increased level of activity, if appropriate.

3. Most commonly occur with SSRIs:
   - Insomnia; agitation. *Administer or instruct client to take dose early in the day. Instruct client to avoid caffeinated food and drinks. Teach relaxation techniques to use before bedtime.
   - Headache. *Administer analgesics as prescribed. Request that physician order another SSRI or another class of antidepressants.
   - Weight loss (may occur early in therapy). *Ensure that client is provided with caloric intake sufficient to maintain desired weight. Caution should be taken in prescribing these drugs for anorectic clients. Weigh client daily or every other day, at the same time, and on the same scale if possible. After prolonged use, some clients may gain weight on SSRIs.
   - Sexual dysfunction. *Men may report abnormal ejaculation or impotence. Women may experience delay or loss of orgasm. If side effect becomes intolerable, a switch to another antidepressant may be necessary.
   - Serotonin syndrome (may occur when two drugs that potentiate serotonergic neurotransmission are used concurrently [see "Interactions"]). *Most frequent symptoms include changes in mental status, restlessness, myoclonus, hyperreflexia, tachycardia, labile blood pressure, diaphoresis, shivering, and tremors. Discontinue offending agent immediately. The physician will prescribe medications to block serotonin receptors, relieve hyperthermia and muscle rigidity, and prevent seizures. Artificial ventilation may be required. The condition will usually resolve on its own within 24 hours once the offending medication has been discontinued. However, if the medication is not discontinued, the condition can progress rapidly to a more serious state and become fatal (Sternbach, 1991).
4. Most commonly occur with MAOIs:
   - Hypertensive crisis. *Hypertensive crisis occurs if the individual consumes foods containing tyramine when receiving MAOI therapy (see Table 10–4). Symptoms of hypertensive crisis include severe occipital headache, palpitations, nausea/vomiting, nuchal rigidity, fever, sweating, marked increase in blood pressure, chest pain, and coma. Treatment of hypertensive crisis: discontinue drug immediately; monitor vital signs; administer short-acting antihypertensive medication as ordered by physician; use external cooling measures to control hyperpyrexia.
5. Miscellaneous side effects:
   - Priapism (with trazodone [Desyrel]). *Priapism is a rare side effect, but it has occurred in some men taking trazodone. If the client complains of prolonged or inappropriate penile erection, withhold medication dosage, and notify the physician immediately. Priapism can become very problematic, requiring surgical intervention and, if not treated successfully, can result in impotence.

Client/Family Education

The client should:

- Continue to take the medication even though the symptoms have not subsided. The therapeutic effect may not be seen for as long as 4 weeks. If after this amount of time no improvement is noted, the physician may prescribe a different medication.
- Use caution when driving or operating dangerous machinery. Drowsiness and dizziness can occur. If these side effects become persistent or interfere with activities of daily living, the client should report them to the physician. Dosage adjustment may be necessary.
- Not stop taking the drug abruptly. To do so might produce withdrawal symptoms, such as nausea, vertigo, insomnia, headache, malaise, and nightmares.
- If taking a tricyclic, use sunscreens and wear protective clothing when spending time outdoors. The skin may be sensitive to sunburn.
- Report occurrence of any of the following symptoms to the physician immediately: sore throat, fever, chills, malaise, unusual bleeding, easy bruising, persistent nausea/vomiting, severe headache, rapid heart rate, difficulty urinating, anorexia/weight loss, seizure activity, stiff or sore neck, and chest pain.
- Rise slowly from a sitting or lying position to prevent a sudden drop in blood pressure.
- Take frequent sips of water, chew sugarless gum, or suck on hard candy if dry mouth is a problem. Good oral care (frequent brushing, flossing) is very important.
- Not consume the following foods or medications when taking MAOIs: aged cheese, wine (especially Chianti), beer, chocolate, colas, coffee, tea, sour cream, beef/chicken livers, canned figs, soy sauce, overripe and fermented foods, pickled herring, preserved sausages, yogurt, yeast products, broad beans, cold remedies, or diet pills. To do so could cause a life-threatening hypertensive crisis.

- Avoid smoking when receiving tricyclic therapy. Smoking increases the metabolism of tricyclics, requiring an adjustment in dosage to achieve the therapeutic effect.
- Not drink alcohol when taking antidepressant therapy. These drugs potentiate the effects of each other.
- Not consume other medications (including over-the-counter medications) without the physician's approval when receiving antidepressant therapy. Many medications contain substances that, in combination with antidepressant medication, could precipitate a life-threatening hypertensive crisis.
- Notify physician immediately if inappropriate or prolonged penile erections occur when taking trazodone (Desyrel). If the erection persists longer than 1 hour, seek emergency room treatment. This condition is rare, but it has occurred in some men who have taken trazodone. If measures are not instituted immediately, impotence can result.
- Not "double up" on medication if a dose of bupropion (Wellbutrin) is missed, unless advised to do so by the physician. Taking bupropion in divided doses will decrease the risk of seizures and other adverse effects.
- Be aware of possible risks of taking antidepressants during pregnancy. Safe use during pregnancy and lactation has not been fully established. These drugs are believed to readily cross the placental barrier; if so, the fetus could experience adverse effects of the drug. Inform the physician immediately if pregnancy occurs, is suspected, or is planned.
- Be aware of the side effects of antidepressants. Refer to written materials furnished by healthcare providers for safe self-administration.
- Carry a card or other identification at all times, describing the medications being taken.

Outcome Criteria/Evaluation

The following criteria may be used for evaluating the effectiveness of therapy with antidepressant medications. The client:

1. Has not harmed self
2. Has not experienced injury caused by side effects such as priapism, hypertensive crisis, photosensitivity, or serotonin syndrome
3. Exhibits vital signs within normal limits
4. Manifests symptoms of improvement in mood (brighter affect, interaction with others, improvement in hygiene, and clear thought and communication patterns)
5. Stays out of room and willingly participates in activities

Mood Stabilizing Agents

Background Assessment Data

For many years, the drug of choice for treatment and management of bipolar mania was lithium carbonate. However, in recent years, a number of investigators and clinicians in practice have achieved satisfactory results with several other medications, alone or in combination with lithium. Table 10–5 provides information about the indication, action, and contraindications and precautions of various medications being used as mood stabilizers.

Interactions

LITHIUM CARBONATE. Increased renal excretion of lithium may occur with acetazolamide, osmotic diuretics, and theophylline. Decreased renal excretion of lithium may occur with nonsteroidal anti-inflammatory drugs and thiazide diuretics. There is an increased risk of neurotoxicity with concurrent use of lithium and carbamazepine, haloperidol, or methyldopa. Concurrent use with fluoxetine or loop diuretics may result in increased serum lithium levels. Increased effects of neuromuscular blocking agents or tricyclic antidepressants and decreased pressor sensitivity of sympathomimetics can occur with concomitant use of lithium. Use of lithium with phenothiazines may result in neurotoxicity, decreased phenothiazine concentrations, or increased lithium concentration. Concurrent use with verapamil may result in decreased lithium levels or lithium toxicity.

CLONAZEPAM. The effects of clonazepam may be increased with concomitant use of CNS depressants, cimetidine, hormonal contraceptives, disulfiram, fluoxetine, isoniazid, ketoconazole, metoprolol, propoxyphene, propranolol, or valproic acid. The effects of clonazepam are decreased by rifampin, barbiturates, theophylline, or phenytoin. Concomitant use may result in increased phenytoin levels and decreased efficacy of levodopa.

CARBAMAZEPINE. The effects of carbamazepine may be increased by verapamil, diltiazem, propoxyphene, erythromycin, clarithromycin, SSRIs, antidepressants, cimetidine, barbiturates, isoniazid, or danazol. The effects of carbamazepine may be

TABLE 10–5 Mood Stabilizing Agents

Classification: Generic (Trade)	Indications	Mechanism of Action	Contraindications/ Precautions	Daily Adult Dosage Range
ANTIMANIC				
Lithium carbonate (Eskalith, Lithane; Lithobid)	Prevention and treatment of manic episodes of bipolar disorder. Also used for bipolar depression. Unlabeled uses: Major depression Neutropenia Cluster or migraine headache prophylaxis Alcohol dependence	Not fully understood, but may enhance reuptake of norepinephrine and serotonin, decreasing the levels in the body, resulting in decreased hyperactivity (may take 1–3 wks for symptoms to subside).	Hypersensitivity. Cardiac or renal disease, dehydration; sodium depletion; brain damage; pregnancy and lactation. Caution with thyroid disorders, diabetes, urinary retention, history of seizures, and with the elderly.	Acute mania: 1800 mg Maintenance: 900–1200 mg
ANTICONVULSANTS				
Clonazepam (Klonopin)	Absence, akinetic, and myoclonic seizures. Unlabeled use: bipolar mania.	Action in the treatment of bipolar disorder is unclear.	Hypersensitivity. Glaucoma, liver disease, lactation. Caution with elderly, liver/renal disease, pregnancy.	0.75–16 mg
Carbamazepine (Tegretol)	Grand mal and psychomotor seizures. Unlabeled uses: bipolar mania, rage reactions, resistant schizophrenia	Action in the treatment of bipolar disorder is unclear.	Hypersensitivity. With MAOIs, lactation. Caution with elderly, liver/renal/cardiac disease, pregnancy.	200–1600 mg
Valproic acid (Depakene; Depakote)	Absence seizures; Unlabeled use: bipolar mania, migraine prophylaxis	Action in the treatment of bipolar disorder is unclear.	Hypersensitivity; liver disease. Caution with elderly, renal/cardiac diseases, pregnancy and lactation.	500–1500 mg
Lamotrigine (Lamictal)	Generalized tonic-clonic seizures; absence and myoclonic seizures; Unlabeled use: bipolar disorder.	Action in the treatment of bipolar disorder is unclear.	Hypersensitivity. Caution with renal and hepatic insufficiency, pregnancy, lactation, and children aged < 16 years	50–200 mg
Gabapentin (Neurontin)	Partial seizures with and without generalization in adults with epilepsy. Unlabeled use: bipolar disorder.	Action in the treatment of bipolar disorder is unclear.	Hypersensitivity. Caution with renal insufficiency, pregnancy, lactation, children, and the elderly.	900–3600 mg
Topiramate (Topamax)	Partial onset seizures. Unlabeled use: bipolar disorder.	Action in the treatment of bipolar disorder is unclear.	Hypersensitivity. Caution with renal and hepatic impairment, pregnancy, lactation, children, and the elderly.	100–200 mg
CALCIUM CHANNEL BLOCKER				
Verapamil (Calan; Isoptin)	Angina, arrhythmias, hypertension. Unlabeled use: bipolar mania, migraine headache prophylaxis.	Action in the treatment of bipolar disorder is unclear.	Hypersensitivity heart block, hypotension, cardiogenic shock, congestive heart failure, pregnancy, lactation. Caution with liver or renal disease, cardiomyopathy, intracranial pressure, the elderly.	160–480 mg
ANTIPSYCHOTIC				
Olanzapine (Zyprexa)	Schizophrenia Bipolar mania	Action in the treatment of bipolar disorder is unclear.	Hypersensitivity children; lactation. Caution with hepatic or cardiovascular disease, history of seizures, comatose or other CNS-depression, prostatic hypertrophy, narrow–angle glaucoma, pregnancy, elderly and debilitated patients	10–20 mg

decreased by felbamate, hydantoins, or phenobarbital. Concurrent use with carbamazepine may decrease levels of corticosteroids, doxycycline, felbamate, quinidine, warfarin, estrogen-containing contraceptives, barbiturates, cyclosporine, benzodiazepines, theophylline, lamotrigine, valproic acid, bupropion, and haloperidol.

VALPROIC ACID. The effects of valproic acid may be increased by chlorpromazine, cimetidine, erythromycin, felbamate, or salicylates. The effects of valproic acid may be decreased by rifampin, carbamazepine, cholestyramine, lamotrigine, phenobarbital, or phenytoin. Concomitant use with valproic acid may increase the effects of tricyclic antidepressants, carbamazepine, CNS depressants, ethosuximide, lamotrigine, phenobarbital, phenytoin, warfarin and other antiplatelet agents, or zidovudine.

LAMOTRIGINE. The effects of lamotrigine are increased by folate inhibitors or valproic acid. The effects of lamotrigine are decreased by primidone, phenobarbital, phenytoin, rifamycin, succinimide, or carbamazepine. Concomitant use with lamotrigine may decrease levels of valproic acid.

GABAPENTIN. Antacids reduce the bioavailability of gabapentin. Coadministration of gabapentin with cimetidine results in a small decrease in renal excretion of gabapentin.

TOPIRAMATE. The effects of topiramate may be decreased with phenytoin, carbamazepine, or valproic acid. Concomitant use of topiramate with alcohol or other CNS depressants can potentiate CNS depression or other cognitive or neuropsychiatric adverse events. A risk of renal stone formation exists with coadministration of topiramate with carbonic anhydrase inhibitors (e.g., acetazolamide or dichlorphenamide). Efficacy of oral contraceptives may be compromised when taken with topiramate. Serum digoxin level is decreased with concomitant topiramate administration.

VERAPAMIL. Additive hypotension can occur with fentanyl, other antihypertensives, nitrates, alcohol, or quinidine. Antihypertensive effects of verapamil may be decreased with nonsteroidal anti-inflammatory drugs. Concurrent use with verapamil may increase serum levels of digoxin. Concomitant use of verapamil with beta-blockers, digoxin, disopyramide, or phenytoin may result in bradycardia, conduction defects, or congestive heart failure. Concurrent use may decrease the metabolism of and increase the risk of toxicity from cyclosporine, prazosin, quinidine, or carbamazepine. Verapamil may decrease the effectiveness of rifampin. Verapamil may increase the muscle-paralyzing effects of nondepolarizing neuromuscular blocking agents. Verapamil effectiveness may be decreased by coadministration with vitamin D compounds and calcium. Verapamil may alter serum lithium levels.

OLANZAPINE. Olanzapine antagonizes the effects of levodopa and dopamine agonists. Concomitant use may produce additive CNS depression with alcohol and other CNS depressants. Use with antihypertensive agents may result in additive hypotensive effects. The effects of olanzapine are decreased with carbamazepine, omeprazole, or rifampin. Decreased clearance of olanzapine occurs with fluvoxamine. Concomitant use with alcohol or diazepam potentiates orthostatic hypotension.

Diagnosis

The following nursing diagnoses may be considered for clients receiving therapy with mood-stabilizing agents:

1. Risk for injury related to manic hyperactivity
2. Risk for self-directed or other-directed violence related to unresolved anger turned inward on the self or outward on the environment
3. Risk for injury related to lithium toxicity
4. Risk for activity intolerance related to side effects of drowsiness and dizziness

Planning/Implementation

The plan of care should include monitoring for side effects of therapy with mood-stabilizing agents and intervening when required to prevent the occurrence of adverse events related to medication administration. Side effects and nursing implications for mood-stabilizing agents are presented in Table 10–6.

LITHIUM TOXICITY. The margin between the therapeutic and toxic levels of lithium carbonate is very narrow. The usual ranges of therapeutic serum concentrations are:

- For acute mania: 1.0 to 1.5 mEq/L
- For maintenance: 0.6 to 1.2 mEq/L

Serum lithium levels should be monitored once or twice a week after initial treatment until dosage and serum levels are stable, then monthly during maintenance therapy. Blood samples should be drawn 12 hours after the last dose.

Symptoms of lithium toxicity begin to appear at blood levels greater than 1.5 mEq/L and are dosage determinate. Symptoms include:

TABLE 10–6 Side Effects and Nursing Implications of Mood Stabilizing Agents

Medication	Side Effects	Nursing Implications
ANTIMANIC		
Lithium carbonate (Eskalith, Lithane)	1. Drowsiness, dizziness, headache	1. Ensure that client does not participate in activities that require alertness, or operate dangerous machinery.
	2. Dry mouth; thirst	2. Provide sugarless candy, ice, frequent sips of water. Ensure that strict oral hygiene is maintained.
	3. GI upset; nausea/vomiting	3. Administer medications with meals to minimize GI upset.
	4. Fine hand tremors	4. Report to physician, who may decrease dosage. Some physicians prescribe a small dose of beta-blocker propranolol to counteract this effect.
	5. Hypotension; arrhythmias; pulse irregularities	5. Monitor vital signs two or three times a day. Physician may decrease dose of medication.
	6. Polyuria; dehydration	6. May subside after initial week or two. Monitor daily intake, output, and weight. Monitor skin turgor daily.
	7. Weight gain	7. Provide instructions for reduced calorie diet. Emphasize importance of maintaining adequate intake of sodium.
ANTICONVULSANTS		
Clonazepam (Klonopin)	1. Nausea/vomiting	1. May give with food or milk to minimize GI upset.
Carbamazepine (Tegretol)	2. Drowsiness; dizziness	2. Ensure that client does not operate dangerous machinery or participate in activities that require alertness.
Valproic acid (Depakene; Depakote)	3. Blood dyscrasias	3. Ensure that client understands the importance of regular blood tests while receiving anticonvulsant therapy.
Gabapentin (Neurontin)	4. Prolonged bleeding time (with valproic acid)	4. Ensure that platelet count and bleeding time are determined before initiation of therapy with valproic acid. Monitor for spontaneous bleeding or bruising.
Lamotrigine (Lamictal)	5. Risk of severe rash (with lamotrigine)	5. Ensure that client is informed to report evidence of skin rash to physician immediately.
Topiramate (Topamax)	6. Decreased efficacy with oral contraceptives (with topiramate)	6. Ensure that client is aware of decreased efficacy of oral contraceptives with concomitant use.
CALCIUM CHANNEL BLOCKER		
Verapamil (Calan; Isoptin)	1. Drowsiness; dizziness	1. Ensure that client does not operate dangerous machinery or participate in activities that require alertness.
	2. Hypotension; bradycardia	2. Take vital signs prior to initiation of therapy and before daily administration of the medication. Physician will provide acceptable parameters for administration. Report marked changes immediately.
	3. Nausea	3. May give with food to minimize GI upset.
	4. Constipation	4. Encourage increased fluid (if not contraindicated) and fiber in the diet.
ANTIPSYCHOTIC		
Olanzapine (Zyprexa)	1. Somnolence, dizziness, asthenia	1. Ensure that client does not operate dangerous machinery or participate in activities that require alertness. Provide assistance as required.
	2. Fever; tachycardia	2. Monitor vital signs regularly. Report changes to physician.
	3. Postural hypotension	3. Instruct client to rise slowly from a lying or sitting position; monitor blood pressure (lying and standing); document and report significant changes.
	4. Dry mouth	4. Provide sugarless candy or gum, ice, and frequent sips of water.
	5. Constipation	5. Order foods high in fiber; encourage increase in physical activity and fluid intake if not contraindicated.
	6. Increased appetite; weight gain	6. Order calorie-controlled diet; provide opportunity for physical exercise; provide diet and exercise instruction.

- **At serum levels of 1.5 to 2.0 mEq/L:** Blurred vision, ataxia, tinnitus, persistent nausea and vomiting, severe diarrhea
- **At serum levels of 2.0 to 3.5 mEq/L:** Excessive output of dilute urine, increasing tremors, muscular irritability, psychomotor retardation, mental confusion, giddiness
- **At serum levels above 3.5 mEq/L:** Impaired consciousness, nystagmus, seizures, coma, oliguria/anuria, arrhythmias, myocardial infarction, cardiovascular collapse

Lithium levels should be monitored before medication administration. The dosage should be withheld and the physician notified if the level reaches 1.5 mEq/L or at the earliest observation or report by the client of even the mildest symptom. If left untreated, lithium toxicity can be life threatening.

Lithium is similar in chemical structure to sodium, behaving in the body in much the same manner and competing at various sites in the body with sodium. If sodium intake is reduced or the body is depleted of its normal sodium (e.g., due to excessive sweating, fever, or diuresis), lithium is reabsorbed by the kidneys, increasing the possibility of toxicity. Therefore, the client must consume a diet adequate in sodium as well as 2,500 to 3,000 mL of fluid per day. Accurate records of intake, output, and client's weight should be kept on a daily basis.

Client/Family Education (for Lithium)

The client should:

- Take medication on a regular basis, even when feeling well. Discontinuation can result in return of symptoms.
- Not drive or operate dangerous machinery until lithium levels are stabilized. Drowsiness and dizziness can occur.
- Not skimp on dietary sodium intake. He or she should choose foods from the food pyramid and avoid "junk" foods. The client should drink 6 to 8 large glasses of water each day and avoid excessive use of beverages containing caffeine (coffee, tea, colas), which promote increased urine output.
- Notify the physician if vomiting or diarrhea occurs. These symptoms can result in sodium loss and an increased risk of toxicity.
- Carry a card or other identification noting that he or she is taking lithium.
- Be aware of appropriate diet should weight gain become a problem. Include adequate sodium and other nutrients, and decrease number of calories.
- Be aware of risks of becoming pregnant when receiving lithium therapy. Use information furnished by healthcare providers regarding methods of contraception. Notify the physician as soon as possible if pregnancy is suspected or planned.
- Be aware of side effects and symptoms associated with toxicity. Notify the physician if any of the following symptoms occur: persistent nausea and vomiting, severe diarrhea, ataxia, blurred vision, tinnitus, excessive output of urine, increasing tremors, or mental confusion.
- Refer to written materials furnished by healthcare providers when receiving self-administered maintenance therapy. Keep appointments for outpatient follow-up; have serum lithium level checked every 1 to 2 months, or as advised by physician.

Client/Family Education (for Anticonvulsants)

The client should:

- Not stop taking drug abruptly. Physician will administer orders for tapering the drug when therapy is to be discontinued.
- Report the following symptoms to the physician immediately: unusual bleeding, spontaneous bruising, sore throat, fever, malaise, dark urine, yellow skin or eyes, or skin rash.
- Not drive or operate dangerous machinery until reaction to the medication has been established.
- Avoid consuming alcoholic beverages and nonprescription medications without approval from physician.
- Carry a card at all times identifying the name of medications being taken.

Client/Family Education (for Calcium Channel Blocker)

The client should:

- Take medication with meals if GI upset occurs.
- Use caution when driving or when operating dangerous machinery. Dizziness, drowsiness, and blurred vision can occur.
- Not abruptly discontinue taking drug. To do so may precipitate cardiovascular problems.
- Report occurrence of any of the following symptoms to physician immediately: irregular heartbeat, shortness of breath, swelling of the hands and feet,

pronounced dizziness, chest pain, profound mood swings, or severe and persistent headache.
- Rise slowly from a sitting or lying position to prevent a sudden drop in blood pressure.
- Not consume other medications (including over-the-counter medications) without physician's approval.
- Carry a card at all times describing medications being taken.

Client/Family Education (for Olanzapine)

The client should:

- Use caution when driving or operating dangerous machinery. Drowsiness and dizziness can occur.
- Report the occurrence of any of the following symptoms to the physician immediately: sore throat, fever, malaise, unusual bleeding, easy bruising, persistent nausea and vomiting, severe headache, rapid heart rate, difficulty urinating, muscle twitching, tremors, darkly colored urine, pale stools, yellow skin or eyes, muscular incoordination, or skin rash.
- Consult dietitian (if weight gain becomes a problem) to establish correct number of calories to maintain appropriate weight and prevent weight gain.
- Ensure that diet has sufficient fiber and fluid to prevent constipation.
- Rise slowly from a sitting or lying position to prevent a sudden drop in blood pressure.
- Take frequent sips of water, chew sugarless gum, or suck on hard candy if dry mouth is a problem. Good oral care (frequent brushing, flossing) is very important.
- Dress warmly in cold weather and avoid extended exposure to very high or low temperatures. Body temperature is harder to maintain with this medication.
- Not drink alcohol when on olanzapine therapy. These drugs potentiate each other's effects.
- Not consume other medications (including over-the-counter products) without the physician's approval. Many medications contain substances that interact with olanzapine in a way that may be harmful.
- Be aware of possible risks of taking olanzapine during pregnancy. Safe use during pregnancy and lactation has not been established. Neuroleptics are thought to readily cross the placental barrier; if so, a fetus could experience adverse effects of the drug. The client should inform the physician immediately if pregnancy occurs, is suspected, or is planned.
- Continue to take the medication, even if feeling well and as though it is not needed. Symptoms may return if medication is discontinued.

Outcome Criteria/Evaluation

The following criteria may be used for evaluating the effectiveness of therapy with mood stabilizing agents. The client:

1. Is maintaining stability of mood
2. Has not harmed self or others
3. Has experienced no injury from hyperactivity
4. Is able to participate in activities without excessive sedation or dizziness
5. Is maintaining appropriate weight
6. Exhibits no signs of lithium toxicity
7. Verbalizes importance of taking medication regularly and reporting for regular laboratory blood tests

Antipsychotic Agents

Background Assessment Data

Indications

Antipsychotic drugs are also called *major tranquilizers* and *neuroleptics*. They are used in the treatment of acute and chronic psychoses, particularly when accompanied by increased psychomotor activity. Selected agents are used as antiemetics (chlorpromazine, perphenazine, prochlorperazine), in the treatment of intractable hiccoughs (chlorpromazine, perphenazine), and for the control of tics and vocal utterances in Tourette's disorder (haloperidol, pimozide). Examples of commonly used antipsychotic agents are presented in Table 10–7.

Action

The exact mechanism of action is not known. These drugs are thought to work by blocking postsynaptic dopamine receptors in the basal ganglia, hypothalamus, limbic system, brainstem, and medulla. Newer medications may exert antipsychotic properties by blocking action on receptors specific to dopamine, serotonin, and other neurotransmitters. Antipsychotic effects may also be related to inhibition of dopamine-mediated transmission of neural impulses at the synapses (see Chapter 3).

TABLE 10–7 Antipsychotic Agents

Chemical Class	Generic (Trade Name)	Daily Dosage Range
Phenothiazines	Chlorpromazine (Thorazine)	40–800 mg
	Fluphenazine (Prolixin)	1–40 mg
	Mesoridazine (Serentil)	30–400 mg
	Perphenazine (Trilafon)	12–64 mg
	Prochlorperazine (Compazine)	15–150 mg
	Thioridazine (Mellaril)	150–800 mg
	Trifluoperazine (Stelazine)	2–40 mg
Thioxanthenes	Thiothixene (Navane)	6–30 mg
Benzisoxazole	Risperidone (Risperdal)	4–16 mg
Butyrophenone	Haloperidol (Haldol)	1–100 mg
Dibenzoxazepine	Loxapine (Loxitane)	20–250 mg
Dihydroindolone	Molindone (Moban)	15–225 mg
Dibenzodiazepine	Clozapine (Clozaril)	300–900 mg
Diphenylbutylpiperidine	Pimozide (Orap)	1–10 mg
Thienobenzodiazepine	Olanzapine (Zyprexa)	5–20 mg
Dibenzothiazepine	Quetiapine (Seroquel)	150–750 mg
Benzothiazolylpiperazine	Ziprasidone (Geodon)	40–160 mg
Dihydrocarbostyril	Aripiprazole (Abilify)	10–30 mg

Contraindications/Precautions

These drugs are contraindicated in clients with known hypersensitivity (cross-sensitivity may exist among phenothiazines). They should not be used when CNS depression is evident, when blood dyscrasias exist, in clients with Parkinson's disease, or those with liver, renal, or cardiac insufficiency.

Caution should be taken in administering these drugs to clients who are elderly, severely ill or debilitated, and to diabetic clients or clients with respiratory insufficiency, prostatic hypertrophy, or intestinal obstruction. Antipsychotics may lower seizure threshold. Individuals should avoid exposure to extremes in temperature when taking antipsychotic medication. Safety in pregnancy and lactation has not been established.

Interactions

Additive anticholinergic effects are observed when antipsychotics are taken concurrently with other drugs that produce these properties (e.g., antihistamines, antidepressants, antiparkinsonian agents). Additive hypotensive effects may occur with beta-adrenergic blocking agents (e.g., propranolol, metoprolol). Antacids and antidiarrheals may decrease absorption of antipsychotics. Barbiturates may increase metabolism and decrease effectiveness of antipsychotics. Additive CNS depression can occur with alcohol, antihistamines, antidepressants, sedative-hypnotics, and anxiolytics.

Diagnosis

The following nursing diagnoses may be considered for clients receiving antipsychotic therapy:

1. Risk for other-directed violence related to panic anxiety and mistrust of others
2. Risk for injury related to medication side effects of sedation, photosensitivity, reduction of seizure threshold, **agranulocytosis, extrapyramidal symptoms, tardive dyskinesia**, and **neuroleptic malignant syndrome**
3. Risk for activity intolerance related to medication side effects of sedation, blurred vision, and weakness
4. Noncompliance with medication regimen related to suspiciousness and mistrust of others

Planning/Implementation

The plan of care should include monitoring for the following side effects from antipsychotic medications. Nursing implications related to each side effect follow the asterisk (*). A profile of side effects comparing various antipsychotic medications is presented in Table 10–8.

1. Anticholinergic effects.
   - Dry mouth. *Provide the client with sugarless candy or gum, ice, frequent sips of water. Ensure that client practices strict oral hygiene.

TABLE 10 – 8 Comparison of Side Effects Among Antipsychotic Agents[1]

Chemical Class	Generic Name	Trade Name	Extrapyramidal Symptoms	Sedation	Anticholinergic	Orthostatic Hypotension	Seizures
Phenothiazines	Chlorpromazine	Thorazine	3	4	3	4	4
	Fluphenazine	Prolixin	5	2	2	2	2
	Mesoridazine	Serentil	2	4	4	4	2
	Perphenazine	Trilafon	4	2	2	2	3
	Prochlorperazine	Compazine	4	3	2	2	4
	Thioridazine	Mellaril	2	4	4	4	1
	Trifluoperazine	Stelazine	4	2	2	2	2
Thioxanthenes	Thiothixene	Navane	4	2	2	2	2
Benzisoxazole	Risperidone	Risperdal	1	1	1	3	1
Butyrophenone	Haloperidol	Haldol	5	1	1	1	1
Dibenzoxazepine	Loxapine	Loxitane	4	3	2	3	4
Dihydroindolone	Molindone	Moban	4	1	2	2	2
Dibenzodiazepine	Clozapine	Clozaril	1	5	5	4	4
Thienobenzo-diazepine	Olanzapine	Zyprexa	1	3	2	1	1
Diphenylbutyl-piperidine	Pimozide	Orap	4	3	2	2	2
Dibenzothiazepine	Quetiapine	Seroquel	1	3	2	1	1
Benzothia-zolylpiperazine	Ziprasidone	Geodon	1	2	1	1	1
Dihydrocarbostyril	Aripiprazole	Abilify	2	2	1	3	2

[1]Key: 1 = Very low
2 = Low
3 = Moderate
4 = High
5 = Very high

Adapted from Schatzberg, Cole, & DeBattista (2003), *Facts and Comparisons* (2003); Marder (1997); and Jibson & Tandon (1996).

- Blurred vision. *Explain that this symptom will most likely subside after a few weeks. Advise client not to drive a car until vision clears. Clear small items from pathway to prevent falls.
- Constipation. *Order foods high in fiber; encourage increase in physical activity and fluid intake if not contraindicated.
- Urinary retention. *Instruct client to report any difficulty urinating; monitor intake and output.

2. Nausea; GI upset. *Tablets or capsules may be administered with food to minimize GI upset. Concentrates may be diluted and administered with fruit juice or other liquid; they should be mixed immediately before administration.
3. Skin rash. *Report appearance of any rash on skin to physician. Avoid spilling any of the liquid concentrate on skin; contact dermatitis can occur with some medications.
4. Sedation. *Discuss with physician the possibility of administering the drug at bedtime. Discuss with physician a possible decrease in dosage or an order for a less sedating drug. Instruct client not to drive or operate dangerous equipment when experiencing sedation.
5. Orthostatic hypotension. *Instruct the client to rise slowly from a lying or sitting position; monitor blood pressure (lying and standing) each shift; document and report significant changes.
6. Photosensitivity. *Ensure that the client wears protective sunscreens, clothing, and sunglasses when spending time outdoors.
7. Hormonal effects.

- Decreased libido, **retrograde ejaculation, gynecomastia** (men). *Provide explanation of the effects and reassurance of their reversibility. If necessary, discuss with physician possibility of ordering alternate medication.
- **Amenorrhea** (women). *Offer reassurance of reversibility; instruct the client to continue use of contraception because amenorrhea does not indicate cessation of ovulation.
- Weight gain. *Weigh client every other day; or-

der calorie-controlled diet; provide opportunity for physical exercise; provide diet and exercise instruction.

8. Electrocardiogram (ECG) changes. ECG changes, including prolongation of the QT interval, are possible with most of the antipsychotics. This is particularly true with ziprasidone (Geodon). Caution is advised in prescribing this medication to individuals with history of arrhythmias. Conditions that produce hypokalemia and/or hypomagnesemia, such as diuretic therapy or diarrhea, should be taken into consideration when prescribing. Routine ECG should be taken before initiation of therapy and periodically during therapy. *Monitor vital signs every shift. Observe for symptoms of dizziness, palpitations, syncope, or weakness.
9. Reduction of seizure threshold. *Closely observe clients with history of seizures. *Note:* This is particularly important with clients taking clozapine (Clozaril). Reportedly, seizures affect 1 to 5 percent of individuals who take this drug, depending on the dosage (Bernstein, 1995).
10. Agranulocytosis. *Relatively rare with most of the antipsychotic drugs. It usually occurs within the first 3 months of treatment. Observe for symptoms of sore throat, fever, and malaise. A complete blood count should be monitored if these symptoms appear. *Exception:* There is a significant risk of agranulocytosis with clozapine (Clozaril). Agranulocytosis is a potentially fatal blood disorder in which the client's white blood cell (WBC) count can drop to extremely low levels. Individuals receiving clozapine therapy are required to have blood levels drawn weekly or biweekly to continue therapy. They are given a 1- or 2-week supply of medication at a time. If the WBC count falls below 3,000 mm^3, or the granulocyte count falls below 1,500 mm^3, clozapine therapy is discontinued. The disorder is reversible if discovered in the early stages. However, the additional required technology of weekly blood tests has made this drug cost-prohibitive for some people.
11. Hypersalivation (with clozapine). *A significant number of clients receiving clozapine (Clozaril) therapy experience extreme salivation. Offer support to the client because this may be an embarrassing situation. It may even be a safety issue (e.g., risk of aspiration) if the problem is very severe.
12. Extrapyramidal symptoms (EPS). *Observe for symptoms and report; administer antiparkinsonian drugs as ordered (Table 10–9).
    - **Pseudoparkinsonism** (tremor, shuffling gait, drooling, rigidity). *Symptoms may appear 1 to 5 days following initiation of antipsychotic medication; occurs most often in women, the elderly, and dehydrated clients.
    - **Akinesia** (muscular weakness). *Same as for pseudoparkinsonism.
    - **Akathisia** (continuous restlessness and fidgeting). *This occurs most frequently in women; symptoms may occur 50 to 60 days after initiation of therapy.
    - **Dystonia** (involuntary muscular movements [spasms] of face, arms, legs, and neck). *This occurs most often in men and in clients younger than 25 years of age.
    - **Oculogyric crisis** (uncontrolled rolling back of the eyes). *This may appear as part of syndrome described as dystonia. It may be mistaken for seizure activity; dystonia and oculogyric crisis should be treated as emergencies. The physician should be contacted, and intravenous benztropine mesylate (Cogentin) is commonly administered. Stay with the client, and offer reassurance and support during this frightening time.
13. Tardive dyskinesia (bizarre facial and tongue movements, stiff neck, and difficulty swallowing). *All clients receiving long-term (months or years)

TABLE 10–9 Antiparkinsonian Agents

Chemical Class	Generic (Trade) Name	Daily Dosage Range
Anticholinergics	Benztropine (Cogentin)	0.5–6 mg
	Biperiden (Akineton)	2–8 mg
	Procyclidine (Kemadrin)	5–20 mg
	Trihexyphenidyl (Artane)	1–15 mg
Antihistamines	Diphenhydramine (Benadryl)	10–400 mg
Dopaminergic agonists	Amantadine (Symmetrel)	200–400 mg
	Bromocriptine (Parlodel)	10–40 mg

antipsychotic therapy are at risk. The symptoms are potentially irreversible. The drug should be withdrawn at the first sign, which is usually vermiform movements of the tongue; prompt action may prevent irreversibility.

14. **Neuroleptic malignant syndrome (NMS).** Symptoms include severe parkinsonian muscle rigidity, hyperpyrexia up to 107°F, tachycardia, tachypnea, fluctuations in blood pressure, diaphoresis, and rapid deterioration of mental status to stupor and coma. *This is a rare but potentially fatal complication of treatment with neuroleptic drugs. Routine assessments should include temperature and observation for parkinsonian symptoms. Onset can occur within hours or even years after drug initiation, and progression is rapid over the following 24 to 72 hours. Discontinue neuroleptic medication immediately. Monitor vital signs, extent of muscle rigidity, intake and output, level of consciousness. The physician may order bromocriptine (Parlodel) or dantrolene (Dantrium) to counteract the effects of neuroleptic malignant syndrome.
15. Hyperglycemia and Diabetes. Studies have suggested an increased risk of treatment-emergent hyperglycemia-related adverse events in clients using atypical antipsychotics (e.g., risperidone, clozepine, olanzapine, quetiapine, ziprasidone, and aripiprazole). The FDA recommends that clients with diabetes starting on atypical antipsychotic drugs be monitored regularly for worsening of glucose control. Clients with risk factors for diabetes should undergo fasting blood glucose testing at the beginning of treatment and periodically thereafter. All clients taking these medications should be monitored for symptoms of hyperglycemia (polydipsia, polyuria, polyphagia, and weakness). If these symptoms appear during treatment, the client should undergo fasting blood glucose testing.

Client/Family Education

The client should:

- Use caution when driving or operating dangerous machinery. Drowsiness and dizziness can occur.
- Not stop taking the drug abruptly after long-term use. To do so might produce withdrawal symptoms, such as nausea, vomiting, dizziness, gastritis, headache, tachycardia, insomnia, tremulousness.
- Use sunscreens and wear protective clothing when spending time outdoors. Skin is susceptible to sunburn, which can occur in as few as 30 minutes.
- Report weekly (if receiving clozapine therapy) to have blood levels drawn and to obtain a weekly supply of the drug.
- Report the occurrence of any of the following symptoms to the physician immediately: sore throat, fever, malaise, unusual bleeding, easy bruising, persistent nausea and vomiting, severe headache, rapid heart rate, difficulty urinating, muscle twitching, tremors, darkly colored urine, excessive urination, excessive thirst, excessive hunger, weakness, pale stools, yellow skin or eyes, muscular incoordination, or skin rash.
- Rise slowly from a sitting or lying position to prevent a sudden drop in blood pressure.
- Take frequent sips of water, chew sugarless gum, or suck on hard candy if dry mouth is a problem. Good oral care (frequent brushing, flossing) is very important.
- Consult physician regarding smoking when on neuroleptic therapy. Smoking increases the metabolism of neuroleptics, requiring an adjustment in dosage to achieve a therapeutic effect.
- Dress warmly in cold weather, and avoid extended exposure to very high or low temperatures. Body temperature is harder to maintain with this medication.
- Not drink alcohol when on neuroleptic therapy. These drugs potentiate each other's effects.
- Not consume other medications (including over-the-counter products) without physician's approval. Many medications contain substances that interact with neuroleptics in a way that may be harmful.
- Be aware of possible risks of taking neuroleptics during pregnancy. Safe use during pregnancy and lactation has not been established. Neuroleptics are thought to readily cross the placental barrier; if so, a fetus could experience adverse effects of the drug. Inform the physician immediately if pregnancy occurs, is suspected, or is planned.
- Be aware of side effects of neuroleptic drugs. Refer to written materials furnished by healthcare providers for safe self-administration.
- Continue to take medication, even if feeling well and as though it is not needed. Symptoms may return if medication is discontinued.
- Carry a card or other identification at all times describing medications being taken.

Outcome Criteria/Evaluation

The following criteria may be used for evaluating the effectiveness of therapy with antipsychotic medications. The client:

1. Has not harmed others
2. Has not experienced injury caused by side effects of lowered seizure threshold or photosensitivity
3. Maintains a WBC count within normal limits
4. Exhibits no symptoms of extrapyramidal side effects, tardive dyskinesia, or neuroleptic malignant syndrome
5. Maintains weight within normal limits
6. Tolerates activity unaltered by the effects of sedation or weakness
7. Takes medication willingly
8. Verbalizes understanding of medication regimen and the importance of regular administration

Antiparkinsonian Agents

Background Assessment Data

Indications

Antiparkinsonian agents are indicated for the treatment of all forms of parkinsonism and for the relief of drug-induced extrapyramidal reactions. Examples of commonly used antiparkinsonian agents are presented in Table 10–9.

Action

The action of these drugs is aimed at restoring the natural balance of two major neurotransmitters in the CNS: acetylcholine and dopamine. The imbalance is a deficiency in dopamine that results in excessive cholinergic activity. Drugs used are anticholinergics (which block the acetylcholine receptor to diminish excess cholinergic effect) or dopaminergic agonists (which increase the content of dopamine in the brain directly by stimulation of dopamine receptors or indirectly by blocking neuronal reuptake of dopamine).

Contraindications/Precautions

These drugs are contraindicated in clients with known hypersensitivity, angle-closure glaucoma, pyloric or duodenal obstruction, peptic ulcers, prostatic hypertrophy, bladder neck obstruction, megaesophagus, megacolon, and myasthenia gravis. Caution should be used in administering to clients with tachycardia, cardiac arrhythmias, hypertension, hypotension, and a tendency toward urinary retention. Caution also should be used in clients who are elderly and debilitated; clients with hepatic, renal, or cardiac insufficiency; and clients exposed to high environmental temperatures.

Interactions

Additive anticholinergic effects and potentially fatal paralytic ileus can occur with other drugs that possess these properties. Additive CNS effects can occur with CNS depressants. Concomitant use of anticholinergics with haloperidol may decrease haloperidol serum concentrations. Coadministration with phenothiazines may result in decreased therapeutic action of phenothiazines and increased incidence of anticholinergic side effects.

Diagnosis

The following nursing diagnoses may be considered for clients receiving therapy with antiparkinsonian agents:

1. Risk for injury related to symptoms of Parkinson's disease or drug-induced EPS
2. Hyperthermia related to anticholinergic effect of decreased sweating
3. Activity intolerance related to side effects of drowsiness, dizziness, ataxia, weakness, confusion
4. Deficient knowledge related to medication regimen

Planning/Implementation

The plan of care should include monitoring for the following side effects from antiparkinsonian agents. Nursing implications related to each side effect follow the asterisk (*).

1. Anticholinergic effects. *These side effects are identical to those produced by antipsychotic drugs. Taking both types of medications compounds these effects. For this reason, the physician may elect to prescribe an antiparkinsonian agent only at the onset of EPS, with orders to be given p.r.n. rather than as routine adjunctive therapy.
   - Dry mouth. *Offer sugarless candy or gum, ice, frequent sips of water. Ensure that client practices strict oral hygiene.
   - Blurred vision. *Explain that this symptom will

most likely subside after a few weeks. Offer to assist with tasks requiring visual acuity.

- Constipation. *Order foods high in fiber; encourage increase in physical activity and fluid intake, if not contraindicated.
- Paralytic ileus. *This is a rare but potentially very serious side effect of anticholinergic drugs. Monitor for abdominal distension, absent bowel sounds, nausea, vomiting, and epigastric pain. Report any of these symptoms to physician immediately.
- Urinary retention. *Instruct client to report any difficulty urinating; monitor intake and output.
- Tachycardia, decreased sweating, elevated temperature. *Assess vital signs each shift; document and report significant changes to physician. Ensure that client remains in cool environment, because the body is unable to cool itself naturally with this medication.

2. Nausea, GI upset. *May administer tablets or capsules with food to minimize GI upset.
3. Sedation, drowsiness, dizziness. *Discuss with physician the possibility of administering the drug at bedtime. Discuss with physician a possible decrease in dosage or an order for a less sedating drug. Instruct the client not to drive or use dangerous equipment when experiencing sedation or dizziness.
4. Exacerbation of psychoses. *Assess for signs of loss of contact with reality. Intervene during a hallucination; talk about real people and real events; reorient the client to reality. Stay with the client during periods of agitation and delirium; remain calm and reassure the client of his or her safety. Discuss with the physician a possible decrease in dosage or change in medication.
5. Orthostatic hypotension. *Instruct client to rise slowly from a lying or sitting position; monitor blood pressure (lying and standing) each shift; document and report significant changes.

Client/Family Education

The client should:

- Take the medication with food if GI upset occurs.
- Use caution when driving or operating dangerous machinery. Drowsiness and dizziness can occur.
- Not stop taking the drug abruptly. To do so might produce unpleasant withdrawal symptoms.
- Report occurrence of any of the following symptoms to the physician immediately: pain or tenderness in area in front of ear; extreme dryness of mouth; difficulty urinating; abdominal pain; constipation; fast, pounding heartbeat; rash; visual disturbances; mental changes.
- Rise slowly from a sitting or lying position to prevent a sudden drop in blood pressure.
- Stay in air-conditioned room when weather is very hot. Perspiration is decreased with antiparkinsonian agents, and the body cannot cool itself as well. There is greater susceptibility to heat stroke. Inform physician if air-conditioned housing is not available.
- Take frequent sips of water, chew sugarless gum, or suck on hard candy if dry mouth is a problem. Good oral care (frequent brushing, flossing) is very important.
- Not drink alcohol when on antiparkinsonian therapy.
- Not consume other medications (including over-the-counter products) without physician's approval. Many medications contain substances that interact with antiparkinsonian agents in a way that may be harmful.
- Be aware of possible risks of taking antiparkinsonian agents during pregnancy. Safe use during pregnancy and lactation has not been fully established. It is thought that antiparkinsonian agents readily cross the placental barrier; if so, fetus could experience adverse effects of the drug. Inform physician immediately if pregnancy occurs, is suspected, or is planned.
- Be aware of side effects of antiparkinsonian agents. Refer to written materials furnished by healthcare providers for safe self-administration.
- Continue to take the medication, even if feeling well and as though it is not needed. Symptoms may return if medication is discontinued.
- Carry a card or other identification at all times describing medications being taken.

Outcome Criteria/Evaluation

The following criteria may be used for evaluating the effectiveness of therapy with CNS stimulants. The client:

1. Has not experienced injury caused by symptoms of Parkinson's disease or drug-related EPS
2. Has not experienced symptoms of hyperthermia
3. Has not experienced intolerance to activity due to side effects of the medication
4. Verbalizes understanding of medication regimen and the importance of regular administration

Sedative-Hypnotics

Background Assessment Data

Indications

Sedative-hypnotics are used in the short-term management of various anxiety states and to treat insomnia. Selected agents are used as anticonvulsants and preoperative sedatives (phenobarbital, pentobarbital, secobarbital) and to reduce anxiety associated with drug withdrawal (chloral hydrate). Examples of commonly used sedative-hypnotics are presented in Table 10–10.

Action

Sedative-hypnotics cause generalized CNS depression. They may produce tolerance with chronic use and have the potential for psychological or physical dependence.

TABLE 10–10 Sedative-Hypnotic Agents

Chemical Class	Generic (Trade) Name	Daily Dosage Range
Barbiturates	Amobarbital (Amytal)	60–200 mg
	Butabarbital (Butisol)	45–120 mg
	Mephobarbital (Mebaral)	32–200 mg
	Pentobarbital (Nembutal)	40–200 mg
	Phenobarbital (Luminal)	30–320 mg
	Secobarbital (Seconal)	90–200 mg
Benzodiazepines	Estazolam (ProSom)	1–2 mg
	Flurazepam (Dalmane)	15–30 mg
	Quazepam (Doral)	7.5–15 mg
	Temazepam (Restoril)	15–30 mg
	Triazolam (Halcion)	0.125–0.5
Miscellaneous	Chloral hydrate (Noctec)	500–1000 mg
	Glutethimide (Doriden)	250–500 mg
	Zaleplon (Sonata)	5–20 mg
	Zolpidem (Ambien)	5–10 mg

Contraindications/Precautions

Sedative-hypnotics are contraindicated in individuals with hypersensitivity to the drug or to any drug within the chemical class. Caution should be used in administering these drugs to clients with hepatic dysfunction or severe renal impairment. They should be used with caution in clients who may be suicidal or who may have been addicted to drugs previously. Hypnotic use should be short-term. Elderly clients may be more sensitive to CNS depressant effects, and dosage reduction may be required.

Interactions

Additive CNS depression can occur when sedative-hypnotics are taken concomitantly with alcohol, antihistamines, antidepressants, phenothiazines, or any other CNS depressants. Barbiturates induce hepatic drug-metabolizing enzymes and can decrease the effectiveness of drugs metabolized by the liver. Sedative-hypnotics should not be used with MAOIs.

Diagnosis

The following nursing diagnoses may be considered for clients receiving therapy with sedative hypnotics:

1. Risk for injury related to abrupt withdrawal from long-term use or decreased mental alertness caused by residual sedation
2. Disturbed sleep pattern related to situational crises, physical condition, or severe level of anxiety
3. Risk for activity intolerance related to side effects of lethargy, drowsiness, and dizziness
4. Risk for acute confusion related to action of the medication on the CNS

Planning/Implementation

Refer to this section in the discussion of antianxiety medications.

Outcome Criteria/Evaluation

The following criteria may be used for evaluating the effectiveness of therapy with sedative-hypnotic medications. The client:

1. Demonstrates a reduction in anxiety, tension, and restless activity
2. Falls asleep within 30 minutes of taking the medication and remains asleep for 6 to 8 hours without interruption
3. Is able to participate in usual activities without residual sedation

4. Experiences no physical injury
5. Exhibits no evidence of confusion
6. Verbalizes understanding of taking the medication on a short-term basis
7. Verbalizes understanding of potential for development of tolerance and dependence with long-term use

Agents for Attention Deficit Hyperactivity Disorder (ADHD)

Background Assessment Data

Indications

The medications in this section are used for ADHD with hyperactivity in children and adults. Examples of commonly used agents for ADHD are presented in Table 10–11.

Action

CNS stimulants increase levels of neurotransmitters (probably norepinephrine, dopamine, and serotonin) in the CNS. They produce CNS and respiratory stimulation, dilated pupils, increased motor activity and mental alertness, diminished sense of fatigue, and brighter spirits. The CNS stimulants discussed in this section include dextroamphetamine sulfate, methamphetamine, amphetamine mixtures, methylphenidate, and pemoline.

Atomoxetine inhibits the reuptake of norepinephrine, and bupropion blocks the uptake of serotonin and norepinephrine and inhibits the reuptake of dopamine. The exact mechanism by which these drugs produce the therapeutic effects in ADHD is unknown. They are not CNS stimulants.

TABLE 10–11 Agents for Attention Deficit Hyperactivity Disorder

Chemical Class	Generic (Trade) Name	Daily Dosage Range
Amphetamines	Dextroamphetamine sulfate (Dexedrine; DextroStat)	5–40 mg
	Methamphetamine (Desoxyn)	5–25 mg
	Amphetamine mixtures (Adderall; Adderall XR)	5–40 mg (XR: 10–30 mg)
Miscellaneous	Methylphenidate (Ritalin)	10–60 mg
	Pemoline (Cylert)	37.5–112.5 mg
	Atomoxetine (Strattera)	> 70 kg: 40–100 mg ≤ 70 kg: 0.5–1.4 mg/kg
	Bupropion (Wellbutrin)	3 mg/kg

Contraindications/Precautions

CNS stimulants are contraindicated in individuals with hypersensitivity to sympathomimetic amines. They should not be used in advanced arteriosclerosis, symptomatic cardiovascular disease, hypertension, hyperthyroidism, glaucoma, agitated or hyperexcitability states, in clients with a history of drug abuse, during or within 14 days of receiving therapy with MAOIs, in children under 3 years of age, and in pregnancy. Atomoxetine and bupropion are contraindicated in clients with hypersensitivity to the drugs or their components, and in concomitant use with, or within 2 weeks of using MAO inhibitors. Atomoxetine is contraindicated in clients with narrow-angle glaucoma. Bupropion is contraindicated in individuals with known or suspected seizure disorder, acute phase of myocardial infarction, and in clients with bulimia or anorexia nervosa.

Caution is advised in using CNS stimulants during lactation; with psychotic children; in Tourette's disorder; in clients with anorexia or insomnia; in elderly, debilitated, or asthenic clients; and in clients with a history of suicidal or homicidal tendencies. Prolonged use may result in tolerance and physical or psychological dependence. Use atomoxetine and bupropion cautiously in clients with urinary retention; hepatic, renal, or cardiovascular disease; suicidal clients; pregnancy and lactation; and elderly and debilitated clients.

Interactions

Use of CNS stimulants within 14 days following administration of MAOIs may result in hypertensive crisis, headache, hyperpyrexia, intracranial hemorrhage, and bradycardia. Insulin requirements may be altered with CNS stimulants. Urine alkalinizers decrease excretion, enhancing the effects of amphetamines; urine acidifiers increase excretion, decreasing the effects. Decreased effects of both drugs can occur when administered concurrently with phenothiazines. With atomoxetine: increased cardiovascular effects with albuterol; increased risk of neuroleptic malignant syndrome when used within 14 days of MAO inhibitors; increased effects of atomoxetine with concomitant use of CYP 2D6 inhibitors (paroxetine, fluoxetine, quinidine). With bupropion: increased risk of seizures with other drugs that lower seizure threshold; acute toxicity of bupropion with concurrent use of MAOIs; hypertension, seizures, and death can occur when used within 14 days of MAOIs.

Diagnosis

The following nursing diagnoses may be considered for clients receiving therapy with agents for ADHD:

1. Risk for injury related to overstimulation and hyperactivity (CNS stimulants) or seizures (possible side effect of bupropion)
2. Risk for suicide secondary to major depression related to abrupt withdrawal after extended use (CNS stimulants)
3. Imbalanced nutrition, less than body requirements, related to side effects of anorexia and weight loss (CNS stimulants)
4. Disturbed sleep pattern related to overstimulation resulting from use of the medication (CNS stimulants) or side effect of insomnia with atomoxetine
5. Nausea related to side effects of atomoxetine or bupropion
6. Pain related to side effect of headache with atomoxetine or bupropion
7. Risk for activity intolerance related to side effects of sedation and dizziness with atomoxetine or bupropion

Planning/Implementation

The plan of care should include monitoring for the following side effects from agents for ADHD. Nursing implications related to each side effect follow the asterisk (*).

1. Overstimulation, restlessness, insomnia (CNS stimulants). *Assess mental status for changes in mood, level of activity, extent of stimulation, and aggressiveness. Ensure that the client is protected from injury. Keep stimuli low and environment as quiet as possible to discourage overstimulation. To prevent insomnia, administer the last dose at least 6 hours before bedtime. Administer sustained-release forms in the morning.
2. Palpitations, tachycardia (CNS stimulants; atomoxetine). *Monitor and record vital signs at regular intervals (two or three times a day) throughout therapy. Report significant changes to the physician immediately.
3. Anorexia, weight loss (CNS stimulants; atomoxetine). *To reduce anorexia, the medication may be administered immediately after meals. The client should be weighed regularly (at least weekly) when receiving therapy with CNS stimulants or atomoxetine because of the potential for anorexia/weight loss and temporary interruption of growth and development.
4. Tolerance, physical and psychological dependence (CNS stimulants). *Tolerance develops rapidly. In children with behavior disorders, a drug "holiday" should be attempted periodically under direction of the physician to determine the effectiveness of the medication and the need for continuation. The drug should not be withdrawn abruptly. To do so could initiate the following syndrome of symptoms: nausea, vomiting, abdominal cramping, headache, fatigue, weakness, mental depression, suicidal ideation, increased dreaming, and psychotic behavior.
5. Nausea and vomiting (atomoxetine and bupropion). *May be taken with food to minimize GI upset.
6. Constipation (atomoxetine and bupropion). *Increase fiber and fluid in diet, if not contraindicated.
7. Potential for seizures (bupropion). *Protect client from injury if seizure should occur. Instruct family and significant others of clients on bupropion therapy how to protect client during a seizure if one should occur. Ensure that doses of the medication are administered at least 8 hours apart.

Client/Family Education

The client should:

- Use caution in driving or operating dangerous machinery. Drowsiness, dizziness, and blurred vision can occur.
- Not stop taking CNS stimulants abruptly. To do so could produce serious withdrawal symptoms.
- Avoid taking CNS stimulants late in the day to prevent insomnia. Take no later than 6 hours before bedtime.
- Not take other medications (including over-the-counter drugs) without physician's approval. Many medications contain substances that, in combination with agents for ADHD, can be harmful.
- Diabetic clients should monitor blood sugar two or

three times a day or as instructed by the physician. Be aware of the need for possible alteration in insulin requirements because of changes in food intake, weight, and activity.

- Avoid consumption of large amounts of caffeinated products (coffee, tea, colas, chocolate), as they may enhance the CNS stimulant effect.
- Notify physician if restlessness, insomnia, anorexia, or dry mouth becomes severe, or if rapid, pounding heartbeat becomes evident.
- Be aware of possible risks of taking agents for ADHD during pregnancy. Safe use during pregnancy and lactation has not been established. Inform the physician immediately if pregnancy is suspected or planned.
- Be aware of potential side effects of agents for ADHD. Refer to written materials furnished by healthcare providers for safe self-administration.
- Carry a card or other identification at all times describing medications being taken.

Outcome Criteria/Evaluation

The following criteria may be used for evaluating the effectiveness of therapy with agents for ADHD. The client:

1. Does not exhibit excessive hyperactivity
2. Has not experienced injury
3. Is maintaining expected parameters of growth and development
4. Verbalizes understanding of safe self-administration and the importance of not withdrawing medication abruptly

SUMMARY

Psychotropic medications are intended to be used as adjunctive therapy to individual or group psychotherapy. *Antianxiety agents* are used in the treatment of anxiety disorders and to alleviate acute anxiety symptoms. The benzodiazepines are the most commonly used group. They are CNS depressants and have a potential for physical and psychological dependence. They should not be discontinued abruptly following long-term use because they can produce a life-threatening withdrawal syndrome. The most common side effects are drowsiness, confusion, and lethargy.

Antidepressants elevate mood and alleviate other symptoms associated with moderate-to-severe depression. These drugs work to increase the concentration of norepinephrine and serotonin in the body. The tricyclics and related drugs accomplish this by blocking the reuptake of these chemicals by the neurons. Another group of antidepressants inhibit MAO, an enzyme that is known to inactivate norepinephrine and serotonin. They are called MAO inhibitors (MAOIs). A third category of drugs blocks neuronal reuptake of serotonin, and has minimal or no effect on reuptake of norepinephrine or dopamine. They are called selective serotonin reuptake inhibitors (SSRIs). Antidepressant medications may take up to 4 weeks to produce the desired effect. The most common side effects of tricyclics are anticholinergic effects, sedation, and orthostatic hypotension. They can also reduce the seizure threshold. MAOIs can cause hypertensive crisis if products containing tyramine are consumed while taking these medications.

The *mood-stabilizing agent* of choice is lithium carbonate. Its mechanism of action is not fully understood, but it is thought to enhance the reuptake of norepinephrine and serotonin in the brain, thereby lowering the levels in the body, resulting in decreased hyperactivity. The most common side effects are dry mouth, GI upset, polyuria, and weight gain. There is a very narrow margin between the therapeutic and toxic levels of lithium. Serum levels must be drawn regularly to monitor for toxicity. Symptoms of lithium toxicity begin to appear at serum levels of approximately 1.5 mEq/L. If left untreated, lithium toxicity can be life-threatening.

Several other medications are being used for stabilizing the mood. Anticonvulsants (carbamazepine, clonazepam, valproic acid, gabapentin, lamotrigine, and topiramate) and the calcium channel blocker, verapamil, have been used with some effectiveness. Their action in the treatment of bipolar mania is not known. Most recently, the Food and Drug Administration has approved the antipsychotic, olanzapine, for the short-term treatment of acute manic episodes.

Antipsychotic drugs are used in the treatment of acute and chronic psychoses. Their action is unknown but is thought to decrease the activity of dopamine in the brain. The phenothiazines are a widely used group. Their most common side effects include anticholinergic effects, sedation, weight gain, reduction in seizure threshold, photosensitivity, and extrapyramidal symptoms. A newer generation of atypical antipsychotic medications, which includes clozapine, risperidone, olanzapine, quetiapine, aripiprazole, and ziprasidone, may have an effect on dopamine, serotonin, and other neurotransmitters. They show promise of greater efficacy with fewer side effects.

Antiparkinsonian agents are used to counteract the extrapyramidal symptoms associated with antipsychotic medications. Antiparkinsonian drugs work to restore the natural balance of acetylcholine and dopamine in the brain. The most common side effects of these drugs are the anticholinergic effects. They may also cause sedation and orthostatic hypotension.

Sedative-hypnotics are used in the management of anxiety states and to treat insomnia. These CNS depressants have the potential for physical and psychological dependence. They are indicated for short-term use only. Side effects and nursing implications are similar to those described for antianxiety medications.

Several medications have been designated as *agents for treatment of ADHD*. These include CNS stimulants that have the potential for physical and psychological dependence. Tolerance develops quickly with CNS stimulants, and they should not be withdrawn abruptly because they can produce serious withdrawal symptoms. The most common side effects are restlessness, anorexia, and insomnia. Other medications that have shown to be effective with ADHD include atomoxetine and bupropion.

TOWNSEND ESSENTIALS

11

CHAPTER

COMPLEMENTARY AND PSYCHOSOCIAL THERAPIES

CHAPTER OUTLINE

KEY TERMS

allopathic medicine
alternative medicine
complementary medicine
acupuncture
acupoints
chiropractic
subluxation
chi
meridians
yoga
psychoanalysis
free association
acupressure
catharsis
abreaction
reality therapy
nonassertive
aggressive
passive-aggressive
cognitive therapy
automatic thoughts

OBJECTIVES

After reading this chapter, the student will be able to:

1. Compare and contrast various types of conventional and alternative therapies.
2. Describe the philosophies behind various complementary therapies, including herbal medicine, acupressure and acupuncture, diet and nutrition, chiropractic medicine, therapeutic touch and massage, yoga, and pet therapy.
3. Discuss the historical background of various complementary therapies.
4. Describe the techniques used in various complementary therapies.
5. Discuss objectives and therapeutic strategies of various psychosocial therapies, including individual psychotherapy, assertiveness training, relaxation therapy, and cognitive therapy.

7. Part of the nurse's continual assessment of the client taking antipsychotic medications is to observe for extrapyramidal symptoms. Examples include:
   a. Muscular weakness, rigidity, tremors, facial spasms.
   b. Dry mouth, blurred vision, urinary retention, orthostatic hypotension.
   c. Amenorrhea, gynecomastia, retrograde ejaculation.
   d. Elevated blood pressure, severe occipital headache, stiff neck.
8. If the foregoing extrapyramidal symptoms should occur, which of the following would be a priority nursing intervention?
   a. Notify the physician immediately.
   b. Administer p.r.n. trihexyphenidyl (Artane).
   c. Withhold the next dose of antipsychotic medication.
   d. Explain to the client that these symptoms are only temporary and will disappear shortly.
9. A concern with children on long-term therapy with CNS stimulants for ADHD is:
   a. Addiction
   b. Weight gain
   c. Tolerance
   d. Growth suppression
10. Doses of bupropion should be administered at least 8 hours apart and never doubled when a dose is missed. The reason for this is:
    a. To prevent orthostatic hypotension.
    b. To prevent seizures.
    c. To prevent hypertensive crisis.
    d. To prevent extrapyramidal symptoms.

REFERENCES

Bernstein, J.G. (1995). Handbook of drug therapy in psychiatry (3rd ed.). St. Louis: Mosby.

Depression Guideline Panel. (1993). Depression in primary care: Vol. 2. Treatment of major depression. Clinical practice guideline, No. 5. Rockville, MD: U.S. Department of Health and Human Services, Public Health Service, Agency for Health Care Policy and Research. AHCPR Pub. No. 93–0551.

Drug facts and comparisons (57th ed.). (2003). St. Louis: Wolters Kluwer.

Haddad, P.M. (2001). Antidepressant discontinuation syndromes: Clinical relevance, prevention, and management. Drug Safety, 24:183–197.

Jibson, M.D., & Tandon, R. (1996). A summary of research findings on the new antipsychotic drugs. The Psychiatric Nursing Forum, 2:i–iii.

Marangell, L.B., Silver, J.M., Goff, D.C., & Yudofsky, S.C. (2003). Psychopharmacology and electroconvulsive therapy. In R.E. Hales & S.C. Yudofsky (Eds.), Textbook of clinical psychiatry (4th ed.). Washington, D.C.: American Psychiatric Publishing.

Marder, S.R. (1997, May). Comparative data on newer antipsychotic drugs. Current Approaches to Psychoses, 6:2–4.

Sadock, B.J., & Sadock, V.A. (2003). Synopsis of psychiatry: Behavioral sciences/clinical psychiatry (9th ed.). Philadelphia: Lippincott Williams & Wilkins.

Sage, D.L. (Producer) (1984). The Brain: Madness. Washington, DC: Public Broadcasting System.

Schatzberg, A.F., Cole, J.O., & DeBattista, C. (2003). Manual of clinical psychopharmacology (4th ed.). Washington, D.C.: American Psychiatric Publishing.

Sternbach, H. (1991, June). The serotonin syndrome. American Journal of Psychiatry, 148:705–713.

Townsend, M.C. (2003). Psychiatric mental health nursing: Concepts of care (4th ed.). Philadelphia: F.A. Davis.

CHAPTER 11

Complementary and Psychosocial Therapies

CHAPTER OUTLINE

KEY TERMS

allopathic medicine
alternative medicine
complementary medicine
acupuncture
acupoints
chiropractic
subluxation
chi
meridians
yoga
psychoanalysis
free association
acupressure
catharsis
abreaction
reality therapy
nonassertive
aggressive
passive-aggressive
cognitive therapy
automatic thoughts

OBJECTIVES

After reading this chapter, the student will be able to:

1. Compare and contrast various types of conventional and alternative therapies.
2. Describe the philosophies behind various complementary therapies, including herbal medicine, acupressure and acupuncture, diet and nutrition, chiropractic medicine, therapeutic touch and massage, yoga, and pet therapy.
3. Discuss the historical background of various complementary therapies.
4. Describe the techniques used in various complementary therapies.
5. Discuss objectives and therapeutic strategies of various psychosocial therapies, including individual psychotherapy, assertiveness training, relaxation therapy, and cognitive therapy.

may have an effect on dopamine, serotonin, and other neurotransmitters. They show promise of greater efficacy with fewer side effects.

Antiparkinsonian agents are used to counteract the extrapyramidal symptoms associated with antipsychotic medications. Antiparkinsonian drugs work to restore the natural balance of acetylcholine and dopamine in the brain. The most common side effects of these drugs are the anticholinergic effects. They may also cause sedation and orthostatic hypotension.

Sedative-hypnotics are used in the management of anxiety states and to treat insomnia. These CNS depressants have the potential for physical and psychological dependence. They are indicated for short-term use only. Side effects and nursing implications are similar to those described for antianxiety medications.

Several medications have been designated as *agents for treatment of ADHD*. These include CNS stimulants that have the potential for physical and psychological dependence. Tolerance develops quickly with CNS stimulants, and they should not be withdrawn abruptly because they can produce serious withdrawal symptoms. The most common side effects are restlessness, anorexia, and insomnia. Other medications that have shown to be effective with ADHD include atomoxetine and bupropion.

REVIEW QUESTIONS

SELF-EXAMINATION/LEARNING EXERCISE

Select the answer that is most appropriate for each of the following questions:

1. Antianxiety medications produce a calming effect by:
   a. Depressing the CNS.
   b. Decreasing levels of norepinephrine and serotonin in the brain.
   c. Decreasing levels of dopamine in the brain.
   d. Inhibiting production of the enzyme MAO.
2. Nancy has a new diagnosis of panic disorder. Dr. S has written a p.r.n. order for alprazolam (Xanax) for when Nancy is feeling anxious. She says to the nurse, "Dr. S prescribed buspirone for my friend's anxiety. Why did he order something different for me?" The nurse's answer is based on which of the following?
   a. Buspirone is not an antianxiety medication.
   b. Alprazolam and buspirone are essentially the same medication, so either is appropriate.
   c. Buspirone has delayed onset-of-action and cannot be used on a p.r.n. basis.
   d. Alprazolam is the only medication that really works for panic disorder.
3. Education for the client who is taking MAOIs should include which of the following?
   a. Fluid and sodium replacement when appropriate, frequent drug blood levels, signs and symptoms of toxicity.
   b. Lifetime of continuous use, possible tardive dyskinesia, advantages of an injection every 2 to 4 weeks.
   c. Short-term use, possible tolerance to beneficial effects, careful tapering of the drug at end of treatment.
   d. Tyramine-restricted diet, prohibitive concurrent use of over-the-counter medications without physician notification.
4. There is a very narrow margin between the therapeutic and toxic levels of lithium carbonate. Symptoms of toxicity are most likely to appear if the serum levels exceed
   a. 0.15 mEq/L
   b. 1.5 mEq/L
   c. 15.0 mEq/L
   d. 150 mEq/L
5. Initial symptoms of lithium toxicity include:
   a. Constipation, dry mouth, drowsiness, oliguria.
   b. Dizziness, thirst, dysuria, arrhythmias.
   c. Ataxia, tinnitus, blurred vision, diarrhea.
   d. Fatigue, vertigo, anuria, weakness.
6. Antipsychotic medications are thought to decrease psychotic symptoms by:
   a. Blocking reuptake of norepinephrine and serotonin.
   b. Blocking the action of dopamine in the brain.
   c. Inhibiting production of the enzyme MAO.
   d. Depressing the CNS.

COMPLEMENTARY THERAPIES

The History of Medicine

2000 BC–Here, eat this root.
1000 AD–That root is heathen. Here, say this prayer.
1850 AD–That prayer is superstition. Here, drink this potion.
1940 AD–That potion is snake oil. Here, swallow this pill.
1985 AD–That pill is ineffective. Here, take this antibiotic.
2000 AD–That antibiotic is ineffective and dangerous. Here, eat this root.

Anonymous

INTRODUCTION

The connection between mind and body, and the influence of each on the other, is well recognized by all clinicians and particularly by psychiatrists. Traditional medicine as it is currently practiced in the United States is based solely on scientific methodology. Traditional medicine, also known as **allopathic medicine**, is the type of medicine historically taught in U.S. medical schools.

The term **alternative medicine** has come to be recognized as practices that differ from the usual traditional practices in the treatment of disease. Surveys have indicated that 42 to 50 percent of the U.S. population has used some form of alternative therapy (Steyer, 2001). More than $25 billion a year is spent on alternative medical therapies in the United States (Sadock & Sadock, 2003).

In 1991, an Office of Alternative Medicine (OAM) was established by the National Institutes of Health (NIH) to study nontraditional therapies and to evaluate their usefulness and their effectiveness. Since that time, the name has been changed to the National Center for Complementary Medicine and Alternative Medicine (NCCAM or CAM). The distinction between the two types is explained in the following manner: **complementary medicine** is used *together* with conventional medicine, and alternative medicine is used *in place of* conventional medicine. The mission statement of the CAM states:

> The NIH OAM facilitates research and evaluation of unconventional medical practices and disseminates this information to the public. (Complementary & Alternative Medicine, 1998)

Although the OAM has not endorsed the methodologies, they have established a list of alternative therapies to be used in practice and for investigative purposes. This list is presented in Table 11–1.

TABLE 11–1 Classification of Alternative Medicine Practices from the NIH Office of Alternative Medicine*

Alternative Systems of Medical Practice	Manual Healing
Acupuncture Anthroposophically extended medicine Ayurveda Community-based healthcare practices Environmental medicine Homeopathic medicine Latin American rural practices Native American practices Natural products Naturopathic medicine Past life therapy Shamanism Tibetan medicine Traditional Oriental medicine	Acupressure Alexander technique Biofield therapeutics Chiropractic medicine Feldenkrais method Massage therapy Osteopathy Reflexology Rolfing Therapeutic touch Trager method Zone therapy
Bioelectromagnetic Applications	**Mind/Body Control**
Blue light treatment and artificial lighting Electroacupuncture Electromagnetic fields Electrostimulation and neuromagnetic stimulation devices Magnetoresonance spectroscopy	Art therapy Biofeedback Counseling Dance therapy Guided imagery Humor therapy Hypnotherapy Meditation Music therapy Prayer therapy Psychotherapy Relaxation techniques Support groups Yoga
Diet, Nutrition, Lifestyle Changes	**Pharmacological & Biological Treatments**
Changes in lifestyle Diet Gerson therapy Macrobiotics Megavitamins Nutritional supplements	Antioxidizing agents Cell treatment Chelation therapy Metabolic therapy Oxidizing agents (ozone, hydrogen peroxide)
Herbal Medicine	
Echinacea (purple coneflower) Ginger rhizome *Ginkgo biloba* extract Ginseng root Wild chrysanthemum flower Witch hazel Yellow dock	

* This list of complementary and alternative medical healthcare practices was developed by the ad hoc advisory panel to the Office of Alternative Medicine (OAM), National Institutes of Health (NIH). It was refined further at a workshop for alternative medicine researchers and practitioners. It was designed for the purposes of discussion and study, and is considered neither complete nor authoritative.

Some health insurance companies and health maintenance organizations appear to be bowing to public pressure by including alternative providers in their networks of providers for treatments such as acupuncture and massage therapy. Chiropractic care has been covered by some third-party payers for many years. Individuals who seek alternative therapy, however, are often reimbursed at lower rates than those who choose traditional practitioners.

Client education is an important part of complementary care. Positive lifestyle changes are encouraged, and practitioners serve as educators as well as treatment specialists. Complementary medicine is viewed as *holistic* healthcare, which deals with not only the physical perspective but also the emotional and spiritual components of the individual. Dr. Tom Coniglione, former professor of medicine at the Oklahoma University Health Sciences Center, states:

> We must look at treating the "total person" in order to be more efficient and balanced within the medical community. Even finding doctors who are well rounded and balanced has become a criterion in the admitting process for medical students. Medicine has changed from just looking at the "scientist perspective of organ and disease" to the total perspective of lifestyle and real impact/results to the patient. This evolution is a progressive and very positive shift in the right direction. (Coniglione, 1998)

Terms such as *harmony* and *balance* are often associated with complementary care. In fact, restoring harmony and balance between body and mind is often the goal of complementary healthcare approaches (Credit, Hartunian, & Nowak, 1998). Although most are not founded in scientific principle, they have been shown to be effective in the treatment of certain disorders and merit further examination as a viable component of holistic healthcare.

COMMONALITIES AND CONTRAST

A number of commonalities and contrasts exist between complementary medicine and conventional healthcare. A summary of these characteristics is presented in Table 11–2.

TYPES OF COMPLEMENTARY THERAPIES

Herbal Medicine

The use of plants to heal is probably as old as humankind. Virtually every culture in the world has relied on herbs and plants to treat illness. Clay tablets from about 4000 BC reveal that the Sumerians had

TABLE 11–2 Commonalities and Contrasts Between Conventional and Complementary Therapies

Conventional	Complementary
Chemotherapy	Plants and other natural products
Curing/treating	Healing/ministering care
Individual viewed as disease category	Individual is viewed as a unique being
End-stage	Hope/hopefulness
Focus is on disease and illness	Focus is on health and wellness
Illness treatment	Health promotion and illness prevention
Nutrition is adjunct and supportive to treatment	Nutrition is the basis of health, wellness, and treatment
Objectivism: person is separate from his/her disease	Subjectivism: person is integral to the illness
Patient	Person
Practitioner as authority	Practitioner as facilitator
Practitioner paternalism/patient dependency	Practitioner as partner/person empowerment
Positivism/materialism: data are physically measurable (through various types of energy systems for screening, diagnosis, and treatment)	Metaphysical: entity is energy system or vital force that utilizes its own vital essences and energy forces to heal itself, prevent illness, and promote health
Reductionistic (emphasis placed on the cellular, organ, or system levels of the body)	Holistic (emphasis placed on treatment of the whole individual in his/her bio-psycho-social-cultural-and-spiritual context)
Specialist care	Self-care
Symptom relief	Alleviation of causative factors
Somatic (biological and physiological) model	Behavioral-psycho-social-spiritual model
Science is only source of knowledge and truth	Multiple sources of knowledge and truth
Technology/invasive	Natural/noninvasive

De Santis, L. In Catalano, J: Nursing Now! Today's Issues, Tomorrow's Trend, (3rd ed.) F. A. Davis Company, Philadelphia, 2003, p. 438. With permission.

apothecaries for dispensing medicinal herbs; the *Pen Tsao*, a Chinese text written around 3000 BC, contained some 1,000 herbal formulas that had probably been used as remedies for thousands of years (Guinness, 1993). When the Pilgrims came to America in the 1600s, they brought with them a variety of herbs to be established and used for medicinal purposes. The new settlers soon discovered that the Native Americans also had their own varieties of plants for healing.

Many people are seeking a return to herbal remedies, because they view these remedies as being less potent than prescription drugs and as being free of adverse side effects. However, because the Food and Drug Administration (FDA) classifies herbal remedies as dietary supplements or food additives, their labels cannot indicate medicinal uses. They are not subject to FDA approval, and they lack uniform standards of quality control.

Several organizations have been established to attempt regulation and control of the herbal industry. They include the Council for Responsible Nutrition, the American Herbal Association, and the American Botanical Council. The Commission E of the German Federal Health Agency is the group responsible for researching and regulating the safety and efficacy of herbs and plant medicines in Germany. All of the Commission E monographs of herbal medicines have been translated into English and compiled into one text (Blumenthal, 1998). This should prove to be an invaluable reference for practitioners of holistic medicine.

Until more extensive testing has been completed on humans and animals, the use of herbal medicines must be approached with caution and responsibility. *The notion that something "natural" is therefore completely safe is a myth.* In fact, some of the plants from which even prescription drugs are derived are highly toxic in their natural state (Guinness, 1993). In addition, because of lack of regulation and standardization, ingredients in these herbal remedies may be adulterated. Their method of manufacture also may alter potency. For example, dried herbs lose potency rapidly because of exposure to air. Guinness (1993) offers the following points for practitioners and individuals contemplating the use of herbal medicines:

1. **Be careful of sources.** Because of the lack of government scrutiny, the purity and potency of the herbal medicines cannot be guaranteed. The buyer must be careful to select reputable brands.
2. **Choose the most reliable forms.** Tinctures and freeze-dried products have been prepared to retard spoilage and prevent loss of potency.
3. **More is not better.** Never take more than the recommended dosages at the suggested intervals. Adverse effects can occur from overdosing with herbal medicines, just as they do with prescription pharmaceuticals.
4. **Monitor physical reactions.** Discontinue the herbal medication at the first sign of allergic or other adverse reaction. Discontinue using it after a reasonable length of time if there seems to be no significant indication that it is producing the desired effect.
5. **Take no risks.** Do not self-medicate with herbal remedies for serious illnesses or injuries. Do not take herbal medications without a physician's approval if you are pregnant or breast-feeding, very young or very old, or taking other medications.

Table 11–3 lists information about common herbal remedies, with possible implications for psychiatric/mental health nursing. Botanical names, medicinal uses, and safety profiles are included.

Acupressure and Acupuncture

Acupressure and **acupuncture** are healing techniques based on the ancient philosophies of traditional Chinese medicine dating back to 3000 BC. The main concept behind Chinese medicine is that healing energy **(chi)** flows through the body along specific pathways called **meridians.** It is believed that these meridians of chi connect various parts of the body similar to the way in which lines on a road map link various locations. The pathways link a conglomerate of points, called **acupoints**. Therefore, it is possible to treat a part of the body distant to another because they are linked by a meridian. Credit, Hartunian, and Nowak (1998) state:

> The goal of traditional Chinese medicine is to keep the body in balance and harmony through the free flow of chi. Disease is a result of blockages in this energy current. (p. 17)

In acupressure, the fingers, thumbs, palms, or elbows are used to apply pressure to the acupoints. This pressure is thought to dissolve any obstructions in the flow of healing energy and to restore the body to a healthier functioning. In acupuncture, hair-thin, sterile, disposable, stainless steel needles are inserted into acupoints to dissolve the obstructions along the

TABLE 11–3 Herbal Remedies

Common Names (Botanical Name)	Medicinal Uses/Possible Action	Safety Profile
Black cohosh (*Cimicifuga racemosa*)	May provide relief of menstrual cramps; improved mood; calming effect. Extracts from the roots are thought to have action similar to estrogen.	Generally considered safe in low doses. Toxic in large doses, causing dizziness, nausea, headaches, stiffness, and trembling. Should not be taken with heart problems, concurrently with antihypertensives, or during pregnancy.
Cascara sagrada (*Rhamnus purshiana*)	Relief of constipation.	Generally recognized as safe; sold as over-the-counter drug in the United States. Should not be used during pregnancy.
Chamomile (*Matricaria chamomilla*)	As a tea, is effective as a mild sedative in the relief of insomnia. May also aid digestion, relieve menstrual cramps, and settle upset stomach.	Generally recognized as safe when consumed in reasonable amounts.
Echinacea (*Echinacea angustifolia* and *Echinacea purpurea*)	Stimulates immune system; may have value in fighting infections and easing the symptoms of colds and flu.	Considered safe in reasonable doses. Observe for side effects of allergic reaction.
Fennel (*Foeniculum vulgare* or *Foeniculum officinale*)	Used to ease stomachaches and to aid digestion. Taken in a tea or in extracts to stimulate the appetites of anorexics (1–2 tsp. seeds steeped in boiling water for making tea).	Generally recognized as safe when consumed in reasonable amounts.
Feverfew (*Tanacetum parthenium*)	Prophylaxis and treatment of migraine headaches. Effective in the fresh leaf or freeze-dried forms (2–3 fresh leaves [or equivalent] per day).	A small percentage of individuals may experience the adverse effect of temporary mouth ulcers. Considered safe in reasonable doses.
Ginger (*Zingiber officinale*)	Ginger tea to ease stomachache and to aid digestion. Two powdered ginger-root capsules have been shown to be effective in preventing motion sickness.	Generally recognized as safe.
Ginkgo (*Ginkgo biloba*)	Used to treat senility, short-term memory loss, and peripheral insufficiency. Has been shown to dilate blood vessels. Usual dosage is 120 mg/day.	Safety has been established with recommended dosages. Possible side effects include headache, gastrointestinal problems, and dizziness. Contraindicated in pregnancy and lactation and in clients with bleeding disorder. Possible compound effect with concomitant use of aspirin or anticoagulants.
Ginseng (*Panax ginseng*)	The ancient Chinese saw this herb as one that increased wisdom and longevity. Current studies support a possible positive effect on the cardiovascular system. Action not known.	Generally considered safe. Side effects may include headache, insomnia, anxiety, skin rashes, diarrhea. Avoid concomitant use with anticoagulants.
Hops (*Humulus lupulus*)	Used in cases of nervousness, mild anxiety, and insomnia. Also may relieve the cramping associated with diarrhea. May be taken as a tea, in extracts, or capsules.	Generally recognized as safe when consumed in recommended dosages.
Kava kava (*Piper methysticum*)	Used to reduce anxiety while promoting mental acuity. Dosage range: 70–210 mg/day.	May cause scaly skin rash when taken at the higher dosage range for long periods. Concurrent use with CNS depressants may produce additive tranquilizing effects. Recent reports of potential for liver damage. FDA is investigating.

Common Names (Botanical Name)	Medicinal Uses/Possible Action	Safety Profile
Passion flower *(Passiflora incarnata)*	Used in tea, capsules, or extracts to treat nervousness and insomnia. Depresses the CNS to produce a mild sedative effect.	Generally recognized as safe in recommended doses.
Peppermint *(Mentha piperita)*	Used as a tea to relieve upset stomachs and headaches and as a mild sedative. Pour boiling water over 1 tbsp. dried leaves and steep to make a tea.	Considered to be safe when consumed in normal quantities.
Psyllium (*Plantago ovata* and *Plantago major*)	Psyllium seeds are a popular bulk laxative commonly used for chronic constipation.	Approved as an over-the-counter drug in the United States.
Skullcap *(Scutellaria lateriflora)*	Used as a sedative for mild anxiety and nervousness.	Considered safe in reasonable amounts.
St. John's wort *(Hypericum perforatum)*	Used in the treatment of mild to moderate depression. May block reuptake of serotonin/norepinephrine and have a mild MAOI effect. Effective dose: 900 mg/day. May also have antiviral, antibacterial, and anti–inflammatory properties.	Generally recognized as safe when taken at recommended dosages. Side effects include mild GI irritation that is lessened with food; photosensitivity when taken in high dosages over long periods. Should not be taken with other psychoactive medications.
Valerian (*Valeriana officinals*)	Used to treat insomnia. Produces restful sleep without morning "hangover." The root may be used to make a tea, or capsules are available in a variety of dosages. Mechanism of action is similar to benzodiazepines, but without addicting properties. Daily dosage range: 100–1000 mg.	Generally recognized as safe when taken at recommended dosages. Side effects may include mild headache or upset stomach. Taking doses higher than recommended may result in severe headache, nausea, morning grogginess, blurry vision. Should not be taken concurrently with CNS depressants.

Adapted from Guinness (1993); Sadock & Sadock (2003); Institute for Natural Resources (1998); Yeager, 1998; and PDR for Herbal Medicines, 2000.

meridians. The needles may be left in place for a specified length of time, they may be rotated, or a mild electric current may be applied. An occasional tingling or numbness is experienced, but little or no pain is associated with the treatment (Credit, Hartunian, & Nowak, 1998).

The Western medical philosophy regarding acupressure and acupuncture is that they stimulate the body's own painkilling chemicals—the morphine-like substances known as *endorphins*. The treatment has been found to be effective in the treatment of asthma, headaches, dysmenorrhea, cervical pain, insomnia, anxiety, depression, substance abuse, stroke rehabilitation, nausea of pregnancy, postoperative and chemotherapy-induced nausea and vomiting, tennis elbow, fibromyalgia, low back pain, and carpal tunnel syndrome (Sadock & Sadock, 2003; NIH, 1997). A recent study suggests that acupuncture may aid in the treatment of cocaine dependence (Avants et al., 2000).

Acupuncture is gaining wide acceptance in the United States by both patients and physicians. This treatment can be administered at the same time other techniques are being used, such as conventional Western techniques, although it is essential that all healthcare providers have knowledge of all treatments being received. Acupuncture should be administered by a physician or an acupuncturist who is board certified by the National Commission for the Certification of Acupuncturists, which requires more than 1,000 hours of acupuncture training. Currently, 34 states and the District of Columbia have set licensure standards for acupuncturists (Natural Healers, 2003).

Diet and Nutrition

The value of nutrition in the healing process has long been underrated. Lutz and Przytulski (2001) state:

> Today many diseases are linked to lifestyle behaviors such as smoking, lack of adequate physical activity, and poor

nutritional habits. Healthcare providers, in their role as educators, emphasize the relationship between lifestyle and risk of disease. Many people, at least in industrialized countries, are increasingly managing their health problems and making personal commitments to lead healthier lives. Nutrition is, in part, a preventive science. Given sufficient resources, how and what one eats is a lifestyle choice. (p. 4)

Individuals select the foods they eat based on a number of factors, not the least of which is enjoyment. Eating must serve social and cultural as well as nutritional needs. The U.S. Departments of Agriculture (USDA) and Health and Human Services (HHS) have collaborated on a set of guidelines to help individuals understand what types of foods to eat and a healthy lifestyle to pursue in order to promote health and prevent disease. Following is a list of these guidelines (USDA/HHS, 2000).

1. **Aim for fitness.** It is important to combine sensible eating with regular physical activity. Individuals who are overweight or obese are at increased risk for high blood pressure, high blood cholesterol, heart disease, stroke, diabetes, and certain types of cancer, arthritis, and respiratory problems. Maintaining a healthy weight should begin in childhood. This means learning to balance the appropriate number of calories with physical activity. The guidelines recommend at least 30 minutes of moderate physical activity every day for adults and 60 minutes daily of moderate physical activity for children. Physical activity and nutrition work together for overall wellness.
2. **Let the pyramid guide your food choices.** No single food can supply all nutrients in the amounts needed for good health. A variety of foods should be selected from the food guide pyramid (Fig. 11–1). Most of the daily servings of food should be selected from the food groups that are closest to the base of the pyramid. A range of servings is suggested for each group of foods. Smaller, sedentary persons should select the lower number of servings. The higher numbers of servings are meant for larger, more active individuals. Table 11–4 provides a summary of information about essential vitamins and minerals.
3. **Choose a variety of whole grains, fruits, and vegetables daily.** Consumption of whole grains, fruits, and vegetables is associated with substantially lower risk for many chronic diseases, including certain types of cancer. These foods are emphasized in this guideline because they are an excellent source of vitamins, minerals, complex carbohydrates (starch and dietary fiber), and, depending on how they are prepared, they are low in fat.
4. **Keep food safe to eat.** It is important to ensure that food is safe from harmful bacteria, viruses, parasites, toxins, and chemical contaminants. Individuals who are most vulnerable to food-borne illnesses include pregnant women, young children, older persons, and people with weakened immune systems or certain chronic illnesses. Ensure that food is fully cooked to a temperature that thoroughly destroys harmful organisms. Do not drink unpasteurized juices or milk. Do not eat raw or partially cooked eggs or foods containing raw eggs or unpasteurized milk. Do not eat raw or undercooked meat, poultry, or fish.
5. **Choose a diet that is low in saturated fat and cholesterol and moderate in total fat.** Heart disease and some types of cancer (e.g., breast and colon) have been linked to high-fat diets. Some dietary fat is required for good health. Fats supply energy and essential fatty acids, and they promote absorption of the fat-soluble vitamins A, D, E, and K. However, fats should comprise no more than 30 percent of the total daily calorie intake. Choose foods with mono- and polyunsaturated fat sources, and keep daily cholesterol intake below 300 mg.

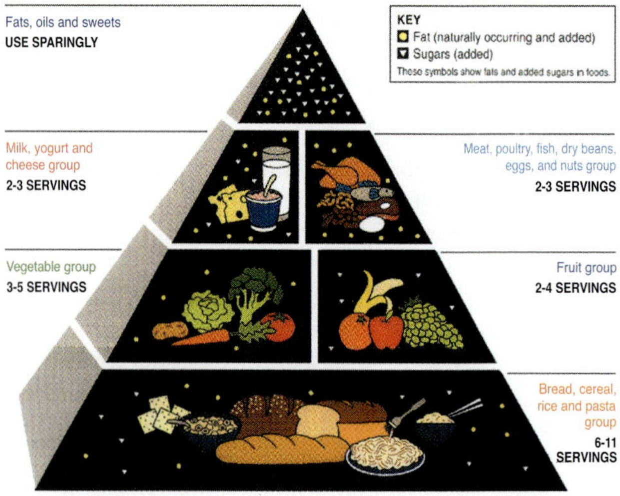

FIGURE 11–1 The Food Guide Pyramid.

TABLE 11–4 Essential Vitamins and Minerals

Vitamin/ Mineral	Function	RDA*	New DRI (UL)**	Food Sources	Comments
Vitamin A	Prevention of night blindness; calcification of growing bones; resistance to infection	Men: 1000 μg Women: 800 μg	Men: 900 μg (3000 μg) Women: 700 μg (3000 μg)	Liver, butter, cheese, whole milk, egg yolk, fish, green leafy vegetables, carrots, pumpkin, sweet potatoes	May be of benefit in prevention of cancer, because of its antioxidant properties, which are associated with control of free radicals that damage DNA and cell membranes.
Vitamin D	Promotes absorption of calcium and phosphorus in the small intestine; prevention of rickets	Men and women: 5 μg	Men and women: 5 μg (50 μg) (5 to 10 for ages 50–70 and 15 for >70)	Fortified milk and dairy products, egg yolk, fish liver oils, liver, oysters; formed in the skin by exposure to sunlight	Without vitamin D, very little dietary calcium can be absorbed.
Vitamin E	An antioxidant that prevents cell membrane destruction	Men: 10 mg Women: 8 mg	Men and women: 15 mg (1000 mg)	Vegetable oils, wheat germ, whole grain or fortified cereals, green leafy vegetables, nuts	As an antioxidant, may have implications in the prevention of Alzheimer's disease, heart disease, breast cancer.
Vitamin K	Synthesis of prothrombin and other clotting factors; normal blood coagulation	Men: 80 μg Women: 65 μg	Men: 120 μg (ND)**** Women: 90 μg (ND)****	Green vegetables (collards, spinach, lettuce, kale, broccoli, brussel sprouts, cabbage) plant oils and margarine	Individuals on anticoagulant therapy should monitor vitamin K intake.
Vitamin C	Formation of collagen in connective tissues; a powerful antioxidant; facilitates iron absorption; aids in the release of epinephrine from the adrenal glands during stress	Men and women: 60 mg	Men: 90 mg (2000 mg) Women: 75 mg (2000 mg)	Citrus fruits, tomatoes, potatoes, green leafy vegetables, strawberries	As an antioxidant, may have implications in the prevention of cancer, cataracts, heart disease. It may stimulate the immune system to fight various types of infection.
Vitamin B_1 (thiamine)	Essential for normal functioning of nervous tissue; coenzyme in carbohydrate metabolism	Men: 1.5 mg Women: 1.1 mg	Men: 1.2 mg (ND)**** Women: 1.1 mg (ND)****	Whole grains, legumes, nuts, egg yolk, meat, green leafy vegetables	Large doses may improve mental performance in people with Alzheimer's disease.
Vitamin B_2 (riboflavin)	Coenzyme in the metabolism of protein and carbohydrate for energy	Men: 1.7 mg Women: 1.3 mg	Men: 1.3 mg (ND)**** Women: 1.1 mg (ND)****	Meat, dairy products, whole or enriched grains, legumes, nuts	May help in the prevention of cataracts; high-dose therapy may be effective in migraine prophylaxis (Schoenen et al., 1998).

(Continued)

TABLE 11–4 Essential Vitamins and Minerals *(Continued)*

Vitamin/ Mineral	Function	RDA*	New DRI (UL)**	Food Sources	Comments
Vitamin B_3 (niacin)	Coenzyme in the metabolism of protein and carbohydrates for energy	Men: 19 mg Women: 15 mg	Men: 16 mg (35 mg) Women: 14 mg (35 mg)	Milk, eggs, meats, legumes, whole grain and enriched cereals, nuts	High doses of niacin have been successful in decreasing levels of cholesterol in some individuals.
Vitamin B_6 (pyridoxine)	Coenzyme in the synthesis and catabolism of amino acids; essential for metabolism of tryptophan to niacin	Men: 2 mg Women: 1.6 mg	Men and women: 1.3 mg (100 mg) After age 50: Men: 1.7 mg Women: 1.5 mg	Meat, fish, grains, legumes, bananas, nuts, white and sweet potatoes	May decrease depression in some individuals by increasing levels of serotonin; deficiencies may contribute to memory problems; also used in the treatment of migraines and premenstrual discomfort.
Vitamin B_{12}	Necessary in the formation of DNA and the production of red blood cells; associated with folic acid metabolism	Men and women: 2 μg	Men and women: 2.4 μg (ND)****	Found in animal products (e.g., meats, eggs, dairy products)	Deficiency may contribute to memory problems. Vegetarians can get this vitamin from fortified foods. Intrinsic factor must be present in the stomach for absorption of vitamin B_{12}.
Folic acid (folate)	Necessary in the formation of DNA and the production of red blood cells	Men: 200 μg Women: 180 μg	Men and women: 400 μg (1000 μg)	Meat; green leafy vegetables; beans; peas; fortified cereals, breads, rice, and pasta	Important in women of childbearing age to prevent fetal neural tube defects; may contribute to prevention of heart disease and colon cancer.
Calcium	Necessary in the formation of bones and teeth, neuron and muscle functioning, blood clotting	Men and women: 800 mg	Men and women: 1000 mg (2500 mg) After age 50: Men and women: 1200 mg	Dairy products, kale, broccoli, spinach, sardines, oysters, salmon	Calcium has been associated with preventing headaches, muscle cramps, osteoporosis, and premenstrual problems. Requires vitamin D for absorption.
Phosphorus	Necessary in the formation of bones and teeth; a component of DNA, RNA, ADP, and ATP; helps control acid-base balance in the blood	Men and women: 800 mg	Men and women: 700 mg (4000 mg)	Milk, cheese, fish, meat, yogurt, ice cream, peas, eggs	

Vitamin/ Mineral	Function	RDA*	New DRI (UL)**	Food Sources	Comments
Magnesium	Protein synthesis and carbohydrate metabolism; muscular relaxation following contraction; bone formation	Men: 350 mg Women: 280 mg	Men: 420 mg (350 mg)*** Women: 320 mg (350 mg)***	Green vegetables, legumes, seafood, milk, nuts, meat	May aid in prevention of asthmatic attacks and migraine headaches. Deficiencies may contribute to insomnia, premenstrual problems.
Iron	Synthesis of hemoglobin and myoglobin; cellular oxidation	Men and women: 10 mg (women who are breast-feeding and those of childbearing age: 15 mg)	Men: 8 mg (45 mg) Women: (45 mg) Childbearing age: 18 mg Over 50: 8 mg Pregnant: 27 mg Breastfeeding: 9 mg	Meat, fish, poultry, eggs, nuts, dark green leafy vegetables, dried fruit, enriched pasta and bread	Iron deficiencies can result in headaches and chronic fatigue.
Iodine	Aids in the synthesis of T_3 and T_4	Men and women: 150 μg	Men and women: 150 μg (1100 μg)	Iodized salt, seafood	Exerts strong controlling influence on overall body metabolism.
Selenium	Works with vitamin E to protect cellular compounds from oxidation	Men: 70 μg Women: 55 μg	Men and women: 55 μg (400 μg)	Seafood, low-fat meats, dairy products, liver	As an antioxidant combined with vitamin E, may have some anti-cancer effect. Deficiency has also been associated with depressed mood.
Zinc	Involved in synthesis of DNA and RNA; energy metabolism and protein synthesis; wound healing; increased immune functioning; necessary for normal smell and taste sensation.	Men: 15 mg Women: 12 mg	Men: 11 mg (40 mg) Women: 8 mg (40 mg)	Meat, seafood, fortified cereals, poultry, eggs, milk	An important source for the prevention of infection and improvement in wound healing.

* Recommended Dietary Allowances, established by the Food and Nutrition Board of the Institute of Medicine, 1989.
** Dietary Reference Intakes (UL), the most recent set of dietary recommendations for adults established by the Food and Nutrition Board of the Institute of Medicine, 1997–2001. UL is the upper limit of intake considered to be safe for use by adults (includes total intake from food, water, and supplements).
*** UL for magnesium applies only to intake from dietary supplements, excluding intake from food and water.
**** ND = Not determined
Adapted from Council for Responsible Nutrition, Washington, D.C. (2001) and U.S. Department of Agriculture (2003).

6. **Choose beverages and foods to moderate your intake of sugars.** Many foods that contain sugars supply unnecessary calories and few nutrients. A significant health problem from eating too much sugar is tooth decay. Scientific evidence indicates that diets high in sugars do not cause hyperactivity or diabetes. A study by Dr. W.B. Grant of the Atmospheric Sciences division of NASA's Langley Research Center reports that sugar may be the highest dietary risk factor for heart disease in women 35 years and older ("Accent on Today's Woman," 1998). He states that, "Fructose metabolizes into triglycerides, then is incorporated into very low density lipoprotein cholesterol." Sugars

should be used in moderation by most healthy people and sparingly by people with low calorie needs.

7. **Choose and prepare foods with less salt.** Sodium and sodium chloride (salt) occur naturally in foods, usually in small amounts. Most foods are prepared with some salt, and some already has been added during processing. In studies with many diverse populations, it has been established that a high intake of salt is associated with high blood pressure. It is therefore important for individuals at risk for high blood pressure to consume less salt in their diets (as well as to increase their physical activity and control their weight). A high salt intake is also thought to increase the amount of calcium excreted in the urine. Loss of calcium can increase the risk of osteoporosis and bone fractures.
8. **If you drink alcoholic beverages, do so in moderation.** High levels of alcohol intake raise the risk for high blood pressure, stroke, heart disease, certain cancers, accidents, violence, suicides, birth defects, and overall mortality. Too much alcohol may cause cirrhosis of the liver, inflammation of the pancreas, and damage to the brain and heart. Heavy drinkers also are at risk of malnutrition because alcohol contains calories that may substitute for those in foods that are more nutritious. The USDA/HHS (2000) report defines "moderation" as:

> ... no more than one drink per day for women and no more than two drinks per day for men. Count as a drink:

- 12 ounces of regular beer (150 calories)
- 5 ounces of wine (100 calories)
- 1.5 ounces of 80-proof distilled spirits (100 calories)

Good nutrition can help with adaptation to the inevitable stresses of life by promoting a healthy body and a feeling of well-being. Knowledge of good nutrition is learned and not necessarily something that comes naturally. Nurses are in an ideal situation for providing individuals with this type of information.

Chiropractic Medicine

Chiropractic medicine is probably the most widely used form of alternative healing in the United States. It was developed in the late 1800s by a self-taught healer named David Palmer. It was later reorganized and expanded by his son, Joshua, a trained practitioner. Palmer's objective was to find a cure for disease and illness that did not rely on drugs, which he considered harmful (Guinness, 1993). Palmer's theory of chiropractic medicine was that energy flows from the brain to all parts of the body through the spinal cord and spinal nerves. When vertebrae of the spinal column become displaced, they may press on a nerve and interfere with the normal nerve transmission. Palmer named the displacement of these vertebrae **subluxation**, and he alleged that the way to restore normal function was to manipulate the vertebrae back into their normal positions. These manipulations are called *adjustments* (Guinness, 1993).

Adjustments are usually performed by hand, although some chiropractors have special treatment tables equipped to facilitate these manipulations (Fig. 11–2). Other processes used to facilitate the outcome of the spinal adjustment by providing muscle relax-

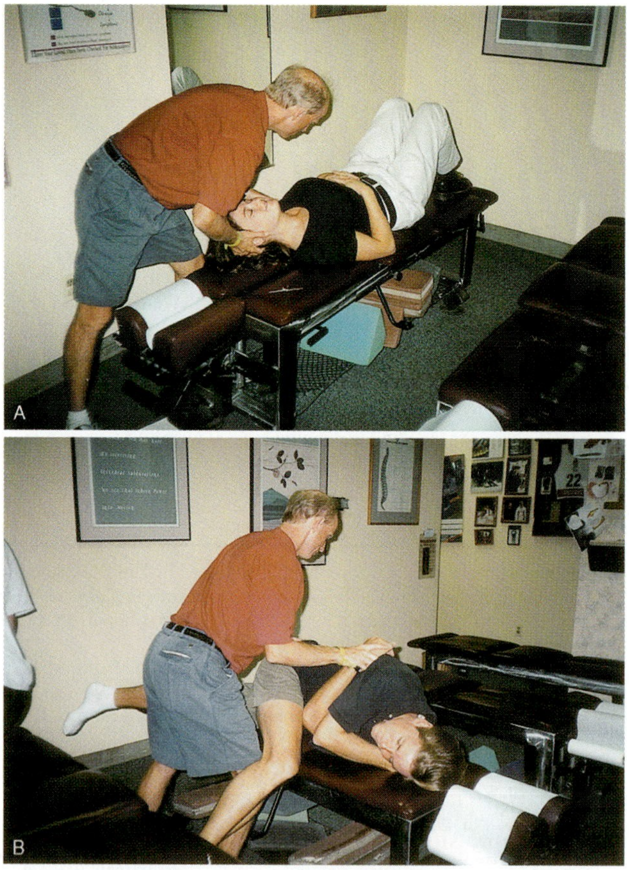

FIGURE 11–2 Chiropractic adjustments. (From Townsend, M.C.: Psychiatric Mental Health Nursing: Concepts of Care, [4th ed.] F.A. Davis Company, Philadelphia, 2003, p. 332.)

ation include massage tables, application of heat or cold, and ultrasound treatments.

The chiropractor takes a medical history and performs a clinical examination, which usually includes x-rays of the spine. Today's chiropractors may practice "straight" therapy; that is, the only therapy provided is that of subluxation adjustments. *Mixer* is a term applied to a chiropractor who combines adjustments with adjunct therapies, such as exercise, heat treatments, or massage.

Individuals seek treatment from chiropractors for many types of ailments and illnesses; the most common is back pain. In addition, chiropractors treat clients with headaches, sciatica, shoulder pain, tennis and golfer's elbow, leg and foot pain, hand and wrist pain, allergies, asthma, stomach disorders, and menstrual problems (Guinness, 1993). Some chiropractors are employed by professional sports teams as their team physicians.

Chiropractors are licensed to practice in all 50 states, and treatment is covered by government and most private insurance plans. They treat over 20 million people in the United States annually (Sadock & Sadock, 2003).

Therapeutic Touch and Massage

Therapeutic Touch

Therapeutic touch was developed in the 1970s by Dolores Krieger, a nurse associated with the New York University School of Nursing. It is based on the philosophy that the human body projects a field of energy. When this field becomes blocked, pain or illness occurs. Practitioners of therapeutic touch use this method to correct the blockages, thereby relieving the discomfort and improving health.

Based on the premise that the energy field extends beyond the surface of the body, the practitioner need not actually touch the client's skin. The therapist's hands are passed over the client's body, remaining 2 to 4 inches from the skin. The goal is to repattern the energy field by performing slow, rhythmic, sweeping hand motions over the entire body (Credit, Hartunian, & Nowak, 1998). Heat should be felt where the energy is blocked. The therapist "massages" the energy field in that area, smoothing it out, and thus correcting the obstruction. Therapeutic touch is thought to reduce pain and anxiety and promote relaxation and health maintenance. It has been useful in the treatment of chronic health conditions.

Massage

Massage is the technique of manipulating the muscles and soft tissues of the body. Chinese physicians prescribed massage for the treatment of disease more than 5,000 years ago. The Eastern style focuses on balancing the body's vital energy (chi) as it flows through pathways (meridians), as described earlier in the discussion of acupressure and acupuncture. The Western style of massage affects muscles, connective tissues (e.g., tendons and ligaments), and the cardiovascular system. Swedish massage, which is probably the best-known Western style, uses a variety of gliding and kneading strokes, along with deep circular movements and vibrations to relax the muscles, improve circulation, and increase mobility (Guinness, 1993).

Massage has been shown to be beneficial in the following conditions: anxiety, chronic back and neck pain, arthritis, sciatica, migraine headaches, muscle spasms, insomnia, pain of labor and delivery, stress-related disorders, and whiplash. Massage is contraindicated in certain conditions, such as high blood pressure, acute infection, osteoporosis, phlebitis, skin conditions, and varicose veins. It also should not be performed over the site of a recent injury, bruise, or burn.

Massage therapists require specialized training in a program accredited by the American Massage Therapy Association and must pass the national certification examination for therapeutic massage and body work.

Yoga

Yoga is thought to have developed in India some 5,000 years ago. It is attributed to an Indian physician and Sanskrit scholar named Patanjali. The ultimate goal of yoga is to unite the human soul with the universal spirit (Guinness, 1993). Yoga has been found to be especially helpful in relieving stress and in improving overall physical and psychological wellness. Proper breathing is a major component of yoga. It is believed that yoga breathing—a deep, diaphragmatic breathing—increases oxygen to brain and body tissues, thereby easing stress and fatigue and boosting energy.

Another component of yoga is meditation. Individuals who practice the meditation and deep breathing associated with yoga find that they are able to achieve a profound feeling of relaxation (Fig. 11–3).

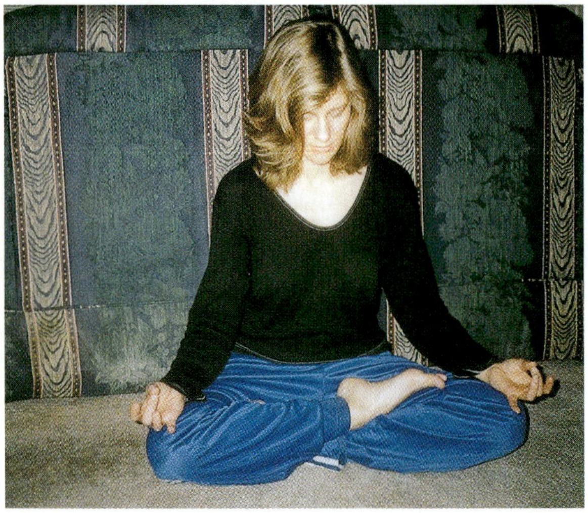

FIGURE 11–3 Achieving relaxation through the practice of yoga.

The most familiar type of yoga practiced in Western countries is hatha yoga. Hatha yoga uses body postures, along with the meditation and breathing exercises, to achieve a balanced, disciplined workout that releases muscle tension, tones the internal organs, and energizes the mind, body, and spirit, so that natural healing can occur (Credit, Hartunian, & Nowak, 1998). The complete routine of poses is designed to work all parts of the body—stretching and toning muscles and keeping joints flexible. Studies have shown that yoga has provided beneficial effects to some individuals with back pain, stress, migraine, insomnia, high blood pressure, rapid heart rate, and limited mobility (Guinness, 1993).

Pet Therapy

The therapeutic value of pets is no longer just theory. Evidence has shown that animals can directly influence a person's mental and physical well-being. Many pet-therapy programs have been established across the country, and the numbers are increasing regularly.

Several studies have provided information about the positive results of human interaction with pets. Some of these include the following:

1. One year following heart attack, clients who have pets have one-fifth the death rate as those who do not (Friedmann & Thomas, 1995).
2. Petting a dog or cat has been shown to lower blood pressure. In one study, volunteers experienced a 7.1-mm Hg drop in systolic and an 8.1-mm Hg decrease in diastolic blood pressure when they talked to and petted their dogs, as opposed to reading aloud or resting quietly (Whitaker, 2000).
3. Bringing a pet into a nursing home or hospital has been shown to enhance a client's mood and social interaction (Sobel & Ornstein, 1996).

Some researchers believe that animals actually may retard the aging process among those who live alone (Fig. 11–4). Loneliness often results in premature death, and having a pet mitigates the effects of loneliness and isolation. Whitaker (2000) suggests:

> Though owning a pet doesn't make you immune to illness, pet owners are, on the whole, healthier than those who don't own pets. Study after study shows that people with pets have fewer minor health problems, require fewer visits to the doctor and less medication, and have fewer risk factors for heart disease, such as high blood pressure or cholesterol levels. (p. 7)

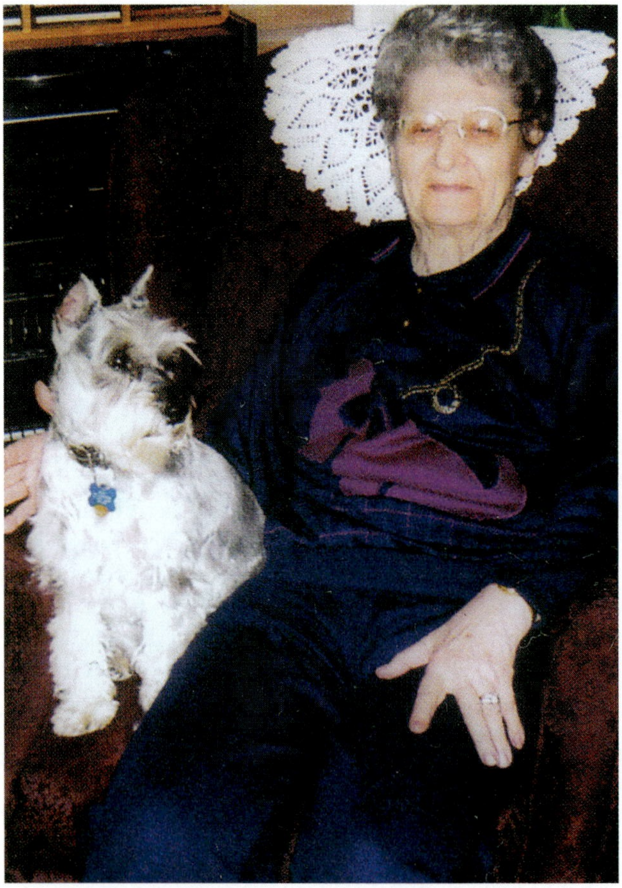

FIGURE 11–4 Healthy aging with pet.

It may never be known precisely why animals affect humans they way they do, but for those who have pets to love, the therapeutic benefits come as no surprise. Pets provide unconditional, nonjudgmental love and affection, which can be the perfect antidote for a depressed mood or a stressful situation. The role of animals in the human healing process still requires more research, but its validity is now widely accepted in both the medical and lay communities.

PSYCHOSOCIAL THERAPIES

Individual Psychotherapy

Individual psychotherapy takes place on a one-to-basis between a client and a therapist. Mental health professionals who usually perform individual psychotherapy include advanced practice registered nurses, psychiatric social workers, psychiatrists, psychologists, and licensed mental health counselors. An agreement is established and, within a therapeutic environment, the therapist assists the client to overcome behavioral symptoms or resolve interpersonal problems. Several models of individual psychotherapy are discussed in this section.

Psychoanalysis

Psychoanalysis is considered by many to be the foundation for individual psychotherapy. It was originated by Freud in the early 20th century (Chapter 2). In psychoanalysis, a major goal is for the client to gain insight and understanding about current relationships and behavior patterns by confronting unconscious conflicts that surface in the transference relationship with the analyst. Psychoanalysis is a lengthy and costly type of treatment. Some of the techniques used in psychoanalysis include the following*:

FREE ASSOCIATION. In free association, the client is allowed to say whatever comes to mind in response to a word that is given by the therapist. For example, the therapist might say "mother" or "blue," and the client would give a response, also typically one word, to each of the words the therapist says. The therapist then looks for a theme or pattern to the client's responses. If the client responds "evil" to the word "mother" or "dead" to the word "blue," the therapist might pick up one potential theme, but if the client responds "kind" and "true" to the words "mother" and "blue," the therapist might hear a completely different theme. The theme may give the therapist an idea of the cause of the client's emotional disturbance.

DREAM ANALYSIS. Freudians believe that behavior is rooted in the unconscious and that dreams are a manifestation of the troubles people repress. Psychoanalysts believe that dreams truly are the mirror to the unconscious. Monitoring and interpreting dreams is an important technique of psychoanalysis. The client is asked to keep a "dream log" by writing in a notebook as much as he or she can remember of both pleasant and particularly disturbing dreams. The dreams are then interpreted in much the same way as free association. Significant people or situations in the dreams are explored with the client, and possible meanings are offered by the therapist.

HYPNOSIS. Hypnotherapy is sometimes used in psychoanalysis as a tool for unlocking the unconscious or for searching further into "past life regression." Hypnosis is very deep relaxation during which the therapist, who has been trained in techniques of trance formation, asks certain questions of the client. Guided imagery also may be used to help the client envision the situation in an effort to find the cause of the problem. At the close of the session, when the individual is still in the trance state, the therapist may offer some posthypnotic suggestions. These typically include positive, affirming statements for the client to think about and to assist the client with changes in behavior he or she wants to accomplish.

CATHARSIS. Sadock and Sadock (2003) define **catharsis** as "the expression of ideas, thoughts, and suppressed material that is accompanied by an emotional response that produces a state of relief in the patient." Catharsis is used in psychoanalysis to allow the client to purge the repressed mental contents from the psyche. Maladaptive symptoms may be resolved by bringing unconscious thoughts and feelings into consciousness. Sometimes the individual not only may recall the painful experience but also actually *relives* it, accompanied by the feelings and emotions associated with the event. This process is called **abreaction**.

Interpersonal Psychotherapy

Interpersonal psychotherapy is a time-limited treatment that was developed for the treatment of major depression. Time-limited psychotherapies (also called brief psychotherapy) have a specific focus, identified goals, and a limited number of sessions, which com-

*This section reprinted with permission from Neeb, K. (2001). Fundamentals of mental health nursing, (2nd ed.) Philadelphia: F.A. Davis.

monly number 5 to 25. Theoretical approaches include psychoanalytic, psychodynamic, interpersonal, and integrative.

Interpersonal psychotherapy (IPT) is based on the concepts of Harry Stack Sullivan, assuming the symptoms and social dysfunction associated with depression (and other psychiatric disorders) are correlated with difficulties in interpersonal relations. The overall goal of IPT is improvement in current interpersonal skills (Sadock & Sadock, 2003). Sessions generally occur weekly for about 12 to 16 weeks.

In the initial sessions, the therapist gathers information by taking a psychiatric history, identifying the major problem, establishing a diagnosis, and, together with the client, outlining the goals of therapy. A plan of action for the remaining therapy sessions defines specific interventions targeted at resolving the identified problem. Sadock and Sadock (2003) state:

> Each session begins with the question "How have things been since we last met?" to focus on current mood states and their association with recent interactions. The basic techniques for handling each problem area are clarifying positive and negative feelings states, identifying past models for relationships, and guiding and encouraging the patient in examining and choosing alternative courses of action. (p. 934)

IPT as monotherapy has been used successfully with mild to moderate major depressive disorder. Studies have shown that in clients with severe or recurrent major depressive disorder, a combination of psychotherapy and pharmacotherapy is better than one alone (Karasu, Gelenberg, & Merriam, 2002). Trials are currently under way to study the efficacy of IPT with social phobia, bipolar disorder, posttraumatic stress disorder, borderline personality disorder, panic disorder, and bulimia. Clinical trials failed to demonstrate efficacy of IPT with substance use disorders (Markowitz, 2003).

Reality Therapy

Reality therapy was developed in the mid-1960s by the American psychiatrist William Glasser. The therapy is based on control theory and suggests all individuals are responsible for the choices they make. It includes the principle that human beings are born with the following five basic needs:

- Power (includes achievement, competence, and accomplishment)
- Belonging (includes social groups as well as families and loved ones)
- Freedom (includes independence and personal autonomy)
- Fun (includes enjoyment and pleasure)
- Survival (includes physiological needs, such as food, shelter, sexual expression)

Personality development is viewed as an attempt to fulfill these five basic needs. Individuals choose behaviors and subsequently discover whether the chosen behaviors are effective or ineffective in satisfying their needs. Glasser and Wubbolding (1995) state, "When [individuals] habitually fail to fulfill their needs effectively, they develop a failure identity characterized by ineffective or out-of-control behaviors."

In reality therapy, emphasis is on the present—the "here and now." Past behavior is addressed only as it influences present choices or future behavior. A primary function of the therapist is to assist the client in dealing with getting needs met in the present. The therapist helps the client identify needs that are not being met, correlate the unmet needs to current ineffective behaviors, and make conscious choices to change to more effective patterns of behavior in an effort to satisfy basic needs.

In reality therapy, psychopathology is viewed in terms of ineffective behaviors. Diagnoses and labels (e.g., neurotic or dysfunctional) are perceived as stereotypical and not particularly useful. The concept of *responsibility* is emphasized. Accepting responsibility for one's own behavior is equated with mental health. An individual who behaves responsibly is able to fulfill his or her basic needs without interfering with others' attempts at need fulfillment. An important part of the therapist's role is serving as a positive role model for responsible behavior.

Glasser and Wubbolding (1995) state:

> Through the skillful use of reality therapy, it is possible to help a person evaluate whether behavioral change is desirable and possible and whether adjusting to the demands of the "real world" would be appropriate and satisfying. If clients decide that change is beneficial to them, they are helped to make better choices designed to maintain or increase their need fulfillment. (p. 294)

Reality therapy can be very self-empowering for a client. Hope is instilled when therapy does not dwell on past failures, and the client is able to look forward toward a change in behavior. Reality therapy promotes the conviction that although an individual is a product of the past, he or she need not continue as its victim.

Relaxation Therapy

Stress is a part of our everyday lives. It can be positive or negative, but it cannot be eliminated. Keeping stress at a manageable level is a lifelong process.

Individuals under stress respond with a physiological arousal that can be dangerous over long periods. Indeed, the stress response has been shown to be a major contributor, directly or indirectly, to coronary heart disease, cancer, lung ailments, accidental injuries, cirrhosis of the liver, and suicide—six of the leading causes of death in the United States.

Relaxation therapy is an effective means of reducing the stress response in some individuals. The amount of anxiety that an individual experiences in response to stress is related to certain predisposing factors, such as characteristics of temperament with which he or she was born, past experiences resulting in learned patterns of responding, and existing conditions, such as health status, coping strategies, and adequate support systems.

Deep relaxation can counteract the physiological and behavioral manifestations of stress. Various methods of relaxation include the following:

DEEP-BREATHING EXERCISES. Tension is released when the lungs are allowed to breathe in as much oxygen as possible. Deep-breathing exercises involve inhaling slowly and deeply through the nose, holding the breath for a few seconds, and then exhaling slowly through the mouth, pursing the lips as if trying to whistle.

PROGRESSIVE RELAXATION. This method of deep-muscle relaxation is based on the premise that the body responds to anxiety-provoking thoughts and events with muscle tension. Each muscle group is tensed for 5 to 7 seconds and then relaxed for 20 to 30 seconds; during relaxation, the individual concentrates on the difference in sensations between the two conditions. Soft, slow background music may facilitate relaxation. A modified version of this technique (called passive progressive relaxation) involves relaxation of the muscles by concentrating on the feeling of relaxation within the muscle, rather than the actual tensing and relaxing of the muscle.

MEDITATION. The goal of meditation is to gain mastery over attention. It brings on a special state of consciousness, as attention is concentrated solely on one thought or object. During meditation, as the individual becomes totally preoccupied with the selected focus, the respiration rate, heart rate, and blood pressure decrease. The overall metabolism declines, and the need for oxygen consumption is reduced.

MENTAL IMAGERY. Mental imagery uses the imagination in an effort to reduce the body's response to stress. The frame of reference is very personal, based on what each individual considers a relaxing environment. The relaxing scenario is most useful when taped and played back at a time when the individual wishes to achieve relaxation.

BIOFEEDBACK. Biofeedback is the use of instrumentation to become aware of processes in the body that usually go unnoticed and to help bring them under voluntary control. Biological conditions, such as muscle tension, skin surface temperature, blood pressure, and heart rate, are monitored by the biofeedback equipment. With special training, the individual learns to use relaxation and voluntary control to modify the biological condition, in turn indicating a modification of the autonomic function it represents. Biofeedback is often used together with other relaxation techniques such as deep breathing, progressive relaxation, and mental imagery.

Assertiveness Training

Assertive behavior helps individuals feel better about themselves by encouraging them to stand up for their own basic human rights. These rights have equal representation for all individuals. However, along with rights come an equal number of responsibilities. Part of being assertive includes living up to these responsibilities.

Assertive behavior increases self-esteem and the ability to develop satisfying interpersonal relationships. This is accomplished through honesty, directness, appropriateness, and respecting one's own rights as well as the rights of others.

Individuals develop patterns of responding in various ways, such as by role modeling, by receiving positive or negative reinforcement, or by conscious choice. These patterns can take the form of nonassertiveness, assertiveness, aggressiveness, or passive-aggressiveness.

Nonassertive individuals seek to please others at the expense of denying their own basic human rights. **Assertive** individuals stand up for their own rights when protecting the rights of others. Those who respond **aggressively** defend their own rights by violating the basic rights of others. Individuals who respond in a **passive-aggressive** manner defend their own rights by expressing resistance to social and occupational demands.

Some important behavioral considerations of assertive behavior include eye contact, body posture, personal distance, physical contact, gestures, facial expression, voice, fluency, timing, listening, thoughts, and content. Various techniques have been developed to assist individuals in the process of becoming more assertive. Some of these include the following:

1. **Standing up for one's basic human rights.**
   Example: "I have the right to express my opinion."
2. **Assuming responsibility for one's own statements.**
   Example: "I *don't want* to go out with you tonight" instead of "I *can't* go out with you tonight." The latter implies a lack of power or ability.
3. **Responding as a "broken record."** Persistently repeating in a calm voice what is wanted.
   Example: Telephone salesperson: "I want to help you save money by changing long-distance services."
   Assertive response: "I don't want to change my long-distance service."
   Telephone salesperson: "I can't believe you don't want to save money!"
   Assertive response: "I don't want to change my long-distance service."
4. **Agreeing assertively.** Assertively accepting negative aspects about oneself. Admitting when an error has been made.
   Example: Ms. Jones: "You sure let that meeting get out of hand. What a waste of time."
   Ms. Smith: "Yes, I didn't do a very good job of conducting the meeting today."
5. **Inquiring assertively.** Seeking additional information about critical statements.
   Example: Male board member: "You made a real fool of yourself at the board meeting last night."
   Female board member: "Oh, really? Just what about my behavior offended you?"
   Male board member: "You were so damned pushy!"
   Female board member: "Were you offended that I spoke up for my beliefs, or was it because my beliefs are in direct opposition to yours?"
6. **Shifting from content to process.** Changing the focus of the communication from discussing the topic at hand to analyzing what is actually going on in the interaction.
   Example: Wife: "Would you please call me if you will be late for dinner?"
   Husband: "Why don't you just get off my back? I always have to account for every minute of my time with you!"
   Wife: "Sounds to me like we need to discuss some other things here. What are you *really* angry about?"
7. **Clouding/fogging.** Concurring with the critic's argument without becoming defensive and without agreeing to change.
   Example: Nurse No. 1: "You make so many mistakes. I don't know how you ever got this job!"
   Nurse No. 2: "You're right. I have made some mistakes since I started this job."
8. **Defusing**. Putting off further discussion with an angry individual until he or she is calmer.
   Example: "You are very angry right now. I don't want to discuss this matter with you when you are so upset. I will discuss it with you in my office at 3 o'clock this afternoon."
9. **Delaying assertively.** Putting off further discussion with another individual until one is calmer.
   Example: "That's a very challenging position you have taken, Mr. Brown. I'll need time to give it some thought. I'll call you later this afternoon."
10. **Responding assertively with irony.**
    Example: Man: "I bet you're one of those so-called 'women's libbers,' aren't you?"
    Woman: "Why yes, I am. Thank you for noticing."

Cognitive Therapy

Cognitive therapy, developed by Aaron Beck, is commonly used in the treatment of mood disorders. In cognitive therapy, the individual is taught to control thought distortions that are considered a factor in the development and maintenance of mood disorders. In the cognitive model, depression is characterized by a triad of negative distortions related to expectations of the environment, self, and future. The environment and activities within it are viewed as unsatisfactory, the self is unrealistically devalued, and the future is perceived as hopeless. In the same model, mania is characterized by a positive cognitive triad—the self is seen as highly valued and powerful, experiences within the environment are viewed as overly positive, and the future is seen as one of unlimited opportunity.

The general goals in cognitive therapy are to obtain symptom relief as quickly as possible, to assist the client in identifying dysfunctional patterns of thinking and behaving, and to guide the client to evidence and logic that effectively tests the validity of the dysfunctional thinking. Therapy focuses on changing "**automatic thoughts**" that occur spontaneously and contribute to the distorted affect. Examples of "automatic thoughts" in depression include the following:

1. **Personalizing**: "I'm the only one who failed."
2. **All or nothing:** "I'm a complete failure."
3. **Mind reading:** "He thinks I'm foolish."
4. **Discounting positives:** "The other questions were so easy. Any dummy could have gotten them right."

Examples of "automatic thoughts" in mania include the following:

1. **Personalizing:** "She's this happy only when she's with me."
2. **All or nothing:** "Everything I do is great."
3. **Mind reading:** "She thinks I'm wonderful."
4. **Discounting negatives:** "None of those mistakes is really important."

The client is asked to describe evidence that both supports and disputes the automatic thought. The logic underlying the inferences is then reviewed with the client. Another technique involves evaluating what would most likely happen if the client's automatic thoughts were true. Implications of consequences are then discussed.

Clients should not become discouraged if one technique seems not to be working. There is no single technique that works with all clients. He or she should be reassured that there are a number of techniques that may be used, and both therapist and client may explore these possibilities. Cognitive therapy has been shown to be an effective treatment for mood disorders, particularly in conjunction with psychopharmacological intervention.

SUMMARY

Alternative medicine includes those practices that differ from the usual traditional ones in the treatment of disease. *Complementary* therapies are those that work in partnership with traditional medical practice. This chapter has presented an overview of several complementary therapies and provided information concerning the appropriateness of their use.

Complementary therapies help the practitioner to view the client in a holistic manner. Most complementary therapies consider the mind and body connection and strive to enhance the body's own natural healing powers. The OAM of the NIH has established a list of alternative therapies to be used in practice and for investigative purposes. More than $25 billion dollars a year is spent on alternative medical therapies in the United States.

This chapter examined herbal medicine, acupressure, acupuncture, diet and nutrition, chiropractic medicine, therapeutic touch, massage, yoga, and pet therapy. Nurses must be familiar with these therapies, as more and more clients seek out the healing properties of these complementary care strategies.

Psychosocial therapies are the tools of practitioners who work in psychiatry. This chapter presented an overview of several psychosocial therapies, including psychoanalysis, interpersonal psychotherapy, reality therapy, relaxation therapy, assertiveness training, and cognitive therapy. Advanced practice psychiatric nurses may use some of these therapies in their practices. It is important for all nurses to understand the concepts associated with these therapies in order to be an effective member of the treatment team.

REVIEW QUESTIONS

SELF-EXAMINATION/LEARNING EXERCISE

Match the following herbs with the uses for which they have been associated:

____	1. Chamomile	a. For mild to moderate depression
____	2. Echinacea	b. To improve memory
____	3. Feverfew	c. To relieve upset stomach
____	4. Ginkgo	d. For insomnia
____	5. Psyllium	e. To stimulate the immune system
____	6. St. John's wort	f. For migraine headache
____	7. Valerian	g. For constipation

8. Which of the following applies to vitamin C?
   a. Coenzyme in protein metabolism; found in meat and dairy products.
   b. Necessary in formation of DNA; found in beans and other legumes.
   c. A powerful antioxidant; found in tomatoes and strawberries.
   d. Necessary for blood clotting; found in whole grains and bananas.

9. Which of the following applies to calcium?
   a. Coenzyme in carbohydrate metabolism; found in whole grains and citrus fruits.
   b. Facilitates iron absorption; found in vegetable oils and liver.
   c. Prevents night blindness; found in egg yolk and cantaloupe.
   d. Important for nerve and muscle functioning; found in dairy products and oysters.

10. Subluxation is a term used by chiropractic medicine to describe:
    a. Displacement of vertebrae in the spine.
    b. Adjustment of displaced vertebrae in the spine.
    c. Interference with the flow of energy from the brain.
    d. Pathways along which energy flows throughout the body.

11. In reality therapy, a primary function of the therapist is:
    a. Assisting the client to deal with getting current needs fulfilled.
    b. Hypnotizing the client to delve into the unconscious.
    c. Analyzing the possible meanings behind the client's dreams.
    d. Taking a psychiatric history and establishing a diagnosis.

12. A fellow worker often borrows small amounts of money from you with the promise that she will pay you back "tomorrow." She currently owes you $15 and has not yet paid back anything that she has borrowed. She asks if she can borrow a couple of dollars for lunch. Which of the following is a *nonassertive* response?
    a. "I've decided not to loan you any more money until you pay me back what you already borrowed."
    b. "I'm so sorry. I only have enough to pay for my own lunch today."
    c. "Get a life, will you? I'm tired of you sponging off me all the time!"
    d. "Sure, here's two dollars." Then to the other workers in the office: "Be sure you never lend Cindy any money. She never pays her debts. I'd be sure never to go to lunch with her if I were you!"

13. Linda always gets very nervous before presenting a sales promotion to the board of directors. She comes to you for assistance. You teach Linda how to perform progressive relaxation exercises. Which of the following would indicate a positive outcome of your intervention?
    a. Linda takes your advice and seeks another, less stressful position.
    b. Linda no longer gets nervous when it is time for her presentation.
    c. Linda decreases pre-presentation stress with relaxation exercises.
    d. Linda makes an appointment with a psychiatrist to pursue psychopharmacological intervention.

14. Nancy's new in-laws came to dinner for the first time. When Nancy's mother-in-law left some food on her place, Nancy thought, "I must be a lousy cook!" This is an example of which type of "automatic thought":
    a. All or nothing
    b. Discounting positives
    c. Catastrophic thinking
    d. Personalizing

INTERNET REFERENCES

a **http://www.herbalgram.org/**

b **http://www.herbmed.org.**

c **http://www.eatright.org/public/**

d **http://www.chiropractic.org/**

e **http://www.pawssf.org/**

f **http://www.holisticmed.com/www/acupuncture.html**

g **http://www.americanyogaassociation.org/**

h **http://www.angelfire.com/ab/brightminds/tReality.html**

REFERENCES

Accent on today's woman: Sugar blues. (1998, August 2). The Sunday Oklahoman.

Avants, S.K., Margolin, A., Holford, T.R., & Kosten, T.R. (2000). A randomized controlled trial of auricular acupuncture for cocaine dependence. Archives of Internal Medicine, 160: 2305–2312.

Blumenthal, M. (Ed.). (1998). The complete German Commission E monographs: Therapeutic guide to herbal medicines. Austin, TX: American Botanical Council.

Complementary and alternative medicine (1998, Spring). Complementary and Alternative Medicine Newsletter, V(2). Silver Spring, MD: Office of Alternative Medicine Clearinghouse.

Coniglione, T. (1998, June). Our doctors must begin looking at the total person. InBalance. Oklahoma City, OK: The Balanced Healing Medical Center.

Council for Responsible Nutrition. (2001). Historical comparison of RDIs, RDAs, and DRIs, 1968 to present. Retrieved September 26, 2003 from http://www.crnusa.org/pdfs/CRNintakes.pdf

Credit, L.P., Hartunian, S.G., & Nowak, M.J. (1998). Your guide to complementary medicine. Garden City Park, NY: Avery Publishing Group.

DeSantis, L. (2003). Alternative and complementary healing practices. In J.T. Catalano (Ed.), Nursing now! Today's issues, tomorrow's trends (3rd ed.). Philadelphia: F.A. Davis.

Friedmann, E., & Thomas, S.A. (1995). Pet ownership, social support, and one-year survival after acute myocardial infarction in the cardiac arrhythmia suppression trial. American Journal of Cardiology, 76:1213.

Glasser, W. & Wubbolding, R.E. (1995). Reality therapy. In R.J. Corsini & D. Wedding (Eds.), Current psychotherapies (5th ed.). Itasca, IL: F.E. Peacock.

Guinness, A.E. (Ed.). (1993). Family guide to natural medicine. Pleasantville, NY: The Reader's Digest Association.

Institute for Natural Resources. (1998). Alternative medicine: An objective view (2nd Ed.). Berkeley, CA: INR.

Karasu, T.B., Gelenberg, A., & Merriam, A. (2002). Practice guideline for the treatment of patients with major depressive disorder. In The American Psychiatric Association practice guidelines for the treatment of psychiatric disorders, compendium 2002. Washington, D.C. American Psychiatric Association.

Lutz, C.A., & Przytulski, K.R. (2001). Nutrition and diet therapy, (3rd ed.) Philadelphia: F.A. Davis.

Markowitz, J.C. (2003). Interpersonal psychotherapy. In R.E. Hales & S.C. Yudofsky (Eds.), Textbook of clinical psychiatry, (4th ed.) Washington, D.C.: American Psychiatric Publishing.

National Institutes of Health (1997, November). NIH consensus report on acupuncture, 15(5).

Natural Healers. (2003). Acupuncture and Oriental Medicine

School and Careers. Retrieved on September 25, 2003, from the World Wide Web at http://www.naturalhealers.com/qa/acupuncture.html?inktomi#q5

PDR for Herbal Medicines (2nd ed.). (2000). Montvale, NJ: Medical Economics Company.

Sadock, B.J., & Sadock, V.A. (2003). Synopsis of psychiatry: Behavioral sciences/clinical psychiatry (9th ed.). Philadelphia: Lippincott Williams & Wilkins.

Schoenen, J., Jacquy, J., & Lenaerts, M. (1998, February). Effectiveness of high-dose riboflavin in migraine prophylaxis: A randomized controlled trial. Neurology (50):466–469.

Sobel, D.S., & Ornstein, R. (1996). The healthy mind, healthy body handbook. Los Altos, CA: DR_X.

Steyer, T.E. (2001). Complementary and alternative medicine: A primer. Family Practice Management, 8:37–42.

U.S. Department of Agriculture (USDA). (2003). Dietary reference intakes (DRI) and recommended dietary allowances (RDA). Food and Nutrition Information Center. Retrieved September 26, 2003, from http://www.nal.usda.gov/fnic/etext/000105.html

U.S. Department of Agriculture & U.S. Department of Health and Human Services (2000). Nutrition and your health: Dietary guidelines for Americans (5th ed.). Washington, D.C.: Author.

Whitaker, J. (2000). Pet owners are a healthy breed. Health & Healing 10:1–8.

Yeager, S. (1998). New foods for healing. Emmaus, PA: Rodale Press.

UNIT THREE

CARE OF CLIENTS WITH PSYCHIATRIC DISORDERS

12

CHAPTER

Delirium, Dementia, and Amnestic Disorders

CHAPTER OUTLINE

KEY TERMS

amnesia
aphasia
apraxia
ataxia
confabulation
delirium
dementia
pseudodementia
primary dementia
secondary dementia

OBJECTIVES

After reading this chapter, the student will be able to:

1. Define and differentiate among *delirium*, *dementia*, and *amnestic disorder*.
2. Discuss etiological implications of delirium, dementia, and amnestic disorders.
3. Describe clinical symptoms and use the information to assess clients with delirium, dementia, and amnestic disorders.
4. Identify nursing diagnoses common to clients with delirium, dementia, and amnestic disorders and select appropriate nursing interventions for each.
5. Identify topics for client and family teaching relevant to these disorders.
6. Discuss criteria for evaluating nursing care of clients with delirium, dementia, and amnestic disorders.
7. Describe various treatment modalities relevant to care of clients with delirium, dementia, and amnestic disorders.

INTRODUCTION

This chapter discusses disorders in which a clinically significant deficit in cognition or memory exists, representing a significant change from a previous level of functioning. The *DSM-IV-TR* (APA, 2000) describes the etiology of these disorders as a general medical condition or a substance, or a combination of these factors.

These disorders were previously identified as *or-*

ganic mental syndromes and disorders. With the publication of the *DSM-IV* (APA, 1994), the name was changed to prevent the implication that *nonorganic* mental disorders do not have a biological basis.

These disorders constitute a large and growing public health problem. Alzheimer's disease, the most common form of dementia, afflicts 5 to 10 percent of all persons in the United States aged 65 years and older. Prevalence increases with age to an estimated 25 to 45 percent of those aged 85 years and older (United States General Accounting Office, 1998). By the year 2050, 14 million people are expected to have this neurodegenerative disease (ADRDA, 2001). After heart disease and cancer, Alzheimer's disease is the third most costly disease to society, accounting for $100 billion in yearly costs (Laraia, 2004). This proliferation is not the result of an "epidemic." It has occurred because more people now survive into the high-risk period for dementia, which is middle age and beyond.

This chapter presents etiological implications, clinical symptoms, and nursing interventions for care of clients with delirium, dementia, and amnestic disorders. The objective is to provide these individuals with the dignity and quality of life they deserve while offering guidance and support to their families or primary caregivers.

DELIRIUM

A **delirium** is characterized by a disturbance of consciousness and a change in cognition that develop rapidly over a short period (APA, 2000). Symptoms of delirium include difficulty sustaining and shifting attention. The person is extremely distractible and must be repeatedly reminded to focus attention. Disorganized thinking prevails and is reflected by speech that is rambling, irrelevant, pressured, and incoherent and that unpredictably switches from subject to subject. Reasoning ability and goal-directed behavior are impaired. Disorientation to time and place is common, and impairment of recent memory is invariably evident. Misperceptions of the environment, including illusions and hallucinations, prevail.

Level of consciousness is often affected, with a disturbance in the sleep-wake cycle. The state of awareness may range from that of hypervigilance to stupor or semicoma. Sleep may fluctuate between hypersomnolence and insomnia. Vivid dreams and nightmares are common.

Psychomotor activity may fluctuate between agitated, purposeless movements (e.g., restlessness, hyperactivity, striking out at nonexistent objects) and a vegetative state resembling catatonic stupor. Various forms of tremor are frequently present.

Emotional instability may be manifested by fear, anxiety, depression, irritability, anger, euphoria, or apathy. These various emotions may be evidenced by crying, calls for help, cursing, muttering, moaning, acts of self-destruction, fearful attempts to flee, or attacks upon others who are falsely viewed as threatening. Autonomic manifestations, such as tachycardia, sweating, flushed face, dilated pupils, and elevated blood pressure, are common.

The symptoms of delirium usually begin quite abruptly (e.g., following a head injury or seizure). At other times, they may be preceded by several hours or days of prodromal symptoms (e.g., restlessness, difficulty thinking clearly, insomnia or hypersomnolence, and nightmares). The slower onset is more common if the underlying etiology is systemic illness or metabolic imbalance.

The duration of delirium is usually brief (e.g., 1 week; rarely more than 1 month) and, upon recovery from the underlying determinant, symptoms usually diminish over a 3- to 7-day period but in some instances may take as long as 2 weeks (Sadock & Sadock, 2003). The age of the client and duration of the delirium influence rate of symptom resolution. Delirium may transition into a more permanent cognitive disorder (e.g., dementia) and is associated with a high mortality rate (Bourgeois, Seaman, & Servis, 2003).

Etiological Implications

The *DSM-IV-TR* (APA, 2000) differentiates between the disorders of delirium by their etiology, although they share a common symptom presentation. Categories of delirium include:

1. Delirium due to a general medical condition
2. Substance-induced delirium
3. Substance-intoxication delirium
4. Substance-withdrawal delirium
5. Delirium due to multiple etiologies

Delirium Due to a General Medical Condition

In this type of delirium, evidence must exist (from history, physical examination, or laboratory findings) to show that the symptoms of delirium are a direct result of the physiological consequences of a general medical condition (APA, 2000). Such conditions include systemic infections, metabolic disorders (e.g., hypoxia, hypercarbia, and hypoglycemia), fluid or electrolyte imbalances, hepatic or renal disease, thiamine deficiency, postoperative states, hypertensive encephalopathy, postictal states, sequelae of head trauma, and others (APA, 2000).

Substance-Induced Delirium

This disorder is characterized by the symptoms of delirium that are attributed to medication side effects or exposure to a toxin. The *DSM-IV-TR* (APA, 2000) lists the following examples of medications that have been reported to result in substance-induced delirium: anesthetics, analgesics, antiasthmatic agents, anticonvulsants, antihistamines, antihypertensive and cardiovascular medications, antimicrobials, antiparkinsonian drugs, corticosteroids, gastrointestinal medications, histamine H_2-receptor antagonists (e.g., cimetidine), immunosuppressive agents, lithium, muscle relaxants, and psychotropic medications with anticholinergic side effects. Toxins reported to cause delirium include organophosphate (anticholinesterase), insecticides, carbon monoxide, and volatile substances such as fuel or organic solvents.

Substance-Intoxication Delirium

With this disorder, the symptoms of delirium may arise within minutes to hours after taking relatively high doses of certain drugs, such as cannabis, cocaine, and hallucinogens. It may take longer periods of sustained intoxication to produce delirium symptoms with alcohol, anxiolytics, or narcotics (APA, 2000).

Substance-Withdrawal Delirium

Withdrawal delirium symptoms develop after reduction or termination of sustained, usually high-dose use of certain substances, such as alcohol, sedatives, hypnotics, or anxiolytics (APA, 2000). The duration of the delirium is directly related to the half-life of the substance involved and may last from a few hours to 2 to 4 weeks.

Delirium Due to Multiple Etiologies

This diagnosis is used when the symptoms of delirium are brought on by more than one etiology. For example, the delirium may be related to more than one general medical condition or it may be due to the combined effects of a general medical condition and substance use (APA, 2000.)

DEMENTIA

Dementia is defined by a "loss of previous levels of cognitive, executive, and memory function in a state of full alertness" (Bourgeois, Seaman, & Servis, 2003). Dementia can be classified as primary or secondary. **Primary dementias** are those, such as Alzheimer's disease, in which the dementia itself is the major sign of some organic brain disease not directly related to any other organic illness. **Secondary dementias** are caused by or related to another disease or condition, such as human immunodeficiency virus (HIV) disease or a cerebral trauma.

In dementia, impairment is evident in abstract thinking, judgment, and impulse control. The conventional rules of social conduct are often disregarded. Behavior may be uninhibited and inappropriate. Personal appearance and hygiene are often neglected.

Language may or may not be affected. Some individuals may have difficulty naming objects, or the language may seem vague and imprecise. In severe forms of dementia, the individual may not speak at all (**aphasia**).

Personality change is common in dementia and may be manifested by an alteration or accentuation of premorbid characteristics. For example, an individual who was previously very socially active may become apathetic and socially isolated. A previously neat person may become markedly untidy in his or her appearance. Conversely, an individual who may have had difficulty trusting others before the illness may exhibit extreme fear and paranoia as manifestations of the dementia.

The reversibility of dementia is a function of the underlying pathology and of the availability and timely application of effective treatment (APA, 2000). Truly reversible dementia occurs in only a small percentage of cases and might be more appropriately termed *temporary* dementia. Reversible dementia can occur as a result of stroke, depression, side effects of certain medications, vitamin or nutritional deficiencies (especially B_{12} or folate), and metabolic disorders (Marchione, 1999). In most clients, dementia runs a progressive, irreversible course.

As the disease progresses, **apraxia**, which is the inability to carry out motor activities despite intact motor function, may develop. The individual may be irritable, moody, or exhibit sudden outbursts over trivial issues. The ability to work or care for personal needs independently will no longer be possible. These individuals can no longer be left alone because they do not comprehend their limitations and are therefore at serious risk for accidents. Wandering away from the home or care setting often becomes a problem.

Several causes have been described for the syndrome of dementia (see section on etiological implications), but dementia of the Alzheimer's type (DAT) accounts for at least two-thirds of all cases of dementia (Kovach & Wilson, 1999). The progressive nature of symptoms associated with DAT has been described according to stages (Hall, 1994; Hall, 1991; Harvard Medical School, 1995a & b; Devanand & Mayeux, 1992; Kovach & Wilson, 1999):

Stage 1. No apparent symptoms. In the first stage of the illness, there is no apparent decline in memory.

Stage 2. Forgetfulness. In this stage, the individual may lose things or forget names of people. Losses in short-term memory are common. The individual is aware of the intellectual decline and may feel ashamed, becoming anxious and depressed, which in turn may worsen the symptoms. Maintaining organization with lists and a structured routine provide some compensation.

Stage 3. Early confusion. As the symptom of confusion begins, there is interference with work performance. The individual may get lost when driving his or her car. Concentration may be interrupted.

Stage 4. Late confusion. At this stage, the individual may forget major events in personal history, such as his or her own child's birthday; experience declining ability to perform tasks, such as shopping and managing personal finances; or be unable to understand current news events. He or she may deny that a problem exists by covering up memory loss with **confabulation** (creating imaginary events to fill in memory gaps). Depression and social withdrawal are common.

Stage 5. Early dementia. In the early stages of dementia, individuals lose the ability to perform activities of daily living (ADLs) independently, such as hygiene, dressing, grooming, and toileting. They may forget addresses, phone numbers, and names of close relatives, and require some assistance to manage on an ongoing basis. Frustration, withdrawal, and self-absorption are common.

Stage 6. Middle dementia. At this stage, the individual may be unable to recall recent major life events or even the name of his or her spouse. Disorientation to surroundings is common, and the person may be unable to recall the day, season, or year. Urinary and fecal incontinence are common. Sleeping becomes a problem. Psychomotor symptoms include wandering, obsessiveness, agitation, and aggression. Symptoms seem to worsen in the late afternoon and evening—a phenomenon termed **sundowning**. Communication becomes more difficult with increasing loss of language skills. Institutional care is usually required at this stage.

Stage 7. Late dementia. In the end stages of DAT, the individual is unable to recognize family members. He or she is most commonly bedfast and aphasic. Problems of immobility, such as decubiti and contractures, may occur.

Kovach and Wilson (1999) describe the late stages of dementia as follows:

> During late-stage dementia, the person becomes more chair-bound or bed-bound. Muscles are rigid and contractures may develop. The person may have very active hands and repetitive movements, grunting, or other vocalizations. There is depressed immune system function and this impairment coupled with immobility may lead to the development of pneumonia, urinary tract infections, sepsis, and pressure ulcers. Appetite decreases and dysphagia is present; aspiration is common. Weight loss generally occurs. Speech and language are severely impaired, with greatly decreased verbal communication. The person may no longer recognize any family members. Bowel and bladder incontinence are present and caregivers need to complete most ADLs for the person. The sleep-wake cycle is greatly altered, and the person spends a lot of time dozing, and appears socially withdrawn and more unaware of the environment or surroundings. Death may be caused by infection, sepsis, or aspiration, although there are not many studies examining cause of death. (p. 352)

Etiological Implications

The *DSM-IV-TR* (APA, 2000) differentiates between the disorders of dementia by their etiology, although they share a common symptom presentation. Categories of dementia include:

1. Dementia of the Alzheimer's type
2. Vascular dementia
3. Dementia due to HIV disease
4. Dementia due to head trauma
5. Dementia due to Parkinson's disease
6. Dementia due to Huntington's disease
7. Dementia due to Pick's disease
8. Dementia due to Creutzfeldt-Jakob disease
9. Dementia due to other general medical conditions
10. Substance-induced persisting dementia
11. Dementia due to multiple etiologies

Dementia of the Alzheimer's Type

This disorder is characterized by the syndrome of symptoms identified as dementia in the *DSM-IV-TR* and in the seven stages described previously. The onset of symptoms is slow and insidious, and the course of the disorder is generally progressive and deteriorating. The *DSM-IV-TR* further categorizes this disorder as *early onset* (first symptoms occurring at age 65 years or younger) or *late onset* (first symptoms occurring after age 65 years) and by the clinical presentation of behavioral disturbance (such as wandering or agitation) superimposed on the dementia.

Refinement of diagnostic criteria now enables clinicians to use specific clinical features to identify the disease with considerable accuracy. Examination by computerized tomography (CT) scan or magnetic resonance imagery (MRI) reveals a degenerative pathology of the brain that includes atrophy, widened cortical sulci, and enlarged cerebral ventricles. Microscopic examinations reveal numerous neurofibrillary tangles and senile plaques in the brains of clients with Alzheimer's disease. These changes apparently occur as a part of the normal aging process. However, in clients with Alzheimer's disease, they are found in dramatically increased numbers, and their profusion is concentrated in the hippocampus and certain parts of the cerebral cortex.

Etiology

The exact cause of Alzheimer's disease is unknown. Several hypotheses have been supported by varying amounts and quality of data. These hypotheses include:

1. **Acetylcholine alterations.** Research has indicated that in the brains of Alzheimer's clients, the enzyme required to produce acetylcholine is dramatically reduced. The reduction seems to be greatest in the areas of the basal forebrain and the nucleus basalis of Meynert (Popkin, 1994). This decrease in production of acetylcholine reduces the amount of the neurotransmitter that is released to cells in the cortex and hippocampus, resulting in a disruption of the cognitive processes.
2. **Accumulation of aluminum.** Several studies have reported higher concentrations of aluminum in the brains of Alzheimer's clients than in those of healthy older persons without dementia. However, high concentrations of aluminum have also been reported in the brains of clients with other types of dementias. Therefore, aluminum as a contributing factor is probably not specific to Alzheimer's disease. The current consensus is that aluminum compounds accumulate only in a brain that is already damaged (Harvard Medical School, 1995a). More research is necessary to determine the role of aluminum in the etiology of all dementias.
3. **Alterations in the immune system.** Several studies have shown that antibodies are produced in the Alzheimer's brain. What the antibodies are produced in response to is unknown. The reactions are actually *auto*antibody production—a reaction against the self—suggesting a possible alteration in the body's immune system as an etiological factor in Alzheimer's disease.
4. **Head trauma.** The etiology of Alzheimer's disease has been associated with serious head trauma (Williams, 1995). Studies have shown that a large number of individuals who had experienced head trauma subsequently (after years) developed Alzheimer's disease. This hypothesis is currently being investigated as a possible cause.
5. **Genetic factors.** There is clearly a familial pattern with some forms of Alzheimer's disease. Some families exhibit a pattern of inheritance that suggests possible autosomal-dominant gene transmission (Sadock & Sadock, 2003). Some studies indicate that early-onset cases are more likely to be familial than late-onset cases and that from one-third to one-half of all cases may be of the genetic form. Some researchers believe that there is a link between Alzheimer's disease and the alteration of a gene found on chromosome 21. People with Down's syndrome who carry an extra copy of chromosome 21 have been found to be unusually susceptible to Alzheimer's disease (Harvard Medical School, 1995a).

Vascular Dementia

In this disorder, the clinical syndrome of dementia is due to significant cerebrovascular disease. The blood vessels of the brain are affected, and progressive intellectual deterioration occurs. Vascular dementia is believed to be the second most common cause of dementia and accounts for about 20 percent of cases (Harvard Medical School, 1995a).

Vascular dementia differs from Alzheimer's disease in that it has a more abrupt onset and runs a highly variable course. Progression of the symptoms occurs in "steps" rather than as a gradual deterioration; that is, at times the dementia seems to clear up, and the individual exhibits lucid thinking. Memory may seem better, and the client may become optimistic that improvement is occurring, only to experience further decline of functioning in a fluctuating pattern of progression. This irregular pattern of decline appears to be an intense source of anxiety for the client.

In vascular dementia, clients suffer the equivalent of small strokes that destroy many areas of the brain. The pattern of deficits is variable, depending on which regions of the brain have been affected (APA, 2000). Certain focal neurological signs are commonly seen with vascular dementia, including weaknesses of the limbs, small-stepped gait, and difficulty with speech.

The disorder is more common in men than in women (APA, 2000). Arvanitakis (2000) states:

> Prognosis for patients with vascular dementia is worse than that for Alzheimer's patients. The three-year mortality rate in cases over the age of 85 years old is quoted at 67 percent, as compared to 42 percent in Alzheimer's disease, and 23 percent in non-demented individuals. However, outcome is ultimately dependent on the underlying risk factors and mechanism of disease, and further studies taking these distinctions into account are warranted.

The diagnosis can be subtyped when the dementia is superimposed with symptoms of delirium, delusions, or depressed mood.

Etiology

The cause of vascular dementia is directly related to an interruption of blood flow to the brain. Symptoms result from death of nerve cells in regions nourished by diseased vessels. Various diseases and conditions that interfere with blood circulation have been implicated.

1. **Arterial hypertension.** High blood pressure is thought to be one of the most significant factors in the etiology of multiple small strokes or cerebral infarcts. Hypertension causes thickening and degeneration of cerebral arterioles, making the small arteries vulnerable to rupture (Phipps et al., 1995).
2. **Cerebral emboli.** Dementia can result from infarcts related to occlusion of blood vessels by debris in the bloodstream. These emboli can arise from diseased heart valves, damage to cells lining the heart, dislodging of clots in large vessels, the release of fat from large bones, or large sudden infusions of air or other gases (Phipps et al., 1995).
3. **Cerebral thrombosis.** Multiple small thrombi may occur in persons whose blood pressure is normal or even below normal if atheromatous changes have occurred in the lining of cerebral arteries (Phipps et al., 1995). This condition causes frequent small and barely perceptible infarcts that can lead to personality changes and cognitive deficits.

Dementia Due to HIV

Infection with HIV-type 1 (HIV-1) produces a dementing illness called HIV-1-associated dementia (HAD) complex. A less severe form, known as HIV-1-associated minor cognitive/motor disorder, also occurs. The severity of symptoms is correlated to the extent of brain pathology. The immune dysfunction associated with HIV disease can lead to brain infections by other organisms, and the HIV-1 also appears to cause dementia directly. In the early stages, neuropsychiatric symptoms may be manifested by barely perceptible changes in a person's normal psychological presentation. Severe cognitive changes, particularly confusion, changes in behavior, and sometimes psychoses, are not uncommon in the later stages.

With the advent of the highly active antiretroviral therapies, incidence rates of HAD have been on the decline. However, it is possible that the prolonged life span of HIV-infected patients taking medications will actually increase the prevalence of HIV dementia in coming years (McArthur, 2003).

Dementia Due to Head Trauma

Serious head trauma can result in symptoms associated with the syndrome of dementia. Amnesia is the most common neurobehavioral symptoms following head trauma, and some permanent disturbance may persist (Wise, Gray, & Seltzer, 1999). Repeated head trauma, such as the type experienced by boxers, can result in *dementia pugilistica*, a syndrome characterized by emotional lability, dysarthria, ataxia, and impulsivity (Sadock & Sadock, 2003).

Dementia Due to Parkinson's Disease

Dementia is observed in as many as 60 percent of clients with Parkinson's disease (Bourgeois, Seaman, & Servis, 2003). In this disease, there is a loss of nerve cells located in the substantia nigra, and dopamine activity is diminished, resulting in involuntary muscle movements, slowness, and rigidity. Tremor in the upper extremities is characteristic. In some instances, the cerebral changes that occur in dementia of Parkinson's disease closely resemble those of Alzheimer's disease.

Dementia Due to Huntington's Disease

Huntington's disease is transmitted as a Mendelian dominant gene. Damage is seen in the areas of the basal ganglia and the cerebral cortex. The onset of symptoms (i.e., involuntary twitching of the limbs or facial muscles) is usually between age 35 and 45 years. The client usually declines into a profound state of dementia and **ataxia**. The average course of the disease to complete incapacitation and death is about 15 years (Nowak & Handford, 1994).

Dementia Due to Pick's Disease

The cause of Pick's disease is unknown, but a genetic factor appears to be involved. The clinical picture is strikingly similar to that of Alzheimer's disease. In fact, diagnosis of Pick's disease is often made on autopsy of a client with clinically diagnosed Alzheimer's disease. Onset of symptoms is usually in middle age, and women are affected more frequently than men (Porth, 1994). Studies reveal that pathology results from atrophy in the frontal and temporal lobes of the brain.

Dementia Due to Creutzfeldt-Jakob Disease

Creutzfeldt-Jakob disease is an uncommon neurodegenerative disease caused by a transmissible agent known as a "slow virus" or prion (APA, 2000). Five to fifteen percent of cases have a genetic component. The clinical presentation is typical of the syndrome of dementia, along with involuntary movements, muscle rigidity, and ataxia. Symptoms may develop at any age in adults, but they typically occur between ages 40 and 60 years. The clinical course is extremely rapid, with progressive deterioration and death within 1 year (Wise, Gray, & Seltzer, 1999).

Dementia Due to Other General Medical Conditions

A number of other general medical conditions can cause dementia. Some of these include endocrine conditions (hypoglycemia, hypothyroidism), pulmonary disease, hepatic or renal failure, cardiopulmonary insufficiency, fluid and electrolyte imbalances, nutritional deficiencies, frontal or temporal lobe lesions, central nervous system (CNS) or systemic infections, uncontrolled epilepsy, and other neurological conditions such as multiple sclerosis (APA, 2000).

Substance-Induced Persisting Dementia

The features associated with this type of dementia are those associated with dementias in general; however, evidence must exist from the history, physical examination, or laboratory findings to show that the deficits are etiologically related to the persisting effects of substance use (APA, 2000). The term *persisting* is used to indicate that the dementia persists long after the effects of substance intoxication or substance withdrawal have subsided. The *DSM-IV-TR* identifies the following types of substances with which persisting dementia is associated:

1. Alcohol
2. Inhalants
3. Sedatives, hypnotics, and anxiolytics
4. Medications: anticonvulsants and intrathecal methotrexate
5. Toxins: lead, mercury, carbon monoxide, organophosphate insecticides, and industrial solvents

The diagnosis is made according to the specific etiological substance involved. For example, if the substance known to cause the dementia is alcohol, the diagnosis is alcohol-induced persisting dementia. If the exact substance presumed to be causing the dementia were unknown, the diagnosis would be unknown substance-induced persisting dementia.

Dementia Due to Multiple Etiologies

This diagnosis is used when the symptoms of dementia are attributed to more than one cause. For example, the dementia may be related to more than one medical condition or to the combined effects of a general medical condition and the long-term use of a substance (APA, 2000).

The etiological factors associated with delirium and dementias are summarized in Table 12–1.

TABLE 12–1 Etiological Factors Implicated in the Development of Delirium and/or Dementia

Biological Factors	Exogenous Factors
Hypoxia: any condition leading to a deficiency of oxygen to the brain	Birth trauma: prolonged labor, damage from use of forceps, other obstetric complications
Nutritional deficiencies: vitamins (particularly B and C); protein; fluid and electrolyte imbalances	Cranial trauma: concussion, contusions, hemorrhage, hematomas
Metabolic disturbances: porphyria; encephalopathies related to hepatic, renal, pancreatic, or pulmonary insufficiencies; hypoglycemia	Volatile inhalant compounds: gasoline, glue, paint, paint thinners, spray paints, cleaning fluids, typewriter correction fluid, varnishes, and lacquers
Endocrine dysfunction: thyroid, parathyroid, adrenal, pancreas, pituitary	Heavy metals: lead, mercury, manganese; other metallic elements: aluminum
Cardiovascular disease: stroke, cardiac insufficiency, atherosclerosis	Organic phosphates: various insecticides
Primary brain disorders: epilepsy, Alzheimer's disease, Pick's disease, Huntington's chorea, multiple sclerosis, Parkinson's disease	Substance abuse/dependence: alcohol, amphetamines, caffeine, cannabis, cocaine, hallucinogens, inhalants, nicotine, opioids, phencyclidine, sedatives, hypnotics, anxiolytics
Infections: encephalitis, meningitis, pneumonia, septicemia, neurosyphilis (dementia paralytica), HIV disease, acute rheumatic fever, Creutzfeldt-Jakob disease	Other medications: anticholinergics, antihistamines, antidepressants, antipsychotics, antiparkinsonians, antihypertensives, steroids, digitalis
Intracranial neoplasms	
Congenital defects: prenatal infections, such as first-trimester maternal rubella	

AMNESTIC DISORDERS

Amnestic disorders are characterized by an inability to learn new information (short-term memory deficit) despite normal attention, and an inability to recall previously learned information (long-term memory deficit). Events from the remote past often are recalled more easily than recently occurring ones. The syndrome differs from dementia in that there is no impairment in abstract thinking or judgment, no other disturbances of higher cortical function, and no personality change.

Profound **amnesia** may result in disorientation to place and time but rarely to self (APA, 2000). The individual may engage in confabulation—the creation of imaginary events to fill in memory gaps.

Some individuals will continue to deny that they have a problem despite evidence to the contrary. Others may acknowledge that a problem exists, but appear unconcerned. Apathy, lack of initiative, and emotional blandness are common. The person may appear friendly and agreeable, but the emotionality is superficial.

The onset of symptoms may be acute or insidious, depending on the pathological process causing the amnestic disorder. Duration and course of the illness may be quite variable, and are correlated with extent and severity of the cause.

Etiological Implications

Amnestic disorders share a common symptom presentation of memory impairment but are differentiated in the *DSM-IV-TR* (APA, 2000) according to etiology:

1. Amnestic disorder due to a general medical condition
2. Substance-induced persisting amnestic disorder

Amnestic Disorder Due to a General Medical Condition

In this type of amnestic disorder, evidence must exist from the history, physical examination, or laboratory findings to show that the memory impairment is the direct physiological consequence of a general medical condition (APA, 2000). The diagnosis is specified further by indicating whether the symptoms are *transient* (present for no more than 1 month) or *chronic* (present for more than 1 month).

General medical conditions that may be associated with amnestic disorder include head trauma, cerebrovascular disease, cerebral neoplastic disease, cerebral anoxia, herpes simplex encephalitis, poorly controlled insulin-dependent diabetes, and surgical intervention to the brain (APA, 2000; Wise, Gray, & Seltzer, 1999).

Transient amnestic syndromes can occur from

epileptic seizures, electroconvulsive therapy, severe migraine, and drug overdose (Wise, Gray, & Seltzer, 1999).

Substance-Induced Persisting Amnestic Disorder

In this disorder, evidence must exist from the history, physical examination, or laboratory findings that the memory impairment is related to the persisting effects of substance use (e.g., a drug of abuse, a medication, or toxin exposure) (APA, 2000). The term *persisting* is used to indicate that the symptoms exist long after the effects of substance intoxication or withdrawal have subsided. The *DSM-IV-TR* identifies the following substances with which amnestic disorder can be associated:

1. Alcohol
2. Sedatives, hypnotics, and anxiolytics
3. Medications: anticonvulsants and intrathecal methotrexate
4. Toxins: lead, mercury, carbon monoxide, organophosphate insecticides, and industrial solvents

The diagnosis is made according to the specific etiological substance involved. For example, if the substance known to be the cause of the amnestic disorder was alcohol, the diagnosis would be alcohol-induced persisting amnestic disorder.

APPLICATION OF THE NURSING PROCESS

Assessment

Nursing assessment of the client with delirium, dementia, or persisting amnesia is based on knowledge of the symptomatology associated with the various disorders described in the beginning of this chapter. Subjective and objective data are gathered by various members of the healthcare team. Clinicians report use of a variety of methods for obtaining assessment information.

The Client History

Nurses play a significant role in acquiring the client history, including the specific mental and physical changes that have occurred and the age at which the changes began. If the client is unable to relate information adequately, the data should be obtained from family members or others who would be aware of the client's physical and psychosocial history.

From the client history, nurses should assess the following areas of concern: (1) type, frequency, and severity of mood swings, personality and behavioral changes, and catastrophic emotional reactions; (2) cognitive changes, such as problems with attention span, thinking process, problem-solving, and memory (recent and remote); (3) language difficulties; (4) orientation to person, place, time, and situation; and (5) appropriateness of social behavior.

The nurse also should obtain information regarding current and past medication usage, history of other drug and alcohol use, and possible exposure to toxins. Knowledge regarding the history of related symptoms or specific illnesses (e.g., Huntington's disease, Alzheimer's disease, Pick's disease, or Parkinson's disease) in other family members might be useful.

Physical Assessment

Assessment of physical systems by both the nurse and the physician has two main emphases: (1) signs of damage to the nervous system and (2) evidence of diseases of other organs that could affect mental function. Diseases of various organ systems can induce confusion, loss of memory, and behavioral changes. These causes must be considered in diagnosing cognitive disorders. In the neurological examination, the client is asked to perform maneuvers or answer questions that are designed to elicit information about the condition of specific parts of the brain or peripheral nerves. Testing will assess mental status and alertness, muscle strength, reflexes, sensory-perception, language skills, and coordination. An example of a mental status examination for a client with dementia is presented in Table 12–2.

A battery of psychological tests may be ordered as part of the diagnostic examination. The results of these tests may be used to make a differential diagnosis between dementia and **pseudodementia** (depression). Depression is the most common mental illness in the elderly, but it is often misdiagnosed and treated inadequately. Cognitive symptoms of depression may mimic dementia, and because of the prevalence of dementia in the elderly, diagnosticians are often too eager to make this diagnosis. A comparison of symptoms of dementia and pseudodementia (depression) is presented in Table 12–3. Nurses can assist in this assessment by carefully observing and documenting these sometimes subtle differences.

TABLE 12–2 Mental Status Examination for Dementia

Patient Name ______________________ **Date** ______________________

Age ____________ **Sex** ____________

Diagnosis ______________________

	Maximum	Client's Score
1. **VERBAL FLUENCY**		
Ask client to name as many animals as he/she can. (Time: 60 seconds) (Score 1 point/2 animals)	10 points	________
2. **COMPREHENSION**		
a. Point to the ceiling	1 point	________
b. Point to your nose and the window	1 point	________
c. Point to your foot, the door, and ceiling	1 point	________
d. Point to the window, your leg, the door, and your thumb	1 point	________
3. **NAMING AND WORD FINDING**		
Ask the client to name the following as you point to them:		
a. Watch stem (winder)	1 point	________
b. Teeth	1 point	________
c. Sole of shoe	1 point	________
d. Buckle of belt	1 point	________
e. Knuckles	1 point	________
4. **ORIENTATION**		
a. Date	2 points	________
b. Day of week	2 points	________
c. Month	1 point	________
d. Year	1 point	________

5. **NEW LEARNING ABILITY**
Tell the client: "I'm going to tell you four words, which I want you to remember." Have the client repeat the four words after they are initially presented, and ask him/her to remember the words for later. Continue with the examination, and at intervals of 5 and 10 minutes, ask the client to recall the words. Three different sets of words are provided here.

		5 min.	10 min.
a. Brown (fun) (grape)	2 points each:	________	________
b. Honesty (loyalty) (happiness)	2 points each:	________	________
c. Tulip (carrot) (stocking)	2 points each:	________	________
d. Eyedropper (ankle) (toothbrush)	2 points each:	________	________

6. **VERBAL STORY FOR IMMEDIATE RECALL**

Tell the client: "I'm going to read you a short story, which I want you to remember. Listen closely to what I read because I will ask you to retell me the story when I finish." Read the story slowly and carefully, without pausing at the slash marks. After completing the paragraph, ask the client to retell the story as accurately as possible. Record the number of correct memories (information within the slashes) and describe confabulation if it is present. (1 point = 1 remembered item [13 maximum points]) — 13 points ________

It was July / and the Rogers / had packed up / their four children / in the station wagon / and were off / on vacation.

They were taking / their yearly trip / to the beach / at Gulf Shores.

This year / they were making / a special / one-day stop / at the aquarium / in New Orleans.

After a long day's drive / they arrived / at the motel / only to discover / that in their excitement / they had left / the twins / and their suitcases / in the front yard.

6. **VISUAL MEMORY (HIDDEN OBJECTS)**

Tell the client that you are going to hide some objects around the office (desk, bed) and you want him/her to remember where they are. Hide four or five common objects (e.g., keys, pen, reflex hammer) in various places in the client's sight. After a delay of several minutes, ask the client to find the objects. (1 point per item found)

a. Coin	1 point	________
b. Pen	1 point	________
c. Comb	1 point	________
d. Key	1 point	________
e. Fork	1 point	________

7. **PAIRED ASSOCIATE LEARNING**

Tell the client that you are going to read a list of words two at a time. The client will be expected to remember the words that belong together (e.g., big—little). When he/she is clear on the directions, read the first list of words at the rate of one pair per second. After reading the first list, test for recall by presenting the first recall list. Give the first word of a pair and ask for the word that was paired it. Correct the incorrect responses and proceed to the next pair. After the first recall has been completed, allow a 10-second delay and continue with the second presentation and recall lists.

Presentation Lists

1	2
a. High—low	a. Good—bad
b. House—income	b. Book—page
c. Good—bad	c. High—low
d. Book—page	d. House—income

Recall Lists

1	2		
a. House________	a. High________	2 points	________
b. Book________	b. Good________	2 points	________
c. High________	c. House________	2 points	________
d. Good________	d. Book________	2 points	________

7. **CONSTRUCTIONAL ABILITY**

Ask client to reconstruct this drawing and to draw the other 2 items: 3 points ________

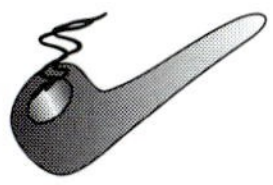

(Continued)

TABLE 12-2 Mental Status Examination for Dementia *(Continued)*

Draw a daisy in a flower pot		3 points	________
Draw a clock with all the numbers and set the clock at 2:30.		3 points	________
10. **WRITTEN COMPLEX CALCULATIONS**			
a. Addition	108 +79	1 point	________
b. Subtraction	605 −86	1 point	________
c. Multiplication	108 ×36	1 point	________
d. Division	43 ⟌ 559	1 point	________
11. **PROVERB INTERPRETATION** Tell the client to explain the following sayings. Record the answers.			
a. Don't cry over spilled milk. ________________________		2 points	________
b. Rome wasn't built in a day. ________________________		2 points	________
c. A drowning man will clutch at a straw. ________________________		2 points	________
d. A golden hammer can break down an iron door. ________________________		2 points	________
e. The hot coal burns, the cold one blackens. ________________________		2 points	________
12. **SIMILARITIES**			
a. Turnip..........cauliflower		2 points	________
b. Car..........airplane		2 points	________
c. Desk..........bookcase		2 points	________
d. Poem..........novel		2 points	________
e. Horse..........apple		2 points	________
	Maximum:	100 points	________

Normal Individuals		Patients with Alzheimer's Disease	
Age Group	**Mean Score (standard deviation)**	**Stage**	**Mean Score (standard deviation)**
40–49	80.9 (9.7)	I	57.2 (9.1)
50–59	82.3 (8.6)	II	37.0 (7.8)
60–69	75.5 (10.5)	III	13.4 (8.1)
70–79	66.9 (9.1)		
80–89	67.9 (11.0)		

Adapted from Strub, R.L. & Black, F. W. *The Mental Status Examination in Neurology*, (4th ed.), Philadelphia: F.A. Davis. With permission.

TABLE 12-3 A Comparison of Dementia and Pseudodementia (Depression)

Symptom Element	Dementia	Pseudodementia (Depression)
Progression of symptoms	Slow	Rapid
Memory	Progressive deficits; recent memory loss greater than remote; may confabulate for memory "gaps"; no complaints of loss	More like forgetfulness; no evidence of progressive deficit; recent and remote loss equal; complaints of deficits; no confabulation (will more likely answer "I don't know")
Orientation	Disoriented to time and place; may wander in search of the familiar	Oriented to time and place; no wandering
Task performance	Consistently poor performance, but struggles to perform	Performance is variable; little effort is put forth
Symptom severity	Worse as the day progresses	Better as the day progresses
Affective distress	Appears unconcerned	Communicates severe distress
Appetite	Unchanged	Diminished
Attention and concentration	Impaired	Intact

Diagnostic Laboratory Evaluations

The nurse also may be required to help the client fulfill the physician's orders for special diagnostic laboratory evaluations. Many of these tests are routinely included with the physical examination and may include evaluation of blood and urine samples to test for various infections; hepatic and renal dysfunction; diabetes or hypoglycemia; electrolyte imbalances; metabolic and endocrine disorders; nutritional deficiencies; and presence of toxic substances, including alcohol and other drugs.

Other diagnostic evaluations may be made by electroencephalogram, which measures and records the brain's electrical activity. With CT scan, an image of the size and shape of the brain can be obtained. A technology called *positron emission tomography* reveals the metabolic activity of the brain, an evaluation some researchers believe is important in the diagnosis of Alzheimer's disease. MRI is used to obtain a computerized image of soft tissue in the body. It provides a sharp detailed picture of the tissues of the brain. A lumbar puncture may be performed to examine the cerebrospinal fluid for evidence of CNS infection or hemorrhage.

Diagnosis/Outcome Identification

Using information collected during the assessment, the nurse completes the client database, from which the selection of appropriate nursing diagnoses is determined. Possible nursing diagnoses for clients with cognitive disorders include:

Risk for trauma related to impairments in cognitive and psychomotor functioning

Risk for suicide related to depressed mood secondary to awareness in decline of mental and/or physical capability

Risk for other-directed violence related to impairment of impulse control; hallucinations

Disturbed thought processes related to cerebral degeneration evidenced by disorientation, confusion, memory deficits, and inaccurate interpretation of the environment

Low self-esteem related to loss of independent functioning evidenced by expressions of shame and self-degradation and progressive social isolation

Self-care deficit related to disorientation, confusion, memory deficits evidenced by inability to fulfill ADLs

The following criteria may be used for measurement of outcomes in the care of the client with cognitive disorders. The client:

1. Has not experienced physical injury
2. Has not harmed self or others
3. Has maintained reality orientation to the best of his or her capability
4. Discusses positive aspects about self and life
5. Fulfills activities of daily living with assistance

Planning/Implementation

Table 12–4 provides a plan of care for the client with a cognitive disorder (irrespective of etiology). Selected nursing diagnoses are presented, along with outcome

TABLE 12–4 Care Plan for the Client with a Cognitive Disorder

Nursing Diagnosis: RISK FOR TRAUMA

Related to: Impairments in cognitive and psychomotor functioning

Outcome Criteria	Nursing Interventions	Rationale
Client will not experience injury.	The following measures may be instituted: a. Arrange furniture and other items in the room to accommodate client's disabilities. b. Store frequently used items within easy access. c. Do not keep bed in an elevated position. Pad siderails and headboard if client has history of seizures. Keep bedrails up when client is in bed (if regulations permit). d. Assign room near nurses' station; observe frequently. e. Assist client with ambulation. f. Keep a dim light on at night. g. If client is a smoker, cigarettes and lighter or matches should be kept at the nurses' station and dispensed only when someone is available to stay with client when he or she is smoking. h. Frequently orient client to place, time, and situation. i. If client is prone to wander, provide an area within which wandering can be carried out safely. j. Soft restraints may be required if client is very disoriented and hyperactive.	To ensure client safety.

Nursing Diagnosis: DISTURBED THOUGHT PROCESSES

Related to: Cerebral degeneration

Evidenced by: Disorientation, confusion, memory deficits, and inaccurate interpretation of the environment

Outcome Criteria	Nursing Interventions	Rationale
Client will interpret the environment accurately and maintain reality orientation to the best of his or her cognitive ability.	1. Frequently orient client to reality. Use clocks and calendars with large numbers that are easy to read. Notes and large, bold signs may be useful as reminders. Allow client to have personal belongings.	1. All of these items serve to help maintain orientation and aid in memory and recognition.
	2. Keep explanations simple. Use face-to-face interaction. Speak slowly and do not shout.	2. These interventions facilitate comprehension. Shouting may create discomfort, and in some instances, may provoke anger.
	3. Discourage rumination or delusional thinking. Talk about real events and real people.	3. Rumination promotes disorientation. Reality orientation increases sense of self-worth and personal dignity.
	4. Monitor for medication side effects.	4. Physiological changes in the elderly can alter the body's response to certain medications. Toxic effects may intensify altered thought processes.

Nursing Diagnosis: SELF-CARE DEFICIT
Related to: Disorientation, confusion, and memory deficits
Evidenced by: Inability to fulfill ADLs

Outcome Criteria	Nursing Interventions	Rationale
Client will accomplish ADLs to the best of his or her ability. Unfulfilled needs will be met by caregivers.	1. Provide a simple, structured environment: a. Identify self-care deficits and provide assistance as required. Promote independent actions as able. b. Allow plenty of time for client to perform tasks. c. Provide guidance and support for independent actions by talking the client through the task one step at a time. d. Provide a structured schedule of activities that does not change from day to day. e. ADLs should follow home routine as closely as possible. f. Provide for consistency in assignment of daily caregivers.	1. To minimize confusion.
	2. Perform ongoing assessment of client's ability to fulfill nutritional needs, ensure personal safety, follow medication regimen, and communicate need for assistance with activities that he or she cannot accomplish independently.	2. Client safety and security are nursing priorities.
	3. Assess prospective caregivers' ability to anticipate and fulfill client's unmet needs. Provide information to assist caregivers with this responsibility. Ensure that caregivers are aware of available community support systems to seek assistance when required. Examples include adult daycare centers, housekeeping and homemaker services, respite–care services, or the local chapter of a national support organization: a. For Parkinson's disease information: National Parkinson Foundation Inc. 1501 NW 9th Ave. Miami, FL 33136 1-800-327-4545 b. For Alzheimer's disease information: Alzheimer's Association 225 N. Michigan Ave., Suite 1700 Chicago, IL 60601-7633 1-800-272-3900	3. To facilitate transition to discharge from treatment center.

criteria, appropriate nursing interventions, and rationales for each.

Client/Family Education

The role of client teacher is important in the psychiatric area, as it is in all areas of nursing. A list of topics for client/family education relevant to cognitive disorders is presented in Table 12–5.

Evaluation

In the final step of the nursing process, reassessment occurs to determine if the nursing interventions have been effective in achieving the intended goals of care. Evaluation of the client with cognitive disorders is based on a series of short-term goals rather than on long-term goals. Resolution of identified problems is unrealistic for this client. Instead, outcomes must be measured in terms of slowing down the process rather

TABLE 12–5 Topics for Client/Family Education Related to Cognitive Disorders

1. Nature of the illness
   a. Possible causes
   b. What to expect
   c. Symptoms
2. Management of the illness
   a. Ways to ensure client safety
   b. How to maintain reality orientation
   c. Providing assistance with ADLs
   d. Nutritional information
   e. Difficult behaviors
   f. Medication administration
   g. Matters related to hygiene and toileting
3. Support services
   a. Financial assistance
   b. Legal assistance
   c. Caregiver support groups
   d. Respite care
   e. Home health care

than stopping or curing the problem. Evaluation questions may include:

1. Has the client experienced injury?
2. Does the client maintain orientation to time, person, place, and situation most of the time?
3. Is the client able to fulfill basic needs? Have those needs unmet by the client been fulfilled by caregivers?
4. Is confusion minimized by familiar objects and a structured, routine schedule of activities?
5. Do the prospective caregivers have information regarding the progression of the client's illness?
6. Do caregivers have information regarding where to go for assistance and support in the care of their loved one?
7. Have the prospective caregivers received instruction in how to promote the client's safety, minimize confusion and disorientation, and cope with difficult client behaviors (hostility, anger, depression, agitation)?

MEDICAL TREATMENT MODALITIES

Delirium

The first step in the treatment of delirium should be the determination and correction of the underlying causes. Additional attention must be given to fluid and electrolyte status, hypoxia, anoxia, and diabetic problems. Staff members should remain with the client at all times to monitor behavior and provide reorientation and assurance. The room should maintain a low level of stimuli.

Some physicians prefer not to prescribe medications for the delirious client, reasoning that additional agents may only compound the syndrome of brain dysfunction (Popkin, 1994). However, the agitation and aggression demonstrated by the delirious client may require chemical and/or mechanical restraint. Choice of specific therapy is made with consideration for the client's clinical condition and the underlying cause of the delirium. Low-dose neuroleptics are the pharmacological treatment of choice in most cases (Trzepacz et al., 2002).

Dementia

Once a definitive diagnosis of dementia has been made, a primary consideration in the treatment of the disorder is the etiology. Focus must be directed to the identification and resolution of potentially reversible processes. Sadock & Sadock (2003) state:

> Once dementia is diagnosed, patients must undergo a complete medical and neurological workup, because 10 to 15 percent of all patients with dementia have a potentially reversible condition if treatment is initiated before permanent brain damage occurs. [Causes of potentially reversible dementia include] hypothyroidism, normal pressure hydrocephalus, and brain tumors. (pp. 339–340)

The need for general supportive care, with provisions for security, stimulation, patience, and nutrition, has been recognized and accepted. A number of pharmaceutical agents have been tried, with varying amounts of success in the treatment of clients with dementia. Some of these drugs are described in the following section according to symptomatology for which they are indicated. (See Chapter 10 for side effects and nursing implications of the psychotropics.)

Cognitive Impairment

The angiotensin-converting enzyme inhibitor physostigmine (Antilirium) has been shown to enhance cognitive functioning in individuals with mild-to-moderate Alzheimer's disease (van Dyck et al., 2000). Use of vasodilators, such as cyclandelate (Cyclan), have resulted in improvements in orientation, communication, and socialization in clients with vascular dementia. Cyclandelate, although still available in Canada, is no longer available in the United States.

Another classification of medications—the cholinesterase inhibitors—is being used for the treatment of mild to moderate cognitive impairment in Alzheimer's disease. Tacrine (Cognex), donepezil (Aricept), rivastigmine (Exelon), and galanthamine (Reminyl) act by elevating acetylcholine concentrations in the cerebral cortex by slowing the degradation of acetylcholine released by still-intact cholinergic neurons. Because their action relies on functionally intact cholinergic neurons, the effects of these medications may lessen as the disease process advances. There is no evidence that cholinesterase inhibitors alter the course of the underlying dementing process.

The Food and Drug Administration recently approved the drug memantine (Namenda) for moderate to severe Alzheimer's disease. Controlled trials have shown promise with this drug in individuals with moderate to severe dementia, who have exhibited improvement in cognitive, social, and motor impairment, and in the ability to participate in ADLs. Memantine is an *N*-methyl D-aspartate antagonist that targets neurotransmitters such as glutamate. Elevated levels of glutamate are associated with neuronal cell death, another process involved in the symptomatology of Alzheimer's disease (Alzheimer's Association, 2003).

Agitation, Aggression, Hallucinations, Thought Disturbances, and Wandering

Antipsychotic medications are used to control agitation, aggression, hallucinations, thought disturbances, and wandering in clients with dementia. The newer antipsychotic medications—risperidone (Risperdal), olanzapine (Zyprexa), quetiapine (Seroquel), and ziprasidone (Geodon)—may be favored because of their lessened propensity to cause anticholinergic and extrapyramidal side effects, although additional research is still needed with geriatric and demented clients (Rabins et al., 2002). Haloperidol (Haldol) is still commonly used because of its proven efficacy in the behaviors associated with dementia, although it carries a higher potentiality of anticholinergic, extrapyramidal, and sedative side effects. The usual adult dosage of any medication must be decreased in elderly individuals.

Depression

Approximately 25 percent of people with Alzheimer's disease also suffer from depression (Johns Hopkins School of Medicine, 2002). Recognizing the symptoms of depression in these individuals is often a challenge. Depression—which affects thinking, memory, sleep, and appetite and interferes with daily life—is sometimes difficult to distinguish from dementia. Clearly, the existence of depression in the client with dementia complicates and worsens the individual's functioning.

Antidepressant medication is sometimes used in treatment of depression in dementia. The selective serotonin reuptake inhibitors—fluoxetine (Prozac), paroxetine (Paxil), sertraline (Zoloft), and citalopram (Celexa)—are now considered by many to be the first-line drug treatment for depression in the elderly because of their favorable side effect profile (Alzheimer Research Forum, 2002; Rabins et al., 2002). Tricyclic antidepressants are avoided because of cardiac side effects and the anticholinergic side effects, which are not tolerated well by the elderly. Trazodone may be a good choice, used at bedtime, for depression and insomnia. Dopaminergic agents (e.g., methylphenidate, amantadine, bromocriptine, and bupropion) may be helpful in the treatment of severe apathy (Rabins et al., 2002).

Anxiety

The progressive loss of mental functioning is a significant source of anxiety in the early stages of dementia. It is important that clients be encouraged to verbalize their feelings and fears associated with this loss. These interventions may be useful in reducing the anxiety of clients with dementia.

Antianxiety medications may be helpful but should not be used routinely or for prolonged periods. The least toxic and most effective of the antianxiety medications are the benzodiazepines. Examples include diazepam (Valium), chlordiazepoxide (Librium), alprazolam (Xanax), lorazepam (Ativan), and oxazepam (Serax). The drugs with shorter half-lives (e.g., lorazepam and oxazepam) are preferred to those longer-acting medications (e.g., diazepam), which promote a higher risk of oversedation and falls. Barbiturates are not appropriate as antianxiety agents because they frequently induce confusion and paradoxical excitement in elderly individuals.

Sleep Disturbances

Sleep problems are common in clients with dementia, and often intensify as the disease progresses.

Wakefulness and nighttime wandering create much distress and anguish in family members who are charged with protection of their loved one. Indeed, sleep disturbances are among the problems that most frequently cause families to place the client in a long-term care facility.

Some physicians treat sleep problems with sedative-hypnotic medications. The benzodiazepines may be useful for some clients but are indicated for relatively brief periods only. Examples include flurazepam (Dalmane), temazepam (Restoril), and triazolam (Halcion). Daytime sedation and cognitive impairment, in addition to paradoxical agitation in elderly clients, are of particular concern with these medications (Mayo Clinic, 2002). The nonbenzodiazepine sedative-hypnotic zolpidem (Ambien), the antidepressant trazodone (Desyrel), and the antihistamine diphenhydramine (Benadryl) are also prescribed. Daytime sedation may also be a problem with these medications. As previously stated, barbiturates should not be used in elderly clients. Sleep problems are usually ongoing, and most clinicians prefer to use medications only to help an individual through a short-term stressful situation. Rising at the same time each morning, eliminating or minimizing afternoon naps, regular physical exercise, proper nutrition, stimulating activities, and retiring at the same time each night are behavioral approaches to sleep problems that may eliminate the need for sleep aids, particularly in the early stages of dementia. Because of the tremendous potential for adverse drug reactions in the elderly, most of whom are already taking multiple medications, pharmacological treatment of insomnia should only be considered as a last resort after every effort at nonpharmacological strategies has been made (Mayo Clinic, 2002).

SUMMARY

This chapter examined a group of disorders that constitute a large and growing public health concern. Cognitive disorders include delirium, dementia, and amnestic disorders.

A delirium is a disturbance of consciousness and a change in cognition that develop rapidly over a short period. Level of consciousness is often affected, and psychomotor activity may fluctuate between agitated purposeless movements and a vegetative state resembling catatonic stupor. The symptoms of delirium usually begin quite abruptly and often are reversible and brief. Delirium may be caused by a general medical condition, substance intoxication or withdrawal, or ingestion of a medication or toxin.

Dementia is a syndrome of acquired, persistent intellectual impairment with compromised function in multiple spheres of mental activity, such as memory, language, visuospatial skills, emotion or personality, and cognition. Symptoms are insidious and develop slowly over time. In most clients, dementia runs a progressive, irreversible course. It may be caused by genetics, cardiovascular disease, infections, neurophysiological disorders, and other general medical conditions.

Amnestic disorders are characterized by an inability to learn new information despite normal attention and an inability to recall previously learned information. Remote past events are often more easily recalled than recent ones. The onset of symptoms may be acute or insidious, depending on the pathological process causing the amnestic disorder. Duration and course of the illness may be quite variable, and are correlated with extent and severity of the cause.

Nursing care of the client with cognitive disorders is presented around the six steps of the nursing process. Objectives of care for the client experiencing an acute syndrome are aimed at eliminating the etiology, promoting client safety, and a return to highest possible functioning. Objectives of care for the client experiencing a chronic, progressive disorder are aimed at preserving the dignity of the individual, promoting deceleration of the symptoms, and maximizing functional capabilities.

Nursing interventions are also directed toward helping the client's family or primary caregivers learn about a chronic, progressive cognitive disorder. Education is provided about the disease process, expectations of client behavioral changes, methods for facilitating care, and sources of assistance and support as they struggle, both physically and emotionally, with the demands brought on by a disease process that is slowly taking their loved one away from them.

INTERNET REFERENCES

- Additional information about Alzheimer's Disease may be located at the following websites:

  a http://www.alz.org

  b http://www.alzheimers.org/index.html

  c http://www.ninds.nih.gov/health_and_medical/disorders/alzheimersdisease_doc.htm

  d http://www.ahcpr.gov/clinic/alzcons.htm

- Information on caregiving can be located at the following website:

  a http://www.aarp.org

- Additional information about medications to treat Alzheimer's disease may be located at the following websites:

  a http://www.fadavis.com/townsend

  b http://www.aafp.org/afp/981001ap/delagarz.html

REVIEW QUESTIONS

SELF-EXAMINATION/LEARNING EXERCISE

Situation: Mrs. G is 67 years old. Her husband brings her to the hospital. He explains that she has become increasingly confused and forgetful. Yesterday, she started a fire in the kitchen when she put some bacon on to fry and went off and forgot it on the stove. Her husband reports that sometimes she seems okay, and sometimes she is completely disoriented. The physician has made an admitting diagnosis of dementia, etiology unknown.

Select the answer that is most appropriate for each of the following questions:

1. Because the etiology of Mrs. G's symptoms is unknown, the physician will attempt to rule out the possibility that a reversible condition exists. An example of a treatable (reversible) form of dementia is one that is caused by which of the following?
   a. Multiple sclerosis
   b. Multiple small brain infarcts
   c. Electrolyte imbalances
   d. HIV disease
2. The physician rules out all reversible etiological factors and diagnoses Mrs. G with dementia of the Alzheimer's type. The cause of this disorder is which of the following?
   a. Multiple small brain infarcts.
   b. Chronic alcohol abuse.
   c. Cerebral abscess.
   d. Unknown.
3. The *primary* nursing intervention in working with Mrs. G is which of the following?
   a. Ensuring that she receives food she likes, to prevent hunger.
   b. Ensuring that the environment is safe, to prevent injury.
   c. Ensuring that she meets the other patients, to prevent social isolation.
   d. Ensuring that she takes care of her own ADLs, to prevent dependence.
4. Some medications have been indicated to decrease the agitation, violence, and bizarre thoughts associated with dementia. Which of the following is a drug suggested for this use?
   a. Risperidone (Risperdal).
   b. Tacrine (Cognex).
   c. Ergoloid (Hydergine).
   d. Diazepam (Valium).
5. Mrs. G says to the nurse, "I have a date tonight. I always have a date on Christmas." Which of the following is the most appropriate response?
   a. "Don't be silly. It's not Christmas, Mrs. G."
   b. "Today is Tuesday, Oct. 21, Mrs. G. We will have supper soon, and then your daughter will come to visit."
   c. "Who is your date with, Mrs. G?"
   d. "I think you need some more medication, Mrs. G. I'll bring it to you now."
6. In addition to disturbances in her cognition and orientation, Mrs. G may also show changes in which of the following?
   a. Hearing, speech, and vision.
   b. Energy, creativity, and coordination.
   c. Personality, speech, and mobility.
   d. Appetite, affect, and attitude.

7. Mrs. G has trouble sleeping and wanders around at night. Which of the following nursing actions would be *best* to promote sleep in Mrs. G?
   a. Ask the doctor to prescribe flurazepam (Dalmane).
   b. Ensure that Mrs. G gets an afternoon nap so she will not be overtired at bedtime.
   c. Make Mrs. G a cup of tea with honey before bedtime.
   d. Ensure that Mrs. G gets regular physical exercise during the day.

8. Mrs. G's daughter says to the nurse, "I read an article about Alzheimer's, and it said the disease is hereditary. Does that mean I'll get it when I'm old?" The nurse bases her response on the knowledge that which of the following factors is *not* associated with increased incidence of dementia of the Alzheimer's type.
   a. Multiple small strokes.
   b. Family history of Alzheimer's disease.
   c. Head trauma.
   d. Advanced age.

9. The physician determines that Mrs. G's dementia is related to cardiovascular disease and changes her diagnosis to vascular dementia. In explaining this disorder to Mrs. G's family, which of the following statements by the nurse is correct?
   a. "She will probably live longer than if her dementia was of the Alzheimer's type."
   b. "Vascular dementia shows step-wise progression. This is why she sometimes seems okay."
   c. "Vascular dementia is caused by plaques and tangles that form in the brain."
   d. "The cause of vascular dementia is unknown."

10. Which of the following interventions is most appropriate in helping Mrs. G with her ADLs?
    a. Perform ADLs for her when she is in the hospital.
    b. Provide her with a written list of activities she is expected to perform.
    c. Tell her that if her morning care is not completed by 9:00 AM, it will be performed for her by the nurse's aide so that Mrs. G can attend group therapy.
    d. Encourage her and give her plenty of time to perform as many of her ADLs as possible independently.

BUILDING YOUR CRITICAL THINKING SKILLS

Joe, a 62-year-old accountant, began having difficulty remembering details necessary to perform his job. He was also having trouble at home, failing to keep his finances straight, and forgetting to pay bills. It became increasingly difficult for him to function properly at work, and eventually he was forced to retire. Cognitive deterioration continued, and behavioral problems soon began. He became stubborn, verbally and physically abusive, and suspicious of almost everyone in his environment. His wife and son convinced him to see a physician, who recommended hospitalization for testing.

At Joe's initial evaluation, he was fully alert and cooperative but obviously anxious and fidgety. He thought he was at his accounting office, and he could not state what year it was. He could not say the names of his parents or siblings, nor did he know who was currently president of the United States. He could not perform simple arithmetic calculations, write a proper sentence, or copy a drawing. He interpreted proverbs concretely and had difficulty stating similarities between related objects.

Laboratory serum studies revealed no abnormalities, but a CT scan showed marked cortical atrophy. The physician's diagnosis was Dementia of the Alzheimer's Type, Early Onset.

Answer the following questions related to Joe:

1. Identify the pertinent assessment data from which nursing care will be devised.
2. What is the primary nursing diagnosis for Joe?
3. How would outcomes be identified?

IMPLICATIONS OF RESEARCH FOR EVIDENCE-BASED PRACTICE

Yaffe, K., Barnes, D., Nevitt, M., Lui, L., and Covinsky, K.: **A prospective study of physical activity and cognitive decline in elderly women: Women who walk.** Archives of Internal Medicine (2001, July 23), 161(14), 1703–1708.

Description of the Study: Subjects included 5,925 predominantly white women, aged 65 and older, and who had completed a mean 13 years of education. They were all without baseline cognitive impairment or physical limitations. Cognitive performance was measured using a modified Mini-Mental State Examination at baseline and 6 to 8 years later. Physical activity was measured by self-reported blocks walked per week and by total kilocalories expended per week in recreation, blocks walked, and stairs climbed. Cognitive decline was defined as a 3-point decline or greater on repeated modified Mini-Mental State Examination.

Results of the Study: Participants were divided into quartiles according to physical activity (median number of blocks walked per week ranged from 7 to 175 per quartile). At follow-up, and after adjustment for age, education level, comorbid conditions, smoking status, estrogen use, and functional limitations, cognitive function had declined significantly less among women in the highest physical activity quartile compared with those in the lowest quartile. For every 1700 kcal/week expended on physical activity, there was a 14 percent decrease in the odds for cognitive decline.

Implications for Nursing Practice: Several studies have suggested that physical activity is positively associated with cognitive function in elderly persons. This study supports this hypothesis. These findings suggest the importance of exercise programs aimed at elderly persons. Nurses must educate their elderly clients about the importance of remaining active. Nurses may also participate in the planning and development of exercise, recreational, and leisure-time activities for the elderly.

REFERENCES

Alzheimer's Association. (2003). Fact sheet: Memantine. Retrieved on October 5, 2003, from http://www.alz.org/ResourceCenter/ByTopic/memantine.htm

Alzheimer Research Forum (2002). Treatment guide: Serotonin reuptake inhibitors. Retrieved on February 10, 2002, from the World Wide Web at http://www.alzforum.org/members/research/treatment_guide/serotonin.html

Alzheimer's Disease and Related Disorders Association (ADRDA). (2001). General Statistics/demographics. Retrieved February 7, 2002, from http://www.alz.org/hc/overview/stats.htm

American Psychiatric Association (APA). (1994). Diagnostic and statistical manual of mental Disorders (4th ed.). Washington, DC: American Psychiatric Association.

APA. (2000). Diagnostic and statistical manual of mental disorders (4th ed.) Text Revision. Washington, DC: American Psychiatric Association.

Arvanitakis, Z. (2000). Dementia and vascular disease. Duval County Medical Society. Retrieved 2-8-02 from http://www.dcmsonline.org/jax-medicine/February 2000/vascdement.htm

Bourgeois, J.A., Seaman, J.S., & Servis, M.E. (2003). Delirium, dementia, and amnestic disorders. In R.E. Hales & S. C. Yudofsky (Eds.), Textbook of clinical psychiatry (4th ed.). Washington, D.C.: American Psychiatric Publishing.

Devanand, D.P., & Mayeux, R. (1992). Alzheimer's disease and other organic causes of mental disorders. In F.I. Kass, J.M. Oldham, & H. Pardes (Eds.), The Columbia University College of Physicians and Surgeons Complete Home Guide to Mental Health. New York: Henry Holt.

Hall, G. R. (1991, October) This hospital patient has Alzheimer's. American Journal of Nursing, 91(10), 44–50.

Hall, G.R. (1994, March). Caring for people with Alzheimer's disease using the conceptual model of progressively lowered stress threshold in the clinical setting. Nursing Clinics of North America, 29(1), 129–141.

Harvard Medical School. (1995a, February). Update on Alzheimer's disease—Part I. The Harvard Mental Health Letter. Boston, MA: Harvard Medical School

Harvard Medical School. (1995b, March). Update on Alzheimer's disease—Part II. The Harvard Mental Health Letter. Boston: Harvard Medical School

Johns Hopkins School of Medicine. (2002). Department of Psychiatry and Behavioral Sciences, Neuropsychiatry and Memory Group. Depression in Alzheimer's disease study. Retrieved on February 9, 2002 from the World Wide Web at http://www.med.jhu.edu/jhhpsychiatry/DIADS.htm

Kovach, C.R. & Wilson, S.A. (1999). Dementia in older adults. In M. Stanley and P. G. Beare (Eds.), Gerontological nursing: A health promotion/protection approach. (2nd ed.). Philadelphia: F.A. Davis.

Laraia, M.T. (2004, January/February). Memantine: First NMDA Receptor antagonist approved for the Treatment of Moderate to Severe Alzheimer's disease. APNA News 16(1): 12–13.

Marchione, M. (1999). Dementia is sometimes temporary, treatable. Journal Sentinel Online. Retrieved February 7, 2002 from http://www.jsonline.com/alive/news/sep99/alzside27092699.asp.

Mayo Clinic Rochester. (2002). Geriatric Medicine, Community Internal Medicine Division. Sleep disorders in the elderly. Retrieved on February 2, 2002 from the World Wide Web at http://www.mayo.edu/geriatrics-rst/Sleep.html

McAllister, T.W. (1992). Neuropsychiatric sequelae of head injuries. Psychiatric Clinics of North America, 15, 395–413.

McArthur, J. (2003). The Geneva Report. Update on neurology: HIV-associated dementia. Retrieved on October 3, 2003 from http://www.hopkins aids.edu/geneva/hilites_mcar_dem.html

Nowak, T.J. & Handford, A.G. (1994). Essentials of pathophysiology. Dubuque, IA: Wm. C. Brown.

Phipps, W.J., Cassmeyer, V. L., Sands, J.K., Lehman, M.K. (1995). Medical-surgical nursing: Concepts and clinical practice (5th ed.). St. Louis: C.V. Mosby.

Popkin, M.K. (1994). Syndromes of brain dysfunction presenting with cognitive impairment or behavioral disturbance: Delirium, dementia, and mental disorders due to a general medical condition. In G. Winokur, & P.J. Clayton (Eds.). The medical basis of psychiatry (2nd ed.). Philadelphia: W.B. Saunders.

Porth, C.M. (1994). Pathophysiology: Concepts of altered health states (4th ed.). Philadelphia: J.B. Lippincott.

Rabins, P., Bland, W., Bright-Long, L., Cohen, E., Katz, I., Rovner, B., Schneider, L., & Blacker, D. (2002). Practice guideline for the treatment of patients with Alzheimer's disease and other dementias of late life. American Psychiatric Association Practice Guidelines for the Treatment of Psychiatric Disorders, Compendium 2002. Washington, D.C.: American Psychiatric Association.

Sadock, B.J. & Sadock, V.A. (2003). Synopsis of psychiatry: behavioral sciences/clinical psychiatry (9th ed.). Philadelphia: Lippincott Williams & Wilkins.

Trzepacz, P., Breitbart, W., Franklin, J., Levenson, J., Martini, D.R., & Wang, P. (2002). Practice guideline for the treatment of patients with delirium. American Psychiatric Association Practice Guidelines for the Treatment of Psychiatric Disorders, Compendium 2002. Washington, D.C.: American Psychiatric Association.

United States General Accounting Office (USGAO). (1998). Alzheimer's disease: Estimates of prevalence in the United States. Washington, DC: USGAO, Publication HEHS 98-16.

van Dyck, C.H., Newhouse, P., Falk, W.E., & Mattes, J.A. (2000). Extended-release physostigmine in Alzheimer's disease: A multicenter, double-blind, 12-week study with dose enrichment. Archives of General Psychiatry, 57(2), 157–164.

Williams, M.E. (1995). Complete guide to aging and health. New York: Harmony Books.

Wise, M.G., Gray, K.F., & Seltzer, B. (1999). Delirium, dementia, and amnestic disorders. In R.E. Hales & S.C. Yudofsky (Eds.), Essentials of clinical psychiatry. Washington, D.C.: American Psychiatric Press.

TOWNSEND ESSENTIALS

13

CHAPTER

SUBSTANCE-RELATED DISORDERS

CHAPTER OUTLINE

KEY TERMS

amphetamines	abuse	ascites	disulfiram (Antabuse)
cannabis	dependence	esophageal varices	substitution therapy
opioids	Wernicke's encephalopathy	hepatic encephalopathy	detoxification
phencyclidine	Korsakoff's psychosis	Alcoholics Anonymous	dual diagnosis

OBJECTIVES

After reading this chapter, the student will be able to:

1. Define *abuse*, *dependence*, *intoxication*, and *withdrawal*.
2. Discuss etiological implications for substance-related disorders.
3. Identify symptomatology and use the information in assessment of clients with various substance-use disorders and substance-induced disorders.
4. Identify nursing diagnoses common to clients with substance-use disorders and substance-induced disorders, and select appropriate nursing interventions for each.
5. Identify topics for client and family teaching that are relevant to substance-use disorders and substance-induced disorders.
6. Describe relevant outcome criteria for evaluating nursing care of clients with substance-use disorders and substance-induced disorders.
7. Describe various modalities relevant to treatment of individuals with substance-use disorders and substance-induced disorders.

INTRODUCTION

The substance-related disorders are composed of two groups: the substance-use disorders (dependence and abuse) and the substance-induced disorders (intoxication, withdrawal, delirium, dementia, amnesia, psychosis, mood disorder, anxiety disorder, sexual dysfunction, and sleep disorders). This chapter discusses dependence, abuse, intoxication, and withdrawal. The remainder of the substance-induced disorders is included in the chapters with which they share symptomatology (e.g., substance-induced mood disorders are included in Chapter 15).

Drugs are a pervasive part of our society. Certain mood-altering substances are quite socially acceptable and are used moderately by many adult Americans. They include alcohol, caffeine, and nicotine. Society has even developed a relative indifference to an occasional abuse of these substances, despite documentation of their negative impact on health.

A large number of substances are produced for medicinal purposes. These include central nervous system (CNS) stimulants (e.g., **amphetamines**), CNS depressants (e.g., sedatives, tranquilizers), as well as numerous over-the-counter preparations designed to relieve nearly every kind of human ailment, real or imagined.

Some illegal substances have achieved a degree of social acceptance by various subcultural groups within our society. These drugs, such as marijuana and hashish, are by no means harmless, and the long-term effects are still being studied. On the other hand, the dangerous effects of other illegal substances (e.g., lysergic acid diethylamide [LSD], **phencyclidine**, cocaine, and heroin) have been well documented.

This chapter discusses the physical and behavioral manifestations and personal and social consequences related to the abuse of or dependency on alcohol, other CNS depressants, CNS stimulants, **opioids**, hallucinogens, and cannabinols. Wide cultural variations in attitudes exist regarding substance consumption and patterns of use. A high prevalence of substance use occurs between the ages of 18 and 24 years. Substance-related disorders are diagnosed more commonly in men than in women, but the gender ratios vary with the class of the substance (American Psychiatric Association [APA], 2000).

Nursing care for substance abuse, dependence, intoxication, and withdrawal is presented in the context of the six steps of the nursing process. Various medical and other treatment modalities are also discussed.

SUBSTANCE-USE DISORDERS

Substance Abuse

Bennett and Woolf (1991) defined substance **abuse** as psychoactive drug use of any class or type, used alone or in combination, that poses significant hazards to health. The *DSM-IV-TR* (APA, 2000) identifies substance abuse as a maladaptive pattern of substance use manifested by recurrent and significant adverse consequences related to repeated use of the substance.

DSM-IV-TR Criteria for Substance Abuse

Substance abuse is described as a maladaptive pattern of substance use leading to clinically significant impairment or distress, as manifested by one (or more) of the following, occurring within a 12-month period:

1. Recurrent substance use resulting in a failure to fulfill major role obligations at work, school, or home (e.g., repeated absences or poor work performance related to substance use; substance-related absences, suspensions, or expulsions from school; neglect of children or household)
2. Recurrent substance use in situations in which it is physically hazardous (e.g., driving an automobile or operating a machine)
3. Recurrent substance-related legal problems (e.g., arrests for disorderly conduct)
4. Continued substance use despite having persistent or recurrent social or interpersonal problems caused or exacerbated by the effects of the substance (e.g., arguments with spouse about consequences of intoxication, physical fights)

Substance Dependence

Physical Dependence

Physical **dependence** on a substance is evidenced by a cluster of cognitive, behavioral, and physiological symptoms indicating that the individual continues use of the substance despite significant substance-related problems (APA, 2000). As this condition develops, the repeated administration of the substance necessitates its continued use to prevent the appearance of unpleasant effects characteristic of the withdrawal syndrome associated with that particular drug. The development of physical dependence is promoted by the phenomenon of *tolerance*. Tolerance is defined as the need for increasingly larger or more frequent doses of a substance in order to obtain the desired effects originally produced by a lower dose.

Psychological Dependence

An individual is considered psychologically dependent on a substance when there is an overwhelming desire to repeat the use of a particular drug to produce pleasure or avoid discomfort (Hermes, 1993). It can be extremely powerful, producing intense craving for a substance as well as its compulsive use.

DSM-IV-TR Criteria for Substance Dependence

At least three of the following characteristics must be present for a diagnosis of substance dependence:

1. Evidence of tolerance, as defined by one of the following: a need for markedly increased amounts of the substance to achieve intoxication or desired effects or markedly diminished effect with continued use of the same amount of the substance.
2. Evidence of withdrawal symptoms, as manifested by one of the following: the characteristic withdrawal syndrome for the substance or the same (or a closely related) substance is taken to relieve or avoid withdrawal symptoms.
3. The substance is often taken in larger amounts or over a longer period than was intended.
4. There is a persistent desire or unsuccessful efforts to cut down or control substance use.
5. A great deal of time is spent in activities necessary to obtain the substance (e.g., visiting multiple doctors or driving long distances), use the substance (e.g., chain-smoking), or recover from its effects.
6. Important social, occupational, or recreational activities are given up or reduced because of substance use.
7. The substance use is continued despite knowledge of having a persistent or recurrent physical or psychological problem that is likely to have been caused or exacerbated by the substance (e.g., current cocaine use despite recognition of cocaine-induced depression, or continued drinking despite recognition that an ulcer was made worse by alcohol consumption).

SUBSTANCE-INDUCED DISORDERS

Substance Intoxication

Substance intoxication is defined as the development of a reversible substance-specific syndrome caused by the recent ingestion of (or exposure to) a substance (APA, 2000). The behavioral changes can be attributed to the physiological effects of the substance on the CNS and develop during or shortly after use of the substance. This category does not apply to nicotine.

DSM-IV-TR Criteria for Substance Intoxication

1. The development of a reversible substance-specific syndrome caused by recent ingestion of (or exposure to) a substance. *Note:* Different substances may produce similar or identical syndromes.
2. Clinically significant maladaptive behavior or psychological changes that are due to the effect of the substance on the CNS (e.g., belligerence, mood lability, cognitive impairment, impaired judgment, impaired social or occupational functioning) and develop during or shortly after use of the substance.
3. The symptoms are not due to a general medical condition and are not better accounted for by another mental disorder.

Substance Withdrawal

Substance withdrawal is the development of a substance-specific maladaptive behavioral change, with physiological and cognitive concomitants, that is due to the cessation of, or reduction in, heavy and prolonged substance use (APA, 2000). Withdrawal is usually, but not always, associated with substance dependence.

DSM-IV-TR Criteria for Substance Withdrawal

1. The development of a substance-specific syndrome caused by the cessation of (or reduction in) heavy and prolonged substance use.
2. The substance-specific syndrome causes clinically significant distress or impairment in social, occupational, or other important areas of functioning.
3. The symptoms are not caused by a general medical condition and are not better accounted for by another mental disorder.

CLASSES OF PSYCHOACTIVE SUBSTANCES

The following 11 classes of psychoactive substances are associated with substance-use and substance-induced disorders. They include:

1. Alcohol
2. Amphetamines and related substances
3. Caffeine
4. **Cannabis**
5. Cocaine
6. Hallucinogens
7. Inhalants
8. Nicotine
9. Opioids
10. Phencyclidine (PCP) and related substances
11. Sedatives, hypnotics, or anxiolytics

ETIOLOGICAL IMPLICATIONS

A number of factors have been implicated in the predisposition to abuse of substances. At present, no single theory can adequately explain the etiology of this problem. No doubt, the interaction between various elements forms a complex collection of determinants that influence a person's susceptibility to abuse substances.

Biological Factors

Genetics

An apparent hereditary factor is involved in the development of substance-use disorders. This is especially evident with alcoholism, and less so with other substances. Children of alcoholics are four times more likely than other children to become alcoholics (American Academy of Child & Adolescent Psychiatry, 1999). Studies with monozygotic and dizygotic twins have also supported the genetic hypothesis. The monozygotic (one egg, genetically identical) twins have twice the rate for concordance of alcoholism compared with dizygotic (two eggs, genetically nonidentical) twins (Franklin & Frances, 1999). Other studies have shown that male biological offspring of alcoholic fathers have a four-times greater incidence of alcoholism than offspring of nonalcoholic fathers. This is true whether the child was reared by the biological parents or by nonalcoholic surrogate parents (Harvard Medical School, 2001)

Biochemical

A second biological hypothesis relates to the possibility that alcohol may produce morphine-like substances in the brain that are responsible for alcohol addiction. These substances are formed by the reaction of biologically active amines (e.g., dopamine, serotonin) with products of alcohol metabolism, such as acetaldehyde (Bennett & Woolf, 1991). Examples of these morphine-like substances include tetrahydropapaveroline and salsolinol. Some tests with animals have shown that injection of these compounds into the brain in small amounts results in patterns of alcohol addiction in animals who had previously avoided even the most dilute alcohol solutions (Behavioral Neuroscience Laboratory, 2002).

Psychological Factors

Developmental Influences

The psychodynamic approach to the etiology of substance abuse focuses on a punitive superego and fixation at the oral stage of psychosexual development (Sadock & Sadock, 2003). Individuals with punitive superegos turn to alcohol to diminish unconscious anxiety. Sadock & Sadock (2003) state, "Anxiety in people fixated at the oral stage may be reduced by taking substances, such as alcohol, by mouth." Alcohol may also serve to increase feelings of power and self-worth in these individuals.

Personality Factors

Certain personality traits are thought to increase a tendency toward addictive behavior. These include low self-esteem, frequent depression, passivity, the inability to relax or to defer gratification, and the inability to communicate effectively (Hermes, 1993).

Substance abuse has also been associated with antisocial personality and depressive response styles. This may be explained by the inability of the individual with antisocial personality to anticipate the aversive consequences of his or her behavior. It is likely an effort on the part of the depressed person to treat the symptoms of discomfort associated with dysphoria. Achievement of relief then provides the positive reinforcement to continue abusing the substance.

Sociocultural Factors

Social Learning

The effects of modeling, imitation, and identification on behavior can be observed from early childhood onward. In relation to drug consumption, the family appears to be an important influence. Various studies have shown that children and adolescents are more likely to use substances if they have parents who provide a model for substance use (Hermes, 1993). Peers often exert a great deal of influence in the life of the child or adolescent who is being encouraged to use substances for the first time. Modeling may continue to be a factor in the use of substances once the individual enters the work force. This is particularly true in the work setting that provides plenty of leisure time with coworkers and where drinking is valued and is used to express group cohesiveness.

Conditioning

Another important learning factor is the effect of the substance itself. Many substances create a pleasurable experience that encourages the user to repeat it. Thus, it is the intrinsically reinforcing properties of addictive drugs that "condition" the individual to seek out their use repeatedly. The environment in which the substance is taken also contributes to the reinforcement. If the environment is pleasurable, substance use is usually increased. Aversive stimuli within an environment are thought to be associated with a decrease in substance use within that environment.

Cultural and Ethnic Influences

Factors within an individual's culture help to establish patterns of substance use by molding attitudes, influencing patterns of consumption based on cultural acceptance, and determining the availability of the substance. For centuries, the French and Italians have considered wine an essential part of the family meal, even for the children. The incidence of alcohol dependency is low, and acute intoxication from alcohol is not common. However, the possibility of chronic physiological effects associated with lifelong alcohol consumption cannot be ignored.

Historically, a high incidence of alcohol dependency has existed within the Native American culture. Native Americans have alcohol dependence rates three times higher than the national average (Newhouse, 1999). Veterans Administration records show that 45 percent of Native American veterans were alcohol dependent, or twice the rate for non-Native American veterans. The Indian Health Service reports that 17 to 19 percent of all Native American deaths are alcohol related, compared with 4.7 percent for the general population (Newhouse, 1999). A number of reasons have been postulated for alcohol abuse among Native Americans: a possible physical cause (difficulty metabolizing alcohol), children modeling their parents' drinking habits, unemployment and poverty, and loss of the traditional Native American religion that some believe have led to the increased use of alcohol to fill the spiritual gap (Newhouse, 1999).

The incidence of alcohol dependence is higher among northern Europeans than southern Europeans. The Finns and the Irish use excessive alcohol consumption for the release of aggression, and the English "pub" is known for its attraction as a social meeting place.

Incidence of alcohol dependence among Asians is relatively low. This may be a result of a possible genetic intolerance of the substance. Some Asians develop unpleasant symptoms, such as flushing, headaches, nausea, and palpitations, when they drink alcohol. Research indicates that this is because of an isoenzyme variant that quickly converts alcohol to acetaldehyde, as well as the absence of an isoenzyme that is needed to oxidize acetaldehyde. This results in a rapid accumulation of acetaldehyde, which produces the unpleasant symptoms (Kibbey, 2002).

THE DYNAMICS OF SUBSTANCE-RELATED DISORDERS

Alcohol Abuse and Dependence

A Profile of the Substance

Alcohol is a natural substance formed by the reaction of fermenting sugar with yeast spores. Although there are many alcohols, the kind in alcoholic beverages is known scientifically as ethyl alcohol and chemically as C_2H_5OH. Its abbreviation, ETOH, is sometimes seen in medical records and in various other documents and publications.

By strict definition, alcohol is classified as a food because it contains calories; however, it has no nutritional value. Different alcoholic beverages are produced by using different sources of sugar for the fermentation process. For example, beer is made from malted barley, wine from grapes or berries, whiskey from malted grains, and rum from molasses. Distilled beverages (e.g., whiskey, scotch, gin, vodka, and other "hard" liquors) derive their name from further concentration of the alcohol through a process called distillation.

The alcohol content varies by type of beverage. For example, most American beers contain 3 to 6 percent alcohol, wine averages 10 to 20 percent, and distilled beverages range from 40 to 50 percent alcohol. The average-sized drink, regardless of beverage, contains a similar amount of alcohol. That is, 12 ounces of beer, 3 to 5 ounces of wine, and a cocktail with 1 ounce of whiskey all contain approximately 0.5 ounce of alcohol. If consumed at the same rate, they all would have an equal effect on the body.

Alcohol exerts a depressant effect on the CNS, resulting in behavioral and mood changes. The effects of alcohol on the CNS are proportional to the alcoholic concentration in the blood. Most states consider that an individual is legally intoxicated with a blood alcohol level of 0.10 g/dL. In October 2000, a federal bill was passed and signed into law imposing a new standard of intoxication of 0.08 g/dL. All states were expected to conform to this new law by 2004 or risk loss of federal highway construction assistance.

The body burns alcohol at about 0.5 ounce per hour, so behavioral changes would not be expected in an individual who slowly consumes only one average-sized drink per hour. Other factors do influence these effects, however, such as individual size and whether the stomach contains food at the time the alcohol is consumed. Alcohol is thought to have a more profound effect when an individual is emotionally stressed or fatigued (National Institute on Alcohol Abuse and Alcoholism [NIAAA], 1997).

Historical Aspects

The use of alcohol can be traced back to the Neolithic Age. Beer and wine are known to have been used around 6400 BC. Although alcohol has little therapeutic value, with the introduction of distillation by the Arabs in the Middle Ages, alchemists believed that alcohol was the answer to all of their ailments. The word "whiskey," meaning "water of life," became widely known.

In America, Native Americans had been drinking beer and wine before the arrival of the first white visitors. Refinement of the distillation process made beverages with high alcohol content readily available. By the early 1800s, one renowned physician of the time, Benjamin Rush, had begun to identify the widespread, excessive, chronic alcohol consumption as a disease and an addiction. The strong religious mores on which this country was founded soon led to a driving force aimed at prohibiting the sale of alcoholic beverages. By the middle of the 19th century, 13 states had passed prohibition laws. The most notable prohibition of major proportions was that in effect in the United States from 1920 to 1933. The mandatory restrictions on national social habits resulted in the creation of profitable underground markets that led to flourishing criminal enterprises. Furthermore, millions of dollars in federal, state, and local revenues from taxes and import duties on alcohol were lost. It is difficult to measure the value of this dollar loss against the human devastation and social costs that occur as a result of alcohol abuse in the United States today.

Patterns of Use/Abuse

Almost half of Americans aged 12 years and older report being current drinkers of alcohol (Substance Abuse and Mental Health Services Administration [SAMHSA], 2002a). Of these individuals, 26 percent are binge drinkers or engage in heavy alcohol use. Why do people drink? Drinking patterns in the United States show that people use alcoholic beverages to enhance the flavor of food with meals; at social gatherings to encourage relaxation and conviviality among the guests; and to promote a feeling of celebration at special occasions such as weddings, birthdays, and anniversaries. An alcoholic beverage (wine) is also used as part of the sacred ritual in some religious ceremonies. Therapeutically, alcohol is the major ingredient in many over-the-counter and prescription medicines that are prepared in concentrated form. Therefore, alcohol can be harmless and enjoyable—sometimes even beneficial—if it is used responsibly and in moderation. Like any other mind-altering drug, however, alcohol has the potential for abuse. Indeed, it is the most widely abused drug in the United States today. The National Council on Alcoholism and Drug Dependence (2002) reports:

> Alcoholism is the third leading cause of death in the United States and is responsible for about 20 percent of the population in mental hospitals and 35 percent of suicides. Nearly 30 percent of teenagers experience negative consequences of alcohol abuse, including alcohol-related accidents and auto crashes, arrests, health problems, and impaired school performance.

Jellinek (1952) outlined four phases through which the alcoholic's pattern of drinking progresses. Some variability among individuals is to be expected within this model of progression.

Phase I. The Prealcoholic Phase. This phase is characterized by the use of alcohol to relieve the everyday stress and tensions of life. As a child, the individual may have observed parents or other adults drinking alcohol and enjoying the effects. The child learns that use of alcohol is an acceptable method of coping with stress. Tolerance develops, and the amount required to achieve the desired effect increases steadily.

Phase II. The Early Alcoholic Phase. This phase begins with blackouts—brief periods of amnesia that occur during or immediately following a period of drinking. Now the alcohol is no longer a source of pleasure or relief for the individual but rather a drug that is *required* by the individual. Other common behaviors include sneaking drinks or secret drinking, preoccupation with drinking and maintaining the supply of alcohol, and rapid gulping of drinks. The individual feels enormous guilt and becomes very defensive about his or her drinking. Excessive use of denial and rationalization is evident.

Phase III. The Crucial Phase. In this phase, the individual has lost control, and physiological dependence is evident. This loss of control has been described as the inability to choose whether or not to drink. Binge drinking, lasting from a few hours to several weeks, is common. These episodes are characterized by sickness, loss of consciousness, squalor, and degradation. In this phase, the individual is extremely ill. Anger and aggression are common manifestations. Drinking is the total focus, and he or she is willing to risk losing everything that was once important in an effort to maintain the addiction. By this phase of the illness, it is common for the individual to have experienced the loss of job, marriage, family, friends and, most especially, self-respect.

Phase IV. The Chronic Phase. This phase is characterized by emotional and physical disintegration. The individual is usually intoxicated more often than he or she is sober. Emotional disintegration is evidenced by profound helplessness and self-pity. Impairment in reality testing may result in psychosis. Life-threatening physical manifestations may be evident in virtually every system of the body. Abstention from alcohol results in a terrifying syndrome of symptoms that include hallucinations, tremors, convulsions, severe agitation, and panic. Depression and ideas of suicide are common.

Effects on the Body

Alcohol can induce a general, nonselective, reversible depression of the CNS. About 20 percent of a single dose of alcohol is absorbed directly and immediately into the bloodstream through the stomach wall. Unlike other "foods," it does not have to be digested. The blood carries it directly to the brain where the alcohol acts on the brain's central control areas, slowing down or depressing brain activity (NIAAA, 1997). The other 80 percent of the alcohol in one drink is processed only slightly more slowly through the upper intestinal tract and into the bloodstream. Only moments after alcohol is consumed, it can be found in all tissues, organs, and secretions of the body. Rapidity of absorption is influenced by various factors. For example, absorption is delayed when the drink is sipped, rather than gulped; when the stomach contains food, rather than being empty; and when the drink is wine or beer, rather than distilled beverages.

At low doses, alcohol produces relaxation, loss of inhibitions, lack of concentration, drowsiness, slurred speech, and sleep. Chronic abuse results in multisystem physiological impairments. These complications include (but are not limited to) those outlined in the following sections.

PERIPHERAL NEUROPATHY. Peripheral neuropathy, characterized by peripheral nerve damage, results in pain, burning, tingling, or prickly sensations of the extremities. Researchers believe it is the direct result of deficiencies in the B vitamins, particularly thiamine. Nutritional deficiencies are common in chronic alcoholics because of insufficient intake of nutrients as well as the toxic effect of alcohol that results in malabsorption of nutrients. The process is reversible with abstinence from alcohol and restoration of nutritional deficiencies. Otherwise, permanent muscle wasting and paralysis can occur.

ALCOHOLIC MYOPATHY. Alcoholic myopathy may occur as an acute or chronic condition. In the acute condition, the individual experiences a sudden onset of muscle pain, swelling, and weakness; a reddish tinge in the urine caused by myoglobin, a breakdown product of muscle excreted in the urine; and a rapid rise in muscle enzymes in the blood (Barclay, 2002). Muscle symptoms are usually generalized, but pain and swelling might selectively involve the calves or other muscle groups. Laboratory studies show elevations of the enzymes creatine phosphokinase (CPK), lactate dehydrogenase (LDH), aldolase, and aspartate aminotransferase (AST). The symptoms of chronic alcoholic myopathy include a gradual wasting and weakness in skeletal muscles. Neither the pain and tenderness nor the elevated muscle enzymes seen in acute myopathy are evident in the chronic condition.

Alcoholic myopathy is thought to be a result of the same B vitamin deficiency that contributes to peripheral neuropathy. Improvement is observed with abstinence from alcohol and the return to a nutritious diet with vitamin supplements.

WERNICKE'S ENCEPHALOPATHY. **Wernicke's encephalopathy** represents the most serious form of thiamine deficiency in alcoholics. Symptoms include paralysis of the ocular muscles, diplopia, ataxia, somnolence, and stupor. If thiamine replacement therapy is not undertaken quickly, death will ensue.

KORSAKOFF'S PSYCHOSIS. **Korsakoff's psychosis** is identified by symptoms of confusion, loss of recent memory, and confabulation in alcoholics. It is frequently encountered in clients recovering from Wernicke's encephalopathy. In the United States, the two disorders are usually considered together and are called *Wernicke-Korsakoff syndrome*. Treatment is with parenteral or oral thiamine replacement.

ALCOHOLIC CARDIOMYOPATHY. The effect of alcohol on the heart is an accumulation of lipids in the myocardial cells resulting in enlargement and a weakened condition. The clinical findings of alcoholic cardiomyopathy generally relate to congestive heart failure or arrhythmia (Schuckit, 2000). Symptoms include decreased exercise tolerance, tachycardia, dyspnea, edema, palpitations, and nonproductive cough. Laboratory studies may show elevation of the enzymes CPK, AST, alanine aminotransferase, and LDH. Changes may be observed by electrocardiogram (ECG), and congestive heart failure may be evident on chest x-ray films.

The treatment is total permanent abstinence from alcohol. Treatment of the congestive heart failure may include rest, oxygen, digitalization, sodium restriction, and diuretics. Prognosis is encouraging if treated in the early stages. The death rate is high for individuals with advanced symptomatology.

ESOPHAGITIS. Esophagitis—inflammation and pain in the esophagus—occurs because of the toxic effects of alcohol on the esophageal mucosa. It also occurs because of frequent vomiting associated with alcohol abuse.

GASTRITIS. The effects of alcohol on the stomach include inflammation of the stomach lining characterized by epigastric distress, nausea, vomiting, and distention. Alcohol breaks down the stomach's protective mucosal barrier, allowing hydrochloric acid to erode the stomach wall. Damage to blood vessels may result in hemorrhage.

PANCREATITIS. This condition may be categorized as *acute* or *chronic*. Acute pancreatitis usually occurs 1 or 2 days after a binge of excessive alcohol consumption. Symptoms include constant, severe epigastric pain; nausea and vomiting; and abdominal distention. The chronic condition leads to pancreatic insufficiency resulting in steatorrhea, malnutrition, weight loss, and diabetes mellitus.

ALCOHOLIC HEPATITIS. Alcoholic hepatitis often follows a severe prolonged bout of drinking, and is usually superimposed on an already damaged liver (Worman, 1998). Clinical manifestations include an enlarged and tender liver, nausea and vomiting, lethargy, anorexia, elevated white blood cell count, and jaundice. **Ascites** and weight loss may be evident in more severe cases. With treatment—which includes strict abstinence from alcohol, proper nutrition, and rest—the individual can completely recover. Severe cases can lead to cirrhosis or **hepatic encephalopathy.**

CIRRHOSIS OF THE LIVER. In the United States, alcohol abuse is the leading cause of liver cirrhosis (Worman, 1998). Cirrhosis is the end-stage of alcoholic liver disease, and results from long-term chronic alcohol abuse. There is widespread destruction of liver cells, which are replaced by fibrous (scar) tissue. Clinical manifestations include nausea and vomiting, anorexia, weight loss, abdominal pain, jaundice, edema, anemia, and blood coagulation abnormalities. Treatment includes abstention from alcohol, correction of malnutrition, and supportive care to prevent complications of the disease. Complications of cirrhosis include:

1. **Portal hypertension.** Elevation of blood pressure through the portal circulation results from defective blood flow through the cirrhotic liver.
2. **Ascites.** Ascites, a condition in which an excessive amount of serous fluid accumulates in the abdominal cavity, occurs in response to portal hypertension. The increased pressure results in the seepage of fluid from the surface of the liver into the abdominal cavity.
3. **Esophageal varices. Esophageal varices** are veins in the esophagus that become distended because of excessive pressure from defective blood flow through the cirrhotic liver. As this pressure in-

creases, these varicosities can rupture, resulting in hemorrhage and sometimes death.

4. **Hepatic encephalopathy.** This serious complication occurs in response to the inability of the diseased liver to convert ammonia to urea for excretion. The continued rise in serum ammonia results in progressively impaired mental functioning, apathy, euphoria or depression, sleep disturbance, increasing confusion, and progression to coma and eventual death. Treatment requires complete abstention from alcohol, temporary elimination of protein from the diet, and reduction of intestinal ammonia using neomycin or lactulose (National Library of Medicine, 2002).

LEUKOPENIA. The production, function, and movement of the white blood cells are impaired in chronic alcoholics. This condition, called leukopenia, places the individual at high risk for contracting infectious diseases as well as for complicated recovery.

THROMBOCYTOPENIA. Platelet production and survival are impaired because of the toxic effects of alcohol. This places the alcoholic at risk for hemorrhage. Abstinence from alcohol rapidly reverses this deficiency.

SEXUAL DYSFUNCTION. Alcohol interferes with the normal production and maintenance of female and male hormones (Virginia Alcohol Safety Action Program [VASAP], 2002). For women, this can mean changes in the menstrual cycles and a decreased or loss of ability to become pregnant. For men, the decreased hormone levels result in a diminished libido, decreased sexual performance, and the development of reactive or absolute impotence over time (VASAP, 2002).

Alcohol Intoxication

Symptoms of alcohol intoxication include disinhibition of sexual or aggressive impulses, mood lability, impaired judgment, impaired social or occupational functioning, slurred speech, incoordination, unsteady gait, nystagmus, and flushed face. Intoxication usually occurs at blood alcohol levels between 100 and 200 mg/dL. Death has been reported at levels ranging from 400 to 700 mg/dL.

Alcohol Withdrawal

Within 4 to 12 hours of cessation of or reduction in heavy and prolonged (several days or longer) alcohol use, the following symptoms may appear: coarse tremor of hands, tongue, or eyelids; nausea or vomiting; malaise or weakness; tachycardia; sweating, elevated blood pressure; anxiety; depressed mood or irritability; transient hallucinations or illusions; headache; and insomnia. A complicated withdrawal syndrome may progress to *alcohol withdrawal delirium.* Onset of delirium is usually on the second or third day following cessation of or reduction in prolonged, heavy alcohol use. Symptoms include those described under the syndrome of delirium (Chapter 12).

Sedative, Hypnotic, or Anxiolytic Abuse and Dependence

A Profile of the Substance

The sedative-hypnotic compounds are drugs of diverse chemical structures that are all capable of inducing varying degrees of CNS depression, from tranquilizing relief of anxiety to anesthesia, coma, and even death. They are generally categorized as (1) barbiturates, (2) nonbarbiturate hypnotics, and (3) antianxiety agents. Effects produced by these substances depend on size of dose and potency of drug administered.

Table 13–1 presents a selected list of drugs included in these categories. Generic names are followed in parentheses by the trade names. Common street names for each category are also included.

Several principles have been identified that apply uniformly to all CNS depressants:

1. **The effects of CNS depressants are additive with one another and with the behavioral state of the user.** For example, when these drugs are used in combination with each other or in combination with alcohol, the depressive effects are compounded. These intense depressive effects are often unpredictable and can even be fatal. Similarly, a person who is mentally depressed or physically fatigued may have an exaggerated response to a dose of the drug that would only slightly affect a person in a normal or excited state.
2. **CNS depressants are capable of producing physiological dependency.** If large doses of CNS depressants are repeatedly administered over a prolonged duration, a period of CNS hyperexcitability occurs on withdrawal of the drug. The response can be quite severe, even leading to convulsions and death.
3. **CNS depressants are capable of producing psychological dependence.** CNS depressants have the potential to generate within the individual a psychic drive for periodic or continuous adminis-

TABLE 13 – 1 Sedative, Hypnotic, and Anxiolytic Drugs

Categories	Generic (Trade) Names	Common Street Names
Barbiturates	Pentobarbital (Nembutal)	Yellow jackets; yellow birds; nembies
	Secobarbital (Seconal)	Red birds; red devils; seggies
	Amobarbital (Amytal)	Blue birds; blue angels
	Secobarbital/amobarbital (Tuinal)	Tooies; jelly beans; rainbows; double-trouble
Nonbarbiturate hypnotics	Ethchlorvynol (Placidyl)	Dyls
	Glutethimide (Doriden)	Gorilla pills, CBs, Cibas, D
	Chloral hydrate (Noctec)	Peter, Mickey
	Triazolam (Halcion)	Sleepers
	Flurazepam (Dalmane)	Sleepers
	Temazepam (Restoril)	Sleepers
Antianxiety agents	Diazepam (Valium)	Vs (color designates strength)
	Chlordiazepoxide (Librium)	Green and whites; roaches
	Meprobamate (Equanil; Miltown)	Dolls; dollies
	Oxazepam (Serax)	
	Alprazolam (Xanax)	
	Lorazepam (Ativan)	
	Clorazepate (Tranxene)	
	Flunitrazepam (Rohypnol)	Date rape drug; roofies, R-2, rope, Mexican Valium

tration of the drug to achieve a maximum level of functioning or feeling of well-being.

4. **Cross-tolerance and cross-dependency may exist between various CNS depressants.** Cross-tolerance is exhibited when one drug results in a lessened response to another drug. Cross-dependence is a condition in which one drug can prevent withdrawal symptoms associated with physical dependence on a different drug (Julien, 2001).

Historical Aspects

Anxiety and insomnia, two of the most common human afflictions, were treated during the 19th century with opiates, bromide salts, chloral hydrate, paraldehyde, and alcohol (Hermes, 1993; Julien, 2001). Because the opiates were known to produce physical dependence, the bromides carried the risk of chronic bromide poisoning, and chloral hydrate and paraldehyde had an objectionable taste and smell, alcohol became the prescribed depressant drug of choice. However, some people refused to use alcohol because they did not like the taste or for moral reasons, and others tended to take more than was prescribed. Therefore, a search for a better sedative drug continued.

Although barbituric acid was first synthesized in 1864, it was not until 1912 that phenobarbital was introduced into medicine as a sedative drug, the first of the structurally classified group of drugs called barbiturates (Julien, 2001). Since that time, more than 2,500 barbiturate derivatives have been synthesized, but currently, less than a dozen remain in medical use. Illicit use of the drugs for recreational purposes grew throughout the 1930s and 1940s.

Efforts to create depressant medications that were not barbiturate derivatives accelerated. By the mid-1950s, the market for depressants had been expanded by the appearance of the nonbarbiturates glutethimide, ethchlorvynol, methyprylon, and meprobamate. Introduction of the benzodiazepines occurred around 1960 with the marketing of chlordiazepoxide (Librium), followed shortly by its derivative diazepam (Valium). The use of these drugs, and others within their group, has grown so rapidly that they have become some of the most widely prescribed medications in clinical use today. Their margin of safety is greater than that of barbiturates and the other nonbarbiturates. However, prolonged use of even moderate doses is likely to result in physical and psychological dependence, with a characteristic syndrome of withdrawal that can be severe.

Patterns of Use/Abuse

Sadock & Sadock (2003) report that about 15 percent of all persons in the United States have had benzodiazepine prescribed by a physician. Of all the drugs used in clinical practice, the sedative-hypnotic-antianxiety drugs are thought to be the most widely prescribed. The *DSM-IV-TR* states:

> In the United States, up to 90 percent of individuals hospitalized for medical care or surgery receive orders for sedative, hypnotic, or anxiolytic medications during their hospital stay, and more than 15 percent of American adults use these medications (usually by prescription) during any one year. (p. 291)

Two patterns of development of dependence and abuse are described. The first pattern is one of an individual whose physician originally prescribed the CNS depressant as treatment for anxiety or insomnia. Independently, the individual has increased the dosage or frequency from that which was prescribed. Use of the medication is justified based on treating symptoms, but as tolerance grows, increasing amounts of the medication are required to produce the desired effect. Substance-seeking behavior is evident as the individual seeks prescriptions from several physicians in order to maintain sufficient supplies.

The second pattern, which the *DSM-IV-TR* reports is more frequent than the first, involves young people in their teens or early 20s who, in the company of their peers, use substances that were obtained illegally. The initial objective is to achieve a feeling of euphoria. The drug is usually used intermittently during recreational gatherings. This pattern of intermittent use leads to regular use and extreme levels of tolerance. Combining use with other substances is not uncommon. Physical and psychological dependence lead to intense substance-seeking behaviors, most often through illegal channels.

Effects on the Body

The sedative-hypnotic compounds induce a general depressant effect. That is, they depress the activity of the brain, nerves, muscles, and heart tissue. They reduce the rate of metabolism in a variety of tissues throughout the body, and in general, they depress any system that uses energy (Julien, 2001). Large doses are required to produce these effects. In lower doses, these drugs appear to be more selective in their depressant actions. Specifically, in lower doses these drugs appear to exert their action on the centers within the brain that are concerned with arousal (e.g., the ascending reticular activating system, in the reticular formation, and the diffuse thalamic projection system).

As stated previously, the sedative-hypnotics are capable of producing all levels of CNS depression—from mild sedation to death. The level is determined by dosage and potency of the drug used. In Figure 13–1, a continuum of the CNS depressant effects is presented to demonstrate how increasing doses of sedative-hypnotic drugs affect behavioral depression.

The primary action of sedative-hypnotics is on nervous tissue. However, large doses may have an effect on other organ systems. Following is a discussion of the physiological effects of sedative-hypnotic/anxiolytic agents.

THE EFFECTS OF SLEEP AND DREAMING. Barbiturate use decreases the amount of sleep time spent in dreaming. During drug withdrawal, dreaming becomes vivid and excessive. Rebound insomnia and increased dreaming (termed *REM rebound*) are not uncommon with abrupt withdrawal from long-term use of these drugs as sleeping aids (Julien, 2001).

RESPIRATORY DEPRESSION. Barbiturates are capable of inhibiting the reticular activating system, resulting in respiratory depression (Sadock & Sadock, 2003). Additive effects can occur with the concurrent use of other CNS depressants, effecting a life-threatening situation.

CARDIOVASCULAR EFFECTS. Hypotension may be a problem with large doses. Only a slight decrease in blood pressure is noted with normal oral dosage.

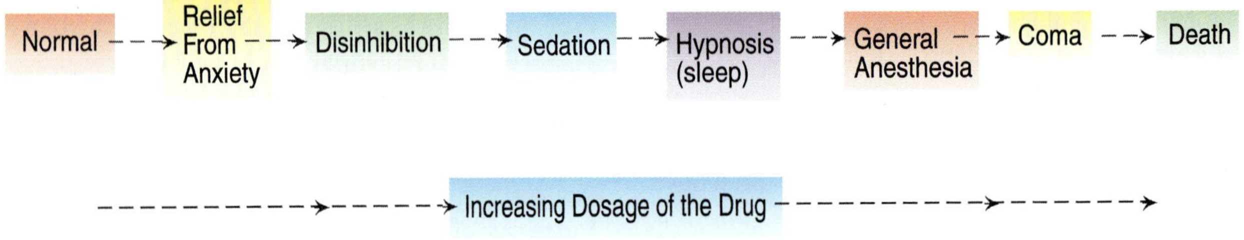

FIGURE 13–1. Continuum of Behavioral Depression

High dosages of barbiturates may result in decreased cardiac output, decreased cerebral blood flow, and direct impairment of myocardial contractility (Habal, 2001).

RENAL FUNCTION. In doses high enough to produce anesthesia, barbiturates may suppress urine function. At the usual sedative-hypnotic dosage, however, there is no evidence that they have any direct action on the kidneys.

HEPATIC EFFECTS. The barbiturates may produce jaundice with doses large enough to produce acute intoxication. Barbiturates stimulate the production of liver enzymes, resulting in a decrease in the plasma levels of both the barbiturates and other drugs metabolized in the liver (Habal, 2001). Preexisting liver disease may predispose an individual to additional liver damage with excessive barbiturate use.

BODY TEMPERATURE. High doses of barbiturates can greatly decrease body temperature. It is not significantly altered with normal dosage levels.

SEXUAL FUNCTIONING. CNS depressants have a tendency to produce a biphasic response. There is an initial increase in libido, presumably from the primary disinhibitory effects of the drug. This initial response is then followed by a decrease in the ability to maintain an erection.

Sedative, Hypnotic, or Anxiolytic Intoxication

The *DSM-IV-TR* (APA, 2000) describes sedative, hypnotic, or anxiolytic intoxication as the presence of clinically significant maladaptive behavioral or psychological changes that develop during, or shortly after, use of one of these substances. These maladaptive changes may include inappropriate sexual or aggressive behavior, mood lability, impaired judgment, or impaired social or occupational functioning. Other symptoms that may develop with excessive use of sedatives, hypnotics, or anxiolytics include slurred speech, incoordination, unsteady gait, nystagmus, impairment in attention or memory, and stupor or coma.

Sedative, Hypnotic, or Anxiolytic Withdrawal

Withdrawal from sedatives, hypnotics, or anxiolytics produces a characteristic syndrome of symptoms that develops after a marked decrease in or cessation of intake after several weeks or more of regular use (APA, 2000). Onset of the symptoms depends on the drug from which the individual is withdrawing. A short-acting anxiolytic (e.g., lorazepam or oxazepam) may produce symptoms within 6 to 8 hours of decreasing blood levels, whereas withdrawal symptoms from substances with longer half-lives (e.g., diazepam) may not develop for more than a week, peak in intensity during the second week, and decrease markedly during the third or fourth week (APA, 2000).

Severe withdrawal is most likely to occur when a substance has been used at high dosages for prolonged periods. However, withdrawal symptoms also have been reported with moderate dosages taken over a relatively short duration. Withdrawal symptoms associated with sedatives, hypnotics, or anxiolytics include autonomic hyperactivity (e.g., sweating or pulse rate greater than 100), increased hand tremor, insomnia, nausea or vomiting, hallucinations, illusions, psychomotor agitation, anxiety, or grand mal seizures.

CNS Stimulant Abuse and Dependence

A Profile of the Substance

The CNS stimulants are identified by the behavioral stimulation and psychomotor agitation that they induce. They differ widely in their molecular structures and in their mechanisms of action. The amount of CNS stimulation caused by a certain drug depends on both the area in the brain or spinal cord that is affected by the drug and the cellular mechanism fundamental to the increased excitability (Byers, 1991).

Groups within this category are classified according to similarities in mechanism of action. The *psychomotor stimulants* induce stimulation by augmentation or potentiation of the neurotransmitters norepinephrine, epinephrine, or dopamine. The *general cellular stimulants* (caffeine and nicotine) exert their action directly on cellular activity. Caffeine inhibits the enzyme phosphodiesterase, allowing increased levels of adenosine 3′,5′-cyclic phosphate, a chemical substance that promotes increased rates of cellular metabolism. Nicotine stimulates ganglionic synapses. This results in increased acetylcholine, which stimulates nerve impulse transmission to the entire autonomic nervous system. A selected list of drugs included in these categories is presented in Table 13–2.

The two most prevalent and widely used stimulants are caffeine and nicotine. Caffeine is readily available in every supermarket and grocery store as a common ingredient in coffee, tea, colas, and chocolate. Nicotine is the primary psychoactive substance found

TABLE 13 – 2 Central Nervous System (CNS) Stimulants

Categories	Generic (Trade) Names	Common Street Names
Amphetamines	Dextroamphetamine (Dexedrine)	Dexies, uppers, truck drivers
	Methamphetamine (Desoxyn)	Meth, speed, crystal, ice
	3,4-methylenedioxyamphetamine (MDMA)[1]	Adam, Ecstasy, Eve, XTC
	Amphetamine + dextroamphetamine (Adderall)	
Nonamphetamine stimulants	Phendimetrazine (Prelu-2)	Diet pills
	Benzphetamine (Didrex)	
	Diethylpropion (Tenuate)	
	Phentermine (Adipex-P; Ionamin)	
	Sibutramine (Meridia)	
	Methylphenidate (Ritalin)	Vitamin R, Skippy, MPH
	Pemoline (Cylert)	
Cocaine	Cocaine hydrochloride	Coke, blow, toot, snow, lady, flake, crack
Caffeine	Coffee, tea, colas, chocolate	Java, mud, brew, cocoa
Nicotine	Cigarettes, cigars, pipe tobacco, snuff	Weeds, fags, butts, chaw, cancer sticks

[1] Also cross-referenced as a hallucinogen

in tobacco products. When used in moderation, these stimulants tend to relieve fatigue and increase alertness. They are a generally accepted part of our culture; however, with increased social awareness regarding the health risks associated with nicotine, its use has become stigmatized in some circles.

The more potent stimulants, because of their potential for physiological dependency, are under regulation by the Controlled Substances Act. These controlled stimulants are available for therapeutic purposes by prescription only; however, they are also clandestinely manufactured and widely distributed on the illicit market.

Historical Aspects

Cocaine is the most potent stimulant derived from natural origin. It is extracted from the leaves of the coca plant, which has been cultivated in the Andean highlands of South America since prehistoric times. Natives of the region chew the leaves of the plant for refreshment and relief from fatigue.

The coca leaves must be mixed with lime to release the cocaine alkaloid. The chemical formula for the pure form of the drug was obtained in 1960. Physicians began using the drug as an anesthetic in eye, nose, and throat surgeries. These therapeutic uses are now obsolete. It has been used therapeutically in the United States in a morphine-cocaine elixir designed to relieve the suffering associated with terminal illness (Bennett & Woolf, 1991).

Cocaine has achieved a degree of acceptability within some social circles. It is illicitly distributed as a white crystalline powder and is often mixed with other ingredients to increase its volume and, therefore, to create more profits. The drug is most commonly "snorted," and chronic users may manifest symptoms that resemble the congested nose of a common cold. The intensely pleasurable effects of the drug create the potential for extraordinary psychological dependency.

Another form of cocaine commonly used in the United States, called "crack," is a cocaine alkaloid that is extracted from its powdered hydrochloride salt by mixing it with sodium bicarbonate and allowing it to dry into small "rocks" (APA, 2000). Because this type of cocaine can be easily vaporized and inhaled, its effects have an extremely rapid onset.

Amphetamine was first prepared in 1887. Various derivatives of the drug soon followed, and clinical use of the drug began in 1927. Amphetamines were used quite extensively for medical purposes through the 1960s, but recognition of their abuse potential has sharply decreased clinical use. Today, they are prescribed only to treat narcolepsy (a rare disorder resulting in an uncontrollable desire for sleep), hyperactivity disorders in children, and in certain cases of obesity. Clandestine production of amphetamines for distribution on the illicit market has become a thriving business.

The earliest history of caffeine is unknown and is shrouded by legend and myth. Caffeine was first discovered in coffee in 1820 and 7 years later in tea. Both beverages have been widely accepted and enjoyed as a "pick-me-up" by many cultures.

Tobacco was used by the aborigines. Introduced in Europe in the middle 16th century, its use grew rapidly and soon became prevalent in the Orient. Tobacco came to America with the settlement of the earliest colonies. Today, it is grown in many countries of the world, and although smoking is decreasing in most industrialized nations, it is increasing in the developing areas (APA, 2000).

Patterns of Use/Abuse

Because of their pleasurable effects, CNS stimulants have a high abuse potential. In 2002, about 2 million Americans were current cocaine users (SAMHSA, 2003). Use was highest among Americans aged 19 to 25 years.

Many individuals who abuse or are dependent on CNS stimulants began using the substance for the appetite-suppressant effect in an attempt at weight control (APA, 2000). Higher and higher doses are consumed in an effort to maintain the pleasurable effects. With continued use, the pleasurable effects diminish, and there is a corresponding increase in dysphoric effects. There is a persistent craving for the substance, however, even in the face of unpleasant adverse effects from continued drug-taking.

CNS stimulant abuse and dependence are usually characterized by episodic or chronic daily, or almost daily, use. Individuals who use the substances on an episodic basis often "binge" on the drug, with very high dosages followed by a day or two of recuperation. This recuperation period is characterized by extremely intense and unpleasant symptoms (called a "crash").

The daily user may take large or small doses and may use the drug several times a day or only at a specific time during the day. The amount consumed usually increases over time as tolerance occurs. Chronic users tend to rely on CNS stimulants to feel more powerful, more confident, and more decisive. They often fall into a pattern of taking "uppers" in the morning and "downers," such as alcohol or sleeping pills, at night.

The average American consumes two cups of coffee (about 200 mg of caffeine) per day. Caffeine is consumed in various amounts by 90 percent of the population. At a level of 500 to 600 mg of daily caffeine consumption, symptoms of anxiety, insomnia, and depression are common. It is also at this level that caffeine dependence and withdrawal can occur. Caffeine consumption is prevalent among children as well as adults. Table 13–3 lists some common sources of caffeine.

Next to caffeine, nicotine, an active ingredient in tobacco, is the most widely used psychoactive substance in U.S. society. Of the U.S. population, more than 30 percent reported current use of a tobacco product in 2002 (SAMHSA, 2003). Since 1964, when the results of the first public health report on smoking were issued, the percentage of total smokers has been on the decline. However, the percentage of women and teenage smokers has declined more slowly than that of adult men. Approximately 400,000 people die annually because of tobacco use, and an estimated 60 percent of the direct healthcare costs in the United States goes to treat tobacco-related illnesses (Sadock & Sadock, 2003).

TABLE 13–3 Common Sources of Caffeine

Source	Caffeine Content (mg)
Food and Beverages	
5–6 oz. brewed coffee	90–125
5–6 oz. instant coffee	60–90
5–6 oz. decaffeinated coffee	3
5–6 oz. brewed tea	70
5–6 oz. instant tea	45
8–12 oz. cola drinks	60
5–6 oz. cocoa	20
8 oz. chocolate milk	2–7
1 oz. chocolate bar	22
Prescription Medications	
APCs (aspirin, phenacetin, caffeine)	32
Cafergot	100
Darvon compound	32
Fiorinal	40
Migralam	100
Over-the-Counter Analgesics	
Anacin, Empirin, Midol, Vanquish	32
Excedrin Migraine (aspirin, acetaminophen, caffeine)	65
Over-the-Counter Stimulants	
No-Doz Tablets	100
Vivarin	200
Caffedrine	250

Effects on the Body

The CNS stimulants are a group of pharmacological agents that are capable of exciting the entire nervous system. This is accomplished by increasing the activity or augmenting the capability of the neurotransmitter agents known to be directly involved in bodily activation and behavioral stimulation. Physiological responses vary markedly according to the potency and dosage of the drug.

CNS EFFECTS. Stimulation of the CNS results in tremor, restlessness, anorexia, insomnia, agitation, and increased motor activity. Amphetamines, nonamphetamine stimulants, and cocaine produce increased alertness, decrease in fatigue, elation and euphoria, and subjective feelings of greater mental agility and muscular power. Chronic use of these drugs may result in compulsive behavior, paranoia, hallucinations, and aggressive behavior (Street Drugs, 2001).

CARDIOVASCULAR/PULMONARY EFFECTS. Amphetamines can induce increased systolic and diastolic blood pressure, increased heart rate, and cardiac arrhythmias (Street Drugs, 2001). These drugs also relax bronchial smooth muscle. Cocaine intoxication typically produces a rise in myocardial demand for oxygen and an increase in heart rate. Severe vasoconstriction may occur and can result in myocardial infarction, ventricular fibrillation, and sudden death. Inhaled cocaine can cause pulmonary hemorrhage, chronic bronchiolitis, and pneumonia. Nasal rhinitis is a result of chronic cocaine snorting.

Caffeine ingestion can result in increased heart rate, palpitations, extrasystoles, and cardiac arrhythmias. Caffeine induces dilation of pulmonary and general systemic blood vessels and constriction of cerebral blood vessels.

Nicotine stimulates the release of epinephrine from the adrenal gland, resulting in constriction of peripheral blood vessels, decreased body temperature, and increased blood pressure (Bennett & Woolf, 1991). Contractions of gastric smooth muscle associated with hunger are inhibited, thereby producing a mild anorectic effect.

GASTROINTESTINAL AND RENAL EFFECTS. Gastrointestinal (GI) effects of amphetamines are somewhat unpredictable; however, a decrease in GI tract motility commonly results in constipation (Bennett & Woolf, 1991). Contraction of the bladder sphincter makes urination difficult. Caffeine exerts a diuretic effect on the kidneys. Nicotine stimulates the hypothalamus to release antidiuretic hormone, reducing the excretion of urine. Because nicotine increases the tone and activity of the bowel, it may occasionally cause diarrhea.

Most CNS stimulants induce a small rise in metabolic rate and various degrees of anorexia. Amphetamines and cocaine can cause a rise in body temperature.

SEXUAL FUNCTIONING. CNS stimulants apparently promote the coital urge in both men and women. Women, more than men, report that stimulants make them feel sexier and have more orgasms. In fact, some men may experience sexual dysfunction with the use of stimulants. For the majority of individuals, however, these drugs exert a powerful aphrodisiac effect, which may be one reason for relapse or continued abuse of the substance (Goldstein, 1994).

CNS Stimulant Intoxication

CNS stimulant intoxication produces maladaptive behavioral and psychological changes that develop during, or shortly after, use of these drugs. Amphetamine and cocaine intoxication typically produce euphoria or affective blunting; changes in sociability; hypervigilance; interpersonal sensitivity; anxiety, tension, or anger; stereotyped behaviors; or impaired judgment. Physical effects include tachycardia or bradycardia, pupillary dilation, elevated or lowered blood pressure, perspiration or chills, nausea or vomiting, weight loss, psychomotor agitation or retardation, muscular weakness, respiratory depression, chest pain, cardiac arrhythmias, confusion, seizures, dyskinesias, dystonias, or coma (APA, 2000).

Intoxication from caffeine usually occurs following consumption in excess of 250 mg. Symptoms include restlessness, nervousness, excitement, insomnia, flushed face, diuresis, GI disturbance, muscle twitching, rambling flow of thoughts and speech, tachycardia or cardiac arrhythmia, periods of inexhaustibility, and psychomotor agitation (APA, 2000).

CNS Stimulant Withdrawal

CNS stimulant withdrawal is the presence of a characteristic withdrawal syndrome that develops within a few hours to several days after cessation of, or reduction in, heavy and prolonged use (APA, 2000). Withdrawal from amphetamines and cocaine causes dysphoria, fatigue, vivid unpleasant dreams, insomnia or hypersomnia, increased appetite, and psychomotor retardation or agitation (APA, 2000). The *DSM-IV-TR* states:

> Marked withdrawal symptoms ("crashing") often follow an episode of intense, high-dose use (a "speed run"). This "crash" is characterized by intense and unpleasant feelings of lassitude and depression, generally requiring several days of rest and recuperation. Weight loss commonly occurs during heavy stimulant use, whereas a marked increase in appetite with rapid weight gain is often observed during withdrawal. Depressive symptoms may last several days to weeks, and may be accompanied by suicidal ideation. (p. 227)

The *DSM-IV-TR* does not include a diagnosis of caffeine withdrawal. However, Sadock & Sadock (2003) state that a number of well-controlled research studies indicate that caffeine withdrawal exists. They cite the following symptoms as typical: headache, fatigue, anxiety, irritability, depression, impaired psychomotor performance, nausea, vomiting, craving for caffeine, and muscle pain and stiffness.

Withdrawal from nicotine results in dysphoric or depressed mood; insomnia; irritability, frustration, or anger; anxiety; difficulty concentrating; restlessness; decreased heart rate; and increased appetite or weight gain (APA, 2000). A mild syndrome of nicotine withdrawal can appear when a smoker switches from regular cigarettes to low-nicotine cigarettes (Sadock & Sadock, 2003).

Inhalant Abuse and Dependence

A Profile of the Substance

Inhalant disorders are induced by inhaling the aliphatic and aromatic hydrocarbons found in substances such as fuels, solvents, adhesives, aerosol propellants, and paint thinners. Specific examples of these substances include gasoline, varnish remover, lighter fluid, airplane glue, rubber cement, cleaning fluid, spray paint, shoe conditioner, and typewriter correction fluid (Sadock & Sadock, 2003).

Patterns of Use/Abuse

Inhalant substances are readily available, legal, and inexpensive. These three factors make inhalants the drug of choice among poor people and among children and young adults. Use may begin by ages 9 to 12 years, and peak in the adolescent years; it is less common after age 35 years (APA, 2000). A national government survey of drug use indicated that 9.7 percent of people in the United States acknowledged ever having used inhalants (SAMHSA, 2003). The highest use was seen in the 12- to 25-year-old age group.

Methods of use include "huffing," a procedure in which a rag soaked with the substance is applied to the mouth and nose and the vapors breathed in. Another common method is called "bagging," in which the substance is placed in a paper or plastic bag and inhaled from the bag by the user. They may also be inhaled directly from the container or sprayed in the mouth or nose.

Sadock & Sadock (2003) report that:

> Inhalant use among adolescents may be most common in those whose parents or older siblings use illegal substances. Inhalant use among adolescents is also associated with an increased likelihood of conduct disorder or antisocial personality disorder. (p. 441)

Tolerance to inhalants has been reported with heavy use. A mild withdrawal syndrome has been documented but does not appear to be clinically significant (APA, 2000).

Children with inhalant disorder may use inhalants several times a week, often on weekends and after school (APA, 2000). Adults with inhalant dependence may use the substance at varying times during each day, or they may binge on the substance during a period of several days.

Effects on the Body

Inhalants are absorbed through the lungs and reach the CNS very rapidly. Inhalants generally act as a CNS depressant (Sadock & Sadock, 2003). The effects are relatively brief, lasting from several minutes to a few hours, depending on the specific substance and amount consumed.

CNS. Inhalants can cause both central and peripheral nervous system damage, which may be permanent (APA, 2000). Neurological deficits such as generalized weakness and peripheral neuropathies may be evident. Other CNS effects that have been reported with heavy inhalant use include cerebral atrophy, cerebellar degeneration, and white-matter lesions resulting in cranial nerve or pyramidal tract signs.

RESPIRATORY EFFECTS. The *DSM-IV-TR* reports the following respiratory effects with inhalant use: upper- or lower-airway irritation, including increased airway resistance; pulmonary hypertension; acute respiratory distress; coughing; sinus discharge; dyspnea; rales; or rhonchi. Rarely, cyanosis may result from pneumonitis or asphyxia. Death may occur from respiratory or cardiovascular depression.

GI EFFECTS. Abdominal pain, nausea, and vomiting may occur. A rash may be present around the individual's nose and mouth. Unusual breath odors are common.

RENAL SYSTEM EFFECTS. Chronic renal failure, hepatorenal syndrome, and proximal renal tubular acidosis have been reported (APA, 2000).

Inhalant Intoxication

The *DSM-IV-TR* defines inhalant intoxication as "clinically significant maladaptive behavioral or psychological changes (e.g., belligerence, assaultiveness, apathy, impaired judgment, impaired social or occupational functioning) that develop during or shortly after, use of or exposure to volatile inhalants." Two or more of the following signs are present:

1. Dizziness
2. Nystagmus
3. Incoordination
4. Slurred speech
5. Unsteady gait
6. Lethargy
7. Depressed reflexes
8. Psychomotor retardation
9. Tremor
10. Generalized muscle weakness
11. Blurred vision or diplopia
12. Stupor or coma
13. Euphoria

The symptoms are not due to a general medical condition and are not better accounted for by another mental disorder.

Opioid Abuse and Dependence

A Profile of the Substance

The term *opioid* refers to a group of compounds that includes opium, opium derivatives, and synthetic substitutes. Opioids exert both a sedative and an analgesic effect, and their major medical uses are for the relief of pain, the treatment of diarrhea, and the relief of coughing. These drugs have addictive qualities; that is, they are capable of inducing tolerance and physiological and psychological dependence.

Opioids are popular drugs of abuse in that they desensitize an individual to both psychological and physiological pain and induce a sense of euphoria. Lethargy and indifference to the environment are common manifestations.

Opioid abusers usually spend much of their time nourishing their habit. Individuals who are opioid dependent are seldom able to hold a steady job that will support their need. They must therefore secure funds from friends, relatives, or whomever they have not yet alienated with their dependency-related behavior. Obtaining funds illegally is common. Common criminal methods are burglary, robbery, prostitution, and selling drugs (Goldstein, 1994).

Methods of administration of opioid drugs include oral, snorting or smoking, and by subcutaneous, intramuscular, and intravenous injection. A selected list of opioid substances is presented in Table 13–4.

Under close supervision, opioids are indispensable in the practice of medicine. They are the most effec-

TABLE 13–4 Opioids and Related Substances

Categories	Generic (Trade) Names	Common Street Names
Opioids of natural origin	Opium (ingredient in various antidiarrheal agents)	Black stuff, poppy, tar, big O
	Morphine (Astramorph; Roxanol)	M, white stuff, Miss Emma
	Codeine (ingredient in various analgesics and cough suppressants)	Terp, schoolboy, syrup, cody
Opioid derivatives	Heroin	H, horse, junk, brown sugar, smack, skag, TNT, Harry
	Hydromorphone (Dilaudid)	DLs, 4s, lords, little D
	Oxycodone (Percodan; OxyContin)	Perks, perkies, Oxy, O.C.
	Hydrocodone (Vicodin)	vike
Synthetic opiate-like drugs	Meperidine (Demerol)	Doctors
	Methadone (Dolophine)	Dollies, done
	Propoxyphene (Darvon)	Pinks and grays
	Pentazocine (Talwin)	Ts
	Fentanyl (Actiq; Duragesic)	Apache, China girl, China white, dance fever, goodfella, jackpot

tive agents known for the relief of intense pain. However, they also induce a pleasurable effect on the CNS that promotes their abuse. The physiological and psychological dependence that occurs with opioids, as well as the development of profound tolerance, contributes to the addict's ongoing quest for more of the substance, regardless of the means.

Historical Aspects

Opium is the Greek word for "juice." In its crude form, opium is a brownish-black, gummy substance obtained from the ripened pods of the opium poppy (Hermes, 1993). References to the use of opiates have been found in the Egyptian, Greek, and Arabian cultures as early as 3000 BC. The drug became widely used both medicinally and recreationally throughout Europe during the 16th and 17th centuries. Most of the opium supply came from China, where the drug was introduced by Arabic traders in the late 17th century. Morphine, the primary active ingredient of opium, was isolated in 1803 by the European chemist Frederich Serturner. Since that time, morphine, rather than crude opium, has been used throughout the world for the medical treatment of pain and diarrhea (Julien, 2001). This process was facilitated in 1853 by the development of the hypodermic syringe, which made it possible to deliver the undiluted morphine quickly into the body for rapid relief from pain.

This development also created a new variety of opiate user in the United States: one who was able to self-administer the drug by injection. During this time, there was also a large influx of Chinese immigrants into the United States, who introduced opium smoking to this country. By the early part of the 20th century, opium addiction was widespread.

In response to the concerns over widespread addiction, in 1914 the U.S. government passed the Harrison Narcotic Act, which created strict controls on the accessibility of opiates. Until that time, these substances had been freely available to the public without a prescription. The Harrison Act banned the use of opiates for other than medicinal purposes and drove the use of heroin underground. To this day, the beneficial uses of these substances are widely acclaimed within the medical profession, but the illicit trafficking of the drugs for recreational purposes continues to resist most efforts aimed at control.

Patterns of Use/Abuse

The development of opioid abuse and dependence may follow one of two typical behavior patterns. The first occurs in the individual who has obtained the drug by prescription from a physician for the relief of a medical problem. Abuse and dependency occur when the individual increases the amount and frequency of use, justifying the behavior as symptom treatment. He or she becomes obsessed with obtaining increasing amounts of the substance, seeking out several physicians in order to replenish and maintain supplies.

The second pattern of behavior associated with abuse and dependency of opioids occurs among individuals who use the drugs for recreational purposes and obtain them from illegal sources. Opioids may be used alone to induce the euphoric effects or in combination with stimulants or other drugs to enhance the euphoria or to counteract the depressant effects of the opioid. Tolerance develops and dependency occurs, leading the individual to procure the substance by whatever means is required in an effort to support the habit. SAMHSA (2003) reports:

> Since the mid-1990s, the prevalence of lifetime heroin use increased for both youths and young adults. From 1995 to 2002, the rate among youths aged 12 to 17 increased from 0.1 to 0.4 percent; among young adults aged 18 to 25, the rate rose from 0.8 to 1.6 percent. During the latter half of the 1990s, the annual number of heroin initiates rose to a level not reached since the late 1970s. In 1974, there were an estimated 246,000 heroin initiates. Between 1988 and 1994, the annual number of new users ranged from 28,000 to 80,000. Between 1995 and 2001, the number of new heroin users was consistently greater than 100,000. Data suggest that there has been a rise in heroin use in recent years, and that this rise has occurred among younger persons who are smoking or sniffing heroin rather than injecting. Some indicators exhibit an overall rise in heroin use, some display a rise in heroin use among youth, college students, and adolescents in small metropolitan areas, and others suggest that new users tend to smoke or sniff rather than inject. In addition, there is some evidence that the time between first use of marijuana and first use of heroin is decreasing.

Effects on the Body

Opiates are sometimes classified as *narcotic analgesics*. They exert their major effects primarily on the CNS, the eyes, and the GI tract (Bennett & Woolf, 1991). Chronic morphine use or acute morphine toxicity is manifested by a syndrome of sedation, chronic constipation, decreased respiratory rate, and pinpoint pupils. Intensity of symptoms is largely dose-dependent. The following physiological effects are common with opioid use.

CNS. All opioids, opioid derivatives, and synthetic opioid-like drugs affect the CNS. Common manifestations include euphoria, mood changes, and mental clouding (Bennett & Woolf, 1991). Other common CNS effects include drowsiness and pain reduction. Pupillary constriction occurs in response to stimulation of the oculomotor nerve. CNS depression of the respiratory centers within the medulla results in respiratory depression. The antitussive response is due to suppression of the cough center within the medulla. The nausea and vomiting commonly associated with opiate ingestion are related to the stimulation of the centers within the medulla that trigger this response.

GI EFFECTS. These drugs exert a profound effect on the GI tract. Both stomach and intestinal tone are increased, whereas peristaltic activity of the intestines is diminished. These effects lead to a marked decrease in the movement of food through the GI tract. This is a notable therapeutic effect in the treatment of severe diarrhea. In fact, no drugs have yet been developed that are more effective than the opioids for this purpose. However, constipation, and even fecal impaction, may be a serious problem for the chronic opioid user.

CARDIOVASCULAR EFFECTS. In therapeutic doses, opioids have minimal effect on the action of the heart. Morphine is used extensively to relieve pulmonary edema and the pain of myocardial infarction in cardiac clients. At high doses, opioids induce hypotension, which may be caused by direct action on the heart or by opioid-induced histamine release.

SEXUAL FUNCTIONING. With heroin, there is decreased sexual pleasure or an indifference to sex (Jernigan, 2002). Retarded ejaculation, impotence, and orgasm failure (in both men and women) may occur. Sexual side effects from opioids appear to be largely influenced by dosage.

Opioid Intoxication

Opioid intoxication constitutes clinically significant maladaptive behavioral or psychological changes that develop during, or shortly after, opioid use (APA, 2000). Symptoms include initial euphoria followed by apathy, dysphoria, psychomotor agitation or retardation, and impaired judgment. Physical symptoms include pupillary constriction (or dilation due to anoxia from severe overdose), drowsiness, slurred speech, and impairment in attention or memory (APA, 2000). Symptoms are consistent with the half-life of most opioid drugs, and usually last for several hours. Severe opioid intoxication can lead to respiratory depression, coma, and even death.

Opioid Withdrawal

Opioid withdrawal produces a syndrome of symptoms that develops after cessation or reduction in heavy and prolonged use of an opiate or related substance. Symptoms include dysphoric mood, nausea or vomiting, muscle aches, lacrimation or rhinorrhea, pupillary dilation, piloerection, sweating, abdominal cramping, diarrhea, yawning, fever, and insomnia. With short-acting drugs such as heroin, withdrawal symptoms occur within 6 to 12 hours after the last dose, peak within 1 to 3 days, and gradually subside over a period of 5 to 7 days (APA, 2000). With longer-acting drugs such as methadone, withdrawal symptoms begin within 1 to 3 days after the last dose and are complete in 10 to 14 days (Sadock & Sadock, 2003). Withdrawal from the ultra-short-acting meperidine begins quickly, reaches a peak in 8 to 12 hours, and is complete in 4 to 5 days (Sadock & Sadock, 2003).

Hallucinogen Abuse and Dependence

A Profile of the Substance

Hallucinogenic substances are capable of distorting an individual's perception of reality. They have the ability to alter sensory perception, induce hallucinations, and for this reason they have sometimes been referred to as "mind expanding." Some of the manifestations have been likened to a psychotic break. The hallucinations experienced by an individual with schizophrenia, however, are most often auditory, whereas substance-induced hallucinations are usually visual (Holbrook, 1991). Perceptual distortions have been reported by some users as a sense of depersonalization (observing oneself having the experience), or being at peace with self and the universe. Others, who describe their experiences as "bad trips," report feelings of panic and a fear of dying or going insane. A common danger reported with hallucinogenic drugs is that of "flashbacks," or a spontaneous recurrence of the hallucinogenic state without ingestion of the drug. These can occur months after the drug was last taken.

Recurrent use can produce tolerance, encouraging users to resort to increasingly higher dosages. No evidence of physical dependence is detectable when the drug is withdrawn; however, recurrent use appears to induce a psychological dependence to the insight-inducing experiences that a user may associate with episodes of hallucinogen use (Sadock & Sadock, 2003). This psychological dependence varies according to the drug, the dose, and the individual user. Hallucinogens are highly unpredictable in the effects they may induce each time they are used.

Many of the hallucinogenic substances have structural similarities. Some are produced synthetically; others are natural products of plants and fungi. A selected list of hallucinogens is presented in Table 13–5.

Historical Aspects

Archeological data obtained with carbon-14 dating suggest that hallucinogens have been used as part of religious ceremonies and at social gatherings by Native Americans for as long as 7,000 years (Goldstein, 1994). Use of the peyote cactus as part of religious ceremonies in the southwestern part of the United States still occurs today, although this ritual use has greatly diminished.

LSD was first synthesized in 1938 by Dr. Albert Hoffman (Holbrook, 1991). It was used as a clinical research tool to investigate the biochemical etiology of schizophrenia. It soon reached the illicit market, however, and its abuse began to overshadow the research effort.

The abuse of hallucinogens reached a peak in the late 1960s, waned during the 1970s, and returned to favor in the 1980s with the so-called designer drugs (e.g., 3,4-methylene-dioxyamphetamine [MDMA] and methoxy-amphetamine [MDA]). One of the most commonly abused hallucinogens today is PCP, even though many of its effects are perceived as undesirable. A number of deaths have been directly attributed to the use of PCP, and numerous accidental deaths have occurred because of overdose and because of the behavioral changes the drug precipitates (Holbrook, 1991).

Several therapeutic uses of LSD have been proposed, including the treatment of chronic alcoholism and the reduction of intractable pain such as occurs in malignant disease. A great deal more research is required regarding the therapeutic uses of LSD. At this time, there is no real evidence of the safety and efficacy of the drug in humans.

Patterns of Use/Abuse

Use of hallucinogens is usually episodic. Because cognitive and perceptual abilities are so markedly affected by these substances, the user must set aside time from normal daily activities for indulging in the consequences. The SAMHSA (2003) reports:

TABLE 13–5 Hallucinogens

Categories	Generic (Trade) Names	Common Street Names
Naturally occurring hallucinogens	Mescaline (the primary active ingredient of the peyote cactus)	Cactus, mesc, mescal, half moon, big chief, bad seed, peyote
	Psilocybin and psilocyn (active ingredients of *Psilocybe* mushrooms)	Magic mushroom, God's flesh, shrooms
	Ololiuqui (morning glory seeds)	Heavenly blue, pearly gates, flying saucers
Synthetic compounds	Lysergic acid diethylamide [LSD] (synthetically produced from a fungal substance found on rye or a chemical substance found in morning glory seeds)	Acid, cube, big D, California sunshine, microdots, blue dots, sugar, orange wedges, peace tablets, purple haze, cupcakes
	Dimethyltryptamine [DMT] and diethyltryptamine [DET] (chemical analogues of tryptamine)	Businessman's trip
	2,5-Dimethoxy-4-methylamphetamine [STP, DOM]	STP (serenity, tranquility, peace)
	Phencyclidine [PCP]	Angel dust, hog, peace pill, rocket fuel
	3,4-Methylenedioxyamphetamine [MDMA][1]	XTC, Ecstasy, Adam, Eve
	Methoxy-amphetamine [MDA]	Love drug

[1] Also cross-referenced as a stimulant.

The prevalence of lifetime hallucinogen use among youths aged 12 to 17 was at its highest level in 2001 (6.1 percent) but declined to 5.7 percent in 2002. Among young adults aged 18 to 25, use increased from 14.3 percent in 1992 to 24.2 percent in 2002. The increase in hallucinogen use in the 1990s appears to have been driven by the use of Ecstasy (i.e., MDMA).

The use of LSD does not lead to the development of physical dependence or withdrawal symptoms (Sadock & Sadock, 2003). However, tolerance does develop quickly and to a high degree. In fact, an individual who uses LSD repeatedly for a period of 3 to 4 days may develop complete tolerance to the drug. Recovery from the tolerance also occurs very rapidly (in 4 to 7 days) so that the individual is able to achieve the desired effect from the drug repeatedly and often.

PCP is usually taken episodically, in binges that can last for several days. However, some chronic users take the substance daily. Physical dependence does not occur with PCP; however, psychological dependence characterized by craving for the drug has been reported in chronic users, as has the slow development of tolerance (Holbrook, 1991). Tolerance apparently develops only with frequent use, such as on a daily basis.

Psilocybin is an ingredient of the *Psilocybe* mushroom indigenous to the United States and Mexico. Ingestion of these mushrooms produces an effect similar to that of LSD but of a shorter duration. This hallucinogenic chemical can now be produced synthetically.

Mescaline is the only hallucinogenic compound used legally for religious purposes today by members of the Native American Church of the United States. It is the primary active ingredient of the peyote cactus. Neither physical nor psychological dependence occurs with the use of mescaline, although tolerance does develop slowly with repeated use (Holbrook, 1991).

Among the very potent hallucinogens of the current drug culture are those that are categorized as derivatives of amphetamines. These include 2,5-dimethoxy-4-methylamphetamine (DOM, STP), MDMA, and MDA. At lower doses, these drugs produce the "high" associated with CNS stimulants. At higher doses, hallucinogenic effects occur. These drugs have existed for many years but were only *rediscovered* in the mid-1980s. Because of the rapid increase in recreational use, the DEA imposed an emergency classification of MDMA as a schedule I drug in 1985.

Effects on the Body

The effects produced by the various hallucinogenics are highly unpredictable. The variety of effects may be related to dosage, the mental state of the individual, and the environment in which the substance is used. Some common effects have been reported (Julien, 2001; APA, 2000; Berger, 2002):

Physiological Effects

- Nausea and vomiting
- Chills
- Pupil dilation
- Increased pulse, blood pressure, and temperature
- Mild dizziness
- Trembling
- Loss of appetite
- Insomnia
- Sweating
- A slowing of respirations
- Elevation in blood sugar

Psychological Effects

- Heightened response to color, texture, and sounds
- Heightened body awareness
- Distortion of vision
- Sense of slowing of time
- All feelings magnified: love, lust, hate, joy, anger, pain, terror, despair
- Fear of losing control
- Paranoia, panic
- Euphoria, bliss
- Projection of self into dreamlike images
- Serenity, peace
- Depersonalization
- Derealization
- Increased libido

The effects of hallucinogens are not always pleasurable for the user. Two types of toxic reactions are known to occur. The first is the *panic reaction*, or "bad trip." Symptoms include an intense level of anxiety, fear, and stimulation. The individual hallucinates and fears going insane. Paranoia and acute psychosis may be evident.

The second type of toxic reaction to hallucinogens is the *flashback*. This phenomenon refers to the transient, spontaneous repetition of a previous LSD-induced experience that occurs in the absence of the substance. Various studies have reported that a range from 15 to 80 percent of hallucinogen users report having experienced flashbacks (Sadock & Sadock, 2003).

Hallucinogen Intoxication

Symptoms of hallucinogen intoxication develop during, or shortly after (within minutes to a few hours) hallucinogen use (APA, 2000). Maladaptive behavioral or psychological changes include marked anxiety or depression, ideas of reference (a type of delusional thinking that all activity within one's environment is "referred to" [about] one's self), fear of losing one's mind, paranoid ideation, and impaired judgment. Perceptual changes occur in a state of full wakefulness and alertness and include intensification of perceptions, depersonalization, derealization, illusions, hallucinations, and synesthesias (APA, 2000). Physical symptoms include pupillary dilation, tachycardia, sweating, palpitations, blurring of vision, tremors, and incoordination (APA, 2000).

Symptoms of PCP intoxication develop within an hour of use (or less when it is smoked, snorted, or used intravenously) (APA, 2000). Specific symptoms are dose related and include belligerence, assaultiveness, impulsiveness, unpredictability, psychomotor agitation, and impaired judgment. Physical symptoms include vertical or horizontal nystagmus, hypertension or tachycardia, numbness or diminished responsiveness to pain, ataxia, dysarthria, muscle rigidity, seizures or coma, and hyperacusis.

Cannabis Abuse and Dependence

A Profile of the Substance

Cannabis is second only to alcohol as the most widely abused drug in the United States. The major psychoactive ingredient of this class of substances is delta-9-tetrahydrocannabinol (THC). It occurs naturally in the plant *Cannabis sativa*, which grows readily in warm climates. Marijuana, the most prevalent type of cannabis preparation, is composed of the dried leaves, stems, and flowers of the plant. Hashish is a more potent concentrate of the resin derived from the flowering tops of the plant. Hash oil is a concentrated form of THC made by boiling hashish in a solvent and filtering out the solid matter (Holbrook, 1991). Cannabis products are usually smoked in the form of loosely rolled cigarettes. Cannabis can also be taken orally when it is prepared in food, but about two to three times the amount of cannabis must be ingested orally to equal the potency of that taken by the inhalation of its smoke (Sadock & Sadock, 2003).

At moderate dosages, cannabis drugs produce effects resembling alcohol and other CNS depressants. By depressing higher brain centers, they release lower centers from inhibitory influences. There has been some controversy in the past over the classification of these substances. They are not narcotics, although they are legally classified as controlled substances. They are not hallucinogens, although in very high dosages they can induce hallucinations. They are not sedative-hypnotics, although they most closely resemble these substances. Like sedative-hypnotics, their action occurs in the ascending reticular activating system.

Psychological dependence has been shown to occur with cannabis and tolerance can occur. Controversy exists about whether physiological dependence occurs with cannabis. Sadock and Sadock (2003) state:

> Withdrawal symptoms in humans are limited to modest increases in irritability, restlessness, insomnia, and anorexia and mild nausea; all these symptoms appear only when a person abruptly stops taking high doses of cannabis. (p. 425)

Common cannabis preparations are presented in Table 13–6.

Historical Aspects

Products of *Cannabis sativa* have been used therapeutically for nearly 5,000 years (Julien, 2001). Cannabis was first used in China and India as an antiseptic and an analgesic. Its use later spread to the Middle East, Africa, and Eastern Europe.

In the United States, medical interest in the use of cannabis arose during the early part of the 19th century. Many articles were published espousing its use

TABLE 13–6 Cannabinoids

Category	Common Preparations	Street Names
Cannabis	Marijuana	Joint, weed, pot, grass, Mary Jane, Texas tea, locoweed, MJ, hay, stick
	Hashish	Hash, bhang, ganja, charas

for many and varied reasons. The drug was almost as commonly used for medicinal purposes as aspirin is today and could be purchased without a prescription in any drugstore. It was purported to have antibacterial and anticonvulsant capabilities, to decrease intraocular pressure, decrease pain, help in the treatment of asthma, increase appetite, and generally raise one's morale.

The drug went out of favor primarily because of the huge variation in potency within batches of medication caused by the variations in the THC content of different plants. Other medications were favored for their greater degree of solubility and faster onset of action than cannabis products. In the late 1920s, an association between marijuana and criminal activity was reported (Holbrook, 1991). A federal law put an end to its legal use in 1937. In the 1960s, marijuana became the symbol of the "antiestablishment" generation, at which time it reached its peak as a drug of abuse.

Research continues concerning the possible therapeutic uses of cannabis. It has been shown to be an effective agent for relieving intraocular pressure in clients with glaucoma. However, lifelong use is often necessary, and the long-term safety and efficacy of these drugs have not been established (Franklin & Frances, 1999).

Cannabis products also have been used in the treatment of nausea and vomiting that accompany cancer chemotherapy. It has been shown in a number of studies to be effective for this purpose when other antinausea medications fail.

Advocates who praise the therapeutic usefulness and support the legalization of the cannabinoids persist within the United States today. Such groups as the Alliance for Cannabis Therapeutics (ACT) and the National Organization for the Reform of Marijuana Laws (NORML) have lobbied extensively to allow disease sufferers easier access to the drug. Currently, 10 states have legalized the medical use of marijuana. The U.S. Drug Enforcement Agency (DEA) (2003) states:

> Legalizing marijuana through the political process bypasses the safeguards established by the Food and Drug Administration (FDA) to protect the public from dangerous or ineffective drugs. Every other prescribed drug must be tested according to scientifically rigorous protocols to ensure that it is safe and effective before it can be sold. The medical marijuana movement and its million-dollar media campaign have helped contribute to the changing attitude among our youth that marijuana use is harmless. Among marijuana's most harmful consequences is its role in leading to the use of other illegal drugs like heroin and cocaine. Long-term studies of students who use drugs show that very few young people use other illegal drugs without first trying marijuana. Although not all people who use marijuana go on to use other drugs, using marijuana sometimes lowers inhibitions about drug use and exposes users to a culture that encourages use of other drugs.

A great deal more research is required to determine the long-term effects of the drug. Until results indicate otherwise, it is safe to assume that the harmful effects of the drug outweigh the benefits.

Patterns of Use/Abuse

In its 2002 National Survey on Drug Use and Health, SAMHSA (2003) reported that an estimated 19.5 million Americans aged 12 years or older were current illicit drug users, meaning they had used an illicit drug during the month before the survey interview. This estimate represents 8.3 percent of the population aged 12 years old or older. Marijuana is the most commonly used illicit drug. In 2002, it was used by 75 percent of current illicit drug users. This constitutes about 14.6 million users of marijuana in the United States in the year 2002.

Many people incorrectly regard cannabis as a substance of low abuse potential. This lack of knowledge has promoted use of the substance by some individuals who believe it is harmless. Tolerance, although it tends to decline rapidly, does occur with chronic use. As tolerance develops, physical dependence also occurs, resulting in a mild withdrawal syndrome (as previously described) upon cessation of drug use.

One controversy that exists regarding marijuana is whether its use leads to the use of other illicit drugs. Sadock and Sadock (2003) state:

> Marijuana is the most widely used illicit drug among high school students. It has been termed a "gateway drug," because the strongest predictor of future cocaine use is frequent marijuana use during adolescence. (p. 1286)

Effects on the Body

Following is a summary of some of the effects that have been attributed to marijuana in recent years. Undoubtedly, as research continues, evidence of additional physiological and psychological effects will be made available.

CARDIOVASCULAR EFFECTS. Cannabis ingestion

induces tachycardia and orthostatic hypotension (National Institutes of Health [NIH], 2003). With the decrease in blood pressure, myocardial oxygen supply is decreased. Tachycardia in turn increases oxygen demand.

RESPIRATORY EFFECTS. Marijuana produces a greater amount of "tar" than its equivalent weight in tobacco. Because of the method by which marijuana is smoked—that is, the smoke is held in the lungs for as long as possible to achieve the desired effect—larger amounts of tar are deposited in the lungs, promoting deleterious effects to the lungs.

Although the initial reaction to the marijuana is bronchodilatation, thereby facilitating respiratory function, chronic use results in obstructive airway disorders (NIH, 2003). Frequent marijuana users often have laryngitis, bronchitis, cough, and hoarseness. Cannabis smoke contains more carcinogens than tobacco smoke; therefore, lung damage and cancer are real risks for heavy users (Goldstein, 1994).

REPRODUCTIVE EFFECTS. Some studies have shown a decrease in levels of serum testosterone and abnormalities in sperm count, motility, and structure correlated with heavy marijuana use (Marijuana and Reproduction, 2002). In women, heavy marijuana use has been correlated with failure to ovulate, difficulty with lactation, and an increased risk of spontaneous abortion.

CNS EFFECTS. Acute CNS effects of marijuana are dose related. Many people report a feeling of being "high"—the equivalent of being "drunk" on alcohol. Symptoms include feelings of euphoria, relaxed inhibitions, disorientation, depersonalization, and relaxation. At higher doses, sensory alterations may occur, including impairment in judgment of time and distance, recent memory, and learning ability. Physiological symptoms may include tremors, muscle rigidity, and conjunctival redness. Toxic effects are generally characterized by panic reactions. Very heavy usage has been shown to precipitate an acute psychosis that is self-limited and short-lived once the drug is removed from the body (Julien, 2001).

Heavy long-term cannabis use is also associated with a syndrome called *amotivational syndrome*. When this syndrome occurs, the individual is preoccupied with using the substance. Symptoms include lethargy, apathy, social and personal deterioration, and lack of motivation. This syndrome appears to be more common in countries in which the most potent preparations are used and where the substance is more freely available than it is in the United States.

SEXUAL FUNCTIONING. Marijuana is reported to enhance the sexual experience in both men and women. The intensified sensory awareness and the subjective slowness of time perception are thought to increase sexual satisfaction. Marijuana also enhances the sexual functioning by releasing inhibitions for certain activities that would normally be restrained.

Cannabis Intoxication

Cannabis intoxication is evidenced by the presence of clinically significant maladaptive behavioral or psychological changes that develop during, or shortly after, cannabis use (APA, 2000). Symptoms include impaired motor coordination, euphoria, anxiety, a sensation of slowed time, and impaired judgment. Physical symptoms include conjunctival injection, increased appetite, dry mouth, and tachycardia. The impairment of motor skills lasts for 8 to 12 hours and interferes with the operation of motor vehicles. These effects are additive to those of alcohol, which is commonly used in combination with cannabis (Sadock & Sadock, 2003).

Tables 13–7 and 13–8 include summaries of the psychoactive substances, including symptoms of intoxication, withdrawal, use, overdose, possible therapeutic uses, and trade and common names by which they may be referred.

APPLICATION OF THE NURSING PROCESS

Assessment

In the pre-introductory phase of relationship development, the nurse must examine his or her feelings about working with a client who abuses substances. If these behaviors are viewed as morally wrong and the nurse has internalized these attitudes from very early in life, it may be very difficult to suppress judgmental feelings. The role that alcohol or other substances has played (or plays) in the life of the nurse most certainly will affect the way in which he or she approaches interaction with the substance-abusing client.

How are attitudes examined? Some individuals may have sufficient ability for introspection to be able to recognize on their own whether they have unresolved issues related to substance abuse. For others, it may be more helpful to discuss these issues in a group situation, where insight may be gained from feedback regarding the perceptions of others.

TABLE 13–7 Psychoactive Substances: A Profile Summary

Class of Drugs	Symptoms of Use	Therapeutic Uses	Symptoms of Overdose	Trade Names	Common Names
CNS Depressants					
Alcohol	Relaxation, loss of inhibitions, lack of concentration, drowsiness, slurred speech, sleep	Antidote for methanol consumption; ingredient in many pharmacological concentrates	Nausea, vomiting; shallow respirations; cold, clammy skin; weak, rapid pulse; coma; possible death	Ethyl alcohol, beer, gin, rum, vodka, bourbon, whiskey, liqueurs, wine, brandy, sherry, champagne	Booze, alcohol, liquor, drinks, cocktails, highballs, nightcaps, moonshine, white lightening, firewater
Other (barbiturates and nonbarbiturates)	Same as alcohol	Relief from anxiety and insomnia; as anticonvulsants and anesthetics	Anxiety, fever, agitation, hallucinations, disorientation, tremors, delirium, convulsions, possible death	Seconal, Nembutal, Amytal Valium Librium Noctec Miltown	Red birds, yellow birds, blue birds Blues/yellows Green & Whites Mickies Downers
CNS Stimulants					
Amphetamines and related drugs	Hyperactivity, agitation, euphoria, insomnia, loss of appetite	Management of narcolepsy, hyperkinesia, and weight control	Cardiac arrhythmias, headache, convulsions, hypertension, rapid heart rate, coma, possible death	Dexedrine, Didrex, Tenuate, Prelu-2, Ritalin, Fastin, Cylert, Meridia, Plegine	Uppers, pep pills, wakeups, bennies, eye-openers, speed, black beauties, sweet As
Cocaine	Euphoria, hyperactivity, restlessness, talkativeness, increased pulse, dilated pupils, rhinitis	Topical anesthetic	Hallucinations, convulsions, pulmonary edema, respiratory failure, coma, cardiac arrest, possible death	Cocaine hydrochloride	Coke, flake, snow, dust, happy dust, gold dust, girl, cecil, C, toot, blow, crack
Opioids	Euphoria, lethargy, drowsiness, lack of motivation, constricted pupils	As analgesics; methadone in substitution therapy; heroin has no therapeutic use	Shallow breathing, slowed pulse, clammy skin, pulmonary edema, respiratory arrest, convulsions, coma, possible death	Heroin Morphine Codeine Dilaudid Demerol Dolophine Percodan Talwin Opium	Snow, stuff, H, harry, horse M, morph, Miss Emma Schoolboy Lords Doctors Dollies Perkies Ts Big O, black stuff
Hallucinogens	Visual hallucinations, disorientation, confusion, paranoid delusions, euphoria, anxiety, panic, increased pulse	LSD has been proposed in the treatment of chronic alcoholism, and in the reduction of intractable pain	Agitation, extreme hyperactivity, violence, hallucinations, psychosis, convulsions, possible death	LSD PCP Mescaline DMT STP	Acid, cube, big D Angel dust, hog, peace pill Mesc Businessman's trip Serenity and peace
Cannabinols	Relaxation, talkativeness, lowered inhibitions, euphoria, mood swings	Marijuana has been used for relief of nausea and vomiting associated with antineoplastic chemotherapy and to reduce eye pressure in glaucoma	Fatigue, paranoia, delusions, hallucinations, possible psychosis	Cannabis Hashish	Marijuana, pot, grass, joint, Mary Jane, MJ Hash, rope, Sweet Lucy

TABLE 13–8 Summary of Symptoms Associated with the Syndromes of Intoxication and Withdrawal

Class of Drugs	Intoxication	Withdrawal	Comments
Alcohol	Aggressiveness, impaired judgment, impaired attention, irritability, euphoria, depression, emotional lability, slurred speech, incoordination, unsteady gait, nystagmus, flushed face	Tremors, nausea/vomiting, malaise, weakness, tachycardia, sweating, elevated blood pressure, anxiety, depressed mood, irritability, hallucinations, headache, insomnia, seizures	Alcohol withdrawal begins within 4–6 hrs after last drink. May progress to delirium tremens on 2nd or 3rd day. Use of Librium or Serax is common for substitution therapy.
Amphetamines and related substances	Fighting, grandiosity, hypervigilance, psychomotor agitation, impaired judgment, tachycardia, pupillary dilation, elevated blood pressure, perspiration or chills, nausea and vomiting	Anxiety, depressed mood, irritability, craving for the substance, fatigue, insomnia or hypersomnia, psychomotor agitation, paranoid and suicidal ideation	Withdrawal symptoms usually peak within 2–4 days, although depression and irritability may persist for months. Tricyclic antidepressants may be used.
Caffeine	Restlessness, nervousness, excitement, insomnia, flushed face, diuresis, GI complaints, muscle twitching, rambling flow of thought and speech, cardiac arrhythmia, periods of inexhaustibility, psychomotor agitation	Headache	Caffeine is contained in coffee, tea, colas, cocoa, chocolate, some over-the-counter analgesics, "cold" preparations, and stimulants.
Cannabis	Euphoria, anxiety, suspiciousness, sensation of slowed time, impaired judgment, social withdrawal, tachycardia, conjunctival redness, increased appetite, hallucinations	Restlessness, irritability, insomnia, loss of appetite	Intoxication occurs immediately and lasts about 3 hours. Oral ingestion is more slowly absorbed and has longer-lasting effects.
Cocaine	Euphoria, fighting, grandiosity, hypervigilance, psychomotor agitation, impaired judgment, tachycardia, elevated blood pressure, pupillary dilation, perspiration or chills, nausea/vomiting, hallucinations, delirium	Depression, anxiety, irritability, fatigue, insomnia or hypersomnia, psychomotor agitation, paranoid or suicidal ideation, apathy, social withdrawal	Large doses of the drug can result in convulsions or death from cardiac arrhythmias or respiratory paralysis.
Inhalants	Belligerence, assaultiveness, apathy, impaired judgment, dizziness, nystagmus, slurred speech, unsteady gait, lethargy, depressed reflexes, tremor, blurred vision, stupor or coma, euphoria, irritation around eyes, throat, and nose		Intoxication occurs within 5 minutes of inhalation. Symptoms last 60–90 min. Large doses can result in death from CNS depression or cardiac arrhythmia.
Nicotine		Craving for the drug, irritability, anger, frustration, anxiety, difficulty concentrating, restlessness, decreased heart rate, increased appetite, weight gain, tremor, headaches, insomnia	Symptoms of withdrawal begin within 24 hours of last drug use and decrease in intensity over days, weeks, or sometimes longer.
Opioids	Euphoria, lethargy, somnolence, apathy, dysphoria, impaired judgment, pupillary constriction, drowsiness, slurred speech, constipation, nausea, decreased respiratory rate and blood pressure	Craving for the drug, nausea/vomiting, muscle aches, lacrimation or rhinorrhea, pupillary dilation, piloerection or sweating, diarrhea, yawning, fever, insomnia	Withdrawal symptoms from heroin appear within 6–8 hours after last dose, reach a peak in the 2nd or 3rd day, and disappear in 7–10 days. Times are shorter with meperidine and longer with methadone.

(Continued)

TABLE 13–8 Summary of Symptoms Associated with the Syndromes of Intoxication and Withdrawal *(Continued)*

Class of Drugs	Intoxication	Withdrawal	Comments
Phencyclidine and related substances	Belligerence, assaultiveness, impulsiveness, psychomotor agitation, impaired judgment, nystagmus, increased heart rate and blood pressure, diminished pain response, ataxia, dysarthria, muscle rigidity, seizures, hyperacusis, delirium		Delirium can occur within 24 hours after use of phencyclidine, or may occur up to a week following recovery from an overdose of the drug.
Sedatives, hypnotics and anxiolytics	Disinhibition of sexual or aggressive impulses, mood lability, impaired judgment, slurred speech, incoordination, unsteady gait, impairment in attention or memory, disorientation, confusion	Nausea/vomiting, malaise, weakness, tachycardia, sweating, anxiety, irritability, orthostatic hypotension, tremor, insomnia, seizures	Withdrawal may progress to delirium, usually within 1 week of last use. Long-acting barbiturates or benzodiazepines may be used in withdrawal substitution therapy.

Whether alone or in a group, the nurse may gain a greater understanding about attitudes and feelings related to substance abuse by responding to the following types of questions. As written here, the questions are specific to alcohol, but could be adapted for any substance.

What are my drinking patterns?
If I drink, why do I drink? When, where, and how much?
If I don't drink, why do I abstain?
Am I comfortable with my drinking patterns?
If I decided not to drink any more, would that be a problem for me?
What did I learn from my parents about drinking?
Have my attitudes changed as an adult?
What are my feelings about people who become intoxicated?
Does it seem more acceptable for some individuals than for others?
Do I ever use terms like "sot," "drunk," or "boozer" to describe some individuals who overindulge, yet overlook it in others?
Do I ever overindulge myself?
Has the use of alcohol (by myself or others) affected my life in any way?
Do I see alcohol/drug abuse as a sign of weakness? A moral problem? An illness?

Unless nurses fully understand and accept their own attitudes and feelings, they cannot be empathetic toward clients' problems. Clients in recovery need to know they are accepted for themselves, regardless of past behaviors. Nurses must be able to separate the client from the behavior and to accept that individual with unconditional positive regard.

Assessment Tools

Nurses are often the individuals who perform the admission interview. A variety of assessment tools is appropriate for use in chemical dependency units. A nursing history and assessment tool was presented in Chapter 6 of this text. With some adaptation, it is an appropriate instrument for creating a database on clients who abuse substances. Table 13–9 presents a drug history and assessment that could be used in conjunction with the general biopsychosocial assessment.

Other screening tools exist for determining whether an individual has a problem with substances. Two such tools developed by the APA for the diagnosis of alcoholism include the Michigan Alcoholism Screening Test and the CAGE Questionnaire (Tables 13–10 and 13–11). Some psychiatric units administer these surveys to all clients who are admitted to help determine if there is a secondary alcoholism problem in addition to the psychiatric problem for which the client is being admitted (sometimes called **dual diagnosis**). It would be possible to adapt these tools to use in diagnosing problems with other drugs as well.

Dual Diagnosis

If it is determined that the client has a coexisting substance disorder and mental illness, he or she may be assigned to a special program that targets both problems. Counseling for the mentally ill person who

TABLE 13-9 Drug History and Assessment*

1. When you were growing up, did anyone in your family drink alcohol or take other kinds of drugs?
2. If so, how did the substance use affect the family situation?
3. When did you have your first drink/drugs?
4. How long have you been drinking/taking drugs on a regular basis?
5. What is your pattern of substance use?
   a. When do you use substances?
   b. What do you use?
   c. How much do you use?
   d. Where are you and with whom when you use substances?
6. When did you have your last drink/drug? What was it and how much did you consume?
7. Does using the substance(s) cause problems for you? Describe. Include family, friends, job, school, other.
8. Have you ever experienced injury as a result of substance use?
9. Have you ever been arrested or incarcerated for drinking/using drugs?
10. Have you ever tried to stop drinking/using drugs? If so, what was the result? Did you experience any physical symptoms, such as tremors, headache, insomnia, sweating, or seizures?
11. Have you ever experienced loss of memory for times when you have been drinking/using drugs?
12. Describe a typical day in your life.
13. Are there any changes you would like to make in your life? If so, what?
14. What plans or ideas do you have for seeing that these changes occur?

* To be used in conjunction with general biopsychosocial nursing history and assessment tool (Chapter 6).

TABLE 13-10 Michigan Alcoholism Screening Test (MAST)

Answer the following questions by placing an X under yes or no.*	**Yes**	**No**
1. Do you enjoy a drink now and then?	0	0
2. Do you feel you are a normal drinker? (By normal we mean you drink less than or as much as most people.)		2
3. Have you ever awakened the morning after some drinking the night before and found that you could not remember a part of the evening?	2	
4. Does your wife, husband, parent, or other near relative ever worry or complain about your drinking?	1	
5. Can you stop drinking without a struggle after one or two drinks?		2
6. Do you ever feel guilty about your drinking?	1	
7. Do friends or relatives think you are a normal drinker?		2
8. Are you able to stop drinking when you want to?		2
9. Have you ever attended a meeting of AA?	5	
10. Have you gotten into physical fights when drinking?	1	
11. Has your drinking ever created problems between you and your wife, husband, a parent, or other relative?	2	
12. Has your wife, husband, or another family member ever gone to anyone for help about your drinking?	2	
13. Have you ever lost friends because of your drinking?	2	
14. Have you ever gotten into trouble at work or school because of drinking?	2	
15. Have you ever lost a job because of drinking?	2	
16. Have you ever neglected your obligations, your family, or your work for 2 or more days in a row because you were drinking?	2	
17. Do you drink before noon fairly often?	1	

(Continued)

TABLE 13-10 Michigan Alcoholism Screening Test (MAST) *(Continued)*

Answer the following questions by placing an X under yes or no.*	**Yes**	**No**
18. Have you ever been told you have liver trouble? Cirrhosis?	2	
19. After heavy drinking have you ever had delirium tremens (DTs) or severe shaking or heard voices or seen things that really were not there?	5	
20. Have you ever gone to anyone for help about your drinking?	5	
21. Have you ever been in a hospital because of drinking?	5	
22. Have you ever been a patient in a psychiatric hospital or on a psychiatric ward of a general hospital where drinking was part of the problem that resulted in hospitalization?	2	
23. Have you ever been seen at a psychiatric or mental health clinic or gone to any doctor, social worker, or clergyman for help with any emotional problem, where drinking was part of the problem?	2	
24. Have you ever been arrested for drunk driving, driving when intoxicated, or driving under the influence of alcoholic beverages? (If yes, how many times?_____)	2 ea	
25. Have you ever been arrested, or taken into custody, even for a few hours, because of other drunk behavior? (If yes, how many times?)	2 ea	

* Items are scored under the response that would indicate a problem with alcohol.
Method of scoring: 0–3 points = no problem with alcohol
4 points = possible problem with alcohol
5 or more = indicates problem with alcohol

From Selzer, M.L.: The Michigan alcohol screening test: The quest for a new diagnostic instrument. American Journal of Psychiatry 1971; 127: 1653–1658.

abuses substances takes a different approach than that which is directed at individuals who abuse substances but are not mentally ill. In the latter, many counselors use direct confrontation of the substance use behaviors. This approach is thought to be detrimental to the treatment of a chronically mentally ill person (Sciacca, 1996). Most dual diagnosis programs take a supportive and nonconfrontational approach.

Peer support groups are an important part of the treatment program. Sciacca (1996) states:

> One of the essential learning experiences is the relationship of the use of drugs or alcohol to each patient's psychiatric symptoms. Group members begin to identify these interaction effects in others and in themselves.

TABLE 13-11 The CAGE Questionnaire

1. Have you ever felt you should *C*ut down on your drinking?
2. Have people *A*nnoyed you by criticizing your drinking?
3. Have you ever felt bad or *G*uilty about your drinking?
4. Have you ever had a drink first thing in the morning to steady your nerves or get rid of a hangover (*E*ye-opener)?

Scoring: 2 or 3 "yes" answers strongly suggest a problem with alochol.

From Mayfield, D., McLeod, G. & Hall, P. (1974), with permission.

Speakers from Alcoholics Anonymous (AA), or other 12-step programs, are often invited to relate experiences to the group. Dual diagnosis clients are sometimes resistant to attending 12-step programs; however, after hearing these speakers, some clients are more amenable to joining these groups.

Substance abuse groups are integrated into regular programming for the psychiatric client with a dual diagnosis. An individual on the psychiatric unit or in a day treatment program will attend a substance abuse group periodically in lieu of another scheduled activity. Topics are directed toward areas that are unique to clients with a mental illness, such as mixing medications with other substances, as well as topics that are common to primary substance abusers. Individuals are encouraged to discuss their personal problems.

Velasco, Meyer, and Lippmann (1997) state:

> The prognosis for patients with psychiatric disorders is typically poorer with accompanying substance abuse than without such problems. For individuals with chemical dependence, the best predictor of improvement is a lessening in severity of concomitant psychiatric symptoms. Improved mental status has a positive impact on the addiction remission potential.

Continued attendance at 12-step group meetings is encouraged upon discharge from treatment. Family involvement is enlisted, and preventive strategies are outlined. Individual case management is common and success is often promoted by this close supervision.

Diagnosis/Outcome Identification

The next step in the nursing process is to identify appropriate nursing diagnoses by analyzing the data collected during the assessment phase. The individual who abuses or is dependent on substances undoubtedly has many unmet physical and emotional needs. Possible nursing diagnoses for clients with substance-related disorders include the following:

Ineffective denial related to weak, underdeveloped ego evidenced by "I don't have a problem with (substance). I can quit any time I want to"

Ineffective coping related to inadequate coping skills and weak ego evidenced by use of substances as a coping mechanism

Imbalanced nutrition: less than body requirements/ deficient fluid volume related to drinking or taking drugs instead of eating, evidenced by loss of weight, pale conjunctiva and mucous membranes, poor skin turgor, electrolyte imbalance, anemias, and other signs and symptoms of malnutrition/dehydration

Risk for infection related to malnutrition and altered immune condition

Low self-esteem related to weak ego, lack of positive feedback evidenced by criticism of self and others and use of substances as a coping mechanism (self-destructive behavior)

Deficient knowledge (effects of substance abuse on the body) related to denial of problems with substances evidenced by abuse of substances

For the client in substance withdrawal, possible nursing diagnoses include:

Risk for injury related to CNS agitation (withdrawal from CNS depressants)

Risk for suicide related to depressed mood (withdrawal from CNS stimulants)

The following criteria may be used for measurement of outcomes in the care of the client with substance related disorders.

The client:

1. Has not experienced physical injury
2. Has not caused harm to self or others
3. Accepts responsibility for own behavior
4. Acknowledges association between personal problems and use of substance(s)
5. Demonstrates more adaptive coping mechanisms that can be used in stressful situations (instead of taking substances)
6. Shows no signs or symptoms of infection or malnutrition
7. Exhibits evidence of increased self-worth by attempting new projects without fear of failure and by demonstrating less defensive behavior toward others
8. Verbalizes importance of abstaining from use of substances in order to maintain optimal wellness

Planning/Implementation

Table 13–12 provides a plan of care for the client with substance-related disorders. Selected nursing diagnoses are presented, along with outcome criteria, appropriate nursing interventions, and rationales for each. Refer to Appendix F for a critical pathway of care for the client in alcohol withdrawal.

Implementation with clients who abuse substances is a long-term process, often beginning with **detoxification** and progressing to total abstinence. The following common major treatment objectives have been identified for clients with substance-use disorders.

Detoxification

1. Provide a safe and supportive environment for the detoxification process.
2. Administer **substitution therapy** as ordered.

Intermediate Care

1. Provide explanations of physical symptoms.
2. Promote understanding and identify the causes of substance dependency.
3. Provide education and assistance in course of treatment to client and family.

Rehabilitation

1. Encourage continued participation in long-term treatment.
2. Promote participation in outpatient support system (e.g., AA).
3. Assist client to identify alternative sources of satisfaction.
4. Provide support for health promotion and maintenance.

TABLE 13–12 Care Plan for the Client with a Substance-Related Disorder

Nursing Diagnosis: INEFFECTIVE DENIAL
Related to: Weak, underdeveloped ego
Evidenced by: Statements indicating no problem with substance use.

Outcome Criteria	Nursing Interventions	Rationale
Client will demonstrate acceptance of responsibility for own behavior and acknowledge association between substance use and personal problems.	1. Develop trust. Convey an attitude of acceptance. Ensure that client understands it is not the *person* but the *behavior* that is unacceptable.	1. Unconditional acceptance promotes dignity and self-worth, qualities that this individual has been trying to achieve with substances.
	2. Correct any misconceptions, such as, "I don't have a drinking problem. I can quit any time I want to." Do this in a matter-of-fact, nonjudgmental manner.	2. These interventions help the client see the condition as an illness that requires help.
	3. Identify recent maladaptive behaviors or situations that have occurred in the client's life, and discuss how use of substances may be a contributing factor. Say, "The lab report shows your blood alcohol level was 250 when you were involved in that automobile accident."	3. The first step in decreasing use of denial is for the client to see the relationship between substance use and personal problems. To confront issues with a caring attitude preserves self-esteem.
	4. Do not allow client to rationalize or blame others for behaviors associated with substance use.	4. This only serves to prolong the denial.

Nursing Diagnosis: INEFFECTIVE COPING
Related to: Inadequate coping skills and weak ego
Evidenced by: Use of substances as coping mechanism

Outcome Criteria	Nursing Interventions	Rationale
Client will be able to verbalize adaptive coping mechanisms to use, instead of substance abuse, in response to stress (and demonstrate, as applicable).	1. Set limits on manipulative behavior. Administer consequences when limits are violated. Obtain routine urine samples for laboratory analysis of substances.	1. Because of weak ego and delayed development, client is unable to establish own limits or delay gratification. Client may obtain substances from various sources when in the hospital.
	2. Explore options available to assist with stress rather than resorting to substance use. Practice these techniques.	2. Because gratification has been closely tied to oral needs, it is unlikely that client is aware of more adaptive coping strategies.
	3. Give positive reinforcement for ability to delay gratification and respond to stress with adaptive coping strategies.	3. Because of weak ego, client needs lots of positive feedback to enhance self-esteem and promote ego development.

Nursing Diagnosis: IMBALANCED NUTRITION: LESS THAN BODY REQUIREMENTS/DEFICIENT FLUID VOLUME
Related to: Use of substances instead of eating
Evidenced by: Loss of weight, pale conjunctiva and mucous membranes, poor skin turgor, electrolyte imbalance, anemias (and/or other signs and symptoms of malnutrition/dehydration)

Outcome Criteria	Nursing Interventions	Rationale
Client will be free of signs/symptoms of malnutrition/dehydration.	1. Parenteral support may be required initially.	1. To correct fluid and electrolyte imbalance, hypoglycemia, and some vitamin deficiencies.
	2. Encourage cessation of smoking.	2. To facilitate repair of damage to GI tract.
	3. Consult dietitian. Determine the number of calories required based on body size and level of activity. Document intake, output and calorie count, and weigh client daily.	3. These interventions are necessary to maintain an ongoing nutritional assessment.

Outcome Criteria	Nursing Interventions	Rationale
	4. Ensure that the amount of protein in the diet is correct for the individual client's condition. Protein intake should be adequate to maintain nitrogen equilibrium, but should be drastically decreased or eliminated if there is potential for hepatic coma.	4. Diseased liver may be incapable of properly metabolizing proteins, resulting in an accumulation of ammonia in the blood that circulates to the brain and can result in altered consciousness.
	5. Sodium may need to be restricted.	5. To minimize fluid retention (e.g., ascites and edema).
	6. Provide foods that are nonirritating to clients with esophageal varices.	6. To avoid irritation and bleeding of these swollen blood vessels.
	7. Provide small frequent feedings of client's favorite foods. Supplement nutritious meals with multiple vitamin and mineral tablet.	7. To encourage intake and facilitate client's achievement of adequate nutrition.

Client/Family Education

The role of client teacher is important in the psychiatric area, as it is in all areas of nursing. A list of topics for client/family education relevant to substance-related disorders is presented in Table 13–13.

TABLE 13–13 Topics for Client/Family Education Related to Substance Use Disorders

Nature of the Illness
1. Effects of (substance) on the body
   a. Alcohol
   b. Other CNS depressants
   c. CNS stimulants
   d. Hallucinogens
   e. Inhalants
   f. Opioids
   g. Cannabinols
2. Ways in which use of (substance) affects life

Management of the Illness
1. Activities to substitute for (substance) in times of stress
2. Relaxation techniques
   a. Progressive relaxation
   b. Tense and relax
   c. Deep breathing
   d. Autogenics
3. Problem-solving skills
4. The essentials of good nutrition

Support Services
1. Financial assistance
2. Legal assistance
3. Alcoholics Anonymous (or other support group specific to another substance)
4. One-to-one support person

Evaluation

The final step of the nursing process involves reassessment to determine if the nursing interventions have been effective in achieving the intended goals of care. Evaluation of the client with a substance-related disorder may be accomplished by using information gathered from the following reassessment questions:

1. Has detoxification occurred without complications?
2. Is the client still in denial?
3. Does the client accept responsibility for his or her own behavior? Has he or she acknowledged a personal problem with substances?
4. Has a correlation been made between personal problems and the use of substances?
5. Does the client still make excuses or blame others for use of substances?
6. Has the client remained substance free during hospitalization?
7. Does the client cooperate with treatment?
8. Does the client refrain from manipulative behavior and violation of limits?
9. Is the client able to verbalize alternative adaptive coping strategies to substitute for substance use? Has the use of these strategies been demonstrated? Does positive reinforcement encourage repetition of these adaptive behaviors?
10. Has nutritional status been restored? Does the client consume diet adequate for his or her size and level of activity? Is the client able to discuss the importance of adequate nutrition?
11. Has the client remained free of infection during hospitalization?

12. Is the client able to verbalize the effects of substance abuse on the body?
13. Does the client verbalize that he or she wants to recover and lead a life free of substances?

TREATMENT MODALITIES FOR SUBSTANCE-RELATED DISORDERS

Alcoholics Anonymous

Alcoholics Anonymous (AA) is a major self-help organization for the treatment of alcoholism. It was founded in 1935 by two alcoholics—a stockbroker, Bill Wilson, and a physician, Dr. Bob Smith—who discovered that they could remain sober through mutual support. This they accomplished not as professionals, but as peers who were able to share their common experiences. Soon they were working with other alcoholics, who in turn worked with others. The movement grew, and remarkably, individuals who had been treated unsuccessfully by professionals were able to maintain sobriety through helping one another.

Today AA chapters exist in virtually every community in the United States. The self-help groups are based on the concept of peer support—acceptance and understanding from others who have experienced the same problems in their lives. The only requirement for membership is a desire on the part of the alcoholic person to stop drinking (AA, 2002a). Each new member is assigned a support person from whom he or she may seek assistance when the temptation to drink occurs.

A survey by the general service office of AA in 1998 (AA, 2002a) revealed the following statistics: members aged 30 and younger comprised 11 percent of the membership; women comprised 34 percent; 88 percent were white; 5 percent were African-American; 4 percent were Hispanic; 2 percent were Native American; and 1 percent were Asian-American and other minorities. The highest percentage (13 percent) represented occupations in the professional and technical fields.

The sole purpose of AA is to help members stay sober. When sobriety has been achieved, they in turn are expected to help other alcoholic persons. The Twelve Steps that embody the philosophy of AA provide specific guidelines on how to attain and maintain sobriety (Table 13–14).

AA accepts alcoholism as an illness and promotes total abstinence as the only cure, emphasizing that the alcoholic person can never safely return to social drinking. They encourage the members to seek sobriety, taking one day at a time. The Twelve Traditions, which are statements of principles that govern the organization, are presented in Table 13–15.

AA has been the model for various other self-help groups associated with abuse or dependency problems. Some of these groups and the memberships for which they are organized are listed in Table 13–16. Nurses need to be fully and accurately informed about available self-help groups and their importance as a treatment resource on the healthcare continuum so that they can use them as a referral source for clients with substance-related disorders.

TABLE 13–14 The Twelve Steps of Alcoholics Anonymous

1. We admitted we were powerless over alcohol—that our lives have become unmanageable.
2. Came to believe that a Power greater than ourselves could restore us to sanity.
3. Made a decision to turn our will and our lives over to the care of God as we understood Him.
4. Made a searching and fearless moral inventory of ourselves.
5. Admitted to God, to ourselves, and to another human being the exact nature of our wrongs.
6. Were entirely ready to have God remove all these defects of character.
7. Humbly asked Him to remove our shortcomings.
8. Made a list of all persons we had harmed and became willing to make amends to them all.
9. Made direct amends to such people whenever possible except when to do so would injure them or others.
10. Continued to take personal inventory and when we were wrong promptly admitted it.
11. Sought through prayer and meditation to improve our conscious contact with God as we understood Him, praying only for knowledge of His will for us and the power to carry that out.
12. Having a spiritual awakening as the result of these steps, we tried to carry this message to alcoholics and to practice these principles in all our affairs.

TABLE 13–15 The Twelve Traditions of Alcoholics Anonymous

1. Our common welfare should come first; personal recovery depends upon AA unity.
2. For our group purpose there is but one ultimate authority—a loving God as He may express Himself in our group conscience. Our leaders are but trusted servants; they do not govern.
3. The one requirement for AA membership is a desire to stop drinking.
4. Each group should be autonomous except in matters affecting other groups or AA as a whole.
5. Each group has but one primary purpose—to carry its message to the alcoholic who still suffers.
6. An AA group ought never endorse, finance, or lend the AA name to any related facility or outside enterprise, lest problems of money, property, and prestige divert us from our primary purpose.
7. Every AA group ought to be fully self-supporting, declining outside contributions.
8. Alcoholics Anonymous should remain forever nonprofessional, but our service centers may employ special workers.
9. Alcoholics Anonymous, as such, ought never be organized; but we may create service boards of committees directly responsible to those they serve.
10. Alcoholics Anonymous has no opinion on outside issues; hence, the Alcoholics Anonymous name ought never be drawn into public controversy.
11. Our public relations policy is based on attraction rather than promotion; we need always maintain personal anonymity at the level of press, radio, and films.
12. Anonymity is the spiritual foundation of all our traditions, ever reminding us to place principles before personalities.

Pharmacotherapy

Disulfiram (Antabuse)

Disulfiram (Antabuse) is a drug that can be administered to individuals who abuse alcohol as a deterrent to drinking. Ingestion of alcohol when disulfiram is in the body results in a syndrome of symptoms that can produce a good deal of discomfort for the individual.

TABLE 13–16 Addiction Self-Help Groups

Group	Membership
Adult Children of Alcoholics (ACOA)	Adults who grew up with an alcoholic in the home
Al-Anon	Families of alcoholics
Alateen	Adolescent children of alcoholics
Children Are People	School-age children with an alcoholic family member
Cocaine Anonymous	Cocaine addicts
Families Anonymous	Parents of children who abuse substances
Fresh Start	Nicotine addicts
Narcotics Anonymous	Narcotic addicts
Nar-Anon	Families of narcotic addicts
Overeaters Anonymous	Food addicts
Pills Anonymous	Polysubstance addicts
Potsmokers Anonymous	Marijuana smokers
Smokers Anonymous	Nicotine addicts
Women for Sobriety	Female alcoholics

It can even result in death if the blood alcohol level is high. The reaction varies according to the sensitivity of the individual and how much alcohol was ingested.

Disulfiram works by inhibiting the enzyme aldehyde dehydrogenase, thereby blocking the oxidation of alcohol at the stage when acetaldehyde is converted to acetate. This results in an accumulation of acetaldehyde in the blood, which is thought to produce the symptoms associated with the disulfiram-alcohol reaction. These symptoms persist as long as alcohol is being metabolized. The rate of alcohol elimination does not appear to be affected.

Symptoms of disulfiram-alcohol reaction can occur within 5 to 10 minutes of ingestion of alcohol. Mild reactions can occur at blood alcohol levels as low as 5 to 10 mg/dL. Symptoms are fully developed at approximately 50 mg/dL and may include flushed skin, throbbing in the head and neck, respiratory difficulty, dizziness, nausea and vomiting, sweating, hyperventilation, tachycardia, hypotension, weakness, blurred vision, and confusion. With a blood alcohol level of approximately 125 to 150 mg/dL, severe reactions can occur, including respiratory depression, cardiovascular collapse, arrhythmias, myocardial infarction, acute congestive heart failure, unconsciousness, convulsions, and death.

Disulfiram should not be administered until it has been ascertained that the client has abstained from alcohol for at least 12 hours. If disulfiram is discontinued, it is important for the client to understand that the sensitivity to alcohol may last for as long as 2 weeks. Consuming alcohol or alcohol-containing substances during this 2-week period could result in the disulfiram-alcohol reaction.

The client receiving disulfiram therapy should be aware of the great number of alcohol-containing substances. These products (e.g., liquid cough and cold preparations, vanilla extract, aftershave lotions, colognes, mouthwash, nail polish removers, and isopropyl alcohol), if ingested or even rubbed on the skin, are capable of producing the symptoms described. The individual must read labels carefully and must inform any doctor, dentist, or other healthcare professional from which assistance is sought that he or she is taking disulfiram. In addition, it is important that the client carry a card explaining participation in disulfiram therapy, possible consequences of the therapy, and symptoms that may indicate an emergency.

Obviously, the client must be assessed carefully before beginning disulfiram therapy. A thorough medical screening is performed before starting therapy, and written informed consent is usually required. The drug is contraindicated for clients who are at high risk for alcohol ingestion. It is also contraindicated for psychotic clients and clients with severe cardiac, renal, or hepatic disease.

Disulfiram therapy is not a cure for alcoholism. It provides a measure of control for the individual who desires to avoid impulse drinking. Clients receiving disulfiram therapy are encouraged to seek other assistance with their problem, such as AA or other support groups, to aid in the recovery process.

Other Medications for Treatment of Alcoholism

The narcotic antagonist naltrexone (ReVia), was approved by the FDA in 1994 for the treatment of alcohol dependence. Naltrexone, which was approved in 1984 for the treatment of heroin abuse, works on the same receptors in the brain that produce the feelings of pleasure when heroin or other opiates bind to them, but it does not produce the "narcotic high" and is not habit forming. Although alcohol does not bind to these same brain receptors, studies have shown that naltrexone works equally well against it (O'Malley et al., 1992; Volpicelli et al., 1992). In comparison to the placebo-treated clients, subjects on naltrexone therapy showed significantly lower overall relapse rates and fewer drinks per drinking day among those clients who did resume drinking. A study with an oral form of nalmefene (Revex) has produced similar results (Mason et al., 1994).

The efficacy of selective serotonin reuptake inhibitors (SSRIs) in the decrease of alcohol craving among alcohol-dependent individuals has yielded mixed results (NIAAA, 1997). A greater degree of success was observed with moderate drinkers than with heavy drinkers.

Counseling

Counseling on a one-to-one basis is often used to help the client who abuses substances. The relationship is goal-directed, and the length of the counseling may vary from weeks to years. The focus is on current reality, active development of a working treatment relationship, environmental manipulation, and strengthening ego assets. The counselor must be warm, kind, and nonjudgmental, yet able to set limits firmly. Najavits and Weiss (1994) state, "The primary characteristic of counselors that influences treatment outcome appears to be interpersonal functioning, including therapists' empathy, genuineness, and respect for patients."

Counseling of the client who abuses substances passes through various phases, each of which is of indeterminate length. In the first phase, an assessment is conducted. Factual data is collected to determine whether the client does indeed have a problem with substances; that is, that substances are regularly impairing effective functioning in a significant life area.

Following the assessment, in the working phase of the relationship, the counselor assists the individual to work on acceptance of the fact that the use of substances causes problems in significant life areas and that he or she is not able to prevent it from occurring. The client states a desire to make changes. The strength of the denial system is determined by the duration and extent of substance-related adverse effects in the person's life. Thus, those individuals with rather minor substance-related problems of recent origin have less difficulty with this stage than those with long-term extensive impairment. The individual also works to gain self-control and abstain from substances.

Once the problem has been identified and sobriety is achieved, the client must have a concrete and workable plan for getting through the early weeks of abstinence. Anticipatory guidance through role-play helps the individual practice how he or she will respond when substances are readily obtainable and the impulse to partake is strong.

Counseling often includes the family or specific family members. In family counseling the therapist tries to help each member see how he or she has affected, and been affected by, the substance abuse behavior. Family strengths are mobilized, and family members are encouraged to move in a positive direction. Referrals are often made to self-help groups such as Al-Anon, Nar-Anon, Alateen, Families Anonymous, and Adult Children of Alcoholics.

Group Therapy

Group therapy with substance abusers has long been regarded as a powerful agent of change. In groups, individuals are able to share their experiences with others who are going through similar problems. They are able to "see themselves in others" and confront their defenses about giving up the substance. They may confront similar attitudes and defenses in others. Groups also give individuals the capacity for communicating needs and feelings directly.

Some groups may be task-oriented education groups in which the leader is charged with presenting material associated with substance abuse and its various effects on the person's life. Other educational groups that may be helpful with individuals who abuse substances include assertiveness techniques and relaxation training. Teaching groups differ from psychotherapy groups, whose focus is more on helping individuals understand and manage difficult feelings and situations, particularly as they relate to use of substances.

Therapy groups and self-help groups such as AA are complementary to each other. Whereas the self-help group focus is on achieving and maintaining sobriety, in the therapy group the individual may learn more adaptive ways of coping, how to deal with problems that may have arisen or were exacerbated by the former substance use, and ways to improve quality of life and to function more effectively without substances.

Psychopharmacology for Substance Intoxication and Substance Withdrawal

Various medications have been used to decrease the intensity of symptoms in an individual who is withdrawing from, or who is experiencing the effects of excessive use of, alcohol and other drugs. **Substitution therapy** may be required to reduce the life-threatening effects of intoxication or withdrawal from some substances. The severity of the withdrawal syndrome depends on the particular drug used, how long it has been used, the dose used, and the rate at which the drug is eliminated from the body (Bennett & Woolf, 1991).

Alcohol

Benzodiazepines are the most widely used group of drugs for substitution therapy in alcohol withdrawal. Chlordiazepoxide (Librium), oxazepam (Serax), and diazepam (Valium) are the most commonly used agents. Because of its ability to decrease the cardiovascular hyperactivity associated with alcohol withdrawal, the benzodiazepine alprazolam (Xanax) is also frequently being used (NIAAA, 1997). The approach to treatment with benzodiazepines for alcohol withdrawal is to start with relatively high doses and reduce the dosage by 20 to 25 percent each day until withdrawal is complete. In clients with liver disease, accumulation of the longer-acting agents (chlordiazepoxide and diazepam) may be problematic, and the use of the shorter-acting benzodiazepine, oxazepam, is more appropriate. Studies have also indicated that control of withdrawal symptoms with benzodiazepines on an "as-needed basis," rather than a fixed schedule, has resulted in the need for lower doses of the medication and less time in treatment (NIAAA, 1997).

Some physicians may order anticonvulsant medication (e.g., carbamazepine, valproic acid, or gabapentin) for management of withdrawal seizures. These drugs are particularly useful in individuals who undergo repeated episodes of alcohol withdrawal. Repeated episodes of withdrawal appear to "kindle" even more serious withdrawal episodes, including the production of withdrawal seizures that can result in brain damage (Julien, 2001). These anticonvulsants have been used successfully in both acute withdrawal and longer-term craving situations.

Multivitamin therapy, in combination with daily injections or oral administration of thiamine, is common protocol. Thiamine is commonly deficient in chronic alcoholics. Replacement therapy is required to prevent neuropathy, confusion, and encephalopathy.

Opioids

Examples of opioids are heroin, morphine, opium, meperidine, codeine, and methadone. Withdrawal symptoms generally begin within 8 to 12 hours after the last opioid dose and become most intense by 36 to 48 hours. The acute phase of withdrawal is over in approximately 10 days; however, symptoms of irritability and restlessness may persist for 2 to 3 months.

Opioid intoxication is treated with narcotic antagonists such as naloxone (Narcan), naltrexone (ReVia), or nalmefene (Revex). Withdrawal therapy includes rest, adequate nutritional support, and methadone substitution. Methadone is given on the first day in a dose sufficient to suppress withdrawal symptoms. The dose is then gradually tapered over a specified time. Federal regulations allow methadone detoxification in licensed facilities to last as long as 180 days (Mirin et al., 2002). As the dose of methadone diminishes, renewed abstinence symptoms may be ameliorated by the addition of clonidine.

In October 2002, the FDA approved two forms of the drug buprenorphine for treating opiate dependence. Buprenorphine is less powerful than methadone but is considered somewhat safer and causes fewer side effects, making it especially attractive for clients who are mildly or moderately addicted. Individuals will be able to access treatment with buprenorphine in office-based settings, providing a choice to methadone clinics. Physicians are deemed qualified to prescribe buprenorphine if they hold an addiction certification from the American Society of Addiction Medicine, the American Academy of Addiction Psychiatry, the APA, or other associations deemed appropriate (Manisses, 2002).

Clonidine (Catapres) also has been used to suppress opiate withdrawal symptoms. As monotherapy, it is not as effective as substitution with methadone, it is nonaddicting, and serves effectively as a bridge to enable the client to stay opiate-free long enough to facilitate termination of methadone maintenance.

Depressants

Substitution therapy for CNS depressant withdrawal (particularly barbiturates) is most commonly with the long-acting barbiturate phenobarbital (Luminal). The dosage required to suppress withdrawal symptoms is administered. When stabilization has been achieved, the dose is gradually decreased by 30 mg/day until withdrawal is complete. Long-acting benzodiazepines are commonly used for substitution therapy when the abused substance is a nonbarbiturate CNS depressant (Ashton, 2002).

Stimulants

Treatment of stimulant intoxication usually begins with minor tranquilizers such as chlordiazepoxide (Librium) and progresses to major tranquilizers such as haloperidol (Haldol). Antipsychotics should be administered with caution because of their propensity to lower seizure threshold (Mack, Franklin, & Frances, 2003). Repeated seizures are treated with intravenous diazepam.

Withdrawal from CNS stimulants is not the medical emergency observed with CNS depressants. Treatment is usually aimed at reducing drug craving and managing severe depression. The client is placed in a quiet atmosphere and allowed to sleep and eat as much as is needed or desired. Suicide precautions may need to be instituted. Antidepressant therapy may be helpful in treating symptoms of depression. Desipramine has been especially successful with symptoms of cocaine withdrawal and abstinence (Mack, Franklin, & Frances, 2003).

Hallucinogens and Cannabinols

Substitution therapy is not required with these drugs. When adverse reactions (e.g., anxiety or panic) occur, benzodiazepines (e.g., diazepam or chlordiazepoxide) may be prescribed to prevent harm to the client or others. Psychotic reactions may be treated with antipsychotic medications.

SUMMARY

An individual is considered to be dependent on a substance when he or she is unable to control its use, even knowing that it interferes with normal functioning; when more and more of the substance is required to produce the desired effects; and when characteristic withdrawal symptoms develop upon cessation or drastic decrease in use of the substance. Abuse is considered when there is continued use of the substance despite having a persistent or recurrent problem that is caused or exacerbated by its use or when the substance is used in physically hazardous situations.

Substance intoxication is defined as the development of a reversible syndrome of maladaptive behavioral or psychological changes that are due to the direct physiological effects of a substance on the CNS and develop during or shortly after ingestion of (or exposure to) a substance. Substance withdrawal is the development of a substance-specific maladaptive behavioral change, with physiological and cognitive concomitants, that is due to the cessation of, or reduction in, heavy and prolonged substance use.

The etiology of substance-use disorders is unknown. Various contributing factors have been implicated, such as genetics, biochemical changes, developmental influences, personality factors, social learning, conditioning, and cultural and ethnic influences.

Seven classes of substances are presented in terms of a profile of the substance, historical aspects, patterns of use and abuse, and effects on the body. These seven classes include alcohol, other CNS depressants, CNS stimulants, opioids, hallucinogens, inhalants, and cannabinols.

The nursing process is presented as the vehicle for delivery of care of the client with a substance-related disorder. The nurse must first examine his or her own feelings regarding personal substance use and the substance use of others. Only the nurse who can be accepting and nonjudgmental of substance-abuse behaviors will be effective in working with these clients. Care of clients with dual diagnoses of mental illness and substance use disorders was discussed.

Treatment modalities for substance-related disorders include self-help groups, deterrent therapy, individual counseling, and group therapy. Substitution pharmacotherapy is frequently implemented with clients experiencing substance intoxication or substance withdrawal. Treatment modalities are implemented on an inpatient basis or in outpatient settings, depending on the severity of the impairment.

REVIEW QUESTIONS

SELF-EXAMINATION/LEARNING EXERCISE

Select the answer that is most appropriate for each of the following questions:

Situation: Mr. White is admitted to the hospital after an extended period of binge alcohol drinking. His wife reports that he has been a heavy drinker for a number of years. Lab reports reveal he has a blood alcohol level of 250 mg/dL. He is placed in the chemical dependency unit for detoxification.

1. When would the first signs of alcohol withdrawal symptoms be expected to occur?
   a. Several hours after the last drink.
   b. Two to three days after the last drink.
   c. Four to five days after the last drink.
   d. Six to seven days after the last drink.

2. Symptoms of alcohol withdrawal include:
   a. Euphoria, hyperactivity, and insomnia.
   b. Depression, suicidal ideation, and hypersomnia.
   c. Diaphoresis, nausea and vomiting, and tremors.
   d. Unsteady gait, nystagmus, and profound disorientation.

3. Which of the following medications is the physician most likely to order for Mr. White during his withdrawal syndrome?
   a. Haloperidol (Haldol).
   b. Chlordiazepoxide (Librium).
   c. Propoxyphene (Darvon).
   d. Phenytoin (Dilantin).

Situation: Dan, age 32 years, has been admitted for inpatient treatment of his alcoholism. He began drinking when he was 15 years old. Through the years, the amount of alcohol he consumes has increased. He and his wife report that for the last 5 years he has consumed at least a pint of bourbon a day. He also drinks beer and wine. He has been sneaking drinks at work, and his effectiveness has started to decline. His boss has told him he must seek treatment or he will be fired. This is his second week in treatment. The first week he experienced an uncomplicated detoxification.

4. Dan states, "I don't have a problem with alcohol. I can handle my booze better than anyone I know. My boss is a jerk! I haven't missed any more days than my coworkers." The nurse's best response is:
   a. "Maybe your boss is mistaken, Dan."
   b. "You are here because your drinking was interfering with your work, Dan."
   c. "Get real, Dan! You're a boozer and you know it!"
   d. "Why do you think your boss sent you here, Dan?"

5. The defense mechanism that Dan is using is:
   a. Denial.
   b. Projection.
   c. Displacement.
   d. Rationalization.

6. Dan's drinking buddies come for a visit, and when they leave, the nurse smells alcohol on Dan's breath. Which of the following would be the best intervention with Dan at this time?

a. Search his room for evidence.
b. Ask, "Have you been drinking alcohol, Dan?"
c. Send a urine specimen from Dan to the lab for drug screening.
d. Tell Dan, "These guys cannot come to the unit to visit you again."

7. Dan begins attendance at AA meetings. Which of the statements by Dan reflects the purpose of this organization?
   a. "They claim they will help me stay sober."
   b. "I'll dry out in AA, then I can have a social drink now and then."
   c. "AA is only for people who have reached the bottom."
   d. "If I lose my job, AA will help me find another."

The following general questions relate to substance abuse:

8. From which of the following symptoms might the nurse identify a chronic cocaine user?
   a. Clear, constricted pupils.
   b. Red, irritated nostrils.
   c. Muscle aches.
   d. Conjunctival redness.
9. An individual who is addicted to heroin is likely to experience which of the following symptoms of withdrawal?
   a. Increased heart rate and blood pressure.
   b. Tremors, insomnia, and seizures.
   c. Incoordination and unsteady gait.
   d. Nausea and vomiting, diarrhea, and diaphoresis.
10. A polysubstance abuser makes the statement, "The green and whites do me good after speed." How might the nurse interpret the statement?
   a. The client abuses amphetamines and anxiolytics.
   b. The client abuses alcohol and cocaine.
   c. The client is psychotic.
   d. The client abuses narcotics and marijuana.

Test Your CRITICAL THINKING SKILLS

Kelly, age 23 years, is a first-year law student. She is engaged to a surgical resident at the local university hospital. She has been struggling to do well in law school because she wants to make her parents, two prominent local attorneys, proud of her. She had never aspired to do anything but go into law, and that is what her parents expected her to do.

Kelly's midterm grades were not as high as she had hoped, so she increased the number of hours of study time, staying awake all night several nights a week to study. She started drinking large amounts of coffee to stay awake, but still found herself falling asleep as she tried to study at the library and in her apartment. As final exams approached, she began to panic that she would not be able to continue the pace of studying she felt she needed in order to make the grades for which she hoped.

One of Kelly's classmates told her that she needed some "speed" to give her that extra energy to study. Her classmate said, "All the kids do it. Hardly anyone I know gets through law school without it." She gave Kelly the name of a source.

Kelly contacted the source, who supplied her with enough amphetamines to see her through final exams. Kelly was excited because she had so much energy, did not require sleep, and was able to study the additional hours she thought she needed for the exams. However, when the results were posted, Kelly had failed two courses and would have to repeat them in summer school if she was to continue with her class in the fall. She continued to replenish her supply of amphetamines from her "contact" until he told her he could not get her anymore. She became frantic, stole a prescription blank from her fiancé, and forged his name for more pills.

She started taking increasing amounts of the medication in order to achieve the "high" she wanted to feel. Her behavior became erratic. Yesterday, her fiancé received a call from a pharmacy to clarify an order for amphetamines that Kelly had written. He insisted that she admit herself to the chemical dependency unit for detoxification.

On the unit, she appears tired, depressed, moves very slowly, and wants to sleep all the time. She keeps saying to the nurse, "I'm a real failure. I'll never be an attorney like my parents. I'm too dumb. I just wish I could die."

Answer the following questions related to Kelly:

1. What is the primary nursing diagnosis for Kelly?
2. Describe important nursing interventions to be implemented with Kelly.
3. In addition to physical safety, what would be the primary short-term goal the nurses would strive to achieve with Kelly?

IMPLICATIONS OF RESEARCH FOR EVIDENCE-BASED PRACTICE

Gaffney, K.F.: **Infant exposure to environmental tobacco smoke.** Journal of Nursing Scholarship (2001) 33 (4), 343–347.

Description of the Study: A review of 10 studies with a range of 100 to more than 1,000 participants was conducted. The studies took place in a variety of healthcare settings in the United States, Australia, and Europe. The studies measured infant exposure to environmental tobacco smoke (ETS). Parents of the infants completed the self-reports that inquired about number of people in the household who smoked and the proximity of the infant to the smoking. The studies focused on children in the first year of life.

Results of the Study: In one of the studies, questionnaire information was supported by hair analysis of the subjects. Median level of hair nicotine was over 1.5 times higher among infants in homes reported by means of questionnaires to have smokers than among those in homes reported to have no smokers. Eight of the 10 studies demonstrated increased risk for poor infant health outcomes associated with ETS exposure. Positive associations were found between infant ETS exposure and gastroesophageal reflux, colic, sudden infant death syndrome, lower respiratory tract infections, ear infections, and altered thyroid function.

Implications for Nursing Practice: The author suggests that nurses may use these results to document the need for identifying mothers who smoke as an important target group for clinical intervention. She states, "This review shows the importance of identifying and assisting mothers who smoke so that this critical proximity with their infants may provide optimal health promotion. Nurses who care for infants as part of the regular health maintenance visits conducted during the first year of life are particularly well-prepared and logically situated to advise and assist these mothers as they initiate the long-term process of smoking cessation."

INTERNET REFERENCES

- Additional information on addictions may be located at the following websites:
  - a http://www.recovery-works.com
  - b http://www.ncbi.nlm.nih.gov
  - c http://www.addictions.org/recoveryworks/
  - d http://www.drugs.indiana.edu

- Additional information on self-help organizations may be located at the following websites:
  - a **http://www.ca.org (Cocaine Anonymous)**
  - b **http://www.aa.org (AA)**
  - c **http://www.delphi.com (Narcotics Anonymous)**

- Additional information about medications for treatment of alcohol and drug dependence may be located at the following websites:
  - a **http://www.fadavis.com/townsend**
  - b **http://www.nlm.nih.gov/medlineplus/**

REFERENCES

Alcoholics Anonymous (AA). (2002a). Analysis of the 1998 survey of the membership of AA. Retrieved February 19, 2002 from http://www.aa.org/english/E_FactFile/P-48_d1.html.

Alcoholics Anonymous. (2002b). The twelve steps of Alcoholics Anonymous. Retrieved on 5-17-04 from http://www.alcoholics-anonymous.org/default/en_services_aa_sub.cfm? subpageid=44&pageid=34

Alcoholics Anonymous. (2002c). A.A. Traditions. Retrieved on 5-17-04 from http://www.alcoholics-anonymous.org/default/en_about_aa_sub.cfm?subpageid=20&pageid=24

American Academy of Child & Adolescent Psychiatry. (1999). Children of alcoholics. Retrieved February 19, 2002, from http://www.aacap.org/publications/factsfam/Alcoholc.htm

American Psychiatric Association (APA). (2000). Diagnostic and statistical manual of mental disorders (4th ed.), Text Revision. Washington, DC: American Psychiatric Association.

Ashton, C.H. (2002). Benzodiazepines: How the work and how to withdraw. Newcastle upon Tyne, UK: University of Newcastle.

Barclay, L.L. (2002). Alcohol-related neurologic disease. Retrieved on February 15, 2002, from http://www2.vhihealthe.com/article/gale/100085011

Behavioral Neuroscience Laboratory. (2002). Tetrahydroisoquinolines and alcohol preference in rats. Retrieved February 14, 2002, from http://www-org.usm.edu/~7Eneurolab/research.htm

Bennett, E.G., & Woolf, D. (1991). Substance abuse: Pharmacologic, developmental, and clinical perspectives (2nd ed.). Albany, NY: Delmar Publishers.

Berger, P.A. (2002). Lysergic acid diethylamide. Encarta Online Encyclopedia. Retrieved February 17, 2002, from http://encarta.msn.com/find/Concise.asp?ti=0564B000

Byers, V.L. (1991). Central nervous system stimulants. In M.M. Kuhn (Ed.), Pharmacotherapeutics: A nursing process approach (2nd ed.). Philadelphia: F.A. Davis.

Franklin, J.E & Frances, R.J. (1999). Alcohol and other psychoactive substance use disorders. In R.E. Hales & S.C. Yudofsky (Eds.), Essentials of clinical psychiatry. Washington, D.C.: American Psychiatric Press.

Goldstein, A. (1994). Addiction: From biology to drug policy. New York: W.H. Freeman.

Habal, R. (2001). Toxicity, barbiturate. Retrieved on October 7, 2003, from http://www.emedicine.com/med/topic207.htm

Harvard Medical School. (2001). Alcohol use and abuse. Boston: Harvard Health Publications.

Hermes, W.J. (1993). Substance abuse. New York: Chelsea House Publishers.

Holbrook, J.M. (1991). Hallucinogens. In E.G. Bennett, & D. Woolf (Eds.), Substance abuse (2nd ed.). Albany, NY: Delmar Publishers.

Jernigan, R. (2002). Heroin. Florida State University School. Retrieved on February 26, 2002, from http://www.fsus.fsu.edu/general/drugs/effects_heroin.html

Julien, R.M. (2001). A primer of drug action: A concise nontechnical guide to the actions, uses, and side effects of psychoactive drugs, Revised & updated (9th ed.). New York: W.H. Freeman.

Kibbey, H. (2002). Genetic influences on alcohol drinking and alcoholism. Indiana University. Retrieved February 14, 2002, from http://www.indiana.edu/~rcapub/v17n3/p18.html

Mack, A.H., Franklin, J.E., & Frances, R.J. (2003). Substance use disorders. In R.E. Hales & S.C. Yudofsky (Eds.), Textbook of Clinical Psychiatry (4th ed.).Washington, D.C.: American Psychiatric Publishing.

Manisses Communications Group. (2002). Will buprenorphine usher in new era for opiate treatment? Alcoholism and Drug Abuse Weekly 14: 1, 6–7.

Marijuana and Reproduction. (2002). Effects on the male and female reproductive systems. Retrieved February, 17, 2002, from http://babyparenting.about.com/library/blmarij1.htm

Mason, G.J., et al. (1994). Double-blind, placebo-controlled pilot study to evaluate the efficacy and safety of oral nalmefene HCl for alcohol dependence. Alcoholism, Clinical and Experimental Research 18:1162–1167.

Mirin, S.M., et al. (2002). Practice guidelines for the treatment of patients with substance use disorders: Alcohol, cocaine, opioids. In the American Psychiatric Association Practice Guidelines for the Treatment of Psychiatric Disorders, Compendium 2002. Washington, D.C.: American Psychiatric Association.

Najavits, L.M., & Weiss, R.D. (1994). Variations in therapist effectiveness in the treatment of patients with substance use disorders: An empirical review. Addiction 89: 679–688.

National Council on Alcoholism and Drug Dependence (2002). All about alcohol. Retrieved February 15, 2002, from http://www.ocnow.com/community/groups/ncadd/All_About_Alcohol.html

National Institute on Alcohol Abuse and Alcoholism (NIAAA)(1997). Ninth special report to the U.S. Congress on alcohol and health. Rockville, MD: The Institute.

National Institutes of Health (NIH) (2003). Workshop on the medical utility of marijuana. Retrieved on October 10, 2003, at http://www.nih.gov/news/medmarijuana/MedicalMarijuana.htm#CLINICAL

National Library of Medicine. (2002). Hepatic encephalopathy. Retrieved on February 15, 2002, from http://www.nlm.nih.gov/medlineplus/ency/article/000302.htm

Newhouse, E. (1999, August 22). Bane of the Blackfeet. Great Falls Tribune Retrieved on February 14, 2002, from http://www.gannett.com/go/difference/greatfalls/pages/part8/blackfeet.html

O'Malley, et al. (1992). Naltrexone and coping skills therapy for alcohol dependence: A controlled study. Archives of General Psychiatry 49:881–887.

Sadock, B.J. & Sadock, V.A. (2003). Synopsis of psychiatry: Behavioral sciences/ clinical psychiatry (9th ed.). Philadelphia: Lippincott Williams & Wilkins.

Schuckit, M.A. (2000). Alcohol and alcoholism. Retrieved on March 10, 2001, from http://psychiatry.medscape.com/HOL/articles/2000/09/hol25/pnt-hol25.html

Sciacca, K. (1996). New initiatives in the treatment of the chronic patient with alcohol/substance use problems. Retrieved on October 10, 2003, from http://users.erols.com/ksciacca/newinit.htm

Street Drugs. (2001). Plymouth, MN: The Publishers Group.

Substance Abuse and Mental Health Services Administration (SAMHSA). (2002a). National household survey on drug abuse, 2000. Retrieved on February 15, 2002, from http://www.samhsa.gov/oas/NHSDA/2kNHSDA/chapter3.htm

Substance Abuse and Mental Health Services Administration (SAMHSA). (2002b). National household survey on drug abuse, 2000. Retrieved on February 17, 2002, from http://www.samhsa.gov/oas/NHSDA/2kNHSDA/chapter2.htm

Substance Abuse and Mental Health Services Administration (SAMHSA). (2003). Office of Applied Studies. 2002 National Survey on Drug Use and Health. Washington, DC: U.S. Department of Health and Human Services.

United States Drug Enforcement Administration (USDEA). (2003). Drug information: Cannabis. Retrieved October 9, 2003, from http://www.dea.gov

Velasco, J., Meyer, A., & Lippmann, S. (1997). How to treat coexistent mental illness and substance abuse. Retrieved October 3, 2003, from http://www.sma.org/smj/97feb3.htm

Virginia Alcohol Safety Action Program (VASAP). (2002). Effects of alcohol on your body. Retrieved on February 15, 2002, from http://www.vasap.state.va.us/Vasap/effects.htm

Volpicelli, J.R, Alterman, A.I., Hayashida, M., & O'Brien, C.P. (1992). Naltrexone in the treatment of alcohol dependence. Archives of General Psychiatry 49:876–880.

Worman, H.J. (1998). Alcoholic liver disease. Columbia University. Retrieved on February 15, 2002 from http://cpmcnet.columbia.edu/dept/gi/alcohol.html

CLASSICAL REFERENCES

Jellinek, E.M. (1952). Phases of alcohol addiction. Quarterly Journal of Studies on Alcohol 13:673–684.

Mayfield, D., McLeod, G., & Hall, P. (1974). The CAGE questionnaire: Validation of a new alcoholism screening instrument. American Journal of Psychiatry, 131:1121–1123.

Seltzer, M.L. (1971). The Michigan Alcoholism Screening Test: The quest for a new diagnostic instrument. American Journal of Psychiatry, 127:1653–1658.

14

CHAPTER

Schizophrenia and Other Psychotic Disorders

CHAPTER OUTLINE

KEY TERMS

delusions
hallucinations
illusion
echolalia
echopraxia
paranoia
religiosity
magical thinking
neuroleptic
neologism
word salad
circumstantiality
tangentiality
perseveration
clang association
catatonic behavior
autism
waxy flexibility
anhedonia
associative looseness
social skills training

OBJECTIVES

After reading this chapter, the student will be able to:

1. Discuss the concepts of schizophrenia and related psychotic disorders.
2. Identify etiological implications in the development of these disorders.
3. Describe various types of schizophrenia and related psychotic disorders.
4. Identify symptomatology associated with these disorders and use this information in client assessment.
5. Formulate nursing diagnoses and goals of care for clients with schizophrenia and other psychotic disorders.
6. Identify topics for client and family teaching relevant to schizophrenia and other psychotic disorders.
7. Describe appropriate nursing interventions for behaviors associated with these disorders.
8. Describe relevant criteria for evaluating nursing care of clients with schizophrenia and related psychotic disorders.
9. Discuss various modalities relevant to treatment of schizophrenia and related psychotic disorders.

INTRODUCTION

The term *schizophrenia* was coined in 1908 by the Swiss psychiatrist Eugen Bleuler. The word was derived from the Greek "skhizo" (split) and "phren" (mind).

Over the years, much debate has surrounded the concept of schizophrenia. Various definitions of the disorder have evolved, and numerous treatment strategies have been proposed, but none have proved to be uniformly effective or sufficient.

Although the controversy lingers, two general factors appear to be gaining acceptance among clinicians. The first is that schizophrenia is probably not a homogeneous disease entity with a single cause but results from a variable combination of genetic predisposition, biochemical dysfunction, physiological factors, and psychosocial stress. The second factor is that there is not now and probably never will be a single treatment that cures the disorder. Instead, effective treatment requires a comprehensive, multidisciplinary effort, including pharmacotherapy and various forms of psychosocial care, such as living skills and **social skills training**, rehabilitation, and family therapy.

Of all the mental illnesses responsible for suffering in society, schizophrenia probably causes more lengthy hospitalizations, more chaos in family life, more exorbitant costs to individuals and governments, and more fears than any other. Because it is such an enormous threat to life and happiness and because its causes are an unsolved puzzle, it has probably been studied more than any other mental disorder.

The following remarks were made by Dr. Laura Hall before the U.S. Congress, at a symposium on schizophrenia research cosponsored by the National Foundation for Brain Research and the National Alliance for the Mentally Ill in March 1996:

> Approximately 1.7 million American adults have the brain disorder schizophrenia. No more than 15 percent of them have a job. They make up more than half of the long-term residents of state and county mental hospitals. They, and others with severe mental illnesses, make up at least one-third of our nation's homeless population. Between 10 and 15 percent of individuals with schizophrenia, commit suicide, usually before age 30. About 8 percent of people in our jails have schizophrenia and are usually housed there for want of appropriate treatment and housing facilities. People with schizophrenia are disproportionately the victims of crime.

This chapter explores various theories of predisposing factors that have been implicated in the development of schizophrenia. Symptomatology associated with different diagnostic categories of the disorder is discussed. Nursing care is presented in the context of the six steps of the nursing process. Various dimensions of medical treatment are explored.

NATURE OF THE DISORDER

Perhaps no psychological disorder is more crippling than schizophrenia. Characteristically, disturbances in thought processes, perception, and affect invariably result in a severe deterioration of social and occupational functioning.

In the United States, the lifetime prevalence of schizophrenia is about 1 percent (Sadock & Sadock, 2003). Societal economic costs are estimated in billions of dollars per year. Symptoms generally appear in late adolescence or early adulthood, although they may occur in middle or late adult life (American Psychiatric Association [APA], 2000). Some studies have indicated that symptoms occur earlier in men than in women. The premorbid personality often indicates social maladjustment or schizoid or other personality disturbances (Black & Andreasen, 1999). This premorbid behavior is often a predictor in the pattern of development of schizophrenia, which can be viewed in four phases.

Phase I: The Schizoid Personality. The *DSM-IV-TR* (APA, 2000) describes this individual as indifferent to social relationships and having a very limited range of emotional experience and expression. They do not enjoy close relationships and prefer to be "loners." They appear cold and aloof. Not all individuals who demonstrate the characteristics of schizoid personality will progress to schizophrenia. However, most individuals with schizophrenia show evidence of having these characteristics in the premorbid condition.

Phase II: The Prodromal Phase. Characteristics of this phase include social withdrawal; impairment in role functioning; behavior that is peculiar or eccentric; neglect of personal hygiene and grooming; blunted or inappropriate affect; disturbances in communication; bizarre ideas; unusual perceptual experiences; and lack of initiative, interests, or energy. The length of this phase is highly variable and may last for many years before deteriorating to the schizophrenic state.

Phase III: Schizophrenia. In the active phase of the disorder, psychotic symptoms are prominent.

Following are the *DSM-IV-TR* (APA, 2000) diagnostic criteria for schizophrenia:

1. **Characteristic Symptoms:** Two (or more) of the following, each present for a significant portion of time during a 1-month period (or less if successfully treated): **delusions, hallucinations,** disorganized speech (e.g., frequent derailment or incoherence), grossly disorganized or **catatonic behavior**, negative symptoms (i.e., affective flattening, alogia, or avolition).
2. **Social/Occupational Dysfunction:** For a significant portion of the time since the onset of the disturbance, one or more major areas of functioning—such as work, interpersonal relations, or self-care—are markedly below the level achieved before the onset (or when the onset is in childhood or adolescence there is failure to achieve expected level of interpersonal, academic, or occupational achievement).
3. **Duration:** Continuous signs of the disturbance persist for at least 6 months. This 6-month period must include at least 1 month of symptoms (or less if successfully treated) that meet criterion 1 (i.e., active-phase symptoms) and may include periods of prodromal or residual symptoms. During these prodromal or residual periods, the signs of the disturbance may be manifested by only negative symptoms, or two or more symptoms listed in criterion 1 present in an attenuated form (e.g., odd beliefs, unusual perceptual experiences).
4. **Schizoaffective and Mood Disorder Exclusion:** Schizoaffective disorder and mood disorder with psychotic features have been ruled out because (1) no major depressive, manic, or mixed episodes have occurred concurrently with the active-phase symptoms; or (2) if mood episodes have occurred during active-phase symptoms, their total duration has been brief relative to the duration of the active and residual periods.
5. **Substance/General Medical Condition Exclusion:** The disturbance is not due to the direct physiological effects of a substance (e.g., a drug of abuse, a medication) or a general medical condition.
6. **Relationship to a Pervasive Developmental Disorder:** If there is a history of autistic disorder or another pervasive developmental disorder, the additional diagnosis of schizophrenia is made only if prominent delusions or hallucinations are also present for at least 1 month (or less if successfully treated).

Phase IV: Residual Phase. Schizophrenia is characterized by periods of remission and exacerbation. A residual phase usually follows an active phase of the illness. Symptoms during the residual phase are similar to those of the prodromal phase, with flat affect and impairment in role functioning being prominent. Residual impairment often increases between episodes of active psychosis.

A return to full premorbid functioning is not common (APA, 2000). However, several factors have been associated with a more positive prognosis. These include good premorbid adjustment, later age at onset, being female, abrupt onset of symptoms precipitated by a stressful event (as opposed to gradual insidious onset of symptoms), associated mood disturbance, brief duration of active-phase symptoms, good interepisode functioning, minimal residual symptoms, absence of structural brain abnormalities, normal neurological functioning, a family history of mood disorder, and no family history of schizophrenia (APA, 2000).

ETIOLOGICAL IMPLICATIONS

The cause of schizophrenia is still uncertain. Most likely no single factor can be implicated in the etiology; rather, the disease probably results from a combination of influences including biological, psychological, and environmental factors.

Biological Influences

Refer to Chapter 3 for a more thorough review of the biological implications of psychiatric illness.

Genetics

The body of evidence for genetic vulnerability to schizophrenia is growing. Studies show that relatives of individuals with schizophrenia have a much higher probability of developing the disease than does the general population. Whereas the lifetime risk for developing schizophrenia is about 1 percent in most population studies, the siblings or offspring of an identified client have a 5 to 10 percent risk of developing schizophrenia (Ho, Black, & Andreasen, 2003).

How schizophrenia is inherited is uncertain. No reliable biological marker has yet been found. It is unknown which genes are important in the vulnerability to schizophrenia or whether one or many genes are implicated. Some individuals have a strong genetic link to the illness, whereas others may have only a weak genetic basis. This theory gives further credence to the notion of multiple causations.

TWIN STUDIES. The rate of schizophrenia among monozygotic (identical) twins is 4 times that of dizygotic (fraternal) twins and almost 50 times that of the general population (Sadock & Sadock, 2003). Identical twins reared apart have the same rate of development of the illness as do those reared together. Because in about half of the cases only one of a pair of monozygotic twins develops schizophrenia, some investigators believe environmental factors interact with genetic ones.

ADOPTION STUDIES. In studies conducted by both American and Danish investigators, adopted children born of schizophrenic mothers were compared with adopted children whose mothers had no psychiatric disorder. It was found that the children who were born of schizophrenic mothers were more likely to develop the illness than the comparison control groups (Black & Andreasen, 1999). Studies also indicate that children born of nonschizophrenic parents, but reared by schizophrenic parents, do not seem to suffer more often from schizophrenia than general controls. These findings provide additional evidence for the genetic basis of schizophrenia.

Biochemical Influences

The oldest and most thoroughly explored biological theory in the explanation of schizophrenia attributes a pathogenic role to abnormal brain biochemistry. Notions of a "chemical disturbance" as an explanation for insanity were suggested by some theorists as early as the mid-19th century.

THE DOPAMINE HYPOTHESIS. This theory suggests that schizophrenia (or schizophrenia-like symptoms) may be caused by an excess of dopamine-dependent neuronal activity in the brain. This excess activity may be related to increased production or release of the substance at nerve terminals, increased receptor sensitivity, too many dopamine receptors, or a combination of these mechanisms (Sadock & Sadock, 2003).

Pharmacological support for this hypothesis exists. Amphetamines, which increase levels of dopamine, induce psychotomimetic symptoms (Sadock & Sadock, 2003). The **neuroleptics** (e.g., chlorpromazine or haloperidol) lower brain levels of dopamine by blocking dopamine receptors, thus reducing the schizophrenic symptoms, including those induced by amphetamines.

Postmortem studies of schizophrenic brains have reported a significant increase in the average number of dopamine receptors in approximately two-thirds of the brains studied. This suggests that an increased dopamine response may not be important in *all* schizophrenic clients. Clients with acute manifestations (e.g., delusions and hallucinations) respond with greater efficacy to neuroleptic drugs than do clients with chronic manifestations (e.g., apathy, poverty of ideas, and loss of drive). The current position, in terms of the dopamine hypothesis, is that manifestations of acute schizophrenia may be related to increased numbers of dopamine receptors in the brain and respond to neuroleptic drugs that block these receptors. Manifestations of chronic schizophrenia are probably unrelated to numbers of dopamine receptors, and neuroleptic drugs are unlikely to be as effective in treating these chronic symptoms.

OTHER BIOCHEMICAL HYPOTHESES. Various other biochemicals have been implicated in the predisposition to schizophrenia. Abnormalities in the neurotransmitters norepinephrine, serotonin, acetylcholine, and gamma-aminobutyric acid and in the neuroregulators, such as prostaglandins and endorphins, have been suggested.

Physiological Influences

A number of physical factors of possible etiological significance have been identified in the medical literature, although their specific mechanisms in the implication of schizophrenia are unclear.

VIRAL INFECTION. Sadock and Sadock (2003) report that epidemiological data indicate a high incidence of schizophrenia after prenatal exposure to influenza. They state:

> Other data supporting a viral hypothesis are an increased number of physical anomalies at birth, an increased rate of pregnancy and birth complications, seasonality of birth consistent with viral infection, geographical clusters of adult cases, and seasonality of hospitalizations. (p. 482)

Other studies have suggested that the exposure is most significant if it occurs during the second trimester of pregnancy (Mednick, 1991). Further research is required into this hypothesis of psychoimmunology as an etiological implication for schizophrenia.

ANATOMICAL ABNORMALITIES. With the use of neuroimaging technologies, structural brain abnormalities have been observed in individuals with schizophrenia. Ventricular enlargement is the most consistent finding; however, sulci enlargement and cerebellar atrophy are also reported (Ho, Black, & Andreasen, 2003). Ho, Black, and Andreasen (2003) state:

> There is substantial evidence to suggest that ventricular enlargement is associated with poor premorbid functioning, negative symptoms, poor response to treatment, and cognitive impairment. CT scan abnormalities may have some clinical significance, but they are not diagnostically specific; similar abnormalities are seen in other disorders such as Alzheimer's disease or alcoholism. (p. 405)

Magnetic resonance imaging (MRI) provides a greater ability to image in multiple planes. Studies with MRI have revealed a possible decrease in cerebral and intracranial size in clients with schizophrenia. Studies have also revealed a decrease in frontal lobe size, but this has been less consistently replicated. MRI has been used to explore possible abnormalities in specific subregions such as the amygdala, hippocampus, temporal lobes, and basal ganglia in the brains of people with schizophrenia.

HISTOLOGICAL CHANGES. Scheibel and his associates (1991) at the University of California at Los Angeles have studied cerebral changes at the microscopic level. In studying brains of clients with schizophrenia, they found a "disordering" or disarray of the pyramidal cells in the area of the hippocampus. This they compared with the normal alignment of the cells in the brains of clients without the disorder. They have hypothesized that this alteration in hippocampal cells occurs during the second trimester of pregnancy and may be related to an influenza virus encountered by the mother during this period. Further research is required to determine the possible link between this birth defect and the development of schizophrenia.

PHYSICAL CONDITIONS. Some studies have reported a link between schizophrenia and epilepsy (particularly temporal lobe), Huntington's chorea, birth trauma, head injury in adulthood, alcohol abuse, cerebral tumor (particularly in the limbic system), cerebrovascular accidents, systemic lupus erythematosus, myxedema, parkinsonism, and Wilson's disease.

Psychological Influences

Early conceptualizations of schizophrenia focused on family relationship factors as major influences in the development of the illness. This probably occurred in light of the conspicuous absence of information related to a biological connection. These early theories related to poor parent-child relationships and dysfunctional family systems as the cause of schizophrenia.

Can family interaction patterns cause schizophrenia? The answer is most probably not. Researchers are now focusing their studies more in terms of schizophrenia as a brain disorder. Nevertheless, Sadock and Sadock (2003) state:

> Clinicians should consider the psychosocial factors affecting schizophrenia. Although, historically, theorists have attributed the development of schizophrenia to psychosocial factors, contemporary clinicians can benefit from using the relevant theories and guidelines of these past observations and hypotheses. Although many psychodynamic theories about the pathogenesis of schizophrenia seem out of date, perceptive clinical observations can help contemporary clinicians understand how the disease may affect a patient's psyche. (p. 483)

Environmental Influences

Sociocultural Factors

Many studies have been conducted that have attempted to link schizophrenia to social class. Indeed, epidemiological statistics have shown that greater numbers of individuals from the lower socioeconomic classes experience symptoms associated with schizophrenia than do those from the higher socioeconomic groups (Ho, Black & Andreasen, 2003). Explanations for this occurrence include the conditions associated with living in poverty, such as congested housing accommodations, inadequate nutrition, absence of prenatal care, few resources for dealing with stressful situations, and feelings of hopelessness for changing one's lifestyle of poverty.

An alternative view is that of the *downward drift hypothesis* (Sadock & Sadock, 2003). This hypothesis relates the schizophrenic's move into, or failure to move out of, the low socioeconomic group to the tendency for social isolation and the segregation of self from others—characteristics of the disease process itself. Proponents of this notion view poor social conditions as a consequence rather than a cause of schizophrenia.

Stressful Life Events

Studies have been conducted in an effort to determine whether psychotic episodes may be precipitated by stressful life events. There is no scientific evidence to indicate that stress causes schizophrenia. However, it is very probable that stress may contribute to the severity and course of the illness. It is known that extreme stress can precipitate psychotic episodes (Sackeim & Mukherjee, 1992). Stress may indeed precipitate symptoms in an individual who possesses a genetic vulnerability to schizophrenia. Sadock and Sadock (2003) state:

> The stress can be biological, environmental, or both. The environmental component can be biological (e.g., an infection) or psychological (e.g., a stressful family situation). (p. 477)

Stressful life events may be associated with exacerbation of schizophrenic symptoms and increased rates of relapse.

Theoretical Integration

The etiology of schizophrenia remains unclear. No single theory or hypothesis has been postulated that substantiates a clear-cut explanation for the disease. Indeed, it seems the more research that is conducted, the more evidence is compiled to support the concept of multiple causation in the development of schizophrenia. The most current theory seems to be that schizophrenia is a biologically based disease, the onset of which is influenced by factors in the environment (internal or external).

TYPES OF SCHIZOPHRENIA AND OTHER PSYCHOTIC DISORDERS

The *DSM-IV-TR* (APA, 2000) identifies various types of schizophrenia and other psychotic disorders. Differential diagnosis is made according to the total symptomatic clinical picture presented.

Disorganized Schizophrenia

This type was previously called *hebephrenic schizophrenia.* Onset of symptoms is usually before age 25 years, and the course is commonly chronic. Behavior is markedly regressive and primitive. Contact with reality is extremely poor. Affect is flat or grossly inappropriate, often with periods of silliness and incongruous giggling. Facial grimaces and bizarre mannerisms are common, and communication is consistently incoherent. Personal appearance is generally neglected, and social impairment is extreme.

Catatonic Schizophrenia

Catatonic schizophrenia is characterized by marked abnormalities in motor behavior and may be manifested in the form of *stupor* or *excitement* (Sadock & Sadock, 2003).

Catatonic stupor is characterized by extreme psychomotor retardation. The individual exhibits a pronounced decrease in spontaneous movements and activity. Mutism (i.e., absence of speech) is common, and negativism (i.e., an apparently motiveless resistance to all instructions or attempts to be moved) may be evident. **Waxy flexibility** may be exhibited. This term describes a type of "posturing," or voluntary assumption of bizarre positions, in which the individual may remain for long periods. Efforts to move the individual may be met with rigid bodily resistance.

Catatonic excitement is manifested by a state of extreme psychomotor agitation. The movements are frenzied and purposeless and are usually accompanied by continuous incoherent verbalizations and shouting. Clients in catatonic excitement urgently require physical and medical control because they are often destructive and violent to others, and their excitement can cause them to injure themselves or to collapse from complete exhaustion.

Catatonic schizophrenia was quite common before the advent of antipsychotic medications for use in psychiatry. The illness is now rare in Europe and North America (Sadock & Sadock, 2003).

Paranoid Schizophrenia

Paranoid schizophrenia is characterized mainly by the presence of delusions of persecution or grandeur and auditory hallucinations related to a single theme. The individual is often tense, suspicious, and guarded, and may be argumentative, hostile, and aggressive. Onset of symptoms is usually later (perhaps in the late 20s or 30s), and less regression of mental faculties, emotional response, and behavior is seen than in the other subtypes of schizophrenia. Social impairment may be minimal, and there is some evidence that prognosis, particularly with regard to occupational functioning and capacity for independent living, is promising (APA, 2000).

Undifferentiated Schizophrenia

Sometimes clients with schizophrenic symptoms do not meet the criteria for any of the subtypes, or they may meet the criteria for more than one subtype. These individuals may be given the diagnosis of undifferentiated schizophrenia. The behavior is clearly psychotic; that is, there is evidence of delusions, hallucinations, incoherence, and bizarre behavior. However, the symptoms cannot be easily classified into any of the previously listed diagnostic categories.

Residual Schizophrenia

This diagnostic category is used when the individual has a history of at least one previous episode of schizophrenia with prominent psychotic symptoms. Residual schizophrenia occurs in an individual who has a chronic form of the disease and is the stage that follows an acute episode (prominent delusions, hallucinations, incoherence, bizarre behavior, and violence). In the residual stage, there is continuing evidence of the illness, although there are no prominent psychotic symptoms. Residual symptoms may include social isolation, eccentric behavior, impairment in personal hygiene and grooming, blunted or inappropriate affect, poverty of or overly elaborate speech, illogical thinking, or apathy.

Schizoaffective Disorder

This disorder is manifested by schizophrenic behaviors, with a strong element of symptomatology associated with the mood disorders (mania or depression). The client may appear depressed, with psychomotor retardation and suicidal ideation, or symptoms may include euphoria, grandiosity, and hyperactivity. However, the decisive factor in the diagnosis of schizoaffective disorder is the presence of characteristic schizophrenic symptoms. For example, in addition to the dysfunctional mood, the individual exhibits bizarre delusions, prominent hallucinations, incoherent speech, catatonic behavior, or blunted or inappropriate affect. The prognosis for schizoaffective disorder is generally better than that for other schizophrenic disorders but worse than that for mood disorders alone (Sadock & Sadock, 2003).

Brief Psychotic Disorder

The essential feature of this disorder is the sudden onset of psychotic symptoms that may or may not be preceded by a severe psychosocial stressor. These symptoms last at least 1 day but less than 1 month, and there is an eventual full return to the premorbid level of functioning (APA, 2000). The individual experiences emotional turmoil, overwhelming perplexity, or confusion. Evidence of impaired reality testing may include incoherent speech, delusions, hallucinations, bizarre behavior, and disorientation. Individuals with preexisting personality disorders (most commonly, histrionic, narcissistic, paranoid, schizotypal, and borderline personality disorders) appear to be susceptible to this disorder (Sadock & Sadock, 2003).

Schizophreniform Disorder

The essential features of this disorder are identical to those of schizophrenia, with the exception that the duration, including prodromal, active, and residual phases, is at least 1 month but less than 6 months (APA, 2000). If the diagnosis is made when the individual is still symptomatic but has been so for less than 6 months, it is qualified as "provisional." The diagnosis is changed to schizophrenia if the clinical picture persists beyond 6 months.

Schizophreniform disorder is thought to have a good prognosis if at least two of the following features are present:

1. Onset of prominent psychotic symptoms within 4 weeks of first noticeable change in usual behavior or functioning
2. Confusion or perplexity at the height of the psychotic episode
3. Good premorbid social and occupational functioning
4. Absence of blunted or flat affect (APA, 2000).

Delusional Disorder

The essential feature of this disorder is the presence of one or more nonbizarre delusions that persist for at least 1 month (APA, 2000). If present at all, hallucinations are not prominent, and apart from the delusions, behavior is not bizarre. The subtype of delusional disorder is based on the predominant delusional theme.

Erotomanic Type

With this type of delusion, the individual believes that someone, usually of a higher status, is in love with him or her. Famous persons are often the subjects of erotomanic delusions. Sometimes the delusion is kept secret, but some individuals may follow, contact, or otherwise try to pursue the object of their delusion.

Grandiose Type

Individuals with grandiose delusions have irrational ideas regarding their own worth, talent, knowledge, or power. They may believe that they have a special relationship with a famous person or even assume the identity of a famous person (believing that the actual person is an imposter). Grandiose delusions of a religious nature may lead to assumption of the identity of a deity or religious leader.

Jealous Type

The content of jealous delusion centers on the idea that the person's sexual partner is unfaithful. The idea is irrational and without cause, but the deluded individual searches for evidence to justify the belief. The sexual partner is confronted (and sometimes physically attacked) regarding the imagined infidelity. The imagined "lover" of the sexual partner may also be the object of the attack. Attempts to restrict the autonomy of the sexual partner in an effort to stop the imagined infidelity are common.

Persecutory Type

In persecutory delusions, which are the most common type, individuals believe they are being malevolently treated in some way. Frequent themes include being conspired against, cheated, spied on, followed, poisoned or drugged, maliciously maligned, harassed, or obstructed in the pursuit of long-term goals (APA, 2000). The individual may obsess about and exaggerate a slight rebuff (real or imagined) until it becomes the focus of a delusional system. Repeated complaints may be directed at legal authorities, lack of satisfaction from which may result in violence toward the object of the delusion.

Somatic Type

Individuals with somatic delusions believe they have some physical defect, disorder, or disease. The *DSM-IV-TR* (APA, 2000) identifies the most common types of somatic delusions as those in which the individual believes that he or she:

1. Emits a foul odor from the skin, mouth, rectum, or vagina
2. Has an infestation of insects in or on the skin
3. Has an internal parasite
4. Has misshapen and ugly body parts
5. Has dysfunctional body parts

Shared Psychotic Disorder

The essential feature of this disorder, also called *folie à deux*, is a delusional system that develops in a second person because of a close relationship with another person who already has a psychotic disorder with prominent delusions (APA, 2000). The person with the primary delusional disorder is usually the dominant person in the relationship, and the delusional thinking is gradually imposed on the more passive partner. This occurs within the context of a long-term close relationship, particularly when the couple has been socially isolated from other people. The course is usually chronic and is more common in women than in men.

Psychotic Disorder Due to a General Medical Condition

The essential features of this disorder are prominent hallucinations and delusions that can be directly attributed to a general medical condition (APA, 2000). The diagnosis is not made if the symptoms occur during the course of a delirium or chronic, progressing dementia. A number of medical conditions can cause psychotic symptoms. Common ones identified by the *DSM-IV-TR* (APA, 2000) are presented in Table 14–1.

Substance-Induced Psychotic Disorder

The essential features of this disorder are the presence of prominent hallucinations and delusions that are

TABLE 14–1 General Medical Conditions that May Cause Psychotic Symptoms

Neurological conditions	Neoplasms Cerebrovascular disease Huntington's disease Epilepsy Auditory nerve injury Deafness Migraine headache CNS infection
Endocrine conditions	Hyperthyroidism Hypothyroidism Hyperparathyroidism Hypoparathyroidism Hypoadrenocorticism
Metabolic conditions	Hypoxia Hypercarbia Hypoglycemia
Autoimmune disorders	Systemic lupus erythematosus
Others	Fluid or electrolyte imbalances Hepatic or renal diseases

judged to be directly attributable to the physiological effects of a substance (i.e., a drug of abuse, a medication, or toxin exposure) (APA, 2000). The diagnosis is made in the absence of reality testing and when history, physical examination, or laboratory findings indicate use of substances. When reality testing has been retained in the presence of substance-induced psychotic symptoms, the diagnosis would be substance-related disorder (Sadock & Sadock, 2003). Substances identified by the *DSM-IV-TR* (APA, 2000) that are believed to induce psychotic disorders are presented in Table 14–2.

TABLE 14–2 Substances that May Cause Psychotic Disorders

Drugs of abuse	Alcohol Amphetamines and related substances Cannabis Cocaine Hallucinogens Inhalants Opioids Phencyclidine and related substances Sedatives, hypnotics, and anxiolytics
Medications	Anesthetics and analgesics Anticholinergic agents Anticonvulsants Antidepressant medication Antihistamines Antihypertensive agents Cardiovascular medications Antimicrobial medications Antiparkinsonian agents Chemotherapeutic agents Corticosteroids Disulfiram Gastrointestinal medications Muscle relaxants Nonsteroidal antiinflammatory agents
Toxins	Anticholinesterase Organophosphate insecticides Nerve gases Carbon monoxide Carbon dioxide Volatile substances (e.g., fuel or paint)

APPLICATION OF THE NURSING PROCESS

Background Assessment Data

In the first step of the nursing process, the nurse gathers a database from which nursing diagnoses are derived and a plan of care is formulated. This first step of the nursing process is extremely important because without an accurate assessment, problem identification, objectives of care, and outcome criteria cannot be accurately determined.

Assessment of the client with schizophrenia may be a complex process, based on information gathered from a number of sources. Clients in an acute episode of their illness are seldom able to make a significant contribution to their history. Data may be obtained from family members, if possible; from old records, if available; or from other individuals who have been in a position to report on the progression of the client's behavior.

The nurse must be familiar with behaviors common to the disorder in order to obtain an adequate assessment of the client with schizophrenia. The *DSM-III-R* (APA, 1987) previously presented behavioral disturbances in eight areas of functioning: content of thought, form of thought, perception, affect, sense of self, volition, impaired interpersonal functioning and relationship to the external world, and psychomotor behavior. These areas of functioning are employed to facilitate the presentation of background information on which to base the initial assessment of the client with schizophrenia. Additional impairments outside the limits of these eight areas are also presented.

Content of Thought

DELUSIONS. Delusions are false personal beliefs that are inconsistent with the person's intelligence or cultural background. The individual continues to have the belief in spite of obvious proof that it is false or irrational. Delusions are subdivided according to their content. Some of the more common ones are listed here.

Delusion of Persecution. The individual feels threatened and believes that others intend harm or persecution toward him or her in some way (e.g., "The FBI has 'bugged' my room and intends to kill me." "I can't take a shower in this bathroom; the nurses have put a camera in there so that they can watch everything I do.").

Delusion of Grandeur. The individual has an exaggerated feeling of importance, power, knowledge, or identity (e.g., "I am Jesus Christ").

Delusion of Reference. All events within the environment are referred by the psychotic person to himself or herself (e.g., "Someone is trying to get a message to me through the articles in this magazine [or newspaper or TV program]; I must break the code so that I can receive the message."). Ideas of reference are less rigid than delusions of reference. An example of an idea of reference is the person irrationally thinking that he or she is being talked about or laughed at by other people.

Delusion of Control or Influence. The individual believes certain objects or persons have control over his or her behavior (e.g., "The dentist put a filling in my tooth; I now receive transmissions through the filling that control what I think and do.").

Somatic Delusion. The individual has a false idea about the functioning of his or her body (e.g., "I'm 70 years old and I will be the oldest person ever to give birth. The doctor says I'm not pregnant, but I know I am.").

Nihilistic Delusion. The individual has a false idea that the self, a part of the self, others, or the world is nonexistent (e.g., "The world no longer exists." "I have no heart.").

RELIGIOSITY. **Religiosity** is an excessive demonstration of or obsession with religious ideas and behavior. Because individuals vary greatly in their religious beliefs and level of spiritual commitment, religiosity is often difficult to assess. The individual with schizophrenia may use religious ideas in an attempt to provide rational meaning and structure to his or her behavior. Religious preoccupation in this vein may therefore be considered a manifestation of the illness. However, clients who derive comfort from their religious beliefs should not be discouraged from employing this means of support. An example of religiosity is the individual who believes the voice he or she hears is God and incessantly searches the Bible for interpretation.

PARANOIA. Individuals with **paranoia** have extreme suspiciousness of others and of their actions or perceived intentions (e.g., "I won't eat this food; I know it has been poisoned.").

MAGICAL THINKING. With **magical thinking,** the person believes that his or her thoughts or behaviors have control over specific situations or people (e.g., the mother who believed if she scolded her son in any way he would be taken away from her). Magical thinking is common in children (e.g., "Step on a crack and you break your mother's back." "An apple a day keeps the doctor away.").

Form of Thought

ASSOCIATIVE LOOSENESS. Thinking is characterized by speech in which ideas shift from one unrelated subject to another. With **associative looseness**, the individual is unaware that the topics are unconnected. When the condition is severe, speech may be incoherent. (For example, "We wanted to take the bus, but the airport took all the traffic. Driving is the ticket when you want to get somewhere. No one needs a ticket to heaven. We have it all in our pockets.")

NEOLOGISMS. The psychotic person invents new words, or **neologisms,** that are meaningless to others but have symbolic meaning to the psychotic person (e.g., "She wanted to give me a ride in her new *uniphorum*.").

CONCRETE THINKING. Concreteness, or literal interpretations of the environment, represents a regression to an earlier level of cognitive development. Abstract thinking is very difficult. For example, the client with schizophrenia has great difficulty describing the abstract meaning of sayings such as "I'm climbing the walls," or "It's raining cats and dogs."

CLANG ASSOCIATIONS. Choice of words is governed by sounds. **Clang associations** often take the form of rhyming; for example, "It is very cold. I am cold and bold. The gold has been sold."

WORD SALAD. A **word salad** is a group of words that are strung together in a random fashion, without any logical connection (e.g., "Most forward action grows life double plays circle uniform.").

CIRCUMSTANTIALITY. With **circumstantiality**, the individual is delayed in reaching the point of a communication because of unnecessary and tedious details. The point or goal is usually met but only with numerous interruptions by the interviewer to keep the person on track of the topic being discussed.

TANGENTIALITY. **Tangentiality** differs from circumstantiality in that the person never really gets to the point of the communication. Unrelated topics are introduced, and the original discussion is lost.

MUTISM. This is an individual's inability or refusal to speak.

PERSEVERATION. The individual who exhibits **perseveration** persistently repeats the same word or idea in response to different questions.

Perception

HALLUCINATIONS. Hallucinations, or false sensory perceptions not associated with real external stimuli, may involve any of the five senses. Types of hallucinations include the following:

Auditory. Auditory hallucinations are false perceptions of sound. Most commonly they are of voices, but the individual may report clicks, rushing noises, music, and other noises. Command hallucinations may place the individual or others in a potentially dangerous situation. "Voices" that issue commands for violence to self or others may or may not be heeded by the psychotic person. Auditory hallucinations are the most common type in psychiatric disorders.

Visual. These are false visual perceptions. They may consist of formed images, such as of people, or of unformed images, such as flashes of light.

Tactile. Tactile hallucinations are false perceptions of the sense of touch, often of something on or under the skin. One specific tactile hallucination is formication, the sensation that something is crawling on or under the skin.

Gustatory. This type is a false perception of taste. Most commonly, gustatory hallucinations are described as unpleasant tastes.

Olfactory. Olfactory hallucinations are false perceptions of the sense of smell.

ILLUSIONS. **Illusions** are misperceptions or misinterpretations of real external stimuli.

Affect

Affect describes the behavior associated with an individual's feeling state or emotional tone.

INAPPROPRIATE AFFECT. Affect is inappropriate when the individual's emotional tone is incongruent with the circumstances (e.g., a young woman who laughs when told of the death of her mother).

BLAND OR FLAT AFFECT. Affect is described as bland when the emotional tone is very weak. The individual with flat affect appears to be void of emotional tone (or overt expression of feelings).

APATHY. The client with schizophrenia often demonstrates an indifference to or disinterest in the environment. The bland or flat affect is a manifestation of the emotional apathy.

Sense of Self

Sense of self describes the uniqueness and individuality a person feels. Because of extremely weak ego boundaries, the individual with schizophrenia lacks this feeling of uniqueness and experiences a great deal of confusion regarding his or her identity.

ECHOLALIA. The client with schizophrenia may repeat words that he or she hears, which is called **echolalia**. This is an attempt to identify with the person speaking. (For instance, the nurse says, "John, it's time for lunch." The client may respond, "It's time for lunch, it's time for lunch" or sometimes, "Lunch, lunch, lunch, lunch").

ECHOPRAXIA. The client who exhibits **echopraxia** may purposelessly imitate movements made by others.

IDENTIFICATION (ON AN UNCONSCIOUS LEVEL) AND IMITATION (ON A CONSCIOUS LEVEL). These ego defense mechanisms are used by schizophrenic individuals and reflect their confusion regarding their self-identity. Because they have difficulty knowing where their ego boundaries end and the other person's begin, their behavior often takes on the form of that which they see in the other person.

DEPERSONALIZATION. The unstable self-identity of an individual with schizophrenia may lead to feelings of unreality (e.g., feeling that one's extremities have changed in size, or a sense of observing oneself from a distance.

Volition

Volition has to do with impairment in the ability to initiate goal-directed activity. In the individual with schizophrenia, this may take the form of inadequate interest, drive, or ability to choose a logical course of action in a given situation.

EMOTIONAL AMBIVALENCE. Ambivalence in the client with schizophrenia refers to the coexistence of opposite emotions toward the same object, person, or situation. These opposing emotions may interfere with the person's ability to make even a very simple decision (e.g., whether to have coffee or tea with lunch). Underlying the ambivalence in the schizophrenic client is the difficulty he or she has in fulfilling a satisfying human relationship. This difficulty is based on the *need-fear dilemma*—the simultaneous need for and fear of intimacy.

IMPAIRED INTERPERSONAL FUNCTIONING AND RELATIONSHIP TO EXTERNAL WORLD. Some clients with acute schizophrenia cling to others and intrude on the personal space of others, exhibiting behaviors that are not socially and culturally acceptable. Impairment in social functioning may also be reflected in social isolation, emotional detachment, and lack of regard for social convention.

AUTISM. **Autism** describes the condition created by the person with schizophrenia who focuses inward on a fantasy world when distorting or excluding the external environment.

DETERIORATED APPEARANCE. Personal grooming and self-care activities may become minimal. The client with schizophrenia may appear disheveled and untidy and may need to be reminded of the need for personal hygiene.

Psychomotor Behavior

ANERGIA. Anergia is a deficiency of energy. The individual with schizophrenia may lack sufficient energy to carry out activities of daily living or to interact with others.

WAXY FLEXIBILITY. Waxy flexibility describes a condition in which the client with schizophrenia allows body parts to be placed in bizarre or uncomfortable positions. Once placed in position, the arm, leg, or head remains in that position for long periods, regardless of how uncomfortable it is for the client. For example, the nurse may position the client's arm in an outward position to take a blood pressure measurement. When the cuff is removed, the client may maintain the arm in the position it was placed to take the reading.

POSTURING. This symptom is manifested by the voluntary assumption of inappropriate or bizarre postures.

PACING AND ROCKING. Pacing back and forth and body rocking (a slow, rhythmic, backward-and-forward swaying of the trunk from the hips, usually when sitting) are common psychomotor behaviors of the client with schizophrenia.

Associated Features

ANHEDONIA. **Anhedonia** is the inability to experience pleasure. This is a particularly distressing symptom that compels some clients to attempt suicide.

REGRESSION. This is the retreat to an earlier level of development. Regression, a primary defense mechanism of schizophrenia, is a dysfunctional attempt to reduce anxiety. It provides the basis for many of the behaviors associated with schizophrenia.

Positive and Negative Symptoms

Some clinicians find it useful to describe symptoms of schizophrenia as positive or negative. Positive symptoms tend to reflect an excess or distortion of normal functions, whereas negative symptoms reflect a diminution or loss of normal functions (APA, 2000). Most clients exhibit a mixture of both types of symptoms.

Positive symptoms are associated with normal brain structures on a CT scan and relatively good responses to treatment. Individuals who exhibit mostly negative symptoms often show structural brain abnormalities on a CT scan and respond poorly to treatment (Sadock & Sadock, 2003). Examples of positive and negative symptoms are presented in Table 14–3.

Diagnosis/Outcome Identification

From analysis of the assessment data, appropriate nursing diagnoses are formulated for the psychotic client and his or her family. From these identified problems, accurate planning of nursing care is executed. Possible nursing diagnoses for clients with psychotic disorders include:

- Disturbed thought processes related to inability to trust, panic anxiety, possible hereditary or biochemical factors, evidenced by delusional thinking; inability to concentrate; impaired volition; inability to problem-solve, abstract, or conceptualize; extreme suspiciousness of others
- Disturbed sensory perception: auditory/visual related to panic anxiety, extreme loneliness and withdrawal into the self, evidenced by inappropriate

TABLE 14–3 Positive and Negative Symptoms of Schizophrenia

Positive Symptoms	Negative Symptoms
Hallucinations	**Affective flattening**
Auditory	Unchanging facial expression
Visual	Poor eye contact
Olfactory	Reduced body language
Gustatory	Inappropriate affect
Tactile	Diminished emotional expression
Delusions	**Alogia (poverty of speech)**
Persecution	Brief, empty responses
Grandeur	Decreased fluency of speech
Reference	Decreased content of speech
Control or influence	**Avolition/apathy**
Somatic	Inability to initiate goal-directed activity
Disorganized thinking/speech	Little or no interest in work or social activities
Loose associations	Impaired grooming/hygiene
Incoherence	**Anhedonia**
Clang associations	Absence of pleasure in social activities
Word salad	Diminished intimacy/sexual interest
Neologisms	**Social isolation**
Concrete thinking	
Echolalia	
Tangentiality	
Circumstantiality	
Disorganized behavior	
Disheveled appearance	
Inappropriate sexual behavior	
Restless, agitated behavior	
Waxy flexibility	

Adapted from *DSM-IV-TR* (APA, 2000) and Sadock & Sadock, 2003.

responses, disordered thought sequencing, rapid mood swings, poor concentration, disorientation

- Social isolation related to inability to trust, panic anxiety, weak ego development, delusional thinking, regression, evidenced by withdrawal, sad dull affect, need-fear dilemma, preoccupation with own thoughts, expression of feelings of rejection or of aloneness imposed by others
- Risk for violence: self-directed or other-directed related to extreme suspiciousness, panic anxiety, catatonic excitement, rage reactions, command hallucinations evidenced by overt and aggressive acts, goal-directed destruction of objects in the environment, self-destructive behavior, or active aggressive suicidal acts
- Impaired verbal communication related to panic anxiety, regression, withdrawal, and disordered, unrealistic thinking evidenced by loose association of ideas, neologisms, word salad, clang association, echolalia, verbalizations that reflect concrete thinking, and poor eye contact
- Self-care deficit related to withdrawal, regression, panic anxiety, perceptual or cognitive impairment, inability to trust, evidenced by difficulty carrying out tasks associated with hygiene, dressing, grooming, eating, and toileting
- Disabled family coping: related to difficulty coping with client's illness evidenced by neglectful care of the client in regard to basic human needs or illness treatment, extreme denial or prolonged overconcern regarding client's illness
- Ineffective health maintenance related to disordered thinking or delusions, evidenced by reported or observed inability to take responsibility for meeting basic health practices in any or all functional pattern areas
- Impaired home-maintenance management related to regression, withdrawal, lack of knowledge or resources, or impaired physical or cognitive functioning, evidenced by unsafe, unclean, disorderly home environment

The following criteria may be used for measurement of outcomes in the care of the client with schizophrenia. The client:

1. Demonstrates an ability to relate satisfactorily with others
2. Recognizes distortions of reality
3. Has not harmed self or others
4. Perceives self realistically
5. Demonstrates the ability to perceive the environment correctly
6. Maintains anxiety at a manageable level
7. Relinquishes the need for delusions and hallucinations
8. Demonstrates the ability to trust others
9. Uses appropriate verbal communication in interactions with others
10. Performs self-care activities independently

Planning/Implementation

Table 14–4 provides a plan of care for the client with schizophrenia. Selected nursing diagnoses are presented, along with outcome criteria, appropriate nursing interventions, and rationales for each. Refer to Appendix F for a critical pathway of care for the client with schizophrenia.

TABLE 14 – 4 Care Plan for the Client with Schizophrenia

Nursing Diagnosis: DISTURBED THOUGHT PROCESSES

Related to: Inability to trust, panic anxiety, possible hereditary or biochemical factors

Evidenced by: Delusional thinking, inability to concentrate, impaired volition, inability to problem solve, abstract, or conceptualize, extreme suspiciousness of others

Outcome Criteria	Nursing Interventions	Rationale
Client will eliminate pattern of delusional thinking. Client will demonstrate trust in others.	1. Convey acceptance of client's need for the false belief, but indicate you do not share the belief.	1. Client must understand that you do not view the idea as real.
	2. Do not argue or deny the belief. Use "reasonable doubt" as a therapeutic technique: "I find that hard to believe."	2. Arguing or denying the belief serves no useful purpose because delusional ideas are not eliminated by this approach, and the development of a trusting relationship may be impeded.
	3. Reinforce and focus on reality. Discourage long ruminations about the irrational thinking. Talk about real events and real people.	3. Discussions that focus on the false ideas are purposeless and useless, and may even aggravate the psychosis.
	4. If client is highly suspicious, the following interventions may help:	4. To decrease client's suspiciousness:
	a. Use same staff as much as possible; be honest and keep all promises.	a. Promotes trust.
	b. Avoid physical contact; avoid laughing, whispering, or talking quietly where client can see but cannot hear what is being said; provide canned food with can opener or serve food family style; avoid competitive activities; use assertive, matter-of-fact, yet friendly approach.	b. Prevents the client from feeling threatened.

Nursing Diagnosis: DISTURBED SENSORY-PERCEPTION: AUDITORY/VISUAL

Related to: Panic anxiety, extreme loneliness and withdrawal into the self

Evidenced by: Inappropriate responses, disordered thought sequencing, rapid mood swings, poor concentration, disorientation

Outcome Criteria	Nursing Interventions	Rationale
Client will be able to define and test reality, eliminating the occurrence of hallucinations.	1. Observe client for signs of hallucinations (listening pose, laughing or talking to self, stopping in midsentence).	1. Early intervention may prevent aggressive response to command hallucinations.
	2. Avoid touching the client without warning.	2. Client may perceive touch as threatening and may respond in an aggressive manner.
	3. An attitude of acceptance will encourage the client to share the content of the hallucination with you.	3. This is important to prevent possible injury to the client or others from command hallucinations.
	4. Do not reinforce the hallucination. Use "the voices" instead of words like "they" that imply validation. Let client know that you do not share the perception. Say, "Even though I realize the voices are real to you, I do not hear any voices."	4. Client must accept the perception as unreal before hallucinations can be eliminated.
	5. Help the client understand the connection between anxiety and hallucinations.	5. If client can learn to interrupt escalating anxiety, hallucinations may be prevented.
	6. Try to distract the client from the hallucination.	6. Involvement in interpersonal activities and explanation of the actual situation will help bring the client back to reality.

Nursing Diagnosis: SOCIAL ISOLATION

Related to: Inability to trust, panic anxiety, weak ego development, delusional thinking, regression

Evidenced by: Withdrawal, sad, dull affect, need-fear dilemma, preoccupation with own thoughts, expression of feelings of rejection or of aloneness imposed by others

Outcome Criteria	Nursing Interventions	Rationale
Client will voluntarily spend time with other clients and staff members in group activities on the unit.	1. Convey an accepting attitude by making brief, frequent contacts. Show unconditional positive regard.	1. An accepting attitude increases feelings of self-worth and facilitates trust.
	2. Offer to be with client during group activities that he or she finds frightening or difficult.	2. The presence of a trusted individual provides emotional security for the client.
	3. Give recognition and positive reinforcement for client's voluntary interactions with others.	3. Positive reinforcement enhances self-esteem and encourages repetition of acceptable behaviors.

Nursing Diagnosis: RISK FOR VIOLENCE: SELF-DIRECTED OR OTHER-DIRECTED

Related to: Extreme suspiciousness, panic anxiety, catatonic excitement, rage reactions, command hallucinations

Evidenced by: Overt and aggressive acts, goal-directed destruction of objects in the environment, self-destructive behavior or active aggressive suicidal acts

Outcome Criteria	Nursing Interventions	Rationale
Client will not harm self or others.	1. Maintain low level of stimuli in client's environment (low lighting, few people, simple decor, low noise level).	1. Anxiety level rises in stimulating environment. Individuals may be perceived as threatening by a suspicious, agitated client.
	2. Observe client behavior frequently. Do this while carrying out routine activities.	2. Observation during routine activities avoids creating suspiciousness on the part of the client. Close observation is necessary so that intervention can occur if required to ensure client (and others') safety.
	3. Remove all dangerous objects from client's environment.	3. Removal of dangerous objects prevents client in an agitated, confused state, from harming self or others.
	4. Redirect violent behavior with physical outlets for the anxiety.	4. Physical exercise is a safe and effective way of relieving pent-up tension.
	5. Staff should maintain a calm attitude toward client.	5. Anxiety is contagious and can be transmitted from staff to client.
	6. Have sufficient staff available to indicate a show of strength to client if it becomes necessary.	6. This shows the client evidence of control over the situation and provides some physical security for staff.
	7. Administer tranquilizing medications as ordered by physician. If client is not calmed by "talking down" or by medication, use of mechanical restraints may be necessary.	7. The avenue of the "least restrictive alternative" must be selected when planning interventions for a violent client.

Nursing Diagnosis: IMPAIRED VERBAL COMMUNICATION

Related to: Panic anxiety; regression; withdrawal; disordered, unrealistic thinking

Evidenced by: Loose association of ideas, neologisms, word salad, clang association, echolalia, verbalizations that reflect concrete thinking, poor eye contact

Outcome Criteria	Nursing Interventions	Rationale
Client will be able to communicate appropriately and comprehensibly by discharge.	1. Attempt to decode incomprehensible communication patterns. Seek validation and clarification by stating, "Is it that you mean… ?" or "I don't understand what you mean by that. Would you please clarify it for me?"	1. These techniques reveal how the client is being perceived by others, while the responsibility for not understanding is accepted by the nurse.

(Continued)

TABLE 14–4 Care Plan for the Client with Schizophrenia *(Continued)*

Outcome Criteria	Nursing Interventions	Rationale
	2. Facilitate trust and understanding by maintaining staff assignments as consistently as possible. The technique of *verbalizing the implied* is used with the client who is mute (unable or unwilling to speak). Example: "That must have been a very difficult time for you when your mother left. You must have felt very alone."	2. This approach conveys empathy and may encourage the client to disclose painful issues.
	3. Anticipate and fulfill client's needs until functional communication pattern returns.	3. Client safety and comfort are nursing priorities.
	4. Orient client to reality as required. Call the client by name. Validate those aspects of communication that help differentiate between what is real and not real.	4. These techniques may facilitate restoration of functional communication patterns in the client.

Nursing Diagnosis: SELF-CARE DEFICIT

Related to: Withdrawal, regression, panic anxiety, perceptual or cognitive impairment, inability to trust

Evidenced by: Difficulty carrying out tasks associated with hygiene, dressing, grooming, eating, toileting

Outcome Criteria	Nursing Interventions	Rationale
Client will demonstrate ability to meet self-care needs independently.	1. Provide assistance with self-care needs as required. Some clients who are severely withdrawn may require total care.	1. Client safety and comfort are nursing priorities.
	2. Encourage client to perform independently as many activities as possible. Provide positive reinforcement for independent accomplishments.	2. Independent accomplishment and positive reinforcement enhance self-esteem and promote repetition of desirable behaviors.
	3. Use concrete communication to show client what is expected. Example: "Pick up the spoon, scoop some mashed potatoes into it, and put it in your mouth."	3. Because concrete thinking prevails, explanations must be provided at the client's concrete level of comprehension.
	4. Creative approaches may need to be taken with the client who is not eating, such as allowing client to open own canned or packaged foods; family-style serving may also be an option.	4. These techniques may be helpful with the client who is paranoid and may be suspicious that he or she is being poisoned with food or medication.
	5. If toileting needs are not being met, establish a structured schedule for the client.	5. A structured schedule will help the client establish a pattern so that he or she can develop a habit of toileting independently.

Nursing Diagnosis: DISABLED FAMILY COPING

Related to: Difficulty coping with client's illness

Evidenced by: Neglectful care of the client in regard to basic human needs or illness treatment, extreme denial or prolonged overconcern regarding client's illness

Outcome Criteria	Nursing Interventions	Rationale
Family will identify more adaptive coping strategies for dealing with client's illness and treatment regimen.	1. Identify level of family functioning. Assess communication patterns, interpersonal relationships between members, role expectations, problem-solving skills, and availability of outside support systems.	1. These factors will help to identify how successful the family is in dealing with stressful situations and areas where assistance is required.
	2. Provide information for the family about the client's illness, what will be required in the treatment regimen, and the long-term prognosis.	2. Knowledge and understanding about what to expect may facilitate the family's ability to successfully integrate the client into the system.
	3. With family members, practice how to respond to bizarre behavior and communication patterns and in the event that the client becomes violent.	3. A plan of action will assist the family to respond adaptively in the face of what they may consider to be a crisis.

Client/Family Education

The role of client teacher is important in the psychiatric area, as it is in all areas of nursing. A list of topics for client/family education relevant to schizophrenia is presented in Table 14–5.

Evaluation

In the final step of the nursing process, a reassessment is conducted in order to determine if the nursing actions have been successful in achieving the objectives of care. Evaluation of the nursing actions for the client with exacerbation of schizophrenic psychosis may be facilitated by gathering information using the following types of questions:

1. Has the client established trust with at least one staff member?
2. Is the anxiety level maintained at a manageable level?
3. Is delusional thinking still prevalent?
4. Is hallucinogenic activity evident? Does the client share content of hallucinations, particularly if commands are heard?
5. Is the client able to interrupt escalating anxiety with adaptive coping mechanisms?
6. Is the client easily agitated?
7. Is the client able to interact with others appropriately?
8. Does the client voluntarily attend therapy activities?
9. Is verbal communication comprehensible?
10. Is the client compliant with medication? Does the client verbalize the importance of taking medication regularly and on a long-term basis? Does he or she verbalize understanding of possible side effects, and when to seek assistance from the physician?
11. Does the client spend time with others rather than isolating self?
12. Is the client able to carry out all activities of daily living independently?
13. Is the client able to verbalize resources from which he or she may seek assistance outside the hospital?
14. Does the family have information regarding support groups in which they may participate, and from which they may seek assistance in dealing with their family member who is ill?
15. If the client lives alone, does he or she have a source for assistance with home maintenance and health management?

TABLE 14–5 Topics for Client/Family Education Related to Schizophrenia

Nature of the Illness
1. What to expect as the illness progresses
2. Symptoms associated with the illness
3. Ways for family to respond to behaviors associated with the illness

Management of the Illness
1. Connection of exacerbation of symptoms to times of stress
2. Appropriate medication management
3. Side effects of medications
4. Importance of not stopping medications
5. When to contact healthcare provider
6. Relaxation techniques
7. Social skills training
8. Daily living skills training

Support Services
1. Financial assistance
2. Legal assistance
3. Caregiver support groups
4. Respite care
5. Home healthcare

TREATMENT MODALITIES FOR SCHIZOPHRENIA AND OTHER PSYCHOTIC DISORDERS

Psychological Treatments

Individual Psychotherapy

Ho, Black, and Andreasen (2003) state:

> Although intensive psychodynamic- and insight-oriented psychotherapy is generally not recommended, the form of individual psychotherapy that psychiatrists employ when providing pharmacological treatment typically involves a synthesis of various psychotherapeutic strategies and interventions. These include problem solving, reality testing, psychoeducation, and supportive and cognitive-behavioral techniques anchored on an empathetic therapeutic alliance with the patient. The goals of such individual psychotherapy are to improve medication compliance, enhance social and occupational functioning, and prevent relapse. (p. 419)

Reality-oriented individual therapy is the most suitable approach to individual psychotherapy for schizophrenia. The primary focus in all cases must reflect efforts to decrease anxiety and increase trust.

Establishing a relationship is often particularly difficult because the individual with schizophrenia is desperately lonely yet defends against kindness, compassion, and trust. He or she is likely to respond to attempts at closeness with suspiciousness, anxiety, aggression, or regression. Successful intervention may best be achieved with honesty, simple directness, and a manner that respects the client's privacy and human dignity. Exaggerated warmth and professions of friendship are likely to be met with confusion and suspicion.

Once a therapeutic interpersonal relationship has been established, reality orientation is maintained through exploration of the client's behavior within relationships. Education is provided to help the client identify sources of real or perceived danger and ways of reacting appropriately. Methods for improving interpersonal communication, emotional expression, and frustration tolerance are attempted.

Individual psychotherapy for clients with schizophrenia is seen as a long-term endeavor that requires patience on the part of the therapist and the ability to accept that a great deal of change may not occur. Some cases report treatment durations of many years before clients regain some extent of independent functioning.

Group Therapy

Group therapy with individuals with schizophrenia has been shown to be effective, particularly with outpatients and when combined with drug treatment. Sadock and Sadock (2003) state:

> Group therapy for people with schizophrenia generally focuses on real-life plans, problems, and relationships. Some investigators doubt that dynamic interpretation and insight therapy are valuable for typical patients with schizophrenia. However, group therapy is effective in reducing social isolation, increasing the sense of cohesiveness, and improving reality testing for patients with schizophrenia. (p. 501)

Group therapy in inpatient settings is less productive. Inpatient treatment usually occurs when symptomatology and social disorganization are at their most intense. At this time, the least amount of stimuli possible is most beneficial for the client. Because group therapy can be an intensive and highly stimulating environment, it may be counterproductive early in treatment.

Group therapy for schizophrenia has been most useful over the long-term course of the illness. The social interaction, sense of cohesiveness, identification, and reality testing achieved within the group setting have proven to be highly therapeutic processes for these clients. Groups led in a supportive manner rather than in an interpretative way appear to be most helpful for schizophrenic clients (Sadock & Sadock, 2003).

Behavior Therapy

Behavior modification has a history of qualified success in reducing the frequency of bizarre, disturbing, and deviant behaviors and increasing appropriate behaviors. Features that have led to the most positive results include:

1. Clearly defining goals and how they will be measured
2. Attaching positive, negative, and aversive reinforcements to adaptive and maladaptive behavior
3. Using simple, concrete instructions and prompts to elicit the desired behavior

Behavior therapy can be a powerful treatment tool for helping clients change undesirable behaviors. In the treatment setting, the therapist can use praise and other positive reinforcements to help the client with schizophrenia reduce the frequency of maladaptive or deviant behaviors. A limitation of this type of treatment is the inability of some individuals with schizophrenia to generalize what they have learned to the community setting following discharge from therapy.

Social Skills Training

Social skills training has become one of the most widely used psychosocial interventions in the treatment of schizophrenia. Scott and Dixon (1995) define psychosocial skills training as:

> ... a class of treatment interventions that uses methods and principles derived from social learning theories to train (or retrain) motor and interpersonal skills and competencies. Complex behaviors are analyzed and broken down into a smaller set of discrete behavioral elements, which are then trained using various core behavioral techniques. These techniques include problem or skill specification, didactic instruction, modeling, role-play or behavioral rehearsal, coaching, feedback, verbal reinforcement, generalization training, and homework.

Social dysfunction is a hallmark of schizophrenia. Indeed, impairment in social functioning is included as one of the defining diagnostic criteria for schizophrenia in the *DSM-IV-TR* (APA, 2000). Considerable attention is now being given to enhancement of social skills in these clients.

The educational procedure in social skills training focuses on role-play. A series of brief scenarios are selected. These should be typical of situations clients experience in their daily lives and be graduated in terms of level of difficulty. The therapist may serve as a role model for some behaviors. For example, "See how I sort of nod my head up and down and look at your face when you talk." The therapist's demonstration is followed by the client's role-playing. Immediate feedback is provided regarding the client's presentation. Only by countless repetitions does the response gradually become smooth and effortless.

Progress is geared toward the client's needs and limitations. The focus is on small units of behavior, and the training proceeds very gradually. Highly threatening issues are avoided, and emphasis is placed on functional skills that are relevant to activities of daily living.

Social Treatment

Milieu Therapy

Some clinicians believe that milieu therapy can be an appropriate treatment for the client with schizophrenia. Research suggests that psychotropic medication is more effective at all levels of care when used along with milieu therapy and that milieu therapy is more successful if used in conjunction with these medications.

Sadock and Sadock (2003) state:

> Most milieu therapy programs emphasize group and social interaction; rules and expectations are mediated by peer pressure for normalization of adaptation. When patients are viewed as responsible human beings, the patient role becomes blurred. Milieu therapy stresses a patient's rights to goals and to have freedom of movement and informal relationship with staff; it also emphasizes interdisciplinary participation and goal-oriented, clear communication. (p. 966)

Individuals with schizophrenia who are treated with milieu therapy alone require longer hospital stays than do those treated with drugs and psychosocial therapy. Other economic considerations, such as the need for a high staff-to-client ratio, in addition to the longer admission, limit the use of milieu therapy in the treatment of schizophrenia.

Family Therapy

Some therapists treat schizophrenia as an illness not only of the client, but of the entire family. Even when families appear to cope well, there is a notable impact on the mental health status of relatives when a family member has the illness. Safier (1997) states:

> When a family member has a serious mental illness, the family must deal with a major upheaval in their lives, a terrible event that causes great pain and grief for the loss of a once-promising child or relationship. (p. 5)

The importance of the expanded role of family in the aftercare of relatives with schizophrenia has been recognized, thereby stimulating interest in family intervention programs designed to support the family system, prevent or delay relapse, and help to maintain the client in the community. These psychoeducational programs treat the family as a resource rather than a stressor, with the focus on concrete problem-solving and specific helping behaviors for coping with stress. Many of these programs recognize a biological basis for the illness and the impact that stress has on the client's ability to function. By providing the family with information about the illness and suggestions for effective coping, psychoeducational programs reduce the likelihood of the client's relapse and the possible emergence of mental illness in previously nonaffected relatives.

Dixon and Lehman (1995) state that although studies of family interventions with schizophrenia differ in their characteristics and methods, they tend to share a common set of assumptions:

1. Schizophrenia is regarded as an illness.
2. The family environment is not implicated in the etiology of the illness.
3. Support is provided and families are enlisted as therapeutic agents.
4. The interventions are part of a treatment package used in conjunction with routine drug treatment and outpatient clinical management.

Lam (1991) outlined the following strategies for intervention with families:

1. Taking a positive approach and establishing a genuine working relationship
2. Providing structure and stability
3. Focusing on the here and now
4. Using family therapy concepts
5. Working on cognitive restructuring
6. Taking a behavioral approach
7. Improving communication

Family therapy typically consists of a brief program of family education about schizophrenia, and a more extended program of family contact designed to reduce overt manifestations of conflict and to alter patterns of family communication and problem solving. The response to this type of therapy has been very dramatic. Ho, Black, and Andreasen (2003) report on several studies, clearly revealing that a more positive outcome in the treatment of the schizophrenic client can be achieved by including the family system in the program of care.

Organic Treatment

Psychopharmacology

Chlorpromazine (Thorazine) was first introduced in the United States in 1952. At that time, it was used in conjunction with barbiturates in surgical anesthesia. With increased use, the drug's psychic properties were recognized, and by 1954 it was marketed as an antipsychotic medication in the United States. The manufacture and sale of other antipsychotic drugs followed in rapid succession. (See Chapter 10 for a detailed discussion of antipsychotic medications.)

Antipsychotic medications are very effective in treating the symptoms of schizophrenia. Unfortunately, substantiated evidence of long-term recovery with antipsychotic medications is notably lacking. *The Merck Manual of Diagnosis and Therapy (MMDT)* (2002) reports:

> Over a short period (1 year), the prognosis of schizophrenia is closely related to how well a person follows a drug treatment plan. Without drug treatment, 70 to 80 percent of the people who have experienced a schizophrenic episode will relapse over the next 12 months and experience a subsequent episode. Drugs taken continuously can reduce the relapse rate to about 30 percent.

The prognosis of schizophrenia is often reported in the paradigm of thirds: One-third of the people achieve significant and lasting improvement. They may never experience another episode of psychosis following the initial occurrence. One-third may achieve some improvement with intermittent relapses and residual disability. Their occupational level may have decreased because of their illness, or they may be socially isolated. Finally, one-third experiences severe and permanent incapacity. They often do not respond to medication and remain chronically ill for much of their lives. Men have poorer outcomes than women do; women respond better to treatment with antipsychotic medications (*MMDT*, 2002).

As mentioned earlier, the efficacy of antipsychotic medications is enhanced by adjunct psychosocial therapy. Because the psychotic manifestations of the illness subside with use of the drugs, clients are generally more cooperative with the psychosocial therapies.

Antipsychotic drugs, also called neuroleptics or major tranquilizers, are effective in the treatment of acute and chronic manifestations of schizophrenia and in maintenance therapy to prevent exacerbation of schizophrenic symptoms. However, because of a number of unpleasant and even dangerous side effects, the advisability of long-term use may be questionable. Common side effects include anticholinergic manifestations (dry mouth, blurred vision, constipation, urinary retention), nausea, gastrointestinal upset, skin rash, sedation, orthostatic hypotension, photosensitivity, decreased libido, retrograde ejaculation, gynecomastia, amenorrhea, weight gain, reduction in seizure threshold, agranulocytosis, extrapyramidal symptoms (pseudoparkinsonism, akinesia, akathisia, dystonia, oculogyric crisis), tardive dyskinesia, and neuroleptic malignant syndrome.

Antiparkinsonian agents may be prescribed to counteract the extrapyramidal symptoms associated with some antipsychotic medications. These drugs are cholinergic blockers, producing the same anticholinergic side effects as the antipsychotic medications. Some physicians routinely prescribe the antiparkinsonian drug to be given on a scheduled basis with the antipsychotic medication. Others prefer to order the drug on an as-needed basis, to be administered only if the neurological symptoms appear, thus reducing the compounded anticholinergic effects of the two drugs together. When the drug is given as needed, it is extremely important for the nurse to be able to recognize the symptoms associated with extrapyramidal side effects so that he or she can administer the antiparkinsonian drug without delay (see Chapter 10). Many physicians are choosing to prescribe the newer atypical antipsychotics (e.g., clozapine, risperidone, olanzapine, sertindole, quetiapine, ziprasidone) that cause few, if any, extrapyramidal symptoms.

For those clients with schizophrenia who do not respond to antipsychotic medications, a number of other pharmacological options have been tried, with various amounts of success. Use of the following medication alternatives have been reported (Sadock & Sadock, 2003; Ho, Black, & Andreasen, 2003):

1. Reserpine, a dopamine receptor antagonist, has been used as an antihypertensive agent and as an antipsychotic. It has produced severe depression in humans and for this reason is now rarely used for either purpose.

2. Lithium carbonate can ameliorate schizophrenic symptoms or suppress episodic violence in clients with schizophrenia but is seldom an adequate drug therapy alone.
3. Carbamazepine ameliorates symptoms in some treatment-resistant psychotic clients, but it alone is not an adequate therapy for schizophrenia.
4. Valium, in high dosages, was shown to control psychotic symptoms of schizophrenia, such as agitation, thought disorder, delusions, and hallucinations. It has also been used to relieve akathisia associated with some antipsychotic medication. The best use of benzodiazepines appears to be as adjunct therapy with antipsychotic medication in the management of psychotic agitation (Ho, Black, & Andreasen, 2003).
5. Propranolol may be useful in controlling temper outbursts in aggressive or violent psychotic clients.

The advent of antipsychotic medications in the 1950s was hailed as a medical breakthrough for psychiatry. At last the physician could do something substantive for the client with schizophrenia. No one knows exactly how the antipsychotic effect is achieved or why it takes several weeks for these effects to be observed. Scientists cannot yet explain why clients do not become tolerant to antipsychotics, or why discontinuing the drug does not make the disease worse than it was before treatment. By studying the action of antipsychotic drugs, however, progress has been made toward understanding what is wrong with the schizophrenic brain. Continual refinement of the research methods and investigation of other transmitter systems may reveal more precisely how the schizophrenic brain differs from the healthy one.

SUMMARY

Of all mental illness, schizophrenia undoubtedly results in the greatest amount of personal, emotional, and social costs. It presents an enormous threat to life and happiness, yet it remains a puzzle to the medical community. In fact, for many years there was little agreement on a definition of schizophrenia. The *DSM-IV-TR* (APA, 2000) identifies specific criteria for diagnosis of the disorder, which were presented in this chapter.

The initial symptoms of schizophrenia most often occur in early adulthood. Development of the disorder can be viewed in four phases: (1) the schizoid personality, (2) the prodromal phase, (3) the active phase of schizophrenia, and (4) the residual phase.

The cause of schizophrenia remains unclear. Research continues, and most contemporary psychiatrists are giving more credence to the biological theories and placing little emphasis on psychosocial influences. Integration of these theories supports the idea that no single factor can be implicated in the etiology, but that the disease most likely results from a combination of influences including genetics, biochemical dysfunction, physiological, and environmental factors.

Various types of schizophrenic and related psychotic disorders have been identified. They are differentiated by their total picture of clinical symptomatology. They include disorganized schizophrenia, catatonic schizophrenia, paranoid schizophrenia, undifferentiated schizophrenia, residual schizophrenia, schizoaffective disorder, brief psychotic disorder, schizophreniform disorder, delusional disorder, shared psychotic disorder, psychotic disorder caused by a general medical condition, and substance-induced psychotic disorder.

Care of the client with schizophrenia was presented in the context of the six steps of the nursing process. Nursing assessment is based on knowledge of symptomatology related to thought content and form, perception, affect, sense of self, volition, impaired interpersonal functioning and relationship to the external world, and psychomotor behavior. Nursing diagnoses were formulated from the assessment data, and a plan of care was developed. Guidelines for evaluation of client outcomes were presented.

Various treatment modalities for schizophrenia were discussed, including individual psychotherapy, group therapy, behavior therapy, social skills training, milieu therapy, family therapy, and psychopharmacology. For the majority of clients, the most effective treatment appears to be a combination of psychotropic medication and psychosocial therapy.

REVIEW QUESTIONS

SELF-EXAMINATION/LEARNING EXERCISE

Situation: Tony is a 20-year-old college dropout who had become increasingly withdrawn, suspicious, and isolated during the past 2 months since his return from out-of-state college. He is brought to the emergency room. His family reports that he has been looking at them strangely as if he did not know them, refusing to talk to anyone, spending a lot of time in his room alone, and refusing all help. The father brought the client to the hospital against his will following a verbal argument during the course of which the client attempted to stab the father with a kitchen knife. The father had successfully subdued him and removed the weapon. On arrival at the emergency room, the client was agitated and exhibiting acutely psychotic symptoms. He reports that "they" told him to kill his father before his father kills him. Verbalizations are often incoherent. Affect is flat, and he continuously scans the environment. He is admitted to the psychiatric unit with a diagnosis of schizophreniform disorder, provisional.

Based on the above situation, select the answer that is most appropriate for each of the following questions:

1. The *initial* nursing intervention for Tony is to:
   a. Give him an injection of Thorazine.
   b. Ensure a safe environment for him and others.
   c. Place him in restraints.
   d. Order him a nutritious diet.
2. The primary goal in working with Tony would be to:
   a. Promote interaction with others.
   b. Decrease his anxiety and increase trust.
   c. Improve his relationship with his parents.
   d. Encourage participation in therapy activities.
3. Orders from the physician include 100 mg chlorpromazine (Thorazine) STAT and then 50 mg b.i.d.; 2 mg benztropine (Cogentin) b.i.d. p.r.n. Why is chlorpromazine ordered?
   a. To reduce extrapyramidal symptoms
   b. To prevent neuroleptic malignant syndrome
   c. To decrease psychotic symptoms
   d. To induce sleep
4. Benztropine was ordered on a p.r.n. basis. Which of the following assessments by the nurse would convey a need for this medication?
   a. The client's level of agitation increases.
   b. The client complains of a sore throat.
   c. The client's skin has a yellowish cast.
   d. The client develops tremors and a shuffling gait.
5. Tony begins to tell the nurse about how the CIA is looking for him and will kill him if they find him. The most appropriate response by the nurse is:
   a. "That's ridiculous, Tony. No one is going to hurt you."
   b. "The CIA isn't interested in people like you, Tony."
   c. "Why do you think the CIA wants to kill you?"
   d. "I find that very hard to believe, Tony."

6. Tony's belief about the CIA is an example of a:
   a. Delusion of persecution
   b. Delusion of reference
   c. Delusion of control or influence
   d. Delusion of grandeur
7. Tony tilts his head to the side, stops talking in midsentence, and listens intently. The nurse recognizes from these signs that Tony is likely experiencing:
   a. Somatic delusions
   b. Catatonic stupor
   c. Auditory hallucinations
   d. Pseudoparkinsonism
8. The most appropriate nursing intervention for the symptom just described is to:
   a. Ask the client to describe his physical symptoms.
   b. Ask the client to describe what he is hearing.
   c. Administer a dose of benztropine.
   d. Call the physician for additional orders.
9. Should Tony suddenly become aggressive and violent on the unit, which of the following approaches would be best for the nurse to use first?
   a. Provide large motor activities to relieve Tony's pent-up tension.
   b. Administer a large dose of sedative to keep Tony calm.
   c. Call for sufficient help to control the situation safely.
   d. Convey to Tony that his behavior is unacceptable and will not be permitted.
10. Tony and his parents attend a weekly family therapy group. The primary focus of this type of group is:
    a. To discuss concrete problem solving and adaptive behaviors for coping with stress
    b. To introduce the family to others with the same problem
    c. To keep the client and family in touch with the healthcare system
    d. To promote family interaction and increase understanding of the illness

INTERNET REFERENCES

- Additional information about schizophrenia may be located at the following websites:
  - a http://www.schizophrenia.com
  - b http://www.nimh.nih.gov
  - c http://schizophrenia.nami.org
  - d http://mentalhealth.com
  - e http://www2.health-center.com
- Additional information about medications to treat schizophrenia may be located at the following websites:
  - a http://www.mentalhealth.com/p30-note.html
  - b http://www.fadavis.com/townsend
  - c http://www.nlm.nih.gov/medlineplus

Test Your Critical Thinking Skills

Sara, a 23-year-old single woman, has just been admitted to the psychiatric unit by her parents. They explain that over the past few months she has become increasingly withdrawn. She stays in her room alone, but lately has been heard talking and laughing to herself.

Sara left home for the first time at age 18 to attend college. She performed well during her first semester, but when she returned after Christmas, she began to accuse her roommate of stealing her possessions. She started writing to her parents that her roommate wanted to kill her and that her roommate was turning everyone against her. She said she feared for her life. She started missing classes and stayed in her bed most of the time. Sometimes she locked herself in her closet. Her parents took her home, and she was hospitalized and diagnosed with paranoid schizophrenia. She has since been maintained on antipsychotic medication and is taking a few classes at the local community college.

Sara tells the admitting nurse that she quit taking her medication 4 weeks ago because the pharmacist who fills the prescriptions is plotting to have her killed. She believes he is trying to poison her. She says she got this information from a television message. As Sara speaks, the nurse notices that she sometimes stops in midsentence and listens; sometimes she cocks her head to the side and moves her lips as though she is talking.

Answer the following questions related to Sara:

1. From the assessment data, what would be the immediate nursing concern in working with Sara?
2. What is the nursing diagnosis related to this concern?
3. What initial interventions must be accomplished before the nurse can be successful in working with Sara?

IMPLICATIONS OF RESEARCH FOR EVIDENCE-BASED PRACTICE

Delaney, C: **Reducing recidivism: Medication versus psychosocial rehabilitation.** Journal of Psychosocial Nursing (1998, November), 36(11), 28–34.

Description of the Study: Because individuals with chronic schizophrenia have high hospital recidivism rates, this study was conducted to gather information that may help these clients become more successful in the community. Sixty persons with lengthy psychiatric histories were voluntary subjects. They were divided into two groups: those on routine medication management and those on medication management in addition to psychosocial support in the form of an outpatient rehabilitation program. The mental health center where the psychosocial support was received provides a wide array of services including outpatient therapy, support housing, partial hospitalization, day treatment, inpatient crisis stabilization, and the "clubhouse," which provides social support and meaningful prevocational training. Clubhouse members may advance their education or develop hobbies. The clubhouse assists members to secure, sustain, and upgrade independent employment.

Results of the Study: At the end of 6 months, it was found that the subjects who were on medication management alone had a higher recidivism rate than those who were on medication management and involved in clubhouse activities. The clubhouse members on medication had 176.49 days out of the hospital in the 6-month period, and the highest recidivism rate was by the patients on medication alone, who had 165.7 days out of the hospital for the same period.

Implications for Nursing Practice: The author of this study states, "Psychosocial rehabilitation clubhouses can decrease inpatient hospitalization in patients with chronic mental illness. Their supportive, vocational, and educational functions are worth the investment in terms of improving quality of life and functioning skills." Establishing and operating these programs is well within the scope of psychiatric nursing practice. These are important implications for nursing in reducing recidivism in this chronic population.

REFERENCES

American Psychiatric Association (APA). (1987). Diagnostic and statistical manual of mental disorders (3rd ed., Revised). Washington, D.C.: American Psychiatric Association.

American Psychiatric Association. (2000). Diagnostic and statistical manual of mental disorders (4th ed.) Text revision. Washington, D.C.: American Psychiatric Association.

Black, D.W., & Andreasen, N.C. (1999). Schizophrenia, schizophreniform disorder, and delusional (paranoid) disorders. In R.E. Hales & S.C. Yudofsky (Eds.), Essentials of Clinical Psychiatry. Washington, DC: American Psychiatric Press.

Dixon, L.B., & Lehman, A.F. (1995). Family interventions for schizophrenia. National Institute of Mental Health. Schizophrenia Bulletin, 21:631–643.

Hall, L.L. (1996). The best of times, the worst of times. Unpublished remarks at symposium on schizophrenia to U.S.

Congress. National Alliance for the Mentally Ill. Retrieved July 31, 2001, from www.schizophrenia.nami.org/schizophrenia/schizophrenia.html

Ho, B.C., Black, D.W., & Andreasen, N.C. (2003). Schizophrenia and other psychotic disorders. In R.E. Hales & S.C. Yudofsky (Eds.), Textbook of clinical psychiatry (4th ed.). Washington, D.C.: American Psychiatric Publishing.

Hollandsworth, J.G. (1990). The physiology of psychological disorders. New York: Plenum Press.

Lam, D.H. (1991). Psychosocial family intervention in schizophrenia: A review of empirical studies. Psychological Medicine, 21:423–441.

Mednick, S.A. (1991). Fetal neural development and adult schizophrenia. The Journal of the California Alliance for the Mentally Ill 2:6–8.

The Merck Manual of Diagnosis and Therapy (MMDT) (2002). Schizophrenia. Retrieved on February 25, 2002, at http://www.merck.com/pubs/mmanual/section15/chapter193/193b.htm

Sackeim, H.A., & Mukherjee, S. (1992). Schizophrenia. In F.I. Kass, J.M. Oldham, & H. Pardes (Eds.), Columbia University College of Physicians and Surgeons complete home guide to mental health. New York: Henry Holt.

Sadock, B.J., & Sadock, V.A. (2003). Synopsis of psychiatry: Behavioral sciences/clinical psychiatry (9th ed.). Philadelphia: Lippincott Williams & Wilkins.

Safier, E. (1997). Our families, the context of our lives. Menninger Perspective, 28:4–9.

Scheibel, A.B. (1991, Summer). Schizophrenia: Cells in disarray. Journal of the California Alliance for the Mentally Ill, 2:9–10.

Scott, J.E., & Dixon, L.B. (1995). Psychological interventions for schizophrenia. National Institute of Mental Health. Schizophrenia Bulletin 21:621–630.

TOWNSEND ESSENTIALS

15

CHAPTER

Mood Disorders

CHAPTER OUTLINE

KEY TERMS

electroconvulsive therapy (ECT)
bipolar disorder
cognitive therapy
cyclothymic disorder
psychomotor retardation
premenstrual dysphoric disorder
postpartum depression
hypomania
mania
melancholia
mood
tyramine
delirious mania

OBJECTIVES

After reading this chapter, the student will be able to:

1. Recount historical perspectives of mood disorders.
2. Discuss epidemiological statistics related to mood disorders.
3. Describe various types of mood disorders.
4. Identify etiological implications in the development of mood disorders.
5. Discuss implications of depression related to developmental stage.
6. Identify symptomatology associated with mood disorders and use this information in client assessment.
7. Formulate nursing diagnoses and goals of care for clients with mood disorders.
8. Identify topics for client and family teaching relevant to mood disorders.
9. Describe appropriate nursing interventions for behaviors associated with mood disorders.
10. Describe relevant criteria for evaluating nursing care of clients with mood disorders.
11. Discuss various modalities relevant to treatment of mood disorders.

INTRODUCTION

Depression is likely the oldest and still one of the most frequently diagnosed psychiatric illnesses. Symptoms of depression have been described almost as far back as there is evidence of written documentation.

An occasional bout with the "blues," a feeling of sadness or downheartedness, is common among healthy people and considered a normal response to everyday disappointments in life. These episodes are short-lived as the individual adapts to the loss, change, or failure (real or perceived) that has been experienced. Pathological depression occurs when adaptation is ineffective.

This chapter focuses on the consequences of dysfunctional grieving as it is manifested by mood disorders. **Mood** describes an individual's sustained emotional tone, which significantly influences behavior, personality, and perception. Mood disorders are classified as depressive or bipolar.

A historical perspective and epidemiological statistics related to mood disorders are presented here. Factors that have been implicated in the etiology of mood disorders provide a framework for studying the dynamics of depression and **bipolar disorder**.

The implications of depression relevant to individuals of various developmental stages are discussed. An explanation of the symptomatology is presented as background knowledge for assessing the client with a mood disorder. Nursing care is described in the context of the six steps of the nursing process. Various medical treatment modalities are explored.

HISTORICAL PERSPECTIVE

Many ancient cultures (e.g., Babylonian, Egyptian, Hebrew) believed in the supernatural or divine origin of depression and **mania**. The Old Testament states in the Book of Samuel that King Saul's depression was inflicted by an "evil spirit" sent from God to "torment" him.

A clearly nondivine point of view regarding depressive and manic states was held by the Greek medical community from the 5th century BC through the 3rd century AD. This represented the thinking of Hippocrates, Celsus, and Galen, among others. They strongly rejected the idea of divine origin and considered the brain to be the seat of all emotional states. Hippocrates believed that **melancholia** was caused by an excess of black bile, a heavily toxic substance produced in the spleen or intestine, which affected the brain.

During the Renaissance, several new theories evolved. Depression was viewed by some as being the result of obstruction of vital air circulation, excessive brooding, or helpless situations beyond the client's control. These strong emotions of depression and mania were reflected in major literary works of the time, including Shakespeare's *King Lear*, *Macbeth*, and *Hamlet*.

In the 19th century, the definition of mania was narrowed down from the concept of total madness to that of a disorder of affect and action. The old notion of melancholia was refurnished with meaning, and emphasis was placed on the primary affective nature of the disorder. Finally, an introduction was made to the possibility of an alternating pattern of affective symptomatology associated with the disorders.

Contemporary thinking has been shaped a great deal by the works of Sigmund Freud, Emil Kraepelin, and Adolf Meyer. Having evolved from these early 20th-century models, current thinking about mood disorders generally encompasses the intrapsychic, behavioral, and biological perspectives. These various perspectives support the notion of multiple causations in the development of mood disorders.

EPIDEMIOLOGY

Major depression is one of the leading causes of disability in the United States. It affects almost 10 percent of the population, or 19 million Americans, in a given year (International Society for Mental Health Online, 2003). During their lifetime, 10 to 25 percent of women and 5 to 12 percent of men will become clinically depressed.

This preponderance has led to the consideration of depression by some researchers as "the common cold of psychiatric disorders" and this generation as an "age of melancholia."

Gender

Studies indicate that the incidence of depressive disorder is higher in women than in men by about 2 to 1. The incidence of bipolar disorder is roughly equal, with a ratio of women to men of 1.2 to 1.

Age

Several studies have shown that the incidence of depression is higher in young women and has a tendency to decrease with age. The opposite has been found in men, with the prevalence of depressive symptoms being lower in younger men and increasing with age (Murphy, 1994). Studies suggest that the median age at onset of bipolar disorder is 18 years in men and 20 years in women (Burke, Burke, & Regier, 1990).

Social Class

Results of studies have indicated an inverse relationship between social class and report of depressive symptoms. Bipolar disorder appears to occur more frequently among the higher social classes, especially professionals and the highly educated (Craig, 1994).

Race

Studies have shown no consistent relationship between race and affective disorder. One problem encountered in reviewing racial comparisons has to do with the socioeconomic class of the race being investigated. Sample populations of nonwhite clients are many times predominantly lower class and are often compared with white populations from middle and upper social classes.

Other studies suggest a second problematic factor in the study of racial comparisons. Clinicians tend to underdiagnose mood disorders and to overdiagnose schizophrenia in clients who have racial or cultural backgrounds different from their own (Sadock & Sadock, 2003). This misdiagnosis may result from language barriers between clients and physicians who are unfamiliar with cultural aspects of nonwhite clients' language and behavior.

Marital Status

The highest incidence of depressive symptoms has been indicated in individuals without close interpersonal relationships and in persons who are divorced or separated (Sadock & Sadock, 2003). When gender and marital status are considered together, the differences reveal lowest rates of depressive symptoms among married men, and the highest by married women and single men. Sadock and Sadock,(2003) state,

> Bipolar I disorder is more common in divorced and single persons than among married persons, but this difference may reflect the early onset and the resulting marital discord characteristic of the disorder. (p. 536)

Seasonality

A number of studies have examined seasonal patterns associated with mood disorders. These studies have revealed two prevalent periods of seasonal involvement: one in the spring (March, April, and May) and one in the fall (September, October, and November). This pattern tends to parallel the seasonal pattern for suicide, which shows a large peak in the spring and a smaller one in October (Goodwin & Jamison, 1990).

TYPES OF MOOD DISORDERS

The *DSM-IV-TR* (American Psychiatric Association [APA], 2000) describes the essential feature of these disorders as a disturbance of mood, characterized by a full or partial manic or depressive syndrome that cannot be attributed to another mental disorder. Mood disorders are classified under two major categories: depressive disorders and bipolar disorders.

Depressive Disorders

Major Depressive Disorder

This disorder is characterized by depressed mood or loss of interest or pleasure in usual activities. Evidence will show impaired social and occupational functioning that has existed for at least 2 weeks, no history of manic behavior, and symptoms that cannot be attributed to use of substances or a general medical condition.

Major depressive disorder may be further classified as follows:

1. **Single episode or recurrent.** A *single episode* specifier is used for an individual's first diagnosis of depression. *Recurrent* is specified when the history reveals two or more episodes of depression.
2. **Mild, moderate, or severe.** These categories are identified by the number and severity of symptoms.
3. **With psychotic features.** The impairment of reality testing is evident. The individual experiences delusions or hallucinations.
4. **With catatonic features.** Identifies the presence of psychomotor disturbances, such as severe **psychomotor retardation**, with or without the presence of waxy flexibility or stupor, or excessive motor activity. The individual may also manifest

symptoms of negativism, mutism, echolalia, or echopraxia.

5. **With melancholic features.** This is a typically severe form of major depressive episode. Symptoms are exaggerated. Even temporary reactivity to usually pleasurable stimuli is absent. History reveals a good response to antidepressant or other somatic therapy.
6. **Chronic.** This classification applies when the current episode of depressed mood has been evident continuously for at least the past 2 years.
7. **With seasonal pattern.** This diagnosis indicates the presence of depressive symptoms during the fall or winter months. This diagnosis is made when the number of seasonal depressive episodes substantially outnumbers the nonseasonal depressive episodes that have occurred over the individual's lifetime (APA, 2000). This disorder has previously been identified in the literature as seasonal affective disorder.
8. **With postpartum onset.** This specifier is used when symptoms of major depression occur within 4 weeks postpartum.

The *DSM-IV-TR* diagnostic criteria for major depressive disorder are presented in Table 15–1.

Dysthymic Disorder

Characteristics of this mood disturbance are similar to, if somewhat milder than, those ascribed to major depressive disorder. Individuals with **dysthymic disorder** describe their mood as sad or "down in the dumps" (APA, 2000). There is no evidence of psychotic symptoms. The essential feature is a chronically depressed mood (or possibly an irritable mood in children or adolescents) for most of the day, more days than not, for at least 2 years (1 year for children and adolescents).

Dysthymic disorder may be further classified as:

1. **Early onset.** Identifies cases of dysthymic disorder when the onset occurs before age 21 years.
2. **Late onset.** Identifies cases of dysthymic disorder when the onset occurs at age 21 years or older.

The *DSM-IV-TR* diagnostic criteria for dysthymic disorder are presented in Table 15–2.

TABLE 15–1 Diagnostic Criteria for Major Depressive Disorder

A. Five (or more) of the following symptoms have been present during the same 2-week period and represent a change from previous functioning; at least one of the symptoms is (1) depressed mood, or (2) loss of interest or pleasure.
   1. Depressed mood most of the day, nearly every day, as indicated by subjective report (e.g., feels sad or empty) or observation made by others (e.g., appears tearful)
      NOTE: In children and adolescents, can be irritable mood
   2. Markedly diminished interest or pleasure in all, or almost all, activities most of the day, nearly every day (as indicated by subjective account or observation made by others)
   3. Significant weight loss when not dieting or weight gain (e.g., a change of more than 5% of body weight in a month), or a decrease or increase in appetite nearly every day
      NOTE: In children, consider failure to make expected weight gains
   4. Insomnia or hypersomnia nearly every day
   5. Psychomotor agitation or retardation nearly every day (observable by others, not merely subjective feelings of restlessness or being slowed down)
   6. Fatigue or loss of energy nearly every day
   7. Feelings of worthlessness or excessive or inappropriate guilt, (which may be delusional) nearly every day (not merely self-reproach or guilt about being sick)
   8. Diminished ability to think or concentrate, or indecisiveness, nearly every day (by subjective account or as observed by others)
   9. Recurrent thoughts of death (not just fear of dying), recurrent suicidal ideation without a specific plan, or a suicide attempt or a specific plan for committing suicide

B. There has never been a manic episode, a mixed episode, or a hypomanic episode that was not substance or treatment induced or due to the direct physiological effects of a general medical condition

C. The symptoms cause clinically significant distress or impairment in social, occupational, or other important areas of functioning

D. The symptoms are not due to the direct physiological effects of a substance (e.g., a drug of abuse or a medication) or a general medical condition (e.g., hypothyroidism)

E. The symptoms are not better accounted for by bereavement (i.e., after the loss of a loved one), the symptoms persist for longer than 2 months, or are characterized by marked functional impairment, morbid preoccupation with worthlessness, suicidal ideation, psychotic symptoms, or psychomotor retardation

American Psychiatric Association, 2000, with permission.

TABLE 15–2 Diagnostic Criteria for Dysthymic Disorder

A. Depressed mood for most of the day, more days than not, as indicated by subjective account or observation by others, for at least 2 years.
NOTE: In children and adolescents, mood can be irritable and duration must be at least 1 year.
B. Presence, while depressed, of two (or more) of the following:
1. Poor appetite or overeating
2. Insomnia or hypersomnia
3. Low energy or fatigue
4. Low self-esteem
5. Poor concentration or difficulty making decisions
6. Feelings of hopelessness
C. During the 2-year period (1 year for children or adolescents) of the disturbance, the person has never been without the symptoms in A or B for more than 2 months at a time.
D. No major depressive disorder has been present during the first 2 years of the disturbance (1 year for children and adolescents).
E. There has never been a manic, mixed, or hypomanic episode, and criteria have never been met for cyclothymic disorder.
F. The disturbance does not occur exclusively during the course of a chronic psychotic disorder, such as schizophrenia or delusional disorder.
G. The symptoms are not due to the direct physiological effects of a substance (e.g., a drug of abuse, a medication) or a general medical condition (e.g., hypothyroidism).
H. The symptoms cause clinically significant distress or impairment in social, occupational, or other important areas of functioning.
Specify if:
Early onset: Before age 21 years
Late onset: Age 21 years or older

American Psychiatric Association, 2000, with permission.

Premenstrual Dysphoric Disorder

The *DSM-IV-TR* (APA, 2000) does not include **premenstrual dysphoric disorder** as an official diagnostic category, but provides a set of research criteria to promote further study of the disorder. The essential features include markedly depressed mood, marked anxiety, mood swings, and decreased interest in activities during the week before menses and subsiding shortly after the onset of menstruation (APA, 2000). The *DSM-IV-TR* research criteria for premenstrual dysphoric disorder are presented in Table 15–3.

TABLE 15–3 Research Criteria for Premenstrual Dysphoric Disorder

A. In most menstrual cycles during the past year, five (or more) of the following symptoms were present for most of the time during the last week of the luteal phase, began to remit within a few days after the onset of the follicular phase, and were absent in the week postmenses, with at least one of the symptoms being 1, 2, 3, or 4:
1. Markedly depressed mood, feelings of hopelessness, or self-deprecating thoughts
2. Marked anxiety, tension, feelings of being "keyed up," or "on edge"
3. Marked affective lability (e.g., feeling suddenly sad or tearful or increased sensitivity to rejection)
4. Persistent and marked anger or irritability or increased interpersonal conflicts
5. Decreased interest in usual activities (e.g., work, school, friends, hobbies)
6. Subjective sense of difficulty in concentrating
7. Lethargy, easy fatigability, or marked lack of energy
8. Marked change in appetite, overeating, or specific food cravings
9. Hypersomnia or insomnia
10. A subjective sense of being overwhelmed or out of control
11. Other physical symptoms, such as breast tenderness or swelling, headaches, joint or muscle pain, a sensation of "bloating," weight gain
B. The disturbance markedly interferes with work or school or with usual social activities and relationships with others (e.g., avoidance of social activities, decreased productivity and efficiency at work or school).
C. The disturbance is not merely an exacerbation of the symptoms of another disorder, such as major depressive disorder, panic disorder, dysthymic disorder, or a personality disorder (although it may be superimposed on any of these disorders).
D. Criteria A, B, and C must be confirmed by prospective daily ratings during at least two consecutive symptomatic cycles.

American Psychiatric Association, 2000, with permission.

Bipolar Disorders

Bipolar disorder is characterized by mood swings from profound depression to extreme euphoria (mania), with intervening periods of normalcy. Delusions or hallucinations may or may not be a part of the clinical picture, and onset of symptoms may reflect a seasonal pattern.

During a manic episode, the mood is elevated, expansive, or irritable. The disturbance is sufficiently severe to cause marked impairment in occupational functioning or in usual social activities or relationships with others or to require hospitalization to prevent harm to self or others. Motor activity is excessive and frenzied. Psychotic features may be present.

A somewhat milder representation of this clinical symptom picture is called **hypomania**. Hypomania is not severe enough to cause marked impairment in social or occupational functioning or to require hospitalization, and it does not include psychotic features. The *DSM-IV-TR* diagnostic criteria for mania are presented in Table 15–4.

The diagnostic picture for depression associated with bipolar disorder is identical to that described for major depressive disorder, with one addition: the client must have a history of one or more manic episodes.

When symptom presentation includes rapidly alternating moods (sadness, irritability, euphoria) accompanied by symptoms associated with both depression and mania, the individual is given a diagnosis of *bipolar disorder, mixed.* This disturbance is severe enough to cause marked impairment in social or occupational functioning or to require hospitalization. Psychotic features may be evident.

Bipolar I Disorder

Bipolar I disorder is the diagnosis given to an individual who is experiencing, or has experienced, a full syndrome of manic or mixed symptoms. The client may also have experienced episodes of depression. This diagnosis is further specified by the current or most recent behavioral episode experienced. For example, the specifier might be a single manic episode (to describe individuals having a first episode of mania) or current (or most recent) manic, hypomanic, mixed, or depressed episode (to describe individuals who have had recurrent mood episodes).

Bipolar II Disorder

This diagnostic category is characterized by recurrent bouts of major depression with episodic occurrence of hypomania. The individual who is assigned this diagnosis may present with symptoms (or history) of depression or hypomania. The client has never experienced an episode that meets the full criteria for mania or mixed symptomatology.

Cyclothymic Disorder

The essential feature of **cyclothymic disorder** is chronic mood disturbance of at least 2-year duration, involving numerous episodes of hypomania and depressed mood of insufficient severity or duration to meet the criteria for bipolar I or bipolar II disorders.

TABLE 15–4 Diagnostic Criteria for Manic Episode

A. A distinct period of abnormally and persistently elevated, expansive, or irritable mood, lasting at least 1 week (or any duration if hospitalization is necessary)

B. During the period of mood disturbance, three (or more) of the following symptoms have persisted (four if the mood is only irritable) and have been present to a significant extent:
   1. Inflated self-esteem or grandiosity
   2. Decreased need for sleep (e.g., feels rested after only 3 hours of sleep)
   3. More talkative than usual or pressure to keep talking
   4. Flight of ideas or subjective experience that thoughts are racing
   5. Distractibility (i.e., attention too easily drawn to unimportant or irrelevant external stimuli)
   6. Increase in goal-directed activity (socially, at work or school, or sexually) or psychomotor agitation
   7. Excessive involvement in pleasurable activities that have a high potential for painful consequences (e.g., engaging in unrestrained buying sprees, sexual indiscretions, or foolish business investments)

C. The mood disturbance is sufficiently severe to cause marked impairment in occupational functioning or in usual social activities or relationships with others, or to necessitate hospitalization to prevent harm to self or others, or there are psychotic features.

D. The symptoms are not due to the direct physiological effects of a substance (e.g., a drug of abuse, a medication, or other treatment) or a general medical condition (e.g., hyperthyroidism).

American Psychiatric Association, 2000, with permission.

TABLE 15–5 Diagnostic Criteria for Cyclothymic Disorder

A. For at least 2 years, the presence of numerous periods with hypomanic symptoms and numerous periods with depressive symptoms that do not meet the criteria for major depressive disorder
NOTE: In children and adolescents, the duration must be at least 1 year.
B. During the 2-year period (1 year in children and adolescents), the person has not been without the symptoms in criterion A for more than 2 months at a time.
C. No major depressive episode, manic episode, or mixed episode has been present during the first 2 years of the disturbance.
D. The symptoms in criterion A are not better accounted for by schizoaffective disorder and are not superimposed on schizophrenia, schizophreniform disorder, delusional disorder, or psychotic disorder not otherwise specified.
E. The symptoms are not due to the direct physiological effects of a substance (e.g., a drug of abuse, a medication) or a general medical condition (e.g., hyperthyroidism).
F. The symptoms cause clinically significant distress or impairment in social, occupational, or other important areas of functioning.

American Psychiatric Association, 2000, with permission.

The individual is never without hypomanic or depressive symptoms for more than 2 months. The *DSM-IV-TR* criteria for cyclothymic disorder are presented in Table 15–5.

Other Mood Disorders

Mood Disorder Due to a General Medical Condition

This disorder is characterized by prominent and persistent disturbance in mood that is judged to be the result of direct physiological effects of a general medical condition (APA, 2000). The mood disturbance may involve depression or elevated, expansive, or irritable mood, and the individual experiences clinically significant distress or impairment in social, occupational, or other important areas of functioning. Types of physiological influences are included in the discussion of etiological implications for mood disorders.

Substance-Induced Mood Disorder

The disturbance of mood associated with this disorder is considered the direct result of physiological effects of a substance (e.g., a drug of abuse, a medication, or toxin exposure). The mood disturbance may involve depression or elevated, expansive, or irritable mood, and causes clinically significant distress or impairment in social, occupational, or other important areas of functioning.

Mood disturbances are associated with *intoxication* from substances such as alcohol, amphetamines, cocaine, hallucinogens, inhalants, opioids, phencyclidine, sedatives, hypnotics, and anxiolytics. Symptoms can occur with *withdrawal* from substances such as alcohol, amphetamines, cocaine, sedatives, hypnotics, and anxiolytics. The following heavy metals and toxins may also cause mood symptoms: gasoline, paint, organophosphate insecticides, nerve gases, carbon monoxide, and carbon dioxide (APA, 2000).

A number of medications have been known to evoke mood symptoms. Classifications include anesthetics, analgesics, anticholinergics, anticonvulsants, antihypertensives, antiparkinsonian agents, antiulcer agents, cardiac medications, oral contraceptives, psychotropic medications, muscle relaxants, steroids, and sulfonamides. Some specific examples are included in the discussion of etiological implications for mood disorders.

DEPRESSIVE DISORDERS

Etiological Implications

Biological Theories

Genetics

Affective illness has been the subject of considerable research on the relevance of hereditary factors. A genetic link has been suggested in numerous studies; however, no definitive mode of genetic transmission has yet to be demonstrated.

TWIN STUDIES. Twin studies suggest a genetic factor in the illness because about 50 percent of monozygotic twins are concordant for the illness (concordant refers to twins who are both affected with the illness). Similar results were revealed in studies of monozygotic twins raised apart. The concordance rate in dizygotic twins is 10 to 25 percent (Sadock & Sadock, 2003).

FAMILY STUDIES. Most family studies have shown that major depression is 1.5 to 3 times more common among first-degree biological relatives of people with the disorder than among the general population (APA, 2000). Indeed, the evidence to support an increased risk of depressive disorder in individuals with a positive family history is quite compelling. It is unlikely that random environmental factors could cause the concentration of illness that is seen within families.

ADOPTION STUDIES. Further support for heritability as an etiological influence in depression comes from studies of the adopted offspring of affectively ill biological parents. Sadock and Sadock (2003) state:

> Adoption studies have shown that the biological children of affected parents remain at increased risk of a mood disorder, even if they are reared in nonaffected, adoptive families. (p. 540)

Biochemical Influences

BIOGENIC AMINES. It has been hypothesized that depressive illness may be related to a deficiency of the neurotransmitters norepinephrine, serotonin, and dopamine at functionally important receptor sites in the brain. Historically, the biogenic amine hypothesis of mood disorders grew out of the observation that reserpine, which depletes the brain of amines, was associated with the development of a depressive syndrome (Winokur, 1994). The catecholamine norepinephrine has been identified as a key component in the mobilization of the body to deal with stressful situations. Neurons that contain serotonin are critically involved in the regulation of many psychobiological functions, such as mood, anxiety, arousal, thinking, cognition, appetite, aggression, and circadian rhythm (Dubovsky & Buzan, 1999). Tryptophan, the amino acid precursor of serotonin, has been shown to enhance the efficacy of antidepressant medications and, on occasion, to be effective as an antidepressant itself. The level of dopamine in the mesolimbic system of the brain is thought to exert a strong influence over human mood and behavior. A diminished supply of these biogenic amines inhibits the transmission of impulses from one neuronal fiber to another, causing a failure of the cells to fire or become charged.

More recently, the biogenic amine hypothesis has been expanded to include another neurotransmitter, acetylcholine. Because cholinergic agents do have profound effects on mood, electroencephalogram, sleep, and neuroendocrine function, it has been suggested that the problem in depression and mania may be an imbalance between the biogenic amines and acetylcholine. Cholinergic transmission is thought to be excessive in depression and inadequate in mania (Dubovsky, Davies, & Dubovsky, 2003).

The precise role that any of the neurotransmitters plays in the etiology of depression is unknown. As the body of research grows, there is no doubt that increased knowledge regarding the biogenic amines will contribute to a greater capacity for understanding and treating affective illness.

Neuroendocrine Disturbances

Neuroendocrine disturbances may play a role in the pathogenesis or persistence of depressive illness. This notion has arisen in view of the marked disturbances in mood observed with the administration of certain hormones or in the presence of spontaneously occurring endocrine disease.

HYPOTHALAMIC-PITUITARY-ADRENOCORTICAL AXIS. In clients who are depressed, the normal system of hormonal inhibition fails, resulting in a hypersecretion of cortisol. This elevated serum cortisol is the basis for the dexamethasone suppression test that is sometimes used to determine if an individual has somatically treatable depression.

HYPOTHALAMIC-PITUITARY-THYROID AXIS. Thyrotropin-releasing factor (TRF) from the hypothalamus stimulates the release of thyroid-stimulating hormone (TSH) from the anterior pituitary gland. In turn, TSH stimulates the thyroid gland. Diminished TSH response to administered TRF is observed in approximately 25 percent of depressed persons. This laboratory test has future potential for identifying clients at high risk for affective illness.

Physiological Influences

Depressive symptoms that occur because of a nonmood disorder or as an adverse effect of certain medications are called *secondary* depression. Secondary depression may be related to medication side effects, neurological disorders, electrolyte or hormonal disturbances, nutritional deficiencies, and other physiological or psychological conditions.

MEDICATION SIDE EFFECTS. A number of drugs, alone or in combination with other medications, can produce a depressive syndrome. Most common among these drugs are those that have a direct effect on the central nervous system. Examples of these include the anxiolytics, antipsychotics, and sedative-hypnotics. Certain antihypertensive medications, such as propranolol and reserpine, have been known to produce depressive symptoms. Depressed mood may also occur with any of the following medications, although the list is by no means all-inclusive (Sadock & Sadock, 2003):

Steroids: prednisone and cortisone
Hormones: estrogen and progesterone
Sedatives: barbiturates and benzodiazepines
Antibacterial and antifungal drugs: ampicillin, cycloserine, tetracycline, and sulfonamides
Antineoplastics: vincristine and zidovudine
Analgesics and anti-inflammatory drugs: opiates, ibuprofen, and phenylbutazone
Antiulcer: cimetidine

NEUROLOGICAL DISORDERS. An individual who has suffered a cardiovascular accident (CVA) may experience a despondency unrelated to the severity of the CVA. These are true mood disorders, and antidepressant drug therapy may be indicated. Brain tumors, particularly in the area of the temporal lobe, often cause symptoms of depression. Agitated depression may be part of the clinical picture associated with Alzheimer's disease, Parkinson's disease, and Huntington's disease. Agitation and restlessness may also represent an underlying depression in the individual with multiple sclerosis.

ELECTROLYTE DISTURBANCES. Excessive levels of sodium bicarbonate or calcium can produce symptoms of depression, as can deficits in magnesium and sodium. Potassium is also implicated in the syndrome of depression. Symptoms have been observed with excesses of potassium in the body and in instances of potassium depletion.

HORMONAL DISTURBANCES. Depression is associated with dysfunction of the adrenal cortex and is commonly observed in both Addison's disease and Cushing's syndrome. Other endocrine conditions that may result in symptoms of depression include hypoparathyroidism, hyperparathyroidism, hypothyroidism, and hyperthyroidism.

An imbalance of the hormones estrogen and progesterone has been implicated in the predisposition to premenstrual dysphoric disorder. It is postulated that excess estrogen or a high estrogen-to-progesterone ratio during the luteal phase of the menstrual cycle is responsible for the symptoms associated with premenstrual syndrome (Sadock & Sadock, 2003).

NUTRITIONAL DEFICIENCIES. Deficiencies in vitamin B_1 (thiamine), vitamin B_6 (pyridoxine), vitamin B_{12}, niacin, vitamin C, iron, folic acid, zinc, calcium, and potassium may produce symptoms of depression (Schimelpfening, 2002).

A number of nutritional alterations have also been implicated in the etiology of premenstrual dysphoric disorder. They include deficiencies in the B vitamins, calcium, magnesium, manganese, vitamin E, and linolenic acid (Frackiewicz & Shiovitz, 2001). Glucose tolerance fluctuations, abnormal fatty acid metabolism, and sensitivity to caffeine and alcohol may also play a role in bringing about the symptoms associated with this disorder. No definitive evidence exists to support any specific nutritional alteration in the etiology of these symptoms.

OTHER PHYSIOLOGICAL CONDITIONS. Other conditions that have been associated with secondary depression include collagen disorders, such as systemic lupus erythematosus (SLE) and polyarteritis nodosa; cardiovascular disease, such as cardiomyopathy, congestive heart failure, myocardial infarction, and CVA (stroke); infections, such as encephalitis, hepatitis, mononucleosis, pneumonia, and syphilis; and metabolic disorders, such as diabetes mellitus and porphyria.

Psychosocial Theories

Psychoanalytical Theory

Freud (1957) presented his classic paper "Mourning and Melancholia" in 1917. He defined the distinguishing features of melancholia as:

> ... a profoundly painful dejection, cessation of interest in the outside world, loss of the capacity to love, inhibition of all activity, and a lowering of the self-regarding feelings to a degree that finds utterances in self-reproaches and self-revilings, and culminates in a delusional expectation of punishment.

He observed that melancholia occurs after the loss of a loved object, actually by death or emotionally by rejection, or by the loss of another abstraction of value to the individual. Freud indicated that in melancholic clients, the depressed person's rage is internally directed because of identification with the lost object (Sadock & Sadock, 2003).

Freud believed that the individual predisposed to melancholia experienced ambivalence in love relationships. He postulated, therefore, that once the loss has been incorporated into the self (ego), the hostile part of the ambivalence that had been felt for the lost object is then turned inward against the ego.

Learning Theory

The model of "learned helplessness" arises out of Seligman's (1973) experiments with dogs. The animals were exposed to electrical stimulation from which they could not escape. Later, when they were given the opportunity to avoid the traumatic experience, they reacted with helplessness and made no attempt to escape. A similar state of helplessness exists in humans who have experienced numerous failures (real or perceived). The individual abandons any further attempt to succeed. Seligman theorized that learned helplessness predisposes individuals to depression by imposing a feeling of lack of control over their life situation. They become depressed because they feel helpless; they have learned that whatever they do is futile. This can be especially damaging very early in life because the sense of mastery over one's environment is an important foundation for future emotional development.

Object Loss Theory

The theory of object loss suggests that depressive illness occurs as a result of having been abandoned by or otherwise separated from a significant other during the first six months of life. Because during this period the mother represents the child's main source of security, she is the "object." The response occurs not only with a physical loss. This absence of attachment, which may be physical or emotional, leads to feelings of helplessness and despair that contribute to lifelong patterns of depression in response to loss.

The concept of "anaclitic depression" was introduced in 1946 by psychiatrist René Spitz to refer to children who became depressed after being separated from their mothers for 3 months or longer during the second 6 months of life (Gale Encyclopedia of Childhood and Adolescence, 1998). The condition included behaviors such as excessive crying, anorexia, withdrawal, psychomotor retardation, stupor, and a generalized impairment in the normal process of growth and development. Some researchers suggest that loss in adult life afflicts people much more severely in the form of depression if the subjects have suffered early childhood loss.

Cognitive Theory

Beck and colleagues (1979) have proposed a theory suggesting that the primary disturbance in depression is cognitive rather than affective. The underlying cause of the depressive affect is seen as cognitive distortions that result in negative, defeated attitudes. Beck identifies three cognitive distortions that he believes serve as the basis for depression:

1. Negative expectations of the environment
2. Negative expectations of the self
3. Negative expectations of the future

These cognitive distortions arise out of a defect in cognitive development, and the individual feels inadequate, worthless, and rejected by others. Outlook for the future is one of pessimism and hopelessness.

Cognitive theorists believe that depression is the product of negative thinking. This is in contrast to the other theorists, who suggest that negative thinking occurs when an individual is depressed. **Cognitive therapy** focuses on helping the individual to alter mood by changing the way he or she thinks. The individual is taught to control negative thought distortions that lead to pessimism, lethargy, procrastination, and low self-esteem (see Chapter 11).

Theoretical Integration

The etiology of depression remains unclear. No single theory or hypothesis has been postulated that substantiates a clear-cut explanation for the disease. Evidence continues to mount in support of multiple causations, recognizing the combined effects of genetic, biochemical, and psychosocial influences on an individual's susceptibility to depression.

Developmental Implications

Childhood

Only in recent years has a consensus developed among investigators identifying major depressive disorder as an entity in children and adolescents that can be identified using criteria similar to those used for adults (Lewis & Volkmar, 1990; APA, 2000). However, it is not uncommon for the symptoms of depression to be manifested differently in childhood, and the picture changes with age (Harvard Medical School, 2002):

1. Up to age 3: Signs may include feeding problems, tantrums, and lack of playfulness and emotional expressiveness.
2. From ages 3 to 5: Common symptoms may include being accident-prone, phobias, and excessive self-reproach for minor infractions.
3. From ages 6 to 8: There may be vague physical complaints and aggressive behavior. They may cling to parents and avoid new people and challenges.
4. At ages 9 to12: Common symptoms include morbid thoughts and excessive worrying. They may

reason that they are depressed because they have disappointed their parents in some way.

Other symptoms of childhood depression may include hyperactivity, delinquency, school problems, psychosomatic complaints, sleeping and eating disturbances, social isolation, and suicidal thoughts or actions.

Children may become depressed for various reasons. In many depressed children, there is a genetic predisposition toward the condition, which is then precipitated by a stressful situation. Common precipitating factors include physical or emotional detachment by the primary caregiver, parental separation or divorce, death of a loved one (person or pet), a move, academic failure, or physical illness. In any event, the common denominator is loss.

The focus of therapy with depressed children is to alleviate the child's symptoms and strengthen the child's coping and adaptive skills, with the hope of possibly preventing future psychological problems. Some studies have shown that untreated childhood depression may lead to subsequent problems in adolescence and adult life. Most children are treated on an outpatient basis. Hospitalization of the depressed child usually occurs only if he or she is actively suicidal, when the home environment precludes adherence to a treatment regimen, or if the child needs to be separated from the home for psychosocial deprivation.

Parental and family therapy are commonly used to help the younger depressed child. Recovery is facilitated by emotional support and guidance to family members. Children older than age 8 years usually participate in family therapy. In some situations, individual treatment may be appropriate for older children. Medications, such as antidepressants or lithium, may be important in the treatment of some children, especially for the more serious and recurrent forms of depression.

Adolescence

Depression may be even harder to recognize in an adolescent than in a younger child. Feelings of sadness, loneliness, anxiety, and hopelessness associated with depression may be perceived as the normal emotional stresses of growing up. Therefore, many young people whose symptoms are attributed to the "normal adjustments" of adolescence do not get the help they need. Depression is a major cause of suicide among teens. During the past three decades, the rate of suicide for ages 15 to 24 years has tripled, and it is the third leading cause of death in this age group (O'Connor, 2002).

Common symptoms of depression in the adolescent are inappropriately expressed anger, aggressiveness, running away, delinquency, social withdrawal, sexual acting out, substance abuse, restlessness, and apathy. Loss of self-esteem, sleeping and eating disturbances, and psychosomatic complaints are also common.

Bipolar disorder, which often emerges during adolescence, is manifested by episodes of impulsivity, irritability, and loss of control, sometimes alternating with periods of withdrawal. These behaviors are often confused with the emotional cycles of adolescence, delaying necessary treatment.

What, then, is the indicator that differentiates mood disorder from the typical stormy behavior of adolescence? A visible manifestation of *behavioral change that lasts for several weeks* is the best clue of a mood disorder. Examples include the normally outgoing and extroverted adolescent who has become withdrawn and antisocial; the good student who previously received consistently high marks but is now failing and skipping classes; and the usually self-confident teenager who is now inappropriately irritable and defensive with others.

Adolescents become depressed for all the same reasons that were discussed in childhood depression. In adolescence, however, depression is a common manifestation of the stress and independence conflicts associated with the normal maturation process. Depression may also be the response to the death of a parent, other relative or friend, or to a breakup with a boyfriend or girlfriend. This perception of abandonment by parents or by one's closest peer relationship is thought to be the most frequent immediate precipitant to adolescent suicide.

Treatment of the depressed adolescent is often conducted on an outpatient basis. Hospitalization may be required in cases of severe depression or threat of imminent suicide, when a family situation is such that treatment cannot be carried out in the home, when the physical condition precludes self-care of biological needs, or when the adolescent has indicated possible harm to self or others in the family.

In addition to supportive psychosocial intervention, antidepressant or lithium therapy is the common modality for treatment of adolescent mood disorders. Various treatments may have to be tried to determine which is most effective.

Senescence

Depression is the most common psychiatric disorder of the elderly, who make up 12.4 percent of the general population of the United States (Administration on Aging, 2002). This is not surprising considering the disproportionate value our society places on youth, vigor, and uninterrupted productivity. These societal attitudes continually nurture the feelings of low self-esteem, helplessness, and hopelessness that become more pervasive and intensive with advanced age. Further, the aging individual's adaptive coping strategies may be seriously challenged by major stressors, such as financial problems, physical illness, changes in bodily functioning, and an increasing awareness of approaching death. The problem is often intensified by the numerous losses individuals experience during this period in life, such as spouse, friends, children, home, and independence. A phenomenon called *bereavement overload* occurs when individuals experience so many losses in their lives that they are not able to resolve one grief response before another one begins. Bereavement overload predisposes elderly individuals to depressive illness.

Although they make up only 12.4 percent of the population, individuals aged 65 and older accounted for 18 percent of all suicides in the United States in 2000 (National Institute of Mental Health [NIMH], 2003). White men aged 85 years and older had the highest number of suicides, with more than 5 times the national rate.

Symptoms of depression in the elderly are not very different from those in younger adults. However, depressive syndromes are often confused by other illnesses associated with the aging process. Symptoms of depression are often misdiagnosed as senile dementia when in fact the memory loss, confused thinking, or apathy symptomatic of senility actually may be due to depression. The early awakening and reduced appetite typical of depression are common among many older people who are not depressed. Compounding this situation is the fact that many medical conditions, such as endocrinological, neurological, nutritional, and metabolic disorders, often present with classic symptoms of depression. Many medications commonly used by the elderly, such as antihypertensives, corticosteroids, and analgesics, also can produce a depressant effect.

Depression does accompany many of the illnesses that afflict older people, such as Parkinson's disease, cancer, arthritis, and the early stages of Alzheimer's disease. Treating depression in these situations can reduce unnecessary suffering and help afflicted individuals cope with their medical problems.

The most effective treatment of depression in the elderly individual is thought to be a combination of psychosocial and biological approaches. Antidepressant medications are administered with consideration for age-related physiological changes in absorption, distribution, elimination, and brain receptor sensitivity. Because of these changes, plasma concentrations of these medications can reach very high levels despite moderate oral doses.

Electroconvulsive therapy (ECT) remains one of the safest and most effective treatments for major depression in the elderly. The response to ECT appears to be slower with advancing age, and the therapeutic effects are of limited duration. However, it may be considered the treatment of choice for the elderly individual who is an acute suicidal risk or is unable to tolerate antidepressant medications.

Other therapeutic approaches include interpersonal, behavioral, cognitive, group, and family psychotherapies. Appropriate treatment of the depressed elderly individual can bring relief from suffering and offer a new lease on life with a feeling of renewed productivity.

Postpartum Depression

The severity of depression in the postpartum period varies from a feeling of the "blues," to moderate depression, to psychotic depression or melancholia. Of women who give birth, approximately 50 to 80 percent experience the "blues" following delivery (Kennedy & Suttenfield, 2002). The incidence of moderate depression is 10 to 16 percent. Severe, or psychotic, depression occurs rarely, in about 1 or 2 out of 1000 postpartum women.

Symptoms of the "maternity blues" include tearfulness, despondency, anxiety, and subjectively impaired concentration appearing in the early puerperium. The symptoms usually begin 3 to 4 days after delivery, worsen by days 5 to 7, and tend to resolve by day 12 (Kennedy & Suttenfield, 2002).

Symptoms of moderate **postpartum depression** have been described as depressed mood varying from day-to-day, with more bad days than good, tending to be worse toward evening and associated with fatigue, irritability, loss of appetite, sleep disturbances, and loss of libido. In addition, the new mother expresses a great deal of concern about her inability to care for her baby. These symptoms begin somewhat later than those described in the "maternity blues," and take from a few weeks to several months to abate.

Postpartum melancholia, or depressive psychosis, is characterized by depressed mood, agitation, indecision, lack of concentration, guilt, and an abnormal attitude toward bodily functions. There may be lack of interest in, or rejection of, the baby, or a morbid fear that the baby may be harmed. Risks of suicide and infanticide should not be overlooked. These symptoms generally develop within 2 to 3 weeks following delivery, but sometimes they occur as early as 48 to 72 hours postpartum (Kennedy & Suttenfield, 2002).

The etiology of postpartum depression remains unclear. "Maternity blues" may be associated with hormonal changes, tryptophan metabolism, or alterations in membrane transport during the early postpartum period. Besides being exposed to these same somatic changes, the woman who experiences moderate-to-severe symptoms probably possesses a vulnerability to depression related to heredity, upbringing, early life experiences, personality, or social circumstances. Some women with this disorder complain of lack of support from their husbands and dissatisfaction with their marriage. Some studies suggest that they are likely to believe that their own parents did not care for them adequately (Harvard Medical School, 1997). The etiology of postpartum depression may very likely be a combination of hormonal, metabolic, and psychosocial influences.

Treatment of postpartum depression varies with the severity of the illness. Psychotic depression may be treated with antidepressant medication, along with supportive psychotherapy, group therapy, and possibly family therapy. Moderate depression may be relieved with supportive psychotherapy and continuing assistance with home management until the symptoms subside. "Maternity blues" usually need no treatment beyond a word of reassurance from the physician or nurse that these feelings are common and will soon pass. A bit of extra support and comfort from significant others also is important.

APPLICATION OF THE NURSING PROCESS TO DEPRESSIVE DISORDERS

Background Assessment Data

Symptomatology of depression can be viewed on a continuum according to severity of the illness. All individuals become depressed from time to time. These are transient symptoms that accompany the everyday disappointments of life. Examples of the disappointments include failing an examination or breaking up with a boyfriend or girlfriend. Transient symptoms of depression subside relatively quickly as the individual advances toward other goals and achievements.

Mild depressive episodes occur when the grief process is triggered in response to the loss of a valued object. This can occur with the loss of a loved one, pet, friend, home, or significant other. As one is able to work through the stages of grief, the loss is accepted, symptoms subside, and activities of daily living are resumed within a few weeks. If this does not occur, grief is prolonged or exaggerated, and symptoms intensify.

Moderate depression occurs when grief is prolonged or exaggerated. The individual becomes fixed in the anger stage of the grief response, and the anger is turned inward on the self. All of the feelings associated with normal grieving are exaggerated out of proportion, and the individual is unable to function without assistance. Dysthymic disorder is an example of moderate depression.

Severe depression is an intensification of the symptoms associated with the moderate level. The individual who is severely depressed may also demonstrate a loss of contact with reality. This level is associated with a complete lack of pleasure in all activities, and ruminations about suicide are common. Major depressive disorder is an example of severe depression. A continuum of depression is presented in Figure 15–1.

Symptoms of depression can be described as alterations in four spheres of human functioning: affective, behavioral, cognitive, and physiological. Alterations within these spheres differ according to extent of severity of symptomatology.

Transient Depression

Symptoms at this level of the continuum are not necessarily dysfunctional. Alterations include:

1. **Affective:** sadness, dejection, feeling downhearted, having the "blues"
2. **Behavioral:** some crying possible
3. **Cognitive:** some difficulty getting mind off one's disappointment
4. **Physiological:** feeling tired and listless

Mild Depression

Symptoms at the mild level of depression are identified by those associated with normal grieving. Alterations at the mild level include:

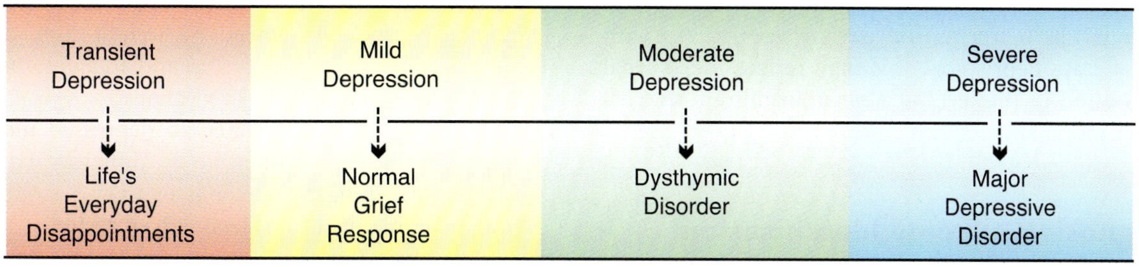

FIGURE 15–1 A continuum of depression.

1. **Affective:** denial of feelings, anger, anxiety, guilt, helplessness, hopelessness, sadness, despondency
2. **Behavioral:** tearfulness, regression, restlessness, agitation, withdrawal
3. **Cognitive:** preoccupation with the loss, self-blame, ambivalence, blaming others
4. **Physiological:** anorexia or overeating, insomnia or hypersomnia, headache, backache, chest pain, or other symptoms associated with the loss of a significant other

Moderate Depression

This level of depression represents a more problematic disturbance. Symptoms associated with dysthymic disorder include:

1. **Affective:** feelings of sadness, dejection, helplessness, powerlessness, hopelessness; gloomy and pessimistic outlook; low self-esteem; difficulty experiencing pleasure in activities
2. **Behavioral:** slowed physical movements (i.e., psychomotor retardation); slumped posture; slowed speech; limited verbalizations, possibly consisting of ruminations about life's failures or regrets; social isolation with a focus on the self; increased use of substances possible; self-destructive behavior possible; decreased interest in personal hygiene and grooming
3. **Cognitive:** retarded thinking processes; difficulty concentrating and directing attention; obsessive and repetitive thoughts, generally portraying pessimism and negativism; verbalizations and behavior reflecting suicidal ideation
4. **Physiological:** anorexia or overeating; insomnia or hypersomnia; sleep disturbances; amenorrhea; decreased libido; headaches; backaches; chest pain; abdominal pain; low energy level; fatigue and listlessness; feeling best early in the morning and continually worse as the day progresses. This may be related to the diurnal variation in the level of neurotransmitters that affect mood and level of activity.

Severe Depression

Severe depression is characterized by an intensification of the symptoms described for moderate depression. Examples of severe depression include major depressive disorder and bipolar depression. Symptoms at the severe level of depression include:

1. **Affective:** feelings of total despair, hopelessness, and worthlessness; flat (unchanging) affect, appearing devoid of emotional tone; prevalent feelings of nothingness and emptiness; apathy; loneliness; sadness; inability to feel pleasure
2. **Behavioral:** psychomotor retardation so severe that physical movement may literally come to a standstill, or psychomotor behavior manifested by rapid, agitated, purposeless movements; slumped posture; sitting in a curled-up position; walking slowly and rigidly; virtually nonexistent communication (when verbalizations do occur, they may reflect delusional thinking); no personal hygiene and grooming; social isolation with no inclination toward interaction with others
3. **Cognitive:** prevalent delusional thinking, with delusions of persecution and somatic delusions being most common; confusion, indecisiveness, and an inability to concentrate; hallucinations reflecting misinterpretations of the environment; excessive self-deprecation, self-blame, and thoughts of suicide. *Note:* Because of the low energy level and retarded thought processes, the individual may be unable to follow through on suicidal ideas. However, the desire is strong at this level.
4. **Physiological:** a general slowdown of the entire body, reflected in sluggish digestion, constipation, and urinary retention; amenorrhea; impotence; diminished libido; anorexia; weight loss; difficulty falling asleep and awakening very early in the

morning; feeling worse early in the morning and somewhat better as the day progresses. As with moderate depression, this may reflect the diurnal variation in the level of neurotransmitters that affect mood and activity.

Diagnosis/Outcome Identification

From the assessment data, the nurse formulates the appropriate nursing diagnoses for the depressed client. From these identified problems, care planning is executed, nursing actions are implemented, and relevant criteria for evaluation are established. Possible nursing diagnoses for depressed clients include:

Risk for suicide related to depressed mood, feelings of worthlessness, anger turned inward on the self, misinterpretations of reality

Dysfunctional grieving related to real or perceived loss, or bereavement overload evidenced by denial of loss, inappropriate expression of anger, idealization of or obsession with the lost object, inability to carry out activities of daily living

Low self-esteem related to learned helplessness, feelings of abandonment by significant other, or impaired cognition fostering negative view of self evidenced by expressions of worthlessness, hypersensitivity to a slight or criticism, and a negative, pessimistic outlook

Powerlessness related to dysfunctional grieving process and a lifestyle of helplessness evidenced by feelings of lack of control over life situation or overdependence on others to fulfill needs

Spiritual distress related to dysfunctional grieving over loss of valued object evidenced by anger toward God, questioning meaning of own existence, or inability to participate in usual religious practices

Social isolation/impaired social interaction related to developmental regression, egocentric behaviors, or fear of rejection or failure of the interaction evidenced by being uncommunicative and withdrawn, seeking to be alone, and dysfunctional interaction with peers, family, or others

Disturbed thought processes related to withdrawal into the self, underdeveloped ego, punitive superego, or impaired cognition fostering negative perception of self or environment evidenced by delusional thinking, confusion, difficulty concentrating, or impaired problem-solving ability

Imbalanced nutrition, less than body requirements related to depressed mood, loss of appetite, or lack of interest in food evidenced by weight loss, poor muscle tone, pale conjunctiva and mucous membranes, poor skin turgor, or weakness

Disturbed sleep pattern related to depressed mood, anxiety, and fears evidenced by difficulty falling asleep, awakening earlier or later than desired, or verbal complaints of not feeling well rested

Self-care deficit (hygiene, grooming) related to depressed mood, or feelings of worthlessness, evidenced by uncombed hair, disheveled clothing, or offensive body odor

The following criteria may be used for measurement of outcomes in the care of the depressed client. The client:

1. Has experienced no physical harm to self
2. Discusses the loss with staff and family members
3. No longer idealize or obsess about the lost object
4. Sets realistic goals for self
5. Is no longer afraid to attempt new activities
6. Is able to identify aspects of self-control over life situation
7. Expresses personal satisfaction and support from spiritual practices
8. Interacts willingly and appropriately with others
9. Is able to maintain reality orientation
10. Is able to concentrate, reason, and solve problems
11. Eats a well-balanced diet with snacks, to prevent weight loss and maintain nutritional status
12. Sleeps 6 to 8 hours per night and reports feeling well rested
13. Bathes, washes and combs hair, and dresses in clean clothing without assistance

Planning/Implementation

Table 15–6 provides a plan of care for the depressed client. Selected nursing diagnoses are presented, along with outcome criteria, appropriate nursing interventions, and rationales for each. A critical pathway for the depressed client may be found in Appendix E.

Client/Family Education

The role of client teacher is important in the psychiatric area, as it is in all areas of nursing. A list of topics for client/family education relevant to depression is presented in Table 15–7.

TABLE 15-6 Care Plan for the Depressed Client

Nursing Diagnosis: RISK FOR SUICIDE

Related to: Depressed mood, feelings of worthlessness, anger turned inward on the self, misinterpretations of reality

Outcome Criteria	Nursing Interventions	Rationale
Client will not harm self	1. Ask client directly: "Have you thought about harming yourself in any way? If so, what do you plan to do? Do you have the means to carry out this plan?"	1. The risk of suicide is greatly increased if the client has developed a plan and particularly if means exist for the client to execute the plan.
	2. Create a safe environment for the client. Remove all potentially harmful objects from client's access (sharp objects, straps, belts, ties, glass items, alcohol). Supervise closely during meals and medication administration. Perform room searches as deemed necessary.	2. Client safety is a nursing priority.
	3. Formulate a short-term verbal or written contract that the client will not harm self. When time is up, make another, and so forth. Secure a promise that the client will seek out staff when feeling suicidal.	3. A degree of the responsibility for his or her safety is given to the client. Increased feelings of self-worth may be experienced when client feels accepted unconditionally regardless of thoughts or behavior.
	4. Maintain close observation of client. Depending on level of suicide precaution, provide one-to-one contact, constant visual observation, or checks every-15-minutes. Place room close to nurse's station; do not assign to private room. Accompany to off-ward activities if attendance is indicated. May need to accompany to bathroom.	4. Close observation is necessary to ensure that client does not harm self in any way. Being alert for suicide and escape attempts facilitates being able to prevent or interrupt harmful behavior.
	5. Maintain special care in administration of medications.	5. Prevents hoarding for overdose or discarding and not taking
	6. Make rounds at frequent, ***irregular*** intervals (especially at night, toward early morning, at change of shift, or other predictably busy times for staff).	6. Prevents staff surveillance from becoming predictable. To be aware of client's location is important, especially when staff is busy, unavailable, and observable
	7. Encourage client to express honest feelings, including anger. Provide hostility release if needed.	7. Depression and suicidal behaviors may be viewed as anger turned inward on the self. If this anger can be verbalized in a nonthreatening environment, the client may be able to eventually resolve these feelings.

Nursing Diagnosis: DYSFUNCTIONAL GRIEVING

Related to: Real or perceived loss; bereavement overload

Evidenced by: Denial of loss, inappropriate expression of anger, idealization of or obsession with lost object, inability to carry out activities of daily living

Outcome Criteria	Nursing Interventions	Rationale
Client will be able to verbalize normal behaviors associated with grieving and begin progression toward resolution.	1. Assess stage of fixation in grief process.	1. Accurate baseline data are required in order to plan accurate care.
	2. Develop trust. Show empathy, concern, and unconditional positive regard.	2. Developing trust provides the basis for a therapeutic relationship.
	3. Explore feelings of anger and help client direct them toward the intended object or person. Promote the use of large motor activities for relieving pent-up tension.	3. Until client can recognize and accept personal feelings regarding the loss, grief work cannot progress. Physical exercise is a safe and effective way of relieving internalized anger.
	4. Teach normal behaviors associated with grieving.	4. Understanding of the grief process will help prevent feelings of guilt generated by these responses.
	5. Help client with honest review of relationship with lost object.	5. Only when the client is able to see both positive and negative aspects related to the lost object will the grieving process be complete.

(Continued)

TABLE 15–6 Care Plan for the Depressed Client *(Continued)*

Nursing Diagnosis: LOW SELF-ESTEEM

Related to: Learned helplessness, feelings of abandonment by significant other, impaired cognition fostering negative view of self

Evidenced by: Expressions of worthlessness, hypersensitivity to slights or criticism, negative, pessimistic outlook

Outcome Criteria	Nursing Interventions	Rationale
Client will be able to attempt new activities without fear of failure. Client will be able to verbalize positive aspects about self.	1. Be accepting of client and spend time with him or her even though pessimism and negativism may seem objectionable. Focus on strengths and accomplishments and minimize failures.	1. Interventions that focus on the positive contribute toward feelings of self-worth.
	2. Promote attendance in therapy groups that offer client simple methods of accomplishment. Encourage client to be as independent as possible.	2. Success and independence promote feelings of self-worth.
	3. Encourage client to recognize areas of change and provide assistance toward this effort.	3. Client will need assistance with problem solving.
	4. Teach assertiveness and communication techniques.	4. Effective communication and assertiveness techniques enhance self-esteem.

Nursing Diagnosis: POWERLESSNESS

Related to: Dysfunctional grieving process, lifestyle of helplessness

Evidenced by: Feelings of lack of control over life situation, overdependence on others to fulfill needs

Outcome Criteria	Nursing Interventions	Rationale
Client will be able to solve problems to take control of life situation.	1. Allow client to participate in goal setting and decision–making regarding own care	1. Providing client with choices will increase his or her feelings of control.
	2. Ensure that goals are realistic and that client is able to identify areas of life situation realistically under his or her control.	2. Realistic goals will avoid setting client up for further failures.
	3. Encourage client to verbalize feelings about areas not within his or her ability to control.	3. Verbalization of unresolved issues may help client accept what cannot be changed.

Nursing Diagnosis: SPIRITUAL DISTRESS

Related to: Dysfunctional grieving over loss of valued object

Evidenced by: Anger toward God, questioning meaning of own existence, inability to participate in usual religious practices

Outcome Criteria	Nursing Interventions	Rationale
Client will express achievement of support and personal satisfaction from spiritual practices.	1. Be accepting and nonjudgmental when client expresses anger and bitterness toward God. Stay with client.	1. The nurse's presence and nonjudgmental attitude increase the client's feelings of self-worth and promote trust in the relationship.
	2. Encourage client to ventilate feelings related to meaning of own existence in the face of current loss.	2. Client may believe he or she cannot go on living without lost object. Catharsis can provide relief and put life back into realistic perspective.
	3. Encourage client as part of grief work to reach out to previous religious practices for support. Encourage client to discuss these practices and how they provided support in the past.	3. Client may find comfort in religious rituals with which he or she is familiar.
	4. Reassure client that he or she is not alone when feeling inadequate in the search for life's answers.	4. Validation of client's feelings and assurance that others share them offers reassurance and an affirmation of acceptability.
	5. Contact spiritual leader of client's choice, if he or she requests.	5. These individuals serve to provide relief from spiritual distress and often can do so when other support persons cannot.

Nursing Diagnosis: HOPELESSNESS

Related to: Absence of support systems and perception of worthlessness

Evidenced by: Verbal cues (despondent content, "I can't"), decreased affect, lack of initiative, suicidal ideas or attempts

Outcome Criteria	Nursing Interventions	Rationale
Client will verbalize a measure of hope and acceptance of life and situations over which he or she has no control.	1. Identify stressors in client's life that precipitated current crisis.	1. Important to identify causative or contributing factors in order to plan appropriate assistance
	2. Determine coping behaviors previously used and client's perception of effectiveness then and now.	2. It is important to identify client's strengths and encourage their use in current crisis.
	3. Encourage client to explore and verbalize feelings and perceptions.	3. Identification of feelings and underlying behaviors helps client to begin process of taking control of own life.
	4. Provide expressions of hope to client in positive, low-key manner, (e.g., "I know you feel you cannot go on, but I believe that things can get better for you. What you are feeling is temporary. It is okay if you don't see it just now. You are very important to the people who care about you.")	4. Even though the client feels hopeless, it is helpful to hear positive expressions from others. The client's current state–of–mind may prevent him or her from identifying anything positive in life. It is important to accept the client's feelings nonjudgmentally and to affirm the individual's personal worth and value.
	5. Help client identify areas of life situation that are under own control.	5. The client's emotional condition may interfere with ability to problem–solve. Assistance may be required to perceive the benefits and consequences of available alternatives accurately.
	6. Identify sources that client may use after discharge when crises occur, or feelings of hopelessness and possible suicidal ideation prevail.	6. Client should be made aware of local suicide hotlines or other local support services from which he or she may seek assistance following discharge from the hospital. A concrete plan provides hope in the face of a crisis.

TABLE 15–7 Topics for Client/Family Education Related to Depression

Nature of the Illness
1. Stages of grief and symptoms associated with each stage
2. What is depression?
3. Why do people get depressed?
4. What are the symptoms of depression?

Management of the Illness
1. Medication management
   a. Nuisance side effects
   b. Side effects to report to physician
   c. Importance of taking regularly
   d. Length of time to take effect
   e. Diet (related to MAOIs)
2. Assertiveness techniques
3. Stress-management techniques
4. Ways to increase self-esteem
5. ECT

Support Services
1. Suicide hotline
2. Support groups
3. Legal and financial assistance

Evaluation of Care for the Depressed Client

In the final step of the nursing process, a reassessment is conducted to determine if the nursing actions have been successful in achieving the objectives of care. Evaluation of the nursing actions for the depressed client may be facilitated by gathering information using the following types of questions:

1. Has self-harm to the individual been avoided?
2. Have suicidal ideations subsided?
3. Does the individual know where to seek assistance outside the hospital when suicidal thoughts occur?
4. Has the client discussed the recent loss with staff and family members?
5. Is he or she able to verbalize feelings and behaviors associated with each stage of the grieving process and recognize own position in the process?
6. Have obsession with and idealization of the lost object subsided?

7. Is anger toward the lost object expressed appropriately?
8. Does client set realistic goals for self?
9. Is he or she able to verbalize positive aspects about self, past accomplishments, and future prospects?
10. Can the client identify areas of life situation over which he or she has control?
11. Is the client able to participate in usual religious practices and feel satisfaction and support from them?
12. Is the client seeking out interaction with others in an appropriate manner?
13. Does the client maintain reality orientation with no evidence of delusional thinking?
14. Is he or she able to concentrate and make decisions concerning own self-care?
15. Is the client selecting and consuming foods sufficiently high in nutrients and calories to maintain weight and nutritional status?
16. Does the client sleep without difficulty and wake feeling rested?
17. Does the client show pride in appearance by attending to personal hygiene and grooming?
18. Have somatic complaints subsided?

BIPOLAR DISORDER (MANIA)

Predisposing Factors

Biological Theories

Genetics

TWIN STUDIES. Twin studies have indicated a concordance rate for bipolar disorder among monozygotic twins at 60 to 80 percent compared to 20 percent in dizygotic twins (Harvard Medical School, 2001). Because monozygotic twins have identical genes and dizygotic twins share only approximately half their genes, this is strong evidence that heredity plays a major role in the etiology of bipolar disorder.

FAMILY STUDIES. Family studies have shown that if one parent has bipolar disorder, the risk that a child will have the disorder is around 28 percent (Dubovsky, Davies, & Dubovsky, 2003). If both parents have the disorder, the risk is 2 to 3 times as great. This has also been shown to be the case in studies of children born to parents with bipolar disorder who were adopted at birth and reared by adoptive parents without evidence of the disorder. These results strongly indicate that genes play a role separate from that of the environment.

Biochemical Influences

BIOGENIC AMINES. Early studies have associated symptoms of depression with a functional deficiency of the biogenic amines norepinephrine, serotonin, and/or dopamine. Mania has been associated with a functional excess of these amines. A recent study at the University of Michigan using a presynaptic marker and positron emission tomography revealed an increased density in the amine-releasing cells in the brains of people with bipolar disorder compared to control subjects (Zubieta et al., 2000). It was hypothesized that these excess cells result in the altered brain chemistry that is associated with the symptoms of bipolar disorder. Some support of this neurotransmitter hypothesis has been demonstrated by the effects of neuroleptic drugs that influence the levels of biogenic amines to produce the desired effect.

ELECTROLYTES. Some studies have suggested possible alterations in normal electrolyte transfer across cell membranes in bipolar disorder resulting in elevated levels of intracellular sodium and calcium (Bohrer, 2001). The link between increased intracellular calcium and symptoms of bipolar disorder may be substantiated by the effectiveness of calcium channel blockers (e.g., verapamil; amlodipine) in some cases of refractory bipolar illness.

Physiological Influences

NEUROANATOMICAL FACTORS. Right-sided lesions in the limbic system, temporobasal areas, basal ganglia, and thalamus have been shown to induce secondary mania (Dubovsky, Davies, & Dubovsky, 2003). Magnetic resonance imaging studies have revealed enlarged third ventricles and subcortical white matter and periventricular hyperintensity in clients with bipolar disorder (Dubovsky & Buzan, 1999).

MEDICATION SIDE EFFECTS. Certain medications used to treat somatic illnesses have been known to trigger a manic response. The most common of these are the steroids, frequently used to treat chronic illnesses such as multiple sclerosis and SLE. Some clients whose first episode of mania occurred during steroid therapy have reported spontaneous recurrence of manic symptoms years later. Amphetamines, antidepressants, and high doses of anticonvulsants and narcotics also have the potential for initiating a manic episode (Dubovsky, Davies, & Dubovsky, 2003).

Psychosocial Theories

The credibility of psychosocial theories has declined in recent years. Conditions such as schizophrenia and bipolar disorder are being viewed by many as diseases of the brain with biological etiologies. The etiology of these illnesses remains unclear, however, and it is possible that both biological and psychosocial factors (such as environmental stressors) are influential (NIMH, 2000).

Kaplan and Sadock (1998) state:

> The causative factors (of mood disorders) can artificially be divided into biological, genetic, and psychosocial, but this division is artificial because the three realms likely interact among themselves. Psychosocial and genetic factors can affect biological factors, such as concentrations of a certain neurotransmitter. Biological and psychosocial factors can also affect gene expression, and biological and genetic factors can affect a person's response to psychosocial factors. (p. 524)

APPLICATION OF THE NURSING PROCESS TO BIPOLAR DISORDER (MANIA)

Background Assessment Data

Symptoms of manic states can be described according to three stages: hypomania, acute mania, and **delirious mania**. Symptoms of mood, cognition and perception, and activity and behavior are presented for each stage.

Stage I: Hypomania

At this stage the disturbance is not sufficiently severe to cause marked impairment in social or occupational functioning or to require hospitalization (APA, 2000).

MOOD. The mood of a hypomanic person is cheerful and expansive. However, there is an underlying irritability that surfaces rapidly when the person's wishes and desires go unfulfilled. The nature of the hypomanic person is very volatile and fluctuating.

COGNITION AND PERCEPTION. Perceptions of the self are exalted—ideas of great worth and ability. Thinking is flighty, with a rapid flow of ideas. Perception of the environment is heightened, but the individual is so easily distracted by irrelevant stimuli that goal-directed activities are difficult.

ACTIVITY AND BEHAVIOR. Hypomanic individuals exhibit increased motor activity. They are perceived as being very extroverted and sociable, and because of this they attract numerous acquaintances. However, they lack the depth of personality and warmth to formulate close friendships. They talk and laugh a lot, usually very loudly and often inappropriately. Increased libido is common. Some individuals experience anorexia and weight loss. The exalted self-perception leads some hypomanics to engage in inappropriate behaviors, such as phoning the president of the United States, or buying huge amounts on a credit card without having the resources to pay.

Stage II: Acute Mania

Symptoms of acute mania may be a progression and intensification of those experienced in hypomania, or may be manifested directly. Most individuals experience marked impairment in functioning and require hospitalization.

MOOD. Acute mania is characterized by euphoria and elation. The person appears to be on a continuous "high." However, the mood is always subject to frequent variation, easily changing to irritability and anger or even to sadness and crying.

COGNITION AND PERCEPTION. Cognition and perception become fragmented and often psychotic in acute mania. Rapid thinking proceeds to racing and disjointed thinking (flight of ideas) and may be manifested by a continuous flow of accelerated, pressured speech (loquaciousness), with abrupt changes from topic to topic. When flight of ideas is severe, speech may be disorganized and incoherent. Distractibility becomes all-pervasive. Attention can be diverted by even the smallest of stimuli. Hallucinations and delusions (usually paranoid and grandiose) are common.

ACTIVITY AND BEHAVIOR. Psychomotor activity is excessive. Sexual interest is increased. There is poor impulse control, and the individual who is normally discreet may become socially and sexually uninhibited. Excessive spending is common. Individuals with acute mania have the ability to manipulate others to carry out their wishes, and if things go wrong, they can skillfully project responsibility for the failure onto others. Energy seems inexhaustible, and the need for sleep is diminished. They may go for many days without sleep and still not feel tired. Hygiene and grooming may be neglected. Dress may be disorganized, flamboyant, or bizarre, and the use of excessive makeup or jewelry is common.

Stage III: Delirious Mania

Delirious mania is a severe form of the disorder characterized by a clouding of consciousness and an intensification of the symptoms associated with acute mania. This condition has become relatively rare since the availability of antipsychotic medication.

MOOD. The mood of the delirious person is very labile. He or she may exhibit feelings of despair, quickly converting to unrestrained merriment and ecstasy or becoming irritable or indifferent to the environment. Panic anxiety may be evident.

COGNITION AND PERCEPTION. Cognition and perception are characterized by a clouding of consciousness, with accompanying confusion, disorientation, and sometimes stupor. Other common manifestations include religiosity, delusions of grandeur or persecution, and auditory or visual hallucinations. The individual is extremely distractible and incoherent.

ACTIVITY AND BEHAVIOR. Psychomotor activity is frenzied and characterized by agitated, purposeless movements. The safety of these individuals is at stake unless this activity is curtailed. Exhaustion, injury to self or others, and eventually death could occur without intervention.

Diagnosis/Outcome Identification

Nursing diagnoses are formulated from the assessment data, and the plan of care is devised. Possible nursing diagnoses for the client with bipolar disorder (mania) include:

Risk for injury related to extreme hyperactivity evidenced by increased agitation and lack of control over purposeless and potentially injurious movements

Risk for violence: self-directed or other-directed related to manic excitement, delusional thinking, hallucinations

Imbalanced nutrition: less than body requirements related to refusal or inability to sit still long enough to eat evidenced by loss of weight, amenorrhea

Disturbed thought processes related to biochemical alterations in the brain evidenced by delusions of grandeur and persecution

Disturbed sensory perception related to biochemical alterations in the brain, possible sleep deprivation, evidenced by auditory and visual hallucinations

Impaired social interaction related to egocentric and narcissistic behavior evidenced by inability to develop satisfying relationships and manipulation of others for own desires

Disturbed sleep pattern related to excessive hyperactivity and agitation, evidenced by difficulty falling asleep and sleeping only short periods

The following criteria may be used for measuring outcomes in the care of the manic client. The client:

1. Exhibits no evidence of physical injury
2. Has not harmed self or others
3. Is no longer exhibiting signs of physical agitation
4. Eats a well-balanced diet with snacks to prevent weight loss and maintain nutritional status
5. Verbalizes an accurate interpretation of the environment
6. Verbalizes that hallucinatory activity has ceased and demonstrates no outward behavior indicating hallucinations
7. Accepts responsibility for own behaviors
8. Does not manipulate others for gratification of own needs
9. Interacts appropriately with others
10. Is able to fall asleep within 30 minutes of retiring
11. Is able to sleep 6 to 8 hours per night without medication

Planning/Implementation

Table 15–8 provides a plan of care for the manic client. Selected nursing diagnoses are presented, along with outcome criteria, appropriate nursing interventions, and rationales for each. A critical pathway for the manic client is included in Appendix E.

Client/Family Education

The role of client-teacher is important in the psychiatric area, as it is in all areas of nursing. A list of topics for client/family education relevant to bipolar disorder is presented in Table 15–9.

Evaluation of Care for the Manic Client

In the final step of the nursing process, a reassessment is conducted to determine if the nursing actions have been successful in achieving the objectives of care. Evaluation of the nursing actions for the manic client may be facilitated by gathering information using the following types of questions.

TABLE 15–8 Care Plan for the Client Experiencing a Manic Episode

Nursing Diagnosis: RISK FOR INJURY
Related to: Extreme hyperactivity
Evidenced by: Increased agitation and lack of control over purposeless and potentially injurious movements

Outcome Criteria	Nursing Interventions	Rationale
Client will not experience injury	1. Reduce environmental stimuli. Assign private room with simple decor, on quiet unit if possible. Keep lighting and noise level low.	1. Client is extremely distractible and responses to even the slightest stimuli are exaggerated. A milieu unit may be too stimulating.
	2. Remove hazardous objects and substances (including smoking materials).	2. Rationality is impaired, and client may harm self inadvertently.
	3. Stay with the client who is hyperactive and agitated.	3. Nurse's presence may offer support and provide feeling of security for the client.
	4. Provide physical activities.	4. Physical activities help relieve pent-up tension.
	5. Administer tranquilizing medication as ordered by physician.	5. Antipsychotics are common and are very effective for providing rapid relief from symptoms of hyperactivity.

Nursing Diagnosis: RISK FOR VIOLENCE: SELF-DIRECTED OR OTHER-DIRECTED
Related to: Manic excitement, delusional thinking, hallucinations

Outcome Criteria	Nursing Interventions	Rationale
Client will not harm self or others	1. Maintain low level of stimuli in client's environment	1. This will minimize anxiety, agitation, and suspiciousness.
	2. Observe client's behavior at least every 15 minutes.	2. This is important so that intervention can occur if required to ensure client's (and others') safety.
	3. Ensure that all sharp objects, glass or mirrored items, belts, ties, smoking materials have been removed from client's environment.	3. These objects must be removed so that client cannot use them to harm self or others.
	4. Redirect violent behavior with physical outlets.	4. Physical activity is good for relieving pent-up tension and hostility.
	5. Maintain and convey a calm attitude to client. Respond matter-of-factly to verbal hostility.	5. Anxiety is contagious and can be transmitted from staff to client.
	6. Have sufficient staff to indicate a show of strength to client if necessary.	6. This conveys evidence of control over the situation and provides some physical security for staff.
	7. Offer tranquilizing medication. If client refuses, use of mechanical restraints may be necessary.	7. Client should be offered an avenue of the "least restrictive alternative."
	8. Medication may then be administered following application of mechanical restraints. Observe client every 15 minutes.	8. This ensures that needs for circulation, nutrition, hydration, and elimination are met. Client safety is a nursing priority.
	9. Remove restraints gradually, one at a time.	9. Gradual removal of restraints minimizes potential for injury to client and staff.

Nursing Diagnosis: IMBALANCED NUTRITION: LESS THAN BODY REQUIREMENTS
Related to: Refusal or inability to sit still long enough to eat
Evidenced by: Weight loss, amenorrhea

Outcome Criteria	Nursing Interventions	Rationale
Client will exhibit no signs or symptoms of malnutrition	1. Provide high-protein, high-calorie, nutritious finger foods and drinks that can be consumed "on the run."	1. Client has difficulty sitting still long enough to eat a meal.
	2. Have juice and snacks on the unit at all times.	2. Nutritious intake is required on a regular basis to compensate for increased caloric requirement as a result of hyperactivity.

(Continued)

TABLE 15-8 Care Plan for the Client Experiencing a Manic Episode *(Continued)*

Outcome Criteria	Nursing Interventions	Rationale
	3. Maintain accurate record of intake, output, calorie count, and weight. Monitor daily laboratory values.	3. These are important nutritional assessment data.
	4. Provide favorite foods.	4. This encourages eating.
	5. Supplement diet with vitamins and minerals.	5. To improve nutritional status.
	6. Walk or sit with client while he or she eats.	6. The nurse's presence offers support and encouragement to client to eat food that will maintain physical wellness.

Nursing Diagnosis: IMPAIRED SOCIAL INTERACTION
Related to: Egocentric and narcissistic behavior
Evidenced by: Inability to develop satisfying relationships and manipulation of others for own desires

Outcome Criteria	Nursing Interventions	Rationale
Client will interact appropriately with others.	1. Recognize that manipulative behaviors help to reduce feelings of insecurity by increasing feelings of power and control.	1. Understanding the motivation behind the behavior may facilitate greater acceptance of the individual.
	2. Set limits on manipulative behaviors. Explain what is expected and the consequences if limits are violated. Terms of the limitations must be agreed on by all staff who will be working with the client.	2. Consequences for violation of limits must be consistently administered, or behavior will not be eliminated.
	3. Ignore attempts by client to argue, bargain, or charm his or her way out of the limit setting.	3. Lack of feedback may decrease these behaviors.
	4. Give positive reinforcement for nonmanipulative behaviors.	4. Positive reinforcement enhances self-esteem and promotes repetition of desirable behaviors.
	5. Discuss consequences of client's behavior and how attempts are made to attribute them to others.	5. Client must accept responsibility for own behavior before adaptive change can occur.
	6. Help client identify positive aspects about self, recognize accomplishments, and feel good about them.	6. As self-esteem is increased, client will feel less need to manipulate others for own gratification.

1. Has the individual avoided personal injury?
2. Has violence to client or others been prevented?
3. Has agitation subsided?
4. Have nutritional status and weight been stabilized? Is the client able to select foods to maintain adequate nutrition?
5. Have delusions and hallucinations ceased? Is the client able to interpret the environment correctly?
6. Is the client able to make decisions about own self-care? Have hygiene and grooming improved?
7. Is behavior socially acceptable? Is client able to interact with others in a satisfactory manner? Has the client stopped manipulating others to fulfill own desires?
8. Is the client able to sleep 6 to 8 hours per night and awaken feeling rested?
9. Does the client understand the importance of maintenance medication therapy? Does he or she understand that symptoms may return if the medication is discontinued?
10. Can the client taking lithium verbalize early signs of lithium toxicity? Does he or she understand the necessity for monthly blood level checks?

TREATMENT MODALITIES FOR MOOD DISORDERS

Psychological Treatments

Individual Psychotherapy

For Depression

Research has documented both the importance of close and satisfactory attachments in the prevention of depression and the role of disrupted attachments in

TABLE 15–9 Topics for Client/Family Education Related to Bipolar Disorder

Nature of the Illness
1. Causes of bipolar disorder
2. Cyclic nature of the illness
3. Symptoms of depression
4. Symptoms of mania

Management of the Illness
1. Medication management
   a. Lithium
   b. Others
      1) Carbamazepine
      2) Valproic acid
      3) Clonazepam
      4) Verapamil
      5) Lamotrigine
      6) Gabapentin
      7) Topiramate
      8) Olanzapine
      9) Risperidone
   c. Side effects
   d. Symptoms of lithium toxicity
   e. Importance of regular blood tests
   f. Adverse effects
   g. Importance of not stopping medication, even when feeling well
2. Assertive techniques
3. Anger management

Support Services
1. Crisis hotline
2. Support groups
3. Individual psychotherapy
4. Legal and financial assistance

the development of depression. With this concept in mind, interpersonal psychotherapy focuses on the client's current interpersonal relations. Interpersonal psychotherapy with the depressed person proceeds through the following phases and interventions:

PHASE I. During the first phase, the client is assessed to determine the extent of the illness. Complete information is then given to the individual regarding the nature of depression, symptom pattern, frequency, clinical course, and alternative treatments. If the level of depression is severe, interpersonal psychotherapy has been shown to be more effective if conducted in combination with antidepressant medication. The client is encouraged to continue working and participating in regular activities during therapy. A mutually agreeable therapeutic contract is negotiated.

PHASE II. Treatment at this phase focuses on helping the client resolve dysfunctional grief reactions. This may include resolving the ambivalence with the lost relationship, serving as a temporary substitute for the lost relationship, and assistance with establishing new relationships. Other areas of treatment focus may include interpersonal disputes between the client and a significant other, difficult role transitions at various developmental life cycles, and correction of interpersonal deficits that may interfere with the client's ability to initiate or sustain interpersonal relationships.

PHASE III. During the final phase of interpersonal psychotherapy, the therapeutic alliance is terminated. With emphasis on reassurance, clarification of emotional states, improvement of interpersonal communication, testing of perceptions, and performance in interpersonal settings, interpersonal psychotherapy has been successful in helping depressed persons recover enhanced social functioning.

For Mania

Manic clients traditionally have been difficult candidates for psychotherapy. They form a therapeutic relationship easily because they are eager to please and grateful for the therapist's interest. However, the relationship often tends to remain shallow and rigid. Some reports have indicated that psychotherapy (in conjunction with medication maintenance treatment) and counseling may be useful with these individuals. Lyness (1997) states:

> Individual or family psychotherapies are often crucial to forming and maintaining the treatment alliances within which compliance issues can be addressed. Psychotherapy also provides the framework for management of ongoing stressors or dysfunctional behavioral patterns that might precipitate or exacerbate the bipolar disorder. (pp. 55–56)

Group Therapy for Depression and Mania

Group therapy forms an important dimension of multimodal treatment of the manic or depressed client. Once an acute phase of the illness is passed, groups can provide an atmosphere in which individuals may discuss issues in their lives that cause, maintain, or arise out of having a serious affective disorder. The element of peer support provides a feeling of security as troublesome or embarrassing issues are discussed and resolved. Some groups have other specific purposes, such as helping to monitor medication-related issues or serving as an avenue for promoting education related to the affective disorder and its treatment.

Support groups help members gain a sense of perspective on their condition and tangibly encourage them to link up with others who have common problems. A sense of hope is conveyed when the individual is able to see that he or she is not alone or unique in experiencing affective illness.

Self-help groups offer another avenue of support for the depressed or manic client. These groups are usually peer-led and are not meant to substitute for, or compete with, professional therapy. They offer supplementary support that frequently enhances compliance with the medical regimen. Examples of self-help groups are the National Depressive and Manic-Depressive Association (NDMDA), Depressives Anonymous, Families of Depressives, Manic and Depressive Support Group, Recovery Inc., and New Images for Widows. Although self-help groups are not psychotherapy groups, they do provide important adjunctive support experiences, which often have therapeutic benefit for participants.

Family Therapy for Depression and Mania

The ultimate objectives in working with families of clients with mood disorders are to resolve the symptoms and initiate or restore adaptive family functioning. As with group therapy, the most effective approach appears to be with a combination of psychotherapeutic and pharmacotherapeutic treatments. Some studies with bipolar disorder have shown that behavioral family treatment combined with medication substantially reduces the relapse rate compared with medication therapy alone.

Sadock and Sadock (2003) state:

> Family therapy is indicated if the disorder jeopardizes the patient's marriage or family functioning or if the mood disorder is promoted or maintained by the family situation. Family therapy examines the role of the mood-disordered member in the overall psychological well-being of the whole family; it also examines the role of the entire family in the maintenance of the patient's symptoms. (p. 565)

Cognitive Therapy for Depression and Mania

In cognitive therapy, the individual is taught to control thought distortions that are considered a factor in the development and maintenance of mood disorders. In the cognitive model, depression is characterized by a triad of negative distortions related to expectations of the environment, self, and future. The environment and activities within it are viewed as unsatisfying, the self is unrealistically devalued, and the future is perceived as hopeless. In the same model, mania is characterized by exaggeratedly positive cognitions and perceptions. The individual perceives the self as highly valued and powerful. Life is experienced with overstated self-assurance, and the future is viewed with unrealistic optimism.

The general goals in cognitive therapy are to obtain symptom relief as quickly as possible, to assist the client in identifying dysfunctional patterns of thinking and behaving, and to guide the client to evidence and logic that effectively test the validity of the dysfunctional thinking. Therapy focuses on changing "automatic thoughts" that occur spontaneously and contribute to the distorted affect. Examples of automatic thoughts in depression include:

1. **Personalizing:** "I'm the only one who failed."
2. **All or nothing:** "I'm a complete failure."
3. **Mind reading:** "He thinks I'm foolish."
4. **Discounting positives:** "The other questions were so easy. Any dummy could have gotten them right."

Examples of automatic thoughts in mania include:

1. **Personalizing:** "She's this happy only when she's with me."
2. **All or nothing:** "Everything I do is great."
3. **Mind reading:** "She thinks I'm wonderful."
4. **Discounting negatives:** "None of those mistakes are really important."

The client is asked to describe evidence that both supports and disputes the automatic thought. The logic underlying the inferences is then reviewed with the client. Another technique involves evaluating what would most likely happen if the client's automatic thoughts were true. Implications of the consequences are then discussed.

Clients should not become discouraged if one technique seems not to be working. No single technique works with all clients. He or she should be reassured that any of a number of techniques may be used, and both therapist and client may explore these possibilities.

Finally, the use of cognitive therapy does not preclude the value of administering medication. Particularly in the treatment of mania, cognitive therapy should be considered a secondary treatment to pharmacological treatment. Cognitive therapy alone has offered encouraging results in the treatment of depression. In fact, the results of several studies with depressed clients show that in some cases cognitive therapy may be equally or even more effective than antidepressant medication (Wright & Thase, 1992; Hollon, DeRubeis, & Evans, 1992).

Organic Treatments

Psychopharmacology

For Depression

For more than 40 years, the tricyclic antidepressants (TCAs) have been widely used to treat depression. Since the initial discovery of their antidepressant properties, the tricyclic drugs have been subjected to hundreds of controlled trials, and their efficacy in treating depressive illness is now firmly established (see Chapter 10 for a detailed discussion of antidepressant medications).

A subsiding of symptoms may not occur for up to 4 weeks after beginning therapy with TCAs. It is important, therefore, for clients to understand that although it may seem the medication is not producing the desired effects, he or she must continue taking it for at least a month to determine efficacy. The greater effectiveness of one medication over another with any given client is not yet fully understood. Choice of drug may be based on symptoms. For example, anxious clients may be started on TCAs with the most sedative properties and clients with psychomotor retardation may be prescribed those antidepressants with the least sedative properties. When possible, selection of the appropriate drug is based on a history of previous responses to antidepressant therapy.

Common side effects of the TCAs include sedation, tachycardia, dry mouth, constipation, urinary retention, blurred vision, orthostatic hypotension, lowering of the seizure threshold, weight gain, and changes in sexual functioning. Elderly individuals may be particularly sensitive to these medications, and adjustments in dosage must be considered. TCAs are absolutely contraindicated in cases of severe heart disease and untreated narrow-angle glaucoma.

Monoamine oxidase inhibitors (MAOIs) have a unique place in the history of antidepressant medications. They were originally used in the treatment of tuberculosis. Evidence that individuals who were treated with the medication experienced a sense of well-being, without bacteriological improvement, led to the discovery of their enzyme inhibition properties and the subsequent hypothesis that monoamines have a function in regulating mood.

Following the initial enthusiasm about MAOIs, they fell into relative disuse for nearly two decades because of a perceived poor risk-to-benefit ratio. Since that time, they have regained acceptance as a viable alternative to TCAs because it has been shown that some individuals respond more beneficially to MAOIs than to any other antidepressant medication.

The greatest concern with using MAOIs is the potential for hypertensive crisis, which is considered a medical emergency. Hypertensive crisis occurs in clients receiving MAOI therapy who consume foods or drugs high in **tyramine** content (see Table 10–3). Typically, symptoms develop within 2 hours after ingestion of a food or drug high in tyramine and include severe occipital and/or temporal pounding headaches with occasional photophobia. Sensations of choking, palpitations, and a feeling of "dread" are common. Marked systolic and diastolic hypertension occurs, sometimes with neck stiffness. In addition to hypertensive crisis, side effects are similar to those associated with the TCAs.

A second generation of antidepressants has been marketed in the United States during the last two decades. These include maprotiline (Ludiomil), amoxapine (Asendin), trazodone (Desyrel), bupropion (Wellbutrin), and mirtazapine (Remeron). Although most of these newer antidepressants were initially touted as being better than drugs used in the past, accumulated evidence and experience have dampened this initial enthusiasm.

Maprotiline, although as effective as the older antidepressants in treating depressive symptoms, carries an increased risk of seizures and greater toxicity in overdose.

Amoxapine, a derivative of the antipsychotic loxapine, is effective in treating psychotic depression, but has a potential for causing neuroleptic malignant syndrome and tardive dyskinesia.

Trazodone is as effective as the older antidepressants and has fewer side effects (the most common being sedation). A relatively rare adverse effect that has been observed with trazodone is priapism (prolonged, painful erection). This is a very problematic condition requiring surgical intervention in some clients.

Bupropion is as effective as the older antidepressants and has notably fewer anticholinergic and cardiovascular side effects. There have been some difficulties in the past, however, with increased risk of seizures, especially in emaciated clients.

Mirtazapine is the newest medication to be included with this group of antidepressants. A great deal has yet to be learned about the safety and efficacy of this drug, although in clinical trials it was associated with several cases of agranulocytosis. Clients taking this medication should be closely monitored for signs and symptoms.

The newest classifications of antidepressants include the selective serotonin reuptake inhibitors

(SSRIs) and the nonselective reuptake inhibitors. The SSRIs include fluoxetine (Prozac), paroxetine (Paxil), sertraline (Zoloft), fluvoxamine (Luvox), citalopram (Celexa), and Escitalopram (Lexapro). The nonselective reuptake inhibitors include venlafaxine (Effexor). These drugs have fewer anticholinergic and cardiovascular side effects than the TCAs and often work faster. Although long-term studies are not yet available, they appear to be just as effective in alleviating symptoms of depression as the older antidepressants.

For Mania

Lithium carbonate is the drug of choice for acute manic episodes and for maintenance therapy to prevent or diminish the intensity of subsequent manic episodes. Its mode of action in the control of manic symptoms is unclear. It has also been indicated for treatment of bipolar depression (see Chapter 10 for a detailed discussion of lithium carbonate).

Common side effects of lithium therapy include drowsiness, dizziness, headache, dry mouth, thirst, gastrointestinal upset, fine hand tremors, pulse irregularities, polyuria, and weight gain. When initiating lithium therapy with an acutely manic individual, physicians commonly order an antipsychotic as well. Because normalization of symptoms with lithium may not be achieved for 1 to 3 weeks, the antipsychotic medication is used to calm the excessive hyperactivity of the manic client until the lithium reaches therapeutic level.

Therapeutic level of lithium carbonate is 1.0 to 1.5 mEq/L for acute mania and 0.6 to 1.2 mEq/L for maintenance therapy. There is a narrow margin between the therapeutic and toxic levels, and lithium levels should be drawn weekly until the therapeutic level is reached, and then monthly during maintenance therapy. Because lithium toxicity is a life-threatening condition, monitoring of lithium levels is critical. The initial symptoms of lithium toxicity include ataxia, blurred vision, severe diarrhea, persistent nausea and vomiting, and tinnitus. Symptoms intensify as toxicity increases and include excessive output of dilute urine, psychomotor retardation, mental confusion, tremors and muscular irritability, seizures, impaired consciousness, oliguria or anuria, arrhythmias, coma, and eventually death.

Pretreatment assessments should include adequacy of renal functioning because 95 percent of ingested lithium is eliminated via the kidneys. Use of lithium during pregnancy is not recommended. Results of studies have indicated a greater number of cardiac anomalies in babies born to mothers who consumed lithium, particularly in the first trimester.

A number of other medications have been tried on an investigational basis in the treatment of mania, with varying degrees of success. Examples include anticonvulsants (carbamazapine, clonazepam, valproic acid, lamotrigine, gabapentin, and topiramate) and calcium channel blockers (verapamil). These drugs have been used as alternate or adjunctive approaches to management of clients with bipolar illness refractory to lithium. Olanzapine (Zyprexa) and risperidone (Risperdal) have recently been approved by the Food and Drug Administration for treatment of mania. It may be given in combination with lithium or, in milder cases, alone.

Electroconvulsive Therapy for Depression and Mania

Electroconvulsive therapy (ECT) is the induction of a grand mal (generalized) seizure through the application of electrical current to the brain. ECT is effective with clients who are acutely suicidal and in the treatment of severe depression, particularly in those clients who are also experiencing psychotic symptoms and those with psychomotor retardation and neurovegetative changes, such as disturbances in sleep, appetite, and energy. It is often considered for treatment only after a trial of therapy with antidepressant medication has proved ineffective.

Episodes of acute mania are occasionally treated with ECT, particularly when the client does not tolerate or fails to respond to lithium or other drug treatment, or when life is threatened by dangerous behavior or exhaustion.

Mechanism of Action

The exact mechanism by which ECT effects a therapeutic response is unknown. Several theories exist, but the one to which the most credibility has been given is the biochemical theory. A number of researchers have demonstrated that electrical stimulation results in significant increases in the circulating levels of several neurotransmitters (Endler & Persad, 1996). These neurotransmitters include serotonin, norepinephrine, and dopamine, the same biogenic amines that are affected by antidepressant medications.

Side Effects

The most common side effects of ECT are temporary memory loss and confusion. Critics of the therapy argue that these changes represent irreversible brain damage. Proponents insist they are temporary and reversible. Marangell, Silver, and Yudofsky (1999) state, "To date, no reliable data have shown permanent memory loss caused by modern ECT." Other researchers have suggested that varying amounts of memory loss may be evident in some clients up to 6 to 7 months following ECT (Popolos, 2002; Sadock & Sadock, 2003).

The controversy continues regarding the choice of unilateral versus bilateral ECT. Studies have shown unilateral placement of the electrodes decreases the amount of memory disturbance. However, unilateral ECT often requires a greater number of treatments to match the efficacy of bilateral ECT in the relief of depression (Marangell, Silver, & Yudofsky, 1999; Barstow, 2002).

Risks Associated with ECT

MORTALITY. Studies indicate that the mortality rate from ECT is about 2 per 100,000 treatments (Marangell, Silver, & Yudofsky, 1999; Sadock & Sadock, 2003). Although the occurrence is rare, the major cause of death with ECT is cardiovascular complications, such as acute myocardial infarction, acute coronary insufficiency, ventricular fibrillation, myocardial rupture, cardiac arrest, cardiovascular collapse, stroke, and ruptured cerebral or aortic aneurysm. Assessment and management of cardiovascular disease *before* treatment are vital in the reduction of morbidity and mortality associated with ECT.

PERMANENT MEMORY LOSS. Marangell, Silver, and Yudofsky (1999) state:

> The initial confusion and cognitive deficits associated with ECT treatment are usually temporary, lasting approximately 30 minutes. Whereas many patients report no problems with their memory, aside from the time immediately surrounding the ECT treatments, others report that their memory is not as good as it was before receiving ECT. To date, no reliable data have shown permanent memory loss caused by modern ECT. Prospective computed tomography and magnetic resonance imaging studies of the brain show no evidence of ECT-induced structural changes. (p. 779)

BRAIN DAMAGE. Brain damage from ECT remains a concern for those who continue to believe in its usefulness and efficacy as a treatment for depression. Critics of the procedure remain adamant in their belief that ECT always results in some amount of immediate brain damage (Endler & Persad, 1996). However, evidence is based largely on animal studies in which the subjects received excessive electrical dosages, and the seizures were unmodified by muscle paralysis and oxygenation (Abrams, 1997). Although this is an area for continuing study, there is no current data to substantiate that ECT produces any permanent changes in brain structure or functioning (Sadock & Sadock, 2003).

Medications

Several medications are associated with ECT. A pretreatment medication, such as atropine sulfate or glycopyrrolate (Robinul), is administered intramuscularly approximately 30 minutes before the treatment. Either medication may be ordered to decrease secretions and counteract the effects of vagal stimulation induced by the ECT.

In the treatment room, the anesthesiologist administers intravenously a short-acting anesthetic, such as thiopental sodium (Pentothal) or methohexital sodium (Brevital). A muscle relaxant, usually succinylcholine chloride (Anectine), is given intravenously to prevent severe muscle contractions during the seizure, thereby reducing the possibility of fractured or dislocated bones. Because succinylcholine paralyzes respiratory muscles as well, the client is oxygenated with pure oxygen before the treatment.

SUICIDE

Information about suicide is presented here because the most suicides are associated with mood disorders. Sadock and Sadock (2003) report, "Almost 95 percent of all people who commit or attempt suicide have a diagnosed mental disorder. Depressive disorders account for 80 percent of this figure."

Epidemiological Factors

Approximately 30,000 persons in the United States end their lives each year by suicide. These statistics have established suicide as the eighth leading cause of death among adults and the third leading cause of death—behind accidents and homicide—among young Americans (aged 15 to 24 years) (Crisis Hotline, 2001). Many more people attempt suicide than succeed, and countless others seriously contemplate the act without carrying it out. Suicide has become a major healthcare problem in the United States today.

Over the years, confusion has existed over the

reality of various notions regarding suicide. Some facts and fables related to suicide are presented in Table 15–10. Risk factors associated with suicide are presented in Table 15–11.

APPLICATION OF THE NURSING PROCESS WITH THE SUICIDAL CLIENT

Assessment

The following items should be considered when conducting a suicidal assessment: demographics, presenting symptoms/medical-psychiatric diagnosis, suicidal ideas or acts, interpersonal support system, analysis of the suicidal crisis, psychiatric/medical/family history, and coping strategies. The Surgeon General, in his "Call to Action to Prevent Suicide," speaks of risk factors and protective factors (United States Public Health Service [USPHS], 1999). Risk factors are associated with a greater potential for suicide and suicidal behavior, whereas protective factors are associated with reduced potential for suicide. These risk and protective factors are outlined in Table 15–12. Table 15–13 presents some additional guidelines for determining the extent of suicide potential.

Demographics

The following demographics are assessed:

Age. Suicide is highest in persons older than 50 years. Adolescents are also at high risk.
Gender. Males are at higher risk than females.
Ethnicity. Caucasians are at higher risk than are Native Americans, who are at higher risk than African-Americans are.
Martial Status. Single, divorced, and widowed persons are at higher risk than married persons.
Socioeconomic Status. Individuals in the highest and lowest socioeconomic classes are at higher risk than those in the middle classes.

TABLE 15–10 Facts and Fables about Suicide

Fables	Facts
People who talk about suicide do not commit suicide. Suicide happens without warning.	Eight out of ten people who kill themselves have given definite clues and warnings about their suicidal intentions. Very subtle clues may be ignored or disregarded by others.
You cannot stop a suicidal person. He/she is fully intent on dying.	Most suicidal people are ambivalent about their feelings regarding living or dying. Most are "gambling with death" and see it as a cry for someone to save them.
Once a person is suicidal, he or she is suicidal forever.	People who want to kill themselves are only suicidal for a limited time. If they are saved from feelings of self-destruction, they can go on to lead normal lives.
Improvement after severe depression means that the suicidal risk is over.	Most suicides occur within about 3 months after the beginning of "improvement," when the individual has the energy to carry out suicidal intentions.
Suicide is inherited, or "runs in families."	Suicide is not inherited. It is an individual matter and can be prevented. However, suicide by a close family member increases an individual's risk factor for suicide.
All suicidal individuals are mentally ill, and suicide is the act of a psychotic person.	Although suicidal persons are extremely unhappy, they are not necessarily psychotic or otherwise mentally ill. They are merely unable, at that point in time, to see an alternative solution to what they consider an unbearable problem.
Suicidal threats and gestures should be considered manipulative or attention-seeking behavior and should not be taken seriously.	All suicidal behavior must be approached with the gravity of the potential act in mind. Attention should be given to the possibility that the individual is issuing a cry for help.
People usually commit suicide by taking an overdose of drugs.	Gunshot wounds are the leading cause of death among suicide victims.
If an individual has attempted suicide, he or she will not do it again.	50%–80% of all people who ultimately kill themselves have a history of a previous attempt.

From Blackburn (1990); Crisis Hotline (2001); USPHS (1999); The Samaritans (2002); and Harvard Medical School (1996).

TABLE 15–11 Risk Factors Associated with Suicide

Risk Factor	Comments
Marital status	The suicide rate for single persons is twice that of married persons. The single, the divorced, and the widowed have rates 4 to 5 times greater than those of the married do.
Gender	Women attempt suicide more, but more men succeed. Successful suicides number about 70% for men and 30% for women. This has to do with the lethality of the means. Although women tend to overdose, men use more lethal means such as firearms.
Age	Suicide rates are positively correlated with age. Rates rise sharply during adolescence, peak between ages 30 and 40, and then level off until age 65, when they rise again for the remaining years.
Religion	Protestants have significantly higher rates of suicide than Catholics and Jews. A strong feeling of cohesiveness within a religious organization seems to be an important factor.
Socioeconomic status	Individuals in the very highest and lowest social classes have higher suicide rates than those in the middle classes. With regard to occupation, suicide rates are higher among physicians, business executives, pharmacists, dentists, lawyers, and engineers. Rates are lowest among farm workers and artisans.
Ethtnicity	Whites are at highest risk for suicide, followed by Native Americans, African-Americans, Hispanic Americans, and Asian Americans.
Psychiatric illness	Individuals with mood disorders are far more likely to commit suicide than those in any other psychiatric or medical risk group. Other disorders that put individuals at risk for suicide include anxiety disorders, substance related disorders, schizophrenia, and borderline personality disorder. Also at risk are individuals with chronic or terminal illness (e.g., multiple sclerosis, AIDS, cancer).

From Sadock & Sadock, 2003; Ghosh, Victor, & Bourgeois, 2003; and Murphy, 1994

Occupation. Professional healthcare personnel and business executives are at highest risk.

Method. Use of firearms presents a significantly higher risk than overdose of substances.

Religion. Protestants are at greater risk than Catholics or Jews.

Family History. Higher risk exists if the individual has a family history of suicide.

TABLE 15–12 Suicide Risk Factors and Protective Factors

Risk Factors	Protective Factors
• Previous suicide attempt • Mental disorders, particularly mood disorders such as depression and bipolar disorder • Concurrent mental, alcohol, and substance abuse disorders • Family history of suicide • Hopelessness • Impulsive and/or aggressive tendencies • Barriers to accessing mental health treatment • Relational, social, work, or financial loss • Physical illness • Easy access to lethal methods, especially guns • Unwillingness to seek help because of stigma attached to mental and substance abuse disorders and/or suicidal thoughts • Influence of significant people—family members, celebrities, peers who have died by suicide—both through direct personal contact or inappropriate media representations • Cultural and religious beliefs—for instance, the belief that suicide is a noble resolution of a personal dilemma • Local epidemics of suicide that have a contagious influence • Isolation—a feeling of being cut off from other people	• Effective and appropriate clinical care for mental, physical, and substance-abuse disorders • Easy access to a variety of clinical interventions and support in seeking help • Restricted access to lethal methods of suicide • Family and community support • Support from ongoing medical and mental healthcare relationships • Learned skills in problem solving, conflict resolution, and nonviolent handling of disputes • Cultural and religious beliefs that discourage suicide and support self-preservation instinct

TABLE 15–13 Assessing the Degree of Suicidal Risk

Behavior	Intensity of Risk: Low	Moderate	High
Anxiety	Mild	Moderate	High or panic
Depression	Mild	Moderate	Severe
Isolation; withdrawal	Some feelings of isolation; no withdrawal	Some feelings of helplessness, hopelessness, and withdrawal	Hopeless, helpless, withdrawn, and self-deprecating
Daily functioning	Fairly good in most activities	Moderately good in some activities	Not good in any activities
Resources	Several	Some	Few or none
Coping strategies being used	Generally constructive	Some that are constructive	Predominantly destructive
Significant others	Several who are available	Few or only one available	Only one or none available
Psychiatric help in past	None, or positive attitude toward	Yes, and moderately satisfied with results	Negative view of help received
Lifestyle	Stable	Moderately stable	Unstable
Alcohol or drug use	Infrequently to excess	Frequently to excess	Continual abuse
Previous suicide attempts	None, or of low lethality	One or more of moderate lethality	Multiple attempts of high lethality
Disorientation; disorganization	None	Some	Marked
Hostility	Little or none	Some	Marked
Suicidal plan	Vague, fleeting thoughts but no plan	Frequent thoughts, occasional ideas about a plan	Frequent or constant thought with a specific plan

Hatton, Corrine L; Valente, Sharon, Suicide: Assessment & Intervention, 2nd Edition, © 1984. Reprinted by permission of Pearson Education, Inc., Upper Saddle River, NJ.

Presenting Symptoms/Medical-Psychiatric Diagnosis

Assessment data must be gathered regarding any psychiatric or physical condition for which the client is being treated. Mood disorders (major depression and bipolar disorders) are the most common disorders that precede suicide. Individuals with substance-use disorders are also at high risk. Other psychiatric disorders in which suicide may be a risk include anxiety disorders, schizophrenia, and borderline and antisocial personality disorders (Medscape Psychiatry, 2001). Other chronic and terminal physical illnesses have also precipitated suicidal acts.

Suicidal Ideas or Acts

How serious is the intent? Does the person have a plan? If so, does he or she have the means? How lethal is the means? Has the individual ever attempted suicide before? These are all questions that must be answered by the person conducting the suicidal assessment.

Individuals may leave both behavioral and verbal clues as to the intent of their act. Examples of behavioral clues include giving away prized possessions, getting financial affairs in order, writing suicide notes, or sudden lifts in mood (may indicate a decision to carry out the intent).

Verbal clues may be both direct and indirect. Examples of direct statements include "I want to die" or "I'm going to kill myself." Examples of indirect statements include "This is the last time you'll see me," "I won't be around much longer for the doctor to have to worry about," or "I don't have anything worth living for anymore."

Other assessments include determining whether the individual has a plan, and if so, whether he or she has the means to carry out that plan. If the person states the suicide will be carried out with a gun, does he or she have access to a gun and bullets? If pills are planned, what kinds of pills are to be used? Are they accessible?

Interpersonal Support System

Does the individual have support persons on whom he or she can rely during a crisis? Lack of a meaningful network of satisfactory relationships may implicate an individual at high risk for suicide during an emotional crisis.

Analysis of the Suicidal Crisis

THE PRECIPITATING STRESSOR. Adverse life events in combination with other risk factors such as depression may lead to suicide (NIMH, 2002). Life stresses accompanied by an increase in emotional disturbance include the loss of a loved person by death or by divorce, problems in major relationships, changes in roles, or serious physical illness.

RELEVANT HISTORY. Has the individual experienced numerous failures or rejections that would increase his or her vulnerability for a dysfunctional response to the current situation?

LIFE-STAGE ISSUES. The ability to tolerate losses and disappointments is often compromised if those losses and disappointments occur during various stages of life in which the individual struggles with developmental issues (e.g., adolescence, midlife).

Psychiatric/Medical/Family History

The individual should be assessed with regard to previous psychiatric treatment for depression, alcoholism, or for previous suicide attempts. Medical history should be obtained to determine presence of chronic, debilitating, or terminal illness. Is there a history of depressive disorder in the family, and has a close relative committed suicide in the past?

Coping Strategies

How has the individual handled previous crises? How does this situation differ from previous ones?

Diagnosis/Outcome Identification

Nursing diagnoses for the suicidal client may include the following:

1. Risk for suicide related to feelings of hopelessness and desperation
2. Hopelessness related to absence of support systems and perception of worthlessness

The following criteria may be used for measurement of outcomes in the care of the suicidal client.

The client:

1. Has experienced no physical harm to self
2. Sets realistic goals for self
3. Expresses some optimism and hope for the future

Planning/Implementation

Refer to Table 15–6 for a plan of care for the suicidal client. Nursing diagnoses are presented, along with outcome criteria, appropriate nursing interventions, and rationales for each.

Intervention with the Outpatient Suicidal Client (or Following Discharge from Inpatient Care)

In some instances, it may be determined that suicidal intent is low and that hospitalization is not required. Instead, the client with suicidal ideation may be treated in an outpatient setting. Guidelines for treatment of the suicidal client on an outpatient basis include the following:

1. The person should not be left alone. Arrangements must be made for the client to stay with family or friends. If this is not possible, hospitalization should be considered.
2. Establish a no-suicide contract with the client. Formulate a written contract that the client will not harm himself or herself in a stated period. For example, the client writes, "I will not harm myself in any way between now and the time of our next counseling session," or "I will call the suicide hotline (or go to the emergency room) if I start to feel like harming myself." When the period of this short-term contract has lapsed, a new contract is negotiated.
3. Enlist the help of family or friends to ensure that the home environment is safe from dangerous items, such as firearms or stockpiled drugs. Give support persons the telephone number of a counselor or emergency contact person in the event that the counselor is not available.
4. Appointments may need to be scheduled daily or every other day at first until the immediate suicidal crisis has subsided.
5. Establish rapport and promote a trusting relationship. It is important for the suicide counselor to become a key person in the client's support system at this time.
6. Be direct. Talk openly and matter-of-factly about suicide. Listen actively and encourage expression of feelings, including anger. Accept the client's feelings in a nonjudgmental manner.
7. Discuss the current crisis in the client's life. Use the problem-solving approach (see Chapter 9). Offer alternatives to suicide. Macnab (1993) suggests the following statements:

> You are incorrect in your belief that suicide is the only and the best solution to your problem. There are alternatives, and they are good. What is more, you will be alive to test them. (p. 265)

8. Help the client identify areas of life situation that are within his or her control and those that cannot be controlled. Discuss feelings associated with these control issues. It is important for the client to feel some control over his or her life situation in order to perceive a measure of self-worth.
9. The physician may prescribe antidepressants for an individual who is experiencing suicidal depression. It is wise to prescribe no more than a 3-day supply of the medication with no refills. The prescription can then be renewed at the client's next counseling session. *Note:* Sadock and Sadock (2003) state:

   > As the depression lifts, patients become energized and are thus able to put their suicidal plans into action. Sometimes, depressed patients, with or without treatment, suddenly appear to be at peace with themselves because they have reached a secret decision to commit suicide. Clinicians should be especially suspicious of such a dramatic clinical change, which may portend a suicide attempt. (p. 921)

10. Macnab (1993) suggests the following steps in crisis counseling with the suicidal client:
    a. Focus on the current crisis and how it can be alleviated. Identify the client's appraisals of how things are, and how things will be. Note how these appraisals change in changing contexts;
    b. Note the client's reactivity to the crisis and how this can be changed. Discuss strategies and procedures for the management of anxiety, anger, and frustration;
    c. Work toward restoration of the client's self-worth, status, morale, and control. Introduce alternatives to suicide;
    d. Rehearse cognitive reconstruction—more positive ways of thinking about the self, events, the past, the present, and the future;
    e. Identify experiences and actions that affirm self-worth and self-efficacy;
    f. Encourage movement toward the new reality, with the coping skills required to manage adaptively;
    g. Be available for ongoing therapeutic support and growth.

Information for Family and Friends of the Suicidal Client

The following suggestions are made for family and friends of an individual who is suicidal:

1. Take any hint of suicide seriously. Anyone expressing suicidal feelings needs immediate attention.
2. Do not keep secrets. If a suicidal person says, "Promise you won't tell anyone," do not make that promise. Suicidal individuals are ambivalent about dying, and suicidal behavior is a cry for help. It is the part of the person that wants to stay alive that tells you about it. Get help for the person and for you. 1-800-SUICIDE is a national hotline that is available 24 hours a day.
3. The Centers for Disease Control and Prevention (CDC, 2002) offer the following suggestions for families and friends of suicidal persons:
   a. Be a good listener. If people express suicidal thoughts or feel depressed, hopeless, or worthless, be supportive. Let them know you are there for them and are willing to help them seek professional help;
   b. Many people find it awkward to put into words how another person's life is important for their own well-being, but it is important to stress that the person's life is important to you and to others. Emphasize in specific terms the ways in which the person's suicide would be devastating to you and to others;
   c. Express concern for individuals who express thoughts about committing suicide. The individual may be withdrawn and reluctant to discuss what he or she is thinking. Acknowledge the person's pain and feelings of hopelessness, and encourage the individual to talk to someone else if he or she does not feel comfortable talking with you;
   d. Familiarize yourself with suicide intervention sources, such as mental health centers and suicide hotlines;
   e. Restrict access to firearms or other means of self-harm;
4. The Mental Health Sanctuary (2001) offers the following tips:
   a. Acknowledge and accept their feelings and be an active listener;
   b. Try to give them hope and remind them that what they are feeling is temporary;
   c. Stay with them. Do not leave them alone. Go to where they are, if necessary;
   d. Show love and encouragement. Hold them, hug them, and touch them. Allow them to cry and express anger;
   e. Help them seek professional help;
   f. Remove any items from the home with which the person may harm himself or herself;
   g. If there are children present, try to remove them from the home. Perhaps other friends or relatives can assist by taking them to their

home. This type of situation can be extremely traumatic for children;

h. DO NOT: judge the person, show anger toward them, provoke guilt in them, discount their feelings, or tell them to "snap out of it." This is a very real and serious situation to suicidal individuals. They are in real pain. They feel the situation is hopeless and there is no other way to resolve it aside from taking their own life.

Intervention with Families and Friends of Suicide Victims

Fraser (1994) states:

> For many people in a post-suicide situation there is a sudden and, for the most part, unexpected shattering of their lives. In addition to the grief and loss associated with the death of a close relative, there is an extra burden for the family members of a suicide victim. Part of that burden is the altered social world in which they suddenly find themselves. Their private sorrow has a public aspect and their grief and adjustment to it must be lived out within a social context that has little in the way of supporting structures for understanding their plight. They must struggle as best they can with their own internal resources, resources which have been severely attenuated by this tragic event.

Suicide of a family member can induce a whole gamut of feelings in the survivors. Macnab (1993) identifies the following symptoms, which may be evident following the suicide of a loved one.

1. A sense of guilt and responsibility
2. Anger, resentment, and rage that can never find its "object"
3. A heightened sense of emotionality, helplessness, failure, and despair
4. A recurring self-searching: "If only I had done something." If only I had not done something." "If only ...."
5. A sense of confusion and search for an explanation: "Why did this happen?" "What does it mean?" "What could have stopped it?" "What will people think?"
6. A sense of inner injury. The family feels wounded. They do not know how they will ever get over it and get on with life.
7. A severe strain is placed on relationships. A sense of impatience, irritability, and anger exists between family members.
8. A heightened vulnerability to illness and disease exists with this added burden of emotional stress.

Strategies for assisting survivors of suicide victims include:

1. Encourage the clients to talk about the suicide, each responding to the others' viewpoints, and reconstructing of events. Share memories.
2. Be aware of any blaming or scapegoating of specific family members. Discuss how each person fits into the family situation, both before and after the suicide.
3. Listen to feelings of guilt and self-persecution. Gently move the individuals toward the reality of the situation.
4. Encourage the family members to discuss individual relationships with the lost loved one. Focus on both positive and negative aspects of the relationships. Gradually, point out the irrationality of any idealized concepts of the deceased person. The family must be able to recognize both positive and negative aspects about the person before grief can be resolved.
5. No two people grieve in the same way. It may appear that some family members are "getting over" the grief faster than others are. All family members must be made to understand that if this occurs, it is not because they "care less," just that they "grieve differently." Variables that enter into this phenomenon include individual past experiences, personal relationship with the deceased person, and individual temperament and coping abilities.
6. Recognize how the suicide has caused disorganization in family coping. Reassess interpersonal relationships in the context of the event. Discuss coping strategies that have been successful in times of stress in the past, and work to reestablish these within the family. Identify new adaptive coping strategies that can be incorporated.
7. Identify resources that provide support: religious beliefs and spiritual counselors, close friends and relatives, survivors of suicide support groups. One on-line connection that puts individuals in contact with survivors groups specific to each state is http://www.afsp.org/survivor/groups.htm. A list of resources that provide information and help for issues regarding suicide is presented in Table 15–14.

Evaluation

Evaluation of the suicidal client is an ongoing process accomplished through continuous reassessment of the client, as well as determination of goal achievement. Once the immediate crisis has been resolved, extended psychotherapy may be indicated. The long-term goals of individual or group psychotherapy for the suicidal client would be for him or her to:

TABLE 15–14 Sources for Information Related to Issues of Suicide

NATIONAL SUICIDE HOTLINE
1-800-SUICIDE
AMERICAN ASSOCIATION OF SUICIDOLOGY
www.suicidology.org
1-202-237-2280
AMERICAN FOUNDATION FOR SUICIDE PREVENTION
www.afsp.org
1-888-333-AFSP
AMERICAN PSYCHIATRIC ASSOCIATION
www.psych.org
1-800-852-8330
AMERICAN PSYCHOLOGICAL ASSOCIATION
www.apa.org
1-800-964-2000
BOYS TOWN
Cares for troubled boys, girls, and families in crisis.
Staff is trained to handle calls related to violence and suicide.
www.boystown.org
1-800-448-3000 (crisis hotline)
1-800-545-5771
CENTERS FOR DISEASE CONTROL AND PREVENTION
NATIONAL CENTER FOR INJURY PREVENTION AND CONTROL
DIVISION OF VIOLENCE PREVENTION
www.cdc.gov/ncipc
1-770-488-4362
THE CENTER FOR MENTAL HEALTH SERVICES
www.mentalhealth.org/highlights/suicide
NATIONAL ALLIANCE FOR THE MENTALLY ILL
www.nami.org
1-800-950-NAMI
NATIONAL DEPRESSIVE AND MANIC-DEPRESSIVE ASSOCIATION (NDMDA)
www.ndmda.org
1-800-82-NDMDA
NATIONAL INSTITUTE OF MENTAL HEALTH
www.nimh.nih.gov
1-800-421-4211
NATIONAL MENTAL HEALTH ASSOCIATION
www.nmha.org
1-800-228-1114
1-800-969-NMHA
THE NATIONAL MENTAL ILLNESS SCREENING PROJECT SUICIDE DIVISION
www.nmisp.org
1-800-573-4433
SUICIDE AWARENESS—VOICES OF EDUCATION
www.save.org
1-612-946-7998
SUICIDE INFORMATION & EDUCATION CENTER
www.siec.ca
1-403-245-3900
SUICIDE PREVENTION ADVOCACY NETWORK
http://spanusa.org
1-888-649-1366

1. Develop and maintain a more positive self-concept.
2. Learn more effective ways to express feelings to others.
3. Achieve successful interpersonal relationships.
4. Feel accepted by others and achieve a sense of belonging.

A suicidal person feels worthless and hopeless. These goals serve to instill a sense of self-worth, and offer a measure of hope and a meaning for living.

SUMMARY

Depression is one of the oldest recognized psychiatric illnesses that is still prevalent today. It is so common, in fact, that it has been referred to as the "common cold of psychiatric disorders."

The cause of depressive disorders is not entirely known. A number of factors, including genetics, biochemical influences, and psychosocial experiences likely enter into the development of the disorder. Secondary depression occurs in response to other physiological disorders. Symptoms occur along a continuum according to the extent of severity from transient to severe. The disorder occurs in all developmental levels, including childhood, adolescence, senescence, and during the puerperium.

Bipolar disorder, mania, is a maladaptive response to loss and has been referred to as the "mirror image of depression." Genetic influences have been strongly implicated in the development of the disorder. Various other physiological factors, such as biochemical and electrolyte alterations, as well as cerebral structural changes, have been implicated. Side effects of certain medications may also induce symptoms of mania. No single theory can explain the etiology of bipolar disorder, and it is likely that the illness is caused by a combination of factors. Symptoms of mania may be observed on a continuum of three phases, each identified by the extent of severity: phase I, hypomania; phase II, acute mania; and phase III, delirious mania.

Suicide is the eighth leading cause of death among

adults and the third leading cause of death among adolescents in the United States today. In assessing risk factors, it is important to consider marital status, gender, age, religion, socioeconomic status, ethnicity, occupation, family history, physical condition, support systems, precipitating stressors, coping strategies, seriousness of intent, and lethality and availability of method.

This chapter presented a plan for care of the suicidal client, including both inpatient and outpatient interventions. Information for family and friends of a suicidal person and suggestions for counseling with families of suicide victims was also included.

Treatment of mood disorders includes individual, group, family, and cognitive therapies. Somatic therapies include psychopharmacology and ECT. Nursing care is accomplished using the six steps of the nursing process.

REVIEW QUESTIONS

SELF-EXAMINATION/LEARNING EXERCISE

Situation: Margaret, age 68 years, was brought to the emergency department of a large regional medical center by her sister-in-law who stated, "She does nothing but sit and stare into space. I can't get her to eat or anything!" Upon assessment, it was found that 6 months ago Margaret's husband of 45 years had died of a massive myocardial infarction. They had no children and had been inseparable. Since her husband's death, Margaret has visited the cemetery every day, changing the flowers often on his grave. She has not removed any of his clothes from the closet or chest of drawers. His shaving materials still occupy the same space in the bathroom. Over the months, Margaret has become increasingly socially isolated. She refuses invitations from friends, preferring instead to make her daily trips to the cemetery. She has lost 15 pounds and her sister-in-law reports that there is very little food in the house. Today she said to her sister-in-law, "I don't really want to live anymore. My life is nothing without Frank." Her sister-in-law became frightened and, with forceful persuasion, was able to convince Margaret she needed to see a doctor. Margaret is admitted to the psychiatric unit.

Based on the above situation, select the answer that is most appropriate for each of the following questions:

1. The *priority* nursing diagnosis for Margaret would be:
   a. Imbalanced nutrition: less than body requirements
   b. Dysfunctional grieving
   c. Risk for suicide
   d. Social isolation
2. The physician orders sertraline (Zoloft) 50 mg b.i.d. for Margaret. After 3 days of the medication, Margaret says to the nurse, "I don't think this medicine is doing any good. I don't feel a bit better." What is the most appropriate response by the nurse?
   a. "Cheer up, Margaret. You have so much to be happy about."
   b. "Sometimes it takes a few weeks for the medicine to bring about an improvement in symptoms."
   c. "I'll report that to the physician, Margaret. Maybe he will order something different."
   d. "Try not to dwell on your symptoms, Margaret. Why don't you join the others down in the dayroom?"

After being stabilized on her medication, Margaret was released from the hospital with directions to continue taking the sertraline as ordered. A week later, her sister-in-law found Margaret in bed and was unable to awaken her. An empty prescription bottle was by her side. She was revived in the emergency department and transferred to the psychiatric unit in a state of severe depression. The physician determines that ECT may help Margaret. Consent is obtained.

3. About 30 minutes before the treatment the nurse administers atropine sulfate 0.4 mg IM. Rationale for this order is:
   a. To decrease secretions and increase heart rate
   b. To relax muscles
   c. To produce a calming effect
   d. To induce anesthesia
4. When Margaret is in the treatment room, the anesthesiologist administers thiopental sodium (Pentothal) followed by IV succinylcholine (Anectine). The purposes of these medications are to:
   a. Decrease secretions and increase heart rate
   b. Prevent nausea and induce a calming effect
   c. Minimize memory loss and stabilize mood
   d. Induce anesthesia and relax muscles

5. After three ECTs, Margaret's mood begins to lift and she tells the nurse, "I feel so much better, but I'm having trouble remembering some things that happened this last week." The nurse's best response would be:

   a. "Don't worry about that. Nothing important happened."
   b. "Memory loss is just something you have to put up with to feel better."
   c. "Memory loss is a side effect of ECT, but it is only temporary. Your memory should return within a few weeks."
   d. "Try to forget about last week, Margaret. You need to look forward from here."

A year later, Margaret presents in the emergency department, once again accompanied by her sister-in-law. This time Margaret is agitated, pacing, demanding, and speaking very loudly. "I didn't want to come here! My sister-in-law is just jealous, and she's trying to make it look like I'm insane!" Upon assessment, the sister-in-law reports that Margaret has become engaged to a 25-year-old construction worker to whom she has willed her sizable inheritance and her home. Margaret loudly praises her fiancé's physique and sexual abilities. She has been spending large sums of money on herself and giving her fiancé $500 a week. The sister-in-law tells the physician, "I know it is Margaret's business what she does with her life, but I'm really worried about her. She is losing weight again. She eats very little and almost never sleeps. I'm afraid she's going to just collapse!" Margaret is once again admitted to the psychiatric unit.

6. The *priority* nursing diagnosis for Margaret is:

   a. Imbalanced nutrition: less than body requirements related to not eating
   b. Risk for injury related to hyperactivity
   c. Disturbed sleep pattern related to agitation
   d. Ineffective coping related to denial of depression

7. One way to promote adequate nutritional intake for Margaret is to:

   a. Sit with her during meals to ensure that she eats everything on her tray.
   b. Have her sister-in-law bring all her food from home, as she knows Margaret's likes and dislikes.
   c. Provide high-calorie, nutritious finger foods and snacks that Margaret can eat "on the run."
   d. Tell Margaret that she will be on room restriction until she starts gaining weight.

8. The physician orders lithium carbonate 600 mg t.i.d. for Margaret. There is a narrow margin between the therapeutic and toxic levels of lithium. Therapeutic range for acute mania is:

   a. 1.0 to 1.5 mEq/L
   b. 10 to 15 mEq/L
   c. 0.5 to 1.0 mEq/L
   d. 5 to 10 mEq/L

9. After an appropriate length of time, the physician determines that Margaret does not respond satisfactorily to lithium therapy. He changes her medication to another drug that has been found to be effective in the treatment of bipolar mania. This drug is:

   a. Molindone (Moban)
   b. Paroxetine (Paxil)
   c. Carbamazepine (Tegretol)
   d. Tranylcypromine (Parnate)

10. Margaret's statement, "My sister-in-law is just jealous, and she's trying to make it look like I'm insane!" is an example of:

    a. A delusion of grandeur
    b. A delusion of persecution
    c. A delusion of reference
    d. A delusion of control or influence

Test Your CRITICAL THINKING SKILLS

Alice, aged 29, had been working in the typing pool of a large corporation for 6 years. Her immediate supervisor recently retired and Alice was promoted to supervisor, in charge of 20 people in the department. Alice was flattered by the promotion but anxious about the additional responsibility of the position. Shortly after the promotion, she overheard two of her former coworkers saying, "Why in the world did they choose her? She's not the best one for the job. I know *I* certainly won't be able to respect her as a boss!" Hearing these comments added to Alice's anxiety and self-doubt.

Shortly after Alice began her new duties, her friends and coworkers noticed a change. She had a great deal of energy and worked long hours on her job. She began to speak very loudly and rapidly. Her roommate noticed that Alice slept very little, yet seldom appeared tired. Every night she would go out to bars and dances. Sometimes she brought men she had just met home to the apartment, something she had never done before. She bought lots of clothes and makeup and had her hair restyled in a more youthful look. She failed to pay her share of the rent and bills but came home with a brand new convertible. She lost her temper and screamed at her roommate to "Mind your own business!" when asked to pay her share.

She became irritable at work, and several of her subordinates reported her behavior to the corporate manager. When the manager confronted Alice about her behavior, she lost control, shouting, cursing, and striking out at anyone and anything that happened to be within her reach. The security officers restrained her and took her to the emergency department of the hospital, where she was admitted to the psychiatric unit. She had no previous history of psychiatric illness.

The psychiatrist assigned a diagnosis of bipolar I disorder and wrote orders for olanzapine (Zyprexa) 15 mg PO STAT, olanzapine 15 mg PO qd, and lithium carbonate 600 mg qid.

Answer the following questions related to Alice:

1. What are the most important considerations with which the nurse who is taking care of Alice should be concerned?
2. Why was Alice given the diagnosis of bipolar I disorder?
3. The doctor should order a lithium level drawn after 4 to 6 days. For what symptoms should the nurse be on the alert?
4. Why did the physician order olanzapine in addition to the lithium carbonate?

IMPLICATIONS OF RESEARCH FOR EVIDENCE BASED PRACTICE

Dimeo, F., Bauer, M., Varahram, I., Proest, G., and Halter, U: **Benefits from Aerobic Exercise in Patients with Major Depression: A Pilot Study.** British Journal of Sports Medicine (2001, April), 35(2), 114–117.

Description of the Study: The literature search for this study revealed that physical activity could reduce the severity of symptoms in depressed patients. Some data suggested that even a single exercise bout might result in substantial mood improvement. This study was conducted to evaluate the short-term effects of a training program on patients with moderate to severe major depression. The study participants included 5 men and 7 women with a mean age of 49 years. They each had been diagnosed with major depressive episode according to the *DSM-IV* criteria. The mean duration of the depressive episode was 35 weeks (range 12 to 96 weeks). Training consisted of walking on a treadmill following an interval-training pattern and was carried out for 30 minutes a day for 10 days. Objective depression scores were measured using the Hamilton Rating Scale for depression. Subjective self-assessment reports were also considered.

Results of the Study: At the end of the training program, there was a clinically relevant and statistically significant reduction in mean depression scores, as follows:

Hamilton Rating scores:	Before: 19.5	After: 13
Self-assessment scores:	Before: 23.2	After: 17.7

Subjective and objective changes in depression scores correlated strongly.

Implications for Nursing Practice: This study concludes that aerobic exercise can produce substantial improvement in mood in patients with major depressive disorders in a short time. Psychiatric nurses can be instrumental in educating depressed clients to these benefits and encourage participation in aerobic exercise programs. They can also be influential in supporting strategy to establish aerobic exercise guidelines and equipment into psychiatric treatment programs.

@ INTERNET REFERENCES

- Additional information about mood disorders, including psychosocial and pharmacological treatment of these disorders may be located at the following websites:
  a **http://www.pslgroup.com/depression.htm**
  b **http://depression.miningco.com/**

c http://www.ndmda.org

d http://www.fadavis.com/townsend

e www.mentalhealth.com/p.html

f www.mhsource.com/bipolar

g www.mhsource.com/depression

h text.nlm.nih.gov/nih/cdc/www/44.html

i www.mental-health-matters.com/mood.html

j www.mentalhelp.net

REFERENCES

Abrams, R. (1997). Electroconvulsive therapy (3rd ed). New York: Oxford University Press.

Administration on Aging. (2002). A profile of older Americans: 2002. Washington, DC: U.S. Department of Health and Human Services.

American Psychiatric Association (APA). (2000). Diagnostic and Statistical manual of mental disorders (4th ed.) Text revision. Washington, D.C.: American Psychiatric Association.

Barstow, D.G. (2002). Electroconvulsive therapy. Gale Encyclopedia of Medicine. Retrieved January 16, 2002, from http://www.findarticles.com/cf_dis/g2601/0004/2601000467/p1/article.jhtml

Blackburn, B. (1990). What you should know about suicide. Dallas, TX: Word Publishing.

Bohrer, G.J. (2001). Going to extremes: The difficulties of living with bipolar illness. Retrieved October 24, 2003, from http://www.nurseweek.com/ce/ce1230a.html

Burke, K.C., Burke, J.D., & Regier, D.A. (1990). Age at onset of selected mental disorders in five community populations. Archives of General Psychiatry, 47,511–518.

Carroll-Ghosh, T., Victor, B.S., & Bourgeois, J.A. (2003). Suicide. In R.E. Hales & S.C. Yudofsky (Eds.), Textbook of Clinical Psychiatry (4th ed.). Washington, DC: American Psychiatric Publishing.

Centers for Disease Control (CDC). (2002). Preventing suicide. Retrieved on January 2, 2002, from http://www.cdc.gov/safeusa/suicide.htm

Craig, T.J. (1994). Epidemiology of psychiatric illness. In G. Winokur & P.J. Clayton (Eds.), The medical basis of psychiatry. Philadelphia: W.B. Saunders.

Crisis Hotline. (2001). Some facts about suicide in the U.S.A. Retrieved December 11, 2001 from http://www.crisishotline.org/strategies/term.html

Dubovsky, S.L. & Buzan, R. (1999). Mood disorders. In R.E. Hales & S.C. Yudofsky (Eds.), Essentials of Clinical Psychiatry. Washington, DC: American Psychiatric Press.

Dubovsky, S. L., Davies, R., & Dubovsky, A.N. (2003). Mood disorders. In R.E. Hales & S.C. Yudofsky (Eds.), Textbook of clinical psychiatry (4th ed.).Washington, D.C.: American Psychiatric Publishing.

Endler, N.E., & Persad, E. (1996). Electroconvulsive therapy—The myths and the realities (2nd ed). Toronto: Hogrefe & Huber Publishers.

Frackiewicz, E.J. & Shiovitz, T.M. (2001). Evaluation and management of premenstrual syndrome. Journal of the American Pharmaceutical Association 41(3), 437–447.

Fraser, M. (1994). What about us?: The legacy of suicide. Retrieved January 6, 2002, from http://www.csu.edu.au/research/crsr/ruralsoc/v4n3p7.htm

Gale Encyclopedia of Childhood and Adolescence. (1998). Anaclitic depression. Retrieved February 28, 2002, from http://www.findarticles.com/cf_dis/g2602/0000/2602000035/p1/article.jhtml

Goodwin, F.K.& Jamison, K.R. (1990). Manic-depressive illness. New York: Oxford University Press.

Harvard Medical School. (2002, February). Depression in Children—Part I. The Harvard Mental Health Letter. Boston, MA: Harvard Medical School Publications Group.

Harvard Medical School. (2001, April). Bipolar disorder—Part I. The Harvard Mental Health Letter. Boston, MA: Harvard Medical School Publications Group.

Harvard Medical School. (1997, September). Postpartum Disorders. The Harvard Mental Health Letter. Boston, MA: Harvard Medical School Publications Group.

Harvard Medical School. (1996, December). Suicide—Part II. The Harvard Mental Health Letter. Boston, MA: Harvard Medical School Publications Group.

Hatten, C.L., & Valente, S.M. (1984). Suicide: Assessment and intervention (2nd ed.). Norwalk, CT: Appleton-Century-Crofts.

Hollon, S.D., DeRubeis, R.J., & Evans, M.D. (1992). Cognitive therapy and pharmacotherapy for depression: singly and in combination. Archives of General Psychiatry, 49, 774–781.

International Society for Mental Health Online [ISMHO]. (2003). All about depression. Retrieved October 23, 2003, from http://www.allaboutdepression.com/gen_01.html#3

Kaplan, H.I., & Sadock, B.J. (1998). Synopsis of psychiatry: Behavioral sciences/clinical psychiatry (8th ed.). Baltimore: Williams & Wilkins

Kennedy, R. & Suttenfield, K. (2002). Postpartum depression. Retrieved March 1, 2002, from http://www.medscape.com/viewarticle/408688

Lewis, M., & Volkmar, F. (1990). Clinical aspects of child and adolescent development. Philadelphia: Lea & Febiger.

Lyness, J.M. (1997). Psychiatric Pearls. Philadelphia: F. A. Davis.

Macnab, F. (1993). Brief psychotherapy: An integrative approach in clinical practice. West Sussex, England: John Wiley & Sons.

Marangell, L.B., Silver, J.M., & Yudofsky, S.C. (1999). Psychopharmacology and electroconvulsive therapy. In R.E. Hales & S.C. Yudofsky (Eds.), Essentials of clinical psychiatry. Washington, D.C.: American Psychiatric Press.

Medscape Psychiatry. (2001). Is suicide always an outcome of illness? Suicide: An overview. Retrieved January 2, 2002, from http://www.medscape.com/Medscape/psychiatry/ClinicalMgmt/CM.v03/CM.v03-03.html

Mental Health Sanctuary. (2001). How to help a suicidal person. Retrieved on December 11, 2001 from http://www.mhsanctuary.com/suicide/sui2.htm

Murphy, C.G. (1994). Suicide and attempted suicide, In G. Winokur, & P.J. Clayton (Eds.), The medical basis of psychiatry (2nd ed.). Philadelphia: W.B. Saunders.

National Institute of Mental Health (NIMH). (2003). Older adults: Depression and suicide facts. Retrieved October 24, 2003 from http://www.nimh.nih.gov

National Institute of Mental Health (NIMH). (2002). In harm's way: Suicide in America. Retrieved January 5, 2002 from http://www.nimh.nih.gov/publicat/harmaway.cfm

National Institute of Mental Health (NIMH). (2000). Bipolar disorder research fact sheet. NIH Publication No. 00-4502. Washington, D.C.: Department of Health and Human Services.

O'Connor, R. (2002). Teen Suicide. Focus Adolescent Services. Retrieved February 28, 2002 from http://www.focusas.com/Suicide.html

Popolos, D. (2002). All about ECT. Retrieved January 12, 2002 from http://www.schizophrenia.com/family/ect1.html

Sadock, B.J. & Sadock, V.A. (2003). Synopsis of psychiatry: Behavioral sciences/ clinical psychiatry (9th ed.). Philadelphia: Lippincott Williams & Wilkins.

Samaritans (The). (2002). Suicide myths and misconceptions. Retrieved on January 2, 2002, from the World Wide Web at http://www.samaritansnyc.org/myths.html

Schimelpfening, N. (2002). A vitamin a day keeps depression away. Retrieved February 28, 2002, from http://depression.about.com/library/weekly/aa051799.htm

U.S. Public Health Service (USPHS). (1999). The Surgeon General's call to action to prevent suicide. Washington, DC: USPHS.

Winokur, G. (1994). Unipolar depression. In G. Winokur and P.J. Clayton (Eds.), The medical basis of psychiatry (2nd ed.). Philadelphia: W.B. Saunders.

Wright, J.H. & Thase, M.E. (1992). Cognitive and biological therapies: a synthesis. Psychiatric Annals, 22, 451–458.

Zubieta, J.K, et al. (2000). High vesicular monoamine transporter binding in asymptomatic bipolar I disorder: Sex differences and cognitive correlates. American Journal of Psychiatry 157: 1619–1628.

CLASSICAL REFERENCES

Beck, A.T., Rush, A.J., Shaw, B.F., & Emery, G. (1979). Cognitive theory of depression. New York: Guilford Press.

Freud, S. (1957). Mourning and melancholia, vol. 14 (standard ed.). London: Hogarth Press. (Original work published 1917.)

Seligman, M.E.P. (1973). Fall into helplessness. Psychology Today, 7, 43–48.[

16

CHAPTER

Townsend Essentials

Anxiety Disorders

CHAPTER OUTLINE

KEY TERMS

agoraphobia
flooding
generalized anxiety disorder
implosion therapy
obsessive-compulsive disorder (OCD)
panic disorder
phobias
post-traumatic stress disorder (PTSD)
ritualistic behavior
specific phobia
social phobia
systematic desensitization

OBJECTIVES

After reading this chapter, the student will be able to:

1. Differentiate among the terms *stress*, *anxiety*, and *fear*.
2. Discuss historical aspects and epidemiological statistics related to anxiety disorders.
3. Differentiate between normal anxiety and psychoneurotic anxiety.
4. Describe various types of anxiety disorders and identify symptomatology associated with each. Use this information in client assessment.
5. Identify etiological factors in the development of anxiety disorders.
6. Formulate nursing diagnoses and outcome criteria for clients with anxiety disorders.
7. Describe appropriate nursing interventions for behaviors associated with anxiety disorders.
8. Identify topics for client and family teaching relevant to anxiety disorders.
9. Evaluate nursing care of clients with anxiety disorders.
10. Discuss various modalities relevant to treatment of anxiety disorders.

INTRODUCTION

The following is an account by singer-songwriter Michael Johnson (1994) relating his experience with performance anxiety:

> You've got your Jolly Roger clothes on, you've got the microphone, the lights are on you, the owner has just told the crowd to shut up, and you are getting that kind of 'show and tell' sickness that you used to get at grade school pageants or college recitals. Suddenly your mouth is so dry that your lips are sticking to your teeth, and you find yourself gesturing oddly with your shoulder and wondering if they think that maybe something unfortunate happened to you and they're trying to cope with the whole thing. It is now, of course, it hits you that you started with the second verse, you're doing a live rewrite, and you have no idea how this song is going to end. Your vocal range has shrunk and your heartbeat is interfering with your vibrato. Your palms are wet and your mouth is dry—a great combination!

Individuals face anxiety on a daily basis. Anxiety, which provides the motivation for achievement, is a necessary force for survival. The term *anxiety* is often used interchangeably with the word *stress;* however, they are not the same. Stress, or more properly, a *stressor*, is an external pressure that is brought to bear on the individual. Anxiety is the subjective emotional response to that stressor. (See Chapter 1 for an overview of anxiety as a psychological response to stress.)

Anxiety may be distinguished from fear in that the former is an emotional process, whereas fear is a cognitive one. Fear involves the intellectual appraisal of a threatening stimulus; anxiety involves the emotional response to that appraisal.

This chapter focuses on disorders that are characterized by exaggerated and often disabling anxiety reactions. Historical aspects and epidemiological statistics are presented. Predisposing factors that have been implicated in the etiology of anxiety disorders provide a framework for studying the dynamics of **phobias, obsessive-compulsive disorder (OCD), generalized anxiety disorder, panic disorder, post-traumatic stress disorder (PTSD)**, and other anxiety disorders. Various theories of causation are presented, although it is most likely that a combination of factors contribute to the etiology of anxiety disorders.

An explanation of the symptomatology is presented as background knowledge for assessing the client with an anxiety disorder. Nursing care is described in the context of the nursing process. Various medical treatment modalities are explored.

HISTORICAL ASPECTS

Individuals have experienced anxiety throughout the ages. Yet anxiety, like fear, was not clearly defined or isolated as a separate entity by psychiatrists or psychologists until the 19th and 20th centuries. In fact, what we now know as anxiety was once solely identified by its physiological symptoms, focusing largely on the cardiovascular system. A myriad of diagnostic terms were used in attempts to identify these symptoms. For example, cardiac neurosis, DaCosta's syndrome, irritable heart, nervous tachycardia, neurocirculatory asthenia, soldier's heart, vasomotor neurosis, and vasoregulatory asthenia are just a few of the names under which anxiety has been concealed over the years (Sadock & Sadock, 2003).

Freud first introduced the term *anxiety neurosis* in 1895. Freud wrote, "I call this syndrome 'anxiety neurosis' because all its components can be grouped round the chief symptom of anxiety" (Freud, 1959). This notion attempted to negate the previous concept of the problem as strictly physical, although it was some time before physicians of internal medicine were ready to accept the psychological implications for the symptoms. In fact, it was not until the years during World War II that the psychological dimensions of these various functional heart conditions were recognized.

For many years, anxiety disorders were viewed as purely psychological or purely biological in nature. In recent years a number of researchers have begun to focus on the interrelatedness of mind and body. Liebowitz (1992) states: "Anxiety disorders provide an excellent example of the complex relationship between mind and body factors in mental illness." It is likely that various factors, including genetic, developmental, environmental, and psychological factors, play a role in the etiology of anxiety disorders.

EPIDEMIOLOGICAL STATISTICS

Anxiety disorders are the most common of all psychiatric illnesses and result in considerable functional impairment and distress (Hollander & Simeon, 2003). Statistics vary widely, but most agree that anxiety disorders are more common in women than in men by at least 2 to 1. Prevalence rates have been given at 1.5 to 5 percent for panic disorder; 2 to 3 percent for OCD; 8 percent for PTSD, and 0.6 to 6 percent for **agoraphobia** (Sadock & Sadock, 2003). A review of the literature reveals a wide range of reports regarding the prevalence of anxiety disorders in children (2 to 43 percent). Epidemiological studies suggest that the symptoms are more prevalent among girls than boys (American Psychiatric Association [APA], 2000) and that minority children and children from low socioeconomic environments may be at greater risk for all emotional illness (Halpern, 1990; Johnson, 1995). Studies of familial patterns suggest that a familial predisposition to anxiety disorders probably exists.

HOW MUCH IS TOO MUCH?

Anxiety is usually considered a normal reaction to a realistic danger or threat to biological integrity or self-concept. Normal anxiety dissipates when the danger or threat is no longer present.

It is difficult to draw a precise line between normal and abnormal anxiety. Normality is determined by societal standards; what is considered normal in Chicago, Illinois may not be considered so in Cairo, Egypt. There may even be regional differences within a country or cultural differences within a region. What criteria then can be used to determine if an individual's anxious response is normal? Anxiety can be considered abnormal or pathological if:

1. It is out of proportion to the situation that is creating it.
   EXAMPLE: Mrs. K witnessed a serious automobile accident 4 weeks ago when she was out driving in her car, and since that time she refuses to drive even to the grocery store a few miles from her house. When he is available, her husband must take her wherever she needs to go.
2. The anxiety interferes with social, occupational, or other important areas of functioning.
   EXAMPLE: Because of the anxiety associated with driving her car, Mrs. K has been forced to quit her job in a downtown bank for lack of transportation.

APPLICATION OF THE NURSING PROCESS

Panic Disorder

Background Assessment Data

This disorder is characterized by recurrent panic attacks, the onset of which are unpredictable, and manifested by intense apprehension, fear, or terror, often associated with feelings of impending doom and accompanied by intense physical discomfort. The symptoms come on unexpectedly; that is, they do not occur immediately before or on exposure to a situation that usually causes anxiety (as in specific phobia). They are not triggered by situations in which the person is the focus of attention (as in social phobia). Organic factors in the role of etiology have been ruled out.

At least four of the following symptoms must be present to identify the presence of a panic attack. When fewer than four symptoms are present, the individual is diagnosed as having a limited-symptom attack.

1. Palpitations, pounding heart, or accelerated heart rate
2. Sweating
3. Trembling or shaking
4. Sensations of shortness of breath or smothering
5. Feeling of choking
6. Chest pain or discomfort
7. Nausea or abdominal distress
8. Feeling dizzy, unsteady, lightheaded, or faint
9. Derealization (feelings of unreality) or depersonalization (being detached from oneself)
10. Fear of losing control or going crazy
11. Fear of dying
12. Paresthesias (numbness or tingling sensations)
13. Chills or hot flashes

The attacks usually last minutes or, more rarely, hours. The individual often experiences some degree of nervousness and apprehension between attacks. Symptoms of depression are common.

The average age of onset of panic disorder is the late 20s. Frequency and severity of the panic attacks vary widely (APA, 2000). Some individuals may have attacks of moderate severity weekly; others may have less severe or limited-symptom attacks several times a week. Still others may experience panic attacks that are separated by weeks or months. The disorder may last for a few weeks or months or for a number of years. Sometimes the individual experiences periods of remission and exacerbation. In times of remission, the person may have recurrent limited-symptom attacks. Panic disorder may or may not be accompanied by agoraphobia.

PANIC DISORDER WITH AGORAPHOBIA. Panic disorder with agoraphobia is characterized by the symptoms described for panic disorder. In addition, the individual experiences a fear of being in places or situations from which escape might be difficult (or embarrassing) or in which help might not be available in the event that a panic attack should occur (APA, 2000). This fear severely restricts travel, and the individual may become nearly or completely housebound or unable to leave the house unaccompanied.

Common agoraphobic situations include being outside the home alone, being in a crowd or standing in a line, being on a bridge, and traveling in a bus, train, or car.

Generalized Anxiety Disorder

Background Assessment Data

Generalized anxiety disorder is characterized by chronic, unrealistic, and excessive anxiety and worry. The symptoms have existed for 6 months or longer and are not attributed to specific organic factors, such as caffeine intoxication or hyperthyroidism.

The *DSM-IV-TR* identifies the following symptoms associated with generalized anxiety disorder. The symptoms must have occurred more days than not for at least 6 months and must cause clinically significant distress or impairment in social, occupational, or other important areas of functioning.

1. Excessive anxiety and worry about a number of events that the individual finds difficult to control
2. Restlessness or feeling keyed up or on edge
3. Being easily fatigued
4. Difficulty concentrating or mind "going blank"
5. Irritability
6. Muscle tension
7. Sleep disturbance (difficulty falling or staying asleep, or restless unsatisfying sleep)

The disorder may begin in childhood or adolescence, but onset is more common after age 20 years. Depressive symptoms and numerous somatic complaints may be a part of the clinical picture. Generalized anxiety disorder tends to be chronic, with frequent stress-related exacerbations and fluctuations in the course of the illness.

Etiological Implications for Panic and Generalized Anxiety Disorders

PSYCHODYNAMIC THEORY. The psychodynamic view focuses on the inability of the ego to intervene when conflict occurs between the id and the superego, producing anxiety. For various reasons (unsatisfactory parent-child relationship; conditional love or provisional gratification), ego development is delayed. When developmental defects in ego function compromise the capacity to modulate anxiety, the individual resorts to unconscious mechanisms to resolve the conflict. Overuse or ineffective use of ego defense mechanisms results in maladaptive responses to anxiety.

COGNITIVE THEORY. The main thesis of the cognitive view is that faulty, distorted, or counterproductive thinking patterns accompany or precede maladaptive behaviors and emotional disorders (Sadock & Sadock, 2003). When there is a disturbance in this central mechanism of cognition, there is a consequent disturbance in feeling and behavior. Because of distorted thinking, anxiety is maintained by erroneous or dysfunctional appraisal of a situation. There is a loss of ability to reason regarding the problem, whether it is physical or interpersonal. The individual feels vulnerable in a given situation, and the distorted thinking results in an irrational appraisal fostering a negative outcome.

BIOLOGICAL ASPECTS. Research investigations into the psychobiological correlation of panic and generalized anxiety disorders have implicated several possibilities.

Genetics. Panic disorder has a strong genetic element (Harvard Medical School, 2001). The concordance rate for identical twins is 30 percent, and the risk for the disorder in a close relative is 10 to 20 percent. The Harvard Medical School (2001) reports:

> A possible hereditary basis is suggested by some new research on a protein called cholecystokinin, which can induce panic attacks when it is injected. In a recent study, investigators found an association between panic disorder and a variant of the gene that controls the manufacture of this protein. (p. 2)

NEUROANATOMICAL. Modern theory on the physiology of emotional states places the key in the lower brain centers, including the limbic system, the diencephalon (thalamus and hypothalamus), and the reticular formation. Structural brain imaging studies in patients with panic disorder have implicated pathological involvement in the temporal lobes, particularly the hippocampus (Sadock & Sadock, 2003).

BIOCHEMICAL. Abnormal elevations of blood lactate have been noted in clients with panic disorder. Likewise, infusion of sodium lactate into clients with anxiety neuroses produced symptoms of panic disorder. Although several laboratories have replicated these findings of increased lactate sensitivity in panic-prone individuals, no specific mechanism that triggers the panic symptoms can be explained (Hollander & Simeon, 2003).

NEUROCHEMICAL. Stronger evidence exists for the involvement of the neurotransmitter norepinephrine in the etiology of panic disorder (Henn, 1994). Norepinephrine is known to mediate arousal, and it causes hyperarousal and anxiety. This fact has been demonstrated by a notable increase in anxiety following the administration of drugs that increase the synaptic availability of norepinephrine, such as yohimbine.

MEDICAL CONDITIONS. The following medical conditions have been associated with individuals who suffer panic and generalized anxiety disorders more frequently than the general population:

1. Abnormalities in the hypothalamic-pituitary-adrenal and hypothalamic-pituitary-thyroid axes
2. Acute myocardial infarction
3. Pheochromocytomas
4. Substance intoxication and withdrawal (cocaine, alcohol, marijuana, opioids)
5. Hypoglycemia
6. Caffeine intoxication
7. Mitral valve prolapse
8. Complex partial seizures

Diagnosis/Outcome Identification

Nursing diagnoses are formulated from the data gathered during the assessment phase and with background knowledge regarding predisposing factors to the disorder. Some common nursing diagnoses for clients with panic disorder and generalized anxiety disorder include:

Panic anxiety related to real or perceived threat to biological integrity or self-concept evidenced by any or all of the physical symptoms identified by the *DSM-IV-TR* as being descriptive of panic or generalized anxiety disorder

Powerlessness related to impaired cognition evidenced by verbal expressions of no control over life situation and nonparticipation in decision-making related to own care or life situation

The following criteria may be used to measure outcomes in the care of the client with panic disorder or generalized anxiety disorder. The client:

1. Is able to recognize signs of escalating anxiety
2. Is able to intervene so that anxiety does not reach the panic level
3. Is able to discuss long-term plan to prevent panic anxiety when stressful situation occurs
4. Practices techniques of relaxation daily
5. Engages in physical exercise three times a week
6. Performs activities of daily living independently
7. Expresses satisfaction for independent functioning
8. Is able to maintain anxiety at manageable level without use of medication
9. Is able to participate in decision-making, thereby maintaining control over life situation
10. Verbalizes acceptance of life situations over which he or she has no control

Planning/Implementation

Table 16–1 provides a plan of care for the client with panic disorder or generalized anxiety disorder. Nursing diagnoses are presented, along with outcome criteria, appropriate nursing interventions, and rationales for each.

Evaluation

Reassessment determines if the nursing actions have been successful in achieving the objectives of care. Evaluation of nursing actions for the client with panic disorder or generalized anxiety disorder may be facilitated by gathering information using the following types of questions:

1. Can the client recognize signs and symptoms of escalating anxiety?
2. Can the client use skills learned to interrupt the escalating anxiety before it reaches the panic level?
3. Can the client demonstrate the activities most appropriate for him or her that can be used to maintain anxiety at a manageable level (e.g., relaxation techniques; physical exercise)?
4. Can the client maintain anxiety at a manageable level without medication?
5. Can the client verbalize a long-term plan for preventing panic anxiety in the face of a stressful situation?
6. Does the client perform activities of daily living independently?
7. Does the client exercise control over life situation by participating in the decision-making process?
8. Can the client verbalize resources outside the hospital from which he or she can seek assistance during times of extreme stress?

Phobias

Background Assessment Data

AGORAPHOBIA WITHOUT HISTORY OF PANIC DISORDER. Agoraphobia without accompanying panic disorder is less common than the type that precipitates panic attacks. In this disorder, there is a fear of being in places or situations from which escape might be difficult or help might not be available if a

TABLE 16–1 Care Plan for the Client with Panic Disorder or Generalized Anxiety Disorder

Nursing Diagnosis: PANIC ANXIETY
Related to: Real or perceived threat to biological integrity or self-concept
Evidenced by: Any or all of the physical symptoms identified by the *DSM-IV-TR*

Outcome Criteria	Nursing Interventions	Rationale
Client will be able to recognize symptoms of onset of anxiety and to intervene before reaching panic level.	1. Stay with the client and offer reassurance of safety and security.	1. The client may fear for his or her life. Presence of a trusted individual provides a feeling of security and assurance of personal safety.
	2. Maintain a calm, nonthreatening, matter-of-fact approach.	2. Anxiety is contagious and may be transferred from staff to client or vice versa. Client develops a feeling of security in the presence of a calm staff person.
	3. Use simple words and brief messages, spoken calmly and clearly, to explain hospital experiences.	3. In an intensely anxious situation, the client is unable to comprehend anything but the most elemental communication.
	4. Keep immediate surroundings low in stimuli (dim lighting, few people, simple decor).	4. A stimulating environment may increase level of anxiety.
	5. Administer tranquilizing medication as ordered by physician. Assess for effectiveness and for side effects.	5. Antianxiety medication provides relief from the immobilizing effects of anxiety.
	6. When level of anxiety has been reduced, explore possible reasons for occurrence.	6. Recognition of precipitating factor(s) is the first step in teaching client to interrupt escalation of anxiety.
	7. Teach signs and symptoms of escalating anxiety, and ways to interrupt its progression (relaxation techniques, deep-breathing exercises, and meditation, or physical exercise, brisk walks, and jogging).	7. Relaxation techniques result in a physiological response opposite that of the anxiety response. Physical activities discharge excess energy in a healthful manner.

Nursing Diagnosis: POWERLESSNESS
Related to: Impaired cognition
Evidenced by: Verbal expressions of no control over life situation and nonparticipation in decision–making related to own care or life situation

Outcome Criteria	Nursing Interventions	Rationale
Client will be able to effectively problem–solve ways to take control of life situation, thereby decreasing feelings of powerlessness and anxiety.	1. Allow client to take as much responsibility as possible for self-care practices. Examples include: a. Allow client to establish own schedule for self-care activities b. Include client in setting goals of care c. Provide client with privacy as need is determined d. Provide positive feedback for decisions made. Respect client's right to make those decisions independently, and refrain from attempting to influence him or her toward those that may seem more logical	1. Providing choices will increase client's feelings of control.
	2. Assist client to set realistic goals.	2. Unrealistic goals set the client up for failure and reinforce feelings of powerlessness.
	3. Help identify areas of life situation that client can control.	3. Client's emotional condition interferes with the ability to solve problems. Assistance is required to perceive the benefits and consequences of available alternatives accurately.
	4. Help client identify areas of life situation that are not within his or her ability to control. Encourage verbalization of feelings related to this inability.	4. This will assist the client to deal with unresolved issues and learn to accept what cannot be changed.

limited symptom attack or panic-like symptoms (rather than full panic attacks) should occur (APA, 2000). It is possible that the individual may have experienced the symptom(s) in the past and is preoccupied with fears of their recurrence. The *DSM-IV-TR* diagnostic criteria for agoraphobia without history of panic disorder are presented in Table 16–2.

Onset of symptoms most commonly occurs in the 20s and 30s and persists for many years. It is diagnosed more commonly in women than in men. Impairment can be severe. In extreme cases, the individual is unable to leave his or her home without being accompanied by a friend or relative. If this is not possible, the person may become totally confined to his or her home.

SOCIAL PHOBIA. **Social phobia** is an excessive fear of a situation where an individual believes he or she may do something embarrassing or be evaluated negatively by others (Noyes & Holt, 1994). The individual has extreme concerns about being exposed to possible scrutiny by others and fears social or performance situations in which embarrassment may occur (APA, 2000). In some instances, the fear may be quite defined, such as the fear of speaking or eating in a public place, fear of using a public restroom, or fear of writing in the presence of others. In other cases, the social phobia may involve general social situations, such as saying things or answering questions in a manner that would provoke laughter on the part of others. Exposure to the phobic situation usually results in feelings of panic anxiety, with sweating, tachycardia, and dyspnea.

Onset of symptoms of this disorder often begins in late childhood or early adolescence and runs a chronic, sometimes lifelong, course. It appears to be equally common among men and women (APA, 2000). Impairment interferes with social or occupational functioning or causes marked distress. The *DSM-IV-TR* diagnostic criteria for social phobia are presented in Table 16–3.

TABLE 16–2 Diagnostic Criteria for Agoraphobia without History of Panic Disorder

A. The presence of agoraphobia related to fear of developing panic-like symptoms. (Agoraphobia: Fear of being in places or situations from which escape might be difficult [or embarrassing] or in which help might not be available in the event of suddenly developing a symptom(s) that could be incapacitating or extremely embarrassing. Examples include: dizziness or falling, depersonalization or derealization, loss of bladder or bowel control, vomiting, or cardiac distress. Because of this fear, the person restricts travel or needs a companion when away from home, or else endures agoraphobic situations despite intense anxiety. Common agoraphobic situations include being outside the home alone, being in a crowd or standing in a line, being on a bridge, and traveling in a bus, train, or car.)
B. Criteria for panic disorder have never been met.
C. The disturbance is not due to the direct physiological effects of a substance (e.g., a drug of abuse, a medication) or a general medical condition.
D. If an associated general medical condition is present, the fear is clearly in excess of that usually associated with the condition.

From the American Psychiatric Association (2000), with permission.

TABLE 16–3 Diagnostic Criteria for Social Phobia

A. A marked and persistent fear of one or more social or performance situations in which the person is exposed to unfamiliar people or to possible scrutiny by others. The individual fears that he or she will act in a way (or show anxiety symptoms) that will be humiliating or embarrassing. **NOTE:** In children, there must be evidence of the capacity for age-appropriate social relationships with familiar people and the anxiety must occur in peer settings, not just in interactions with adults.
B. Exposure to the feared social situation almost invariably provokes anxiety, which may take the form of a situationally bound or situationally predisposed panic attack. **NOTE:** In children, the anxiety may be expressed by crying, tantrums, freezing, or shrinking from social situations with unfamiliar people.
C. The person recognizes that the fear is excessive or unreasonable. **NOTE:** In children, this feature may be absent.
D. The feared social or performance situations are avoided or else are endured with intense anxiety or distress.
E. The avoidance, anxious anticipation, or distress in the feared social or performance situation(s) interferes significantly with the person's normal routine, occupational (academic) functioning, or social activities or relationships, or there is marked distress about having the phobia.
F. In individuals under age 18 years, the duration is at least 6 months.
G. The fear or avoidance is not due to the direct physiological effects of a substance (e.g., a drug of abuse, a medication) or a general medical condition and is not better accounted for by another mental disorder (e.g., panic disorder with or without agoraphobia, separation anxiety disorder, body dysmorphic disorder, a pervasive developmental disorder, or schizoid personality disorder).
H. If a general medical condition or another mental disorder is present, the fear in criterion A is unrelated to it (e.g., the fear is not of stuttering, trembling in Parkinson's disease, or exhibiting abnormal eating behavior in anorexia nervosa or bulimia nervosa).

The diagnosis is further specified as generalized if the fears include most social situations.

From the American Psychiatric Association (2000), with permission.

SPECIFIC PHOBIA. Specific phobia was formerly called simple phobia. The essential feature of this disorder is a marked, persistent, and excessive or unreasonable fear when in the presence of, or when anticipating an encounter with, a specific object or situation (APA, 2000).

Specific phobias frequently occur concurrently with other anxiety disorders, but they are rarely the focus of clinical attention in these situations (APA, 2000). Treatment is generally aimed at the primary diagnosis because it usually produces the greatest distress and interferes with functioning more so than does a specific phobia.

The phobic person may be no more (or less) anxious than another person until exposed to the phobic object or situation. Exposure to the phobic stimulus produces overwhelming symptoms of panic, including palpitations, sweating, dizziness, and difficulty breathing. In fact, these symptoms may occur in response to the individual merely thinking about the phobic stimulus. Invariably the person recognizes that his or her fear is excessive or unreasonable, but is powerless to change, even though the individual may occasionally endure the phobic stimulus when experiencing intense anxiety.

Phobias may begin at almost any age. Those that begin in childhood often disappear without treatment, but those that begin or persist into adulthood usually require assistance with therapy. The disorder is diagnosed more often in women than in men.

Although the disorder is common among the general population, people seldom seek treatment unless the phobia interferes with their ability to function. Obviously the individual who has a fear of snakes, but who lives on the 23rd floor of an urban, high-rise apartment building, is not likely to be bothered by the phobia unless he or she decides to move to an area where snakes are prevalent. On the other hand, a fear of elevators may very well interfere with this individual's daily functioning.

Specific phobias have been classified according to the phobic stimulus. A list of some of the more common ones appears in Table 16–4. This list is by no means all-inclusive. People can become phobic about almost any object or situation, and anyone with a little knowledge of Greek or Latin can produce a phobia classification, thereby making possibilities for the list almost infinite.

The *DSM-IV-TR* identifies subtypes of the most common specific phobias. They include the following:

TABLE 16–4 Classifications of Specific Phobias

Classification	Fear
Acrophobia	Height
Ailurophobia	Cats
Algophobia	Pain
Anthophobia	Flowers
Anthropophobia	People
Aquaphobia	Water
Arachnophobia	Spiders
Astraphobia	Lightning
Belonephobia	Needles
Brontophobia	Thunder
Claustrophobia	Closed spaces
Cynophobia	Dogs
Dementophobia	Insanity
Equinophobia	Horses
Gamophobia	Marriage
Herpetophobia	Lizards, reptiles
Homophobia	Homosexuality
Murophobia	Mice
Mysophobia	Dirt, germs, contamination
Numerophobia	Numbers
Nyctophobia	Darkness
Ochophobia	Riding in a car
Ophidiophobia	Snakes
Pyrophobia	Fire
Scoleciphobia	Worms
Siderodromophobia	Railroads or train travel
Taphephobia	Being buried alive
Thanatophobia	Death
Trichophobia	Hair
Triskaidekaphobia	The number 13
Xenophobia	Strangers
Zoophobia	Animals

1. **Animal type**. This subtype would be identified as part of the diagnosis if the fear were of animals or insects.
2. **Natural environment type**. Examples of this subtype include objects or situations that occur within the natural environment, such as heights, storms, or water.
3. **Blood-injection-injury type**. This diagnosis should be specified if the fear is of seeing blood or an injury or of receiving an injection or other invasive medical or dental procedure.
4. **Situational type.** This subtype is designated if the fear is of a specific situation, such as public transportation, tunnels, bridges, elevators, flying, driving, or enclosed places.
5. **Other type**. This category covers all other excessive or irrational fears. It may include fear of con-

TABLE 16–5 Diagnostic Criteria for Specific Phobia

A. Marked and persistent fear that is excessive or unreasonable cued by the presence or anticipation of a specific object or situation (e.g., flying, heights, animals, receiving an injection, seeing blood).
B. Exposure to the phobic stimulus almost invariably provokes an immediate anxiety response, which may take the form of a situationally bound or situationally predisposed panic attack. **NOTE:** In children, the anxiety may be expressed by crying, tantrums, freezing, or clinging.
C. The person recognizes that the fear is excessive or unreasonable. **NOTE:** In children, this feature may be absent.
D. The phobic situation(s) is avoided or else is endured with intense anxiety or distress.
E. The avoidance, anxious anticipation, or distress in the feared situation(s) interferes significantly with the person's normal routine, occupational (or academic) functioning, or social activities or relationships, or there is marked distress about having the phobia.
F. In individuals under 18 years, the duration is at least 6 months.
G. The anxiety, panic attacks, or phobic avoidance associated with the specific object or situation are not better accounted for by another mental disorder.

The diagnosis may be further specified as:
Animal type
Natural environment type (e.g., heights, storms, water)
Blood-injection-injury type
Situational type (e.g., airplanes, elevators, enclosed places)
Other type

From the American Psychiatric Association (2000), with permission.

tracting a serious illness, fear of situations that might lead to vomiting or choking, fear of loud noises, or fear of driving.

The *DSM-IV-TR* diagnostic criteria for specific phobia are presented in Table 16–5.

Etiological Implications for Phobias

The cause of phobias is unknown; however, various theories exist that may offer insight into the etiology.

PSYCHOANALYTICAL THEORY. Freud believed that phobias develop when a child experiences normal incestuous feelings toward the opposite-sex parent (Oedipal complex) and fears aggression from the same-sex parent (castration anxiety). To protect themselves, these children *repress* this fear of hostility from the father and *displace* it onto something safer and more neutral, which becomes the phobic stimulus. The phobic stimulus becomes the symbol for the father, but the child does not realize this.

Modern-day psychoanalysts believe in the same concept of phobic development, but believe that castration anxiety is not the sole source of phobias. They believe that other unconscious fears may also be expressed in a symbolic manner as phobias. For example, a female child who was sexually abused by an adult male family friend when he was taking her for a ride in his boat grew up with an intense, irrational fear of all water vessels. Psychoanalytical theory postulates that fear of the man was repressed and displaced onto boats. Boats then became an unconscious symbol for the feared person but one that the young girl viewed as safer since her fear of boats prevented her from having to confront the real fear.

LEARNING THEORY. Classic conditioning in the case of phobias may be explained as follows: a stressful stimulus produces the "unconditioned" response of fear. When the stressful stimulus is repeatedly paired with a harmless object, eventually the harmless object alone produces a "conditioned" response: fear. This becomes a phobia when the individual consciously avoids the harmless object to escape fear.

Some learning theorists hold that fears are conditioned responses and, thus, they are learned by imposing rewards for certain behaviors. In the instance of phobias, when the individual avoids the phobic object, he or she escapes fear, which is indeed a powerful reward.

Phobias also may be acquired by direct learning or imitation (modeling) (e.g., a mother who exhibits fear toward an object will provide a model for the child, who may also develop a phobia of the same object).

COGNITIVE THEORY. Cognitive theorists espouse that anxiety is the product of faulty cognitions or anxiety-inducing self-instructions. Two types of faulty thinking have been investigated: negative self-statements and irrational beliefs. Cognitive theorists believe that some individuals engage in negative and irrational thinking that produces anxiety reactions. The individual begins to seek out avoidance behaviors to prevent the anxiety reactions, and phobias result.

Somewhat related to the cognitive theory is the involvement of locus of control. Johnson and Sarason (1978) suggested that individuals with internal locus of control and those with external locus of control might respond differently to life change. These researchers proposed that locus of control orientation may be an important variable in the development of phobias. Individuals with an external control orienta-

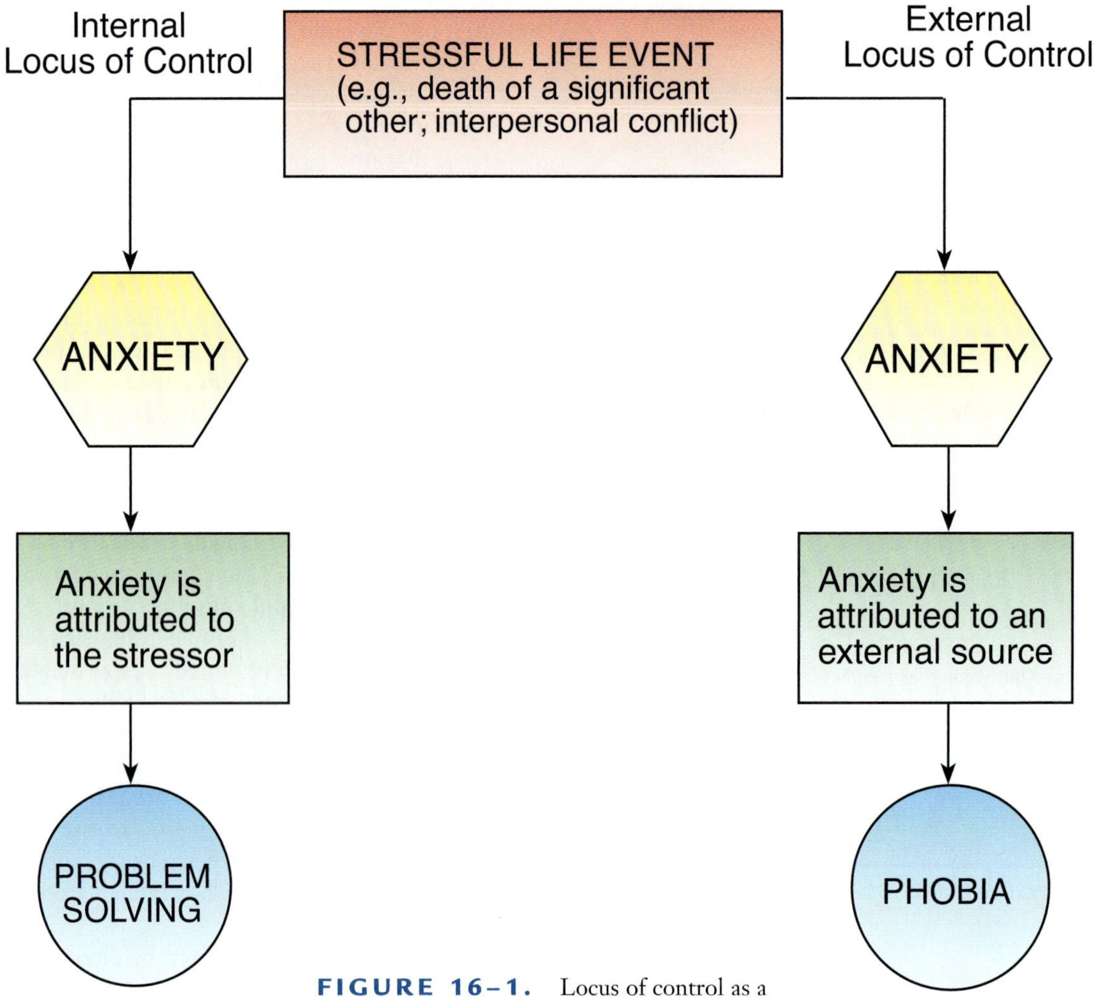

FIGURE 16–1. Locus of control as a variable in the etiology of phobias.

tion experiencing anxiety attacks in a stressful period are likely to mislabel the anxiety and attribute it to external sources (e.g., crowded areas) or to a disease (e.g., heart attack). They may perceive the experienced anxiety as being outside of their control. Figure 16–1 depicts a graphic model of the relationship between locus of control and the development of phobias.

Biological Aspects

TEMPERAMENT. More than 50 percent of children experience normal fears and anxieties before they are 18 years old (Gale Encyclopedia of Childhood and Adolescence, 1998). Most infants are afraid of loud noises. Common fears of toddlers and preschoolers include strangers, animals, darkness, and being separated from parents or attachment figures. During the school-age years, there is fear of death and anxiety about school achievement. Fears of social rejection and sexual anxieties are common among adolescents.

Innate fears represent a part of the overall characteristics or tendencies with which one is born that influence how he or she responds throughout life to specific situations. Innate fears usually do not reach phobic intensity but may have the capacity for such development if reinforced by events in later life. For example, a 4-year-old girl is afraid of dogs. By age 5, however, she has overcome her fear and plays with her own dog and the neighbors' dogs without fear. Then, when she is 19, she is bitten by a stray dog and develops a dog phobia.

LIFE EXPERIENCES. Certain early experiences may set the stage for phobic reactions later in life. Some researchers believe that phobias, particularly specific phobias, are symbolic of original anxiety-producing objects or situations that have been repressed. Examples include:

1. A child who is punished by being locked in a closet develops a phobia for elevators or other closed places.
2. A child who falls down a flight of stairs develops a phobia for high places.
3. A young woman who, as a child, survived a plane crash in which both her parents were killed has a phobia of airplanes.

Diagnosis/Outcome Identification

Nursing diagnoses are formulated from the data gathered during the assessment phase and with background knowledge regarding predisposing factors to the disorder. Some common nursing diagnoses for clients with phobias include:

Fear related to causing embarrassment to self in front of others; to being in a place from which one is unable to escape; or to a specific stimulus, evidenced by behavior directed toward avoidance of the feared object or situation

Social isolation related to fears of being in a place from which one is unable to escape, evidenced by staying alone, refusing to leave room or home

The following criteria may be used for measurement of outcomes in the care of the client with phobic disorders. The client:

1. Functions adaptively in the presence of the phobic object or situation without experiencing panic anxiety.
2. Demonstrates techniques that can be used to maintain anxiety at a manageable level.
3. Voluntarily attends group activities and interacts with peers.
4. Discusses feelings that may have contributed to irrational fears.
5. Verbalizes a future plan of action for responding in the presence of the phobic object or situation without developing panic anxiety.

Planning/Implementation

Table 16–6 provides a plan of care for the client with phobic disorder. Nursing diagnoses are presented,

TABLE 16–6 Care Plan for Clients with Phobic Disorders

Nursing Diagnosis: FEAR

Related to: Causing embarrassment to self in front of others, being in a place from which one is unable to escape, or to a specific stimulus

Evidenced by: Behavior directed toward avoidance of the feared object or situation

Outcome Criteria	Nursing Interventions	Rationale
Client will be able to function in presence of phobic object or situation without experiencing panic anxiety.	1. Reassure client that he or she is safe.	1. At the panic level of anxiety, client may fear for his or her own life.
	2. Explore client's perception of the threat to physical integrity or threat to self-concept.	2. It is important to understand client's perception of the phobic object or situation to assist with the desensitization process.
	3. Discuss reality of the situation with client to recognize aspects that can be changed and those that cannot.	3. Client must accept the reality of the situation (aspects that cannot change) before the work of reducing the fear can progress.
	4. Include client in making decisions related to selection of alternative coping strategies. (e.g., client may choose either to avoid the phobic stimulus or to attempt to eliminate the fear associated with it.)	4. Allowing the client choices provides a measure of control and serves to increase feelings of self-worth.
	5. If client elects to work on elimination of the fear, techniques of desensitization or implosion therapy may be employed. (see explanation of these techniques under Treatment Modalities at the end of this chapter.)	5. Fear is decreased as the physical and psychological sensations diminish in response to repeated exposure to the phobic stimulus under nonthreatening conditions.
	6. Encourage client to explore underlying feelings that may be contributing to irrational fears and to face them rather than suppress them.	6. Exploring underlying feelings may help the client to confront unresolved conflicts and develop more adaptive coping abilities.

(Continued)

TABLE 16–6 Care Plan for Clients with Phobic Disorders *(Continued)*

Nursing Diagnosis: SOCIAL ISOLATION
Related to: Fears of being in a place from which one is unable to escape
Evidenced by: Staying alone; refusing to leave room or home

Outcome Criteria	Nursing Interventions	Rationale
Client will voluntarily participate in group activities with peers.	1. Convey an accepting attitude and unconditional positive regard. Make brief, frequent contacts. Be honest and keep all promises.	1. These interventions increase feelings of self-worth and facilitate a trusting relationship.
	2. Attend group activities with client if it may be frightening for him or her.	2. The presence of a trusted individual provides emotional security.
	3. Be cautious with touch. Allow client extra space and an avenue for exit if anxiety becomes overwhelming.	3. A person in panic anxiety may perceive touch as threatening.
	4. Administer tranquilizing medications as ordered by physician. Monitor for effectiveness and adverse side effects.	4. Antianxiety medications, such as diazepam, chlordiazepoxide, or alprazolam help to reduce level of anxiety in most individuals, thereby facilitating interactions with others.
	5. Discuss with client signs and symptoms of increasing anxiety and techniques to interrupt the response (e.g., relaxation exercises, "thought stopping").	5. Maladaptive behaviors, such as withdrawal and suspiciousness, are manifested during times of increased anxiety.
	6. Give recognition and positive reinforcement for voluntary interactions with others.	6. This enhances self-esteem and encourages repetition of acceptable behaviors.

along with outcome criteria, appropriate nursing interventions, and rationales for each.

Evaluation

Reassessment is conducted to determine if the nursing actions have been successful in achieving the objectives of care. Evaluation of the nursing actions for the client with a phobic disorder may be facilitated by gathering information using the following types of questions:

1. Can the client discuss the phobic object or situation without becoming anxious?
2. Can the client function in the presence of the phobic object or situation without experiencing panic anxiety?
3. Does the client voluntarily leave the room or home to attend group activities?
4. Is the client able to verbalize the signs and symptoms of escalating anxiety?
5. Is the client able to demonstrate techniques that he or she may use to prevent the anxiety from escalating to the panic level?
6. Can the client verbalize the thinking process that promoted the irrational fears?
7. Is the client capable of creating change in his or her life to confront (or eliminate, or avoid) the phobic situation?
8. Is the client able to verbalize resources outside the hospital from which he or she can seek assistance during times of extreme stress?

Obsessive-Compulsive Disorder

Background Assessment Data

The *DSM-IV-TR* describes obsessive-compulsive disorder (OCD) as recurrent obsessions or compulsions that are severe enough to be time-consuming or to cause marked distress or significant impairment (APA, 2000). *Obsessions* are defined as unwanted, intrusive, persistent ideas, thoughts, impulses, or images that cause marked anxiety or distress. The most common ones include repeated thoughts about contamination, repeated doubts, a need to have things in a particular order, aggressive or horrific impulses, and sexual imagery (APA, 2000).

Compulsions denote unwanted repetitive behavior patterns or mental acts (e.g., praying, counting, repeating words silently) that are intended to reduce anxiety, not to provide pleasure or gratification (APA, 2000). They may be performed in response to an obsession or in a stereotyped fashion. The individual recognizes that the behavior is excessive or unreasonable but, because of the feeling of relief from discomfort that it promotes, he or she is compelled to continue the act. The most common compulsions involve washing and cleaning, counting, checking, requesting or demanding assurances, repeating actions, and ordering (APA, 2000). The *DSM-IV-TR* diagnostic criteria for OCD are presented in Table 16–7.

The disorder is equally common among men and women. It may begin in childhood, but more often begins in adolescence or early adulthood. The course is usually chronic and may be complicated by depression or substance abuse. Single people are affected by OCD more often than are married people (Sadock & Sadock, 2003).

TABLE 16 – 7 Diagnostic Criteria for Obsessive-Compulsive Disorder (OCD)

A. Either obsessions or compulsions:
Obsessions as defined by 1, 2, 3, and 4:
1. Recurrent and persistent thoughts, impulses, or images that are experienced, at some time during the disturbance, as intrusive and inappropriate and that cause marked anxiety or distress.
2. The thoughts, impulses, or images are not simply excessive worries about real-life problems.
3. The person attempts to ignore or suppress such thoughts, impulses, or images, or to neutralize them with some other thought or action.
4. The person recognizes that the obsessional thoughts, impulses, or images are a product of his or her own mind (not imposed from without as in thought insertion).

Compulsions as defined by 1 and 2:
1. Repetitive behaviors (e.g., hand washing, ordering, checking) or mental acts (e.g., praying, counting, repeating words silently) that the person feels driven to perform in response to an obsession, or according to rules that must be applied rigidly.
2. The behaviors or mental acts are aimed at preventing or reducing distress or preventing some dreaded event or situation; however, these behaviors or mental acts are not connected in a realistic way with what they are designed to neutralize or prevent or are clearly excessive.

B. At some point during the course of the disorder, the person has recognized that the obsessions or compulsions are excessive or unreasonable. **NOTE:** This does not apply to children.

C. The obsessions or compulsions cause marked distress, are time-consuming (take more than 1 hr/day), or significantly interfere with the person's normal routine, occupational (or academic) functioning, or usual social activities or relationships.

D. If another axis I disorder is present, the content of the obsessions or compulsions is not restricted to it (e.g., preoccupation with food in the presence of an eating disorder; hair pulling in the presence of trichotillomania; concern with appearance in the presence of body dysmorphic disorder; preoccupation with having a serious illness in the presence of hypochondriasis; preoccupation with sexual urges or fantasies in the presence of a paraphilia; or guilty ruminations in the presence of major depressive disorder).

E. This disturbance is not due to the direct physiological effects of a substance (e.g., drug of abuse, a medication) or a general medical condition.

From the American Psychiatric Association (2000), with permission.

Etiological Implications for Obsessive-Compulsive Disorder

PSYCHOANALYTICAL THEORY. Psychoanalytical theorists propose that individuals with OCD have weak, underdeveloped egos (for any of a variety of reasons: unsatisfactory parent-child relationship, conditional love, or provisional gratification). The psychoanalytical concept views clients with OCD as having regressed to earlier developmental stages of the infantile superego—the harsh, exacting, punitive characteristics of which now reappear as part of the psychopathology. Regression to the pre-Oedipal anal-sadistic phase, combined with use of specific ego defense mechanisms (isolation, undoing, displacement, reaction formation), produces the clinical symptoms of obsessions and compulsions (Kaplan & Sadock, 1998). Aggressive impulses (common during the anal-sadistic developmental phase) are channeled into thoughts and behaviors that prevent the feelings of aggression from surfacing and producing intense anxiety fraught with guilt (generated by the punitive superego).

LEARNING THEORY. Learning theorists explain obsessive-compulsive behavior as a conditioned response to a traumatic event. The traumatic event produces anxiety and discomfort, and the individual learns to prevent the anxiety and discomfort by avoiding the situation with which they are associated. This type of learning is called *passive avoidance* (staying away from the source). When passive avoidance is not possible, the individual learns to engage in behaviors that provide relief from the anxiety and discomfort associated with the traumatic situation. This type of learning is called *active avoidance* and describes the behavior pattern of the individual with OCD (Sadock, & Sadock, 2003).

According to this classic conditioning interpretation, a traumatic event should mark the beginning of the obsessive-compulsive behaviors. However, in a significant number of cases, the onset of the behavior is gradual, and the clients relate the onset of their problems to stress in general rather than to one or more traumatic events.

BIOLOGICAL ASPECTS. Recent findings suggest that neurobiological disturbances may play a role in the pathogenesis and maintenance of OCD.

Neuroanatomy. Abnormalities in various regions of the brain have been implicated in the neurobiology of OCD. Functional neuroimaging techniques have shown abnormal metabolic rates in the basal ganglia and orbitofrontal cortex of individuals with OCD (MacKenzie, 1994).

Physiology. Electrophysiological studies, sleep electroencephalogram studies, and neuroendocrine studies have suggested that there are commonalities between depressive disorders and OCD (Sadock & Sadock, 2003). Neuroendocrine commonalities were suggested in studies in which about one-third of OCD clients show nonsuppression on the dexamethasone-suppression test and decreased growth hormone secretion with clonidine infusions.

Biochemical. A number of studies have implicated the neurotransmitter serotonin as influential in the etiology of obsessive-compulsive behaviors. Drugs that have been used successfully in alleviating the symptoms of OCD are clomipramine and the selective serotonin reuptake inhibitors (SSRIs), all of which are believed to block the neuronal reuptake of serotonin, thereby potentiating serotoninergic activity in the central nervous system.

Diagnosis/Outcome Identification

Nursing diagnoses are formulated from the data gathered during the assessment phase and with background knowledge regarding predisposing factors to the disorder. Some common nursing diagnoses for clients with OCD include:

Ineffective coping related to underdeveloped ego, punitive superego; avoidance learning; possible biochemical changes; evidenced by **ritualistic behavior** and/or obsessive thoughts

Ineffective role performance related to need to perform rituals evidenced by inability to fulfill usual patterns of responsibility

The following criteria may be used to measure outcomes in the care of the client with OCD. The client:

1. Is able to maintain anxiety at a manageable level without resorting to the use of ritualistic behavior
2. Is able to perform activities of daily living independently
3. Verbalizes understanding of relationship between anxiety and ritualistic behavior
4. Verbalizes specific situations that in the past have provoked anxiety and resulted in seeking relief through rituals
5. Demonstrates more adaptive coping strategies to deal with stress, such as thought stopping, relaxation techniques, and physical exercise
6. Is able to resume role-related responsibilities because of decreased need for ritualistic behaviors

Planning/Implementation

Table 16–8 provides a plan of care for the client with OCD. Nursing diagnoses are presented, along with outcome criteria, appropriate nursing interventions, and rationales for each.

Evaluation

Reassessment is conducted in order to determine if the nursing actions have been successful in achieving the objectives of care. Evaluation of the nursing actions for the client with OCD may be facilitated by gathering information using the following types of questions:

1. Can the client refrain from performing rituals when anxiety level rises?
2. Can the client demonstrate substitute behaviors to maintain anxiety at a manageable level?
3. Does the client recognize the relationship between escalating anxiety and the dependence on ritualistic behaviors for relief?
4. Can the client verbalize situations that occurred in the past during which this strategy was used?
5. Can the client verbalize a plan of action for dealing with these stressful situations in the future?
6. Can client perform self-care activities independently?
7. Can the client demonstrate an ability to fulfill role-related responsibilities?
8. Can the client verbalize resources from which he or she can seek assistance during times of extreme stress?

Post-Traumatic Stress Disorder

Background Assessment Data

Post-traumatic stress disorder (PTSD) is described by the *DSM-IV-TR* as the development of characteristic

TABLE 16–8 Care Plan for the Client with Obsessive-Compulsive Disorder

Nursing Diagnosis: INEFFECTIVE COPING
Related to: Underdeveloped ego, punitive superego, avoidance learning, possible biochemical changes
Evidenced by: Ritualistic behavior or obsessive thoughts

Outcome Criteria	Nursing Interventions	Rationale
Client will demonstrate ability to cope effectively without resorting to obsessive-compulsive behaviors or increased dependency.	1. Work with client to determine types of situations that increase anxiety and result in ritualistic behaviors.	1. Recognition of precipitating factors is the first step in teaching the client to interrupt the escalating anxiety.
	2. Initially meet the client's dependency needs as required. Encourage independence and give positive reinforcement for independent behaviors.	2. Sudden and complete elimination of all avenues for dependency would create intense anxiety on the part of the client. Positive reinforcement enhances self-esteem and encourages repetition of desired behaviors.
	3. In the beginning of treatment, allow plenty of time for rituals. Do not be judgmental or verbalize disapproval of the behavior.	3. To deny client this activity may precipitate panic anxiety.
	4. Support client's efforts to explore the meaning and purpose of the behavior.	4. Client may be unaware of the relationship between emotional problems and compulsive behaviors. Recognition is important before change can occur.
	5. Provide structured schedule of activities for client, including adequate time for completion of rituals.	5. Structure provides a feeling of security for the anxious client.
	6. Gradually begin to limit amount of time allotted for ritualistic behavior as client becomes more involved in unit activities.	6. Anxiety is minimized when client is able to replace ritualistic behaviors with more adaptive ones.
	7. Give positive reinforcement for nonritualistic behaviors.	7. Positive reinforcement enhances self-esteem and encourages repetition of desired behaviors.
	8. Help client learn ways of interrupting obsessive thoughts and ritualistic behavior with techniques such as thought stopping, relaxation, and physical exercise.	8. Knowledge and practice of coping techniques that are more adaptive will help client change and let go of maladaptive responses to anxiety.

Nursing Diagnosis: INEFFECTIVE ROLE PERFORMANCE
Related to: Need to perform rituals
Evidenced by: Inability to fulfill usual patterns of responsibility

Outcome Criteria	Nursing Interventions	Rationale
Client will be able to resume role-related responsibilities.	1. Determine client's previous role within the family and extent to which this role is altered by the illness. Identify roles of other family members.	1. This is important assessment data for formulating an appropriate plan of care.
	2. Discuss client's perception of role expectations.	2. Determine if client's perception of his or her role expectations are realistic.
	3. Encourage client to discuss conflicts evident within the family system. Identify how client and other family members have responded to this conflict.	3. Identifying specific stressors, as well as adaptive and maladaptive responses within the system, is necessary before assistance can be provided in an effort to create change.
	4. Explore available options for changes or adjustments in role. Practice through role–play.	4. Planning and rehearsal of potential role transitions can reduce anxiety.
	5. Encourage family participation in the development of plans to effect positive change, and work to resolve the cause of the anxiety from which the client seeks relief through use of ritualistic behaviors.	5. Input from the individuals who will be directly involved in the change will increase the likelihood of a positive outcome.
	6. Give client lots of positive reinforcement for ability to resume role responsibilities by decreasing need for ritualistic behaviors.	6. Positive reinforcement enhances self-esteem and promotes repetition of desired behaviors

symptoms following exposure to an extreme traumatic stressor involving a personal threat to physical integrity or to the physical integrity of others. The symptoms may occur after learning about unexpected or violent death, serious harm, or threat of death or injury of a family member or other close associate (APA, 2000). These symptoms are not related to common experiences such as uncomplicated bereavement, marital conflict, or chronic illness but are associated with events that would be markedly distressing to almost anyone. The individual may experience the trauma alone or in the presence of others. Examples of some experiences that may produce this type of response include participation in military combat, experiencing violent personal assault, being kidnapped or taken hostage, being tortured, being incarcerated as a prisoner of war, experiencing natural or manmade disasters, surviving severe automobile accidents, or being diagnosed with a life-threatening illness (APA, 2000).

Characteristic symptoms include reexperiencing the traumatic event, a sustained high level of anxiety or arousal, or a general numbing of responsiveness. Intrusive recollections or nightmares of the event are common. Some individuals may be unable to remember certain aspects of the trauma.

Symptoms of depression are common with this disorder and may be severe enough to warrant a diagnosis of a depressive disorder. In the case of a life-threatening trauma shared with others, survivors often describe painful guilt feelings about surviving when others did not, or about the things they had to do to survive (APA, 2000). Substance abuse is common.

The full symptom picture must be present for more than 1 month and cause significant interference with social, occupational, and other areas of functioning. If the symptoms have not been present for more than 1 month, the diagnosis assigned is acute stress disorder (APA, 2000).

The disorder can occur at any age. Symptoms may begin in the first 3 months after the trauma, or there may be a delay of several months or even years. The *DSM-IV-TR* diagnostic criteria for PTSD are presented in Table 16–9.

Studies reveal lifetime prevalence for PTSD of approximately 8 percent of the adult population in the United States (APA, 2000). About 30 percent of Vietnam veterans have experienced PTSD, and an additional 25 percent encountered subclinical forms of the disorder (Sadock & Sadock, 2003).

Etiological Implications for Post-Traumatic Stress Disorder

Reports of symptoms and syndromes with PTSD-like features have existed in writing throughout the centuries. In the early part of the 20th century, traumatic

TABLE 16–9 Diagnostic Criteria for Post-Traumatic Stress Disorder

A. The person has been exposed to a traumatic event in which both of the following were present:
   1. The person experienced, witnessed, or was confronted with an event or events that involved actual or threatened death or serious injury, or a threat to the physical integrity of self or others.
   2. The person's response involved intense fear, helplessness, or horror. **NOTE:** In children, this may be expressed instead by disorganized or agitated behavior.

B. The traumatic event is persistently reexperienced in one (or more) of the following ways:
   1. Recurrent and intrusive distressing recollections of the event, including images, thoughts, or perceptions. **NOTE:** In young children, repetitive play may occur in which themes or aspects of the trauma are expressed.
   2. Recurrent distressing dreams of the event. **NOTE:** In children, there may be frightening dreams without recognizable content.
   3. Acting or feeling as if the traumatic event were recurring (includes a sense of reliving the experience, illusions, hallucinations, and dissociative flashback episodes, including those that occur on awakening or when intoxicated). **NOTE:** In young children, trauma-specific reenactment may occur.
   4. Intense psychological distress at exposure to internal or external cues that symbolize or resemble an aspect of the traumatic event.
   5. Physiological reactivity on exposure to internal or external cues that symbolize or resemble an aspect of the traumatic event.

C. Persistent avoidance of stimuli associated with the trauma and numbing of general responsiveness (not present before the trauma), as indicated by three (or more) of the following:
   1. Efforts to avoid thoughts, feelings, or conversations associated with the trauma
   2. Efforts to avoid activities, places, or people that arouse recollections of the trauma
   3. Inability to recall an important aspect of the trauma
   4. Markedly diminished interest or participation in significant activities
   5. Feeling of detachment or estrangement from others
   6. Restricted range of affect (e.g., unable to have loving feelings)
   7. Sense of a foreshortened future (e.g., does not expect to have a career, marriage, children, or a normal life span)

D. Persistent symptoms of increased arousal (not present before the trauma), as indicated by two (or more) of the following:
   1. Difficulty falling or staying asleep
   2. Irritability or outbursts of anger
   3. Difficulty concentrating
   4. Hypervigilance
   5. Exaggerated startle response

E. Duration of the disturbance more than 1 month.

F. Disturbance that causes clinically significant distress or impairment in social, occupational, or other important areas of functioning. Specify if acute (symptoms less than 3 months), chronic (symptoms 3 months or more), or delayed onset (onset of symptoms at least 6 months after the stressor).

From the American Psychiatric Association (2000), with permission.

neurosis was viewed as the ego's inability to master the extent of disorganization brought about by a traumatic experience. Very little was written about post-traumatic neurosis during the years between 1950 and 1970. This absence was followed in the 1970s and 1980s with an explosion in the amount of research and writing on the subject. Peterson, Prout, and Schwarz (1991) have stated:

> Clearly, the psychological casualties of the Vietnam War were largely responsible for the renewed interest in post-traumatic neurosis. Most of the early papers on post-traumatic neurosis were about Vietnam veterans.

Indeed, the category of PTSD did not appear until the third edition of the *Diagnostic and Statistical Manual of Mental Disorders (DSM-III)* in 1980 after a need was indicated by increasing numbers of problems with Vietnam veterans and victims of multiple disasters.

PSYCHOSOCIAL THEORY. Green, Wilson, and Lindy (1985) have proposed an etiological model of PTSD that has become widely accepted. This theory seeks to explain why certain persons exposed to massive trauma develop PTSD and others do not. Variables include characteristics that relate to (1) the traumatic experience, (2) the individual, and (3) the recovery environment.

THE TRAUMATIC EXPERIENCE. Specific characteristics relating to the trauma have been identified as crucial elements in the determination of an individual's long-term response to stress. They include:

1. Severity and duration of the stressor
2. Extent of anticipatory preparation
3. Exposure to death
4. Numbers affected by life threat
5. Amount of control over recurrence
6. Location where the trauma was experienced (e.g., familiar surroundings, at home, in a foreign country)

THE INDIVIDUAL. Variables that are considered important in determining an individual's response to trauma include:

1. Degree of ego-strength
2. Effectiveness of coping resources
3. Presence of preexisting psychopathology
4. Outcomes of previous experiences with stress/trauma
5. Behavioral tendencies (temperament)
6. Current psychosocial developmental stage
7. Demographic factors (e.g., age, socioeconomic status, education)

THE RECOVERY ENVIRONMENT. It has been suggested that the quality of the environment in which the individual attempts to work through the traumatic experience is correlated with outcome. Environmental variables include:

1. Availability of social supports
2. The cohesiveness and protectiveness of family and friends
3. The attitudes of society regarding the experience
4. Cultural and subcultural influences

Peterson and associates (1991) suggest that the recovery environment for Vietnam veterans and rape victims has often been less supportive than that for disaster victims or the victims of assault or other crimes. In research with Vietnam veterans, it was shown that the best predictors of PTSD were the severity of the stressor and the amount of psychosocial isolation in the recovery environment.

LEARNING THEORY. Learning theorists view negative reinforcement as behavior that leads to a reduction in an aversive experience. This reduction of the undesirable experience is the reinforcement that enhances the repetition of the behavior. The avoidance behaviors and psychic numbing in response to a trauma are mediated by negative reinforcement (behaviors that decrease the emotional pain of the trauma). Behavioral disturbances, such as anger and aggression and drug and alcohol abuse, are the behavioral patterns that are reinforced by their capacity to reduce objectionable feelings.

COGNITIVE THEORY. These models take into consideration the cognitive appraisal of an event and focus on assumptions that an individual makes about the world. Epstein (1990) outlines three fundamental beliefs that most people construct in a personal theory of reality. They include:

1. The world is benevolent and a source of joy.
2. The world is meaningful and controllable.
3. The self is worthy (e.g., lovable, good, and competent).

As life situations occur, some disequilibrium is expected to occur until accommodation for the change has been made, and it has become assimilated into one's personal theory of reality. An individual is vulnerable to PTSD when the fundamental beliefs are invalidated by a trauma that cannot be comprehended and a sense of helplessness and hopelessness prevail. One's appraisal of the environment can be drastically altered.

BIOLOGICAL ASPECTS. It has been suggested that an individual who has experienced previous trauma is more likely to develop symptoms after a stressful life event (Hollander & Simeon, 2003). These individuals with previous traumatic experiences may be more likely to become exposed to future traumas because they can be inclined to reactivate the behaviors associated with the original trauma.

Hollander and Simeon (2003) also report on studies that suggest an endogenous opioid peptide response may assist in the maintenance of chronic PTSD. The hypothesis supports a type of "addiction to the trauma," which is explained in the following manner.

Opioids, including endogenous opioid peptides, have the following psychoactive properties:

1. Tranquilizing action
2. Reduction of rage/aggression
3. Reduction of paranoia
4. Reduction of feelings of inadequacy
5. Antidepressant action

These studies suggest that physiological arousal initiated by reexposure to trauma-like situations enhances production of endogenous opioid peptides and results in increased feelings of comfort and control. When the stressor terminates, the individual may experience opioid withdrawal, the symptoms of which bear strong resemblance to those of PTSD.

Diagnosis/Outcome Identification

Nursing diagnoses are formulated from the data gathered during the assessment phase and with background knowledge regarding predisposing factors to the disorder. Some common nursing diagnoses for clients with PTSD include:

Post-trauma syndrome related to distressing event considered to be outside the range of usual human experience evidenced by flashbacks, intrusive recollections, nightmares, psychological numbness related to the event, dissociation, or amnesia

Dysfunctional grieving related to loss of self as perceived before the trauma or other actual or perceived losses incurred during or after the event, evidenced by irritability and explosiveness, self-destructiveness, substance abuse, verbalization of survival guilt, or guilt about behavior required for survival

The following criteria may be used for measurement of outcomes in the care of the client with PTSD. The client:

1. Can acknowledge the traumatic event and the impact it has had on his or her life
2. Is experiencing fewer flashbacks, intrusive recollections, and nightmares than he or she was on admission (or at the beginning of therapy)
3. Can demonstrate adaptive coping strategies (e.g., relaxation techniques, mental imagery, music, art)
4. Can concentrate and has made realistic goals for the future
5. Includes significant others in the recovery process and willingly accepts their support
6. Verbalizes no ideas or intent of self-harm
7. Has worked through feelings of survivor's guilt
8. Gets enough sleep to avoid risk of injury
9. Verbalizes community resources from which he or she may seek assistance in times of stress
10. Attends support group for individuals who have recovered or are recovering from similar traumatic experiences
11. Verbalizes desire to put the trauma in the past and progress with his or her life

Planning/Implementation

Table 16–10 provides a plan of care for the client with PTSD. Nursing diagnoses are presented, along with

TABLE 16–10 Care Plan for the Client with Post-Traumatic Stress Disorder

Nursing Diagnosis: POST–TRAUMA SYNDROME

Related to: Distressing event considered outside the range of usual human experience

Evidenced by: Flashbacks, intrusive recollections, nightmares, psychological numbness related to the event, dissociation, or amnesia

Outcome Criteria	Nursing Interventions	Rationale
The client will integrate the traumatic experience into his or her persona, renew significant relationships, and establish meaningful goals for the future.	1. a. Assign the same staff as often as possible. b. Use a nonthreatening, matter-of-fact, but friendly approach. c. Respect client's wishes regarding interaction with individuals of opposite sex at this time (especially important if the trauma was rape). d. Be consistent; keep all promises; convey acceptance; spend time with client.	1. All of these interventions serve to facilitate a trusting relationship.
	2. Stay with client during periods of flashbacks and nightmares. Offer reassurance of safety and security and assure client that these symptoms are common following a trauma of the magnitude he or she has experienced.	2. Presence of a trusted individual may calm fears for personal safety and reassure client that he or she is not "going crazy."
	3. Obtain accurate history from significant others about the trauma and the client's specific response.	3. Various types of traumas elicit different responses in clients (e.g., human-engendered traumas often generate a greater amount of humiliation and guilt in victims than trauma associated with natural disasters).
	4. Encourage the client to talk about the trauma at his or her own pace. Provide a nonthreatening, private environment, and include a significant other if the client wishes. Acknowledge and validate client's feelings as they are expressed.	4. This debriefing process is the first step in the progression toward resolution.
	5. Discuss coping strategies used in response to the trauma and those used during stressful situations in the past. Determine those that have been most helpful, and discuss alternative strategies for the future. Include available support systems, including religious and cultural influences. Identify maladaptive coping strategies (e.g., substance use, psychosomatic responses) and practice adaptive coping strategies for future post–trauma responses.	5. Resolution of the post-trauma response is largely dependent on the effectiveness of the coping strategies employed.
	6. Assist the individual to try to comprehend the trauma if possible. Discuss feelings of vulnerability and the individual's "place" in the world following the trauma.	6. Post-trauma response is largely a function of the shattering of basic beliefs the victim holds about self and world. Assimilation of the event into one's persona requires that some meaning associated with the event be incorporated into the basic beliefs, which will affect how the individual eventually comes to reappraise self and world (Epstein, 1990).

(Continued)

TABLE 16 – 10 Care Plan for the Client with Post-Traumatic Stress Disorder *(Continued)*

Nursing Diagnosis: DYSFUNCTIONAL GRIEVING

Related to: Loss of self as perceived prior to the trauma or other actual/perceived losses incurred during/following the event

Evidenced by: Irritability and explosiveness, self-destructiveness, substance abuse, verbalization of survival guilt or guilt about behavior required for survival

Outcome Criteria	Nursing Interventions	Rationale
Client will demonstrate progress in dealing with stages of grief and will verbalize a sense of optimism and hope for the future.	1. Acknowledge feelings of guilt or self-blame that client may express.	1. Guilt at having survived a trauma in which others died is common. The client needs to discuss these feelings and recognize that he or she is not responsible for what happened but must take responsibility for own recovery.
	2. Assess stage of grief in which the client is fixed. Discuss normalcy of feelings and behaviors related to stages of grief.	2. Knowledge of grief stage is necessary for accurate intervention. Guilt may be generated if client believes it is unacceptable to have these feelings. Knowing they are normal can provide a sense of relief.
	3. Assess impact of the trauma on client's ability to resume regular activities of daily living. Consider employment, marital relationship, and sleep patterns.	3. Following a trauma, individuals are at high risk for physical injury because of disruption in their ability to concentrate and problem–solve and because of inadequate sleep. Isolation and avoidance behaviors may interfere with interpersonal relatedness.
	4. Assess for self-destructive ideas and behavior.	4. The trauma may result in feelings of hopelessness and worthlessness, leading to high risk for suicide.
	5. Assess for maladaptive coping strategies, such as substance abuse.	5. These behaviors interfere with and delay the recovery process.
	6. Identify available community resources from which the individual may seek assistance if problems with dysfunctional grieving persist.	6. Support groups for victims of various types of traumas exist within most communities. The presence of support systems in the recovery environment has been identified as a major predictor in the successful recovery from trauma.

outcome criteria, appropriate nursing interventions, and rationales for each. A critical pathway for the post-trauma client may be found in Appendix E.

Evaluation

Reassessment is conducted in order to determine if the nursing actions have been successful in achieving the objectives of care. Evaluation of the nursing actions for the client with PTSD may be facilitated by gathering information using the following types of questions:

1. Can the client discuss the traumatic event without experiencing panic anxiety?
2. Does the client voluntarily discuss the traumatic event?
3. Can the client discuss changes that have occurred in his or her life because of the traumatic event?
4. Does the client have "flashbacks?"
5. Can the client sleep without medication?
6. Does the client have nightmares?
7. Has the client learned new, adaptive coping strategies for assistance with recovery?

8. Can the client demonstrate successful use of these new coping strategies in times of stress?
9. Can the client verbalize stages of grief and the normal behaviors associated with each?
10. Can he or she recognize own position in the grieving process?
11. Is guilt being alleviated?
12. Has the client maintained or regained satisfactory relationships with significant others?
13. Can the client look to the future with optimism?
14. Does the client attend a regular support group for victims of similar traumatic experiences?
15. Does the client have a plan of action for dealing with symptoms, if they return?

Anxiety Disorder Due to a General Medical Condition

Background Assessment Data

The symptoms of this disorder are recognized as the direct physiological consequence of a general medical condition. Symptoms may include prominent generalized anxiety symptoms, panic attacks, or obsessions or compulsions (APA, 2000). History, physical examination, or laboratory findings must be evident to substantiate the diagnosis.

The *DSM-IV-TR* (APA, 2000) lists the following types and examples of medical conditions that may cause anxiety symptoms:

Endocrine conditions: hyperthyroidism and hypothyroidism, pheochromocytoma, hypoglycemia, hyperadrenocorticism

Cardiovascular conditions: congestive heart failure, pulmonary embolism, arrhythmia

Respiratory conditions: chronic obstructive pulmonary disease, pneumonia, hyperventilation

Metabolic conditions: vitamin B_{12} deficiency, porphyria

Neurological conditions: neoplasms, vestibular dysfunction, encephalitis

Care of clients with this disorder must take into consideration the underlying cause of the anxiety. Holistic nursing care is essential to ensure that the client's physiological and psychosocial needs are met. Nursing actions appropriate for the specific medical condition must be considered. Actions for dealing with the symptoms of anxiety were discussed previously.

Substance-Induced Anxiety Disorder

Background Assessment Data

The *DSM-IV-TR* (APA, 2000) describes the essential features of this disorder as prominent anxiety symptoms that are judged to be due to the direct physiological effects of a substance (i.e., a drug of abuse, a medication, or toxin exposure). The symptoms may occur during substance intoxication or withdrawal, and they may involve prominent anxiety, panic attacks, phobias, or obsessions or compulsions. Diagnosis of this disorder is made only if the anxiety symptoms are in excess of those usually associated with the intoxication or withdrawal syndrome and warrant independent clinical attention. Evidence of intoxication or withdrawal must be available from history, physical examination, or laboratory findings to substantiate the diagnosis. See Chapter 13 for a discussion of the types of substances that may produce these symptoms.

Nursing care of the client with substance-induced anxiety disorder must take into consideration the nature of the substance and the context in which the symptoms occur (i.e., intoxication or withdrawal) (see Chapter 13). Nursing actions for dealing with anxiety symptoms were discussed previously.

TREATMENT MODALITIES

Individual Psychotherapy

Most clients experience a marked lessening of anxiety when given the opportunity to discuss their difficulties with a concerned and sympathetic therapist. Sadock and Sadock (2003) state:

> [Insight-oriented psychotherapy] focuses on helping patients understand the hypothesized unconscious meaning of the anxiety, the symbolism of the avoided situation, the need to repress impulses, and the secondary gains of the symptoms. (p. 608)
>
> With continuous and regular contact with an interested, sympathetic, and encouraging professional person, patients may be able to function by virtue of this help, without which their symptoms would incapacitate them. (p. 623)

The psychotherapist also can use logical and rational explanations to increase the client's understanding about various situations that create anxiety in his or her life. Educational topics for client and family are presented in Table 16–11.

TABLE 16 – 11 Topics for Client/Family Education Related to Anxiety Disorders

Nature of the Illness
1. What is anxiety?
2. To what might it be related?
3. What is OCD?
4. What is PTSD?
5. Symptoms of anxiety disorders.

Management of the Illness
1. Medication management:
   - Possible adverse effects
   - Length of time to take effect
   - What to expect from the medication
     a. For panic disorder and generalized anxiety disorder
        (1) Benzodiazepines
        (2) Buspirone (Buspar)
        (3) Tricyclics
        (4) SSRIs
        (5) Propranolol
        (6) Clonidine
     b. For phobic disorders
        (1) Benzodiazepines
        (2) Tricyclics
        (3) Propranolol
        (4) SSRIs
     c. For OCD
        (1) SSRIs
        (2) Clomipramine
     d. For PTSD
        (1) Tricyclics
        (2) SSRIs
        (3) MAOIs
        (4) Trazodone
        (5) Propranolol
        (6) Carbamazepine
        (7) Valproic acid
        (8) Lithium carbonate
2. Stress management
   a. Teach ways to interrupt escalating anxiety
      (1) Relaxation techniques
         (a) Progressive muscle relaxation
         (b) Imagery
         (c) Music
         (d) Meditation
         (e) Yoga
         (f) Physical exercise

Support Services
1. Crisis hotline
2. Support groups
3. Individual psychotherapy

Cognitive Therapy

The cognitive model relates how individuals respond in stressful situations to their subjective cognitive appraisal of the event. Anxiety is experienced when the cognitive appraisal is one of danger with which the individual perceives that he or she is unable to cope. Impaired cognition can contribute to anxiety disorders when the individual's appraisals are chronically negative. Automatic negative appraisals provoke self-doubts, negative evaluations, and negative predictions. Anxiety is maintained by this dysfunctional appraisal of a situation.

Cognitive therapy strives to assist the individual to reduce anxiety responses by altering cognitive distortions. Anxiety is described as being the result of exaggerated, *automatic* thinking.

Cognitive therapy for anxiety is brief and time-limited, usually lasting from 5 to 20 sessions. Brief therapy discourages the client's dependency on the therapist, which is prevalent in anxiety disorders, and encourages the client's self-sufficiency.

A sound therapeutic relationship is a necessary condition for effective cognitive therapy. The client must be able to talk openly about fears and feelings for the therapeutic process to occur. A major part of treatment consists of encouraging the client to face frightening situations and to be able to view them realistically, and talking about them is one way of achieving this. Treatment is a collaborative effort between client and therapist.

Rather than offering suggestions and explanations, the therapist uses questions to encourage the client to correct his or her anxiety-producing thoughts. The client is encouraged to become aware of the thoughts, examine them for cognitive distortions, substitute more balanced thoughts, and eventually develop new patterns of thinking.

Cognitive therapy is structured and orderly, which is important for the anxious client who is often confused and lacks self-assurance. The focus is on solving current problems. Together, the client and therapist work to identify and correct maladaptive thoughts and behaviors that maintain a problem and block its solution.

Cognitive therapy is based on education. The premise is that one develops anxiety because he or she has learned inappropriate ways of handling life experiences. The belief is that with practice individuals can learn effective ways of responding to these experiences. Homework assignments, a central feature of cognitive therapy, provide an experimental, problem-solving approach to overcoming long-held anxieties. Through fulfillment of these personal "experiments," the effectiveness of specific strategies and techniques is determined.

Behavior Therapy

Two common forms of behavior therapy include **systematic desensitization** and **implosion therapy (flooding)**. They are commonly used to treat clients with phobic disorders and to modify stereotyped behavior of clients with PTSD (Embry, 1990). They also are effective in a variety of other anxiety-producing situations.

Systematic Desensitization

In systematic desensitization, the client is gradually exposed to the phobic stimulus, either in a real or an imagined situation. The concept was introduced by Joseph Wolpe in 1958 and is based on behavioral conditioning principles. Emphasis is placed on reciprocal inhibition or counterconditioning.

Reciprocal inhibition is described as the restriction of anxiety prior to the effort of reducing avoidance behavior. The rationale behind this concept is that because relaxation is antagonistic to anxiety, individuals cannot be anxious and relaxed at the same time.

Systematic desensitization with reciprocal inhibition involves two main elements:

1. Training in relaxation techniques
2. Progressive exposure to a hierarchy of fear stimuli when in the relaxed state

The individual is instructed in the art of relaxation using techniques most effective for him or her (e.g., progressive relaxation, mental imagery, tense and relax, meditation). When the individual has mastered the relaxation technique, exposure to the phobic stimulus is initiated. He or she is asked to present a hierarchal arrangement of situations pertaining to the phobic stimulus in order ranging from most disturbing to least disturbing. When in a state of maximum relaxation, the client may be asked to imagine the phobic stimulus. Initial exposure is focused on a concept of the phobic stimulus that produces the least amount of fear or anxiety. In subsequent sessions, the individual is gradually exposed to stimuli that are more fearful. Sessions may be executed in fantasy, in real-life (*in vivo*) situations, or sometimes in a combination of both.

> **CASE STUDY**
>
> John was afraid to ride on elevators. He had been known to climb 24 flights of stairs in an office building to avoid riding the elevator. John's own insurance office had plans for moving the company to a high-rise building soon, with offices on the 32nd floor. John sought assistance from a therapist who employed systematic desensitization for this problem. He was taught to achieve a sense of calmness and well-being by using a combination of mental imagery and progressive relaxation techniques. In the relaxed state, John was initially instructed to imagine the entry level of his office building, with a clear image of the bank of elevators. In subsequent sessions, and always in the relaxed state, John progressed to images of walking onto an elevator, having the elevator door close after he had entered, riding the elevator to the 32nd floor, and emerging from the elevator once the doors were opened. The progression included being accompanied in the activities by the therapist and eventually accomplishing them alone.
>
> Therapy for John also included *in vivo* sessions in which he was exposed to the phobic stimulus in real-life situations (always after achieving a state of relaxation). This technique, combining imagined and *in vivo* procedures, proved very successful for John, and his employment in the high-rise complex was no longer in jeopardy because of claustrophobia.

Implosion Therapy (Flooding)

Implosion therapy, or *flooding*, is a therapeutic process in which the client must imagine situations or participate in real-life situations that he or she finds extremely frightening for a prolonged period of time. Relaxation training is not a part of this technique. Plenty of time must be allowed for these sessions because brief periods may be ineffective or even harmful. A session is terminated when the client responds with considerably less anxiety than at the beginning of the session.

In flooding, the therapist "floods" the client with information concerning situations that trigger anxiety in him or her. The therapist describes anxiety-provoking situations in vivid detail and is guided by the client's response; the more anxiety provoked, the more expedient is the therapeutic endeavor. The same theme is continued as long as it arouses anxiety. The therapy is continued until a topic no longer elicits inappropriate anxiety on the part of the client. Sadock and Sadock (2003) state:

> Many patients refuse flooding because of the psychological discomfort involved. It is also contraindicated in patients for whom intense anxiety would be hazardous (e.g., patients with heart disease or fragile psychological adaptation). The technique works best with specific phobias. (p. 952)

Group/Family Therapy

Group therapy has been strongly advocated for clients with PTSD. It has proved especially effective with Vietnam veterans (Sadock & Sadock, 2003). The importance of being able to share their experiences with empathetic fellow veterans, to talk about problems in social adaptation, and to discuss options for managing their aggression toward others has been emphasized. Some groups are informal and leaderless, such as veterans' "rap" groups, and some are led by experienced group therapists that may have had some first-hand experience with the trauma. Some groups involve family members, thereby recognizing that the symptoms of PTSD may also severely affect them. Hollander and Simeon (2003) state:

> Because of past experiences, [clients with PTSD] are often mistrustful and reluctant to depend on authority figures, whereas the identification, support, and hopefulness of peer settings can facilitate therapeutic change. (p. 606)

Psychopharmacology

For Panic and Generalized Anxiety Disorders

ANXIOLYTICS. The benzodiazepines have been used with success in the treatment of generalized anxiety disorder. They can be prescribed on an as-needed basis when the client is feeling particularly anxious. Alprazolam, lorazepam, and clonazepam have been particularly effective in the treatment of panic disorder. The major risks with benzodiazepine therapy are physical dependence and tolerance, which may encourage abuse. Because withdrawal symptoms can be life-threatening, clients must be warned against abrupt discontinuation of the drug and should be tapered off the medication at the end of therapy.

The antianxiety agent, buspirone (Buspar), is effective in about 60 to 80 percent of clients with generalized anxiety disorder (Sadock & Sadock, 2003). One disadvantage of buspirone is its 10- to 14-day delay in alleviating symptoms. However, the benefit of lack of physical dependence and tolerance with buspirone may make it the drug of choice in the treatment of generalized anxiety disorder.

ANTIDEPRESSANTS. Several antidepressants are effective as major antianxiety agents. The tricyclics clomipramine and imipramine have been used with success in clients experiencing panic disorder. However, since the advent of SSRIs, the tricyclics are less widely used because of their tendency to produce severe side effects at the high doses required to relieve symptoms of panic disorder (Sadock & Sadock, 2003).

The SSRIs have been effective in the treatment of panic disorder. Paroxetine and sertraline have been approved by the Food and Drug Administration (FDA) for this purpose. The dosage of these drugs must be titrated slowly because clients with panic disorder appear to be sensitive to the overstimulation caused by SSRIs.

The use of antidepressants in the treatment of generalized anxiety disorder is still being investigated. Some success has been reported with the tricyclic imipramine and with the SSRIs. The FDA has recently approved paroxetine and venlafaxine-extended release in the treatment of generalized anxiety disorder.

ANTIHYPERTENSIVE AGENTS. Several studies have called attention to the effectiveness of beta-blockers (e.g., propranolol) and alpha$_2$-receptor agonists (e.g., clonidine) in the amelioration of anxiety symptoms (Hollander & Simeon, 2003). Propranolol has potent effects on the somatic manifestations of anxiety (e.g., palpitations, tremors), with less dramatic effects on the psychic component of anxiety. It appears to be most effective in the treatment of acute situational anxiety (e.g., performance anxiety; test anxiety), but it is not the first-line drug of choice in the treatment of panic disorder and generalized anxiety disorder.

Clonidine is effective in blocking the acute anxiety effects in conditions such as opioid and nicotine withdrawal. However, it has had limited usefulness in the long-term treatment of panic and generalized anxiety disorders, particularly because of the development of tolerance to its antianxiety effects.

For Phobic Disorders

ANXIOLYTICS. The benzodiazepines have been successful in the treatment of social phobia (Hollander & Simeon, 2003). Controlled studies have shown the efficacy of alprazolam and clonazepam in reducing the symptoms of social anxiety. They both are well tolerated and have a rapid onset of action. However, because of their potential for abuse and dependence, they are not considered first-line choice of treatment for social phobia.

ANTIDEPRESSANTS. The tricyclic imipramine and the monoamine oxidase inhibitor (MAOI) phenelzine are effective in diminishing symptoms of agoraphobia and social phobias. In recent years, the SSRIs have become the first-line treatment of choice for social phobia. Paroxetine was recently approved by the FDA for this purpose, and open trials with the other SSRIs have shown promise. Additional clinical trials have also indicated efficacy with other antidepressants, including nefazodone, venlafaxine, and bupropion.

ANTIHYPERTENSIVE AGENTS. The beta-blockers, propranolol and atenolol, have been tried with success in clients experiencing anticipatory performance anxiety or "stage fright" (Hollander & Simeon, 2003). This type of phobic response produces symptoms such as sweaty palms, racing pulse, trembling hands, dry mouth, labored breathing, nausea, and memory loss. The beta-blockers appear to be quite effective in reducing these symptoms in some individuals.

For Obsessive-Compulsive Disorder

ANTIDEPRESSANTS. The SSRIs fluoxetine, paroxetine, sertraline, and fluvoxamine have been approved by the FDA for the treatment of OCD. Doses in excess of what is effective for treating depression may be required for OCD. Common side effects include sleep disturbances, headache, and restlessness. These effects are often transient and are less troublesome than those of the tricyclics.

The tricyclic antidepressant clomipramine was the first drug approved by the FDA in the treatment of OCD. Clomipramine is more selective for serotonin reuptake than any of the other tricyclics. Its efficacy in the treatment of OCD is well established, although the adverse effects, such as those associated with all the tricyclics, may make it less desirable than the SSRIs.

For Post-Traumatic Stress Disorder

ANTIDEPRESSANTS. The SSRIs are now considered first-line treatment of choice for PTSD because of their efficacy, tolerability, and safety ratings (Sadock & Sadock, 2003). Paroxetine and sertraline have been approved by the FDA for this purpose. The tricyclic antidepressants (e.g., amitriptyline and imipramine), the MAOIs (e.g., phenelzine), and trazodone have also been effective in the treatment of PTSD.

ANXIOLYTICS. Alprazolam has been prescribed for PTSD clients for its antidepressant and antipanic effects. Other benzodiazepines have also been used, despite the absence of controlled studies demonstrating their efficacy in PTSD. Kaplan and Sadock (1998) state:

> Although some anecdotal reports point to the effectiveness of alprazolam in PTSD, the use of this drug is complicated by the high association of substance-related disorders in patients with the disorder and by the emergence of withdrawal symptoms on discontinuation of the drug. (p. 622)

One study with buspirone showed significant reduction in PTSD symptoms (Sadock & Sadock, 2003). Further controlled trials with this drug are needed to validate its efficacy in treating PTSD.

ANTIHYPERTENSIVES. The beta-blocker propranolol and the alpha$_2$-receptor agonist clonidine have been successful in alleviating some of the symptoms associated with PTSD. In clinical trials, marked reductions in nightmares, intrusive recollections, hypervigilance, insomnia, startle responses, and angry outbursts were reported with the use of these drugs (Hollander & Simeon, 2003).

OTHER DRUGS. Carbamazepine, valproate, and lithium carbonate have been reported to alleviate symptoms of intrusive recollections, flashbacks, nightmares, impulsivity, irritability, and violent behavior in PTSD clients. Sadock and Sadock (2003) report that little positive evidence exists concerning the use of antipsychotics in PTSD. They suggest that these drugs "should be reserved for the short-term control of severe aggression and agitation."

SUMMARY

Anxiety is a necessary force for survival and has been experienced by humanity throughout the ages. It was first described as a physiological disorder and identified by its physical symptoms, particularly the cardiac symptoms. The psychological implications for the symptoms were not recognized until the early 1900s.

Anxiety is considered a normal reaction to a realistic danger or threat to biological integrity or self-concept. Normality of the anxiety experienced in response to a stressor is defined by societal and cultural standards.

Anxiety disorders are more common in women than in men by at least two to one. Studies of familial patterns suggest that a familial predisposition to anxiety disorders probably exists.

The *DSM-IV-TR* identifies several broad categories of anxiety disorders. They include panic and generalized anxiety disorders, phobic disorders, OCD, PTSD, anxiety disorder due to a general medical condition, and substance-induced anxiety disorder. A number of elements, including psychosocial factors, biological influences, and learning experiences most likely contribute to the development of these disorders.

Treatment of anxiety disorders includes individual psychotherapy, cognitive therapy, behavior therapy, group and family therapy, and psychopharmacology. Common behavior therapies include systematic desensitization and implosion therapy (flooding). Nursing care is accomplished using the six steps of the nursing process.

Nurses encounter clients experiencing anxiety in virtually all types of healthcare settings. Nurses should be able to recognize the symptoms of anxiety and help clients understand that these symptoms are normal and acceptable.

Clients with anxiety disorders are seen in all types of medical and psychiatric facilities. Nurses help clients to gain insight and increase self-awareness in relation to their illness. Intervention focuses on assisting clients to learn techniques with which they may interrupt the escalation of anxiety before it reaches unmanageable proportions. Maladaptive behavior patterns are replaced by new, more adaptive, coping skills.

REVIEW QUESTIONS

SELF-EXAMINATION/LEARNING EXERCISE

For each situation, select the answer that is most appropriate for the questions that follow.

Situation: Ms. T. has been diagnosed with agoraphobia.

1. Which behavior would be most characteristic of this disorder?
   a. Ms. T. experiences panic anxiety when she encounters snakes.
   b. Ms. T. refuses to fly in an airplane.
   c. Ms. T. will not eat in a public place.
   d. Ms. T. stays in her home for fear of being in a place from which she cannot escape.
2. The therapist who works with Ms. T. would likely choose which of the following therapies for her?
   a. 10 mg Valium q.i.d.
   b. Group therapy with other agoraphobics
   c. Facing her fear in gradual step progression
   d. Hypnosis
3. Should the therapist choose to use implosion therapy, Ms. T. would be:
   a. Taught relaxation exercises
   b. Subjected to graded intensities of the fear
   c. Instructed to stop the therapeutic session as soon as anxiety is experienced
   d. Presented with massive exposure to a variety of stimuli associated with the phobic object/situation

Situation: Sandy is a 29-year-old woman who has been admitted to the psychiatric unit with a diagnosis of OCD. She spends many hours, day and night, washing her hands.

4. The most likely reason Sandy washes her hands so much is that it:
   a. Relieves her anxiety
   b. Reduces the probability of infection
   c. Gives her a feeling of control over her life
   d. Increases her self-concept
5. The *initial* care plan for Sandy would include which of the following nursing interventions?
   a. Keep Sandy's bathroom locked so she cannot wash her hands all the time.
   b. Structure Sandy's schedule so that she has plenty of time for washing her hands.
   c. Put Sandy in isolation until she promises to stop washing her hands so much.
   d. Explain Sandy's behavior to her, since she is probably unaware that it is maladaptive.
6. On Sandy's fourth hospital day, she says to the nurse, "I'm feeling better now. I feel comfortable on this unit, and I'm not ill-at-ease with the staff or other patients anymore." In light of this change, which nursing intervention is most appropriate?
   a. Give attention to the ritualistic behaviors each time they occur and point out their inappropriateness.
   b. Ignore the ritualistic behaviors, and they will be eliminated for lack of reinforcement.
   c. Set limits on the amount of time Sandy may engage in the ritualistic behavior.
   d. Continue to allow Sandy all the time she wants to carry out the ritualistic behavior.

Situation: John is a 28-year-old high-school science teacher whose army reserve unit was called to fight in Operation Desert Storm. John did not want to fight. He admits that he joined the reserves to help pay off his college loans. In Saudi Arabia, he participated in combat and witnessed the wounding of several from his unit, as well as the death of his best friend. He has been experiencing flashbacks, intrusive recollections, and nightmares. His wife reports he is afraid to go to sleep, and his work is suffering. Sometimes he just sits as though he is in a trance. John is diagnosed with PTSD.

7. John says to the nurse, "I can't figure out why God took my buddy instead of me." From this statement, the nurse assesses which of the following in John?
   a. Repressed anger
   b. Survivor's guilt
   c. Intrusive thoughts
   d. Spiritual distress

8. John experiences a nightmare during his first night in the hospital. He explains to the nurse that he was dreaming about gunfire all around and people being killed. The nurse's most appropriate initial intervention is:
   a. Administer alprazolam as ordered p.r.n. for anxiety.
   b. Call the physician and report the incident.
   c. Stay with John and reassure him of his safety.
   d. Have John listen to a tape of relaxation exercises.

9. Which of the following therapy regimens would most appropriately be ordered for John?
   a. Paroxetine and group therapy
   b. Diazepam and implosion therapy
   c. Alprazolam and behavior therapy
   d. Carbamazepine and cognitive therapy

10. Which of the following may be influential in the predisposition to PTSD?
    a. Unsatisfactory parent/child relationship
    b. Excess of the neurotransmitter serotonin
    c. Distorted, negative cognitions
    d. Severity of the stressor and availability of support systems

INTERNET REFERENCES

- Additional information about anxiety disorders and medications to treat these disorders may be located at the following websites:
  - a http://www.adaa.org
  - b http://www.mentalhealth.com
  - c http://www.psychweb.com/disorders/index.htm
  - d http://www.nimh.nih.gov/
  - e http://www.psychiatrymatters.md/index.asp?sec=sres&criteria=anxiolytics
  - f http://www.fadavis.com/townsend

Test Your CRITICAL THINKING SKILLS

Sarah, aged 25, was taken to the emergency room by her friends. They were at a dinner party when Sarah suddenly clasped her chest and started having difficulty breathing. She complained of nausea and was perspiring profusely. She had calmed down some by the time they reached the hospital. She denied any pain, and electrocardiogram and laboratory results were unremarkable.

Sarah told the admitting nurse that she had a history of these "attacks." She began having them in her sophomore year of college. She knew her parents had expectations that she should follow in their example and become an attorney. They also expected her to earn grades that would promote acceptance by a top Ivy League university. Sarah experienced her first attack when she made a "B" in English during her third semester of college. Since that time, she has experienced these symptoms sporadically, often in conjunction with her perception of the need to excel. She graduated with top honors from Harvard.

Last week Sarah was promoted within her law firm. She was assigned her first solo case of representing a couple whose baby had died at birth and who were suing the physician for malpractice. She has experienced these panic symptoms daily for the past week, stating, "I feel like I'm going crazy!"

Sarah is transferred to the psychiatric unit. The psychiatrist diagnoses panic disorder without agoraphobia.

Answer the following questions related to Sarah:

1. What would be the priority nursing diagnosis for Sarah?
2. What is the priority nursing intervention with Sarah?
3. What medical treatment might you expect the physician to prescribe?

IMPLICATIONS OF RESEARCH FOR EVIDENCE-BASED PRACTICE

Johnson, J.G., Cohen, P., Pine, D.S., Klein, D.F., Kasen, S., & Brook, J.S: **Association between cigarette smoking and anxiety disorders during adolescence and early adulthood.** Journal of the American Medical Association (2000, November 8), 284(18), 2348–2351.

Description of the Study: The main objective of this study was to investigate the longitudinal association between cigarette smoking and anxiety disorders among adolescents and young adults. The study sample included 688 teenagers (51 percent female and 49 percent male) from upstate New York. The youths were interviewed at a mean age of 16 years, during the years 1985 to 1986, and again at a mean age of 22 years, during the years 1991 to 1993. At age 16, 6 percent of the participants smoked 20 or more cigarettes a day. The number increased to 15 percent by age 22.

Results of the Study: Of the participants who smoked 20 cigarettes or more a day during adolescence, a significant number developed an anxiety disorder during young adulthood: 20.5 percent developed generalized anxiety disorder, 10.3 percent developed agoraphobia, and 7.7 percent developed panic disorder. According to the researchers, cigarette smoking does not appear to increase the risk of developing OCD or social anxiety disorder.

Implications for Nursing Practice: The results of this study present just one more reason why adolescents should be encouraged not to smoke or not to begin smoking. The implications for nursing practice are serious. Nurses can initiate and become involved in educational programs to discourage cigarette smoking. Many negative health concerns are related to smoking, and this study provides additional information to include in educational programs designed specifically for adolescents.

REFERENCES

American Psychiatric Association (APA). (2000). Diagnostic and statistical manual of mental disorders (4th ed.) Text revision. Washington DC: American Psychiatric Association.

Embry, C.K. (1990). Psychotherapeutic interventions in chronic post-traumatic stress disorder. In M.E. Wolf & A.D. Mosnaim (Eds.), Post-traumatic stress disorder: Etiology, phenomenology, and treatment. Washington, DC: American Psychiatric Press.

Epstein, S. (1990). Beliefs and symptoms in maladaptive resolutions of the traumatic neurosis. In Ozer, et al. (Eds.), Perspectives on personality (Vol. 3). London: Jessica Kingsley.

Gale Encyclopedia of Childhood and Adolescence (1998). Fear. Retrieved March 3, 2002 from http://www.findarticles.com/cf_dls/g2602/0002/2602000246/p1/article.jhtml

Green, B.L., Wilson, J.P., & Lindy, J.D. (1985). Conceptualizing posttraumatic stress disorder: A psychosocial framework. In C.R. Figley (Ed.). Trauma and its wake: The study and treatment of posttraumatic stress disorder. New York: Brunner/Mazel.

Halpern, R. (1990). Poverty and early childhood parenting: Toward a framework for intervention. American Journal of Orthopsychiatry, 60(1), 6–8.

Harvard Medical School (2001, March). Panic disorder. The Harvard Mental Health Letter. Boston, MA: Harvard Medical School Publications Group.

Henn, F.A. (1994). The neurobiologic basis of psychiatric illness. In G. Winokur & P.J. Clayton (Eds.), The medical basis of psychiatry (2nd ed.). Philadelphia: W.B. Saunders.

Hollander, E. & Simeon, D. (2003). Anxiety disorders. In R.E. Hales & S.C. Yudofsky (Eds.), Textbook of Clinical Psychiatry (4th ed.). Washington, DC: American Psychiatric Press.

Johnson, B.S. (1995). Mental health of children, adolescents, and families. In B.S. Johnson (Ed.), Child, adolescent & family psychiatric nursing. Philadelphia: J.B. Lippincott.

Johnson, M. (1994, May/June). Stage fright. From Performing

songwriter 1(6). Retrieved March 2, 2002 from http://www.mjblue.com/pfright.html

Kaplan, H.I. and Sadock, B.J. (1998). Synopsis of Psychiatry: Behavioral sciences/clinical psychiatry (8th ed.). Baltimore: Williams & Wilkins.

Liebowitz, M.R. (1992). Anxiety and anxiety disorders. In F.I. Kass, J.M. Oldham, & H. Pardes (Eds.), The Columbia University College of Physicians and Surgeons complete home guide to mental health. New York: Henry Holt.

MacKenzie, T.B. (1994). Obsessive-compulsive neurosis. In G. Winokur & P.J. Clayton (Eds.), The medical basis of psychiatry (2nd ed.). Philadelphia: W.B. Saunders.

Peterson, K.C., Prout, M.F., & Schwarz, R.A. (1991). Post-traumatic stress disorder: A clinician's guide. New York: Plenum Press.

Sadock, B.J. & Sadock, V.A. (2003). Synopsis of psychiatry: Behavioral sciences/clinical psychiatry (9th ed.). Philadelphia: Lippincott Williams & Wilkins.

CLASSICAL REFERENCES

Freud, S. (1959). On the grounds for detaching a particular syndrome from neurasthenia under the description 'anxiety neurosis.' In The standard edition of the complete psychological works of Sigmund Freud (Vol. 3). London: Hogarth Press.

Johnson, J.H. & Sarason, I.B. (1978). Life stress, depression, and anxiety: Internal-external control as moderator variable. Journal of Psychosomatic Research, 22, 205–208.

CHAPTER 17

Anxiety-Related Disorders

CHAPTER OUTLINE

KEY TERMS

autoimmune
psychophysiological
type B personality
abreaction
derealization
fugue
anosmia
hypochondriasis
primary gain
secondary gain
tertiary gain
carcinogen
type A personality
type C personality
amnesia
depersonalization
integration
aphonia
hysteria
la belle indifference
pseudocyesis
somatization

OBJECTIVES

After reading this chapter, the student will be able to:

1. Discuss historical aspects and epidemiological statistics related to psychophysiological, somatoform, and dissociative disorders.
2. Describe various types of psychophysiological, somatoform, and dissociative disorders and identify symptomatology associated with each; use this information in client assessment.
3. Identify etiological implications in the development of psychophysiological, somatoform, and dissociative disorders.
4. Formulate nursing diagnoses and goals of care for clients with psychophysiological, somatoform, and dissociative disorders.
5. Describe appropriate nursing interventions for behaviors associated with psychophysiological, somatoform, and dissociative disorders.
6. Evaluate the nursing care of clients with psychophysiological, somatoform, and dissociative disorders.
7. Discuss various modalities relevant to treatment of psychophysiological, somatoform, and dissociative disorders.

INTRODUCTION

Psychophysiological responses to anxiety are those in which it has been determined that psychological factors contribute to the initiation or exacerbation of the physical condition. With these responses, evidence *does* exist to support the presence of organic pathology or a known pathophysiological process. The *DSM-IV-TR* (American Psychiatric Association [APA], 2000) states that certain psychological factors can influence the development or exacerbation of, or delayed recovery from, various medical conditions. These psychological factors include:

1. Mental disorders (e.g., major depressive disorder)
2. Psychological symptoms (e.g., depressed mood or anxiety)
3. Personality traits or coping style (e.g., denial of need for medical care)
4. Maladaptive health behaviors (e.g., smoking or overeating)
5. Stress-related physiological responses (e.g., tension headaches)
6. Other unspecified psychological factors (e.g., interpersonal or cultural factors)

Somatoform disorders are characterized by physical symptoms suggesting medical disease but without demonstrable organic pathology or known pathophysiological mechanism to account for them. They are classified as mental disorders because pathophysiological processes are not demonstrable or understandable by existing laboratory procedures, and there is evidence or strong presumption that psychological factors are the major cause of the symptoms. Lack of evidence of organic pathology is the major difference between somatoform disorders and psychophysiological disorders. **Somatization** refers to all those mechanisms by which anxiety is translated into physical illness or bodily complaints.

Dissociative disorders are defined by a disruption in the usually integrated functions of consciousness, memory, identity, or perception of the environment (APA, 2000). Dissociative responses occur when anxiety becomes overwhelming and the personality becomes disorganized. Defense mechanisms that normally govern consciousness, identity, and memory break down, and behavior occurs with little or no participation on the part of the conscious personality.

This chapter focuses on disorders characterized by moderate to severe anxiety that has been repressed and is being expressed in the form of physiological symptoms and dissociative behaviors. Historical and epidemiological statistics are presented. Factors that have been implicated in the etiology of these responses provide a framework for studying the dynamics of psychophysiological, somatoform, and dissociative disorders. An explanation of the symptomatology of these disorders is presented as background knowledge for assessing the client, and nursing care is described in the context of the nursing process. Various medical treatment modalities are explored.

HISTORICAL ASPECTS

For more than a century, physicians have agreed that in some disorders there is an interaction between emotional and physical factors. Four general types of reaction to stress have been identified. These reactions parallel Peplau's (1963) four levels of anxiety (see Chapter 1). These reactions are:

1. *The normal reaction,* in which there is increased alertness and a mobilization of defenses for action
2. *The psychophysiological reaction,* in which the defenses fail and the response is translated into somatic symptoms
3. *The neurotic reaction,* in which the anxiety is so great that the defense becomes ineffective and neurotic symptoms develop
4. *The psychotic reaction,* in which loss of control results in misperception of the environment

Along the continuum of anxiety, psychophysiological disorders occur at the moderate-to-severe level.

Hans Selye (1976) studied the physiological response of a biological system to change imposed on it. He found that, regardless of the stressor, the biological entity responded with a predictable syndrome of physical symptoms. In this aroused state, the individual garners the strength to face the stress and mobilizes the defenses to resolve it. However, if the defenses fail and the stressor is not quickly resolved, the body remains in this aroused state indefinitely, becoming susceptible to psychophysiological illness.

Historically, somatoform disorders have been identified as *hysterical neuroses.* The term **hysteria** describes a polysymptomatic disorder that usually begins in adolescence (rarely after the 20s), chiefly affects women, and is characterized by recurrent, multiple somatic complaints. The concept of hysteria is at least 4,000 years old and probably originated in Egypt. The name has been in use since the time of Hippocrates.

Over the years, symptoms of hysterical neuroses have been associated with witchcraft, demonology and sorcery, dysfunction of the nervous system, and unexpressed emotion. Somatoform disorders are thought to occur in response to repressed severe anxiety. Freud observed that, under hypnosis, clients with hysterical neurosis could recall past memories and emotional experiences that would relieve their symptoms. This led to his proposal that unexpressed emotion can be "converted" into physical symptoms.

Freud (1962) viewed dissociation as a type of repression—an active defense mechanism used to remove threatening or unacceptable mental contents from conscious awareness. He also described the defense of splitting of the ego in the management of incompatible mental contents. Despite the fact that the study of dissociative processes dates back to the 19th century, scientists still know remarkably little about the phenomena. Questions remain unanswered: Are dissociative disorders psychopathological processes or ego-protective devices? Are dissociative processes under voluntary control, or are they an unconscious effort? Maldonado and Spiegel (2003) state:

> These disorders have much to teach us about the way humans adapt to traumatic stress, and about information processing in the brain. (p. 709)

EPIDEMIOLOGICAL STATISTICS

Epidemiological statistics related to psychophysiological disorders will be presented with each disorder described. Virtually any organic disorder can be considered psychophysiological. Sadock and Sadock (2003) state, "... psychological or behavioral factors play a role in almost every medical condition". A list of some (although certainly not all) psychophysiological disorders is presented in Table 17–1.

The lifetime prevalence of somatization disorder in the general population is estimated to be 0.2 to 2 percent in women and 0.2 percent in men (Sadock & Sadock, 2003). Lifetime prevalence rates of conversion disorder vary widely. Statistics within the general population have ranged from 5 to 30 percent. **Hypochondriasis** affects 1 to 5 percent of the general population (APA, 2000). All somatoform disorders are more common in women than in men, with the exception of hypochondriasis, which affects women and men equally. Somatization and conversion disorders are more common in the poorly educated, in rural areas, and in individuals from the lower socioeconomic groups (Sadock & Sadock, 2003).

TABLE 17–1 Examples of Psychophysiological Disorders

Acne	Immune disease (e.g., MS, SLE)
Amenorrhea	Impotence
Angina pectoris	Irritable bowel syndrome
Asthma	Migraine headache
Cancer	Nausea and vomiting
Cardiospasm	Neurodermatitis
Coronary heart disease	Obesity
Duodenal ulcer	Pylorospasm
Dysmenorrhea	Regional enteritis
Enuresis	Rheumatoid arthritis
Essential hypertension	Sacroiliac pain
Gastric ulcer	Skin disease (e.g., psoriasis)
Herpes	Tension headache
Hyperglycemia	Tuberculosis
Hyperthyroidism	Ulcerative colitis
Hypoglycemia	

Modified from APA (2000); Sadock & Sadock (2003); and Pelletier (1992).

Dissociative disorders are thought to be quite rare. **Amnesia** is the most common dissociative symptom, and it appears in almost all the dissociative disorders (Sadock & Sadock, 2003). Dissociative **fugue** is rare and occurs most often under conditions of war, natural disasters, or intense psychosocial stress. Sadock and Sadock (2003) report that perhaps as many as 5 percent of all patients with psychiatric disorders meet the criteria for dissociative identity disorder (DID). The disorder occurs from three to nine times more frequently in women than in men (APA, 2000). Symptoms of **depersonalization** may occur at some time in up to half of all adults, particularly in the event of severe psychosocial stress (APA, 2000).

APPLICATION OF THE NURSING PROCESS

I. Background Assessment Data - Types of Psychophysiological Disorders

Asthma

Asthma is a syndrome of airflow limitation characterized by increased responsiveness of the tracheobronchial tree to various stimuli and manifested by airway smooth muscle contraction, hypersecretion of mucus, and inflammation (Anderson, 1991). It affects 12 to 15 million Americans, including approximately 10 to 12 percent of children under age 18 (Cleveland Clinic, 2001). Asthma may occur at any age, although it is more common in individuals under age 40.

Etiological Influences

1. **Hereditary factors.** Hereditary factors may play a role in the etiology of asthma. People who have a family history of asthma have an increased risk of developing the disease. Asthma also appears to be more common in families that have individuals with hay fever or eczema.
2. **Allergies.** A number of agents have been implicated in precipitation of asthmatic attacks, including aspirin, dust, food additives, cigarette smoke, and environmental pollutants. Other factors that may precipitate an attack include exercise and cold air.
3. **Psychosocial influences.** Individuals with asthma are characterized as having excessive dependency needs, although no specific personality type has been identified (Sadock & Sadock, 2003). Individuals with asthma have been associated with certain personality characteristics, including fears, emotional lability, increased anxiety, and depression (Sadock & Sadock, 2003; Levenson, 2003).

Medical Treatment Modalities

The most commonly prescribed medications for asthma are bronchodilators and corticosteroids, usually from a metered-dose inhaler. Bronchodilators increase the airway diameter, and corticosteroids reduce the inflammatory response. Some clients also may be candidates for short- or long-term psychotherapy. The internist or family physician maintains care of the physical component of the client's illness, whereas the psychotherapist focuses on attitudes, emotions, and helping the client to progress with the separation-individuation process. The psychological aspects are kept separate from the physical aspects of the illness so that the therapeutic relationship is not destroyed if the client suffers an asthmatic attack during psychotherapy.

Cancer

Cancer is a malignant neoplasm in which the basic structure and activity of the cells have become deranged, usually because of changes in the DNA. These mutated cells grow wildly and rapidly and lose their similarity to the original cells. The malignant cells spread to other areas by invading surrounding tissues and by entering the blood and lymphatic system. If left untreated, the malignant neoplasms usually result in death.

Cancer is the second leading cause of death in the United States. However, 5-year survival rates have increased because of early diagnosis and treatment and the improvement of treatment modalities for most cancers. The largest number of deaths from cancer in both men and women is attributed to cancer of the lung (National Cancer Institute, 2002a). The incidence and mortality rates for cancer are higher for African-Americans than for Caucasians and lower in Latinos than for both African-Americans and Caucasians (National Cancer Institute, 2002b). Cancer has been called a "disease of the aging," as the likelihood of developing cancer increases with age.

Etiological Influences

1. **Hereditary factors.** Certain cancers, such as those of the stomach, breast, colon, kidney, uterus, and lung tend to occur in a familial pattern. Whether this indicates an inherited susceptibility or common exposure to an etiological factor is unknown.
2. **Environmental factors.** Exposure to occupational or environmental **carcinogens** may lead to specific cancers. Examples include cigarette smoke, aniline dye, radium, asphalt, arsenic, chromate, uranium, and asbestos. Various drugs have been implicated in the onset of cancer. They include immunosuppressive agents, diethylstilbestrol, oral contraceptives, cytotoxic agents, and radioisotopes. Certain viruses have been implicated as a causative factor of cancer in some animals. However, the role of viruses in the etiology of cancer in humans has not been definitely established.
3. **Psychosocial influences.** Hafen and associates (1996) report on specific characteristics that have been associated with individuals who develop cancer. The term **type C personality** has been coined to describe these characteristics. Cancer has sometimes been called the "nice guy's disease." Common characteristics that were found to be associated with type C personality include repression of negative emotions, passivity, apologetic, and overly cooperative. Other researchers who have

studied these characteristics identify the following profile for the type C personality:

- Suppresses anger and hostility to an extreme (experiences these emotions but does not express them)
- Exhibits a calm, placid exterior
- Commonly feels depressed and in despair
- Low self-esteem; low self-worth
- Puts others' needs before their own
- Has a tendency toward self-pity (acts as the martyr)
- Sets unrealistic standards and is inflexible in the enforcement of these standards
- Resents others for perceived "wrongs," although others are never aware of these feelings

Levenson (2003) reports on a number of studies that provide support, as well as a lack of support, for several psychological factors associated with the onset and progression of cancer. Depression has been linked to a higher-than-normal risk of developing cancer, as well as death from the disease. The ability to express one's emotions rather than repress them has been shown to have an association with a more positive cancer prognosis. A lack of closeness with parents and less satisfactory interpersonal relationships have been linked to later development of cancer. Variables of positive relationships have been associated with increased survival rates.

Some studies have been conducted in an effort to determine if there is a link between psychosocial stress and the onset of cancer symptoms. Results suggest a positive correlation between the effects of stress and the induction and growth of neoplastic tumors in extensive work with experimental animals and in more limited studies with humans. Biopsychosocial events appear to reduce immunological competence at a critical time and may allow a mutant cell to thrive and grow (Pelletier, 1992).

Medical Treatment Modalities

Surgery, radiation therapy, and chemotherapy are the treatments of choice to control or cure cancer or to provide palliative measures when a cure is not possible. Psychotherapy may help those possibly cancer-prone individuals with type C characteristics. He or she must learn to express the feelings and emotions that have been suppressed. Psychotherapy also may be of benefit to patients with cancer. Some studies indicate a decrease in mortality rate in cancer patients who experience a reduction of anxiety, depression, and traumatic stress (Levenson, 2003).

Coronary Heart Disease

Coronary heart disease (CHD) is defined as myocardial impairment caused by an imbalance between coronary blood flow and myocardial oxygen requirements resulting from changes in the coronary circulation (Woods, Underhill, & Cowan, 1991). It is the leading cause of death in the United States. Five million people have CHD. It is more prevalent in men than in women, although the number of women with CHD is increasing, probably because of greater social and economic pressures on women and changes in their lifestyles. The incidence of CHD is higher in older individuals and in the affluent (Abraham, 1995).

Etiological Influences

1. **Hereditary factors.** A family history of CHD increases an individual's risk of developing the disease. It is not known whether there is a direct genetic link or if the risk is related more to environmental lifestyle patterns. Other risk factors that may have a genetic component include high serum lipoprotein levels (particularly cholesterol and triglycerides), hypertension, and diabetes mellitus.
2. **Environmental factors.** Various lifestyle habits have been implicated as risk factors for CHD. The association between cigarette smoking and CHD has now been clearly established. Obesity, defined as body mass index (weight/height^2) of 30 or greater, has also been associated with increased risk of developing CHD. Sedentary lifestyle has been implicated as a risk factor. It is thought that physical exercise offers some protection by helping to maintain lower blood pressure, helping with weight maintenance, and increasing levels of high-density lipoproteins (Sobel & Ornstein, 1996).
3. **Psychosocial influences.** Friedman and Rosenman (1974) have conducted the most comprehensive research to date in the area of personality and CHD. They developed a detailed profile of the CHD-prone individual, which they identified as **type A personality.** They also studied personality characteristics of individuals who experienced stress in a different manner and seemed less prone to CHD. This personality profile was called **type B personality.**

Friedman and Rosenman identified two character traits that, when occurring together, automatically classify an individual as type A personality. These two traits are excessive competitive drive and a chronic, continual sense of time urgency. Additional type A characteristics include:

- Easily aroused hostility that is usually kept under control but flares up unexpectedly, often when others would consider it unwarranted
- Very aggressive and ambitious, concentrating almost exclusively on his or her career
- Having no time for hobbies and, during any leisure time, feeling guilty relaxing as if wasting time
- Seldom feeling satisfied with accomplishments; always feeling must do more
- Measuring achievements in numbers produced and dollars earned
- Continually struggling to achieve and feeling there is never enough time (time becomes the enemy of the type A personality)
- Appearing to be very extroverted and social; often dominating conversation; outgoing personality often concealing a deep-seated insecurity about own worth
- Driving ambition and need to win (leads the type A personality to undertake all activities, including recreational, with the same competitive drive; becomes aggressive when putting undue pressure to compete on self)

People with type B personalities are not the opposite of those with type A; they are only different from them. Those with type B personality are not less successful than those with type A personality. They may perform every bit as well on their jobs—maybe better. Those with type B do not feel the constant sense of time urgency that those with type A feel. They can function under time pressure when it is required, but it is not a pervasive part of their lives as it is with those type A individuals. The ambition of type B individuals is probably based on goals that have been well thought out. There is not the constant need for competition and comparison with peers. Self-worth often comes from goals other than material and social success. Individuals with type B personality recognize and accept both strengths and limitations. They view leisure as a time to relax, and they do so without feeling guilty. They take the time to consider alternatives and to think things through before deciding or acting. These characteristics often result in creative output by persons with type B personality. Those with type A are prone to making more errors because of their impulsivity (i.e., acting before thinking things through). In Friedman and Rosenman's study, type A behavior was clearly a contributing factor to CHD.

Medical Treatment Modalities

Intervention with chemotherapeutic agents is common in the treatment of CHD. Vasodilators (e.g., nitroglycerin) to increase coronary tissue perfusion, beta-blockers (e.g., propranolol) and calcium channel blockers (e.g., verapamil) to treat angina and hypertension, and antihyperlipidemic agents (e.g., clofibrate, pravachol) to lower serum lipid levels are commonly prescribed. For clients with significant obstruction of the major coronary arteries, surgical intervention with coronary artery bypass grafting or percutaneous transluminal coronary angioplasty may be attempted.

Various techniques, such as progressive relaxation, autohypnosis, meditation, biofeedback, and group therapy, have been tried (with mixed results) in an attempt to modify the type A behavior pattern associated with CHD. Positive outcomes in the reduction of type A behaviors have been observed with combinations of education, interpersonal counseling, and behavior modification therapy. Hafen and associates (1996) report that 18 controlled studies have now shown that the toxic, hostile parts of type A personality (and even the excessive busyness) can indeed be transformed into safer behaviors.

Peptic Ulcer

Peptic ulcers are an erosion of the mucosal wall in the esophagus, stomach, duodenum, or jejunum. Deeper lesions may penetrate the mucosal layer and extend into the muscular layers of the intestinal wall (Simmons & Heitkemper, 1991).

Peptic ulcers occur four times more frequently in men than in women. Peak ages have traditionally been identified as 40 to 50 years, although these ages are increasing. Within these vulnerable age groups, peptic ulcers are estimated to affect up to 10 percent of the general population (Sands, 1995a).

Etiological Influences

1. **Hereditary factors.** There appears to be a hereditary predisposition to peptic ulcer disease, because a person with a family member with ulcer disease has three times the risk of developing an ulcer compared with the general population (Simmons &

Heitkemper, 1991). The ulcer itself occurs because of an imbalance in the secretion of hydrochloric acid and the mucosal resistance factors. Any factor that stimulates higher-than-normal hydrochloric acid secretion can promote the development of peptic ulcers.

2. **Environmental factors.** Cigarette smoking and regular use of aspirin have been strongly implicated in the etiology of peptic ulcer disease. Other agents such as alcohol, steroids, and nonsteroidal anti-inflammatory drugs (NSAIDs) are also ulcerogenic in that they can cause damage to the gastric mucosal barrier. Gastric ulcers have also been associated with infection by the bacterium *Helicobacter pylori.* It is possible that the reduced immune response related to psychosocial stress results in vulnerability to *H. pylori* infection (Sadock & Sadock, 2003).
3. **Psychosocial influences.** Studies have observed increased gastric secretion and motility in the presence of hostility, resentment, guilt, and frustration (Hafen et al., 1996). Some psychodynamic investigators have related the link between ulcers and stress to an unfulfilled dependency need in ulcer-prone individuals. These individuals tend to have an unhealthy attachment to others, and although they are dependent by nature, they perceive that they have few people on whom they can depend in times of crisis. They are excessive worriers and seem to have more times of crises than most people, possibly because they are such pessimists and always seem to expect the worst from a situation (Hafen et al., 1996). Anxiety and depression are common among ulcer-prone individuals.

Medical Treatment Modalities

Pharmacological interventions for peptic ulcer include antacids to neutralize gastric acid, antisecretory agents (e.g., histamine H_2 antagonists [cimetidine and ranitidine] and proton pump inhibitors [omeprazole, esomeprazole, and lansoprazole]), cytoprotective agents to coat ulcerated mucosal tissue and inhibit pepsin activity, and antibiotics and anti-infectives to treat *H. pylori* infection. A reduction or elimination from the diet of spicy foods, caffeine, and alcohol is recommended. Smoking and the intake of aspirin and NSAIDs should be avoided. Psychotherapy with ulcer clients focuses on troublesome conflicts such as passivity, dependency, aggression, anger, and frustration. These need to be addressed in treatment, respecting the client's defensive structure and need for support and reassurance. Studies have indicated greater improvement and less recurrence among individuals who were treated with a combination of chemotherapy and psychotherapy than in those who received chemotherapy alone.

Essential Hypertension

Essential hypertension is the persistent elevation of blood pressure for which there is no apparent cause or associated underlying disease (Cunningham, 1991). It is a major cause of cerebrovascular accident (stroke), cardiac disease, and renal failure. Twenty-five percent of the adult population in the United States is hypertensive, a condition characterized by a blood pressure of 140/90 mm Hg or higher (American Heart Association, 2002). Because hypertension is often asymptomatic, it is estimated that 50 percent of persons with hypertension do not know they have it (Walsh, 1995). The disorder is more common in men than in women and is twice as prevalent in the African-American population as it is in the Caucasian population.

Etiological Influences

1. **Hereditary factors.** Individuals who have a positive family history of hypertension are at greater risk of developing the disorder than those who do not.
2. **Physiological influences.** Physiological influences that have been implicated in the etiology of essential hypertension include an imbalance of circulating vasoconstrictors (e.g., angiotensin) and vasodilators (e.g., prostaglandins), increased sympathetic nervous system activity resulting in increased vasoconstriction, and impairment of sodium and water excretion (Cunningham, 1991).
3. **Environmental factors.** Obesity and cigarette smoking have been implicated as contributing factors to essential hypertension.
4. **Psychosocial influences.** Kaplan and Sadock (1998) offer the following psychodynamic explanation of the individual with essential hypertension:

> People with hypertension appear to be congenial, compliant, and compulsive. Although their anger is not expressed openly, they have much inhibited rage, which they handle poorly. There may be a familial genetic predisposition to hypertension; that is, when chronic stress occurs in a genetically predisposed compulsive personality who has repressed and suppressed rage, hypertension may result. (p. 803)

Medical Treatment Modalities

Treatment of individuals with essential hypertension is directed toward lowering blood pressure through lifestyle changes, pharmacological therapy, or both. Dietary modifications include restriction of sodium, caffeine, alcohol, and saturated fats. Weight reduction may also be necessary. Individuals with hypertension should not smoke. Increased physical activity, particularly aerobic-type exercise, has been shown to lower blood pressure in hypertensive individuals. Pharmacological intervention may be with a diuretic, beta-blocker, calcium channel blocker, or angiotensin-converting enzyme inhibitor.

Relaxation techniques, such as meditation, yoga, hypnosis, and biofeedback reduce blood pressure in some individuals. They are especially useful for individuals with higher initial pressures and as adjunctive therapy to pharmacological treatment. Supportive psychotherapy during which the individual is encouraged to express honest feelings, particularly anger, may also be helpful.

Migraine Headache

Migraine headache is a vascular event in which pain arises from the scalp, its blood vessels, and its muscles; from the dura mater and its venous sinuses; and from the blood vessels at the base of the brain (Schenk, 1995). Pain most commonly originates in the muscles of the face, neck, and head; the blood vessels; and the dura mater. The blood vessels dilate and become congested with blood. Pain results from the exertion of pressure on nerves that lie in or around these congested blood vessels.

Migraine headaches can occur at any age, but commonly begin in persons between ages 16 and 30 years. They are more common in women than in men and often are associated with various phases of the menstrual cycle. Approximately 5 percent of the general population suffers from migraine headaches.

Etiological Influences

1. **Hereditary factors.** Heredity appears to play an important role in the etiology of migraine headaches. It is common for individuals from several generations within the same family to experience the disorder. Occasionally members of one or two generations are spared, but it is common to track a history of headaches in aunts, uncles, cousins, or grandparents.
2. **Environmental factors.** Some foods, beverages, and drugs can precipitate migraine in certain individuals. These substances include caffeine, chocolate, aged cheese, vinegar, organ meats, alcoholic beverages, sour cream, yogurt, aspartame, citrus fruits, bananas, raisins, avocados, onions, smoked meats, monosodium glutamate, and products preserved with nitrites. Drugs that lower blood pressure, particularly reserpine and hydralazine, have been known to trigger migraine headaches.

   Some people experience attacks only during or after physical exertion. This may be caused by the chemical or blood vessel changes that occur during physical exertion or by the depletion of certain biological substances that may occur after exercise. Various other factors that have been implicated in the development of migraine headaches include cigarette smoking, bright lights, changes in the weather, high elevations, oral contraceptives, altered sleep patterns, and skipping meals.
3. **Psychosocial influences.** Certain characteristics have been identified as "the migraine personality." Migraine sufferers have been described as perfectionistic, overly conscientious, and somewhat inflexible. They may be meticulously neat and tidy, compulsive, and are often very hard workers. They are usually quite intelligent, exacting, and place a very high premium on success, setting high (sometimes unrealistic) expectations on themselves and others. Delegation of responsibility is difficult, as they feel no one can perform the task as well as they can. Classically, there is repressed or suppressed anger. The individual experiences hostility and anger but cannot express these feelings openly. Some researchers have identified the migraine personality as a clone of the type A personality (Hafen, et al., 1996).

Emotions play a critical role in the precipitation of migraine headaches. An individual experiencing emotional stress may develop a migraine headache in response to the secondary gains received from assuming the sick role. Migraine headaches therefore may provide a means of escape for dealing with the stressful situation. Other individuals experience migraine attacks only *after* the emotionally distressing event has passed or lessened. This has been called "let-down" headache and can be one of the influential factors in provoking the weekend or holiday migraine, when the anxiety has been relieved and the individual finally relaxes (Robbins & Lang, 1995).

Medical Treatment Modalities

Pharmacological intervention for migraine headache is directed toward prevention with drugs such as propranolol, amitriptyline, fluoxetine, verapamil, divalproex sodium, or venlafaxine. Once a migraine attack has begun, some physicians will administer an injection of a narcotic, such as meperidine or codeine, which blocks the pain and allows the individual to sleep until the attack subsides. A newer class of drugs, the serotonin receptor agonists (sumatriptan, naratriptan, zolmitriptan, and rizatriptan), which are available in oral, injectable, and inhalant forms, has been shown to be effective in interrupting migraine attacks. Various drugs related to ergotamine tartrate are prescribed to be taken at the first sign of onset of a migraine attack. They are ineffective once the attack has begun. Psychotherapy may be necessary in some instances, both to help relieve unresolved anger and to help modify some of the characteristics associated with "migraine personality." Biofeedback, regular physical exercise (unless it is known to trigger migraine attacks), relaxation training, behavior therapy, and diet modification have been reported to be useful for some individuals.

Rheumatoid Arthritis

Rheumatoid arthritis is a disease characterized by chronic musculoskeletal pain caused by inflammatory disease of the joints (Sadock & Sadock, 2003). It is a *systemic* disease and may be manifested by lesions of the major organs of the body. Rheumatoid arthritis is more prevalent in women than in men by a ratio of 2:1 or 3:1. It affects 1 to 3 percent of the population in the United States, with an estimated 200,000 cases diagnosed annually. The disease is characterized by periods of remission and exacerbation.

Etiological Influences

1. **Hereditary factors.** Heredity appears to be influential in the predisposition to rheumatoid arthritis. The serum protein rheumatoid factor is found in at least half of rheumatoid arthritics and frequently in their close relatives (Pelletier, 1992). It is an inherited characteristic and increases vulnerability to the disease. Although the rheumatoid factor is present in clients with other autoimmune diseases, it is rare in the population at large. It is postulated that rheumatoid arthritis may be an *autoimmune* disease. If so, it may be related to a dysfunctional immune mechanism and initiated by an infectious process. The antibodies that form because of the infection instead are directed against the self in an **autoimmune** response that results in tissue damage.
2. **Psychosocial influences.** The notion that certain personality traits were associated with rheumatoid arthritis has lost credibility (Levenson, 2003). Clients with rheumatoid arthritis were thought to be self-sacrificing, masochistic, conforming, self-conscious, inhibited, and perfectionistic because of their inability to express feelings of anger.

Some evidence suggests that emotionally traumatic life events, such as the loss of a key person by death or separation, often precede the first symptoms of rheumatoid arthritis and precipitate its onset in some individuals. Thus, emotional decompensation in predisposed individuals may result in the onset or exacerbation of rheumatoid arthritis. Levenson (2003) states,

> Although the early view of rheumatoid arthritis as a classic psychosomatic disorder has been discarded, the consensus in the rheumatological literature is that psychological factors are important, but their relations with illness in rheumatoid arthritis are complex. (p. 644)

Medical Treatment Modalities

Pharmacological treatment for rheumatoid arthritis is with aspirin, NSAIDs, antirheumatic agents (e.g., gold, penicillamine), corticosteroids (e.g., prednisone), and antineoplastic agents (e.g., methotrexate). Surgery may be required for some individuals with severe deformities, significant functional disabilities, or poorly controlled pain. Psychotherapy may help individuals cope and adapt to the chronicity of this condition. Denial of the illness is a common initial response to diagnosis. Over time, a number of adaptive processes, including resignation, episodic anger, sadness, and anxiety, may occur. Clients may blame themselves or believe that the disease is the result of past behaviors. Depression may need to be treated separately.

Ulcerative Colitis

Ulcerative colitis is a chronic inflammatory ulcerative disease of the colon and is usually associated with bloody diarrhea (Sadock & Sadock, 2003). An estimated 250,000 Americans have ulcerative colitis (National Digestive Diseases Information Clearinghouse, 2002). It can occur at any age but is most prevalent between the ages of 15 and 40 years. Ulcerative colitis affects males and females equally. The disease is prevalent in Caucasians and rare in African-Americans and Native Americans. There is a high incidence of ulcerative colitis in American and European Jews (Sands, 1995b).

Etiological Influences

1. **Hereditary factors.** A genetic factor may be involved in the development because individuals who have a family member with ulcerative colitis are at greater risk than the general population. The possibility that ulcerative colitis may be an autoimmune disease has generated a great deal of research interest. High rates of anticolon antibodies are found in relatives of ulcerative colitis clients. Das (2002) reports on research being conducted at the Robert Wood Johnson University Medical School, which reveals that ulcerative colitis is an autoimmune response to the protein tropomyosin that is present in the epithelial cells of the colon. He also states that the immune response may be triggered by some type of bacterial infection within the colon.
2. **Psychosocial influences.** Sadock and Sadock (2003) state,

> Studies of patients with ulcerative colitis have shown a predominance of obsessive-compulsive traits. They are neat, orderly, punctual, and have difficulty expressing anger. (p. 827)

Onset or exacerbation of ulcerative colitis has been associated with stressful life events or psychological trauma. The altered immune status that accompanies psychological stress may be an influencing factor in predisposed individuals.

Medical Treatment Modalities

Nutritional therapy is a primary focus in treatment of ulcerative colitis. Although there are no general restrictions on diet, clients must avoid foods that they identify as irritating. Pharmacological treatment may include sulfasalazine, which appears to have both anti-inflammatory and antimicrobial properties. Severe forms of the disease are treated with corticosteroids. Antidiarrheals and antispasmodics provide symptomatic relief. Surgery to remove the colon may be necessary for ulcerative colitis intractable to medical management or when complications of the disease occur. Because emotions and stress have been known to play a role in exacerbation of the illness, psychological support may help to decrease the frequency of these attacks by helping the individual to recognize the stressors that precipitate exacerbations and identify more adaptive ways of coping. The person with ulcerative colitis often feels a lack of control over his or her life. Psychological support may help the client cope with feelings of insecurity, dependency, and depression. It is important for the individual to express feelings of repressed or suppressed anger.

Diagnosis/Outcome Identification

Nursing diagnoses are formulated from the data gathered during the assessment phase and with background knowledge regarding etiological implications for the disorder. Some common nursing diagnoses for clients with specific psychophysiological disorders include:

Asthma
Ineffective airway clearance
Activity intolerance
Anxiety (severe)
Cancer
Fear
Anticipatory grieving
Disturbed body image
Coronary Heart Disease
Pain
Fear
Activity intolerance
Peptic Ulcer Disease
Pain
Impaired tissue integrity
Hypertension
Risk for ineffective tissue perfusion
Risk for sexual dysfunction
Migraine Headache
Pain
Ineffective role performance
Rheumatoid Arthritis
Pain
Self-care deficit
Activity intolerance
Ulcerative Colitis
Pain
Diarrhea
Risk for imbalanced nutrition: Less than body requirements

Some nursing diagnoses common to the general category of psychological factors affecting medical condition include:

Ineffective coping related to repressed anxiety and inadequate coping methods, evidenced by initiation or exacerbation of physical illness

Deficient knowledge related to psychological factors affecting medical condition, evidenced by statements such as "I don't know why the doctor put me on the psychiatric unit; I have a physical problem."

Low self-esteem related to unmet dependency needs, evidenced by self-negating verbalizations and demanding sick-role behaviors

Ineffective role performance related to physical illness accompanied by real or perceived disabling symptoms, evidenced by changes in usual patterns of responsibility

The following criteria may be used for measurement of outcomes in the care of the client with a psychophysiological disorder. The client:

1. Denies pain or other physical complaint
2. Demonstrates the ability to perform more adaptive coping strategies in the face of stressful situations
3. Verbalizes stressful situations that have led to or worsened physical symptoms in the past
4. Verbalizes a plan to cope with stressful situations in an effort to prevent exacerbation of physical symptoms
5. Performs activities of daily living independently

Planning/Implementation

In Table 17–2, selected nursing diagnoses common to the general category are presented in a plan of care. Nursing diagnoses are included, along with outcome criteria, appropriate nursing interventions, and rationales for each.

TABLE 17–2 Care Plan for the Client with a Psychophysiological Disorder

Nursing Diagnosis: INEFFECTIVE COPING
Related to: Repressed anxiety and inadequate coping methods
Evidenced by: Initiation or exacerbation of physical illness

Outcome Criteria	Nursing Interventions	Rationale
Client will achieve physical wellness and demonstrate the ability to prevent exacerbation of physical symptoms as a coping mechanism in response to stress.	1. Perform thorough physical assessment.	1. Physical assessment is necessary to determine specific care required for client's physical condition.
	2. Monitor laboratory values, vital signs, intake and output, and other assessments.	2. This is necessary to maintain an accurate ongoing appraisal.
	3. Together with the client, identify goals of care and ways in which he or she may best achieve those goals. Client may need assistance with problem solving.	3. Personal involvement in his or her own care provides a feeling of control and increases chances for positive outcomes.
	4. Encourage client to discuss current life situations that he or she perceives as stressful and the feelings associated with each.	4. Verbalization of true feelings in a nonthreatening environment may help client come to terms with unresolved issues.
	5. During client's discussion, note times during which a sense of powerlessness or loss of control over life situations emerges. Focus on these times and discuss ways in which the client may maintain a feeling of control.	5. A sense of self-worth develops and is maintained when an individual feels power over his or her own life situations.
	6. As client becomes able to discuss feelings more openly, assist him or her, in a nonthreatening manner, to relate certain feelings to the appearance of physical symptoms.	6. Client may be unaware of the relationship between physical symptoms and emotional problems.

(Continued)

TABLE 17 – 2 Care Plan for the Client with a Psychophysiological Disorder *(Continued)*

Outcome Criteria	Nursing Interventions	Rationale
	7. Discuss stressful times when physical symptoms did not appear and the adaptive coping strategies that were used during those situations. Therapy is facilitated by identifying areas of strength and using them to the client's benefit. Provide positive reinforcement for adaptive coping mechanisms used. Suggest alternative coping strategies, but allow client to determine which can best be incorporated into his or her lifestyle.	7. Positive reinforcement enhances self-esteem and encourages repetition of desired behaviors. Client may require assistance with problem solving but must be allowed and encouraged to make decisions independently.
	8. Help client to identify a resource within the community (friend, significant other, group) to use as a support system for the expression of feelings.	8. A positive support system may help to prevent maladaptive coping through physical illness.

Nursing Diagnosis: DEFICIENT KNOWLEDGE

Related to: Psychological factors affecting medical condition

Evidenced by: Statements such as "I don't know why the doctor put me on the psychiatric unit. I have a physical problem."

Outcome Criteria	Nursing Interventions	Rationale
Client will be able to verbalize psychological factors affecting his or her physical condition.	1. Assess client's level of knowledge regarding effects of psychological problems on the body.	1. An adequate database is necessary for the development of an effective teaching plan.
	2. Assess client's level of anxiety and readiness to learn.	2. Learning does not occur beyond the moderate level of anxiety.
	3. Discuss physical examinations and laboratory tests that have been conducted. Explain purpose and results of each.	3. Client has the right to know about and accept or refuse any medical treatment.
	4. Explore feelings and fears held by client. Go slowly. These feelings may have been suppressed or repressed for so long that their disclosure may be a very painful experience. Be supportive.	4. Expression of feelings in the presence of a trusted individual and in a nonthreatening environment may encourage the individual to confront unresolved feelings.
	5. Have client keep a diary of appearance, duration, and intensity of physical symptoms. A separate record of situations that the client finds especially stressful should also be kept.	5. Comparison of these records may provide objective data from which to observe the relationship between physical symptoms and stress.
	6. Help client identify needs that are being met through the sick role. Together, formulate more adaptive means for fulfilling these needs. Practice by role-playing.	6. Repetition through practice serves to reduce discomfort in the actual situation.
	7. Provide instruction in assertiveness techniques, especially the ability to recognize the differences among passive, assertive, and aggressive behaviors and the importance of respecting the rights of others while protecting one's own basic rights.	7. These skills will preserve client's self-esteem and improve his or her ability to form satisfactory interpersonal relationships.
	8. Discuss adaptive methods of stress management, such as relaxation techniques, physical exercise, meditation, breathing exercises, and autogenics.	8. Use of these adaptive techniques may decrease appearance of physical symptoms in response to stress.

Client/Family Education

The role of client teacher is important in the psychiatric area, as it is in all areas of nursing. A list of topics for client and family education relevant to psychological factors that affect the medical condition is presented in Table 17–3.

Evaluation

Reassessment is conducted to determine if the nursing actions have been successful in achieving the objectives of care. Evaluation of the nursing actions for the client with a psychophysiological disorder may be facilitated by gathering information using the following types of questions.

1. Does the client complain of pain or other physical symptoms?
2. Are the physical symptoms interfering with role responsibilities?
3. Does the client verbalize that physical symptoms have been relieved?
4. Can the client carry out activities of daily living independently?
5. Can the client verbalize alternative coping strategies for dealing with stress?
6. Can the client demonstrate the ability to use these more adaptive coping strategies in the face of stress?
7. Does client recognize which types of stressful situations or maladaptive health behaviors exacerbate physical symptoms?
8. Can the client correlate the appearance of the physical symptoms with a stressful situation or maladaptive health behavior?
9. Can the client verbalize unfulfilled needs for which the sick role may be compensating?
10. Can the client verbalize alternative ways to fulfill these needs?
11. Can the client verbalize resources to which he or she may go when feeling the need for assistance in times of stress?

TABLE 17–3 Topics for Client/Family Education Related to Psychological Factors Affecting Medical Condition

Nature of the Illness

1. Provide information to the client about specific disease process:
   a. Asthma
   b. Cancer
   c. Coronary heart disease
   d. Peptic ulcer
   e. Essential hypertension
   f. Migraine headache
   g. Rheumatoid arthritis
   h. Ulcerative colitis
   i. Other
2. Discuss psychological implications of exacerbation or delayed healing

Management of the Illness

1. Discuss ways to identify onset of escalating anxiety
2. Discuss ways to interrupt escalating anxiety:
   a. Assertive techniques
   b. Relaxation techniques
   c. Physical activities
   d. Talking with trusted individual
   e. Meditation
3. Discuss pain management
4. Discuss how family can prevent reinforcing the illness
5. Pharmacology:
   a. Discuss why physician has prescribed certain medications
   b. Discuss possible side effects of medications
   c. Provide printed information about what symptoms to report to physician
6. Discuss medical treatment modalities of the illness
7. Discuss possible lifestyle changes related to the illness

Support Services

1. Support groups
2. Individual psychotherapy
3. Biofeedback

II. Background Assessment Data—Types of Somatoform Disorders

Somatization Disorder

Somatization disorder is a syndrome of multiple somatic symptoms that cannot be explained medically and are associated with psychosocial distress and long-term seeking of assistance from healthcare professionals. Symptoms may be vague, dramatized, or exaggerated in their presentation. The disorder is chronic, with symptoms beginning before age 30. The symptoms are identified as pain (in at least four different sites), gastrointestinal symptoms (e.g., nausea, vomiting, diarrhea), sexual symptoms (e.g., irregular menses, erectile or ejaculatory dysfunction), and symptoms suggestive of a neurological condition (e.g., paralysis, blindness, deafness) (APA, 2000). Anxiety and depression are frequently manifested, and suicidal threats and attempts are common.

The disorder usually runs a fluctuating course, with periods of remission and exacerbation. Clients often receive medical care from several physicians, sometimes concurrently, leading to the possibility of dangerous combinations of treatments (APA, 2000). They have a tendency to seek relief through overmedicating with prescribed analgesics or antianxiety agents. Drug abuse and dependence are common complications of somatization disorder. When suicide results, it is usually in association with substance abuse (Sadock & Sadock, 2003).

It has been suggested that, in somatization disorder, there may be some overlapping of personality characteristics and features associated with histrionic personality disorder. These symptoms include heightened emotionality, impressionistic thought and speech, seductiveness, strong dependency needs, and a preoccupation with symptoms and the self.

Pain Disorder

The essential feature of pain disorder is severe and prolonged pain that causes clinically significant distress or impairment in social, occupational, or other important areas of functioning (APA, 2000). This diagnosis is made when psychological factors have been judged to have a major role in the onset, severity, exacerbation, or maintenance of the pain, even when the physical examination reveals pathology that is associated with the pain. Psychological implications in the etiology of the pain complaint may be evidenced by the correlation of a stressful situation with the onset of the symptom. Additional psychological implications may be supported by the facts that (1) appearance of the pain enables the client to avoid some unpleasant activity [**primary gain**]; and (2) the pain promotes emotional support or attention that the client might not otherwise receive [**secondary gain**].

Characteristic behaviors include frequent visits to physicians in an effort to obtain relief, excessive use of analgesics, and requests for surgery (Sadock & Sadock, 2003). Symptoms of depression are common and often severe enough to warrant a diagnosis of major depression. Dependence on addictive substances is a common complication of pain disorder.

Hypochondriasis

Hypochondriasis is defined as a person's preoccupation with the fear of contracting, or the belief of having, a serious disease (Sadock & Sadock, 2003). The fear becomes disabling and persists despite appropriate reassurance that no organic pathology can be detected. Occasionally medical disease may be present, but in the individual with hypochondriasis, the symptoms are excessive in relation to the extent of pathology.

The preoccupation may be with a specific organ or disease (e.g., cardiac disease), with bodily functions (e.g., peristalsis or heartbeat), or even with minor physical alterations (e.g., a small sore or an occasional cough) (APA, 2000). Individuals with hypochondriasis may become convinced that a rapid heart rate indicates they have heart disease or that the small sore is skin cancer. They are profoundly preoccupied with their bodies and are aware of even the slightest change in feeling or sensation. However, their response to these small changes is usually unrealistic and exaggerated.

Individuals with hypochondriasis often have a long history of "doctor shopping" and are convinced that they are not receiving proper treatment. Anxiety and depression are common, and obsessive-compulsive traits frequently accompany the disorder. Social and occupational functioning may be impaired because of the disorder.

Individuals with hypochondriasis are so convinced that their symptoms are related to organic pathology that they adamantly reject, and are often irritated by, any implication that stress or psychosocial factors play any role in their condition. They are so apprehensive and fearful that they become alarmed at the slightest intimation of serious illness. Even reading about a disease or hearing that someone they know has been diagnosed with an illness precipitates alarm on their part.

Conversion Disorder

Conversion disorder is a loss of or change in body function resulting from a psychological conflict, the physical symptoms of which cannot be explained by any known medical disorder or pathophysiological mechanism. Clients are unaware of the psychological basis and are therefore unable to control their symptoms.

Conversion symptoms affect voluntary motor or sensory functioning suggestive of neurological disease and are therefore sometimes called "pseudoneurological" (APA, 2000). Examples include paralysis, **aphonia**, seizures, coordination disturbance, difficulty swallowing, urinary retention, akinesia, blindness, deafness, double vision, **anosmia**, loss of pain sensation, and hallucinations. **Pseudocyesis** (false pregnancy) is a conversion symptom and may represent a strong desire to be pregnant (Cloninger, 1994).

Precipitation of conversion symptoms must be explained by psychological factors, and this may be evidenced by the presence of primary or secondary gain. When an individual achieves *primary gain*, the conversion symptoms enable avoidance of difficult situations or unpleasant activities about which he or she is anxious. Conversion symptoms promote *secondary gain* as a way to obtain attention or support that might not otherwise be forthcoming.

The symptom usually occurs after a situation that produces extreme psychological stress for the individual. The symptom appears suddenly, and often the person expresses a relative lack of concern that is out of keeping with the severity of the impairment (APA, 2000). This lack of concern is identified as **la belle indifference** and is often a clue to the physician that the problem may be psychological rather than physical. Other individuals, however, may present symptoms in a dramatic or histrionic fashion (APA, 2000).

Most conversion symptoms resolve within a few days or weeks. About 75 percent of people who experience conversion symptoms never experience another episode, but 25 percent have additional episodes during periods of stress (Sadock & Sadock, 2003). Symptoms of blindness, aphonia, and paralysis are associated with a good prognosis, whereas seizures and tremor are associated with poorer prognosis (APA, 2000).

Body Dysmorphic Disorder

This disorder, formerly called dysmorphophobia, is characterized by the exaggerated belief that the body is deformed or defective in some specific way. The most common complaints involve imagined or slight flaws of the face or head, such as thinning hair, acne, wrinkles, scars, vascular markings, facial swelling or asymmetry, or excessive facial hair (APA, 2000). Other complaints may have to do with some aspect of the nose, ears, eyes, mouth, lips, or teeth. Some clients may present with complaints involving other parts of the body, and in some instances a true defect is present. However, the significance of the defect is unrealistically exaggerated and the concern is grossly excessive.

Symptoms of depression and characteristics associated with obsessive-compulsive personality are common in individuals with body dysmorphic disorder. Social and occupational impairment may occur because of the excessive anxiety experienced by the individual in relation to the imagined defect. The person's medical history may reflect numerous visits to plastic surgeons and dermatologists in an unrelenting drive to correct the imagined defect. He or she may undergo unnecessary surgical procedures toward this effort.

The etiology of body dysmorphic disorder is unknown. In some clients, the disorder is attributable to another pervasive psychiatric disorder, such as schizophrenia, major mood disorder, or anxiety disorder. This has been supported by the responsiveness of the condition to the serotonin-specific drugs (Sadock & Sadock, 2003).

Etiological Implications for Somatoform Disorders

GENETIC. Studies have shown an increased incidence of somatization disorder, conversion disorder, and hypochondriasis in first-degree relatives, implying a possible inheritable predisposition (Sadock & Sadock, 2003; Yutzy, 2003; Soares & Grossman, 2001).

BIOCHEMICAL. Decreased levels of serotonin and endorphins may play a role in the etiology of pain disorder. Serotonin is probably the main neurotransmitter involved in inhibiting the firing of afferent pain fibers. The deficiency of endorphins seems to correlate with an increase of incoming sensory (pain) stimuli (Sadock & Sadock, 2003).

PSYCHODYNAMIC. Some psychodynamicists view hypochondriasis as an ego defense mechanism. Physical complaints are the expression of low self-esteem and feelings of worthlessness, because it is easier to feel something is wrong with the body than to feel something is wrong with the self. Another view of hypochondriasis (as well as pain disorder) is related to a defense against guilt. The individual views the self as "bad," based on real or imagined past misconduct, and views physical suffering as the deserved punishment required for atonement.

The psychodynamic theory of conversion disorder proposes that emotions associated with a traumatic event, which the individual cannot express because of moral or ethical unacceptability, are "converted" into physical symptoms. The unacceptable emotions are repressed and converted to a somatic hysterical symptom that is symbolic in some way of the original emotional trauma.

FAMILY DYNAMICS. Some families have difficulty expressing emotions openly and resolving conflicts verbally. When this occurs, the child may become ill, and a shift in focus is made from the open conflict to the child's illness, leaving unresolved the underlying issues that the family cannot confront openly. Thus, somatization by the child brings some stability to the family, as harmony replaces discord and the child's welfare becomes the common concern. The child in turn receives positive reinforcement for the illness.

LEARNING THEORY. Somatic complaints are often reinforced when the sick role relieves the individual from the need to deal with a stressful situation, whether it is within society or within the family. The sick person learns that he or she may avoid stressful obligations, postpone unwelcome challenges, and be excused from troublesome duties (primary gain); become the prominent focus of attention because of the illness (secondary gain), or relieve conflict within the family as concern is shifted to the ill person and away from the real issue (**tertiary gain**). These types of positive reinforcement virtually guarantee repetition of the response.

Past experience with serious or life-threatening physical illness, be it personal or that of a close family member, can predispose an individual to hypochondriasis. Once an individual has experienced a threat to biological integrity, he or she may develop a fear of recurrence. The fear of recurring illness generates an exaggerated response to minor physical changes, leading to hypochondriacal behaviors.

Diagnosis/Outcome Identification

Nursing diagnoses are formulated from the data gathered during the assessment phase and with background knowledge regarding etiological implications for the illness. Some common nursing diagnoses for clients with somatoform disorders include:

Ineffective coping related to repressed anxiety and unmet dependency needs evidenced by verbalization of numerous physical complaints in the absence of any pathophysiological evidence; focus on the self and physical symptoms (somatization disorder)

Chronic pain related to repressed anxiety and learned maladaptive coping skills evidenced by verbal complaints of pain, with evidence of psychological contributing factors, and excessive use of analgesics (pain disorder)

Fear (of having a serious disease) related to experience with life-threatening illness of self or significant others evidenced by preoccupation with and unrealistic interpretation of bodily signs and sensations (hypochondriasis)

Disturbed sensory perception related to repressed severe anxiety evidenced by loss or alteration in physical functioning, without evidence of organic pathology; la belle indifference (conversion disorder)

Disturbed body image related to repressed severe anxiety evidenced by preoccupation with imagined defect; verbalizations that are out of proportion to any actual physical abnormality that may exist; and numerous visits to plastic surgeons or dermatologists seeking relief (body dysmorphic disorder)

The following criteria may be used for measurement of outcomes in the care of the client with somatoform disorders. The client:

1. Effectively uses adaptive coping strategies during stressful situations without resorting to physical symptoms
2. Verbalizes relief from pain and demonstrates adaptive coping strategies during stressful situations to prevent the onset of pain
3. Interprets bodily sensations rationally; verbalizes understanding of the significance the irrational fear held for him or her; and has decreased the number and frequency of physical complaints
4. Is free of physical disability and is able to verbalize understanding of the correlation between the loss of or alteration in function and extreme emotional stress
5. Verbalizes a realistic perception of his or her appearance and expresses feelings that reflect a positive body image

Planning/Implementation

Table 17–4 provides a plan of care for the client with a somatoform disorder. Nursing diagnoses are presented, along with outcome criteria, appropriate nursing interventions, and rationales for each.

Evaluation

Reassessment is conducted to determine if the nursing actions have been successful in achieving the objectives of care. Evaluation of the nursing actions for the client with a somatoform disorder may be facilitated by gathering information using the following types of questions:

1. Can the client recognize signs and symptoms of escalating anxiety?
2. Can the client intervene with adaptive coping strategies to interrupt the escalating anxiety before physical symptoms are exacerbated?

TABLE 17–4 Care Plan for the Client With a Somatoform Disorder

Nursing Diagnosis: INEFFECTIVE COPING

Related to: Repressed anxiety and unmet dependency needs

Evidenced by: Verbalization of numerous physical complaints in the absence of any pathophysiological evidence; total focus on the self, and physical symptoms

Outcome Criteria	Nursing Interventions	Rationale
Client will demonstrate ability to cope with stress by means other than preoccupation with physical symptoms.	1. Monitor physician's ongoing assessments, laboratory reports, and other data to maintain assurance that possibility of organic pathology is clearly ruled out. Review findings with client.	1. Accurate medical assessment is vital for the provision of adequate and appropriate care. Honest explanation may help client understand psychological implications.
	2. Recognize and accept that the physical complaint is real to the client, even though no organic etiology can be identified.	2. Denial of the client's feelings is nontherapeutic and interferes with establishment of a trusting relationship.
	3. Identify what the physical symptoms are providing for the client: increased dependency, attention, distraction from other problems.	3. Identification of underlying motivation is important in assisting the client with problem resolution.
	4. Initially, fulfill the client's most urgent dependency needs, but gradually withdraw attention to physical symptoms. Minimize time given in response to physical complaints.	4. Anxiety and maladaptive behaviors will increase if dependency needs are ignored initially. Gradual withdrawal of positive reinforcement will discourage repetition of maladaptive behaviors.
	5. Explain to client that any new physical complaints will be referred to the physician and give no further attention to them. Ensure physician's assessment of the complaint.	5. The possibility of organic pathology must always be considered. Failure to do so could jeopardize client safety.
	6. Encourage client to verbalize fears and anxieties. Explain that attention will be withdrawn if rumination about physical complaints begins. Follow through.	6. Without consistency of limit–setting, change will not occur.
	7. Discuss possible alternative coping strategies client may use in response to stress (e.g., relaxation exercises, physical activities, assertiveness skills). Give positive reinforcement for use of these alternatives.	7. Client may need help with problem solving. Positive reinforcement encourages repetition.
	8. Help client identify ways to achieve recognition from others without resorting to physical complaints.	8. Positive recognition from others enhances self-esteem and minimizes the need for attention through maladaptive behaviors.

Nursing Diagnosis: CHRONIC PAIN

Related to: Repressed anxiety and learned maladaptive coping skills

Evidenced by: Verbal complaints of pain, with evidence of contributing psychological factors, and excessive use of analgesics

Outcome Criteria	Nursing Interventions	Rationale
Client will verbalize relief from pain and demonstrate more adaptive coping strategies for dealing with life situation.	1. Monitor physician's ongoing assessments and laboratory reports.	1. Organic pathology must be clearly ruled out.
	2. Recognize and accept that the pain is real to the client even though no organic etiology can be identified.	2. Denying the client's feelings is nontherapeutic and hinders the development of a trusting relationship.
	3. Observe and record the duration and intensity of the pain. Note factors that precipitate the onset of pain.	3. Identification of the precipitating stressor is important for assessment and care planning.
	4. Provide pain medication as prescribed by physician.	4. Client comfort and safety are nursing priorities.
	5. Provide nursing comfort measures (e.g., backrub, warm bath, heating pad) with a matter-of-fact approach that does not reinforce the pain behavior.	5. Comfort measures may provide some relief from pain. Secondary gains from physical symptoms may prolong maladaptive behaviors.
	6. Offer attention at times when client is not focusing on pain.	6. Positive reinforcement encourages repetition of adaptive behaviors.
	7. Identify activities that serve to distract client from focus on self and pain.	7. These distracters serve in a therapeutic manner as a transition from focus on self and pain to focus on unresolved psychological issues that may be contributing to the pain.

(Continued)

TABLE 17 – 4 Care Plan for the Client With a Somatoform Disorder *(Continued)*

Outcome Criteria	Nursing Interventions	Rationale
	8. Encourage verbalization of feelings. Explore meaning that pain holds for client. Help client connect symptoms of pain to times of increased anxiety and to identify specific situations that cause anxiety to rise.	8. Verbalization of feelings in a nonthreatening environment facilitates expression and resolution of disturbing emotional issues.
	9. Encourage client to identify alternative methods of coping with stress.	9. Alternative stress management techniques may avert the use of pain as a maladaptive response to stress.
	10. Explore ways to intervene as symptoms begin to intensify (e.g., visual or auditory distractions, mental imagery, deep-breathing exercises, application of hot or cold compresses, relaxation exercises).	10. These techniques are adaptive ways of preventing the pain from becoming disabling.
	11. Provide positive reinforcement for times when client is not focusing on pain.	11. Positive reinforcement, in the form of the nurse's presence and attention, may encourage a continuation of more adaptive behaviors.

Nursing Diagnosis: FEAR (OF HAVING A SERIOUS DISEASE)
Related to: Past experience with life-threatening illness of self or significant others
Evidenced by: Preoccupation with and unrealistic interpretation of bodily signs and sensations

Outcome Criteria	Nursing Interventions	Rationale
Client will verbalize irrationality of fear and interpret bodily sensations correctly.	1. Monitor physician's ongoing assessments and laboratory reports.	1. Organic pathology must be clearly ruled out.
	2. Refer all new physical complaints to physician.	2. To assume that all physical complaints are hypochondriacal would place client's safety in jeopardy.
	3. Assess function client's illness is fulfilling (e.g., unfulfilled needs for dependency, nurturing, caring, attention, or control).	3. This information may provide insight into reasons for maladaptive behavior and provide direction for planning client care.
	4. Identify times during which preoccupation with physical symptoms escalates. Determine extent of correlation of physical complaints with times of increased anxiety.	4. Client is unaware of the psychosocial implications of the physical complaints. Knowledge of the relationship is the first step in the process for creating change.
	5. Convey empathy. Let client know that you understand how a specific symptom may conjure up fears of previous life-threatening illness.	5. Unconditional acceptance and empathy promote a therapeutic nurse/client relationship.
	6. Initially allow client a limited amount of time (e.g., 10 minutes each hour) to discuss physical symptoms.	6. Because this has been his or her primary method of coping for so long, complete prohibition of this activity would likely raise client's anxiety level significantly, exacerbating the hypochondriacal behavior.
	7. Help client determine what techniques may be most useful to implement when fear and anxiety are exacerbated (e.g., relaxation techniques, mental imagery, thought-stopping techniques, physical exercise).	7. All of these techniques are effective to reduce anxiety and may assist client in the transition from focusing on fear of physical illness to the discussion of honest feelings.
	8. Gradually increase the limit on amount of time spent each hour in discussing physical symptoms. If client violates the limits, withdraw attention.	8. Lack of positive reinforcement may help to extinguish maladaptive behavior.
	9. Encourage client to discuss feelings associated with fear of serious illness.	9. Verbalization of feelings in a nonthreatening environment facilitates expression and resolution of disturbing emotional issues. When the client can express feelings directly, there is less need to express them through physical symptoms.
	10. Role-play the client's plan for dealing with the fear the next time it assumes control and before it becomes disabling through the exacerbation of physical symptoms.	10. Anxiety and fears are minimized when client has achieved a degree of comfort through practicing a plan for dealing with stressful situations in the future.

Nursing Diagnosis: DISTURBED SENSORY PERCEPTION

Related to: Repressed severe anxiety

Evidenced by: Loss or alteration in physical functioning, without evidence of organic pathology; "la belle indifference"

Outcome Criteria	Nursing Interventions	Rationale
Client will demonstrate recovery of lost or altered function.	1. Monitor physician's ongoing assessments, laboratory reports, and other data to ensure organic pathology is clearly ruled out.	1. Failure to do so may jeopardize client safety.
	2. Identify primary or secondary gains that the physical symptom is providing for the client (e.g., increased dependency, attention, protection from a stressful event).	2. Primary and secondary gains are etiological factors and may be used to assist in problem resolution.
	3. Do not focus on the disability, and encourage client to be as independent as possible. Intervene only when client requires assistance.	3. Positive reinforcement would encourage continual use of the maladaptive response to achieve secondary gains, such as dependency.
	4. Do not allow the client to use the disability as a manipulative tool to avoid participation in therapeutic activities. Withdraw attention if client continues to focus on physical limitation.	4. Lack of reinforcement may help to extinguish the maladaptive response.
	5. Encourage client to verbalize fears and anxieties. Help identify physical symptoms as a coping mechanism that is used in times of extreme stress.	5. Clients with conversion disorder are usually unaware of the psychological implications of their illness.
	6. Help client identify coping mechanisms to use when faced with stressful situations, rather than retreating from reality with a physical disability.	6. Client needs assistance with problem solving at this severe level of anxiety.
	7. Give positive reinforcement for identification or demonstration of alternative, more adaptive coping strategies.	7. Positive reinforcement enhances self-esteem and encourages repetition of desirable behaviors.

Nursing Diagnosis: DISTURBED BODY IMAGE

Related to: Repressed severe anxiety

Evidenced by: Preoccupation with imagined defect; verbalizations that are out of proportion to any actual physical abnormality that may exist; numerous visits to plastic surgeons or dermatologists seeking relief

Outcome Criteria	Nursing Interventions	Rationale
Client will verbalize realistic perception of body appearance.	1. Assess client's perception of body image. Keep in mind that this image is real to the client.	1. Assessment information is necessary in developing an accurate plan of care. Denial of the client's feelings impedes the development of a trusting, therapeutic relationship.
	2. Help client to see that body image is distorted or out of proportion in relation to the significance of an actual physical anomaly.	2. Recognition that a misperception exists is necessary before the client can accept reality and reduce the significance of the imagined defect.
	3. Encourage verbalization of fears and anxieties associated with identified stressful life situations. Discuss alternative adaptive coping strategies.	3. Verbalization of feelings with a trusted individual may help the client come to terms with unresolved issues. Knowledge of alternative coping strategies may help the client respond to stress more adaptively in the future.
	4. Involve client in activities that reinforce a positive sense of self not based on appearance.	4. When the client is able to develop self-satisfaction based on accomplishments and unconditional acceptance, significance of the imagined defect or minor physical anomaly will diminish.
	5. Make referrals to support groups for individuals with similar histories (e.g., Adult Children of Alcoholics, Victims of Incest, Survivors of Suicide, Adults Abused as Children).	5. Having a support group of understanding, empathic peers can help the client accept the reality of the situation, correct distorted perceptions, and make adaptive life changes.

3. Can the client verbalize an understanding of the correlation between physical symptoms and times of escalating anxiety?
4. Does the client have a plan for dealing with increased stress to prevent exacerbation of physical symptoms?
5. Does the client demonstrate a decrease in ruminations about physical symptoms?
6. Have fears of serious illness diminished?
7. Does the client demonstrate full recovery from previous loss or alteration of physical functioning?
8. Does the client verbalize a realistic perception and satisfactory acceptance of personal appearance?

MEDICAL TREATMENT MODALITIES FOR SOMATOFORM DISORDERS

Individual Psychotherapy

The goal of psychotherapy is to help clients develop healthy and adaptive behaviors, encourage them to move beyond their somatization, and manage their lives more effectively. The focus is on personal and social difficulties that the client is experiencing in daily life as well as the achievement of practical solutions for these difficulties.

Treatment is initiated with a complete physical examination to rule out organic pathology. Once this has been ensured, the physician turns attention to the client's social and personal problems and away from the somatic complaints.

Group Psychotherapy

Group therapy may be helpful for somatoform disorders because it provides a setting where clients can share their experiences of illness, learn to verbalize thoughts and feelings, and be confronted by group members and leaders when they reject responsibility for maladaptive behaviors. It has been reported to be the treatment of choice for both somatization disorder and hypochondriasis, in part because it provides the social support and social interaction that these clients need.

Behavior Therapy

Behavior therapy is more likely to be successful in instances when secondary gain is prominent. This may involve working with the client's family or significant others who may be perpetuating the physical symptoms by rewarding passivity and dependency and being overly solicitous and helpful. Behavioral therapy focuses on teaching these individuals to reward the client's autonomy, self-sufficiency, and independence. This process becomes more difficult when the client is markedly regressed and the sick role well established.

Psychopharmacology

Antidepressants, such as tricyclics and selective serotonin reuptake inhibitors (SSRIs), are often used with somatoform pain disorder. Among the tricyclics reported to have analgesic effect are amitriptyline (Elavil), nortriptyline (Aventyl), imipramine (Tofranil), desipramine (Norpramin), clomipramine (Anafranil), and doxepin (Sinequan) (King, 1999). They often provide pain relief at a dosage below that used to treat depression. The SSRIs paroxetine (Paxil), fluoxetine (Prozac), sertraline (Zoloft), and fluvoxamine (Luvox) have been studied for their analgesic effects, but have been found to be somewhat less efficacious than the tricyclics with which they were compared (King, 1999).

Anticonvulsants such as phenytoin (Dilantin), carbamazepine (Tegretol), and clonazepam (Klonopin) have been reported to be effective in treating neuropathic and neuralgic pain, at least for short periods. Their efficacy in other somatoform pain disorders is less clear.

Pharmacological therapy also seems to be effective in the treatment of body dysmorphic disorder. The most positive results have been with clomipramine (Anafranil) and fluoxetine (Prozac), which have been shown to reduce symptoms in more than 50 percent of clients with body dysmorphic disorder (Sadock & Sadock, 2003).

III. Background Assessment Data - Types of Dissociative Disorders

Dissociative Amnesia

Dissociative amnesia is an inability to recall important personal information, usually of a traumatic or stressful nature, that is too extensive to be explained by ordinary forgetfulness and is not related to the direct effect of substance use or a neurological or other general medical condition (APA, 2000). Five types of recall disturbance have been described. In the following examples, the individual is involved in a traumatic automobile accident in which a loved one is killed.

1. **Localized amnesia.** The inability to recall all incidents associated with the traumatic event for a specific time following the event (usually a few hours to a few days).
   Example: The individual cannot recall events of the automobile accident and events occurring during a period after the accident (a few hours to a few days).
2. **Selective amnesia.** The inability to recall only certain incidents associated with a traumatic event for a specific period after the event.
   Example: The individual may not remember events associated with the impact of the accident but may remember being taken away in the ambulance.
3. **Continuous amnesia.** The inability to recall events occurring after a specific time up to and including the present.
   Example: The individual cannot remember events associated with the automobile accident and anything that has occurred since. The individual cannot form new memories although he or she is apparently alert and aware.
4. **Generalized amnesia.** The rare phenomenon in which an individual is not able to recall personal identity or anything that has happened during his or her lifetime.
5. **Systematized amnesia.** With this type of amnesia, the individual cannot remember events that relate to a specific category of information (e.g., one's family) or to one particular person or event.

The individual with amnesia usually appears alert and may give no indication to observers that anything is wrong, although at the onset of the episode there may be a brief period of disorganization or clouding of consciousness (Sadock & Sadock, 2003). Clients suffering from amnesia are often brought to general hospital emergency departments by police who have found them wandering confusedly around the streets. Onset of an amnestic episode usually follows severe psychosocial stress. Termination is typically abrupt and followed by complete recovery. Recurrences are unusual.

Dissociative Fugue

The characteristic feature of dissociative fugue is a sudden, unexpected travel away from home or customary place of daily activities, with inability to recall some or all of one's past (APA, 2000). An individual in a fugue state cannot recall personal identity and often assumes a new identity. Sadock and Sadock (2003) state:

> During [the fugue], they have complete amnesia for their past lives and associations, but unlike patients with dissociative amnesia, they are generally unaware that they have forgotten anything. Only when they suddenly return to their former selves do they recall the time antedating the onset of the fugue, but then they remain amnestic for the period of the fugue itself. (p. 680)

Individuals in a fugue state do not appear to be behaving in any way out of the ordinary. Contacts with other people are minimal. The assumed identity may be simple and incomplete or complex and elaborate. If a complex identity is established, the individual may engage in intricate interpersonal and occupational activities. A divergent perception regarding the assumption of a new identity in dissociative fugue is reported by Spiegel and Maldonado (1999):

> It was thought that the assumption of a new identity was typical of dissociative fugue. However, [studies have documented] that in the majority of cases there is a loss of personal identity but no clear assumption of a new identity. (p. 457)

Clients with dissociative fugue have often been picked up by police when found wandering in a confused and frightened condition after emerging from the fugue in unfamiliar surroundings. They are usually taken to the emergency department of a general hospital and, upon assessment, are able to provide details of their earlier life, but have no recall after the beginning of the fugue state. Information from other sources usually reveals severe psychological stress or excessive alcohol use precipitated the fugue behavior. Duration is usually brief—hours to days or, more rarely, months—and recovery is rapid and complete. Recurrences are not common.

Dissociative Identity Disorder

Dissociative identity disorder (DID) was formerly called multiple personality disorder. This disorder is characterized by the existence of two or more personalities in a single individual. Only one of the personalities is evident at any given moment, and one of them is dominant most of the time over the course of the disorder. Each personality is unique and composed of a complex set of memories, behavior patterns, and social relationships that surface during the dominant interval. The transition from one personality to another is usually sudden, often dramatic, and usually precipitated by stress. The *DSM-IV-TR* (APA, 2000) states:

> The time required to switch from one identity to another is usually a matter of seconds, but, less frequently, may be gradual. Behavior that may be frequently associated with identity switches include rapid blinking, facial changes, changes in voice or demeanor, or disruption in the individual's train of thought. (p. 527)

Before therapy, the original personality usually has no knowledge of the other personalities, but when there are two or more subpersonalities, they are usually aware of each other's existence. Most often, the various subpersonalities have different names, but they may be unnamed and may be of a different sex, race, and age. The various personalities are usually disparate and may even appear to be the exact opposite of the original personality. For example, a normally shy, socially withdrawn, faithful husband may become a gregarious womanizer and heavy drinker with the emergence of another personality.

Generally, there is amnesia regarding the events that took place when another personality was in the dominant position. Often, however, one personality is not bound by such amnesia and retains complete awareness of the existence, qualities, and activities of the other personalities (Sadock & Sadock, 2003). Subpersonalities that are amnestic for other subpersonalities experience the periods when others are dominant as "lost time" or blackouts. They may "wake up" in unfamiliar situations with no idea where they are, how they got there, or who the people around them are. They may frequently be accused of lying when they deny remembering or being responsible for events or actions that occurred when another personality controlled the body.

Dissociative identity disorder is not always incapacitating. Some individuals with DID maintain responsible positions, complete graduate degrees, and are successful spouses and parents before diagnosis and during treatment. Before they are diagnosed with DID, many individuals are misdiagnosed with depression, borderline and antisocial personality disorders, schizophrenia, epilepsy, or bipolar disorder.

Depersonalization Disorder

Depersonalization disorder is characterized by a temporary change in the quality of self-awareness, which often takes the form of feelings of unreality, changes in body image, feelings of detachment from the environment, or a sense of observing oneself from outside the body. Depersonalization (a disturbance in the perception of oneself) is differentiated from **derealization**, which describes an alteration in the perception of the external environment. Both of these phenomena also occur in a variety of psychiatric illnesses such as schizophrenia, depression, anxiety states, and organic mental disorders. As previously stated, the symptom of depersonalization is very common. It is estimated that approximately half of all adults experience transient episodes of depersonalization (APA, 2000). The diagnosis of depersonalization disorder is made only if the symptom causes significant distress or impairment in functioning.

The *DSM-IV-TR* describes this disorder as the persistence or recurrence of episodes of depersonalization characterized by a feeling of detachment or estrangement from one's self (APA, 2000). There may be a mechanical or dreamlike feeling or a belief that the body's physical characteristics have changed. If derealization is present, objects in the environment are perceived as altered in size or shape. Other people in the environment may seem automated or mechanical.

These altered perceptions are experienced as disturbing and are often accompanied by anxiety, depression, fear of going insane, obsessive thoughts, somatic complaints, and disturbance in the subjective sense of time (APA, 2000). The disorder occurs at least twice as often in women as in men and is a disorder of younger people, rarely occurring in individuals older than 40 years of age (Sadock & Sadock, 2003).

Etiological Implications for Dissociative Disorders

GENETICS. The *DSM-IV-TR* suggests that DID is more common in first-degree relatives of people with the disorder than in the general population. The disorder is often seen in more than one generation of a family.

NEUROBIOLOGICAL. Some clinicians have suggested a possible correlation between neurological alterations and dissociative disorders. Although available information is inadequate, dissociative amnesia and dissociative fugue may be related to neurophysiological dysfunction. Areas of the brain that have been associated with memory include the hippocampus, the mammillary bodies, the dorsomedial thalamus, and the inferior temporal cortices (Waziri, 1994).

Cloninger (1994) cites studies from which he reports the following:

> Dissociative reactions may be precipitated by excessive cortical arousal, which in turn triggers reactive inhibition of signals at synapses in sensorimotor pathways by way of negative feedback relationships between the cerebral cortex and the brainstem reticular formation. (p. 182)

Some studies have suggested a possible link between DID and certain neurological conditions, such as temporal lobe epilepsy and severe migraine headaches. Electroencephalographic abnormalities have been observed in some clients with DID (Sadock & Sadock, 2003).

PSYCHODYNAMIC THEORY. Freud (1962) believed that dissociative behaviors occurred when individuals repressed distressing mental contents from conscious awareness. He believed that the unconscious was a dynamic entity in which repressed mental contents were stored and unavailable to conscious recall. Current psychodynamic explanations of dissociation are based on Freud's concepts. The repression of mental contents is perceived as a coping mechanism for protecting the client from emotional pain that has arisen from disturbing external circumstances or anxiety-provoking internal urges and feelings (Cloninger, 1994). In the case of depersonalization, the pain and anxiety are expressed as feelings of unreality or detachment from the environment of the painful situation.

PSYCHOLOGICAL TRAUMA. A growing body of evidence points to the etiology of DID as a set of traumatic experiences that overwhelms the individual's capacity to cope by any means other than dissociation. These experiences usually take the form of severe physical, sexual, or psychological abuse by a parent or significant other in the child's life. DID is thought to serve as a survival strategy for the child in this traumatic environment, where he or she creates a new being who is able to endure the overwhelming pain of reality, and the primary self can then escape awareness of the pain. Each new personality has at its nucleus a means of responding without anxiety and distress to various painful or dangerous stimuli.

Diagnosis/Outcome Identification

Nursing diagnoses are formulated from the data gathered during the assessment phase and with background knowledge regarding etiological implications for the disorder. Some common nursing diagnoses for clients with dissociative disorders include:

Disturbed thought processes related to severe psychological stress and repression of anxiety, evidenced by loss of memory (dissociative amnesia)

Ineffective coping related to severe psychosocial stressor or substance abuse and repressed severe anxiety, evidenced by sudden travel away from home with inability to recall previous identity (dissociative fugue)

Disturbed personal identity related to childhood trauma/abuse evidenced by the presence of more than one personality within the individual (dissociative identity disorder)

Disturbed sensory perception (visual/kinesthetic) related to severe psychological stress and repression of anxiety evidenced by alteration in the perception or experience of the self or the environment (depersonalization disorder)

The following criteria may be used for measurement of outcomes in the care of the client with a dissociative disorder. The client:

1. Can recall events associated with a traumatic or stressful situation
2. Can recall all events of past life
3. Can verbalize the extreme anxiety that precipitated the dissociation
4. Can demonstrate more adaptive coping strategies to avert dissociative behaviors in the face of severe anxiety
5. Verbalizes understanding of the existence of multiple personalities and the purposes they serve
6. Is able to maintain a sense of reality during stressful situations

Planning/Implementation

Table 17–5 provides a plan of care for the client with a dissociative disorder. Nursing diagnoses are included, along with outcome criteria, appropriate nursing interventions, and rationales.

Evaluation

Reassessment is conducted in order to determine if the nursing actions have been successful in achieving the objectives of care. Evaluation of the nursing actions for the client with a dissociative disorder may be

TABLE 17–5 Care Plan for the Client With a Dissociative Disorder

Nursing Diagnosis: DISTURBED THOUGHT PROCESSES

Related to: Severe psychological stress and repression of anxiety

Evidenced by: Loss of Memory

Outcome Criteria	Nursing Interventions	Rationale
Client will recover deficits in memory and develop more adaptive coping mechanisms to deal with stress.	1. Obtain as much information as possible about the client from family and significant others if possible. Consider likes, dislikes, important people, activities, music, and pets.	1. A comprehensive baseline assessment is important for the development of an effective plan of care.
	2. Do not flood client with data regarding his or her past life.	2. Individuals who are exposed to painful information from which the amnesia is providing protection may decompensate even further into a psychotic state.
	3. Expose client to stimuli that represent pleasant experiences from the past, such as smells associated with enjoyable activities, beloved pets, and music known to have been pleasurable. As memory begins to return, engage client in activities that may provide additional stimulation.	3. Recall may occur during activities that simulate life experiences.
	4. Encourage client to discuss situations that have been especially stressful and to explore the feelings associated with those times.	4. Verbalization of feelings in a nonthreatening environment may help client come to terms with unresolved issues that may be contributing to the dissociative process.
	5. Identify specific conflicts that remain unresolved, and assist client to identify possible solutions. Provide instruction regarding more adaptive ways to respond to anxiety.	5. Unless these underlying conflicts are resolved, any improvement in coping behaviors must be viewed as temporary.

Nursing Diagnosis: INEFFECTIVE COPING

Related to: Severe psychosocial stressor or substance abuse and repressed severe anxiety

Evidenced by: Sudden travel away from home with inability to recall previous identity

Outcome Criteria	Nursing Interventions	Rationale
Client will demonstrate more adaptive ways of coping in stressful situations than resorting to dissociation.	1. Reassure client of safety and security through your presence. Dissociative behaviors may be frightening to the client.	1. Presence of a trusted individual provides feeling of security and assurance of freedom from harm.
	2. Identify stressor that precipitated severe anxiety.	2. This information is necessary for the development of an effective plan of client care and problem resolution.
	3. Explore feelings that client experienced in response to the stressor. Help client understand that the disequilibrium felt is acceptable in times of severe stress.	3. Client's self-esteem is preserved by the knowledge that others may experience these behaviors under similar circumstances.
	4. As anxiety level decreases and memory returns, use exploration and an accepting, nonthreatening environment to encourage client to identify repressed traumatic experiences that contribute to chronic anxiety.	4. Client must confront and deal with painful issues to achieve resolution.
	5. Have client identify methods of coping with stress in the past and determine whether the response was adaptive or maladaptive.	5. In times of extreme anxiety, client is unable to evaluate appropriateness of response. This information is necessary for client to develop a plan of action for the future.
	6. Help client define more adaptive coping strategies. Make suggestions of alternatives that might be tried. Examine benefits and consequences of each alternative. Assist client in the selection of those that are most appropriate.	6. Depending on current level of anxiety, client may require assistance with problem solving and decision making.
	7. Provide positive reinforcement for client's attempts to change.	7. Positive reinforcement enhances self-esteem and encourages repetition of desired behaviors.
	8. Identify community resources individual may use for support if past maladaptive coping patterns return.	8. Knowledge alone that this type of support exists may provide the client with a feeling of security. Use of the resources may help to keep the client from decompensating.

Nursing Diagnosis: DISTURBED PERSONAL IDENTITY
Related to: Childhood trauma/abuse
Evidenced by: The presence of more than one personality within the individual

Outcome Criteria	Nursing Interventions	Rationale
Client will verbalize understanding about the existence of multiple personalities in the self, the reason for their existence, and the importance of eventual integration of the personalities into one.	1. The nurse must develop a trusting relationship with the original personality and with each of the subpersonalities.	1. Trust is the basis of a therapeutic relationship. Each of the personalities views itself as a separate entity and must initially be treated as such.
	2. Help client understand the existence of the subpersonalities and the need each serves in the personal identity of the individual.	2. Client may initially be unaware of the dissociative response. Knowledge of the needs each personality fulfills is the first step in the integration process.
	3. Help client identify stressful situations that precipitate transition from one personality to another. Carefully observe and record these transitions.	3. Identification of stressors is required to assist client in responding more adaptively and to eliminate the need for transition to another personality.
	4. Use nursing interventions necessary to deal with maladaptive behaviors associated with individual subpersonalities. For example, if one personality is suicidal, precautions must be taken to guard against client's self-harm. If another personality has a tendency toward physical hostility, precautions must be taken to protect others.	4. The safety of client and others is a nursing priority.
	5. Help subpersonalities to understand that their "being" will not be destroyed but will be integrated into a unified identity within the individual.	5. Because subpersonalities function as separate entities, the idea of total elimination generates fear and defensiveness.
	6. Provide support during disclosure of painful experiences and reassurance when client becomes discouraged with lengthy treatment.	6. Positive reinforcement may encourage repetition of desirable behaviors.

Nursing Diagnosis: DISTURBED SENSORY PERCEPTION (VISUAL/KINESTHETIC)
Related to: Severe psychological stress and repression of anxiety
Evidenced by: Alteration in the perception or experience of the self or the environment

Outcome Criteria	Nursing Interventions	Rationale
Client will demonstrate the ability to perceive stimuli correctly and maintain a sense of reality during stressful situations.	1. Provide support and encouragement during times of depersonalization. Clients manifesting these symptoms may express fear and anxiety at experiencing such behaviors. They do not understand the response and may express a fear of going insane.	1. Support and encouragement from a trusted individual provide a feeling of security when fears and anxieties are manifested.
	2. Explain the depersonalization behaviors and the purpose they usually serve for the client.	2. This knowledge may help to minimize fears and anxieties associated with their occurrence.
	3. Explain the relationship between severe anxiety and depersonalization behaviors. Help relate these behaviors to times of severe psychological stress that client has experienced.	3. The client may be unaware that the occurrence of depersonalization behaviors is related to severe anxiety. Knowledge of this relationship is the first step in the process of behavioral change.
	4. Explore past experiences and possibly repressed painful situations, such as trauma or abuse.	4. Traumatic experiences may predispose individuals to dissociative disorders.
	5. Discuss these painful experiences with client, and encourage him or her to deal with the feelings associated with these situations. Work to resolve the conflicts these repressed feelings have nurtured.	5. Conflict resolution will serve to decrease the need for the dissociative response to anxiety.
	6. Discuss ways the client may more adaptively respond to stress, and use role-play to practice these new methods.	6. Having practiced through role-play helps to prepare client to face stressful situations by using these new behaviors when they occur in real life.

facilitated by gathering information using the following types of questions:

1. Has the client's memory been restored?
2. Can the client connect occurrence of psychological stress to loss of memory?
3. Does the client discuss fears and anxieties with members of the staff in an effort toward resolution?
4. Can the client discuss the presence of various personalities within the self?
5. Can he or she verbalize why these personalities exist?
6. Can the client verbalize situations that precipitate transition from one personality to another?
7. Can the client maintain a sense of reality during stressful situations?
8. Can the client verbalize a correlation between stressful situations and the onset of depersonalization behaviors?
9. Can the client demonstrate more adaptive coping strategies for dealing with stress without resorting to dissociation?

MEDICAL TREATMENT MODALITIES

Dissociative Amnesia

Many cases of dissociative amnesia resolve spontaneously when the individual is removed from the stressful situation. For other more refractory conditions, intravenous administration of amobarbital is useful in the retrieval of lost memories. Most clinicians recommend supportive psychotherapy also to reinforce adjustment to the psychological impact of the retrieved memories and the emotions associated with them.

In some instances, psychotherapy is used as the primary treatment. Techniques of persuasion and free or directed association are used to help the client remember. In other cases, hypnosis may be required to mobilize the memories. Once the memories are obtained through hypnosis, psychotherapy may be employed to help the client integrate the memories into his or her conscious state (Sadock & Sadock, 2003).

Dissociative Fugue

Recovery from dissociative fugue is usually rapid, spontaneous, and complete. Treatment is similar to that of dissociative amnesia (Sadock & Sadock, 2003). In some instances, manipulation of the environment or psychotherapeutic support may help to diminish stress or help the client adapt to stress in the future.

When the fugue is prolonged, techniques of gentle encouragement, persuasion, or directed association may be helpful, alone or in combination with hypnosis or amobarbital interviews.

Dissociative Identity Disorder

The goal of therapy for the client with DID is to optimize the client's function and potential. The achievement of **integration** (a blending of all the personalities into one) is usually considered desirable, but in some cases, resolution or a smooth collaboration among the subpersonalities may be all that is realistic (Kluft, 1991).

Intensive, long-term psychotherapy with the DID client is directed toward uncovering the underlying psychological conflicts, helping him or her gain insight into these conflicts, and striving to synthesize the various identities into one integrated personality. Clients are assisted to recall past traumas in detail. They must mentally reexperience the abuse that caused their illness. This process, called **abreaction**, or "remembering with feeling," is so painful that clients sometimes scream, sob, and flail about, just as they did during the actual event (Gupta, 1990).

During therapy, each personality is actively explored and encouraged to become aware of the others across previously amnestic barriers. Traumatic memories associated with the different personality manifestations, especially those related to childhood abuse, are examined.

Kluft (1991) identifies the following elements of therapy for the person with DID:

1. Establish an atmosphere of safety and security in which to initiate treatment.
2. Identify the relationships among subpersonalities, and work with each personality equally.
3. Provide each personality with information about its role in the dissociated system.
4. Encourage awareness, communication, empathy, and cooperation among personalities.
5. Process events associated with the origins of the disorder.
6. Incorporate new coping skills to replace dissociation behaviors.
7. Do not assume that the course of treatment will be smooth. The course of treatment is often difficult and anxiety provoking to client and therapist alike,

especially when aggressive or suicidal personalities are in the dominant role. When this occurs, it may be necessary to hospitalize the client for brief periods until emotional stabilization has been achieved.

When integration is achieved, the individual becomes a total of all the feelings, experiences, memories, skills, and talents that were previously in the command of the various personalities. He or she learns how to function effectively without the necessity for creating new personalities to cope with life. This is possible only after years of intense psychotherapy, and even then, recovery is often incomplete.

Depersonalization Disorder

Information about the treatment of depersonalization disorder is sparse and inconclusive. Various regimens have been tried, although none have proven widely successful. Anxiolytics provide symptomatic relief if anxiety is an important element of the clinical condition (Sadock & Sadock, 2003). If other psychiatric disorders, such as schizophrenia, are evident, they too may be treated pharmacologically. A study by Simeon, Stein, and Hollander (1998) found the antidepressant clomipramine (Anafranil) to be a promising pharmacological treatment for primary depersonalization disorder. For clients with evident intrapsychic conflict, analytically oriented insight psychotherapy may be useful. Specific recommendations for the management of depersonalization disorder must await extensive clinical investigation.

SUMMARY

Psychophysiological disorders, somatoform disorders, and dissociative disorders are associated with anxiety that occurs at the moderate to severe level. The anxiety is repressed and manifested in the form of symptoms and behaviors associated with these disorders.

Psychophysiological disorders are those in which psychological factors contribute to the initiation or exacerbation of the physical condition. There is evidence of demonstrable organic pathology, or a known pathophysiological process involved. The *DSM-IV-TR* (APA, 2000) identifies this category as "psychological factors affecting medical condition." Types of psychological factors identified by the *DSM-IV-TR* include mental disorders, psychological symptoms, personality traits or coping styles, maladaptive health behaviors, stress-related physiological responses, and others.

Virtually any organic disorder can be considered psychophysiological. The following disorders were discussed in this chapter:

- Asthma
- Cancer
- Coronary heart disease
- Essential hypertension
- Migraine headache
- Peptic ulcer disease
- Rheumatoid arthritis
- Ulcerative colitis

Somatoform disorders, known historically as hysteria, affect about 1 percent of the female population. Types of somatoform disorders include somatization disorder, pain disorder, hypochondriasis, conversion disorder, and body dysmorphic disorder.

Somatization disorder is manifested by physical symptoms that may be vague, dramatized, or exaggerated in their presentation. No evidence of organic pathology can be identified. In pain disorder, the predominant symptom is pain for which either there is no medical explanation or for which the symptom is exaggerated out of proportion to what would be the expected reaction. Hypochondriasis is an unrealistic preoccupation with fear of having a serious illness. This disorder may follow a personal experience, or the experience of a close family member with serious or life-threatening illness.

The individual with conversion disorder experiences a loss of or alteration in bodily functioning, unsubstantiated by medical or pathophysiological explanation. Psychological factors are evident by the primary or secondary gains the individual achieves from experiencing the physiological manifestation. A relative lack of concern regarding the symptom is identified as "la belle indifference."

Body dysmorphic disorder, formerly called dysmorphophobia, is the exaggerated belief that the body is deformed or defective in some way. It may be related to serious psychiatric illness.

A dissociative response has been described as a defense mechanism to protect the ego in the face of overwhelming anxiety. Dissociative responses result in an alteration in the normally integrative functions of identity, memory, or consciousness. Classification of dissociative disorders includes dissociative amnesia,

a. "I don't want to hear about another physical complaint. You know they are all in your head. It's time for group therapy now."
b. "Let's sit down here together and you can tell me about this new pain you are experiencing. You'll just have to miss group therapy today."
c. "I will report this pain to your physician. In the meantime, group therapy starts in 5 minutes. You must leave now to be on time."
d. "I will call your physician and see if he will order a new pain medication for your side. The one you have now doesn't seem to provide relief. Why don't you get some rest for now?"

Situation: Ellen, age 32 years, was diagnosed as having DID at age 28. Since that time she has been in therapy with a psychiatrist, who has detected the presence of 12 personalities and identified a history of childhood abuse. Yesterday, Beth, the personality with suicidal ideations, swallowed a bottle of 20 alprazolam (Xanax) pills. Ellen's roommate found her when she returned from work and called the emergency medical service. She was stabilized in the emergency department, and 48 hours later, she was transferred to the psychiatric unit.

12. The primary nursing diagnosis for Ellen would be:
    a. Disturbed personal identity related to childhood abuse
    b. Disturbed sensory perception related to repressed anxiety
    c. Disturbed thought processes related to memory deficit
    d. Risk for suicide related to unresolved grief

13. In establishing trust with Ellen, the nurse must:
    a. Try to relate to Ellen as though she did not have multiple personalities
    b. Establish a relationship with each of the personalities separately
    c. Ignore behaviors that Ellen attributes to Beth
    d. Explain to Ellen that he or she will work with her only if she maintains the status of the primary personality

14. The ultimate goal of therapy for Ellen is:
    a. Integration of the personalities into one
    b. For her to have the ability to switch from one personality to another voluntarily
    c. For her to select which personality she wants to be her dominant self
    d. For her to recognize that the various personalities exist

15. Which of the following is an appropriate nursing intervention for controlling the behavior of the "suicidal personality," Beth?
    a. When Beth emerges, put the client in restraints.
    b. Keep Ellen in isolation during her hospitalization.
    c. Make a verbal contract with Ellen that Beth will do no harm.
    d. Elicit the help of another, strong-willed personality to help control Beth's behavior.

REVIEW QUESTIONS

SELF-EXAMINATION/LEARNING EXERCISE

Match each of the following psychophysiological disorders to the psychosocial profile with which it has been associated:

_______ 1. Asthma	a. Competitive; aggressive; ambitious; no time for leisure; never satisfied with accomplishments; easily aroused hostility
_______ 2. Cancer	b. Obsessive-compulsive by nature; anxious; rigid; excessively neat; repressed anger; depression is common
_______ 3. Coronary heart disease	c. Excessive dependency needs; personality traits include many fears, emotional lability, anxiety, and depression
_______ 4. Peptic ulcer disease	d. Unfulfilled dependency needs; excessive worriers; anxiety and depression common; increased gastric secretion in presence of hostility and frustration
_______ 5. Essential hypertension	e. Perfectionistic; somewhat rigid; compulsive; sets unrealistic expectations; suppresses or represses anger
_______ 6. Migraine headache	f. "The nice guy"; suppresses anger; low self-esteem; depression is common; feelings of hopelessness
_______ 7. Rheumatoid arthritis	g. Appears to be congenial and compliant; does not express anger openly, but suppresses a great deal of internal rage
_______ 8. Ulcerative colitis	h. Self-sacrificing; inhibited; perfectionistic; repressed anger; onset of symptoms may be associated with loss of a loved one

Select the answer that is most appropriate for each of the following questions:

Situation: Lorraine is a frequent visitor to the outpatient clinic. She has been diagnosed with somatization disorder.

9. Which of the following symptom profiles would you expect when assessing Lorraine?
   a. Multiple somatic symptoms in several body systems
   b. Fear of having a serious disease
   c. Loss or alteration in sensorimotor functioning
   d. Belief that her body is deformed or defective in some way

10. Nursing care for Lorraine would focus on helping her to:
   a. Eliminate the stress in her life
   b. Discontinue her numerous physical complaints
   c. Take her medication only as prescribed
   d. Learn more adaptive coping strategies

11. Lorraine tells the nurse about a pain in her side. She says she has not experienced it before. Which is the most appropriate response by the nurse?

a. "I don't want to hear about another physical complaint. You know they are all in your head. It's time for group therapy now."
b. "Let's sit down here together and you can tell me about this new pain you are experiencing. You'll just have to miss group therapy today."
c. "I will report this pain to your physician. In the meantime, group therapy starts in 5 minutes. You must leave now to be on time."
d. "I will call your physician and see if he will order a new pain medication for your side. The one you have now doesn't seem to provide relief. Why don't you get some rest for now?"

Situation: Ellen, age 32 years, was diagnosed as having DID at age 28. Since that time she has been in therapy with a psychiatrist, who has detected the presence of 12 personalities and identified a history of childhood abuse. Yesterday, Beth, the personality with suicidal ideations, swallowed a bottle of 20 alprazolam (Xanax) pills. Ellen's roommate found her when she returned from work and called the emergency medical service. She was stabilized in the emergency department, and 48 hours later, she was transferred to the psychiatric unit.

12. The primary nursing diagnosis for Ellen would be:
    a. Disturbed personal identity related to childhood abuse
    b. Disturbed sensory perception related to repressed anxiety
    c. Disturbed thought processes related to memory deficit
    d. Risk for suicide related to unresolved grief

13. In establishing trust with Ellen, the nurse must:
    a. Try to relate to Ellen as though she did not have multiple personalities
    b. Establish a relationship with each of the personalities separately
    c. Ignore behaviors that Ellen attributes to Beth
    d. Explain to Ellen that he or she will work with her only if she maintains the status of the primary personality

14. The ultimate goal of therapy for Ellen is:
    a. Integration of the personalities into one
    b. For her to have the ability to switch from one personality to another voluntarily
    c. For her to select which personality she wants to be her dominant self
    d. For her to recognize that the various personalities exist

15. Which of the following is an appropriate nursing intervention for controlling the behavior of the "suicidal personality," Beth?
    a. When Beth emerges, put the client in restraints.
    b. Keep Ellen in isolation during her hospitalization.
    c. Make a verbal contract with Ellen that Beth will do no harm.
    d. Elicit the help of another, strong-willed personality to help control Beth's behavior.

especially when aggressive or suicidal personalities are in the dominant role. When this occurs, it may be necessary to hospitalize the client for brief periods until emotional stabilization has been achieved.

When integration is achieved, the individual becomes a total of all the feelings, experiences, memories, skills, and talents that were previously in the command of the various personalities. He or she learns how to function effectively without the necessity for creating new personalities to cope with life. This is possible only after years of intense psychotherapy, and even then, recovery is often incomplete.

Depersonalization Disorder

Information about the treatment of depersonalization disorder is sparse and inconclusive. Various regimens have been tried, although none have proven widely successful. Anxiolytics provide symptomatic relief if anxiety is an important element of the clinical condition (Sadock & Sadock, 2003). If other psychiatric disorders, such as schizophrenia, are evident, they too may be treated pharmacologically. A study by Simeon, Stein, and Hollander (1998) found the antidepressant clomipramine (Anafranil) to be a promising pharmacological treatment for primary depersonalization disorder. For clients with evident intrapsychic conflict, analytically oriented insight psychotherapy may be useful. Specific recommendations for the management of depersonalization disorder must await extensive clinical investigation.

SUMMARY

Psychophysiological disorders, somatoform disorders, and dissociative disorders are associated with anxiety that occurs at the moderate to severe level. The anxiety is repressed and manifested in the form of symptoms and behaviors associated with these disorders.

Psychophysiological disorders are those in which psychological factors contribute to the initiation or exacerbation of the physical condition. There is evidence of demonstrable organic pathology, or a known pathophysiological process involved. The *DSM-IV-TR* (APA, 2000) identifies this category as "psychological factors affecting medical condition." Types of psychological factors identified by the *DSM-IV-TR* include mental disorders, psychological symptoms, personality traits or coping styles, maladaptive health behaviors, stress-related physiological responses, and others.

Virtually any organic disorder can be considered psychophysiological. The following disorders were discussed in this chapter:

- Asthma
- Cancer
- Coronary heart disease
- Essential hypertension
- Migraine headache
- Peptic ulcer disease
- Rheumatoid arthritis
- Ulcerative colitis

Somatoform disorders, known historically as hysteria, affect about 1 percent of the female population. Types of somatoform disorders include somatization disorder, pain disorder, hypochondriasis, conversion disorder, and body dysmorphic disorder.

Somatization disorder is manifested by physical symptoms that may be vague, dramatized, or exaggerated in their presentation. No evidence of organic pathology can be identified. In pain disorder, the predominant symptom is pain for which either there is no medical explanation or for which the symptom is exaggerated out of proportion to what would be the expected reaction. Hypochondriasis is an unrealistic preoccupation with fear of having a serious illness. This disorder may follow a personal experience, or the experience of a close family member with serious or life-threatening illness.

The individual with conversion disorder experiences a loss of or alteration in bodily functioning, unsubstantiated by medical or pathophysiological explanation. Psychological factors are evident by the primary or secondary gains the individual achieves from experiencing the physiological manifestation. A relative lack of concern regarding the symptom is identified as "la belle indifference."

Body dysmorphic disorder, formerly called dysmorphophobia, is the exaggerated belief that the body is deformed or defective in some way. It may be related to serious psychiatric illness.

A dissociative response has been described as a defense mechanism to protect the ego in the face of overwhelming anxiety. Dissociative responses result in an alteration in the normally integrative functions of identity, memory, or consciousness. Classification of dissociative disorders includes dissociative amnesia, dissociative fugue, dissociative identity disorder, and depersonalization disorder.

The individual with dissociative amnesia is unable to recall important personal information that is too extensive to be explained by ordinary forgetfulness. Dissociative fugue is characterized by a sudden, unexpected travel away from home with an inability to recall the past, including personal identity. Duration of the fugue is usually brief, and once it is over the individual recovers memory of the past life but is amnestic for the time covered by the fugue. The prominent feature of DID is the existence of two or more personalities within a single individual. An individual may have many personalities, each of which serves a purpose for that individual of enduring painful stimuli that the original personality is too weak to face. Depersonalization disorder is characterized by an alteration in the perception of oneself (sometimes described as a feeling of having separated from the body and watching the activities of the self from a distance).

Nursing care of individuals with anxiety-related disorders is accomplished using the steps of the nursing process. Background assessment data was presented, along with nursing diagnoses common to each disorder. Interventions appropriate to each nursing diagnosis and relevant outcome criteria for each were included. An overview of current medical treatment modalities was discussed.

Nurses can assist clients with these disorders by helping them to understand their problem, and identify and establish new, more adaptive behavior patterns.

Test Your CRITICAL THINKING SKILLS

Sam was admitted to the psychiatric unit from the emergency department of a general hospital in the Midwest. The owner of a local bar called the police when Sam suddenly seemed to "lose control. He just went ballistic." The police reported that Sam did not know where he was or how he got there. He kept saying, "My name is John Brown, and I live in Philadelphia." When the police ran an identity check on Sam, they found that he was indeed John Brown from Philadelphia and his wife had reported him missing a month ago. Mrs. Brown explained that about 12 months before his disappearance, her husband, who was a shop supervisor at a large manufacturing plant, had been having considerable difficulty at work. He had been passed over for a promotion, and his supervisor had been very critical of his work. Several of his staff had left the company for other jobs, and without enough help, Sam had been unable to meet shop deadlines. Work stress made him very difficult to live with at home. Previously an easygoing, extroverted individual, he became withdrawn and extremely critical of his wife and children. Immediately preceding his disappearance, he had had a violent argument with his 18-year-old son, who called Sam a "loser" and stormed out of the house to stay with some friends. Sam disappeared the following day. The psychiatrist assigns a diagnosis of dissociative fugue.

Answer the following questions related to Sam:

1. Describe the *priority* nursing intervention with Sam as he is admitted to the psychiatric unit.
2. What approach should be taken to help Sam with his problem?
3. What is the long-term goal of therapy for Sam?

IMPLICATIONS OF RESEARCH FOR EVIDENCE BASED PRACTICE

Ford, D.E., Mead, L.A., Chang, P.P., Cooper-Patrick, L., Wang, N.Y., & Klag, M.J: **Depression is a risk factor for coronary artery disease in men: The precursor study.** Archives of Internal Medicine (1998, July 13); 158:1422–1426.

Description of the Study: This study was conducted to determine if clinical depression is an independent risk factor for coronary artery disease. The subjects included 1,190 male Johns Hopkins medical students enrolled between 1948 and 1964. The subjects were followed through 1995 and assessed on family history, health behaviors, and clinical depression. At baseline, the subjects showed no significant differences in the prevalence of known cardiac risk factors. Follow-up studies for cardiovascular disease were assessed with reviews of annual questionnaires, National Death Index searches, medical records, death certificates, and autopsy reports.

Results of the Study: The cumulative incidence of clinical depression in the medical students at 40 years of follow up (assessed by self-reported symptoms, diagnoses, and treatments) was 12 percent. Multivariate analyses indicated that the men who reported clinical depression were twice as likely to develop coronary heart disease or suffer a myocardial infarction (MI) than the nondepressed men. The increased risk for MI was shown to persist for up to 10 years after onset of the first depressive episode.

Implications for Nursing Practice: The authors state that several studies have found depression to be an important predictor of poor outcome after the onset of coronary artery disease. This study finds that clinical depression may be an independent risk factor for coronary artery disease. The actual mechanism by which this occurs is speculative. It has been suggested that changes in the autonomic nervous system and increased platelet reactivity that occurs in clinical depression may play a role. The results of this study provide justification for consideration of clinical depression in the prevention and treatment of coronary artery disease in men. Nurses working in cardiology and other medical-surgical areas should include assessment for depression in their initial interviews. Treatment of depression may decrease risk of cardiac disease in some individuals.

INTERNET REFERENCES

- Additional information about psychophysiological disorders discussed in this chapter may be located at the following websites:

a http://www.nci.nih.gov

b http://www.cancer.org

c http://www.americanheart.org/

d http://www.headaches.org/

e http://www.pslgroup.com/ASTHMA.HTM

f http://www.gastro.org/

g http://www.pslgroup.com/HYPERTENSION.HTM

h http://content.health.msn.com/condition_center/rha

i http://www.niddk.nih.gov/health/digest/pubs/colitis/colitis.htm

- Additional information about somatoform disorders may be located at the following websites:

  a http://www.psyweb.com/Mdisord/somatd.html

  b http://www.uib.no/med/avd/med_a/gastro/wilhelms/hypochon.html

  c http://www.emedicine.com/EMERG/topic112.htm

  d http://www.findarticles.com/cf_dis/g2601/0012/2601001276/p1/article.jhtml

- Additional information about dissociative disorders may be located at the following websites:

  a http://www.human-nature.com/odmh/dissociative.html

  b http://www.nami.org/helpline/dissoc.htm

  c http://www.voiceofwomen.com/VOW2_11950/center.html

  d http://www.issd.org/

  e http://www.findarticles.com/cf_dis/g2601/0004/2601000438/p1/article.jhtml

REFERENCES

Abraham, T. (1995). Management of persons with dysrhythmias and coronary artery disease. In W. J. Phipps, V.L. Cassmeyer, J.K. Sands, & M.K. Lehman (Eds.), Medical-surgical nursing (5th ed.). St. Louis: Mosby.

American Heart Association (2002). Blood pressure levels. Retrieved April 13, 2002 from http://216.185.112.5/presenter.jhtml?identifier=4450.

American Psychiatric Association (APA). (2000). Diagnostic and statistical manual of mental disorders (4th ed.) Text revision. Washington, DC: American Psychiatric Association.

Anderson, K.L. (1991). Obstructive respiratory disorders. In M.L. Patrick, S.L. Woods, R.F. Craven, J.S. Rokovsky, & P.M. Bruno (Eds.), Medical-surgical nursing (2nd ed.). Philadelphia: J.B. Lippincott.

Cleveland Clinic. (2001). What is asthma? Retrieved March 31, 2002 from http://content.health.msn.com/content/article/1660.51094?z=1660_51062_6507_00_03

Cloninger, C.R. (1994). Somatoform and dissociative disorders. In G.Winokur & P.J. Clayton (Eds.), The medical basis of psychiatry (2nd ed.). Philadelphia: W.B. Saunders.

Cunningham, S.L. (1991). Hypertension. In M.L. Patrick, S.L. Woods, R.F. Craven, J.S. Rokovsky, & P.M. Bruno (Eds.), Medical-surgical nursing (2nd ed.). Philadelphia: J.B. Lippincott.

Das, K. (2002). Ulcerative colitis research: In search of the target autoantigen(s). Retrieved on April 2, 2002 from http://ibd.patientcommunity.com/features/das.cfm

Gupta, N.E. (1990, March). Who am I? Ladies Home Journal, CVII (3): 161, 233–237.

Hafen, B.Q., Karren, K.J., Frandsen, K.J., & Smith, N.L. (1996). Mind/body health: The effects of attitudes, emotions, and relationships. Boston: Allyn & Bacon.

Kaplan, H.I. & Sadock, B.J. (1998). Synopsis of psychiatry: Behavioral sciences/clinical psychiatry (8th ed.). Baltimore: Williams & Wilkins.

King, S. A. (1999). Pain disorders. In R.E. Hales and S.C. Yudofsky (Eds.), Essentials of clinical psychiatry. Washington, DC: American Psychiatric Press.

Kluft, R.P. (1991). Multiple personality disorder. In A. Tasman & S.M. Goldfinger (Eds.), American Psychiatric Press review of psychiatry, Vol. 10. Washington, DC: American Psychiatric Press.

Levenson, J. L. (2003). Psychological factors affecting medical conditions. In R.E. Hales & S.C. Yudofsky (Eds.), Textbook of clinical psychiatry (4th ed). Washington, DC: American Psychiatric Publishing.

Maldonado, J.R. & Spiegel, D. (2003). Dissociative Disorders. In R.E. Hales & S.C. Yudofsky (Eds.), Textbook of clinical psychiatry (4th ed.). Washington, DC: American Psychiatric Publishing.

National Cancer Institute (2002a). U.S. Cancer Death Rate 1992–1998: All races, both sexes. Retrieved April 1, 2002 from http://newscenter.cancer.gov/pressreleases/reportq&a.html

National Cancer Institute (2002b). Racial and ethnic patterns of cancer in the United States. Retrieved April 1, 2002 from http://seer.cancer.gov/Publications/REPoC/allsites.pdf

National Digestive Diseases Information Clearinghouse (2002). Ulcerative Colitis. Retrieved April 2, 2002 from http://www.niddk.nih.gov/health/digest/pubs/colitis/colitis.htm

Pelletier, K.R. (1992). Mind as healer, mind as slayer. New York: Dell.

Robbins, L. & Lang, S.S. (1995). Headache help. Boston: Houghton Mifflin.

Sadock, B.J. & Sadock, V.A. (2003). Synopsis of psychiatry: Behavioral sciences/clinical psychiatry (9th ed.). Philadelphia: Lippincott Williams & Wilkins.

Sands, J.K. (1995a). Management of persons with problems of the stomach and duodenum. In W.J. Phipps, V.L. Cassmeyer, J.K. Sands, & M.K. Lehman (Eds.), Medical-surgical nursing (5th ed.). St. Louis: Mosby.

Sands, J.K. (1995b). Management of persons with problems of the intestines. In W.J. Phipps, V.L. Cassmeyer, J.K. Sands, & M.K. Lehman (Eds.), Medical-surgical nursing (5th ed.). St. Louis: Mosby.

Schenk, E. (1995). Management of persons with problems of the brain. In W.J. Phipps, V.L. Cassmeyer, J.K. Sands, & M.K. Lehman (Eds.), Medical-surgical nursing (5th ed.). St. Louis: Mosby.

Simmons, L.M. & Heitkemper, M. (1991). Ulcers of the gastrointestinal tract. In M.L. Patrick, S.L. Woods, R.F. Craven, J.S. Rokovsky, & P. M. Bruno (Eds.), Medical-surgical nursing (2nd ed.). Philadelphia: J.B. Lippincott.

Soares, N. and Grossman, L. (2001, September 14). Somatoform disorder: Conversion. Emedicine Journal, 2(9). Retrieved March 15, 2002 from http://www.emedicine.com/PED/topic2780.htm

Sobel, D.S. & Ornstein, R. (1996). The healthy mind healthy body handbook. New York: Patient Education Media.

Spiegel, D. & Maldonado, J.R. (1999). Dissociative disorders. In R.E. Hales & S.C. Yudofsky (Eds.), Essentials of clinical psychiatry. Washington, DC: American Psychiatric Press.
Walsh, M.E. (1995). Management of persons with vascular problems. In W.J. Phipps, V.L. Cassmeyer, J.K. Sands, & M.K. Lehman (Eds.), Medical-surgical nursing (5th ed.). St. Louis: Mosby.
Waziri, R. (1994). The amnestic syndrome. In G. Winokur and P.J. Clayton (Eds.), The medical basis of psychiatry (2nd ed.). Philadelphia: W.B. Saunders.
Woods, S.L., Underhill, S.L., & Cowan, M. (1991). Coronary heart disease: Myocardial ischemia and infarction. In M.L. Patrick, S.L. Woods, R.F. Craven, J.S. Rokovsky, & P. M. Bruno (Eds.), Medical-surgical nursing (2nd ed.). Philadelphia: J.B. Lippincott.
Yutzy, S.H. (2003). Somatoform disorders. In R.E. Hales & S.C. Yudofsky (Eds.), Textbook of clinical psychiatry (4th ed.). Washington, DC: American Psychiatric Publishing.

CLASSICAL REFERENCES

Freud, S. (1962). The neuro-psychoses of defense. In J. Strachey (Ed.), Standard edition of the complete psychological works of Sigmund Freud, vol. 3. London: Hogarth Press. (Original work published 1984).
Friedman, M. & Rosenman, R.H. (1974). Type A behavior and your heart. New York: Alfred A. Knopf.
Peplau, H. (1963). A working definition of anxiety. In S. Burd & M. Marshall (Eds.), Some clinical approaches to psychiatric nursing. New York: Macmillan.
Selye, H. (1976). The stress of life. New York: McGraw-Hill.

18

CHAPTER

Disorders of Human Sexuality

CHAPTER OUTLINE

KEY TERMS

anorgasmia
dyspareunia
exhibitionism
fetishism
frotteurism
voyeurism
homosexuality
lesbian
masochism
paraphilia
orgasm
pedophilia
premature ejaculation
retarded ejaculation
sadism
sensate focus
transsexualism
transvestic fetishism
vaginismus

OBJECTIVES

After reading this chapter, the student will be able to:

1. Describe developmental processes associated with human sexuality.
2. Discuss historical and epidemiological aspects of paraphilias and sexual dysfunction disorders.
3. Identify various types of paraphilias and sexual dysfunction disorders.
4. Discuss etiological implications of paraphilias and sexual dysfunction disorders.
5. Formulate nursing diagnoses and goals of care for clients with sexual disorders.
6. Identify appropriate nursing interventions for clients with sexual disorders.
7. Evaluate care of clients with sexual disorders.
8. Describe various medical treatment modalities for clients with sexual disorders.
9. Discuss variations in sexual orientation.
10. Identify various types of sexually transmitted diseases and discuss the consequences of each.

INTRODUCTION

Human beings are sexual beings. Sexuality is a basic human need and an innate part of the total personality. It influences our thoughts, actions, and interactions, and it is involved in aspects of physical and mental health.

Society's attitude toward sexuality is changing. Clients are more open to seeking assistance in matters that pertain to sexuality. Although not all nurses need to be educated as sex therapists, they can readily integrate information on sexuality into the care they give by focusing on preventive, therapeutic, and educational interventions to assist individuals to attain, regain, or maintain sexual wellness.

This chapter focuses on disorders associated with sexual functioning. Primary consideration is given to the categories of **paraphilias** and sexual dysfunction as classified in the *DSM-IV-TR* (American Psychiatric Association [APA], 2000). An overview of human sexual development throughout the life span is presented. Historical and epidemiological information associated with sexual disorders is included. Predisposing factors that have been implicated in the etiology of sexual disorders provide a framework for studying the dynamics of these disorders. Various medical treatment modalities are explored. A discussion of variations in sexual orientation is included. Various types of sexually transmitted diseases (STDs) are described, and an explanation of the consequences of each is presented.

Symptomatology of each disorder is presented as background knowledge for assessing clients with sexual disorders. A tool for acquiring a sexual history is included. Nursing care is described in the context of the nursing process.

DEVELOPMENT OF HUMAN SEXUALITY

Birth Through Age 12

Although the sexual identity of an infant is determined before birth by chromosomal factors and physical appearance of the genitals, postnatal factors can greatly influence the way developing children perceive themselves sexually. Masculinity and femininity, as well as gender roles, are for the most part culturally defined. For example, differentiation of roles may be initiated at birth by painting a child's room pink or blue and by clothing the child in frilly, delicate dresses or tough, sturdy rompers.

It is common for infants to touch and explore their genitals. In fact, research on infantile sexuality indicates that both male and female infants are capable of sexual arousal and **orgasm** (Reinisch, 1990).

By age 2 or 2–1/2 years, children know what gender they are. They know that they are like the parent of the same gender and different from the parent of the opposite gender and from other children of the opposite gender. They become acutely aware of anatomical sex differences during this time (Clunn, 1991).

By age 4 or 5, children engage in heterosexual play. "Playing doctor" can be a popular game at this age. In this way, children form a concept of marriage to a member of the opposite gender.

Children increasingly gain experience with masturbation during childhood, although certainly not all children masturbate during this period. Most children begin self-exploration and genital self-stimulation at about 15 to 19 months of age (Sadock & Sadock, 2003).

Late childhood and preadolescence may be characterized by homosexual play (Reinisch, 1990). Generally, the activity involves no more than touching the other's genitals. Girls at this age become interested in menstruation, and both sexes are interested in learning about fertility, pregnancy, and birth. Interest in the opposite sex increases. Children of this age become self-conscious about their bodies and are concerned with physical attractiveness.

Children ages 10 to 12 are preoccupied with pubertal changes and the beginnings of romantic interest in the opposite gender. Prepubescent boys may engage in group sexual activities such as genital exhibition or group masturbation. Homosexual sex play is common. Prepubescent girls may engage in some genital exhibition, but they are usually not as preoccupied with the genitalia as are boys of this age (Reinisch, 1990).

Adolescence

Adolescence represents acceleration in terms of biological changes and psychosocial and sexual development. This time of turmoil is nurtured by awakening endocrine forces and a new set of psychosocial tasks to undertake (Bell, 1998). Included in these tasks are issues relating to sexuality, such as how to deal with new or more powerful sexual feelings, whether to participate in various types of sexual behavior, how to recognize love, how to prevent unwanted pregnancy, and how to define age-appropriate sex roles.

Biologically, puberty begins for the female adolescent with breast enlargement, widening of the hips, and growth of pubic and ancillary hair. The onset of menstruation usually occurs between the ages of 11 and 13 years. In the male adolescent, growth of pubic hair and enlargement of the testicles begin at 12 to 16 years of age. Penile growth and the ability to ejaculate usually occur from the ages of 13 to 17. There is a marked growth of the body between ages 11 and 17, accompanied by the growth of body and facial hair, increased muscle mass, and a deeper voice.

Sexuality is slower to develop in the female than in the male adolescent. Women show steady increases in sexual responsiveness that peak in their middle 20s or early 30s. Sexual maturity for men is usually reached in the late teens, but their sexual drive remains high through young adulthood (Murray & Zentner, 2001). Masturbation is a common sexual activity among male adolescents. Approximately 60 to 90 percent of adolescent boys and 40 percent of adolescent girls masturbate (Slap, 1998).

Many individuals have their first experience with sexual intercourse during the adolescent years. Although studies indicate a variety of statistics related to incidence of adolescent coitus, three notable trends have become evident during the past two decades. According to Sadock and Sadock (2003), the trends are as follows:

1. More adolescents are engaging in premarital intercourse.
2. The incidence of premarital intercourse for girls has increased.
3. The average age of first intercourse is decreasing.

The American culture has ambivalent feelings toward adolescent sexuality. Psychosexual development is desired, but most parents want to avoid anything that may encourage teenage sex. The rise in number of cases of STDs, some of which are life-threatening, also contributes to fears associated with unprotected sexual activity in all age groups.

Adulthood

This period of the life cycle begins at approximately 20 years of age and continues to age 65. Sexuality associated with ages 65 and older is discussed in Chapter 23.

Marital Sex

Choosing a marital partner or developing a sexual relationship with another individual is one of the major tasks in the early years of this life-cycle stage. Current cultural perspective reflects that the institution of marriage has survived. Approximately 80 to 90 percent of all people in the United States marry, and of those who divorce, a high percentage remarries. Intimacy in marriage is one of the most common forms of sexual expression for adults. The average American couple has coitus about 2 or 3 times per week when they are in their 20s, with the frequency gradually declining to about once weekly for those aged 45 and over (Sinclair Intimacy Institute, 2002). Many adults continue to masturbate even though they are married and have ready access to heterosexual sex. This behavior is perfectly normal, although it often evokes feelings of guilt and may be kept secret.

Extramarital Sex

Approximately 20 to 30 percent of men have extramarital sex at some time during their marriages compared with about 15 to 20 percent of women (McCarthy & McCarthy, 1998). Although the incidence of extramarital sex for men seems to be holding constant, some evidence exists to suggest that the incidence for women may be increasing.

Although attitudes toward premarital sex have changed substantially during the last several decades, attitudes toward extramarital sex have remained relatively stable. Most women and men say they believe sexual exclusivity should be a goal in marriage, although they were less certain about what would happen if their partner did not live up to that ideal. Some studies place the incidence of divorce caused by infidelity or adultery at around 20 percent of all divorce cases (Reinisch, 1990).

Sex and the Single Person

Attitudes about sexual intimacy among singles—never married, divorced, or widowed—vary from individual to individual. Some single people settle for any kind of relationship, casual or committed, that they believe will enrich their lives. Others deny any desire for marriage or sexual intimacy, cherishing instead the independence they retain by being "unattached." Still others may search desperately for a spouse, with the desperation increasing as the years wear on.

Most divorced men and women return to having an active sex life following separation from their spouse. More widowed men than widowed women return to an active sex life after the loss of their partner. This may have to do in part with the fact that men choose women partners younger than themselves and because widows outnumber widowers by 4 to 1 (Administration on Aging, 2002).

The "Middle" Years—40 to 65

With the advent of the middle years, a decrease in hormonal production initiates a number of changes in the sex organs as well as the rest of the body. The average age of onset of menopause for the woman is around 50, although changes can be noted from about 40 to 60 years of age. Approximately 1 percent of women experience symptoms as early as age 35 (Murray & Zentner, 2001). The decrease in estrogen can result in loss of vaginal lubrication, making intercourse painful. Other symptoms may include insomnia, "hot flashes," headaches, heart palpitations, and depression. Hormonal supplements may alleviate some of these symptoms, although controversy currently exists within the medical community regarding the safety of hormone replacement therapy.

With the decrease of androgen production during these years, men also experience sexual changes. The amount of ejaculate may decrease, and ejaculation may be less forceful. The testes decrease in size, and erections may be less frequent and less rigid. By age 50, the refractory period increases, and men may require 8 to 24 hours after orgasm before another erection can be achieved.

Biological drives decrease, and interest in sexual activity may decrease during these "middle" years. Although men need longer stimulation to reach orgasm and intensity of pleasure may decrease, women stabilize at the same level of sexual activity as at the previous stage in the life cycle and often have a greater capacity for orgasm in middle adulthood than in young adulthood (Sadock & Sadock, 2003). Murray and Zentner (2001) state,

> The enjoyment of sexual relations in younger years, rather than the frequency, is a key factor for maintenance of desire and activity in women, whereas frequency of relations and enjoyment are important factors for men. (p. 690)

SEXUAL DISORDERS

Paraphilias

The term **paraphilia** is used to identify repetitive or preferred sexual fantasies or behaviors that involve any of the following:

1. The preference for use of a nonhuman object
2. Repetitive sexual activity with humans that involves real or simulated suffering or humiliation
3. Repetitive sexual activity with nonconsenting partners

The *DSM-IV-TR* specifies that these sexual fantasies or behaviors are recurrent over a period of at least 6 months and cause the individual significant clinical distress or impairment in social, occupational, or other important areas of functioning (APA, 2000).

Historical Aspects

Historically, some restrictions on human sexual expression have always existed. Under the code of Orthodox Judaism, masturbation was punishable by death. In ancient Catholicism it was considered a carnal sin. In the late 19th century, masturbation was viewed as a major cause of insanity.

The sexual exploitation of children was condemned in ancient cultures, as it continues to be today. Incest remains the one taboo that crosses cultural barriers. It was punishable by death in Babylonia, Judea, and ancient China, and offenders were given the death penalty as late as 1650 in England.

Oral-genital, anal, homosexual, and animal sexual contacts were viewed by the early Christian church as unnatural and were considered greater transgressions than extramarital sexual activity because they did not lead to biological reproduction. Today, of these church-condemned behaviors, only sex with animals (zoophilia) retains the classification as paraphilia in the *DSM-IV-TR.*

Epidemiological Statistics

Relatively few data exist on the prevalence or course of the paraphilias. Most available information has been obtained from studies of incarcerated sex offenders. Another source of information has been from outpatient psychiatric services for paraphiliacs outside the criminal justice system.

Because few paraphiliacs experience personal distress from their behavior, most individuals come for treatment because of pressure from their partners or the authorities (Becker & Johnson, 2003). Data suggest that most people with paraphilias who seek outpatient treatment do so for **pedophilia** (45 percent), **exhibitionism** (25 percent), or **voyeurism** (12 percent).

Most individuals with paraphilias are men, and more than 50 percent of these individuals develop the onset of their paraphilic arousal before age 18 (Sadock & Sadock, 2003). The behavior peaks between ages 15 and 25 and gradually declines so that, by age 50, the occurrence of paraphilic acts is very low, except for those paraphilic behaviors that occur in isolation or with a cooperative partner. Some individuals with these disorders experience multiple paraphilias.

Types of Paraphilias

The following types of paraphilias are identified by the *DSM-IV-TR:*

EXHIBITIONISM. Exhibitionism is characterized by recurrent, intense, sexual urges, behaviors, or sexually arousing fantasies, of at least a 6-month duration, involving the exposure of one's genitals to an unsuspecting stranger (APA, 2000). Masturbation may occur during the exhibitionism. In almost 100 percent of cases of exhibitionism, the perpetrators are men and the victims are women (Sadock & Sadock, 2003).

The urges for genital exposure intensify when the exhibitionist has excessive free time or is under significant stress. Most people who engage in exhibitionism have rewarding sexual relationships with adult partners but concomitantly expose themselves to others.

FETISHISM. **Fetishism** involves recurrent, intense, sexual urges or behaviors, or sexually arousing fantasies, of at least a 6-month duration, involving the use of nonliving objects (APA, 2000). The sexual focus is commonly on objects intimately associated with the human body (e.g., shoes, gloves, stockings) (Sadock & Sadock, 2003). The fetish object is usually used during masturbation or incorporated into sexual activity with another person in order to produce sexual excitation.

When the fetish involves cross-dressing, the disorder is called **transvestic fetishism**. The individual is a heterosexual man who keeps a collection of women's clothing that he intermittently uses to dress in when alone. The sexual arousal may be produced by an accompanying fantasy of the individual as a woman with female genitalia, or merely by the view of himself fully clothed as a woman without attention to the genitalia (APA, 2000).

Requirement of the fetish object for sexual arousal may become so intense in some individuals that to be without it may result in impotence. Onset of the disorder usually occurs during adolescence.

The disorder is chronic, and the complication arises when the individual becomes progressively more intensely aroused by sexual behaviors that exclude a sexual partner. The person with the fetish and his partner may become so distant that the partner eventually terminates the relationship.

FROTTEURISM. **Frotteurism** is the recurrent preoccupation with intense sexual urges, behaviors, or fantasies of at least a 6-month duration involving touching and rubbing against a nonconsenting person (APA, 2000). Sexual excitement is derived from the actual touching or rubbing, not from the coercive nature of the act. Almost without exception, the gender of the frotteur is male.

The individual usually chooses to commit the act in crowded places, such as on buses or subways during rush hour. In this way, he can provide rationalization for his behavior, should someone complain, and can more easily escape arrest. The frotteur waits in a crowd until he identifies a victim, then he follows her and allows the rush of the crowd to push him against her. He fantasizes a relationship with his victim when rubbing his genitals against her thighs and buttocks or touching her genitalia or breasts with his hands. He often escapes detection because of the victim's initial shock and denial that such an act has been committed in a public place.

PEDOPHILIA. The *DSM-IV-TR* describes the essential feature of pedophilia as recurrent sexual urges, behaviors, or sexually arousing fantasies, of at least 6-months duration, involving sexual activity with a prepubescent child. The age of the molester is at least 16, and he or she is at least 5 years older than the child is. This category of paraphilia is the most common of sexual assaults.

Most child molestations involve genital fondling or oral sex. Vaginal or anal penetration of the child is most common in cases of incest. Others may limit their activity to undressing the child and looking, exposing themselves, masturbating in the presence of the child, or gently touching and fondling the child (APA, 2000). Onset usually occurs during adolescence, and the disorder often runs a chronic course, particularly with male pedophiles who demonstrate a preference for little boys.

SEXUAL MASOCHISM. The identifying feature of sexual **masochism** is recurrent, intense, sexual urges, behaviors, or sexually arousing fantasies, of at least a 6-month duration, involving the act (real, not simulated) of being humiliated, beaten, bound, or otherwise made to suffer (APA, 2000). These masochistic activities may be fantasized (e.g., being raped) and may be performed alone (e.g., self-inflicted pain) or with a partner (e.g., being restrained, spanked, or beaten by the partner). Some masochistic activities have resulted in death, in particular those that involve sexual arousal by oxygen deprivation. The disorder is usually chronic and can progress to the point at which the individual cannot achieve sexual satisfaction without masochistic fantasies or activities.

SEXUAL SADISM. The *DSM-IV-TR* identifies the essential feature of sexual **sadism** as recurrent, intense, sexual urges, behaviors, or sexually arousing fantasies, of at least a 6-month duration, involving acts (real, not simulated) in which the psychological or physical suffering (including humiliation) of the victim is sexually exciting to the person (APA, 2000). The sadistic activities may be fantasized or acted on with a consenting or nonconsenting partner. In all instances, sexual excitation occurs in response to the suffering of the victim. Examples of sadistic acts include restraint, beating, burning, rape, cutting, torture, and even killing.

The course of the disorder is usually chronic, with the severity of the sadistic acts often increasing over time. Activities with nonconsenting partners are usually terminated by legal apprehension.

VOYEURISM. This disorder is identified by recurrent, intense, sexual urges, behaviors, or sexually arousing fantasies, of at least a 6-month duration, involving the act of observing an unsuspecting person who is naked, in the process of disrobing, or engaging in sexual activity (APA, 2000). Sexual excitement is achieved through the act of looking, and no contact with the person is attempted. Masturbation usually accompanies the "window peeping" but may occur later as the individual fantasizes about the voyeuristic act.

Onset of voyeuristic behavior is usually before age 15, and the disorder is often chronic. Most voyeurs enjoy satisfying sexual relationships with an adult partner. Few apprehensions occur because most targets of voyeurism are unaware that they are being observed.

Etiological Implications for Paraphilias

BIOLOGICAL FACTORS. Various studies have implicated several organic factors in the etiology of paraphilias. Destruction of parts of the limbic system in animals has been shown to cause hypersexual behavior (Becker & Johnson, 2003). Temporal lobe diseases, such as psychomotor seizures or temporal lobe tumors, have been implicated in some individuals with paraphilias. Abnormal levels of androgens also may contribute to inappropriate sexual arousal. The majority of studies have involved violent sex offenders, and the results cannot accurately be generalized.

PSYCHOANALYTICAL THEORY. The psychoanalytical approach defines a paraphiliac as one who has failed the normal developmental process toward heterosexual adjustment (Sadock & Sadock, 2003). This occurs when the individual fails to resolve the Oedipal crisis and identifies with the parent of the opposite gender or selects an inappropriate object for libido cathexis. Becker and Johnson (2003) offer the following explanation:

> Severe castration anxiety during the Oedipal phase of development leads to the substitution of a symbolic object (inanimate or an anatomic part) for the mother, as in fetishism and transvestitism. Similarly, anxiety over arousal to the mother can lead to the choice of "safe," inappropriate sexual partners, as in pedophilia and zoophilia, or safe sexual behaviors in which there is no sexual contact, as in exhibitionism and voyeurism. (p. 758)

BEHAVIORAL THEORY. The behavioral model hypothesizes that whether or not an individual engages in paraphiliac behavior depends on the type of reinforcement he or she receives following the behavior. The initial act may be committed for various reasons. Some examples include recalling memories of experiences from an individual's early life (especially the first shared sexual experience), modeling behavior of others who have carried out paraphilic acts, mimicking sexual behavior depicted in the media, and recalling past trauma such as one's own molestation (Sadock & Sadock, 2003).

Once the initial act has been committed, the paraphiliac consciously evaluates the behavior and decides whether or not to repeat it. Fear of punishment, or perceived harm or injury to the victim, or a lack of pleasure derived from the experience, may lead to a nonrecurrent act. However, when negative consequences do not occur, when the act itself is highly pleasurable, or when the paraphiliac immediately escapes and thereby avoids seeing negative consequences experienced by the victim, the activity is more likely to be repeated.

THEORETICAL INTEGRATION. Marshall and Barbaree (1990) contend that one model alone is not sufficient to explain the etiology of paraphilias. They suggest that an integration of learning experiences, sociocultural factors, and biological processes must occur to account for these deviant sexual behaviors. A combination of biological inheritance, hormonal variations, poor parenting, sociocultural attitudes, and aspects of the learning paradigm previously described probably provides the most comprehensive etiological explanation for paraphilias to date (Abel, Rouleau, & Osborn, 1994).

Medical Treatment Modalities

BIOLOGICAL TREATMENT. Biological treatment of individuals with paraphilias has focused on blocking or decreasing the level of circulating androgens. The most extensively used of the antiandrogenic medications are the progestin derivatives that block testosterone synthesis or block androgen receptors (Becker & Johnson, 2003). They do not influence the direction of sexual drive toward appropriate adult partners. Instead, they act to decrease libido, and thus break the individual's pattern of compulsive deviant sexual behavior (Becker & Johnson, 2003). They are not meant to be the sole source of treatment and work best when given in conjunction with participation in individual or group psychotherapy.

PSYCHOANALYTICAL THERAPY. Psychoanalytical approaches have been tried in the treatment of paraphilias. In this type of therapy, the therapist helps the client to identify unresolved conflicts and traumas from early childhood. The therapy focuses on helping the individual resolve these early conflicts, thus relieving the anxiety that prevents him or her from forming appropriate sexual relationships. In turn, the individual has no further need for paraphilic fantasies.

BEHAVIORAL THERAPY. Aversion techniques have been used to modify undesirable behavior. Aversion therapy methods in the treatment of paraphilias involve pairing noxious stimuli, such as electric shocks and bad odors, with the impulse, which then diminishes. Behavioral therapy also includes skills training and cognitive restructuring in an effort to change the individual's maladaptive beliefs (Becker & Johnson, 2003).

Other behavioral approaches to decreasing inappropriate sexual arousal have included covert sensitization and satiation. With covert sensitization, the individual combines inappropriate sexual fantasies with aversive, anxiety-provoking scenes under the guidance of the therapist (Becker & Johnson, 2003). Satiation is a technique in which the postorgasmic individual repeatedly fantasizes deviant behaviors to the point of saturation with the deviant stimuli, consequently making the fantasies and behavior unexciting.

Role of the Nurse

Treatment of the person with a paraphilia is often very frustrating for both the client and the therapist. Most individuals with paraphilias deny that they have a problem and seek psychiatric care only after their inappropriate behavior comes to the attention of others. In secondary prevention, the focus is to diagnose and treat the problem as early as possible to minimize difficulties. These individuals should be referred to specialists who are accustomed to working with this special population.

Nursing may best become involved in the primary prevention process. The focus of primary prevention in sexual disorders is to intervene in home life or other facets of childhood in an effort to prevent problems from developing. An additional concern of primary prevention is to assist in the development of adaptive coping strategies to deal with stressful life situations.

Three major components of sexual development have been identified: (1) gender identity (one's sense of maleness or femaleness); (2) sexual responsiveness (arousal to appropriate stimuli); and (3) the ability to establish relationships with others. A disturbance in one or more of these components may lead to a variety of sexual deviations.

Different developmental components seem to be disturbed in the various sexual deviations. For example, gender identity may be disturbed in transvestitism or transsexualism. The second component, sexual responsiveness to appropriate stimuli, is disturbed in the case of the fetishist. In the case of the exhibitionist or the frotteur, the ability to form relationships may be disturbed.

Nurses can participate in the regular evaluation of these developmental components to ensure that as children mature, their development in each of these three components is healthy, thereby preventing deviant sexual behaviors. Nurses who work in pediatrics, psychiatry, public health, ambulatory clinics, schools, and any other facility requiring contact with children must be knowledgeable about human sexual development. Accurate assessment and early intervention by these nurses can contribute a great deal toward primary prevention of sexual disorders.

Sexual Dysfunctions

The Sexual Response Cycle

Because sexual dysfunctions occur as disturbances in any of the phases of the sexual response cycle, an understanding of anatomy and physiology is a prerequisite to considerations of pathology and treatment.

Phase I: Desire. During this phase, the desire to have sexual activity occurs in response to verbal, physical, or visual stimulation. Sexual fantasies can also bring about this desire.

Phase II. Excitement. This is the phase of sexual arousal and erotic pleasure. Physiological changes occur. The male responds with penile tumescence and erection. Female changes include vasocongestion in the pelvis, vaginal lubrication, and expansion and swelling of the external genitalia (APA, 2000).

Phase III. Orgasm. Orgasm is identified as a peaking of sexual pleasure, with release of sexual tension and rhythmic contraction of the perineal muscles and reproductive organs (APA, 2000). Orgasm in women is marked by simultaneous rhythmic contractions of the uterus, the lower third of the vagina, and the anal sphincter. In the man, a forceful emission of semen occurs in response to rhythmic spasms of the prostate, seminal vesicles, vas, and urethra (APA, 2000; Sadock & Sadock, 2003).

Phase IV: Resolution. If orgasm has occurred, this phase is characterized by disgorgement of blood from the genitalia (detumescence) creating a sense of general relaxation, well-being, and muscular relaxation. If orgasm does not occur, resolution may take 2 to 6 hours and be associated with irritability and discomfort (Sadock & Sadock, 2003).

After orgasm, men experience a refractory period that may last from a few minutes to many hours, during which time they cannot be stimulated to further orgasm. Commonly, the length of the refractory period increases with age. Women experience no refractory period and may be able to respond to additional stimulation almost immediately (APA, 2000).

Historical and Epidemiological Aspects Related to Sexual Dysfunction

Concurrent with the cultural changes occurring during the sexual revolution of the 1960s and 1970s came an increase in scientific research into sexual physiology and sexual dysfunctions. Masters and Johnson (1966; 1970) pioneered this work with their studies on human sexual response and the treatment of sexual dysfunctions. Spear (2001) reports:

> Sex therapy, the treatment of sexual disorders, has evolved from early studies on sexual behavior made over 50 years ago. During these 50 years, the approach to sex therapy has changed immensely. When William Masters and Virginia Johnson published *Human Sexual Inadequacy* in 1970, the sexual revolution, born in the 1960s, was not yet in full force. Due in part to the development of the oral contraceptive known as 'the pill' and the rise in the politics of feminism, society began to take a different, more open view of sexuality. The rise in sex therapy addressed [sexual] issues as they had never been addressed before, in the privacy of a doctor's office.

Sexual dysfunction consists of an impairment or disturbance in any of the phases of the sexual response cycle. No one knows exactly how many people experience sexual dysfunctions. Knowledge exists only about those who seek some kind of treatment for the problem, and their number may be few compared with those who have a dysfunction but suffer quietly and never seek therapy.

In 1970, Masters and Johnson reported that 50 percent of all American couples suffer from some type of sexual dysfunction. In 1984, Robins and associates estimated that 24 percent of the U.S. population would experience a sexual dysfunction at some time in their lives. The *DSM-IV-TR* reports on the most comprehensive survey to date, conducted on a representative sample of the U.S. population between ages 18 and 59, regarding the prevalence of the various sexual dysfunctions. The data are presented in Table 18–1.

Types of Sexual Dysfunction

Sexual Desire Disorders

HYPOACTIVE SEXUAL DESIRE DISORDER. This disorder is defined by the *DSM-IV-TR* (APA, 2000) as a persistent or recurrent deficiency or absence of sexual fantasies and desire for sexual activity. The diagnosis of deficiency or absence is made by the clinician taking into account factors that affect sexual functioning, such as age and the context of the person's life.

An individual's absolute level of sexual desire may not be the problem; rather, the problem may be a discrepancy between the partners' levels. The conflict may occur if one partner wants to have sexual relations

TABLE 18–1 Estimates of Prevalence Rates* for Sexual Dysfunctions

Disorder	Men (%)	Women (%)
Dyspareunia	3	15
Orgasm problems	10	25
Hypoactive sexual desire	—	33
Premature ejaculation	27	—
Arousal problems	—	20
Erectile difficulties	10	—

*Prevalence rate refers to an estimate of the number of people who have a disorder at any given time.
Adapted from the *DSM-IV-TR* (APA, 2000).

more often than the other does. Care must be taken not to label one partner as pathological when the problem actually lies in the discrepancy of sexual desire between the partners.

An estimated 20 percent of the total population has hypoactive sexual desire disorder (Sadock & Sadock, 2003). The complaint is more common in women than in men.

SEXUAL AVERSION DISORDER. This disorder is characterized by a persistent or recurrent extreme aversion to, and avoidance of, all (or almost all) genital sexual contact with a sexual partner (APA, 2000). Whereas individuals displaying hypoactive desire are often neutral or indifferent toward sexual interaction, sexual aversion implies anxiety, fear, or disgust in sexual situations.

Sexual Arousal Disorders

FEMALE SEXUAL AROUSAL DISORDER. Female sexual arousal disorder is identified in the *DSM-IV-TR* as a persistent or recurrent inability to attain, or to maintain until completion of the sexual activity, an adequate lubrication/swelling response of sexual excitement.

MALE ERECTILE DISORDER. Male erectile disorder is characterized by persistent or recurrent inability to attain, or to maintain until completion of the sexual activity, an adequate erection (APA, 2000). *Primary erectile dysfunction* refers to cases in which the man has never been able to have intercourse; *secondary erectile dysfunction* refers to cases in which the man has difficulty getting or maintaining an erection but has been able to have vaginal or anal intercourse at least once.

Orgasmic Disorders

FEMALE ORGASMIC DISORDER. Female orgasmic disorder is defined by the *DSM-IV-TR* as persistent or recurrent delay in, or absence of, orgasm following a normal sexual excitement phase. This condition is sometimes referred to as **anorgasmia**. Women who can achieve orgasm through noncoital clitoral stimulation but are not able to experience it during coitus in the absence of manual clitoral stimulation are not necessarily categorized as anorgasmic (Sadock & Sadock, 2003).

A woman is considered to have *primary orgasmic dysfunction* when she has never experienced orgasm by any kind of stimulation. *Secondary orgasmic dysfunction* exists if the woman has experienced at least one orgasm, regardless of the means of stimulation, but no longer does so.

MALE ORGASMIC DISORDER. Male orgasmic disorder, sometimes referred to as **retarded ejaculation**, is characterized by persistent or recurrent delay in, or absence of, orgasm following a normal sexual excitement phase during sexual activity that the clinician, taking into account the person's age, judges to be adequate in focus, intensity, and duration (APA, 2000). With this disorder, the man is unable to ejaculate, even though he has a firm erection and has had more than adequate stimulation. The severity of the problem may range from occasional problems ejaculating (*secondary disorder*) to a history of never having experienced an orgasm (*primary disorder*). In the most common version, the man cannot ejaculate during coitus but may be able to ejaculate by means of other types of stimulation.

PREMATURE EJACULATION. The *DSM-IV-TR* describes **premature ejaculation** as persistent or recurrent ejaculation with minimal sexual stimulation before, on, or shortly after penetration and before the person wishes it. Diagnosis should take into account factors that affect duration of the excitement phase, such as age, novelty of the sexual partner or situation, and recent frequency of sexual activity (APA, 2000).

An estimated 27 percent of the male population has this dysfunction, and 35 to 40 percent of men treated for sexual disorders have premature ejaculation as the chief complaint (Sadock & Sadock, 2003; Becker & Johnson, 2003). It is particularly common among young men who have a very high sex drive and have not yet learned to control ejaculation.

Sexual Pain Disorders

DYSPAREUNIA. **Dyspareunia** is recurrent or persistent genital pain associated with sexual intercourse in a man or a woman (APA, 2000). It is not caused by **vaginismus**, lack of lubrication, other general medical condition, or physiological effects of substance use. In women, the pain may be felt in the vagina, around the vaginal entrance and clitoris, or deep in the pelvis. In men, the pain is felt in the penis. Dyspareunia makes intercourse very unpleasant and may even lead to abstention from sexual activity.

Prevalence studies of dyspareunia have provided estimates of 15 percent in women and 3 percent in men (APA, 2000). Dyspareunia in men is often associated with urinary tract infection, with pain being experienced during urination as well as during ejaculation.

VAGINISMUS. Vaginismus is an involuntary constriction of the outer one-third of the vagina that prevents penile insertion and intercourse (APA, 2000).

Vaginismus is less prevalent than female orgasmic disorder, and most often afflicts highly educated women and those in the high socioeconomic groups (Sadock & Sadock, 2003). It is estimated that 12 to 17 percent of women presenting to sexual therapy clinics do so with the complaint of vaginismus (Leiblum, 1999).

SEXUAL DYSFUNCTION DUE TO A GENERAL MEDICAL CONDITION AND SUBSTANCE-INDUCED SEXUAL DYSFUNCTION. With these disorders, the sexual dysfunction is judged to be caused by the direct physiological effects of a general medical condition or use of a substance. The dysfunction may involve pain, impaired desire, impaired arousal, or impaired orgasm. Types of medical conditions that are associated with sexual dysfunction include neurological (e.g., multiple sclerosis, neuropathy), endocrine (e.g., diabetes mellitus, thyroid dysfunctions), vascular (e.g., atherosclerosis), and genitourinary (e.g., testicular disease, urethral or vaginal infections). Substances that can interfere with sexual functioning include alcohol, amphetamines, cocaine, opioids, sedatives, hypnotics, anxiolytics, antidepressants, antipsychotics, antihypertensives, and others.

Etiological Implications for Sexual Dysfunction

Biological Factors

SEXUAL DESIRE DISORDERS. Studies have correlated decreased levels of serum testosterone with hypoactive sexual desire disorder in men (Merck Manual, 2002a). Evidence also exists that suggests a relationship between serum testosterone and increased female libido (Leiblum, 1999). Diminished libido has been observed in both men and women with elevated levels of serum prolactin (Walling, 2000). Various medications have also been implicated in the etiology of hypoactive sexual desire disorder. Some examples include antihypertensives, antipsychotics, antidepressants, anxiolytics, and anticonvulsants. Alcohol and cocaine have also been associated with impaired desire, especially after chronic use.

SEXUAL AROUSAL DISORDERS. Postmenopausal women require a longer period of stimulation for lubrication to occur, and there is generally less vaginal transudate after menopause (Reinisch, 1990). Various medications, particularly those with antihistaminic and anticholinergic properties, may also contribute to decreased ability for arousal in women. Arteriosclerosis is a common cause of male erectile disorder resulting from arterial insufficiency (Goldberg, 1998). Various neurological disorders can contribute to erectile dysfunctions as well. The most common neurologically based cause may be diabetes, which places men at high risk for neuropathy (Wincze & Carey, 1991). Others include temporal lobe epilepsy and multiple sclerosis. Trauma (e.g., spinal cord injury, pelvic cancer surgery) can also result in erectile dysfunction. Several medications have been implicated in the etiology of this disorder, including antihypertensives, antipsychotics, antidepressants, and anxiolytics. Chronic use of alcohol has also been shown to be a contributing factor.

ORGASMIC DISORDERS. Results of research on the increased ability to achieve orgasm in posthysterectomy women by administering an estrogen-androgen hormone combination have been mixed (Wincze & Carey, 1991). Although the hormone replacement did influence sexual desire and arousal, effects on orgasmic response remain unclear. Drugs, particularly selective serotonin reuptake inhibitors, may inhibit orgasm (Merck Manual, 2002b). Medical conditions, such as depression, hypothyroidism, and diabetes mellitus, may cause decreased sexual arousal and orgasm.

Biological factors associated with inhibited male orgasm include surgery of the genitourinary tract (e.g., prostatectomy), various neurological disorders (e.g., Parkinson's disease), and other diseases (e.g., diabetes mellitus). Medications that have been implicated include antihypertensives, antidepressants, and antipsychotics (Merck Manual, 2002a). Transient cases of the disorder may occur with excessive alcohol intake.

Although premature ejaculation is commonly caused by psychological factors, general medical conditions or substance use may also be contributing influences. Particularly in cases of secondary dysfunction, in which a man at one time had ejaculatory control but later lost it, physical factors may be involved. Examples include a local infection such as prostatitis or a degenerative neural disorder such as multiple sclerosis.

SEXUAL PAIN DISORDERS. A number of organic factors can contribute to painful intercourse in women, including intact hymen, episiotomy scar, vaginal or urinary tract infection, ligament injuries, endometriosis, or ovarian cysts or tumors. Painful intercourse in men may also be caused by various organic factors. For example, infection caused by poor hygiene under the foreskin of an uncircumcised man can cause pain. Phimosis, a condition in which the foreskin cannot be pulled back, can also cause painful intercourse. An allergic reaction to various vaginal spermicides or irritation caused by vaginal infections may be a contributing factor. Finally, various prostate problems may cause pain on ejaculation.

Psychosocial Factors

SEXUAL DESIRE DISORDERS. Phillips (2000) identified a number of individual and relationship factors that may contribute to hypoactive sexual desire disorder. Individual causes include religious orthodoxy, sexual identity conflicts, past sexual abuse, financial, family, or job problems, depression, and aging-related concerns (e.g., changes in physical appearance). Among the relationship causes are interpersonal conflicts; current physical, verbal, or sexual abuse; extramarital affairs, and desire or practices that differ from partner.

Regarding sexual aversion disorder, Leiblum (1999) states:

> Many clinicians believe that this disorder might best be viewed as a phobia and removed from the sexual desire category. In general, sexual aversion is associated with a history of sexual or gynecologic trauma.

SEXUAL AROUSAL DISORDERS. A number of psychological factors have been cited as possible impediments to female arousal. They include doubt, guilt, fear, anxiety, shame, conflict, embarrassment, tension, disgust, irritation, resentment, grief, hostility toward partner, and a puritanical or moralistic upbringing. It is well documented that sexual abuse is a significant risk factor for desire and arousal disorders in women (Lieblum, 1999).

Problems with male sexual arousal may be related to chronic stress, anxiety, or depression (Sadock & Sadock, 2003). Developmental factors that hinder the ability to be intimate, that lead to a feeling of inadequacy or distrust, or that develop a sense of being unloving or unlovable may also result in impotence. Relationship factors that may affect erectile functioning include lack of attraction to one's partner, anger toward one's partner, or being in a relationship that is not characterized by trust (Wincze & Carey, 1991). Unfortunately, regardless of the etiology of the impotence, once it occurs, the man may become increasingly anxious about his next sexual encounter. This anticipatory anxiety about achieving and maintaining an erection may then perpetuate the problem.

ORGASMIC DISORDERS. Numerous psychological factors are associated with inhibited female orgasm. They include fears of becoming pregnant, rejection by the sexual partner, damage to the vagina, hostility toward men, and feelings of guilt regarding sexual impulses (Sadock & Sadock, 2003). Negative cultural conditioning ("nice girls don't enjoy sex") may also influence the adult female's sexual response. Various developmental factors also have relevance to orgasmic dysfunction. Examples include childhood exposure to rigid religious orthodoxy, negative family attitudes toward nudity and sex, and traumatic sexual experiences during childhood or adolescence, such as incest or rape (Phillips, 2000; Clayton, 2002).

Psychological factors are also associated with inhibited male orgasm. In the primary disorder (in which the man has never experienced orgasm), the man often comes from a rigid, puritanical background. He perceives sex as sinful and the genitals as dirty, and he may have conscious or unconscious incest wishes and guilt (Sadock & Sadock, 2003). In the case of secondary disorder (previously experienced orgasms that have now stopped), interpersonal difficulties are usually implicated. There may be some ambivalence about commitment, fear of pregnancy, or unexpressed hostility.

Premature ejaculation may be related to a lack of physical awareness on the part of a sexually inexperienced man. The ability to control ejaculation occurs as a gradual maturing process with a sexual partner in which foreplay becomes more give-and-take "pleasuring," rather than strictly goal oriented. The man becomes aware of the sensations and learns to delay the point of ejaculatory inevitability. Relationship problems such as a stressful marriage, negative cultural conditioning, anxiety over intimacy, and lack of comfort in the sexual relationship may also contribute to this disorder (Sadock & Sadock, 2003).

SEXUAL PAIN DISORDERS. Vaginismus may occur in response to having experienced dyspareunia (painful intercourse) for various organic reasons stated in the "biological factors" section. Involuntary constriction within the vagina occurs in response to anticipatory pain, making intercourse impossible. The diagnosis does not apply if the cause of the vaginismus is determined to be organic (Sadock & Sadock, 2003). A variety of psychosocial factors has been implicated including negative childhood conditioning of sex as dirty, sinful, and shameful. Early traumatic sexual experiences (e.g., rape or incest) may also cause vaginismus. Other factors that may be important in the etiology of vaginismus include homosexual orientation, traumatic experience with an early pelvic examination, pregnancy phobia, STD phobia, or cancer phobia (Phillips, 2000; Leiblum, 1999; Dreyfus, 1998; Sadock & Sadock, 2003).

Application of the Nursing Process to Sexual Disorders

ASSESSMENT. Most assessment tools for taking a general nursing history contain some questions devoted to sexuality. Many nurses feel uncomfortable obtaining information about the subject. However, accurate data must be collected if problems are to be identified and resolutions attempted. Sexual health is an integral part of physical and emotional well-being. The nursing history is incomplete if items directed toward sexuality are not included.

Indeed, most nurses are not required to obtain a sexual history as in depth as the one presented in this chapter. However, certain clients require a more extensive sexual history than that which is included in the general nursing history. These include clients who have medical or surgical conditions that may affect their sexuality; clients with infertility problems, STDs, or complaints of sexual inadequacy; clients who are pregnant, or have gynecological problems; those seeking information on abortion or family planning; and individuals in premarital, marital, and psychiatric counseling.

The best approach for taking a sexual history is a nondirective one; that is, it is best to use the sexual history outline as a guideline but allow the interview to progress in a less restrictive manner than the outline permits (with one question immediately following the other). The order of the questions should be adjusted according to the client's needs as they are identified during the interview. A nondirective approach allows time for the client to interject information related to feelings or concerns about his or her sexuality.

The language used should be understandable to the client. If he or she uses terminology that is unfamiliar, ask for clarification. Take level of education and cultural influences into consideration.

The nurse's attitude must convey warmth, openness, honesty, and objectivity. Personal feelings, attitudes, and values should not interfere with acceptance of the client. The nurse must remain nonjudgmental. This is conveyed by listening in an interested matter-of-fact manner, without overreaction to any information the client may present.

The content outline for a sexual history presented in Table 18–2 is not intended to be used as a rigid questionnaire but as a guideline from which the nurse may select appropriate topics for gathering information about the client's sexuality. The outline should be individualized according to client needs.

DIAGNOSIS/OUTCOME IDENTIFICATION. Nursing diagnoses are formulated from the data gathered during the assessment phase and with back-

TABLE 18–2 Sexual History: Content Outline

I. Identification data
   - A. Client
     1. Age
     2. Gender
     3. Marital status
   - B. Parents
     1. Ages
     2. Dates of death and ages at death
     3. Birthplace
     4. Marital status
     5. Religion
     6. Education
     7. Occupation
     8. Congeniality
     9. Demonstration of affection
     10. Feelings toward parents
   - C. Siblings (same information as above)
   - D. Marital partner (same information as above)
   - E. Children
     1. Ages
     2. Gender
     3. Strengths
     4. Identified problems

II. Childhood sexuality
   - A. Family attitudes about sex
     1. Parents' openness about sex
     2. Parents' attitudes about nudity
   - B. Learning about sex
     1. Asking parents about sex
     2. Information volunteered by parents
     3. At what age and how did client learn about: pregnancy, birth, intercourse, masturbation, nocturnal emissions, menstruation, homosexuality, STDs
   - C. Childhood sex activity
     1. First sight of nude body:
        - a. Same gender
        - b. Opposite gender
     2. First genital self-stimulation
        - a. Age
        - b. Feelings
        - c. Consequences
     3. First sexual exploration at play with another child
        - a. Age (of self and other child)
        - b. Gender of other child
        - c. Nature of the activity
        - d. Feelings and consequences

(Continued)

TABLE 18 – 2 Sexual History: Content Outline *(Continued)*

4. Sexual activity with older persons
   a. Age (of self and other person)
   b. Gender of other person
   c. Nature of the activity
   d. Client willingness to participate
   e. Feelings and consequences

D. Did you ever see your parents (or others) having intercourse? Describe your feelings.

E. Childhood sexual theories or myths:
   1. Thoughts about conception and birth
   2. Roles of male/female genitals and other body parts in sexuality

III. Onset of adolescence
- A. In girls:
  1. Information about menstruation:
     a. How received; from whom
     b. Age received
     c. Feelings
  2. Age
     a. Of first period
     b. When breasts began to develop
     c. At appearance of ancillary and pubic hair
  3. Menstruation
     a. Regularity; discomfort; duration
     b. Feelings about first period
- B. In boys:
  1. Information about puberty:
     a. How received; from whom
     b. Age received
     c. Feelings
  2. Age:
     a. Of appearance of ancillary and pubic hair
     b. Change of voice
     c. First orgasm (with or without ejaculation); emotional reaction

IV. Orgastic experiences
- A. Nocturnal emissions (male) or orgasms (female) during sleep.
  1. Frequency
- B. Masturbation
  1. Age begun; ever punished?
  2. Frequency; methods used
  3. Marital partner's knowledge
  4. Practiced with others? Spouse?
  5. Emotional reactions
  6. Accompanying fantasies
- C. Necking and petting ("making out")
  1. Age when begun
  2. Frequency
  3. Number of partners
  4. Types of activity
- D. Premarital intercourse
  1. Frequency
  2. Relationship with and number of partners
  3. Contraceptives used
  4. Feelings
- E. Orgasmic frequency
  1. Past
  2. Present

V. Feelings about self as masculine/feminine
- A. The male client:
  1. Does he feel masculine?
  2. Accepted by peers?
  3. Sexually adequate?
  4. Feelings/concerns about body:
     a. Size
     b. Appearance
     c. Function
- B. The female client:
  1. Does she feel feminine?
  2. Accepted by peers?
  3. Sexually adequate?
  4. Feelings/concerns about body:
     a. Size
     b. Appearance
     c. Function

VI. Sexual fantasies and dreams
- A. Nature of sex dreams
- B. Nature of fantasies
  1. During masturbation
  2. During intercourse

VII. Dating
- A. Age and feelings about:
  1. First date
  2. First kissing
  3. First petting or "making out"
  4. First going steady

VIII. Engagement
- A. Age
- B. Sex activity during engagement period:
  1. With fiance
  2. With others

IX. Marriage
- A. Date of marriage
- B. Age at marriage: Spouse:
- C. Spouse's occupation
- D. Previous marriages: Spouse:
- E. Reason for termination of previous marriages:
  Client: Spouse:
- F. Children from previous marriages:
  Client: Spouse:
- G. Wedding trip (honeymoon):
  1. Where? How long?
  2. Pleasant or unpleasant?
  3. Sexual considerations?
- H. Sex in marriage:
  1. General satisfaction/dissatisfaction.
  2. Thoughts about spouse's general satisfaction/dissatisfaction
- I. Pregnancies
  1. Number: Ages of couple:

2. Results (normal birth; cesarean delivery; miscarriage; abortion)
3. Planned or unplanned
4. Effects on sexual adjustment
5. Sex of child wanted or unwanted

X. Extramarital sex
  A. Emotional attachments
    1. Number; frequency; feelings
  B. Sexual intercourse
    1. Number; frequency; feelings
  C. Postmarital masturbation
    1. Frequency; feelings
  D. Postmarital homosexuality
    1. Frequency; feelings
  E. Multiple sex ("swinging")
    1. Frequency; feelings

XI. Sex after widowhood, separation, or divorce:
  A. Outlet
    1. Orgasms in sleep
    2. Masturbation
    3. Petting
    4. Intercourse
    5. Homosexuality
    6. Other
  B. Frequency; feelings

XII. Sexual variations and disorders:
  A. Homosexuality
    1. First experience; describe circumstances
    2. Frequency since adolescence
  B. Sexual contact with animals
    1. First experience; describe nature of contact
    2. Frequency and recent contact
    3. Feelings
  C. Voyeurism
    1. Describe types of observation experienced
    2. Feelings
  D. Exhibitionism
    1. To whom? When?
    2. Feelings
  E. Fetishes; transvestitism
    1. Nature of fetish
    2. Nature of transvestite activity
    3. Feelings
  F. Sadomasochism
    1. Nature of activity
    2. Sexual response
    3. Frequency; recency
    4. Consequences
  G. Seduction and rape
    1. Has client seduced/raped another?
    2. Has client ever been seduced/raped?
  H. Incest
    1. Nature of the sexual activity
    2. With whom?
    3. When occurred? Frequency; recency.
    4. Consequences
  I. Prostitution
    1. Has client ever accepted/paid money for sex?
    2. Type of sexual activity engaged in.
    3. Feelings about prostitution.

XIII. Certain effects of sex activities
  A. STDs
    1. Age at learning about STDs
    2. Type of STD contracted
    3. Age and treatment received.
  B. Illegitimate pregnancy
    1. At what age(s)
    2. Outcome of the pregnancy(ies)
    3. Feelings
  C. Abortion
    1. Why performed?
    2. At what age(s)?
    3. How often?
    4. Before or after marriage?
    5. Circumstance: who, where, how?
    6. Feelings about abortion: at the time; in retrospect; anniversary reaction.

XIV. Use of erotic material
  A. Personal response to erotic material
    1. Sexual pleasure—arousal
    2. Mild pleasure
    3. Disinterest; disgust
  B. Use in connection with sexual activity
    1. Type and frequency of use
    2. To accompany what type of sexual activity

Adapted from an outline prepared by the Group for Advancement of Psychiatry, based on the Sexual Performance Evaluation Questionnaire of the Marriage Council of Philadelphia. Used with permission.

ground knowledge regarding predisposing factors to the disorder. The following nursing diagnoses may be used for the client with sexual disorders:

Sexual dysfunction related to depression and conflict in relationship evidenced by loss of sexual desire

Ineffective sexuality patterns related to conflicts with sexual orientation or variant preferences, evidenced by expressed dissatisfaction with sexual behaviors (e.g., voyeurism, transvestitism)

The following criteria may be used for measurement of outcomes in the care of the client with sexual disorders. The client:

1. Can correlate stressful situations that decrease sexual desire
2. Can communicate with partner about sexual situation without discomfort
3. Can verbalize ways to enhance sexual desire
4. Verbalizes resumption of sexual activity at level satisfactory to self and partner
5. Can correlate variant behaviors with times of stress

6. Can verbalize fears about abnormality and inappropriateness of sexual behaviors
7. Expresses desire to change variant sexual behavior
8. Participates and cooperates with extended plan of behavior modification
9. Expresses satisfaction with own sexuality pattern

PLANNING/IMPLEMENTATION. Table 18–3 provides a plan of care for the client with sexual disorders. Nursing diagnoses are presented, along with outcome criteria, appropriate nursing interventions, and rationales.

CLIENT/FAMILY EDUCATION. The role of client teacher is important in the psychiatric area, as it is in all areas of nursing. A list of topics for client and family education relevant to sexual disorders is presented in Table 18–4.

EVALUATION. Reassessment is necessary to determine if selected interventions have been successful in helping the client overcome problems with sexual functioning. Evaluation may be facilitated by gathering information using the following types of questions.

For the client with sexual dysfunction:

1. Has the client identified life situations that promote feelings of depression and decreased sexual desire?
2. Can he or she verbalize ways to deal with this stress?
3. Can the client satisfactorily communicate with sexual partner about the problem?
4. Have the client and sexual partner identified ways to enhance sexual desire and the achievement of sexual satisfaction for both?
5. Are client and partner seeking assistance with relationship conflict?
6. Do both partners agree on what the major problem is? Are they motivated to attempt change?
7. Do client and partner verbalize an increase in sexual satisfaction?

For the client with variant sexual behaviors:

1. Can the client correlate an increase in variant sexual behavior to times of severe stress?
2. Has the client been able to identify those stressful situations and verbalize alternative ways to deal with them?
3. Does the client express a desire to change variant sexual behavior and a willingness to cooperate with extended therapy to do so?

TABLE 18–3 Care Plan for the Client With a Sexual Disorder

Nursing Diagnoses: SEXUAL DYSFUNCTION
Related to: Depression and conflict in relationship; biological or psychological contributing factors to the disorder
Evidenced by: Loss of sexual desire or ability to perform

Outcome Criteria	Nursing Interventions	Rationale
Client identifies stressors that contribute to loss of sexual desire. Client resumes sexual activity at level satisfactory to self and partner.	1. Assess client's sexual history and previous level of satisfaction in sexual relationship.	1. Client history establishes a database from which to work and provides a foundation for goal setting.
	2. Assess client's perception of the problem.	2. Client's idea of what constitutes a problem may differ from that of the nurse. It is the client's perception on which the goals of care must be established.
	3. Help client determine time dimension associated with the onset of the problem and discuss what was happening in life situation at that time.	3. Stress in all areas of life will affect sexual functioning. Client may be unaware of correlation between stress and sexual dysfunction.
	4. Assess client's level of energy.	4. Fatigue decreases client's desire and enthusiasm for participation in sexual activity.
	5. Review medication regimen; observe for side effects.	5. Many medications can affect libido. Evaluation of drug and individual response is important to ascertain whether drug is responsible for the problem.
	6. Provide information regarding sexuality and sexual functioning.	6. Increasing knowledge and correcting misconceptions can decrease feelings of powerlessness and anxiety and facilitate problem resolution.
	7. Refer for additional counseling or sex therapy if required.	7. Client and partner may need additional or more in-depth assistance if problems in sexual relationship are severe or remain unresolved.

Nursing Diagnosis: INEFFECTIVE SEXUALITY PATTERNS
Related to: Conflicts with sexual orientation or variant preferences
Evidenced by: Expressed dissatisfaction with sexual behaviors (e.g., voyeurism, transvestism)

Outcome Criteria	Nursing Interventions	Rationale
Client will express satisfaction with own sexuality pattern.	1. Take sexual history, noting client's expression of areas of dissatisfaction with sexual pattern.	1. Knowledge of what client perceives as the problem is essential for providing the type of assistance he or she may need.
	2. Assess areas of stress in client's life and examine relationship with sexual partner.	2. Sexual variant behaviors are often associated with added stress in the client's life.
	3. Note cultural, social, ethnic, racial, and religious factors that may contribute to conflicts regarding variant sexual practices.	3. Client may be unaware of the influence these factors exert in creating feelings of shame and guilt.
	4. Be accepting and nonjudgmental.	4. Sexuality is a very personal and sensitive subject. The client is more likely to share this information if he or she does not fear being judged by the nurse.
	5. Assist therapist in plan of behavior modification to help client decrease variant behaviors.	5. Individuals with paraphilias are treated by specialists who have experience in modifying variant sexual behaviors. Nurses can intervene by providing assistance with implementation of the plan for behavior modification.
	6. Teach client that sexuality is a normal human response and is not synonymous with any one sexual act; that it involves complex interrelationships among self-concept, body image, personal history, family, cultural influences, and all interactions with others (Vande Vusse & Simandl, 1992).	6. If client feels abnormal or unlike everyone else, the self-concept is likely to be very low—even worthless. Helping him or her to see that feelings and motivations are common, even though the behavior is variant, may help to increase feelings of self-worth and desire to change behavior.

TABLE 18–4 Topics for Client/Family Education Related to Sexual Disorders

Nature of the Illness
1. The human sexual response cycle
2. What is "normal" and "abnormal?"
3. Types of sexual dysfunctions
4. Causes of sexual dysfunctions
5. Types of paraphilias
6. Causes of paraphilias
7. Symptoms associated with sexual dysfunctions and paraphilias

Management of the Disorder
1. Teach practices and ways of sexual expression.
2. Teach relaxation techniques.
3. Teach side effects of medications that may be contributing to sexual dysfunction.
4. Teach effects of alcohol consumption on sexual functioning.
5. Teach about STDs (see Table 18–5).

Support Services
1. Provide appropriate referral for assistance from sex therapist.
2. One national association to which many qualified sex therapists belong is:
American Association of Sex Educators, Counselors and Therapists
435 N. Michigan Avenue, Suite 1717
Chicago, IL 60611–4067
(312) 644–0828

4. Does the client express an understanding about the normalcy of sexual feelings, aside from the inappropriateness of his or her behavior?
5. Are expressions of increased self-worth evident?

Treatment Modalities for Sexual Dysfunctions

Sexual Desire Disorders

HYPOACTIVE SEXUAL DESIRE DISORDER. Hypoactive sexual desire disorder has been treated in both men and women with the administration of testosterone. The masculinizing side effects make this approach unacceptable to women, and the evidence that it increases libido in men is inconclusive. Becker and Johnson (2003) describe the most effective treatment as a combination of cognitive therapy to deal with maladaptive beliefs; behavioral treatment, such as exercises to enhance sexual pleasuring and communication; and relationship therapy to deal with the individual's use of sex as a method of control.

Low sexual desire is often the result of partner incompatibility. If this is the case, the therapist may choose to shift from the sexual issue to helping a couple identify and deal with their incompatibility (Wincze & Carey, 1991).

SEXUAL AVERSION DISORDER. Systematic desensitization (see Chapter 16) is often the treatment of choice for sexual aversion disorder, to reduce the client's fear and avoidance of sex (Becker & Johnson, 2003). Gradual exposure, under relaxed conditions, to imagined and actual sexual situations decreases the amount of anxiety generated by these experiences. Successful treatment of sexual phobias has also been reported using tricyclic medications and psychosexual therapy aimed at developing insight into unconscious conflicts.

Sexual Arousal Disorders

FEMALE SEXUAL AROUSAL DISORDER. The goal of treatment for female sexual arousal disorder is to reduce the anxiety associated with sexual activity. Masters and Johnson (1970) reported successful results using their behaviorally oriented **sensate focus** exercises to treat this disorder. The objective is to reduce the goal-oriented demands of intercourse on both the man and the woman, thus reducing performance pressures and anxiety associated with possible failure. Regarding sensate focus, Kaplan (1987) states:

> The term "sensate focus," invented by Masters and Johnson, is a rather clumsy term for a simple and beautiful activity. It means that the couple desists from intercourse and orgasm for several days or weeks during which time they gently caress each other's bodies and genitals. I prefer the term "pleasuring" (which was also introduced into the literature by Masters and Johnson). Many authorities believe that these exercises are among their most significant clinical innovations. (p. 29)

The couple is instructed to take turns caressing each other's bodies. Initially, they are to avoid touching breasts and genitals, and to focus on the sensations of being touched. The caressing progresses to include touching of the breasts and genitals, to touching each other simultaneously, and eventually to include intercourse. Kaplan (1987) states, "Sensate focus is a learning experience whereby pleasurable responses are reinforced and sexual anxiety is diminished because the fear of failure is removed." (p. 33)

MALE ERECTILE DISORDER. Sensate focus has been used effectively for male erectile disorder as well. Clinicians widely agree that even when significant organic factors have been identified, psychological factors may also be present and must be considered in treatment (Wincze & Carey, 1991).

Group therapy, hypnotherapy, and systematic desensitization have also been used successfully in reducing the anxiety that may contribute to erectile difficulties. Psychodynamic interventions may help alleviate intrapsychic conflicts contributing to performance anxiety (Becker & Johnson, 2003).

Various medications, including testosterone and yohimbine, have been used to treat male erectile dysfunction. Penile injections of papaverine or prostaglandin have been used to produce an erection lasting from 1 to 4 hours (Abel, Rouleau, & Osborn, 1994).

A medication approved by the U. S. Food and Drug Administration (FDA) in 1998 for the treatment of erectile dysfunction is sildenafil (Viagra). Sildenafil blocks the action of phosphodiesterase, an enzyme that breaks down cyclic guanosine monophosphate, a compound that is required to produce an erection. This action only occurs, however, in the presence of nitric oxide, which is released during sexual arousal. Sildenafil does not result in sexual arousal. It works to achieve penile erection in the presence of sexual arousal. In research trials, sildenafil was effective in improving erections for 63 to 82 percent of men who took 25- to 100-mg dosages. Adverse effects include headache, facial flushing, indigestion, nasal congestion, dizziness, and visual changes (color tinges and blurred vision that was mild and temporary in nature) (Goldberg, 1998). Two additional drugs in the same classification, vardenafil (Levitra) and tadalafil (Cialis), received FDA approval in fall 2003. Two other oral medications for erectile dysfunction, apomorphine and phentolamine, are being investigated at this time. Phentolamine is also used in combination with papaverine in an injectable form. Both of these medications increase blood flow to the penis, resulting in an erection.

For erectile dysfunction refractory to other treatment methods, penile prostheses may be implanted. Two basic types are currently available: a bendable silicone implant and an inflatable device. The bendable variety requires a relatively simple surgical technique for insertion of silicone rods into the erectile areas of the penis. This results in a perpetual state of semierection for the client. The inflatable penile prosthesis produces an erection only when desired, and the appearance of the penis in both the flaccid and erect states is completely normal. Potential candidates for penile implantation should undergo careful psychological and physical screening. Although penile implants do not enable the client to recover the ability to ejaculate or to have an orgasm, men with prosthetic devices have generally reported satisfaction with their subsequent sexual functioning (Kaplan & Sadock, 1998).

FEMALE ORGASMIC DISORDER. Because anxiety may contribute to the lack of orgasmic ability in women, sensate focus is often advised to reduce anxiety, increase awareness of physical sensations, and transfer communications skills from the verbal to the nonverbal domain. Phillips (2000) provides the following description of therapy for the anorgasmic woman:

> Treatment relies on maximizing stimulation and minimizing inhibition. Stimulation may include masturbation with prolonged stimulation (initially up to one hour) and/or the use of a vibrator as needed, and muscular control of sexual tension (alternating contraction and relaxation of the pelvic muscles during high sexual arousal). The latter is similar to Kegel exercises. Methods to minimize inhibition include distraction by "spectatoring" (observing oneself from a third-party perspective), fantasizing, or listening to music.

Treatment for secondary anorgasmia (in which the client has had orgasms in the past, but is now unable to achieve them) focuses on the couple and their relationship. Therapy with both partners is essential to the success of this disorder.

MALE ORGASMIC DISORDER. Treatment for male orgasmic disorder is similar to that described for the anorgasmic woman. A combination of sensate focus and masturbatory training has been used with a high degree of success in the Masters and Johnson clinic. Treatment for male orgasmic disorder usually includes the sexual partner.

Premature Ejaculation. Masters, Johnson, and Kolodny (1995) developed a highly successful technique for the treatment of premature ejaculation. Sensate focus is used, with progression to genital stimulation. When the man reaches the point of imminent ejaculation, the woman is instructed to apply the "squeeze" technique: applying pressure at the base of the glans penis with her thumb and first two fingers. Pressure is held for 4 seconds and then released. This technique is continued until the man is no longer on the verge of ejaculating. This technique is practiced during subsequent periods of sexual stimulation.

Sexual Pain Disorders

DYSPAREUNIA. Treatment for the pain of intercourse begins with a thorough physical and gynecological examination. When organic pathology has been eliminated, the client's fears and anxieties underlying sexual functioning are investigated (Becker & Johnson, 2003). Systematic desensitization has been used successfully to decrease fears and anxieties associated with painful intercourse.

VAGINISMUS. Treatment of this disorder begins with education of the woman and her sexual partner regarding the anatomy and physiology of the disorder (i.e., what exactly is occurring during the vaginismus reflex and possible etiologies). The involuntary nature of the disorder is stressed in an effort to alleviate the perception on the part of the sexual partner that this occurrence is an act of willful withholding by the woman.

The second phase of treatment involves systematic desensitization. The client is taught a series of tensing and relaxing exercises aimed at relaxation of the pelvic musculature. Relaxation of the pelvic muscles is followed by a procedure involving the systematic insertion of dilators of graduated sizes until the woman is able to accept the penis into the vagina without discomfort. This physical therapy, combined with treatment of identified relationship problems, has been used by the Masters and Johnson clinic with considerable success (Masters, Johnson, & Kolodny, 1995).

VARIATIONS IN SEXUAL ORIENTATION

Homosexuality

Homosexual activity occurs under some circumstances in probably all known human cultures and all mammalian species for which it has been studied. The term **homosexuality** is derived from the Greek root *homo* meaning "same" and refers to sexual preference for individuals of the same gender. It may be applied in a general way to homosexuals of both genders, but is often used to specifically denote male homosexuality. The term **lesbianism**, used to identify female homosexuality, is traced to the Greek poet Sappho who lived on the island of Lesbos and is known for the love poems she wrote to other women. Most homosexuals prefer the term "gay," as it is less derogatory in its lack of emphasis on the sexual aspects of the orientation. A heterosexual is referred to as "straight."

The psychiatric community in general does not consider consensual homosexuality to be a mental disturbance (Sadock & Sadock, 2003). The concept of homosexuality as a disturbance in sexual orientation no longer appears in the *DSM*. Instead, the *DSM-IV-TR* (APA, 2000) is concerned only with the individual who experiences "persistent and marked distress about his or her sexual orientation."

Many members of American culture disapprove of homosexuality. In a survey by *The Washington Post*, Harvard University, and the Henry J. Kaiser Family

Foundation (1998), 53 percent of those surveyed responded that they believed sexual relations between two adults of the same sex was always wrong. Some experts believe American attitudes toward homosexuals can best be described as homophobic. *Homophobia* is defined as a negative attitude toward or fear of homosexuality or homosexuals (Sadock & Sadock, 2003). It may be indicative of a deep-seated insecurity about one's own gender identity. Homophobic behaviors include extreme prejudice against, abhorrence of, and discomfort around homosexuals. These behaviors are usually rationalized by religious, moral, or legal considerations.

Relationship patterns are as varied among homosexuals as they are among heterosexuals. Some homosexuals may remain with one partner for an extended period, even for a lifetime, whereas others prefer not to make a commitment, and "play the field" instead.

No one knows for sure why people become homosexual or heterosexual. Various theories have been proposed regarding the issue, but no single etiological factor has consistently emerged. Many contributing factors likely influence the development of sexual orientation.

Etiological Implications

BIOLOGICAL THEORIES. A study by Bailey and Pillard (1991) has shown a 52 percent concordance for homosexual orientation in monozygotic twins and 22 percent in dizygotic twins. The data were significant and suggest the possibility of a heritable trait. Sadock and Sadock (2003) state:

> Gay men show a familial distribution; they have more brothers who are gay than do heterosexual men. One study found that 33 out of 40 pairs of gay brothers shared a genetic marker on the bottom half of the X chromosome. (p. 698)

A number of studies have been conducted to determine whether or not there is a hormonal influence in the etiology of homosexuality. It has been hypothesized that levels of testosterone may be lower and levels of estrogen higher in homosexual men than in heterosexual men. Results have been inconsistent. It has also been suggested that exposure to inappropriate levels of androgens during the critical fetal period of sexual differentiation may contribute to homosexual orientation (Sadock & Sadock, 2003). This hypothesis lacks definitive evidence, and conclusions regarding its validity remain tentative.

PSYCHOSOCIAL THEORIES. Freud (1930) believed that all humans are inherently bisexual, with the capacity for both heterosexual and homosexual behavior. He theorized all individuals go through a homoerotic phase as children. Thus, if homosexuality occurs later in life, it is due to arrest of normal psychosexual development. He also believed homosexuality could occur as a result of pathological family relationships in which the child adopts a negative Oedipal position; that is, there is sexualized attachment to the parent of the same gender and identification with the parent of the opposite gender.

Some theories suggest that a dysfunctional family pattern may have an etiological influence in the development of homosexuality. These "nurture" theories focus on the parent-child relationship and, most specifically, the relationship with the same-gender parent. Homosexual men often have a dominant supportive mother and a weak, remote, or hostile father (Saunders & Pickering, 1997). Lesbians may have had a dysfunctional mother-daughter relationship. Both subsequently try to meet their unmet same-gender needs through sexual relationships.

These theories of family dynamics have been disputed by some clinicians who believe that parents have very little influence on the outcome of their children's sexual-partner orientation (Reinisch, 1990).

Special Concerns

People with homosexual preferences have problems that are similar to those of their heterosexual counterparts. Considerations of attractiveness and finding a partner and concerns about sexual adequacy are common to both. STDs are epidemic among sexually active individuals of all sexual orientations. Of particular concern is acquired immunodeficiency syndrome (AIDS), which was considered a "gay disease" for the first few years of the epidemic. AIDS is a fatal viral illness that, initially in the western world, was indeed largely transmitted by male homosexual activity. Although AIDS is now known to spread through contaminated blood products, the sharing of needles by intravenous drug users, and heterosexual contact, some individuals still believe AIDS is God's way of punishing homosexuals. These societal attitudes are considered by many homosexuals to be their greatest burden.

Some homosexuals live in fear of the discovery of their sexual orientation; they fear being rejected by parents and significant others. They experience a great deal of cognitive dissonance related to the disparity between their overt behavior and their inner feelings. Social sanctions still exist in some areas against homosexuals with regard to employment, housing, and public accommodations. The Human Rights Commission protects homosexuals; however, discrimination is still widespread.

Nurses must examine their personal attitudes and feelings about homosexuality. They must be able to recognize when negative feelings are compromising the care they give. Increasing numbers of homosexuals are being honest about their sexual orientation. Healthcare workers must ensure that these individuals receive care with dignity, which is the right of all human beings. Nurses who have come to terms with their own feelings about homosexuality are better able to separate the person from the behavior. Acceptance of alternative sexual orientation is not an essential component of nursing; unconditional acceptance of the individual is.

Transsexualism

Transsexualism is a disorder of gender identity or gender dysphoria (unhappiness or dissatisfaction with one's gender) of the most extreme variety. An individual, despite having the anatomical characteristics of a given gender, has the self-perception of being of the opposite gender. The disorder is relatively rare, with an estimated prevalence of 1 in 30,000 for men and 1 in 100,000 for women (Sadock & Sadock, 2003).

The *DSM-IV-TR* does not identify transsexualism as a specific disorder, choosing instead to discuss the broader category of *gender identity disorder*; however, transsexualism is included in the 10th revision of the *International Classification of Diseases (ICD-10)*.

Individuals with this disorder do not feel comfortable wearing the clothes of their assigned gender and often engage in cross-dressing. They may find their own genitals repugnant and may repeatedly submit requests to the healthcare system for hormonal and surgical gender reassignment. Depression and anxiety are common and are often attributed by the individual to inability to live in the desired gender role.

Etiological Implications

BIOLOGICAL THEORIES. Several studies have been conducted to determine if sex hormone levels are abnormal in individuals with gender dysphoria. In some studies, decreased levels of testosterone were found in male transsexuals, and abnormally high levels of testosterone were found in female transsexuals, but the results have been inconsistent (Becker & Johnson, 2003).

As with homosexuality, there has been some speculation that gender-disordered individuals may be exposed to inappropriate hormones during the prenatal period, which can result in a genetic woman or a genetic man possessing the qualities and perception of the opposite gender. Evidence that prenatal exposure to these hormones predisposes to transsexualism, however, remains inconclusive.

PSYCHOSOCIAL THEORIES. It is generally accepted that transsexualism has physiological origins. However, some clinicians believe that the etiology is based on a combination of biological and environmental factors, particularly family dynamics.

Special Concerns

Treatment of the transsexual is a complex process. The true transsexual intensely desires to have the genitalia and physical appearance of the assigned gender changed to conform to his or her gender identity. This change requires a great deal more than surgical alteration of physical features. In most cases, the individual must undergo extensive psychological testing and counseling, as well as live in the role of the desired gender for up to 2 years before surgery.

Hormonal treatment is initiated during this period. Male clients receive estrogens, which results in a redistribution of body fat in a more "feminine" pattern, enlargement of the breasts, a softening of the skin, and reduction in body hair. Females receive testosterone, which also causes a redistribution of body fat, growth of facial and body hair, enlargement of the clitoris, and deepening of the voice (Becker & Johnson, 2003). Amenorrhea usually occurs within a few months.

Surgical treatment for the male-to-female transsexual involves removal of the penis and testes and creation of an artificial vagina. Care is taken to preserve sensory nerves in the area so that the individual may continue to experience sexual stimulation.

Surgical treatment for the female-to-male transsexual is more complex and usually less successful (Reinisch, 1990). A mastectomy and sometimes a hysterectomy are performed. A penis and scrotum are constructed from tissues in the genital and abdominal area, and the vaginal orifice is closed. A penile implant is used to attain erection. Both men and women continue to receive maintenance hormone therapy following surgery. Satisfaction with the results is high, and most consider the pain and discomfort worthwhile. Sadock and Sadock (2003) state:

> Outcome studies are highly variable in terms of how success is defined and measured (for example, successful intercourse and body image satisfaction). About 70 percent of male-to-female and 80 percent of female-to-male reassignment surgery patients report satisfactory results. (p. 737)

Nursing care of the post–sex-reassignment surgical client is similar to that of most other postsurgical clients. Particular attention is given to maintaining comfort, preventing infection, preserving integrity of the surgical site, maintaining elimination, and meeting nutritional needs. Psychosocial needs may have to do with body image, fears and insecurities about relating to others, and being accepted in the new gender role. Meeting these needs can begin with nursing in a nonthreatening, nonjudgmental healing atmosphere.

Bisexuality

A bisexual person is not exclusively heterosexual or homosexual; he or she engages in sexual activity with members of both genders. Bisexuals are also sometimes referred to as ambisexual.

Bisexuality is more common than exclusive homosexuality. Statistics suggest that approximately 75 percent of all men are exclusively heterosexual and only 2 percent are exclusively homosexual, leaving a relatively large percentage that have engaged in sexual activity with both men and women.

A diversity of sexual preferences exists among bisexuals. Some individuals prefer men and women equally, whereas others prefer one gender but also accept sexual activity with the other gender. Some bisexuals may alternate between homosexual and heterosexual activity for long periods; others may have both a male and a female lover at the same time. Whereas some individuals maintain their bisexual orientation throughout their lives, others may become exclusively homosexual or heterosexual.

Etiological Implications

Little research exists on the etiology of bisexuality. Freud (1930) believed that all humans are inherently bisexual; that is, he believed that all individuals have the capacity for both heterosexual and homosexual interactions.

Much research on the development of homosexuality rests on the assumption that it is somehow determined by pathological conditions in childhood. Many heterosexual individuals, however, have their first homosexual encounter later in life. It is unlikely that an initial homosexual encounter that occurs in the 30s or 40s was determined by a pathological condition that occurred when the individual was 3 or 4 years old. Some encounters, too, are based solely on the situation, such as the heterosexual man who engages in homosexual behavior when in prison and then returns to heterosexuality following his release. This behavior most likely was determined by circumstances rather than a pathological process that occurred in childhood.

Gender identity (determining whether one is male or female) is usually established by the age of 2 to 3 years (Sadock & Sadock, 2003). Sexual identity (determining whether one is heterosexual or homosexual or both) may continue to evolve throughout one's lifetime.

SEXUALLY TRANSMITTED DISEASES

Phipps (1995) defines STDs as diseases that usually are or can be transmitted from one person to another through intimate contact with the genitalia, mouth, or rectum. They may be transmitted from one person to another through heterosexual or homosexual contact, and external genital evidence of pathology may or may not be manifested.

STDs are at epidemic levels in the United States. Individuals are beginning an active sex life at an earlier age. More women are sexually active than ever before. The social changes that may have contributed to the increase in STDs are sometimes referred to as the three Ps: permissiveness, promiscuity, and the pill. The widespread knowledge that antibiotics were available to cure infections and the availability of the pill to prevent pregnancy resulted in significant increases in promiscuity and the subsequent exposure to and spread of STDs.

A primary nursing responsibility in STD control is education that is aimed at prevention of the disease. Nurses must know which diseases are most prevalent, how they are transmitted, their signs and symptoms, available treatment, and consequences of avoiding treatment (Table 18-5). They must teach this information to clients in hospitals and clinics and take an active role in programs of education in the community. Early education is important in order to decrease the spread of STDs.

STDs have a particularly emotive significance because they can be transmitted between sexual partners. Consequently, STDs carry strong connotations of illicit sex and considerable social stigma, as well as potentially disastrous medical consequences. Feelings of guilt in clients with STDs can be overwhelming. These individuals need strong support to overcome not only the physical difficulties but also the social and emotional ones associated with having this type of illness.

Prevention of STDs is the ideal goal, but early detection and appropriate treatment continue to be con-

TABLE 18–5 Sexually Transmitted Diseases

Disease	Organism of Transmission	Method of Transmission	Signs and Symptoms	Available Treatment	Potential Complications
Gonorrhea	*Neisseria gonorrhoeae (bacterium)*	Vaginal sex; anal sex; genital-oral sex; via hand moistened with infected secretions and placed in contact with mucous membranes (e.g., the eyes)	Males: urethritis; dysuria, purulent discharge from urethra; proctitis; pharyngitis. Females: initially asymptomatic. Progresses to infection of cervix, urethra, and fallopian tubes.	Tetracycline; penicillin G; amoxicillin; ampicillin; spectinomycin	Men: sterility from orchitis or epididymitis. Women: chronic pelvic inflammatory disease; infertility; ectopic pregnancy; blindness from gonococcal conjunctivitis.
Syphilis	*Treponema pallidum (spirochete)*	Vaginal sex; anal sex; genital-oral sex; via contact of infected secretions with intact mucous membranes or abraded skin.	Primary stage: painless chancre on penis, vulva, vagina, mouth, anus, or other point of contact with mucous membranes or abraded skin. Secondary stage: rash, headache, anorexia, weight loss, fever, sore throat, body aches, anemia.	Long-acting penicillin G; tetracycline; erythromycin	Latent stage: lasts many years; no symptoms but can be passed on to fetus. Tertiary stage: blindness, heart disease, insanity, ulcerated lesions on skin, mucous membranes, or internal organs.
Chlamydial infection	*Chlamydia trachomatis* (intracellular bacterium)	Vaginal sex; anal sex; via hand moistened with infected secretions and placed in contact with mucous membranes.	Women: cervicitis (asymptomatic or may have discharge, dysuria, soreness, bleeding) Men: urethral discharge and dysuria.	Tetracycline; erythromycin	Scarring in the fallopian tubes; ectopic pregnancy; infertility.
Genital herpes	Herpes simplex virus, type 1 or type 2	Vaginal sex; anal sex; genital-oral sex; skin-to-skin contact with infected areas; to newborn through vaginal delivery.	Blistery lesions in the genital area causing pain, itching, burning. Also vaginal or urethral discharge, fever, headache, malaise, and myalgias.	Acyclovir applied directly to the area provides symptomatic relief. No cure.	Recurrences are possible. Potential complications include: meningitis, encephalitis, urethral strictures. Possible risk of cervical cancer.
Genital warts	*Condyloma acuminatum* (human papilloma virus)	Vaginal sex; anal sex; skin-to-skin contact with infected areas.	Cauliflower–like warts that appear on penis or scrotum in men, and labia, vaginal walls, or cervix in women. Mild itching may occur.	Application of fluorouracil; cryotherapy; electrocautery; surgical removal.	Recurrences are possible. Possible increased risk of cervical cancer.

(Continued)

TABLE 18–5 Sexually Transmitted Diseases *(Continued)*

Disease	Organism of Transmission	Method of Transmission	Signs and Symptoms	Available Treatment	Potential Complications
Hepatitis B	Hepatitis B virus	Vaginal sex; anal sex; genital-oral sex; contact with infectious blood or blood products; contact of infectious secretions with mucous membranes or abraded skin.	Malaise, anorexia, nausea/vomiting, fever, headache, mild pain in right upper quadrant of abdomen, jaundice.	No cure. Treatment involves supportive care; bedrest for extended period. Medications generally have not been found to be useful.	Complications include chronic hepatitis; cirrhosis; liver cancer.
AIDS	Human immunodeficiency virus (HIV)	Exchange of body fluids via: anal sex; vaginal sex; genital-oral sex; shared use of needles during drug use. Skin-to-skin contact when there are open sores on the skin. Transfusion with contaminated blood. Perinatal transmission: during delivery and through breast milk.	May be asymptomatic for as long as 10 years following infection with HIV. Early signs of AIDS include severe weight loss, diarrhea, fever, night sweats, or the presence of a persistent opportunistic infection (e.g., herpes or candidiasis).	No cure. Antiretroviral medication used to slow growth of the virus. Other medications given for symptomatic relief.	Regardless of treatment, AIDS is eventually fatal. New medications have dramatically increased the time from diagnosis to death, and research continues in drug treatments and vaccine development.

sidered a realistic objective. Nurses are in an excellent position to provide the education required for prevention, as well as the physical treatment and social and emotional support to assist clients with STDs regain and maintain optimal wellness.

SUMMARY

This chapter has provided information related to the development of sexuality throughout the life cycle. Normal sexual response patterns were described in an effort to provide background information for the recognition and treatment of sexual disorders.

The *DSM-IV-TR* identifies two major categories of sexual disorders: paraphilias and sexual dysfunctions. Paraphilias are a group of behaviors involving sexual activity with nonhuman objects, or with nonconsenting partners, or that involve suffering to others. Types of paraphilias include exhibitionism, fetishism, frotteurism, pedophilia, sexual masochism or sadism, and voyeurism.

Sexual dysfunctions are disturbances that occur in any of the phases of the normal human sexual response cycle. They include sexual desire disorders, sexual arousal disorders, orgasmic disorders, and sexual pain disorders.

Etiological implications and symptomatology for each of these sexual disorders were presented as background assessment data. A content outline for obtaining a sexual history was included. The delivery of nursing care was described in the context of the nursing process.

A description of current medical treatment modalities for each of the sexual disorders was presented. Alternative sexual orientations, including homosexuality, transsexualism, and bisexuality, were discussed. Finally, information on the transmission, signs and symptoms, treatment, and potential complications of the most prevalent STDs was suggested as material for use in programs of education targeted for decreasing the spread of sexually transmitted diseases.

Human sexuality influences all aspects of physical and mental health. Clients are becoming more open to discussing matters pertaining to sexuality, and it is therefore important for nurses to integrate information on sexuality into the care they give. This can be done by focusing on preventive, therapeutic, and educational interventions to assist individuals to attain, regain, or maintain sexual wellness.

REVIEW QUESTIONS

SELF-EXAMINATION/LEARNING EXERCISE

Select the answer that is most appropriate for each of the following questions:

1. Janice, aged 24, and her husband are seeking treatment at the sex therapy clinic. They have been married for 3 weeks and have never had sexual intercourse together. Pain and vaginal tightness prevent penile entry. Sexual history reveals Janice was raped when she was 15 years old. The physician would most likely assign which of the following diagnoses to Janice?
   a. Dyspareunia
   b. Vaginismus
   c. Anorgasmia
   d. Sexual aversion disorder
2. The most appropriate nursing diagnosis for Janice would be:
   a. Pain related to vaginal constriction.
   b. Ineffective sexuality patterns related to inability to have vaginal intercourse.
   c. Sexual dysfunction related to history of sexual trauma.
   d. Dysfunctional grieving related to loss of self-esteem because of rape.
3. The first phase of treatment may be initiated by the nurse. It would include which of the following?
   a. Sensate focus exercises
   b. Tense and relaxation exercises
   c. Systematic desensitization
   d. Education about the disorder
4. The second phase of treatment includes which of the following?
   a. Gradual dilation of the vagina
   b. Sensate focus exercises
   c. Hypnotherapy
   d. Administration of minor tranquilizers
5. Statistically, the outcome of therapy for Janice and her husband is likely:
   a. To be unsuccessful
   b. To be very successful
   c. To be of very long duration
   d. To result in divorce

Match each of the paraphilias listed on the left with its correct behavioral description from the column on the right:

______ 6. Exhibitionism	a. Tom watches his neighbor through her window each night as she undresses for bed. Later he fantasizes about having sex with her.
______ 7. Transvestic fetishism	b. Frank drives his car up to a strange woman, stops, and asks her for directions. As she is explaining, he reveals his erect penis to her.

_______ 8. Voyeurism	c. Tim, aged 17, babysits for his 11-year-old neighbor, Jeff. Six months ago, Tim began fondling Jeff's genitals. They now engage in mutual masturbation each time they are together.
_______ 9. Frotteurism	d. John is 32 years old. He buys women's clothing at the thrift shop. Sometimes he dresses as a woman and goes to a singles' bar. He becomes sexually excited as he fantasizes about men being attracted to him as a woman.
_______ 10. Pedophilia	e. Fred rides a crowded subway every day. He stands beside a woman he views as very attractive. Just as the subway is about to stop, he places his hand on her breast and rubs his genitals against her buttock. As the door opens, he dashes out and away. Later he fantasizes she is in love with him.

Test Your CRITICAL THINKING SKILLS

Linda was hospitalized on the psychiatric unit for depression. During her nursing assessment interview, she stated, "According to my husband, I can't do anything right—not even have sex." When asked to explain further, Linda said she and her husband had been married for 17 years. She said that in the beginning, they had experienced a mutually satisfying sexual relationship and "made love" two or three times a week. Their daughter was born after they had been married 2 years, followed 2 years later by the birth of their son. They now have two teenagers (ages 15 and 13) who, by Linda's admission, require a great deal of her time and energy. She says, "I'm too tired for sex. Besides, the kids might hear. I would be so embarrassed if they did. I walked in on my parents having sex once when I was a teenager, and I thought I would die! My parents never mentioned it. It was just as if it never happened! It was so awful! However, sex is just so important to my husband, though, and we haven't had sex in months. We argue all the time about it. I'm afraid it's going to break us up."

Answer the following questions related to Linda:

1. What would be the primary nursing diagnosis for Linda?
2. What interventions might the nurse include in the treatment plan for Linda?
3. What would be a realistic goal for which Linda might strive?

IMPLICATIONS OF RESEARCH FOR EVIDENCE-BASED PRACTICE

Keller, M.L., Duerst, B.L., and Zimmerman, J: **Adolescents views of sexual decision-making.** IMAGE: Journal of Nursing Scholarship (1996, Summer); 28(2):125–130.

Description of the Study: Because large numbers of adolescents continue, despite intensive educational efforts, to engage in behaviors that place them at high risk for sexually transmitted diseases (STDs), this study was undertaken in an attempt to determine reasons adolescents give for abstinence, engaging in safer sex (intercourse with a condom) or unprotected intercourse. The sample included 62 male and 53 female students enrolled in the health or social science classes of six rural school districts in Wisconsin. Average age was 17.5 years. Respondents completed a study questionnaire in which they responded to a vignette in which a teenage couple became sexually aroused. They were to choose an ending to the vignette in one of three ways: the couple abstains from intercourse, the couple has sexual intercourse using a condom, or the couple has sexual intercourse without using a condom. The subjects were then asked to give reasons why they chose the particular ending, and possible feelings associated with all three choices from the perspective of the couple in the vignette.

Results of the Study: By a large margin, most of the subjects chose an ending in which the couple had sexual intercourse. Forty-three percent chose the outcome of intercourse with a condom; 33 percent chose the ending of unprotected sexual intercourse; and 23 percent chose the abstinence ending. Reasons given for response of intercourse with a condom included responsibility, safety, and "people expect to use condoms these days." Reasons given for outcome of unprotected sexual intercourse included, "it's what usually happens," no condom available, and loss of control. The most frequent reason given for choosing the abstinence ending was that "the couple did not know each other well enough to have sexual intercourse."

Implications for Nursing Practice: The authors suggest that data from this study suggest the importance of helping adolescents know that they have control over a situation. Unprotected sex was attributed to loss of control and being "swept away by desire." A second aspect might be to use fear-inducing strategies. Reasons given for abstinence and use of condoms included fear about pregnancy and STDs. Reinforcement of the legitimacy of these fears can be part of an educational intervention by nurses to motivate teens to engage in desirable behaviors. The ability to help adolescents think about the *positive* consequences of safer sex was also a consideration for nursing intervention.

INTERNET REFERENCES

- Additional information about sexual disorders may be located at the following websites:
  - a http://www.sexualhealth.com/
  - b http://www-hsl.mcmaster.ca/tomflem/sexual.html
  - c http://www.priory.com/sex.htm
- Additional information about gender identity disorders may be located at the following websites:
  - a http://www.avitale.com/
  - b http://eserver.org/gender/
  - c http://www.findarticles.com/cf_dis/g2699/0001/2699000148/p1/article.jhtml
- Additional information about STDs may be located at the following websites:
  - a http://www.cdc.gov/nchstp/dstd/dstdp.html
  - b http://www.niaid.nih.gov/factsheets/stdinfo.htm

REFERENCES

Abel, G.G., Rouleau, J.L., & Osborn, C.A. (1994). Sexual disorders. In G. Winokur & P.J. Clayton (Eds.), The medical basis of psychiatry (2nd ed.). Philadelphia: W.B. Saunders.

Administration on Aging. (2002). A profile of older Americans: 2002. Washington, DC: U.S. Department of Health and Human Services.

American Psychiatric Association (APA). (2000). Diagnostic and statistical manual of mental disorders (4th ed.) Text revision. Washington, DC: American Psychiatric Association.

Bailey, J.M. & Pillard, R.C. (1991). A genetic study of male sexual orientation. Archives of General Psychiatry, 48, 1089–1096.

Becker, J.V. & Johnson, B.R. (2003). Sexual and gender identity disorders. In R.E. Hales & S.C. Yudofsky (Eds.), Textbook of psychiatry (4th ed.) Washington, DC: American Psychiatric Publishing.

Bell, R. (1998). Changing bodies, changing lives (3rd ed.). New York: Random House.

Clayton, A.H. (2002). Sexual dysfunction. In S.G. Kornstein & A.H. Clayton (Eds.), Women's mental health. New York: The Guilford Press.

Clunn, P. (1991). Child psychiatric nursing. St.Louis: Mosby.

Dreyfus, E.A. (1998). Sexuality and sex therapy: When there is

sexual dysfunction. Retrieved March 22, 2002, from http://www.shpm.com/articles/sex/sexther2.html
Goldberg, K.A. (1998). Viagra: The potency pill. Lincolnwood, IL: Publications International.
Kaplan, H.I. & Sadock, B.J. (1998). Synopsis of psychiatry: Behavioral sciences/clinical psychiatry (8th ed.).Baltimore: Williams & Wilkins.
Kaplan, H.S. (1987). Manual of sex therapy (2nd ed.). New York: Brunner/Mazel.
Kaplan, H.S. (1979). Disorders of sexual desire and other new concepts and techniques in sex therapy. New York: Brunner/Mazel.
Leiblum, S.R. (1999). Sexual problems and dysfunction: Epidemiology, classification, and risk factors. The Journal of Gender-Specific Medicine, 2(5):41–45.
Marshall, W.L. & Barbaree, H.E. (1990). An integrated theory of the etiology of sexual offending. In W.L. Marshall, D.R. Laws, & H.E. Barbaree (Eds.), Handbook of sexual assault: Issues, theories, and treatment of the offender. New York: Plenum Press.
Masters, W.H., Johnson, V.E., & Kolodny, R.C. (1995). Human sexuality (5th ed.). New York: Longman.
McCarthy, B. & McCarthy, E. (1998). Couple sexual awareness. New York: Carroll & Graf.
Merck Manual. (2002a). Sexual dysfunctions. Retrieved March 22, 2002, from http://www.merck.com/pubs/mmanual/section15/chapter192/192b.htm
Merck Manual. (2002b). Female orgasmic disorder. Retrieved March 22, 2002, from http://www.merck.com/pubs/mmanual/section18/chapter243/243c.htm
Murray R.B. & Zentner, J.P. (2001). Health promotion strategies through the life span (7th ed.). Upper Saddle River, NJ: Prentice Hall.
Phillips, N.A. (2000, July 1). Female sexual dysfunction: Evaluation and treatment. American Family Physician, 62(1):127–136, 141–142.
Phipps, W.J. (1995). Management of persons with sexually transmitted diseases. In W.J. Phipps, V.L. Cassmeyer, J.K. Sands, & M.K. Lehman (Eds.), Medical-surgical nursing: Concepts and clinical practice (5th ed.). St. Louis: Mosby.
Reinisch, J.M. (1990). The Kinsey Institute new report on sex. New York: St. Martin's Press.
Robins, L.N., et al. (1984). Lifetime prevalence of specific psychiatric disorders in three sites. Archives of General Psychiatry, 41, 949–958.
Sadock, B.J. & Sadock, V.A. (2003). Synopsis of psychiatry: Behavioral sciences/clinical psychiatry (9th ed.). Philadelphia: Lippincott Williams & Wilkins.
Sands, J. K. (1995). Human sexuality. In W.J. Phipps, V.L. Cassmeyer, J.K. Sands, & M.K. Lehman (Eds.), Medical-surgical nursing: Concepts and clinical practice (5th ed.). St.Louis: Mosby.
Saunders, P. & Pickering, R. (1997). The causes of homosexuality. Retrieved March 24, 2002, from http://www.cmf.org.uk/pubs/nucleus/nucoct97/cause.htm
Sinclair Intimacy Institute. (2002). Sexual dysfunction in the United States. Retrieved March 20, 2002, from http://www.intimacyinstitute.com/about/research/
Slap, G.B. (1998). Masturbation. In the Gale Encyclopedia of Childhood and Adolescence. Retrieved on March 20, 2002, from http://www.findarticles.com/Cf_dis/g2602/0003/2602000366/p1/article.jhtml
Spear, J. (2001). Changing attitudes towards sex. Gale Encyclopedia of Psychology (2nd ed.). Retrieved on March 22, 2002, from http://www.findarticles.com/cf_dis/g2699/0003/2699000313/p1/article.jhtml
VandeVusse, L. & Simandl, G. (1992). Sexuality patterns, altered. In K.V. Gettrust & P.D. Brabec (Eds.), Nursing diagnosis in clinical practice: Guides for care planning. Albany, NY: Delmar.
Walling, A.D. (2000, March 15). When to measure prolactin levels. American Family Physician. Retrieved March 22, 2002, from http://www.findarticles.com/cf_0/m3225/6_61/61432859/p1/article.jhtml
The Washington Post, Harvard University, and the Henry J. Kaiser Family Foundation (1998). A sense of moral decline. Washington, DC: Washington Post.
Wincze, J.P. & Carey, M.P. (1991). Sexual dysfunction: A guide for assessment and treatment. New York: The Guilford Press.

CLASSICAL REFERENCES

Freud, S. (1930). Three contributions to the theory of sex (4th ed.). New York: Nervous and Mental Disease Publishing.
Masters, W.H. & Johnson, V.E. (1966). Human sexual response. Boston: Little, Brown.
Masters, W.H. & Johnson, V.E. (1970). Human sexual inadequacy. Boston: Little, Brown.

19

CHAPTER

Eating Disorders

CHAPTER OUTLINE

KEY TERMS

amenorrhea
binging
purging
body image
emaciated
anorexia nervosa
obesity
anorexiants
bulimia nervosa

OBJECTIVES

After reading this chapter, the student will be able to:

1. Identify and differentiate among the various eating disorders.
2. Discuss epidemiological statistics related to eating disorders.
3. Describe symptomatology associated with anorexia nervosa, bulimia nervosa, and obesity, and use the information in client assessment.
4. Identify etiological implications in the development of eating disorders.
5. Formulate nursing diagnoses and outcomes of care for clients with eating disorders.
6. Describe appropriate interventions for behaviors associated with eating disorders.
7. Evaluate the nursing care of clients with eating disorders.
8. Discuss various modalities relevant to treatment of eating disorders.

INTRODUCTION

Nutrition is required to sustain life, and most individuals acquire nutrients from eating food; however, nutrition and life sustenance are not the only reasons most people eat food. Indeed, in an affluent culture, life sustenance may not even be a consideration. It is sometimes difficult to remember that many people within this affluent American culture, as well as all over the world, are starving from lack of food.

The hypothalamus contains the appetite regulation center within the brain. This complex neural system regulates the body's ability to recognize when it is hungry and when it has been sated. Halmi (2003) states:

> Eating behavior is now known to reflect an interaction between an organism's physiological state and environmental conditions. Salient physiological variables include the balance of various neuropeptides and neurotransmitters, metabolic state, metabolic rate, condition of the

> gastrointestinal tract, amount of storage tissue, and sensory receptors for taste and smell. Environmental conditions include features of the food such as taste, texture, novelty, accessibility, and nutritional composition, and other external conditions such as ambient temperature, presence of other people, and stress. (p. 1001)

Society and culture have a great deal of influence on eating behaviors. Eating is a social activity; seldom does an event of any social significance occur without the presence of food. Yet, society and culture also influence how people (and in particular, women) must look. History reveals a regularity of fluctuation in what society has considered desirable in the human female body. Archives and historical paintings reveal the fashionableness and desirability of the plump, full-figured women of the 16th and 17th centuries. Beauty in the Victorian era was characterized by a slender, wan appearance that continued through the flapper era of the 1920s. During the depression era and World War II, the full-bodied woman was again admired, only to be superseded in the late 1960s by the image of the superthin models propagated by the media, which remains the ideal of today. As it has been said, "A woman can't be too rich or too thin." Eating disorders, as we know them, can dispute this quote.

This chapter explores the disorders associated with undereating and overeating. Because psychological or behavioral factors play a potential role in the presentation of these disorders, they fall well within the realm of psychiatry and psychiatric nursing. Epidemiological statistics are presented along with predisposing factors that have been implicated in the etiology of anorexia nervosa, bulimia nervosa, and obesity. An explanation of the symptomatology is presented as background knowledge for assessing the client with an eating disorder. Nursing care is described in the context of the nursing process. Various treatment modalities are explored.

EPIDEMIOLOGICAL FACTORS

The incidence of **anorexia nervosa** has increased in the past 30 years both in the United States and in Western Europe (Halmi, 2003). Studies indicate a prevalence rate among young women in the United States of approximately 0.5 to 1 percent (Sadock & Sadock, 2003). Anorexia nervosa occurs predominantly in females aged 12 to 30 years. Less than 10 percent of the cases are males (APA, 2000). Anorexia nervosa was once believed to be more prevalent in the higher socioeconomic classes, but evidence is lacking to support this hypothesis.

Bulimia nervosa is more prevalent than anorexia nervosa. Estimates of the disorder range from 1 to 3 percent of young women (Sadock & Sadock, 2003). Onset of bulimia nervosa commonly occurs in late adolescence or early adulthood. Cross-cultural research suggests that bulimia nervosa occurs primarily in societies that place emphasis on thinness as the model of attractiveness for women and where an abundance of food is available (Eckert & Mitchell, 1994).

Obesity has been defined as a body mass index (BMI) (weight/height^2) of 30 or greater. In 1997, almost 1 in 5 adults (18.8 percent of men and 19.3 percent of women) were obese (National center for Health Statistics, 2001). Obesity is more common in black women than in white women and more common in white men than in black men. The prevalence among lower socioeconomic classes is six times that in upper socioeconomic classes, and there is an inverse relationship between obesity and level of education (National Center for Health Statistics, 2001). Approximately 0.1 percent of the population is categorized as "morbidly" obese, which is defined by the National Institutes of Health (NIH) as a BMI greater than 40 kg/m^2 (Long, 1995).

APPLICATION OF THE NURSING PROCESS

Background Assessment Data (Symptomatology)

Anorexia Nervosa

This disorder is characterized by a morbid fear of obesity. Symptoms include gross distortion of **body image**, preoccupation with food, and refusal to eat. The term *anorexia* is actually a misnomer. It was initially believed that anorexics did not experience sensations of hunger. However, research indicates that they do indeed suffer from pangs of hunger, and it is only with food intake of less than 200 calories per day that hunger sensations actually cease.

The distortion in body image is manifested by the individual's perception of being "fat" when he or she is obviously underweight or even **emaciated**. Weight loss is usually accomplished by reduction in food intake and often extensive exercising. Self-induced vomiting and the abuse of laxatives or diuretics also may occur.

Weight loss is marked. For example, the individual may present for healthcare services weighing less than 85 percent of expected weight. Other symptoms include hypothermia, bradycardia, hypotension, edema, lanugo, and a variety of metabolic changes. **Amenorrhea** usually follows weight loss but in some instances may precede it (APA, 2000).

There may be an obsession with food. For example, these individuals may hoard or conceal food, talk about food and recipes at great length, or prepare elaborate meals for others, only to restrict themselves to a limited amount of low-calorie food intake. Compulsive behaviors, such as hand washing, also may be present. Age at onset is usually early to late adolescence. It is estimated to occur in approximately 0.5 to 1 percent of adolescent females and is 10 to 20 times more common in females than in males (Sadock & Sadock, 2003). Psychosexual development is generally delayed.

Feelings of depression and anxiety often accompany this disorder. In fact, some studies have suggested a possible interrelationship between eating disorders and affective disorders. Table 19–1 outlines the *DSM-IV-TR* (APA, 2000) diagnostic criteria for anorexia nervosa.

TABLE 19 – 1 Diagnostic Criteria for Anorexia Nervosa

A. Refusal to maintain body weight at or above a minimally normal weight for age and height (e.g., weight loss leading to maintenance of body weight less than 85% of that expected; or failure to make expected weight gain during period of growth, leading to body weight less than 85% of that expected)
B. Intense fear of gaining weight or becoming fat, even though underweight
C. Disturbance in the way one's body weight or shape is experienced, undue influence of body weight or shape on self-evaluation, or denial of the seriousness of the current low body weight
D. In postmenarchal females, amenorrhea; that is, the absence of at least three consecutive menstrual cycles. (A woman is considered to have amenorrhea if her periods occur only following hormone, [e.g., estrogen] administration.)

Specify type:

Restricting Type: During the current episode of anorexia nervosa, the person has not regularly engaged in binge eating or purging behavior (i.e., self-induced vomiting or the misuse of laxatives, diuretics, or enemas)

Binge-Eating/Purging Type: During the current episode of anorexia nervosa, the person has regularly engaged in binge-eating or purging behavior (i.e., self-induced vomiting or the misuse of laxatives, diuretics, or enemas).

From the American Psychiatric Association (2000), with permission.

Bulimia Nervosa

Bulimia nervosa is an episodic, uncontrolled, compulsive, rapid ingestion of large quantities of food over a short time (**binging**), followed by inappropriate compensatory behaviors to rid the body of the excess calories. The food consumed during a binge often has a high caloric content, a sweet taste, and a soft or smooth texture that can be eaten rapidly, sometimes even without being chewed (Sadock & Sadock, 2003). The binging episodes often occur in secret and are usually only terminated by abdominal discomfort, sleep, social interruption, or self-induced vomiting. Although the eating binges may bring pleasure when they are occurring, self-degradation and depressed mood commonly follow.

To rid the body of the excessive calories, the individual may engage in **purging** behaviors (self-induced vomiting or the misuse of laxatives, diuretics, or enemas) or other inappropriate compensatory behaviors, such as fasting or excessive exercise. There is a persistent overconcern with personal appearance, particularly regarding how they believe others perceive them. Weight fluctuations are common because of the alternating binges and fasts. However, most individuals with bulimia are within a normal weight range—some slightly underweight, some slightly overweight.

Excessive vomiting and laxative/diuretic abuse may lead to problems with dehydration and electrolyte imbalance. Gastric acid in the vomitus also contributes to the erosion of tooth enamel. In rare instances, the individual may experience tears in the gastric or esophageal mucosa.

Some people with this disorder are subject to mood disorders, anxiety disorders, substance abuse or dependence, most frequently involving amphetamines or alcohol (APA, 2000). Diagnostic criteria for bulimia nervosa are presented in Table 19–2.

Etiological Implications for Anorexia Nervosa and Bulimia Nervosa

Biological Influences

Genetics

A hereditary predisposition to eating disorders has been hypothesized based on family histories and an

TABLE 19–2 Diagnostic Criteria for Bulimia Nervosa

A. Recurrent episodes of binge eating. An episode of binge eating is characterized by both of the following:
   1. Eating, in a discrete period of time (e.g., within any 2-hour period), an amount of food that is definitely larger than most people would eat during a similar period of time and under similar circumstances.
   2. A sense of lack of control over eating during the episode (e.g., a feeling that one cannot stop eating or control what or how much one is eating).

B. Recurrent inappropriate compensatory behavior in order to prevent weight gain, such as self-induced vomiting; misuse of laxatives, diuretics, enemas, or other medications; fasting; or excessive exercise.

C. The binge eating and inappropriate compensatory behaviors both occur, on average, at least twice a week for 3 months.

D. Self-evaluation is unduly influenced by body shape and weight.

E. The disturbance does not occur exclusively during episodes of anorexia nervosa.

Specify type:

Purging type: During the current episode of bulimia nervosa, the person has regularly engaged in self-induced vomiting or the misuse of laxatives, diuretics, or enemas.

Nonpurging type: During the current episode of bulimia nervosa, the person has used other inappropriate compensatory behaviors, such as fasting or excessive exercise, but has not regularly engaged in self-induced vomiting or the misuse of laxatives, diuretics, or enemas.

SOURCE: From the American Psychiatric Association (2000), with permission.

apparent association with other disorders for which the likelihood of genetic influences exists. Anorexia nervosa is more common among sisters and mothers of those with the disorder than among the general population. Several studies have reported a higher than expected frequency of mood disorders among first-degree biological relatives of people with anorexia nervosa and bulimia nervosa and of substance abuse and dependence in relatives of individuals with bulimia nervosa (APA, 2000).

Neuroendocrine Abnormalities

Some speculation has occurred regarding a primary hypothalamic dysfunction in anorexia nervosa. Studies consistent with this theory have revealed elevated cerebrospinal fluid cortisol levels and a possible impairment of dopaminergic regulation in individuals with anorexia (Eckert & Mitchell, 1994). Additional evidence in the etiological implication of hypothalamic dysfunction is gathered from the fact that many people with anorexia experience amenorrhea before the onset of starvation and significant weight loss.

Neurochemical Influences

Neurochemical influences in bulimia may be associated with the neurotransmitters serotonin and norepinephrine (Sadock & Sadock, 2003). This hypothesis has been supported by the positive response these individuals have shown to therapy with the selective serotonin reuptake inhibitors (SSRIs). Some studies have found high levels of endogenous opioids in the spinal fluid of clients with anorexia, promoting the speculation that these chemicals may contribute to denial of hunger (Sadock & Sadock, 2003; Harvard Mental Health Letter, 1997). Some of these individuals have been shown to gain weight when given naloxone, an opioid antagonist.

Psychodynamic Influences

Psychodynamic theories suggest that eating disorders result from very early and profound disturbances in mother-infant interactions. The result is retarded ego development in the child and an unfulfilled sense of separation-individuation. This problem is compounded when the mother responds to the child's physical and emotional needs with food. Manifestations include a disturbance in body identity and a distortion in body image. When events occur that threaten the vulnerable ego, feelings emerge of lack of control over one's body (self). Behaviors associated with food and eating serve to provide feelings of control over one's life.

Family Influences

Conflict Avoidance

In the theory of the family as a system, psychosomatic symptoms, including anorexia nervosa, are reinforced in an effort to avoid spousal conflict. Parents are able to deny marital conflict by defining the sick child as the family problem. In these families, there is an unhealthy involvement between the members (enmeshment); the members strive at all costs to maintain "appearances"; and the parents endeavor to retain the child in the dependent position. Conflict avoidance may be a strong factor in the interpersonal dynamics of some families in which children develop eating disorders.

Elements of Power and Control

The issue of control may become the overriding factor in the family of the client with an eating disorder. These families often consist of a passive father, a domineering mother, and an overly dependent child. A high value is placed on perfectionism in this family, and the child feels he or she must satisfy these standards. Parental criticism promotes an increase in obsessive and perfectionistic behavior on the part of the child, who continues to seek love, approval, and recognition. The child eventually begins to feel helpless and ambivalent toward the parents. In adolescence, these distorted eating patterns may represent a rebellion against the parents, viewed by the child as a means of gaining and remaining in control. The symptoms are often triggered by a stressor that the adolescent perceives as a loss of control in some aspect of his or her life.

Obesity

Obesity is not classified as a psychiatric disorder in the *DSM-IV-TR*, but because of the strong emotional factors associated with the condition, it may be considered under "Psychological Factors Affecting Medical Condition."

A third category of eating disorder is also being considered by the APA. Research criteria for binge-eating disorder (BED) are presented in the *DSM-IV-TR* (see Table 19–3). Obesity is a factor in BED because the individual binges on large amounts of food but does not engage in behaviors to rid the body of the excess calories. The following formula is used to determine extent of obesity in an individual:

$$\text{Body mass index} = \frac{\text{Weight (kg)}}{\text{Height (m)}^2}$$

The BMI range for normal weight is 20 to 24.9. Studies by the National Center for Health Statistics indicate that *overweight* is defined as a BMI of 25.0 to 29.9 (based on U.S. Dietary Guidelines for Americans). Based on criteria of the World Health Organization, *obesity* is defined as a BMI of 30.0 or greater. These guidelines, which were released by the National Heart, Lung, and Blood Institute in June 1998, have been received by the medical community with a great deal of controversy. This change in guidelines increased the number of individuals in the United States considered obese from one-third to approximately one-half. The average American woman has a BMI of 26, and fashion models typically have BMIs of 18 (America's Health Network, 1998). Table 19–4 presents an example of some BMIs based on weight (in pounds) and height (in inches).

Obese people often present with hyperlipidemia, particularly elevated triglyceride and cholesterol levels. They commonly have hyperglycemia and are at risk for developing diabetes mellitus. Osteoarthritis may be evident resulting from trauma to weight-bearing joints. Workload on the heart and lungs is increased, often leading to symptoms of angina or respiratory insufficiency (Long, 1995).

TABLE 19 – 3 Research Criteria for Binge-Eating Disorder

A. Recurrent episodes of binge eating. An episode of binge eating is characterized by both of the following:
   (1) Eating, in a discrete period of time (e.g., within any 2-hour period), an amount of food that is definitely larger than most people would eat in a similar period of time under similar circumstances
   (2) A sense of lack of control over eating during the episode (e.g., a feeling that one cannot stop eating or control what or how much one is eating)

B. The binge-eating episodes are associated with three (or more) of the following:
   (1) Eating much more rapidly than normal
   (2) Eating until feeling uncomfortably full
   (3) Eating large amounts of food when not feeling physically hungry
   (4) Eating alone because of being embarrassed by how much one is eating
   (5) Feeling disgusted with oneself, depressed, or very guilty after overeating

C. Marked distress regarding binge eating is present.

D. The binge eating occurs, on average, at least 2 days a week for 6 months.
   Note: The method of determining frequency differs from that used for bulimia nervosa; future research should address whether the preferred method of setting a frequency threshold is counting the number of days on which binges occur or counting the number of episodes of binge eating.

E. The binge eating is not associated with the regular use of inappropriate compensatory behaviors (e.g., purging, fasting, excessive exercise) and does not occur exclusively during the course of anorexia nervosa or bulimia nervosa.

From the American Psychiatric Association (2000), with permission.

TABLE 19–4 Body Mass Index (BMI) Chart

To use this table, find the appropriate height in the left-hand column. Move across to a given weight. The number at the top of the column is the BMI at that height and weight. Pounds have been rounded off.

BMI HEIGHT (INCHES)	19	20	21	22	23	24	25	26	27	28	29	30	31	32	33	34	35	36	37	38	39	40
	BODY WEIGHT (POUNDS)																					
58	91	96	100	105	110	115	119	124	129	134	138	143	148	153	158	162	167	172	177	181	186	191
59	94	99	104	109	114	119	124	128	133	138	143	148	153	158	163	168	173	178	183	188	193	198
60	97	102	107	112	118	123	128	133	138	143	148	153	158	163	168	174	179	184	189	194	199	204
61	100	106	111	116	122	127	132	137	143	148	153	158	164	169	174	180	185	190	195	201	206	211
62	104	109	115	120	126	131	136	142	147	153	158	164	169	175	180	186	191	196	202	207	213	218
63	107	113	118	124	130	135	141	146	152	158	163	169	175	180	186	191	197	203	208	214	220	225
64	110	116	122	128	134	140	145	151	157	163	169	174	180	186	192	197	204	209	215	221	227	232
65	114	120	126	132	138	144	150	156	162	168	174	180	186	192	198	204	210	216	222	228	234	240
66	118	124	130	136	142	148	155	161	167	173	179	186	192	198	204	210	216	223	229	235	241	247
67	121	127	134	140	146	153	159	166	172	178	185	191	198	204	211	217	223	230	236	242	249	255
68	125	131	138	144	151	158	164	171	177	184	190	197	203	210	216	223	230	236	243	249	256	262
69	128	135	142	149	155	162	169	176	182	189	196	203	209	216	223	230	236	243	250	257	263	270
70	132	139	146	153	160	167	174	181	188	195	202	209	216	222	229	236	243	250	257	264	271	278
71	136	143	150	157	165	172	179	186	196	200	208	215	222	229	236	243	250	257	265	272	279	286
72	140	147	154	162	169	177	184	191	199	206	213	221	228	235	242	250	258	265	272	279	287	294
73	144	151	159	166	174	182	189	197	204	212	219	227	235	242	250	257	265	272	280	288	295	302
74	148	155	163	171	179	186	194	202	210	218	225	233	241	249	256	264	272	280	287	295	303	311
75	152	160	168	176	184	192	200	208	216	224	232	240	248	256	264	272	279	287	295	303	311	319
76	156	164	172	180	189	197	205	213	221	230	238	246	254	263	271	279	287	295	304	312	320	328

National Heart, Lung & Blood Institute, a division of the National Institutes of Health (1998).

Etiological Implications for Obesity

Biological Influences

Genetics

Genetics have been implicated in the development of obesity in that 80 percent of offspring of two obese parents are obese (Halmi, 2003). Studies of twins and adoptees reared by normal and overweight parents have supported this implication of heredity as a factor.

Physiological Factors

Lesions in the appetite and satiety centers in the hypothalamus may contribute to overeating and lead to obesity. Hypothyroidism is a problem that interferes with basal metabolism and may lead to weight gain. Weight gain can also occur in response to the decreased insulin production of diabetes mellitus and the increased cortisone production of Cushing's disease.

Lifestyle Factors

On an elementary level, obesity can be viewed as an ingestion of a greater number of calories than are expended. Weight gain occurs when caloric intake exceeds caloric output in terms of basal metabolism and physical activity. Many overweight individuals lead sedentary lifestyles, making it very difficult to burn off calories.

Psychosocial Influences

The psychoanalytical view of obesity proposes that obese individuals have unresolved dependency needs and are fixed in the oral stage of psychosexual development. The symptoms of obesity are viewed as depressive equivalents, attempts to regain "lost" or frustrated nurturance and caring. Liberman (1994) states:

> Overeating can be an attempt to compensate for unfulfilled needs, like an insatiable desire for impossible love, constant feelings of emptiness, lack of self-esteem and

feelings of insecurity. This mechanism is common to people rejected by mothers who neglected their feeding or who faked genuine and positive feelings replacing them with over-protection, offering food to compensate for, or substitute non-existent affection. What is at stake here is seeking in food the "good mother" image and the possibility of being nurtured by unconditional love.

Diagnosis/Outcome Identification

Based on the data collected during the nursing assessment, possible nursing diagnoses for the client with eating disorders include:

Imbalanced nutrition: less than body requirements related to refusal to eat

Deficient fluid volume (risk for or actual) related to decreased fluid intake; self-induced vomiting; laxative and/or diuretic abuse

Ineffective denial related to retarded ego development and fear of losing the only aspect of life over which he or she perceives some control (eating)

Imbalanced nutrition: more than body requirements related to compulsive overeating

Disturbed body image/low self-esteem related to retarded ego development, dysfunctional family system, or feelings of dissatisfaction with body appearance

Anxiety (moderate to severe) related to feelings of helplessness and lack of control over life events

The following criteria may be used for measurement of outcomes in the care of clients with eating disorders. The client:

1. Has achieved and maintained at least 80 percent of expected body weight
2. Has vital signs, blood pressure, and laboratory serum studies within normal limits
3. Verbalizes importance of adequate nutrition
4. Verbalizes knowledge regarding consequences of fluid loss caused by self-induced vomiting (or laxative/diuretic abuse) and importance of adequate fluid intake
5. Verbalizes events that precipitate anxiety and demonstrates techniques for its reduction
6. Verbalizes ways in which he or she may gain more control of the environment and thereby reduce feelings of helplessness
7. Expresses interest in welfare of others and less preoccupation with own appearance
8. Verbalizes that image of body as "fat" was misperception and demonstrates ability to take control of own life without resorting to maladaptive eating behaviors (anorexia nervosa)
9. Has established a healthy pattern of eating for weight control, and weight loss toward a desired goal is progressing
10. Verbalizes plans for future maintenance of weight control

Planning/Implementation

Tables 19–5 and 19–6 provide plans of care for clients with eating disorders. Nursing diagnoses are presented, along with outcome criteria, appropriate nursing interventions, and rationales. A critical pathway of care for the client with anorexia nervosa may be found in Appendix E.

Client/Family Education

The role of client teacher is important in the psychiatric area, as it is in all areas of nursing. A list of topics for client/family education relevant to eating disorders is presented in Table 19–7.

Evaluation

Evaluation of the client with an eating disorder requires a reassessment of the behaviors for which the client sought treatment. Behavioral change will be required on both the part of the client and family members. The following types of questions may provide assistance in gathering data required for evaluating whether the nursing interventions have been effective in achieving the goals of therapy.

For Anorexia or Bulimia

1. Has the client steadily gained 2 to 3 pounds per week to at least 80 percent of body weight for age and size?
2. Is the client free of signs and symptoms of malnutrition and dehydration?
3. Does the client consume adequate calories as determined by the dietitian?
4. Have there been any attempts to stash food from tray to discard later?
5. Have there been any attempts to self-induce vomiting?
6. Has the client admitted that a problem exists and that eating behaviors are maladaptive?
7. Have behaviors aimed at manipulating the environment been discontinued?

TABLE 19–5 Care Plan for Client With Eating Disorders: Anorexia Nervosa and Bulimia Nervosa

Nursing Diagnoses: IMBALANCED NUTRITION; LESS THAN BODY REQUIREMENTS; DEFICIENT FLUID VOLUME (RISK FOR OR ACTUAL)

Related to: Refusal to eat/drink; self-induced vomiting; abuse of laxatives/diuretics

Evidenced by: Loss of weight, poor muscle tone and skin turgor, lanugo, bradycardia, hypotension, cardiac arrhythmias, pale, dry mucous membranes

Outcome Criteria	Nursing Interventions	Rationale
Client will achieve 80% of target body weight and be free of signs and symptoms of malnutrition/dehydration.	1. Dietitian will determine number of calories required to provide adequate nutrition and realistic weight gain.	1. Adequate calories are required to allow a weight gain of 2–3 lb/wk.
	2. Explain to the client that privileges and restrictions will be based on compliance with treatment and direct weight gain. Do not focus on food and eating.	2. The real issues have little to do with food or eating patterns. Focus on the control issues that have precipitated these behaviors.
	3. Weigh client daily, immediately upon arising and following first voiding. Always use same scale, if possible. Keep strict record of intake and output. Assess skin turgor and integrity regularly. Assess moistness and color of oral mucous membranes.	3. These assessments are important measurements of nutritional status and provide guidelines for treatment.
	4. Stay with client during established time for meals (usually 30 min) and for at least 1 hr following meals.	4. Lengthy mealtimes put excessive focus on food and eating and provide client with attention and reinforcement. The hour following meals may be used to discard food stashed from tray or to engage in self-induced vomiting.
	5. If weight loss occurs, initiate restrictions. Client must understand that if nutritional status deteriorates, tube feedings will begin. This is implemented in a matter-of-fact, nonpunitive way.	5. Restrictions and limits must be established and carried out consistently to avoid power struggles, to encourage client compliance with therapy, and to ensure client safety.

Nursing Diagnosis: INEFFECTIVE DENIAL

Related to: Retarded ego development and fear of losing the only aspect of life over which client perceives some control (eating)

Evidenced by: Inability to admit the impact of maladaptive eating behaviors on life pattern

Outcome Criteria	Nursing Interventions	Rationale
Client will verbalize understanding that eating behaviors are maladaptive and demonstrate the ability to cope with issues of control in a more adaptive manner.	1. Develop a trusting relationship. Convey positive regard.	1. Trust and unconditional acceptance promote dignity and self-worth and provide a strong foundation for a therapeutic relationship.
	2. Avoid arguing or bargaining with the client who is resistant to treatment. State matter-of-factly which behaviors are unacceptable and how privileges will be restricted for noncompliance.	2. The person who is denying a problem and who has a weak ego will use manipulation to achieve control. Consistency and firmness by staff will decrease use of these behaviors.
	3. Encourage client to verbalize feelings regarding role within the family and issues related to dependence/independence, intense need for achievement, and sexuality. Help client recognize ways to gain control over these problematic areas of life.	3. When client feels control over major life issues, the need to gain control through maladaptive eating behaviors will diminish.

Nursing Diagnosis: DISTURBED BODY IMAGE/LOW SELF-ESTEEM

Related to: Retarded ego development and dysfunctional family system

Evidenced by: Distorted body image, difficulty accepting positive reinforcement, depressed mood, and self-deprecating thoughts

Outcome Criteria	Nursing Interventions	Rationale
Client will acknowledge misperception of body image as "fat" and verbalize positive self-attributes.	1. Help client to develop a realistic perception of body image and relationship with food. Compare specific measurement of the client's body with the client's perceived calculations.	1. There may be a large discrepancy between the actual body size and the client's perception of body size. Client needs to recognize that the misperception of body image is unhealthy and that maintaining control through maladaptive eating behaviors is dangerous—even life threatening.
	2. Promote feelings of control within the environment through participation and independent decision-making. Through positive feedback, help client learn to accept self as is, including weaknesses as well as strengths.	2. Client must come to understand that he or she is a capable, autonomous individual who can perform outside the family unit and who is not expected to be perfect. Control of his or her life must be achieved in other ways besides dieting and weight loss.
	3. Help client realize that perfection is unrealistic, and explore this need with him or her.	3. As client begins to feel better about self, identifies positive self-attributes, and develops the ability to accept certain personal inadequacies, the need for unrealistic achievement should diminish.

TABLE 19–6 Care Plan for the Client with an Eating Disorder: Obesity

Nursing Diagnosis: IMBALANCED NUTRITION: MORE THAN BODY REQUIREMENTS

Related to: Compulsive Overeating

Evidenced by: Weight of more than 20% over expected body weight for age and height; BMI>30

Outcome Criteria	Nursing Interventions	Rationale
Client will demonstrate change in eating patterns resulting in a steady weight loss.	1. Encourage the client to keep a diary of food intake.	1. A food diary provides the opportunity for client to gain a realistic picture of the amount of food ingested and provides a database on which to tailor the dietary program.
	2. Discuss feelings and emotions associated with eating.	2. This helps to identify when client is eating to satisfy an emotional need rather than a physiological one.
	3. With input from the client, formulate an eating plan that includes food from the basic food groups with emphasis on low-fat intake. It is helpful to keep the plan as similar to client's usual eating pattern as possible.	3. Diet must eliminate calories while maintaining adequate nutrition. Client is more likely to stay on the eating plan if he or she is able to participate in its creation and it deviates as little as possible from usual types of foods.
	4. Identify realistic increment goals for weekly weight loss.	4. Reasonable weight loss (1–2 lb/wk) results in more lasting effects. Excessive, rapid weight loss may result in fatigue and irritability and ultimately lead to failure in meeting goals for weight loss. Motivation is more easily sustained by meeting "stair-step" goals.

(Continued)

TABLE 19-6 Care Plan for the Client with an Eating Disorder: Obesity *(Continued)*

Outcome Criteria	Nursing Interventions	Rationale
	5. Plan progressive exercise program tailored to individual goals and choice.	5. Exercise may enhance weight loss by burning calories and reducing appetite, increasing energy, toning muscles, and enhancing sense of well-being and accomplishment. Walking is an excellent choice for overweight individuals.
	6. Discuss the probability of reaching plateaus when weight remains stable for extended periods.	6. Client should know this is likely to happen as changes in metabolism occur. Plateaus cause frustration, and client may need additional support during these times to remain on the weight loss program.
	7. Administer medications to assist with weight loss if ordered by physician.	7. Appetite-suppressant drugs (e.g., sibutramine) and others that have weight loss as a side effect (e.g., fluoxetine) may be helpful to someone who is morbidly obese. They should be used for this purpose for only a short period while the individual attempts to adjust to the new pattern of eating.

Nursing Diagnosis: DISTURBED BODY IMAGE/LOW SELF-ESTEEM
Related to: Dissatisfaction with appearance
Evidenced by: Verbalization of negative feelings about the way he or she looks and desire to lose weight

Outcome Criteria	Nursing Interventions	Rationale
Client will begin to accept self based on self-attributes rather than on appearance, while actively pursuing weight loss as desired.	1. Assess client's feelings and attitudes about being obese.	1. Obesity and compulsive eating behaviors may have deep-rooted psychological implications, such as compensation for lack of love and nurturing or a defense against intimacy.
	2. Ensure that the client has privacy during self-care activities.	2. The obese individual may be sensitive or self-conscious about his or her body.
	3. Have client recall coping patterns related to food in family of origin and explore how these may affect current situation.	3. Parents are role models for their children. Maladaptive eating behaviors are learned within the family system and are supported through positive reinforcement. Food may be substituted by the parent for affection and love, and eating is associated with a feeling of satisfaction, becoming the primary defense.
	4. Determine client's motivation for weight loss and set goals.	4. The individual may harbor repressed feelings of hostility, which may be expressed inward on the self. Because of a poor self-concept, the person often has difficulty with relationships. When the motivation is to lose weight for someone else, successful weight loss is less likely to occur.
	5. Help client identify positive self-attributes. Focus on strengths and past accomplishments unrelated to physical appearance.	5. It is important that self-esteem not be tied solely to size of the body. Client needs to recognize that obesity need not interfere with positive feelings regarding self-concept and self-worth.
	6. Refer client to support or therapy group.	6. Support groups can provide companionship, increase motivation, decrease loneliness and social ostracism, and give practical solutions to common problems. Group therapy can be helpful in dealing with underlying psychological concerns.

TABLE 19-7 Topics for Client/Family Education Related to Eating Disorders

Nature of the Illness
1. Symptoms of anorexia nervosa
2. Symptoms of bulimia nervosa
3. What constitutes obesity?
4. Causes of eating disorders
5. Effects of the illness or condition on the body

Management of the Illness
1. Principles of nutrition (foods for maintenance of wellness)
2. Ways client may feel in control of life (aside from eating)
3. Importance of expressing fears and feelings, rather than holding them inside
4. Alternative coping strategies (to maladaptive eating behaviors)
5. For the obese client:
   a. How to plan a reduced-calorie, nutritious diet
   b. How to read food content labels
   c. How to establish a realistic weight loss plan
   d. How to establish a planned program of physical activity
6. Correct administration of prescribed medications (e.g., antidepressants, anorexiants)
7. Indication for and side effects of prescribed medications
8. Relaxation techniques
9. Problem-solving skills

Support Services
1. Weight Watchers International
2. Overeaters Anonymous
3. National Association of Anorexia Nervosa and Associated Disorders (ANAD)
   P.O. Box 7
   Highland Park, IL 60035
   (847) 831-3438
4. The American Anorexia/Bulimia Association, Inc.
   165 W. 46th St., Suite 1108
   New York, NY 10036
   (212) 575-6200

8. Is the client willing to discuss the real issues concerning family roles, sexuality, dependence/independence, and the need for achievement?
9. Does the client understand how he or she has used maladaptive eating behaviors in an effort to achieve a feeling of some control over life events?
10. Has the client acknowledged that perception of body image as "fat" is incorrect?

For Obesity

1. Has the client shown a steady weight loss since starting the new eating plan?
2. Does he or she verbalize a plan to help stay on the new eating plan?
3. Does the client verbalize positive self-attributes not associated with body size or appearance?

For Anorexia, Bulimia, and Obesity

1. Has the client been able to develop a more realistic perception of body image?
2. Has the client acknowledged that past self-expectations may have been unrealistic?
3. Does client accept self as less than perfect?
4. Has the client developed adaptive coping strategies to deal with stress without resorting to maladaptive eating behaviors?

TREATMENT MODALITIES

The immediate aim of treatment in eating disorders is to restore the client's nutritional status. Complications of emaciation, dehydration, and electrolyte imbalance can lead to death. Once the physical condition is no longer life-threatening, other treatment modalities may be initiated.

Behavior Modification

Efforts to change the maladaptive eating behaviors of clients with anorexia and bulimia have become the widely accepted treatment. The importance of instituting a behavior modification program with these clients is to ensure that the program does not "control" them. Issues of control are central to the etiology of these disorders, and in order for the program to be successful, the client must perceive that he or she is in control of the treatment.

Successes have been observed when the client is allowed to contract for privileges based on weight gain. The client has input into the care plan and can clearly see what the treatment choices are. The client has control over eating, over the amount of exercise pursued, and even over whether or not to induce vomiting. Goals of therapy, along with the responsibilities of each for goal achievement, are agreed on by client and staff.

Staff and client also agree on a system of rewards and privileges that can be earned by the client, who is given ultimate control. He or she has a choice of whether or not to abide by the contract—a choice of whether or not to gain weight—and a choice of whether or not to earn the desired privilege.

Individual Therapy

Although individual psychotherapy is not the therapy of choice for eating disorders, it can be helpful when underlying psychological problems are contributing to the maladaptive behaviors. In supportive psychotherapy, the therapist encourages the client to explore unresolved conflicts and to recognize the maladaptive eating behaviors as defense mechanisms used to ease the emotional pain. The goals are to resolve the personal issues and establish more adaptive coping strategies for dealing with stressful situations.

Family Therapy

Eckert and Mitchell (1994) state:

> Counseling of family members is a necessary component of an effective treatment program. This involves educating the family about the disorder, assessing the family's impact on maintaining the disorder, and assisting in methods to promote normal functioning of the patient. (p. 199)

In many instances, eating disorders may be considered *family* disorders, and resolution cannot be achieved until dynamics within the family have improved. Family therapy deals with education of the members about the disorder's manifestations, possible etiology, and prescribed treatment. Support is given to family members as they deal with feelings of guilt associated with the perception that they may have contributed to the onset of the disorder. Support is also given as they deal with the social stigma of having a family member with emotional problems.

In some instances, when the dysfunctional family dynamics are related to conflict avoidance, the family may be noncompliant with therapy as they attempt to maintain equilibrium by keeping a member in the sick role. When this occurs, it is essential to focus on the functional operations within the family and to help them manage conflict and create change.

Referrals are made to local support groups for families of individuals with eating disorders. Resolution and growth can sometimes be achieved through interaction with others who are experiencing or have experienced the numerous problems of living with a family member with an eating disorder.

Psychopharmacology

There are no medications specifically indicated for eating disorders. Various medications have been prescribed for associated symptoms, such as anxiety and depression. Halmi, Mitchell, and Rigotti (1995) report on the use of fluoxetine (Prozac), sertraline (Zoloft), and clomipramine (Anafranil) for clients with anorexia nervosa. Cyproheptadine (Periactin) has been used as an appetite stimulant; and antipsychotics such as chlorpromazine (Thorazine), and lithium carbonate have also been used to treat anorexia nervosa in selected clients.

Fluoxetine (Prozac) has been found to be useful in the treatment of bulimia nervosa (Walsh, et al., 2000). A dosage of 60 mg a day (triple the usual antidepressant dosage) was found to be most effective with bulimic clients. It is possible that fluoxetine, an SSRI, may decrease the craving for carbohydrates, thereby decreasing the incidence of binge eating, which is often associated with consumption of large amounts of carbohydrates. Other antidepressants, such as imipramine (Tofranil), desipramine (Norpramin), trazodone (Desyrel), and phenelzine (Nardil), also have been shown to be effective in controlled treatment studies (Halmi, 2003; Halmi, Mitchell, & Rigotti, 1995). Fluoxetine has also been successful in treating clients who are overweight, possibly for the same reason that was explained for bulimic clients. The effective dosage for promoting weight loss is 60 mg a day. Sadock and Sadock (2003) state:

> Sympathomimetics are used in the treatment of obesity because of their anorexia-inducing effects. Because tolerance develops for the anorectic effects and because of the drugs' high abuse potential, their use for this indication is limited. (p. 1118)

Withdrawal from **anorexiants** may result in a rebound weight gain and, in some clients, a concomitant lethargy and depression. Two anorexiants that were once widely used, fenfluramine and dexfenfluramine, have been removed from the market because of their association with serious heart and lung disease.

A medication for treating obesity, called sibutramine (Meridia), became available in March 1998. It has been suggested only for individuals who have a significant amount of weight to lose. The mechanism of action in the control of appetite appears to occur by inhibiting the neurotransmitters serotonin and norepinephrine. Common side effects include headache, dry mouth, constipation, and insomnia. More troublesome side effects include increased blood pressure, rapid heart rate, and seizures. Some concern has recently been expressed about possible cardiac disease associated with the use of sibutramine. Some individuals have claimed a number of cardiovascular-related deaths in association with use of the drug. This claim is currently unsubstantiated. Caution must be taken in prescribing this medication for an individual with a history of cardiac disease.

SUMMARY

The incidence of eating disorders has continued to increase over the past 30 years. Individuals with anorexia nervosa, a disorder that is characterized by a morbid fear of obesity and a gross distortion of body image, literally can starve themselves to death. The individual believes he or she is fat even when emaciated. The disorder is commonly accompanied by depression and anxiety.

Bulimia nervosa is an eating disorder characterized by the consumption of huge amounts of food, usually in a short period, and often in secret. Tension is relieved and pleasure felt during the time of the binge, but it is soon followed by feelings of guilt and depression. Individuals with this disorder "purge" themselves of the excessive intake with self-induced vomiting, or the misuse of laxatives, diuretics, or enemas. They also are subject to mood and anxiety disorders.

Compulsive eating can result in obesity, which is defined by the NIH as a BMI of 30. Obesity predisposes the individual to many health concerns, and at the morbid level (a BMI of 40.0), the weight alone can contribute to increases in morbidity and mortality.

This chapter explored the etiological factors associated with these three eating disorders. Symptomatology was identified as background assessment data. Nursing care was presented in the context of the six steps of the nursing process. Care plans for anorexia/bulimia and obesity were included. The treatment modalities of behavior modification, individual psychotherapy, family therapy, and psychopharmacology were discussed.

REVIEW QUESTIONS

SELF-EXAMINATION/LEARNING EXERCISE

Select the answer that is most appropriate for each of the following questions:

1. Some obese individuals take amphetamines to suppress appetite and help them lose weight. Which of the following is an adverse effect associated with use of amphetamines that makes this practice undesirable?
   a. Bradycardia
   b. Amenorrhea
   c. Tolerance
   d. Convulsions
2. Psychoanalytically, the theory of obesity relates to the individual's unconscious equation of food with:
   a. Nurturance and caring
   b. Power and control
   c. Autonomy and emotional growth
   d. Strength and endurance
3. From a physiological point of view, the *most common* cause of obesity is probably:
   a. Lack of nutritional education
   b. More calories consumed than expended
   c. Impaired endocrine functioning
   d. Low basal metabolic rate
4. Nancy, aged 14, has just been admitted to the psychiatric unit for anorexia nervosa. She is emaciated and refusing to eat. What is the primary nursing diagnosis for Nancy?
   a. Dysfunctional grieving
   b. Imbalanced nutrition: less than body requirements
   c. Interrupted family processes
   d. Anxiety (severe)
5. Which of the following physical manifestations would you expect to assess in Nancy?
   a. Tachycardia, hypertension, hyperthermia
   b. Bradycardia, hypertension, hyperthermia
   c. Bradycardia, hypotension, hypothermia
   d. Tachycardia, hypotension, hypothermia
6. Nancy continues to refuse to eat. What is the most appropriate response by the nurse?
   a. "You know that if you don't eat, you will die."
   b. "If you continue to refuse to take food orally, you will be fed through a nasogastric tube."
   c. "You might as well leave if you are not going to follow your therapy regimen."
   d. "You don't have to eat if you don't want to. It is your choice."
7. Which medication might you expect the physician to prescribe for Nancy?
   a. Chlorpromazine (Thorazine)
   b. Diazepam (Valium)
   c. Fluoxetine (Prozac)
   d. Carbamazepine (Tegretol)

8. Jane is hospitalized on the psychiatric unit. She has a history and current diagnosis of bulimia nervosa. Which of the following symptoms would be congruent with Jane's diagnosis?
   a. Binging, purging, obesity, hyperkalemia
   b. Binging, purging, normal weight, hypokalemia
   c. Binging, laxative abuse, amenorrhea, severe weight loss
   d. Binging, purging, severe weight loss, hyperkalemia
9. Jane has stopped vomiting in the hospital and tells the nurse she is afraid she is going to gain weight. Which is the most appropriate response by the nurse?
   a. "Don't worry. The dietitian will ensure you don't get too many calories in your diet."
   b. "Don't worry about your weight. We are going to work on other problems when you are in the hospital."
   c. "I understand that you are concerned about your weight, but I want you to tell me about your recent invitation to join the National Honor Society. That's quite an accomplishment."
   d. "You are not fat, and the staff will ensure that you do not gain weight when you are in the hospital, because we know that is important to you."
10. The binging episode is thought to involve:
    a. A release of tension, followed by feelings of depression
    b. Feelings of fear, followed by feelings of relief
    c. Unmet dependency needs and a way to gain attention
    d. Feelings of euphoria, excitement, and self-gratification

Test Your CRITICAL THINKING SKILLS

Janice, a high school sophomore, wanted desperately to become a cheerleader. She practiced endlessly before tryouts, but she was not selected. A week later, her boyfriend, Roy, broke up with her to date another girl. Janice, who was 5 feet 3 inches tall and weighed 110 pounds, decided it was because she was too fat. She began to exercise at every possible moment. She skipped meals, and tried to keep her daily consumption to no more than 300 calories. She lost a great deal of weight but became very weak. She felt cold all of the time and wore sweaters in the warm weather. She collapsed during her physical education class at school and was rushed to the emergency department. On admission, she weighed 90 pounds. She was emaciated and anemic. The physician admitted her with a diagnosis of anorexia nervosa.

Answer the following questions about Janice:

1. What will be the *primary* consideration in her care?
2. How will treatment be directed toward helping her gain weight?
3. How will the nurse know if Janice is using self-induced vomiting to rid herself of food consumed at meals?

IMPLICATIONS OF RESEARCH FOR EVIDENCE BASED PRACTICE

Whitaker, R.C., Wright, J.A., Pepe, M.S., Seidel, K.D., and Dietz, W.H: **Predicting obesity in young adulthood from childhood and parental obesity.** New England Journal of Medicine (1997, September 25), 337: 869–873.

Description of the Study: This study investigated the risk of obesity in young adulthood associated with both obesity in childhood and obesity in one or both parents. The study included 854 subjects born at a health maintenance organization in Washington State between 1965 and 1971. Subjects' and parents' health records were reviewed. Childhood obesity was defined as a body-mass index (BMI) at or above the 85th percentile for age and sex, and obesity in adulthood was defined as a BMI $\geq$ 27.8 for men and $\geq$ 27.3 for women. Follow-up occurred when the subjects were between ages 21 and 29 years.

Results of the Study: In young adulthood, 35 percent (135 subjects) were obese. Among those subjects who were obese during childhood, the following data were collected:

- Obese at age 1 or 2 years without obese parents: 8 percent were obese in young adulthood
- Obese at age 10 to 14 years with at least 1 obese parent: 79 percent obese in young adulthood

Results indicated that obese children younger than age 3 years without obese parents were at low risk for obesity in adulthood, but among older children, obesity is an increasingly important predictor of adult obesity, regardless of whether the parents are obese. Parental obesity was found to more than double the risk of adult obesity among both obese and non-obese children less than 10 years of age.

Implications for Nursing Practice: Nurses are in a position to help identify individuals at high risk for obesity. Nurses may be instrumental in establishing screening programs to identify individuals in need of assistance with weight reduction and nutritional education. A number of health problems (e.g., heart disease, diabetes, hypertension) are associated with obesity, and a great need exists to help individuals establish nutritional weight loss programs within the community. Fifty-eight million Americans (ages 20 through 74 years) are overweight. Nurses face a challenge to assist these individuals in an effort to improve nutritional and health status.

IMPLICATIONS OF RESEARCH FOR EVIDENCE BASED PRACTICE

Sullivan, P.F., Bulik, C.M., Fear, J.L., and Pickering, A: **Outcome of anorexia nervosa: a case control study.** American Journal of Psychiatry (1998, July), 155: 9399–946.

Description of the Study: The objective of this study was to try to improve knowledge related to outcomes of treatment of anorexia nervosa. Participants included 70 female patients referred to an eating disorders service between January 1, 1981, and December 31, 1984. The comparison group was a random community sample of 98. All subjects were interviewed with a structured diagnostic instrument.

Results of the Study: Ten percent of the patients continued to meet the criteria for anorexia nervosa an average of 12 years after the initial diagnosis. Among those who no longer met the criteria 12 years later, relatively low body weight and cognitive features characteristic of anorexia nervosa (e.g., perfectionism; compulsiveness) persisted. The rates of lifetime comorbid major depression, alcohol dependence, and a number of anxiety disorders were very high.

Implications for Nursing Practice: The authors suggest that in this era of managed care/brief treatment, too often therapeutic approaches for anorexia nervosa focus on weight gain and neglect to detect associated psychological features and comorbidity. This study has implications for nursing to ensure that the emotional component of the disease is not overlooked. Anorexia nervosa can be considered a family illness, and for this reason, the entire family should be considered for therapy. Treating the individual weight problem alone and neglecting the psychological component of the disease can lead to a chronic situation that also can include comorbid psychiatric illnesses.

INTERNET REFERENCES

- Additional information about anorexia nervosa and bulimia nervosa may be located at the following websites:
  - a http://www.aabainc.org
  - b http://www.psych.org/public_info/eatingdisorders52201.cfm
  - c http://www.mentalhealth.com/dis/p20-et01.html
  - d http://www.anred.com/
  - e http://www.mentalhealth.com/dis/p20-et02.html

f http://www.nimh.nih.gov/publicat/eatdis.htm

g http://medlineplus.nlm.nih.gov/medlineplus/eatingdisorders.html

- Additional information about obesity may be located at the following websites:

a http://www.shapeup.org/

b http://www.obesity.org/

c http://medlineplus.nlm.nih.gov/medlineplus/obesity.html

d http://www.asbp.org/

e http://www.niddk.nih.gov/health/nutrit/pubs/binge.htm

REFERENCES

American Psychiatric Association (APA). (2000). Diagnostic and statistical manual of mental disorders (4th ed.) Text revision. Washington, DC: American Psychiatric Association.

America's Health Network. (1998). Easy answer to weight-loss in America? Fat Chance! Retrieved July 10, 1998 from http://www.ahn.com/community/wellness/authors/twinkle/fatchance/htm

Eckert, E.D & Mitchell, J.E. (1994). Anorexia nervosa and bulimia nervosa. In G. Winokur & P.J. Clayton (Eds.), The medical basis of psychiatry (2nd ed.). Philadelphia: WB Saunders.

Halmi, K.A. (2003). Eating disorders: Anorexia nervosa, bulimia nervosa, and obesity. In R.E. Hales & S.C. Yudofsky (Eds.), Textbook of clinical psychiatry (4th ed.). Washington, DC: American Psychiatric Publishing.

Halmi, KA., Mitchell, J.E., & Rigotti, N.A. (1995). Recognizing and treating eating disorders. Contemporary Nurse Practitioner, 1(1), 26–39.

Harvard Mental Health Letter (1997, October). Eating disorders—Part I. Boston, MA: Harvard Medical School Health Publications Group.

Liberman, M. (1994). Eating disorders and myths: A study of the symbolic meaning of eating disorders. Retrieved November 18, 2003 from http://www.cgjungpage.org/articles/mlibereatdis.html

Long, B.C. (1995). Healthy life-styles: Nutrition, exercise, rest and sleep. In W.J. Phipps, V.L. Cassmeyer, J.K. Sands, & M.K. Lehman (Eds.), Medical-surgical nursing: concepts and clinical practice (5th ed.). St. Louis: Mosby.

National Center for Health Statistics, Division of Data Services, U.S. Department of Health and Human Services. (2001). Prevalence of overweight and obesity among adults in the United States. Retrieved September 2, 2001 from http://www.cdc.gov/nchs/products/pubs/pubd/hestats/3and4/overweight.htm.

National Heart, Lung, & Blood Institute. (1998). Body mass index (BMI) chart. Bethesda, MD: National Institute of Health.

Sadock, B.J. & Sadock, V.A. (2003). Synopsis of psychiatry: Behavioral sciences/clinical psychiatry (9th ed.). Philadelphia: Lippincott Williams & Wilkins.

Walsh, T., Agras, W.S., Devlin, M.J., Fairburn, C.G., Wilson, G..T., Kahn, C., & Chally, M.K. (2000, August). Fluoxetine for bulimia nervosa following poor response to psychotherapy. The American Journal of Psychiatry 157:1332–1334.

20
CHAPTER

Personality Disorders

CHAPTER OUTLINE

KEY TERMS

histrionic
narcissism
object constancy
passive-aggressive
personality
schizoid
schizotypal
splitting

OBJECTIVES

After reading this chapter, the student will be able to:

1. Define *personality*.
2. Compare stages of personality development according to Sullivan, Erikson, and Mahler.
3. Identify various types of personality disorders.
4. Discuss historical and epidemiological statistics related to various personality disorders.
5. Describe symptomatology associated with borderline personality disorder and antisocial personality disorder, and use these data in client assessment.
6. Identify etiological implications for borderline personality disorder and antisocial personality disorder.
7. Formulate nursing diagnoses and goals of care for clients with borderline personality disorder and antisocial personality disorder.
8. Describe appropriate nursing interventions for behaviors associated with borderline personality disorder and antisocial personality disorder.
9. Evaluate nursing care of clients with borderline personality disorder and antisocial personality disorder.
10. Discuss various modalities relevant to treatment of personality disorders.

INTRODUCTION

The word **personality** is derived from the Greek term *persona*. It was used originally to describe the theatrical mask worn by some dramatic actors at the time. Over the years, it lost its connotation of pretense and illusion and came to represent the person behind the mask—the "real" person. Kaplan and Sadock (1998) define personality as:

> ... a person's characteristic totality of emotional and behavioral traits apparent in ordinary life, a totality that is usually stable and predictable. (p. 775)

The *DSM-IV-TR* (American Psychiatric Association [APA], 2000) defines personality *traits* as "enduring patterns of perceiving, relating to, and thinking about the environment and oneself that are exhibited in a wide range of social and personal contexts." Personality *disorders* occur when these traits become inflexible and maladaptive and cause significant functional impairment or subjective distress. These disorders are coded on axis II of the multiaxial diagnostic system used by the APA (see Chapter 1 for an explanation of this system). Virtually all individuals exhibit some behaviors associated with the various personality disorders from time to time. It is only when significant functional impairment occurs in response to these personality characteristics that the individual is thought to have a personality disorder.

Personality development occurs in response to a number of biological and psychological influences. These variables include (but are not limited to) heredity, temperament, experiential learning, and social interaction. A number of theorists have attempted to provide information about personality development. Most suggest that it occurs in an orderly, steplike fashion. These stages overlap, however, as maturation occurs at different rates in different individuals. The theories of Sullivan (1953), Erikson (1963), and Mahler (Mahler, Pine, & Bergman, 1975) were presented at length in Chapter 2. The stages of personality development according to these three theorists are compared in Table 20–1. The nurse should understand "normal" personality development before learning about what is considered dysfunctional.

TABLE 20–1 Comparison of Personality Development—Sullivan, Erikson, and Mahler

MAJOR DEVELOPMENTAL TASKS AND DESIGNATED AGES

Sullivan	*Erikson*	*Mahler*
Birth to 18 months: Relief from anxiety through oral gratification of needs.	Birth to 18 months: To develop a basic trust in the mothering figure and be able to generalize it to others.	Birth to 1 month: Fulfillment of basic needs for survival and comfort
18 months to 6 years: Learning to experience a delay in personal gratification without undue anxiety.	18 months to 3 years: To gain some self-control and independence within the environment.	1 to 5 months: Developing awareness of external source of need fulfillment.
6 to 9 years: Learning to form satisfactory peer relationships.	3 to 6 years: To develop a sense of purpose and the ability to initiate and direct own activities.	5 to 10 months: Commencement of a primary recognition of separateness from the mothering figure.
9 to 12 years: Learning to form satisfactory relationships with persons of the same sex; the initiation of feelings of affection for another person.	6 to 12 years: To achieve a sense of self-confidence by learning, competing, performing successfully, and receiving recognition from significant others, peers, and acquaintances.	10 to 16 months: Increased independence through locomotor functioning; increased sense of separateness of self.
12 to 14 years: Learning to form satisfactory relationships with persons of the opposite sex; developing a sense of identity.	12 to 20 years: To integrate the tasks mastered in the previous stages into a secure sense of self.	16 to 24 months: Acute awareness of separateness of self; learning to seek "emotional refueling" from mothering figure to maintain feeling of security.

(Continued)

TABLE 20-1 Comparison of Personality Development—Sullivan, Erikson, and Mahler *(Continued)*

Sullivan	*Erikson*	*Mahler*
14 to 21 years: Establishing self-identity; experiences satisfying relationships; working to develop a lasting, intimate opposite-sex relationship.	20 to 30 years: To form an intense, lasting relationship or a commitment to another person, a cause, an institution, or a creative effort. 30 to 65 years: To achieve the life goals established for oneself, while also considering the welfare of future generations. 65 years to death: To review one's life and derive meaning from both positive and negative events, while achieving a positive sense of self-worth.	24 to 36 months: Sense of separateness established on the way to object constancy, able to internalize a sustained image of loved object/person when it is out of sight; resolution of separation anxiety.

Historical and epidemiological aspects of personality disorders are discussed in this chapter. Predisposing factors that have been implicated in the etiology of personality disorders are presented. Symptomatology is explained to provide background knowledge for assessing clients with personality disorders.

Individuals with personality disorders are not often treated in acute care settings for the personality disorder as their primary psychiatric diagnosis. However, many clients with other psychiatric and medical diagnoses manifest symptoms of personality disorders. Nurses are likely to encounter clients with these personality characteristics frequently in all healthcare settings.

Nurses working in psychiatric settings may often encounter clients with borderline and antisocial personality characteristics. The behavior of borderline clients is very unstable, and hospitalization is often required because of attempts at self-injury. The client with antisocial personality disorder may enter the psychiatric arena because of judicially ordered evaluation. Psychiatric intervention may be an alternative to imprisonment for antisocial behavior if it is deemed potentially helpful.

Nursing care of clients with borderline personality disorder or antisocial personality disorder is presented in this chapter in the context of the nursing process. Various medical treatment modalities for personality disorders are explored.

HISTORICAL ASPECTS

The concept of a personality disorder has been present throughout the history of medicine (Phillips, Yen, & Gunderson, 2003). In the 4th century B.C., Hippocrates concluded that all disease stemmed from an excess or imbalance among four bodily humors: yellow bile, black bile, blood, and phlegm. Hippocrates identified four fundamental personality styles that he concluded stemmed from excesses in the four humors: the irritable and hostile choleric (yellow bile); the pessimistic melancholic (black bile); the overly optimistic and extraverted sanguine (blood); and the apathetic phlegmatic (phlegm).

Within the profession of medicine, the first recognition that personality disorders, apart from psychosis, were cause for their own special concern was in 1801, with the recognition that an individual can behave irrationally even when the powers of intellect are intact. Nineteenth-century psychiatrists embraced the term *moral insanity*, the concept of which defines what we know today as personality disorders.

A major difficulty for psychiatrists has been the establishment of a classification of personality disorders. The *DSM-IV-TR* provides specific criteria for diagnosing these disorders. The *DSM-IV-TR* groups the personality disorders into three clusters. These clusters, and the disorders classified under each, are described as follows:

1. Cluster A: behaviors described as odd or eccentric:

   a. Paranoid personality disorder
   b. Schizoid personality disorder
   c. Schizotypal personality disorder
2. Cluster B: behaviors described as dramatic, emotional, or erratic:
   a. Antisocial personality disorder
   b. Borderline personality disorder
   c. Histrionic personality disorder
   d. Narcissistic personality disorder
3. Cluster C: behaviors described as anxious or fearful:
   a. Avoidant personality disorder
   b. Dependent personality disorder
   c. Obsessive-compulsive personality disorder

Note: The third edition of the *DSM* included **passive-aggressive** personality disorder in cluster C. In the *DSM-IV-TR,* this disorder has been included in the section on "Criteria Provided for Further Study." For purposes of this text, passive-aggressive personality disorder will be described with the cluster C disorders.

Historically, individuals with personality disorders have been labeled as "bad" or "immoral" and as deviants in the range of normal personality dimensions. The events and sequences that result in pathology of the personality are complicated and difficult to unravel. Continued study is needed to facilitate understanding of this complex behavioral phenomenon.

TYPES OF PERSONALITY DISORDERS

Paranoid Personality Disorder

Definition and Epidemiological Statistics

The *DSM-IV-TR* defines paranoid personality disorder as "a pervasive distrust and suspiciousness of others such that their motives are interpreted as malevolent, beginning by early adulthood and present in a variety of contexts" (APA, 2000). Sadock and Sadock (2003) identify the characteristic feature as a long-standing suspiciousness and mistrust of people in general. Prevalence is difficult to establish because individuals with the disorder seldom seek assistance for their problem or require hospitalization. When they present for treatment at the insistence of others, they may be able to pull themselves together sufficiently so that their behavior does not appear maladaptive. The disorder is more commonly diagnosed in men than in women.

Clinical Picture

Individuals with paranoid personality disorder are constantly on guard, hypervigilant, and ready for any real or imagined threat. They appear tense and irritable. They have developed a hard exterior and become immune or insensitive to the feelings of others. They avoid interactions with other people, lest they be forced to relinquish some of their own power. They always feel that others are there to take advantage of them.

They are extremely oversensitive and tend to misinterpret even minute cues within the environment, magnifying and distorting them into thoughts of trickery and deception. Because they trust no one, they are constantly "testing" the honesty of others. Their intimidating manner provokes almost everyone with whom they come in contact into exasperation and anger.

Individuals with paranoid personality disorder maintain their self-esteem by attributing their shortcomings to others. They do not accept responsibility for their own behaviors and feelings and project this responsibility onto others. They are envious and hostile toward others who are highly successful and believe the only reason they are not as successful is because they have been treated unfairly. People who are paranoid are extremely vulnerable and constantly on the defensive. Any real or imagined threat can release hostility and anger that is fueled by animosities from the past. The desire for reprisal and vindication is so intense that a possible loss of control can result in aggression and violence. These outbursts are usually brief, and the paranoid person soon regains the external control, rationalizes the behavior, and reconstructs the defenses central to his or her personality pattern.

Etiological Implications

Research has indicated a possible hereditary link in paranoid personality disorder. Studies have revealed a higher incidence of paranoid personality disorder among relatives of clients with schizophrenia than among control subjects (Sadock & Sadock, 2003).

Psychosocially, people with paranoid personality disorder may have been subjected to parental antagonism and harassment. They likely served as scapegoats for displaced parental aggression and gradually relinquished all hope of affection and approval. They learned to perceive the world as harsh and unkind, a place calling for protective vigilance and mistrust. They entered the world with "chip-on-the-shoulder" attitudes and met with many rebuffs and rejections. Anticipating humiliation and betrayal by others, the paranoid person learned to attack first.

Schizoid Personality Disorder

Definition and Epidemiological Statistics

Schizoid personality disorder is characterized primarily by a profound defect in the ability to form personal relationships or to respond to others in any meaningful, emotional way (Phillips, Yen, & Gunderson, 2003). These individuals display a lifelong pattern of social withdrawal, and their discomfort with human interaction is apparent. Prevalence of schizoid personality disorder within the general population has been estimated at between 3 and 7.5 percent. Significant numbers of people with the disorder are never observed in a clinical setting. Sex ratio of the disorder is unknown, although it is diagnosed more frequently in men.

Clinical Picture

Persons with schizoid personality disorder appear cold, aloof, and indifferent to others. They prefer to work in isolation and are unsociable, with little need or desire for emotional ties (Sadock & Sadock, 2003). They are able to invest enormous affective energy in intellectual pursuits.

In the presence of others, they appear shy, anxious, or uneasy. They are inappropriately serious about everything and have difficulty acting in a lighthearted manner. Their behavior and conversation exhibit little or no spontaneity. Typically, they are unable to experience pleasure, and their affect is commonly bland and constricted.

Etiological Implications

Although the role of heredity in the etiology of schizoid personality disorder is unclear, the feature of introversion appears to be a highly inheritable characteristic (Phillips, Yen, & Gunderson, 2003). Further studies are required before definitive statements can be made.

Psychosocially, the development of schizoid personality is probably influenced by early interactional patterns that the person found to be cold and unsatisfying. The childhoods of these individuals have often been characterized as bleak, cold, and notably lacking empathy and nurturing. A child brought up with this type of parenting may become a schizoid adult if that child possesses a temperamental disposition that is shy, anxious, and introverted. Phillips, Yen, and Gunderson (2003) state:

> Clinicians have noted that schizoid personality disorder occurs in adults who experienced cold, neglectful, and ungratifying relationships in early childhood, which leads these persons to assume that relationships are not valuable or worth pursuing. (pp. 812–813)

Schizotypal Personality Disorder

Definition and Epidemiological Statistics

Individuals with **schizotypal** personality disorder were once described as "latent schizophrenics." Their behavior is odd and eccentric but does not decompensate to the level of schizophrenia. Schizotypal personality is a graver form of the pathologically less severe schizoid personality pattern. Studies indicate that approximately 3 percent of the population has this disorder (APA, 2000).

Clinical Picture

Individuals with schizotypal personality disorder are aloof and isolated and behave in a bland and apathetic manner. Magical thinking, ideas of reference, illusions, and depersonalization are part of their everyday world. Examples include superstitiousness; belief in clairvoyance, telepathy, or "sixth sense"; and beliefs that "others can feel my feelings" (APA, 2000).

The speech pattern is sometimes bizarre. People with this disorder often cannot orient their thoughts logically and become lost in personal irrelevancies and tangential asides that seem vague, digressive, and not pertinent to the topic at hand. This feature of their personality only further alienates them from others.

Under stress, these individuals may decompensate and demonstrate psychotic symptoms, such as delusional thoughts, hallucinations, or bizarre behaviors, but they are usually of brief duration (Sadock & Sadock, 2003). They often talk or gesture to themselves, as if "living in their own world." Their affect is bland or inappropriate, such as expressing silly laughter when discussing his or her problems (Phillips, Yen, & Gunderson, 2003).

Etiological Implications

Some evidence suggests that schizotypal personality disorder is more common among the first-degree biological relatives of people with schizophrenia than among the general population, indicating a possible hereditary factor (APA, 2000). Although speculative, other biogenic factors that may contribute to the development of this disorder include anatomical deficits or neurochemical dysfunctions resulting in diminished activation, minimal pleasure-pain sensibilities, and impaired cognitive functions. These biological etiological factors give support to the close link between schizotypal personality disorder and schizophrenia and are considered when classifying schizotypal personality disorder with schizophrenia rather than with the personality disorders in the *International Classification of Diseases (ICD-10)* (Phillips, Yen, & Gunderson, 2003).

The early family dynamics of the individual with schizotypal personality disorder may have been characterized by indifference, impassivity, or formality, leading to a pattern of discomfort with personal affection and closeness. Early on, affective deficits made them unattractive and unrewarding social companions. They were likely shunned, overlooked, rejected, and humiliated by others, resulting in feelings of low self-esteem and a marked distrust of interpersonal relations. Having failed repeatedly to cope with these adversities, they began to withdraw and reduce contact with individuals and situations that evoked sadness and humiliation. Their new inner world provided them with a more significant and potentially rewarding existence than that experienced in reality.

Antisocial Personality Disorder

Definition and Epidemiological Statistics

Antisocial personality disorder is a pattern of socially irresponsible, exploitative, and guiltless behavior that reflects a disregard for the rights of others (Phillips, Yen, & Gunderson, 2003). These individuals exploit and manipulate others for personal gain and have a general disregard for the law. They have difficulty sustaining consistent employment and in developing stable relationships. It is one of the oldest and best researched of the personality disorders and has been included in all editions of the *Diagnostic and Statistical Manual of Mental Disorders*. In the United States, prevalence estimates range from 3 percent in men to about 1 percent in women (APA, 2000). The disorder is more common among the lower socioeconomic classes, particularly so among highly mobile residents of impoverished urban areas (Sadock & Sadock, 2003). The *ICD-10* identifies this disorder as *dissocial personality disorder*.

Note: The clinical picture, etiological implications, nursing diagnoses, and interventions for care of clients with antisocial personality disorder are presented later in this chapter.

Borderline Personality Disorder

Definition and Epidemiological Statistics

Borderline personality disorder is characterized by a pattern of intense and chaotic relationships, with affective instability and fluctuating attitudes toward other people. These individuals are impulsive, directly and indirectly self-destructive, and lack a clear sense of identity. Prevalence estimates of borderline personality range from 2 to 3 percent of the population. It is the most common form of personality disorder, occurring in every culture (Phillips, Yen, & Gunderson, 2003). It is twice as common in women as in men (Sadock & Sadock, 2003). The *ICD-10* identifies this disorder as *emotionally unstable personality disorder*.

Note: The clinical picture, etiological implications, nursing diagnoses, and interventions for care of clients with borderline personality disorder are presented later in this chapter.

Histrionic Personality Disorder

Definition and Epidemiological Statistics

Histrionic personality disorder is characterized by colorful, dramatic, and extroverted behavior in excitable, emotional people (Sadock & Sadock, 2003). They have difficulty maintaining long-lasting relationships, although they require constant affirmation of approval and acceptance from others. Prevalence of the disorder is thought to be about 2 to 3 percent, and it is more common in women than in men.

Clinical Picture

People with histrionic personality disorder tend to be self-dramatizing, attention seeking, overly gregarious, and seductive. They use manipulative and exhibitionistic behaviors in their demands to be the center of attention. People with histrionic personality disorder often demonstrate, in mild pathological form, what our society tends to foster and admire in its members: to be well liked, successful, popular, extroverted, attractive, and sociable. However, beneath these surface characteristics is a driven quality—an all-consuming need for approval and a desperate striving to be conspicuous and to evoke affection or attract attention at all costs. Failure to evoke the attention and approval they seek often results in dejection and anxiety.

Individuals with this disorder are highly distractible and flighty by nature. They have difficulty paying attention to detail. They can portray themselves as carefree and sophisticated on the one hand and as inhibited and naive on the other. They tend to be highly suggestible, impressionable, and easily influenced by others. They are strongly dependent.

Interpersonal relationships are fleeting and superficial. The person with histrionic personality disorder, having failed throughout life to develop the richness of inner feelings and lacking resources on which to draw, lacks the ability to provide another with genuinely sustained affection. Somatic complaints are common in these individuals, and fleeting episodes of psychosis may occur during periods of extreme stress.

Etiological Implications

Neurobiological correlates have been proposed in the predisposition to histrionic personality disorder. Pfohl (1994) reports on a possible link to the dopaminergic neurotransmitter system. He states that the basic histrionic personality dimension of novelty seeking, which includes impulsiveness, excitability, and disorderliness, may be associated with low basal dopaminergic activity. Heredity also may be a factor because the disorder is apparently more common among first-degree biological relatives of people with the disorder than in the general population.

Phillips, Yen, and Gunderson (2003) report on research that suggests that the behavioral characteristics of histrionic personality disorder may be associated with a biogenetically determined temperament. From this perspective, histrionic personality disorder would arise out of "an extreme variation of temperamental disposition."

From a psychosocial perspective, learning experiences may contribute to the development of histrionic personality disorder. The child may have learned that positive reinforcement was contingent on the ability to perform parentally approved and admired behaviors. It is likely that the child rarely received positive or negative feedback. Parental acceptance and approval came inconsistently and only when the behaviors met parental expectations. Hannig (2002) states:

> The root causes [of histrionic personality disorder] surround an un-bonded mother relationship and an abusive paternal relationship. When a child is not the center of a parent's attention, neglect, lack of bonding, and deprivation leave one starving for attention, approval, praise, and reassurance.

Narcissistic Personality Disorder

Definition and Epidemiological Statistics

Persons with narcissistic personality disorder have an exaggerated sense of self-worth. They lack empathy and are hypersensitive to the evaluation of others. They believe that they have the inalienable right to receive special consideration and that their desire is sufficient justification for possessing whatever they seek.

This diagnosis appeared for the first time in the third edition of the *Diagnostic and Statistical Manual of Mental Disorders*. However, the concept of **narcissism** has its roots in the 19th century. It was viewed by early psychoanalysts as a normal phase of psychosexual development. The *DSM-IV-TR* (APA, 2000) estimates that the disorder occurs in 2 to 16 percent of the clinical population and less than 1 percent of the general population. It is diagnosed more often in men than in women.

Clinical Picture

Individuals with narcissistic personality disorder appear to lack humility, being overly self-centered and exploiting others to fulfill their own desires. They often do not conceive of their behavior as being inappropriate or objectionable. Because they view themselves as "superior" beings, they believe they are entitled to special rights and privileges.

Although often grounded in grandiose distortions of reality, their mood is usually optimistic, relaxed, cheerful, and carefree. This mood can easily change, however, because of their fragile self-esteem. If they do not meet self-expectations, do not receive the positive feedback they expect from others, or draw criticism from others, they may respond with rage, shame, humiliation, or dejection. They may turn inward and fantasize rationalizations that convince them of their continued stature and perfection.

The exploitation of others for self-gratification results in impaired interpersonal relationships. In selecting a mate, narcissistic individuals frequently choose a person who will provide them with the praise and positive feedback that they require and who will not ask much from their partner in return.

Etiological Implications

Several psychodynamic theories exist regarding the predisposition to narcissistic personality disorder. Phillips, Yen, and Gunderson (2003) suggest that, as children, these individuals had their fears, failures, or dependency needs responded to with criticism, disdain, or neglect. They grow up with contempt for these behaviors in themselves and others and are unable to view others as sources of comfort and support. They project an image of invulnerability and self-sufficiency that conceals their true sense of emptiness and contributes to their inability to feel deeply.

Mark (2002) suggests that the parents of individuals with narcissistic personality disorder were often narcissistic themselves. The parents were demanding, perfectionistic, and critical, and they placed unrealistic expectations on the child. Children model their parents' behavior, giving way to the adult narcissist. Mark (2002) also suggests that the parents may have subjected the child to physical or emotional abuse or neglect.

Narcissism may also develop from an environment in which parents attempt to live their lives vicariously through their child. They expect the child to achieve the things they did not achieve, possess that which they did not possess, and have life better and easier than they did. The child is not subjected to the requirements and restrictions that may have dominated the parents' lives, and thereby grows up believing he or she is above that which is required for everyone else. Mark (2002) states:

> [Some] researchers believe that parents who over-indulge their children or who provide indiscriminate praise and those who do not set limits as to what is appropriate in their children's behavior can also produce adults who will suffer from narcissistic personality disorder. The message here appears to be inconsistency—inconsistency in parenting—the child does not know where to turn or how to behave appropriately; they do not know what is reality and what is fantasy. This of course is a major aspect of the symptoms of narcissistic personality disorder—sufferers tend to shun reality.

Avoidant Personality Disorder

Definition and Epidemiological Statistics

The individual with avoidant personality disorder is extremely sensitive to rejection and because of this may lead a socially withdrawn life. It is not that he or she is asocial; in fact, there may be a strong desire for companionship. The extreme shyness and fear of rejection, however, create needs for unusually strong guarantees of uncritical acceptance (Sadock & Sadock, 2003). Prevalence of the disorder in the general population is between 0.5 and 1 percent, and it appears to be equally common in men and women (APA, 2000).

Clinical Picture

Individuals with this disorder are awkward and uncomfortable in social situations. From a distance, others may perceive them as timid, withdrawn, or perhaps cold and strange. Those who have closer relationships with them, however, soon learn of their sensitivities, touchiness, evasiveness, and mistrustful qualities.

Their speech is usually slow and constrained, with frequent hesitations, fragmentary thought sequences, and occasional confused and irrelevant digressions. They are often lonely and express feelings of being unwanted. They view others as critical, betraying, and humiliating. They desire to have close relationships but avoid them because of their fear of being rejected. Depression, anxiety, and anger at oneself for failing to develop social relations are commonly experienced.

Etiological Implications

It is possible that there is a hereditary influence with avoidant personality disorder because it seems to occur more frequently in certain families (Rettew & Jellinek, 2002). Some infants who exhibit traits of hyperirritability, crankiness, tension, and withdrawal behaviors may possess a temperamental disposition toward an avoidant pattern.

The primary psychosocial predisposing influence to avoidant personality disorder is parental rejection and censure, which is often reinforced by peers (Phillips, Yen, & Gunderson, 2003). These children are often reared in a family in which they are belittled, abandoned, and criticized, such that any natural optimism is extinguished and replaced with feelings of low self-worth and social alienation. They learn to be suspicious and to view the world as hostile and dangerous.

Dependent Personality Disorder

Definition and Epidemiological Statistics

Dependent personality disorder is characterized by "a pervasive and excessive need to be taken care of that leads to submissive and clinging behavior and fears of separation" (APA, 2000). These characteristics are evident in the tendency to allow others to make decisions, to feel helpless when alone, to act submissively, to subordinate needs to others, to tolerate mistreatment by others, to demean oneself to gain acceptance, and to fail to function adequately in situations that require assertive or dominant behavior.

The disorder is relatively common. Sadock and Sadock (2003) discuss the results of one study of personality disorders in which 2.5 percent of the sample were diagnosed with dependent personality disorder. It is more common in women than in men and more common in the youngest children of a family.

Clinical Picture

Individuals with dependent personality disorder have a notable lack of self-confidence that is often apparent in their posture, voice, and mannerisms. They are typically passive and acquiescent to the desires of others. They are overly generous and thoughtful and underplay their own attractiveness and achievements. They may appear to others to "see the world through rose-colored glasses," but when alone, they may feel pessimistic, discouraged, and dejected. Others are not made aware of these feelings; their "suffering" is done in silence.

Individuals with dependent personality disorder assume the passive and submissive role in relationships. They are willing to let others make their important decisions. Should the dependent relationship end, they feel helpless and fearful because they feel incapable of caring for themselves (Phillips, Yen, & Gunderson, 2003). They may hastily and indiscriminately attempt to establish another relationship with someone they believe can provide them with the nurturance and guidance they need.

They avoid positions of responsibility and become anxious when forced into them. They have feelings of low self-worth and are easily hurt by criticism and disapproval. They will do almost anything, even if it is unpleasant or demeaning, to earn the acceptance of others.

Etiological Implications

An infant may be genetically predisposed to a dependent temperament. Twin studies measuring submissiveness have shown a higher correlation between identical twins than in fraternal twins (Phillips, Yen, & Gunderson, 2003).

Psychosocially, dependency is fostered in infancy when stimulation and nurturance are experienced exclusively from one source. The infant becomes attached to one source to the exclusion of all others. If this exclusive attachment continues as the child grows, the dependency is nurtured. A problem may arise when parents become overprotective and discourage independent behaviors on the part of the child. Parents who make new experiences unnecessarily easy for the child and refuse to allow him or her to learn by experience encourage their child to give up efforts at achieving autonomy. Dependent behaviors may be subtly rewarded in this environment, and the child may come to fear a loss of love or attachment from the parental figure if independent behaviors are attempted.

Obsessive-Compulsive Personality Disorder

Definition and Epidemiological Statistics

Individuals with obsessive-compulsive personality disorder are very serious and formal and have difficulty expressing emotions. They are overly disciplined, perfectionistic, and preoccupied with rules. They are inflexible about the way in which things must be done and have a devotion to productivity to the exclusion of personal pleasure. An intense fear of making mistakes leads to difficulty with decision-making. The disorder is relatively common and occurs more often in men than in women. In the family constellation, it appears to be most common in oldest children.

Clinical Picture

Individuals with obsessive-compulsive personality disorder are inflexible and lack spontaneity. They are meticulous and work diligently and patiently at tasks that require accuracy and discipline. They are especially concerned with matters of organization and efficiency and tend to be rigid and unbending about rules and procedures.

Social behavior tends to be polite and formal. Individuals with this disorder are very "rank-conscious," a characteristic that is reflected in their contrasting behaviors with "superiors" as opposed to "inferiors." They can be very solicitous to and ingratiating with authority figures. However, with subordinates the compulsive person is autocratic and condemnatory, often appearing pompous and self-righteous.

People with obsessive-compulsive personality disorder typify the "bureaucratic personality," the so-called company man. They see themselves as conscientious, loyal, dependable, and responsible and are contemptuous of people whose behavior they consider frivolous and impulsive. Emotional behavior is considered immature and irresponsible.

Although on the surface these individuals appear to be calm and controlled, underneath this exterior lies a great deal of ambivalence, conflict, and hostility. Individuals with this disorder commonly use the defense mechanism of reaction formation. Not daring to expose their true feelings of defiance and anger, they withhold these feelings so strongly that the opposite feelings come forth. The defenses of isolation, intellectualization, rationalization, and undoing are also commonly evident (Phillips, Yen, & Gunderson, 2003).

Etiological Implications

In the psychoanalytical view, the parenting style in which the individual with obsessive-compulsive personality disorder was reared is one of overcontrol. These parents expect their children to live up to their imposed standards of conduct and condemn them if they do not. Praise for positive behaviors is bestowed on the child with much less frequency than punishment for undesirable behaviors. In this environment, individuals become experts in learning what they must *not* do to avoid punishment and condemnation rather than what they *can* do to achieve attention and praise. They learn to heed rigid restrictions and rules. Positive achievements are expected, taken for granted, and only occasionally acknowledged by their parents, whose comments and judgments are limited to pointing out transgressions and infractions of rules.

Passive-Aggressive Personality Disorder

Definition and Epidemiological Statistics

The *DSM-IV-TR* defines this disorder as a pervasive pattern of negativistic attitudes and passive resistance to demands for adequate performance in social and occupational situations that begins by early adulthood and occurs in a variety of contexts. The name of the disorder is based on the assumption that such people are passively expressing covert aggression. Passive-aggressive disorder has been included in all editions of the *Diagnostic and Statistical Manual of Mental Disorders*, and although no statistics exist that speak to its prevalence, the syndrome appears to be relatively common.

Clinical Picture

Pfohl (1994) describes the passive-aggressive personality in the following manner:

> Passive-aggressive personality disorder is characterized by passive resistance and general obstructiveness in response to the expectations of others. Such individuals would rarely be assertive enough to openly disagree with a treatment plan but may express disagreement indirectly by 'losing' a prescription or 'forgetting' the psychotherapy homework assignment. (p. 427)

Passive-aggressive individuals feel cheated and unappreciated. They believe that life has been unkind to them, and they express envy and resentment over the "easy life" that they perceive others having. When they feel another has wronged them, they may go to great lengths to seek retribution, or "get even," but always in a subtle and passive manner rather than discussing their feelings with the offending individual. As a tactic of interpersonal behavior, passive-aggressive individuals commonly switch among the roles of the martyr, the affronted, the aggrieved, the misunderstood, the contrite, the guilt-ridden, the sickly, and the overworked. In this way, they are able to vent their anger and resentment subtly, while gaining the attention, reassurance, and dependency they crave.

Etiological Implications

Contradictory parental attitudes and behavior are implicated in the predisposition to passive-aggressive personality disorder. In the family dynamics, at any moment and without provocation, these children may receive the kindness and support they crave or hostility and rejection. Parental responses are inconsistent and unpredictable, and these children internalize the conflicting attitudes toward themselves and others. For example, they do not know whether to think of themselves as competent or incompetent and are unsure as to whether they love or hate those on whom they depend. Double-bind communication may also be exhibited in these families. Expressions of concern and affection may be verbalized, only to be negated and undone through subtle and devious behavioral manifestations. This *approach-avoidance* pattern is modeled by the children, who then become equally equivocal and ambivalent in their own thinking and actions.

Through this type of environment, children learn to control their anger for fear of provoking parental withdrawal and not receiving love and support—even on an inconsistent basis. Overtly the child appears polite and undemanding; hostility and inefficiency are manifested only covertly and indirectly.

APPLICATION OF THE NURSING PROCESS

Borderline Personality Disorder

Background Assessment Data

Historically, there has been a group of clients who did not classically conform to standard categories of neuroses or psychoses. The designation "borderline" was introduced to identify the clients who seemed to fall on the border between the two categories. Other terminology that has been used in an attempt to identify this disorder includes *ambulatory schizophrenia*, *pseudoneurotic schizophrenia*, and *emotionally unstable personality*. When the term *borderline* was first proposed for inclusion in the third edition of the *DSM*, some psychiatrists feared it might be used as a "wastebasket" diagnosis for difficult-to-treat clients. However, a specific set of criteria has been established for diagnosing what has been described as "a consistent and stable course of unstable behavior" (Table 20–2).

TABLE 20–2 Diagnostic Criteria for Borderline Personality Disorder

A pervasive pattern of instability of interpersonal relationships, self-image, and affect, and marked impulsivity beginning by early adulthood and present in a variety of contexts, as indicated by five (or more) of the following:

1. Frantic efforts to avoid real or imagined abandonment (*Note:* Do not include suicidal or self-mutilating behavior covered in criterion 5).
2. A pattern of unstable and intense interpersonal relationships characterized by alternating between extremes of idealization and devaluation.
3. Identity disturbance: markedly and persistently unstable self-image or sense of self
4. Impulsivity in at least two areas that are potentially self-damaging (e.g., spending, sex, substance abuse, reckless driving, binge eating)
   Note: Do not include suicidal or self-mutilating behavior covered in criterion 5.
5. Recurrent suicidal behavior, gestures, or threats, or self-mutilating behavior
6. Affective instability due to marked reactivity of mood (e.g., intense episodic dysphoria, irritability, or anxiety, usually lasting a few hours and only rarely more than a few days)
7. Chronic feelings of emptiness
8. Inappropriate, intense anger, or difficulty controlling anger (e.g., frequent displays of temper, constant anger, recurrent physical fights)
9. Transient, stress-related paranoid ideation or severe dissociative symptoms

From the APA (2000), with permission.

Clinical Picture

Individuals with borderline personality disorder always seem to be in a state of crisis. Their affect is one of extreme intensity, and their behavior reflects frequent changeability. These changes can occur within days, hours, or even minutes. Often these individuals exhibit a single, dominant affective tone, such as depression, which may give way periodically to anxious agitation or inappropriate outbursts of anger.

CHRONIC DEPRESSION. Depression is so common in clients with this disorder that before the inclusion of borderline personality disorder in the *DSM*, many of these clients were diagnosed as depressed. Depression occurs in response to feelings of abandonment by the mother in early childhood (see "Etiological Implications"). Underlying the depression is a sense of rage that is sporadically turned inward on the self and externally on the environment. Seldom is the individual aware of the true source of these feelings until well into long-term therapy.

INABILITY TO BE ALONE. Because of this chronic fear of abandonment, clients with borderline personality disorder have little tolerance for being alone. They prefer a frantic search for companionship, no matter how unsatisfactory, to sitting with feelings of loneliness, emptiness, and boredom (Sadock & Sadock, 2003).

Patterns of Interaction

CLINGING AND DISTANCING. The client with borderline personality disorder commonly exhibits a pattern of interaction with others that is characterized by clinging and distancing behaviors. When clients are clinging to another individual, they may exhibit helpless, dependent, or even childlike behaviors. They overidealize a single individual with whom they want to spend all their time, with whom they express a frequent need to talk, or from whom they seek constant reassurance. Acting-out behaviors, even self-mutilation, may result when they cannot be with this chosen individual. Distancing behaviors are characterized by hostility, anger, and devaluation of others, arising from a feeling of discomfort with closeness.

Distancing behaviors also occur in response to separations, confrontations, or attempts to limit certain behaviors. Devaluation of others is manifested by discrediting or undermining their strengths and personal significance.

SPLITTING. **Splitting** is a primitive ego defense mechanism that is common in people with borderline personality disorder. It arises from their lack of achievement of **object constancy** and is manifested in an inability to integrate and accept both positive and negative feelings. In their view, people—including themselves—and life situations are all good or all bad. For example, if a caregiver is nurturing and supportive, he or she is lovingly idealized. Should the nurturing relationship be threatened in any way (e.g., the caregiver must move because of his or her job), the individual is devalued, and the idealized image changes from beneficent caregiver to one of hateful and cruel persecutor (Phillips, Yen, & Gunderson, 2003).

MANIPULATION. In their efforts to prevent the separation they so desperately fear, clients with this disorder become masters of manipulation. Virtually any behavior becomes an acceptable means of achieving the desired result: relief from separation anxiety. Playing one individual against another is a common ploy to allay these fears of abandonment.

SELF-DESTRUCTIVE BEHAVIORS. Repetitive, self-mutilative behaviors are classic manifestations of borderline personality disorder. Although these acts can be fatal, most commonly they are manipulative gestures designed to elicit a rescue response from significant others. Suicide attempts are relatively common and often result from feelings of abandonment following separation from a significant other. The endeavor is often attempted, however, incorporating a measure of "safety" into the plan (e.g., swallowing pills in an area where the person will surely be discovered by others; or swallowing pills and making a phone call to report the deed to someone).

Other types of destructive behaviors include cutting, scratching, and burning. Various theories abound regarding why these individuals are able to inflict pain on themselves. One hypothesis suggests they may have higher levels of endorphins in their bodies, thereby increasing their threshold for pain. Another theory relates to the individual's personal identity disturbance. It proposes that since much of the self-mutilating behaviors take place when the individual is in a state of depersonalization and derealization, he or she does not initially feel the pain. They continue the mutilation until pain is felt in an effort to counteract the feelings of unreality. Some clients with borderline personality disorder have reported that "... to feel pain is better than to feel nothing." Pain validates their existence.

IMPULSIVITY. Individuals with borderline personality disorder have poor impulse control based on primary process functioning. Impulsive behaviors associated with borderline personality disorder include substance abuse, gambling, promiscuity, reckless driving, and binging and purging (APA, 2000). Many times these acting-out behaviors occur in response to real or perceived feelings of abandonment.

Etiological Implications

According to Mahler's theory of object relations (Mahler, Pine, & Bergman, 1975), the infant passes through six phases from birth to 36 months, when a sense of separateness from the parenting figure is finally established. These phases include:

Phase 1 (birth to 1 month), autistic phase. During this period, the baby spends most of his or her time in a half-waking, half-sleeping state. The main goal is fulfillment of needs for survival and comfort.

Phase 2 (1 to 5 months), symbiotic phase. At this time, there is a type of psychic fusion of mother and child. The child views the self as an extension of the parenting figure, although there is a developing awareness of external sources of need fulfillment.

Phase 3 (5 to 10 months), differentiation phase. The child is beginning to recognize that there is separateness between the self and the parenting figure.

Phase 4 (10 to 16 months), practicing phase. This phase is characterized by increased locomotor functioning and the ability to explore the environment independently. A sense of separateness of the self is increased.

Phase 5 (16 to 24 months), rapprochement phase. Awareness of separateness of the self becomes acute. This is frightening to the child, who wants to regain some lost closeness but not return to symbiosis. The child wants the mother there as needed for "emotional refueling" and to maintain feelings of security.

Phase 6 (24 to 36 months), on the way to object constancy phase. In this phase, the child completes the individuation process and learns to relate to objects in an effective, constant manner. A sense of separateness is established, and the child is able to internalize a sustained image of the loved object or person when out of sight. Separation anxiety is resolved.

The individual with borderline personality disorder becomes fixed in the rapprochement phase of development. This occurs when the child shows increasing separation and autonomy. The mother, who feels secure in the relationship as long as the child is dependent, begins to feel threatened by the child's increasing independence. The mother may indeed be experiencing her own fears of abandonment. In response to separation behaviors, the mother withdraws the emotional support or "refueling" that is so vitally needed during this phase for the child to feel secure. Instead, the mother rewards clinging, dependent behaviors and punishes (withholding emotional support) independent behaviors. With his or her sense of emotional survival at stake, the child learns to behave in a manner that satisfies the parental wishes. An internal conflict develops within the child, based on fear of abandonment. He or she wants to achieve independence common to this stage of development but fears that mother will withdraw emotional support as a result. This unresolved fear of abandonment remains with the child into adulthood. Unresolved grief for the nurturing they failed to receive results in internalized rage that manifests itself in the depression so common in those with borderline personality disorder.

Diagnosis/Outcome Identification

Nursing diagnoses are formulated from the data gathered during the assessment phase and with background knowledge regarding etiological implications for the disorder. Some common nursing diagnoses for the client with borderline personality disorder include:

Risk for self-mutilation related to parental emotional deprivation (unresolved fears of abandonment)

Dysfunctional grieving related to maternal deprivation during rapprochement phase of development (internalized as a loss, with fixation in anger stage of grieving process), evidenced by depressed mood, acting-out behaviors

Impaired social interaction related to extreme fears of abandonment and engulfment evidenced by alternating clinging and distancing behaviors

Disturbed personal identity related to underdeveloped ego evidenced by feelings of depersonalization and derealization

Anxiety (severe to panic) related to unconscious conflicts based on fear of abandonment evidenced by transient psychotic symptoms (disorganized thinking; misinterpretation of the environment)

Chronic low self-esteem related to lack of positive feedback evidenced by manipulation of others and inability to tolerate being alone

The following criteria may be used for measurement of outcomes in the care of clients with borderline personality disorder. The client:

1. Has not harmed self
2. Seeks out staff when desire for self-mutilation is strong
3. Is able to identify true source of anger
4. Expresses anger appropriately
5. Relates to more than one staff member
6. Completes activities of daily living independently
7. Does not manipulate one staff member against the other in order to fulfill own desires

Planning/Implementation

In Table 20–3, selected nursing diagnoses common to the client with borderline personality disorder are presented in a plan of care. Outcome criteria along with appropriate nursing interventions and rationales are included for each.

Evaluation

Reassessment is conducted to determine if the nursing actions have been successful in achieving the objectives of care. Evaluation of the nursing actions for the client with borderline personality disorder may be facilitated by gathering information using the following types of questions:

1. Has the client been able to seek out staff when feeling the desire for self-harm?
2. Has the client avoided self-harm?
3. Can the client correlate times of desire for self-harm to times of evaluation in level of anxiety?
4. Can the client discuss feelings with staff (particularly feelings of depression and anger)?
5. Can the client identify the true source toward which the anger is directed?
6. Can the client verbalize understanding of the basis for his or her anger?
7. Can the client express anger appropriately?
8. Can the client function independently?
9. Can the client relate to more than one staff member?

TABLE 20-3 Care Plan for the Client with Borderline Personality Disorder

Nursing Diagnosis: RISK FOR SELF-MUTILATION

Related to: Parental emotional deprivation (unresolved fears of abandonment)

Outcome Criteria	Nursing Interventions	Rationale
Client will not harm self.	1. Observe client's behavior frequently. Do this through routine activities and interactions; avoid appearing watchful and suspicious.	1. Close observation is required so that intervention can occur if required to ensure client's (and others') safety.
	2. Secure a verbal contract from client that he or she will seek out a staff member when the urge for self-mutilation is felt.	2. Discussing feelings of self-harm with a trusted individual provides a degree of relief to the client. A contract gets the subject out in the open and places some of the responsibility for his or her safety with the client. An attitude of acceptance of the client as a worthwhile individual is conveyed.
	3. If self-mutilation occurs, care for client's wounds in a matter-of-fact manner. Do not give positive reinforcement to this behavior by offering sympathy or additional attention.	3. Lack of attention to the maladaptive behavior may decrease repetition of its use.
	4. Encourage client to talk about feelings he or she was having just before this behavior occurred.	4. To problem solve the situation with the client, knowledge of the precipitating factors is important.
	5. Act as a role model for appropriate expression of angry feelings, and give positive reinforcement to client when attempts to conform are made.	5. It is vital that the client expresses angry feelings because suicide and other self-destructive behaviors are often viewed as a response to anger turned inward on the self.
	6. Remove all dangerous objects from client's environment.	6. Client safety is a nursing priority.
	7. If warranted by high acuity of the situation, staff may need to be assigned on a one-to-one basis.	7. Because of their extreme fear of abandonment, clients with this disorder should not be left alone at a stressful time as it may cause an acute rise in anxiety and agitation levels.

Nursing Diagnosis: DYSFUNCTIONAL GRIEVING

Related to: Maternal deprivation during rapprochement phase of development (internalized as a loss, with fixation in anger stage of grieving process)

Evidenced by: Depressed mood, acting-out behaviors

Outcome Criteria	Nursing Interventions	Rationale
Client will be able to identify true source of anger, accept ownership of the feelings, and express them in a socially acceptable manner in an effort to initiate progression through the grief process.	1. Convey an accepting attitude—one that creates a nonthreatening environment for the client to express feelings. Be honest and keep all promises.	1. An accepting attitude conveys to the client that you believe he or she is a worthwhile person. Trust is enhanced.
	2. Identify the function that anger, frustration, and rage serve for the client. Allow him or her to express these feelings within reason.	2. Verbalization of feelings in a nonthreatening environment may help client come to terms with unresolved issues.
	3. Encourage client to discharge pent-up anger through participation in large motor activities (e.g., brisk walks, jogging, physical exercises, volleyball, punching bag, exercise bike).	3. Physical exercise provides a safe and effective method for discharging pent-up tension.
	4. Explore with client the true source of the anger. This is a painful therapy that often leads to regression as the client deals with the feelings of early abandonment.	4. Reconciliation of the feelings associated with this stage is necessary before progression through the grieving process can continue.
	5. As anger is displaced onto the nurse or therapist, caution must be taken to guard against the negative effects of countertransference (see Chapter 5). These are very difficult clients having the capacity for eliciting a whole array of negative feelings from the therapist.	5. The existence of negative feelings by the nurse or therapist must be acknowledged, but they must not be allowed to interfere with the therapeutic process.

(Continued)

TABLE 20–3 Care Plan for the Client with Borderline Personality Disorder *(Continued)*

Outcome Criteria	Nursing Interventions	Rationale
	6. Explain the behaviors associated with the normal grieving process. Help the client recognize his or her position in this process.	6. Knowledge of the acceptability of the feelings associated with normal grieving may help to relieve some of the guilt that these responses generate.
	7. Help client to understand appropriate ways to express anger. Give positive reinforcement for behaviors used to express anger appropriately. Act as a role model.	7. Positive reinforcement enhances self-esteem and encourages repetition of desirable behaviors.
	8. Set limits on acting-out behaviors and explain consequences of violation of those limits. Be supportive yet consistent and firm in caring for this client.	8. Client lacks sufficient self-control to limit maladaptive behaviors, so assistance is required from staff. Without consistency on the part of all staff members working with this client, a positive outcome will not be achieved.

Nursing Diagnosis: IMPAIRED SOCIAL INTERACTION
Related to: Extreme fears of abandonment and engulfment
Evidenced by: Alternating clinging and distancing behaviors and staff splitting

Outcome Criteria	Nursing Interventions	Rationale
Client will exhibit no evidence of splitting or clinging and distancing behaviors in relationships with staff and/or peers.	1. Encourage client to examine these behaviors (to recognize that they are occurring).	1. Client may be unaware of splitting or of clinging and distancing pattern of interaction with others. Recognition must occur before change can occur.
	2. Help client realize that you will be available, without reinforcing dependent behaviors.	2. Knowledge of your availability may provide needed security for the client.
	3. Give positive reinforcement for independent behaviors.	3. Positive reinforcement enhances self-esteem and encourages repetition of desirable behaviors.
	4. Rotate staff members who work with the client in order to avoid client developing dependence on particular individuals.	4. Client must learn to relate to more than one staff member in an effort to decrease use of splitting and diminish fears of abandonment.
	5. Explore feelings that relate to fears of abandonment and engulfment with client. Help client understand that clinging and distancing behaviors are engendered by these fears.	5. Exploration of feelings with a trusted individual may help client come to terms with unresolved issues.
	6. Help client understand how these behaviors interfere with satisfactory relationships.	6. Client may be unaware of others' perception of him or her and why these behaviors are not acceptable to others.
	7. Assist client to work toward achievement of object constancy. Be available, without promoting dependency.	7. This may help client resolve fears of abandonment and develop the ability to establish satisfactory intimate relationships.

10. Can the client verbalize the knowledge that the staff members will return and are not abandoning the client when leaving for the day?
11. Can the client separate from the staff in an appropriate manner?
12. Can the client delay gratification and refrain from manipulating others in order to fulfill own desires?
13. Can the client verbalize resources within the community from whom he or she may seek assistance in times of extreme stress?

Antisocial Personality Disorder

Background Assessment Data

In the *DSM-I*, antisocial behavior was categorized as a "sociopathic or psychopathic" reaction that was symptomatic of any of several underlying personality disorders. The *DSM-II* represented it as a distinct personality type, a distinction that has been retained in subsequent editions. The *DSM-IV-TR* diagnostic criteria for antisocial personality disorder are presented in Table 20–4.

TABLE 20–4 Diagnostic Criteria for Antisocial Personality Disorder

A. A pervasive pattern of disregard for and violation of the rights of others occurring since age 15 years, as indicated by three (or more) of the following:
  1. Failure to conform to social norms with respect to lawful behaviors as indicated by repeatedly performing acts that are grounds for arrest
  2. Deceitfulness, as indicated by repeated lying, use of aliases, or conning others for personal profit or pleasure
  3. Impulsivity or failure to plan
  4. Irritability and aggressiveness, as indicated by repeated physical fights or assaults
  5. Reckless disregard for safety of self or others
  6. Consistent irresponsibility, as indicated by repeated failure to sustain consistent work behavior or honor financial obligations
  7. Lack of remorse, as indicated by being indifferent to or rationalizing having hurt, mistreated, or stolen from another

B. The individual is at least 18 years old.

C. Evidence of conduct disorder with onset before age 15 years

D. The occurrence of antisocial behavior is not exclusively during the course of schizophrenia or a manic episode

From the APA (2000), with permission.

Individuals with antisocial personality disorder are not seen often in most clinical settings, and when they are, it is commonly a way to avoid legal consequences. Sometimes they are admitted to the healthcare system by court order for psychological evaluation. However, most frequently these individuals may be encountered in prisons, jails, and rehabilitation services.

Clinical Picture

Phillips, Yen, and Gunderson (2003) describe antisocial personality disorder as a pattern of socially irresponsible, exploitative, and guiltless behavior that reflects a disregard for the rights of others. These individuals exploit and manipulate others for personal gain and have a general disregard for the law. They have difficulty sustaining consistent employment and in developing stable relationships. They appear cold and callous, often intimidating others with their brusque and belligerent manner. They tend to be argumentative and, at times, cruel and malicious. They lack warmth and compassion and are often suspicious of these qualities in others.

Individuals with antisocial personality have a very low tolerance for frustration, act impetuously, and are unable to delay gratification. They are restless and easily bored, often taking chances and seeking thrills, acting as if they were immune to danger.

When things go their way, individuals with this disorder act cheerful, even gracious and charming. Because of their low tolerance for frustration, this pleasant exterior can change very quickly. When what they desire now is challenged, they are likely to become furious and vindictive. Easily provoked to attack, their first inclination is to demean and dominate. They believe that "good guys come in last," and show contempt for the weak and underprivileged. They exploit others to fulfill their own desires, showing no trace of shame or guilt for their behavior.

Individuals with antisocial personalities see themselves as victims, using projection as the primary ego defense mechanism. They do not accept responsibility for the consequences of their behavior. Gorman, Sultan, and Raines (1996) state:

> These individuals have come to suspect that any person or institution may try to control them, rendering them powerless and vulnerable to attack. (p. 228)

In their own minds, this perception justifies their malicious behavior, lest they be the recipient of unjust persecution and hostility from others.

Satisfying interpersonal relationships are not possible because individuals with antisocial personalities have learned to place their trust only in themselves. They have a philosophy that "everyone is out to 'help number one' and that one should stop at nothing to avoid being pushed around" (APA, 2000).

One of the most distinctive characteristics of individuals with antisocial personalities is their tendency to ignore conventional authority and rules. They act as though established social norms and guidelines for self-discipline and cooperative behavior do not apply to them. They are flagrant in their disrespect for the law and for the rights of others.

Etiological Implications

BIOLOGICAL INFLUENCES. The *DSM-IV-TR* reports that antisocial personality is more common among first-degree biological relatives of those with the disorder than among the general population (APA, 2000). Cadoret (1994) reports on studies that implicate the role of genetics in antisocial personality disorder. These studies of families of individuals with antisocial personality show higher numbers of relatives with antisocial personality or alcoholism than are found in the general population. Additional studies have shown that children of parents with antisocial behavior are more likely to be diagnosed with antisocial personality, even when they are separated at birth from biological parents and reared by individuals without the disorder.

Characteristics associated with temperament in the newborn may be significant in the predisposition to antisocial personality. Parents who bring their children with behavior disorders to clinics often report that the child displayed temper tantrums from infancy and would become furious when awaiting a bottle or diaper change. As these children mature, they commonly develop a bullying attitude toward other children. Parents report that they are undaunted by punishment and generally quite unmanageable. They are daring and foolhardy in their willingness to chance physical harm, and they seem unaffected by pain.

Mannuzza and associates (1998) identified attention-deficit hyperactivity disorder and conduct disorder during prepuberty as predisposing factors to antisocial personality disorder.

Although these biogenetic influences may describe some familial pattern to the development of antisocial personality disorder, no basic pathology process has yet been determined as an etiological factor. Cadoret (1994) states:

> Whereas abnormalities of electroencephalography or autonomic nervous system reactivity have been described more frequently in antisocial populations, many antisocials still do not show such abnormalities. Any basic structural, biochemical, or functional abnormality eludes us at present. (p. 212)

FAMILY DYNAMICS. Antisocial personality disorder frequently arises from a chaotic home environment (Cadoret, 1994). Parental deprivation during the first 5 years of life appears to be a critical predisposing factor in the development of antisocial personality disorder. Separation due to parental delinquency appears to be more highly correlated with the disorder than is parental loss from other causes. The presence or intermittent appearance of inconsistent impulsive parents, not the loss of a consistent parent, is environmentally *most* damaging.

Studies have shown that individuals with antisocial personality disorder often have been severely physically abused in childhood. The abuse contributes to the development of antisocial behavior in several ways. First, it provides a model for behavior. Second, it may result in injury to the child's central nervous system, thereby impairing the child's ability to function appropriately. Finally, it engenders rage in the victimized child, which is then displaced onto others in the environment.

A number of factors associated with disordered family functioning have been implicated in the development of antisocial personality (Cadoret, 1994; Phillips, Yen, & Gunderson, 2003). The following circumstances may influence the predisposition to antisocial personality disorder:

1. Absence of parental discipline
2. Extreme poverty
3. Removal from the home
4. Growing up without parental figures of both sexes
5. Erratic and inconsistent methods of discipline
6. Being "rescued" each time he or she is in trouble (never having to suffer the consequences of one's own behavior)
7. Maternal deprivation

Diagnosis/Outcome Identification

Nursing diagnoses are formulated from the data gathered during the assessment phase and with background knowledge regarding predisposing factors to the disorder. Some common nursing diagnoses for the client with antisocial personality disorder include:

Risk for other-directed violence related to rage reactions, negative role-modeling, inability to tolerate frustration

Defensive coping related to dysfunctional family system, evidenced by disregard for societal norms and laws, absence of guilty feelings, or inability to delay gratification

Chronic low self-esteem related to repeated negative feedback resulting in diminished self-worth, evidenced by manipulation of others to fulfill own desires or inability to form close, personal relationships

Impaired social interaction related to negative role modeling and low self-esteem, evidenced by inability to develop a satisfactory, enduring, intimate relationship with another

Deficient knowledge (self-care activities to achieve and maintain optimal wellness) related to lack of interest in learning and denial of need for information, evidenced by demonstration of inability to take responsibility for meeting basic health practices

The following criteria may be used to measure outcomes in the care of the client with antisocial personality disorder. The client:

1. Discusses angry feelings with staff and in group sessions

2. Has not harmed self or others
3. Can rechannel hostility into socially acceptable behaviors
4. Follows rules and regulations of the milieu environment
5. Can verbalize which of his or her behaviors are not acceptable
6. Shows regard for the rights of others by delaying gratification of own desires when appropriate
7. Does not manipulate others in an attempt to increase feelings of self-worth
8. Verbalizes understanding of knowledge required to maintain basic health needs

Planning/Implementation

Table 20–5 presents a care plan of selected nursing diagnoses common to the client with antisocial person-

TABLE 20–5 Care Plan for the Client with Antisocial Personality Disorder

Nursing Diagnosis: RISK FOR OTHER-DIRECTED VIOLENCE

Related to: Rage reactions, negative role-modeling, inability to tolerate frustration

Outcome Criteria	Nursing Interventions	Rationale
Client will not harm self or others.	1. Convey an accepting attitude toward this client. Feelings of rejection are undoubtedly familiar to him or her. Work on development of trust. Be honest, keep all promises, and convey the message that it is not ***him*** or ***her*** but the ***behavior*** that is unacceptable.	1. An attitude of acceptance promotes feelings of self-worth. Trust is the basis on which a therapeutic relationship is established.
	2. Maintain low level of stimuli in client's environment (low lighting, few people, simple decor, low noise level).	2. A stimulating environment may increase agitation and promote aggressive behavior.
	3. Observe client's behavior frequently during routine activities and interactions; avoid appearing watchful and suspicious.	3. Close observation is required so that intervention can occur if required to ensure client's (and others') safety.
	4. Remove all dangerous objects from client's environment.	4. Client safety is a nursing priority.
	5. Help client identify the true object of his or her hostility.	5. Because of weak ego development, client may be misusing the defense mechanism of displacement. Helping him or her recognize this in a nonthreatening manner may help reveal unresolved issues so that they may be confronted.
	6. Encourage client to verbalize hostile feelings gradually.	6. Verbalization of feelings in a nonthreatening environment may help client come to terms with unresolved issues.
	7. Explore with client alternative ways of handling frustration (e.g., large motor skills that channel hostile energy into socially acceptable behaviors).	7. Physically demanding activity helps to relieve pent-up tension.
	8. Staff should maintain and convey a calm attitude.	8. Anxiety is contagious and can be transferred from staff to client. A calm attitude provides client with a feeling of safety and security.
	9. Have sufficient staff available to present a show of strength to client if necessary.	9. This conveys to client evidence of control over the situation and provides some physical security for staff.
	10. Administer tranquilizing medications as ordered by physician or request an order if necessary. Monitor for effectiveness and for adverse side effects.	10. Antianxiety agents (e.g., diazepam, chlordiazepoxide, oxazepam) produce a calming effect and may help to allay hostile behaviors (**Note:** Medications are not often prescribed for clients with this disorder because of these individuals' strong susceptibility to addictions.)

(Continued)

TABLE 20–5 Care Plan for the Client with Antisocial Personality Disorder *(Continued)*

Outcome Criteria	Nursing Interventions	Rationale
	11. If client is not calmed by "talking down" or by medication, use of mechanical restraints may be necessary. Be sure to have sufficient staff available to assist. Follow protocol established by the institution in executing this intervention. The Joint Commission on Accreditation of Healthcare Organizations requires that the physician reevaluate and issue a new order for restraints every 4 hours for adults aged 18 and older. If the client has previously refused medication, administer it after restraints have been applied. Most states consider this intervention appropriate in emergency situations or in the event that a client is likely to harm self or others. Never use restraints as a punitive measure; they should only be used as a protective measure for a client who is out of control. Observe the client in restraints every 15 min (or according to institutional policy). Ensure that circulation to extremities is not compromised (check temperature, color, pulses). Assist client with needs related to nutrition, hydration, and elimination. Position client so that comfort is facilitated and aspiration can be prevented.	11. Client safety is a nursing priority.
	12. As agitation decreases, assess client's readiness for restraint removal or reduction. Remove one restraint at a time, while assessing client's response.	12. This minimizes risk of injury to client and staff.

Nursing Diagnosis: DEFENSIVE COPING
Related to: Dysfunctional family system
Evidenced by: Disregard for societal norms and laws, absence of guilty feelings, inability to delay gratification

Outcome Criteria	Nursing Interventions	Rationale
Client will be able to follow rules and delay personal gratification.	1. From the onset, client should be made aware of which behaviors are acceptable and which are not. Explain consequences of violation of the limits. A consequence must involve something of value to the client. All staff must be consistent in enforcing these limits. Consequences should be administered in a matter-of-fact manner immediately following the infraction.	1. Because client cannot (or will not) impose own limits on maladaptive behaviors, they must be delineated and enforced by staff. Undesirable consequences may help to decrease repetition of these behaviors.
	2. Do not attempt to coax or convince client to do the "right thing." Do not use the words "You should (or shouldn't)..."; instead, use "You will be expected to...". The ideal would be for client to eventually internalize societal norms, beginning with this step-by-step, "either/or" approach (***either*** you do [don't do] this, ***or*** this will occur).	2. Explanations must be concise, concrete, and clear, with little or no capacity for misinterpretation.
	3. Provide positive feedback or reward for acceptable behaviors.	3. Positive reinforcement enhances self-esteem and encourages repetition of desirable behaviors.
	4. Begin to increase the length of time requirement for acceptable behavior to achieve the reward. For example, 2 hours of acceptable behavior may be exchanged for a phone call, 4 hours for 2 hours of television; 1 day of acceptable behavior for a recreational therapy bowling activity and 5 days for a weekend pass.	4. This type of intervention may assist the client in learning to delay gratification.

Outcome Criteria	Nursing Interventions	Rationale
	5. A milieu unit provides the appropriate environment for the client with antisocial personality.	5. The democratic approach, with specific rules and regulations, community meetings, and group therapy sessions, emulates the type of societal situation in which the client must learn to live. Feedback from peers is often more effective than confrontation from an authority figure. The client learns to follow the rules of the group as a positive step in the progression toward internalizing the rules of society.
	6. Help client to gain insight into his or her own behaviors. Often these individuals rationalize to such an extent that they deny that what they have done is wrong (e.g., "The owner of this store has so much money, he'll never miss the little bit I take. He has everything, and I have nothing. It's not fair! I deserve to have some of what he has.").	6. Client must come to understand that certain behaviors will not be tolerated within the society and that severe consequences will be imposed upon those individuals who refuse to comply. Client must ***want*** to become a productive member of society before he or she can be helped.
	7. Talk about past behaviors with client. Discuss behaviors that are acceptable by society and those which are not. Help client identify ways in which he or she has exploited others. Encourage client to explore how he or she would feel if the circumstances were reversed.	7. An attempt may be made to enlighten the client to the sensitivity of others by promoting self-awareness in an effort to help the client gain insight into his or her own behavior.
	8. Throughout the relationship with the client, maintain an attitude of "It is not ***you*** but your ***behavior*** that is unacceptable."	8. An attitude of acceptance promotes feelings of dignity and self-worth.

ality disorder. Outcome criteria, appropriate nursing interventions, and rationales are included for each.

Evaluation

Reassessment is conducted to determine if the nursing actions have been successful in achieving the objectives of care. Evaluation of the nursing actions for the client with antisocial personality disorder may be facilitated by gathering information using the following types of questions:

1. Does the client recognize when anger is getting out of control?
2. Can the client seek out staff instead of expressing anger in an appropriate manner?
3. Can the client use other sources for rechanneling anger (e.g., physical activities)?
4. Has harm to others been avoided?
5. Can the client follow rules and regulations of the milieu with little or no reminding?
6. Can the client verbalize which behaviors are appropriate and which are not?
7. Does the client express a desire to change?
8. Can the client delay gratifying own desires in deference to those of others when appropriate?
9. Does the client manipulate others in an attempt to have his or her own desires fulfilled?
10. Does the client fulfill activities of daily living willingly and independently?
11. Can the client verbalize methods of achieving and maintaining optimal wellness?
12. Can the client verbalize community resources from which he or she can seek assistance with daily living and healthcare needs when required?

TREATMENT MODALITIES

Few would argue that treatment of individuals with personality disorders is difficult and, in some instances, may even seem impossible. Personality characteristics are learned very early in life and perhaps may even be genetic. It is not surprising, then, that these enduring patterns of behavior may take years to change, if change occurs. Phillips, Yen, and Gunderson (2003) state:

> Because personality disorders consist of deeply ingrained attitudes and behavior patterns that consolidate during development and have endured since early adulthood, they have always been believed to be very resistant to change. Moreover, treatment efforts are further confounded by the degree to which patients with a personality disorder do not recognize their maladaptive personality traits as undesirable or needing to be changed. (p. 809)

Most clinicians believe it best to strive for lessening the inflexibility of the maladaptive traits and reducing their interference with everyday functioning and meaningful relationships. Little research exists to guide the decision of which therapy is most appropriate in the treatment of personality disorders. Selection of intervention is generally based on the area of greatest dysfunction, such as cognition, affect, behavior, or interpersonal relations. Following is a brief description of various types of therapies and the disorders to which they are customarily suited.

Interpersonal Psychotherapy

Depending on the therapeutic goals, interpersonal psychotherapy with personality disorders is brief and time-limited, or it may involve long-term exploratory psychotherapy. Interpersonal psychotherapy may be particularly appropriate because personality disorders largely reflect problems in interpersonal style.

Long-term psychotherapy attempts to understand and modify the maladjusted behaviors, cognition, and affects of clients with personality disorders that dominate their personal lives and relationships (Tyrer & Stein, 1993). The core element of treatment is the establishment of an empathic therapist-client relationship, based on collaboration and guided discovery in which the therapist functions as a role model for the client.

Interpersonal psychotherapy is suggested for clients with paranoid, schizoid, schizotypal, borderline, dependent, narcissistic, and obsessive-compulsive personality disorders.

Psychoanalytical Psychotherapy

The treatment of choice for individuals with histrionic personality disorder has been psychoanalytical psychotherapy (Phillips, Yen, & Gunderson, 2003). Treatment focuses on the unconscious motivation for seeking total satisfaction from others and for being unable to commit oneself to a stable, meaningful relationship.

Milieu or Group Therapy

This treatment is especially appropriate for individuals with antisocial personality disorder, who respond to support and feedback from peers. In milieu or group therapy, feedback from peers is more effective than in one-to-one interaction with a therapist. Group therapy—particularly homogeneous supportive groups that emphasize the development of social skills—may be helpful in overcoming social anxiety and developing interpersonal trust and rapport in clients with avoidant personality disorder (Phillips, Yen, & Gunderson, 2003). Feminist consciousness-raising groups can be useful in helping dependent clients struggling with social-role stereotypes.

Cognitive/Behavioral Therapy

Behavioral strategies offer reinforcement for positive change. Social skills training and assertiveness training teach alternative ways to deal with frustration. Cognitive strategies help the client recognize and correct inaccurate internal mental schemata. This type of therapy may be useful for clients with obsessive-compulsive, passive-aggressive, antisocial, and avoidant personality disorders.

Psychopharmacology

Psychopharmacology may be helpful in some instances. Although these drugs have no effect in the direct treatment of the disorder itself, some symptomatic relief can be achieved. Antipsychotic medications are helpful in the treatment of psychotic decompensations experienced by clients with paranoid, schizotypal, or borderline personality disorders (Sanislow & McGlashan, 1998).

A variety of pharmacological interventions have been used with borderline personality disorder. The selective serotonin reuptake inhibitors (SSRIs) and monoamine oxidase inhibitors have been successful in decreasing impulsivity and self-destructive acts in these clients (Phillips, Yen, & Gunderson, 2003). The SSRIs also have been successful in reducing anger, impulsiveness, and mood instability in clients with borderline personality disorder (Salzman, 1996). Antipsychotics have resulted in improvement in illusions, ideas of reference, paranoid thinking, anxiety, and hostility in some clients.

Lithium carbonate and propranolol (Inderal) may be useful for the violent episodes observed in clients with antisocial personality disorder (Cadoret, 1994). Caution must be given to prescribing medications outside the structured setting because of the high risk for substance abuse by these individuals.

For the client with avoidant personality disorder, anxiolytics are sometimes helpful whenever previously avoided behavior is being attempted. The mere possession of the medication may be reassurance enough to help the client through the stressful period. Antidepressants, such as sertraline (Zoloft) and paroxetine (Paxil), may be useful with these clients if panic disorder develops.

SUMMARY

Clients with personality disorders are undoubtedly some of the most difficult ones healthcare workers are likely to encounter. Personality characteristics are formed very early in life and are difficult, if not impossible, to change. In fact, some clinicians believe the therapeutic approach is not to try to change the characteristics but rather to decrease the inflexibility of the maladaptive traits and reduce their interference with everyday functioning and meaningful relationships.

This chapter presents a review of the development of personality according to Sullivan, Erikson, and Mahler. The stages identified by these theorists represent the "normal" progression and establish a foundation for studying dysfunctional patterns.

The concept of a personality disorder has been present throughout the history of medicine. Problems have arisen in the attempt to establish a classification system for these disorders. The *DSM-IV-TR* groups them into three clusters. Cluster A (behaviors described as odd or eccentric) includes paranoid, schizoid, and schizotypal personality disorders. Cluster B (behaviors described as dramatic, emotional, or erratic) includes antisocial, borderline, histrionic, and narcissistic personality disorders. Cluster C (behaviors described as anxious or fearful) includes avoidant, dependent, and obsessive-compulsive disorders. Passive-aggressive personality disorder, which the *DSM-IV-TR* includes in "Criteria Provided for Further Study," was included with the cluster C disorders.

Nursing care of the client with a personality disorder is accomplished using the steps of the nursing process. Background assessment data were presented along with information regarding possible etiological implications for each disorder. An overview of current medical treatment modalities for each disorder was presented.

Care of clients with borderline personality disorder and antisocial personality disorder was described at length. Individuals with borderline personality disorder may enter the healthcare system because of their instability and frequent attempts at self-destructive behavior. The individual with antisocial personality disorder may become part of the healthcare system to avoid legal consequences or because of a court order for psychological evaluation. Nursing diagnoses common to each disorder were presented along with appropriate interventions and relevant outcome criteria for each.

Nurses who work in all types of clinical settings should be familiar with the characteristics associated with personality-disordered individuals. Nurses working in psychiatry must be knowledgeable about appropriate intervention with these clients, for it is unlikely that they will encounter a greater professional challenge than these clients present.

INTERNET REFERENCES

- Additional information about personality disorders may be located at the following Web sites:
  - a http://www.mentalhealth.com/dis/p20-pe04.html
  - b http://www.mentalhealth.com/dis/p20-pe08.html
  - c http://www.mentalhealth.com/dis/p20-pe05.html
  - d http://www.mentalhealth.com/dis/p20-pe09.html
  - e http://www.mentalhealth.com/dis/p20-pe06.html
  - f http://www.mentalhealth.com/dis/p20-pe07.html
  - g http://www.mentalhealth.com/dis/p20-pe10.html
  - h http://www.mentalhealth.com/dis/p20-pe01.html
  - i http://www.mentalhealth.com/dis/p20-pe02.html
  - j http://www.mentalhealth.com/dis/p20-pe03.html
  - k http://www.mentalhealth.com/p13.html#Per
  - l http://www.nimh.nih.gov/publicat/bpd.cfm

REVIEW QUESTIONS

SELF-EXAMINATION/LEARNING EXERCISE

Select the answer that is most appropriate for each of the following questions:

1. Kim has a diagnosis of borderline personality disorder. She often exhibits alternating clinging and distancing behaviors. The most appropriate nursing intervention with this type of behavior would be to:
   a. Encourage Kim to establish trust in one staff person, with whom all therapeutic interaction should take place.
   b. Secure a verbal contract from Kim that she will discontinue these behaviors.
   c. Withdraw attention if these behaviors continue.
   d. Rotate staff members who work with Kim so that she will learn to relate to more than one person.
2. Kim manipulates the staff in an effort to fulfill her own desires. All of the following may be examples of manipulative behaviors in the borderline client *except*:
   a. Refusal to stay in room alone, stating, "It's so lonely."
   b. Asking Nurse Jones for cigarettes after 30 minutes, knowing the assigned nurse has explained she must wait 1 hour.
   c. Stating to Nurse Jones, "I really like having you for my nurse. You're the best one around here."
   d. Cutting arms with razor blade after discussing dismissal plans with physician.
3. "Splitting" by the client with borderline personality disorder denotes:
   a. Evidence of precocious development
   b. A primitive defense mechanism in which the client sees objects as all good or all bad
   c. A brief psychotic episode in which the client loses contact with reality
   d. Two distinct personalities within the borderline client
4. According to Margaret Mahler, predisposition to borderline personality disorder occurs when developmental tasks go unfulfilled in which of the following phases?
   a. Autistic phase, during which the child's needs for security and comfort go unfulfilled
   b. Symbiotic phase, during which the child fails to bond with the mother
   c. Differentiation phase, during which the child fails to recognize separateness between self and mother
   d. Rapprochement phase, during which the mother withdraws emotional support in response to the child's increasing independence

Situation: Jack was arrested for breaking into a jewelry store and stealing thousands of dollars worth of diamonds. At his arraignment, the judge ordered a psychological evaluation. He has just been admitted by court order to the locked unit. Based on a long history of maladaptive behavior, he has been given the diagnosis of antisocial personality disorder.

5. Which of the following characteristics would you expect to assess in Jack?
   a. Lack of guilt for wrongdoing
   b. Insight into his own behavior
   c. Ability to learn from experiences
   d. Compliance with authority

6. Milieu therapy is a good choice for clients with antisocial personality disorder because it:
   a. Provides a system of punishment and rewards for behavior modification
   b. Emulates a social community in which the client may learn to live harmoniously with others
   c. Provides mostly one-to-one interaction between the client and therapist
   d. Provides a structured setting in which the clients have very little input into the planning of their care

7. In evaluating Jack's progress, which of the following behaviors would be considered the most significant indication of positive change?
   a. Jack got angry only once in group this week.
   b. Jack was able to wait a whole hour for a cigarette without verbally abusing the staff.
   c. On his own initiative, Jack sent a note of apology to a man he had injured in a recent fight.
   d. Jack stated that he would no longer start any more fights.

8. Donna and Katie work in the secretarial pool of a large organization. It is 30 minutes until quitting time when a supervisor hands Katie a job that will take an hour and says he wants it done before she leaves. She then says to Donna, "I can't stay over! I'm meeting Bill at 5:00 PM! Be a doll, Donna. Do this job for me!" Donna agrees, although silently she is furious at Katie since this is the third time this has happened in 2 weeks. Katie leaves and Donna says to herself, "This is crazy. I'm not finishing this job for her. Let's see how she likes getting in trouble for a change." Donna leaves without finishing the job. This is an example of which type of personality characteristic?
   a. Antisocial
   b. Paranoid
   c. Passive-aggressive
   d. Obsessive-compulsive

9. Carol is a new nursing graduate being oriented on a medical/surgical unit by the head nurse, Mrs. Carey. When Carol describes a new technique she has learned for positioning immobile clients, Mrs. Carey states, "What are you trying to do ... tell me how to do my job? We have always done it this way on this unit, and we will continue to do it this way until I say differently!" This is an example of which type of personality characteristic?
   a. Antisocial
   b. Paranoid
   c. Passive-aggressive
   d. Obsessive-compulsive

10. Which of the following behavioral patterns is characteristic of individuals with histrionic personality disorder?
    a. Belittling themselves and their abilities
    b. Overreacting inappropriately to minor stimuli
    c. Suspicious and mistrustful of others
    d. A lifelong pattern of social withdrawal

Test Your CRITICAL THINKING SKILLS

Lana, aged 32, was diagnosed with borderline personality disorder when she was 26 years old. Her husband took her to the emergency department when he walked into the bathroom and found her cutting her legs with a razor blade. At that time, assessment revealed that Lana had a long history of self-mutilation, which she had carefully hidden from her husband and others. Lana began long-term psychoanalytical psychotherapy on an outpatient basis. Therapy revealed that Lana had been physically and sexually abused as a child by both her mother and her father, both now deceased. She admitted to having chronic depression, and her husband related episodes of rage reactions. Lana has been hospitalized on the psychiatric unit for a week because of suicidal ideations. After making a no-suicide contract with the staff, she is allowed to leave the unit on pass to keep a dental appointment that she made a number of weeks ago. She has just returned to the unit and says to her nurse, "I just took 20 Desyrel when I was sitting in my car in the parking lot."

Answer the following questions related to Lana:

1. The nurse is well acquainted with Lana and believes this is a manipulative gesture. How should the nurse handle this situation?
2. What is the priority nursing diagnosis for Lana?
3. Lana likes to "split" the staff into "good guys" and "bad guys." What is the most important intervention for splitting by a person with borderline personality disorder?

IMPLICATIONS OF RESEARCH FOR EVIDENCE BASED PRACTICE

Zanarini, M.C., and Frankenburg, F.R.: **Olanzapine treatment of female borderline personality disorder patients: A double blind, placebo-controlled pilot study.** Journal of Clinical Psychiatry (2001, November), 62(11): 849–854.

Description of the Study: The intent of this study was to compare the efficacy and safety of olanzapine versus placebo in the treatment of women meeting the criteria for borderline personality disorder (BPD). Subjects included 28 women meeting the "Revised Diagnostic Interview for Borderlines" and the *DSM-IV* criteria for BPD. The subjects were randomly assigned, 19 to olanzapine and 9 to placebo. Treatment duration was 6 months. Outcomes were self-reported on the "Symptom Checklist-90," and changes were measured in anxiety, depression, paranoia, anger/hostility, and interpersonal sensitivity.

Results of the Study: Olanzapine was associated with a significantly greater rate of improvement over time than placebo in all of the symptom areas studied except depression. Weight gain was modest but higher in the olanzapine group than in the placebo group. No serious movement disorders were noted.

Implications for Nursing Practice: Olanzapine appears to be a safe and effective agent in the treatment of women meeting the criteria for BPD. Nurses who work with individuals who have BPD should be familiar with this medication and understand the nursing implications associated with its administration. The implications of this study are particularly significant for nurses who have prescriptive authority and treat clients with BPD.

REFERENCES

American Psychiatric Association (APA) (2000). Diagnostic and statistical manual of mental disorders. (4th ed.) Text revision. Washington, DC: American Psychiatric Association.

Cadoret, R. (1994). Antisocial personality. In G. Winokur & P.J. Clayton (Eds.), The medical basis of psychiatry. Philadelphia: WB Saunders.

Gorman, L., Sultan, D.F., & Raines, M.L. (1996). Davis's manual of psychosocial nursing for general patient care. Philadelphia: FA Davis.

Hannig, P.J. (2002). Histrionic personality disorder: A brief profile. Retrieved April 5, 2002, from http://www.nvo.com/psych_help/nss-folder/publicfolder/ Histrionic%20Personality.htm

Kaplan, H.I., & Sadock, B.J. (1998). Synopsis of psychiatry: Behavioral sciences/clinical psychiatry (8th ed.). Baltimore: Williams & Wilkins.

Mannuzza, S., Klein, R.G., Bessler, A., Malloy, P., & LaPadula, M. (1998, April). Adult psychiatric status of hyperactive boys grown up. American Journal of Psychiatry, 155, 493–498.

Mark, R. (2002). How to deal with narcissistic personality disorder. Retrieved April 5, 2002, from http://wiwi.essortment.com/narcissisticp_rwmn.htm

Pfohl, B. (1994). Personality disorders. In G. Winokur & P.J. Clayton (Eds.), The medical basis of psychiatry (2nd ed.). Philadelphia: WB Saunders.

Phillips, K.A., Yen, S., & Gunderson, J.G. (2003). Personality disorders. In R.E. Hales & S.C. Yudofsky (Eds.), Textbook of clinical psychiatry (4th ed.).Washington, DC: American Psychiatric Publishing.

Rettew, D.C., & Jellinek, M.S. (2002). Personality disorder: Avoidant personality. Retrieved April 5, 2002, from http://www.emedicine.com/PED/topic189.htm

Sadock, B.J., & Sadock, V.A. (2003). Synopsis of psychiatry: Behavioral sciences/clinical psychiatry (9th ed.). Philadelphia: Lippincott Williams & Wilkins.
Salzman, C. (1996). What drug treatments are available for borderline personality disorder? The Harvard Mental Health Letter, 13(3), 8.
Sanislow, C.A., & McGlashan, T.H. (1998). Treatment outcome of personality disorders. Canadian Journal of Psychiatry, 43: 237–250.
Tyrer, P. & Stein, G. (1993). Personality disorder reviewed. London, England: Royal College of Psychiatrists.

CLASSICAL REFERENCES

Erikson, E. (1963). Childhood and society (2nd ed.). New York: WW Norton.
Mahler, M., Pine, F., & Bergman, A. (1975). The psychological birth of the human infant. New York: Basic Books.
Sullivan, H.S. (1953). The interpersonal theory of psychiatry. New York: WW Norton.

INTRODUCTION

This chapter examines various disorders in which the symptoms usually first become evident during infancy, childhood, or adolescence. That is not to say that some of the disorders discussed in this chapter do not appear later in life or that symptoms associated with other disorders, such as major depression or schizophrenia, do not appear in childhood or adolescence. The basic concepts of care are applied to treatment in those instances, with consideration of the variances in age and developmental level.

Developmental theories were discussed in Chapter 2. Any nurse working with children or adolescents should be knowledgeable about "normal" stages of growth and development. The developmental process is one that is invariably fraught with frustrations and difficulties. Behavioral responses are individual and idiosyncratic. They are, indeed, *human* responses.

Whether a child's behavior indicates emotional problems is often difficult to determine. The *DSM-IV-TR* (American Psychiatric Association [APA], 2000) includes the following criteria among many of its diagnostic categories. An emotional problem exists if the behavioral manifestations:

- Are not age-appropriate
- Deviate from cultural norms
- Create deficits or impairments in adaptive functioning

This chapter focuses on the nursing process in care of clients with mental retardation, autistic disorder, attention-deficit/hyperactivity disorder, conduct disorder, oppositional defiant disorder, Tourette's disorder, and separation anxiety disorder. Additional treatment modalities are included.

MENTAL RETARDATION

Mental retardation is defined by deficits in general intellectual functioning and adaptive functioning (APA, 2000). General intellectual functioning is measured by an individual's performance on intelligence quotient (IQ) tests. Adaptive functioning refers to the person's ability to adapt to the requirements of daily living and the expectations of his or her age and cultural group. The *DSM-IV-TR* identifies criteria for mental retardation as IQ of 70 or below, with deficits or impairments in communication, self-care, home living, social/interpersonal skills, use of community resources, self-direction, functional academic skills, work, leisure, health, and safety.

Etiological Implications

The *DSM-IV-TR* (APA, 2000) states that the etiology of mental retardation may be primarily biological or psychosocial or some combination of both. In approximately 30 to 40 percent of individuals seen in clinical settings, the etiology cannot be determined. Five major predisposing factors have been identified.

Hereditary Factors

Hereditary factors are implicated as the cause in approximately 5 percent of the cases. These factors include inborn errors of metabolism, such as Tay-Sachs disease, phenylketonuria, and hyperglycinemia. Also included are chromosomal disorders, such as Down syndrome and Klinefelter's syndrome, and single-gene abnormalities, such as tuberous sclerosis and neurofibromatosis.

Early Alterations in Embryonic Development

Prenatal factors that result in early alterations in embryonic development account for approximately 30 percent of mental retardation cases. Damages may occur in response to toxicity associated with maternal ingestion of alcohol or other drugs. Maternal illnesses and infections during pregnancy (e.g., rubella, cytomegalovirus) and complications of pregnancy (e.g., toxemia, uncontrolled diabetes) also can result in congenital mental retardation (Sadock & Sadock, 2003).

Pregnancy and Perinatal Factors

Approximately 10 percent of cases of mental retardation are the result of factors that occur during pregnancy (e.g., fetal malnutrition, viral and other infections, and prematurity) or during the birth process. Examples of the latter include trauma to the head incurred during the process of birth, placenta previa or premature separation of the placenta, and prolapse of the umbilical cord.

General Medical Conditions Acquired in Infancy or Childhood

General medical conditions acquired during infancy or childhood account for approximately 5 percent

21
CHAPTER

Children and Adolescents

CHAPTER OUTLINE

KEY TERMS

aggression
autistic disorder
temperament
impulsivity
negativism
clinging
palilalia
echolalia

OBJECTIVES

After reading this chapter, the student will be able to:

1. Identify psychiatric disorders usually first diagnosed in infancy, childhood, or adolescence.
2. Discuss etiological implications for mental retardation, autistic disorder, attention-deficit/hyperactivity disorder (ADHD), conduct disorder, oppositional defiant disorder, Tourette's disorder, and separation anxiety disorder.
3. Identify symptomatology and use the information in the assessment of clients with the aforementioned disorders.
4. Identify nursing diagnoses common to clients with these disorders and select appropriate nursing interventions for each.
5. Discuss relevant criteria for evaluating nursing care of clients with selected infant, childhood, and adolescent psychiatric disorders.
6. Describe treatment modalities relevant to selected disorders of infancy, childhood, and adolescence.

INTRODUCTION

This chapter examines various disorders in which the symptoms usually first become evident during infancy, childhood, or adolescence. That is not to say that some of the disorders discussed in this chapter do not appear later in life or that symptoms associated with other disorders, such as major depression or schizophrenia, do not appear in childhood or adolescence. The basic concepts of care are applied to treatment in those instances, with consideration of the variances in age and developmental level.

Developmental theories were discussed in Chapter 2. Any nurse working with children or adolescents should be knowledgeable about "normal" stages of growth and development. The developmental process is one that is invariably fraught with frustrations and difficulties. Behavioral responses are individual and idiosyncratic. They are, indeed, *human* responses.

Whether a child's behavior indicates emotional problems is often difficult to determine. The *DSM-IV-TR* (American Psychiatric Association [APA], 2000) includes the following criteria among many of its diagnostic categories. An emotional problem exists if the behavioral manifestations:

- Are not age-appropriate
- Deviate from cultural norms
- Create deficits or impairments in adaptive functioning

This chapter focuses on the nursing process in care of clients with mental retardation, autistic disorder, attention-deficit/hyperactivity disorder, conduct disorder, oppositional defiant disorder, Tourette's disorder, and separation anxiety disorder. Additional treatment modalities are included.

MENTAL RETARDATION

Mental retardation is defined by deficits in general intellectual functioning and adaptive functioning (APA, 2000). General intellectual functioning is measured by an individual's performance on intelligence quotient (IQ) tests. Adaptive functioning refers to the person's ability to adapt to the requirements of daily living and the expectations of his or her age and cultural group. The *DSM-IV-TR* identifies criteria for mental retardation as IQ of 70 or below, with deficits or impairments in communication, self-care, home living, social/interpersonal skills, use of community resources, self-direction, functional academic skills, work, leisure, health, and safety.

Etiological Implications

The *DSM-IV-TR* (APA, 2000) states that the etiology of mental retardation may be primarily biological or psychosocial or some combination of both. In approximately 30 to 40 percent of individuals seen in clinical settings, the etiology cannot be determined. Five major predisposing factors have been identified.

Hereditary Factors

Hereditary factors are implicated as the cause in approximately 5 percent of the cases. These factors include inborn errors of metabolism, such as Tay-Sachs disease, phenylketonuria, and hyperglycinemia. Also included are chromosomal disorders, such as Down syndrome and Klinefelter's syndrome, and single-gene abnormalities, such as tuberous sclerosis and neurofibromatosis.

Early Alterations in Embryonic Development

Prenatal factors that result in early alterations in embryonic development account for approximately 30 percent of mental retardation cases. Damages may occur in response to toxicity associated with maternal ingestion of alcohol or other drugs. Maternal illnesses and infections during pregnancy (e.g., rubella, cytomegalovirus) and complications of pregnancy (e.g., toxemia, uncontrolled diabetes) also can result in congenital mental retardation (Sadock & Sadock, 2003).

Pregnancy and Perinatal Factors

Approximately 10 percent of cases of mental retardation are the result of factors that occur during pregnancy (e.g., fetal malnutrition, viral and other infections, and prematurity) or during the birth process. Examples of the latter include trauma to the head incurred during the process of birth, placenta previa or premature separation of the placenta, and prolapse of the umbilical cord.

General Medical Conditions Acquired in Infancy or Childhood

General medical conditions acquired during infancy or childhood account for approximately 5 percent

UNIT FOUR

PSYCHIATRIC/ MENTAL HEALTH NURSING OF SPECIAL POPULATIONS

Sadock, B.J., & Sadock, V.A. (2003). Synopsis of psychiatry: Behavioral sciences/clinical psychiatry (9th ed.). Philadelphia: Lippincott Williams & Wilkins.
Salzman, C. (1996). What drug treatments are available for borderline personality disorder? The Harvard Mental Health Letter, 13(3), 8.
Sanislow, C.A., & McGlashan, T.H. (1998). Treatment outcome of personality disorders. Canadian Journal of Psychiatry, 43: 237–250.
Tyrer, P. & Stein, G. (1993). Personality disorder reviewed. London, England: Royal College of Psychiatrists.

CLASSICAL REFERENCES

Erikson, E. (1963). Childhood and society (2nd ed.). New York: WW Norton.
Mahler, M., Pine, F., & Bergman, A. (1975). The psychological birth of the human infant. New York: Basic Books.
Sullivan, H.S. (1953). The interpersonal theory of psychiatry. New York: WW Norton.

of cases of mental retardation. They include infections, such as meningitis and encephalitis; poisonings, such as from insecticides, medications, and lead; and physical trauma, such as head injuries, asphyxiation, and hyperpyrexia (Sadock & Sadock, 2003).

Environmental Influences and Other Mental Disorders

Between 15 and 20 percent of cases of mental retardation are attributed to deprivation of nurturance and social, linguistic, and other stimulation and to severe mental disorders, such as autistic disorder (APA, 2000).

Recognition of the cause and period of inception provides information regarding what to expect in terms of behavior and potential. However, each child is different, and consideration must be given on an individual basis in every case.

Application of the Nursing Process to Mental Retardation

Background Assessment Data (Symptomatology)

The extent of severity of mental retardation is identified by the client's IQ level. Four levels have been delineated: mild, moderate, severe, and profound. The various behavioral manifestations and abilities associated with each of these levels of retardation are outlined in Table 21–1.

Nurses should assess and focus on each client's strengths and individual abilities. Knowledge regarding level of independence in the performance of self-care activities is essential to the development of an adequate plan for the provision of nursing care.

Diagnosis/Outcome Identification

Selection of appropriate nursing diagnoses for the mentally retarded client depends largely on the extent

TABLE 21–1 Developmental Characteristics of Mental Retardation by Degree of Severity

Level (IQ)	Ability to Perform Self-Care Activities	Cognitive/ Educational Capabilities	Social/ Communication Capabilities	Psychomotor Capabilities
Mild (50–70)	Capable of independent living, with assistance during times of stress.	Capable of academic skills to sixth-grade level. As adult can achieve vocational skills for minimum self-support.	Capable of developing social skills. Functions well in a structured, sheltered setting.	Psychomotor skills usually not affected, although may have some slight problems with coordination.
Moderate (35–49)	Can perform some activities independently. Requires supervision.	Capable of academic skill to second-grade level. As adult may be able to contribute to own support in sheltered workshop.	May experience some limitation in speech communication. Difficulty adhering to social convention may interfere with peer relationships.	Motor development is fair. Vocational capabilities may be limited to unskilled gross motor activities.
Severe (20–34)	May be trained in elementary hygiene skills. Requires complete supervision.	Unable to benefit from academic or vocational training. Profits from systematic habit training.	Minimal verbal skills. Wants and needs often communicated by acting-out behaviors.	Poor psychomotor development. Only able to perform simple tasks under close supervision.
Profound (below 20)	No capacity for independent functioning. Requires constant aid and supervision.	Unable to profit from academic or vocational training. May respond to minimal training in self-help if presented in the close context of a one-to-one relationship.	Little, if any, speech development. No capacity for socialization skills.	Lack of ability for both fine and gross motor movements. Requires constant supervision and care. May be associated with other physical disorders.

Adapted from American Psychiatric Association (2000) and Sadock and Sadock (2003).

of severity of the condition and the client's capabilities. Possible nursing diagnoses include:

Risk for injury related to altered physical mobility or aggressive behavior
Self-care deficit related to altered physical mobility or lack of maturity
Impaired verbal communication related to developmental alteration
Impaired social interaction related to speech deficiencies or difficulty adhering to conventional social behavior
Delayed growth and development related to isolation from significant others; inadequate environmental stimulation; hereditary factors
Anxiety (moderate to severe) related to hospitalization and absence of familiar surroundings
Defensive coping related to feelings of powerlessness and threat to self-esteem
Ineffective coping related to inadequate coping skills secondary to developmental delay

The following criteria may be used for measurement of outcomes in the care of the client with mental retardation. The client:

1. Has experienced no physical harm
2. Has had self-care needs fulfilled
3. Interacts with others in a socially appropriate manner
4. Has maintained anxiety at a manageable level
5. Is able to accept direction without becoming defensive
6. Demonstrates adaptive coping skills in response to stressful situations

Planning/Implementation

Table 21–2 provides a plan of care for the child with mental retardation, using selected nursing diagnoses, outcome criteria, and appropriate nursing interventions and rationales.

Although this plan of care is directed toward the individual client, it is essential that family members or primary caregivers participate in the ongoing care of the client with mental retardation. They need to receive information regarding the scope of the condition, realistic expectations and client potentials, methods for modifying behavior as required, and community resources from which they may seek assistance and support.

TABLE 21–2 Care Plan for the Child With Mental Retardation

Nursing Diagnosis: RISK FOR INJURY
Related to: Altered physical mobility or aggressive behavior

Outcome Criteria	Nursing Interventions	Rationale
Client will not experience injury.	1. Create a safe environment for the client. 2. Ensure that small items are removed from area where client will be ambulating and sharp items are out of reach. 3. Store items that client uses frequently within easy reach. 4. Pad siderails and headboard of client with history of seizures. 5. Prevent physical aggression and acting out behaviors by learning to recognize signs that client is becoming agitated.	1–5. Client safety is a nursing priority.

Nursing Diagnosis: SELF-CARE DEFICIT
Related to: Altered physical mobility or lack of maturity

Outcome Criteria	Nursing Interventions	Rationale
Client will be able to participate in aspects of self-care.	1. Identify aspects of self-care that may be within the client's capabilities. Work on one aspect of self-care at a time. Provide simple, concrete explanations. Offer positive feedback for efforts. 2. When one aspect of self-care has been mastered to the best of the client's ability, move on to another. Encourage independence but intervene when client is unable to perform.	1. Positive reinforcement enhances self-esteem and encourages repetition of desirable behaviors. 2. Client comfort and safety are nursing priorities.

Nursing Diagnosis: IMPAIRED VERBAL COMMUNICATION

Related to: Developmental alteration

Outcome Criteria	Nursing Interventions	Rationale
Client will be able to communicate needs and desires to staff.	1. Maintain consistency of staff assignment over time.	1. Consistency of staff assignments facilitates trust and the ability to understand client's actions and communications.
	2. Anticipate and fulfill client's needs until satisfactory communication patterns are established. Learn (from family, if possible) special words client uses that are different from the norm. Identify nonverbal gestures or signals that client may use to convey needs if verbal communication is absent. Practice these communications skills repeatedly.	2. Some children with mental retardation, particularly at the severe level, can only learn by systematic habit training.

Nursing Diagnosis: IMPAIRED SOCIAL INTERACTION

Related to: Speech deficiencies or difficulty adhering to conventional social behavior

Outcome Criteria	Nursing Interventions	Rationale
Client will be able to interact with others using behaviors that are socially acceptable and appropriate to developmental level.	1. Remain with client during initial interactions with others on the unit. 2. Explain to other clients the meaning behind some of the client's nonverbal gestures and signals. Use simple language to explain to client which behaviors are acceptable and which are not. Establish a procedure for behavior modification with rewards for appropriate behaviors and aversive reinforcement for inappropriate behaviors.	1. Presence of a trusted individual provides a feeling of security. 2. Positive, negative, and aversive reinforcements can contribute to desired changes in behavior. These privileges and penalties are individually determined as staff learns the likes and dislikes of the client.

Evaluation

Evaluation of care given to the client with mental retardation should reflect positive behavioral changes. Evaluation is accomplished by determining if the goals of care have been met through implementation of the nursing actions selected. The nurse reassesses the plan and makes changes where required. Reassessment data may include information gathered by asking the following questions:

1. Have nursing actions providing for the client's safety been sufficient to prevent injury?
2. Have all of the client's self-care needs been fulfilled? Can he or she fulfill some of these needs independently?
3. Has the client been able to communicate needs and desires so that he or she can be understood?
4. Has the client learned to interact appropriately with others?
5. When regressive behaviors surface, can the client accept constructive feedback and discontinue the inappropriate behavior?
6. Has anxiety been maintained at a manageable level?
7. Has the client learned new coping skills through behavior modification? Does the client demonstrate evidence of increased self-esteem because of the accomplishment of these new skills and adaptive behaviors?
8. Have primary caregivers been taught realistic expectations of the client's behavior and methods for attempting to modify unacceptable behaviors?
9. Have primary caregivers been given information regarding various resources from which they can seek assistance and support within the community?

AUTISTIC DISORDER

Autistic disorder is characterized by a withdrawal of the child into the self and into a fantasy world of his or her own creation. The child has markedly abnormal or impaired development in social interaction and communication and a markedly restricted repertoire of activity and interests (APA, 2000). Activities and interests are restricted and may be considered somewhat bizarre.

The disorder is relatively rare and occurs four to five times more often in boys than in girls. Onset of the disorder occurs before age 3, and in most cases it runs a chronic course, with symptoms persisting into adulthood.

Etiological Implications

Biological Factors

NEUROLOGICAL IMPLICATIONS. It is generally accepted that autism is caused by abnormalities in brain structures or functions (National Institute of Mental Health [NIMH], 2002). Abnormalities have been found in the area of the amygdala, which is known to help regulate aspects of social and emotional behavior. Elevated levels of serotonin have also been found in a number of people with autism. Magnetic resonance imagery (MRI) has been used to study brain activity of children with autistic disorder, revealing markedly less activity in the parietal areas and the corpus callosum than in their peers unaffected by the disorder (NIMH, 2002).

Popper and associates (2003) identify early developmental problems such as postnatal neurological infections, congenital rubella, phenylketonuria, and fragile X syndrome as possible implications in the predisposition to autistic disorder. Several studies have also implicated various structural and functional abnormalities in the brain. These include ventricular enlargement, left temporal lobe abnormalities, and increased glucose metabolism. Popper and associates (2003) state: "The neurobiological dysfunction appears to be quite diffuse, and no clear primary deficit is found in most autistic individuals."

Genetics

Recent research has revealed strong evidence that genetic factors may play a significant role in the etiology of autism (Popper et al., 2003). Studies have shown that parents who have one child with autism are at increased risk for having more than one child with autism (NIMH, 2002). Other studies with both monozygotic and dizygotic twins also have provided evidence of a genetic involvement. Research into how genetic factors influence the development of autistic disorder is now being conducted.

Application of the Nursing Process to Autistic Disorder

Background Assessment Data (Symptomatology)

IMPAIRMENT IN SOCIAL INTERACTION. Children with autistic disorder do not form interpersonal relationships with others. They do not respond to or show interest in people. As infants, they may have an aversion to affection and physical contact. As toddlers, the attachment to a significant adult may be absent or manifested as exaggerated adherence behaviors. In childhood, there is failure to develop cooperative play, imaginative play, and friendships. Those children with minimal handicaps may eventually progress to the point of recognizing other children as part of their environment, if only in a passive manner.

IMPAIRMENT IN COMMUNICATION AND IMAGINATIVE ACTIVITY. Both verbal and nonverbal skills are affected. Language may be totally absent or characterized by immature structure or idiosyncratic utterances whose meaning is clear only to those who are familiar with the child's past experiences. Nonverbal communication, such as facial expression or gestures, is often absent or socially inappropriate. The pattern of imaginative play is often restricted and stereotypical.

RESTRICTED ACTIVITIES AND INTERESTS. Even minor changes in the environment are met with resistance or sometimes with hysterical responses. Attachment to or extreme fascination with objects that move or spin (e.g., fans) is common. Routine may become an obsession, with minor alterations in routine leading to marked distress. Stereotyped body movements (hand-clapping, rocking, whole-body swaying) and verbalizations (repetition of words or phrases) are typical. Diet abnormalities may include eating only a few specific foods or consuming an excessive amount of fluids. Behaviors that are self-injurious, such as head banging or biting the hands or arms, may be evident.

Diagnosis Outcome Identification

Based on data collected during the nursing assessment, possible nursing diagnoses for the client with autistic disorder include:

Risk for self-mutilation related to neurological alterations

Impaired social interaction related to inability to trust; neurological alterations

Impaired verbal communication related to withdrawal into the self; inadequate sensory stimulation; neurological alterations

Disturbed personal identity inadequate sensory stimulation; neurological alterations

The following criteria may be used for measurement of outcomes in the care of the client with autistic disorder. The client:

1. Exhibits no evidence of self-harm
2. Interacts appropriately with at least one staff member

3. Demonstrates trust in at least one staff member
4. Is able to communicate so that he or she can be understood by at least one staff member
5. Demonstrates behaviors that indicate he or she has begun the separation/individuation process

Planning/Implementation

Table 21–3 provides a plan of care for the child with autistic disorder, including selected nursing diagnoses, outcome criteria, and appropriate nursing interventions and rationales.

Evaluation

Evaluation of care for the child with autistic disorder reflects whether the nursing actions have been effective in achieving the established goals. The nursing process calls for reassessment of the plan. Questions for gathering reassessment data may include:

TABLE 21–3 Care Plan for the Child With Autistic Disorder

Nursing Diagnosis: RISK FOR SELF-MUTILATION
Related to: Neurological alterations

Outcome Criteria	Nursing Interventions	Rationale
Client will not harm self.	1. Work with the child on a one-to-one basis.	1. One-to-one interaction facilitates trust.
	2. Try to determine if the self-mutilative behavior occurs in response to increasing anxiety, and if so, to what the anxiety may be attributed.	2. Mutilative behaviors may be averted if the cause can be determined and alleviated.
	3. Try to intervene with a diversion or replacement activity and offer nursing attention to the child as anxiety level starts to rise.	3. Diversion and replacement activities may provide needed feelings of security and substitute for self-mutilative behaviors.
	4. Protect the child when self-mutilative behaviors occur. Devices such as helmets padded hand mitts, or arm covers may provide protection when the risk for self-harm exists.	4. Client safety is a priority nursing intervention.

Nursing Diagnosis: IMPAIRED SOCIAL INTERACTION
Related to: Inability to trust; neurological alterations

Outcome Criteria	Nursing Interventions	Rationale
Client will initiate social interactions with caregiver.	1. Assign a limited number of caregivers to the child. Ensure that warmth, acceptance, and availability are conveyed.	1. Warmth, acceptance, and availability, along with consistency of assignment, enhance the establishment and maintenance of a trusting relationship.
	2. Provide child with familiar objects, such as familiar toys or a blanket. Support child's attempts to interact with others.	2. Familiar objects and presence of a trusted individual provide security during times of distress.
	3. Give positive reinforcement for eye contact with something acceptable to the child (e.g., food, familiar object). Gradually replace with social reinforcement (e.g., touch, smiling, hugging).	3. Being able to establish eye contact is essential to the child's ability to form satisfactory interpersonal relationships.

Nursing Diagnosis: IMPAIRED VERBAL COMMUNICATION
Related to: Withdrawal into the self; inadequate sensory stimulation; neurological alterations.

Outcome Criteria	Nursing Interventions	Rationale
Client will establish a means of communicating needs and desires to others.	1. Maintain consistency in assignment of caregivers.	1. Consistency facilitates trust and enhances the caregiver's ability to understand the child's attempts to communicate.
	2. Anticipate and fulfill the child's needs until communication can be established.	2. Anticipating needs helps to minimize frustration while the child is learning communication skills.
	3. Seek clarification and validation.	3. Validation ensures that the intended message has been conveyed.
	4. Give positive reinforcement when eye contact is used to convey nonverbal expressions.	4. Positive reinforcement increases self-esteem and encourages repetition.

(Continued)

TABLE 21–3 Care Plan for the Child With Autistic Disorder *(Continued)*

Nursing Diagnosis: DISTURBED PERSONAL IDENTITY

Related to: Inadequate sensory stimulation; neurological alterations

Outcome Criteria	Nursing Interventions	Rationale
Client will name own body parts as separate and individual from those of others.	1. Assist child to recognize separateness during self-care activities, such as dressing and feeding.	1. Recognition of body parts during dressing and feeding increases the child's awareness of self as separate from others.
	2. Assist the child in learning to name own body parts. This can be facilitated by the use of mirrors, drawings, and pictures of the child. Encourage appropriate touching of, and being touched by, others.	2. All of these activities may help increase the child's awareness of self as separate from others.

1. Has the child been able to establish trust with at least *one* caregiver?
2. Have the nursing actions directed toward preventing mutilative behaviors been effective in protecting the client from self-harm?
3. Has the child attempted to interact with others? Has he or she received positive reinforcement for these efforts?
4. Has eye contact improved?
5. Has the child established a means of communicating his or her needs and desires to others? Have all self-care needs been met?
6. Does the child demonstrate an awareness of self as separate from others? Can he or she name own body parts and body parts of caregiver?
7. Can he or she accept touch from others? Does he or she willingly and appropriately touch others?

ATTENTION-DEFICIT/HYPERACTIVITY DISORDER

The essential feature of ADHD is a persistent pattern of inattention and/or hyperactivity-**impulsivity** that is more frequent and severe than is typically observed in individuals at a comparable level of development (APA, 2000). These children are highly distractible and unable to contain stimuli. Motor activity is excessive, and movements are random and impulsive. Onset of the disorder is difficult to diagnose in children younger than age 4 years because their characteristic behavior is much more variable than that of older children. Frequently the disorder is not recognized until the child enters school. It is four to nine times more common in boys than in girls and may occur in as many as 3 to 7 percent of school-age children (APA, 2000). The *DSM-IV-TR* further categorizes the disorder into the following subtypes:

1. **ADHD, combined type**. This subtype is used if at least six symptoms of inattention and at least six symptoms of hyperactivity-impulsivity have persisted for at least 6 months. Most children and adolescents with the disorder have the combined type. It is not known whether the same is true of adults with the disorder.
2. **ADHD, predominantly inattentive type**. This subtype is used if at least six symptoms of inattention (but fewer than six symptoms of hyperactivity-impulsivity) have persisted for at least 6 months.
3. **ADHD, predominantly hyperactive-impulsive type**. This subtype is used if at least six symptoms of hyperactivity-impulsivity (but fewer than six symptoms of inattention) have persisted for at least 6 months. In many cases, inattention still may be a significant clinical feature.

Etiological Implications

Biological Influences

GENETICS. A number of studies have revealed supportive evidence of genetic influences in the etiology of ADHD. Results have indicated that a large number of parents of hyperactive children showed signs of hyperactivity during their own childhoods; that hyperactive children are more likely than children with more typical behavior to have siblings who are also hyperactive; and that when one twin of an identical twin pair has the disorder, the other is likely to have it too (National Institute of Mental Health [NIMH], 2000).

BIOCHEMICAL THEORY. Although it is believed that certain neurotransmitters—particularly dopamine, norepinephrine, and possibly serotonin—are involved in producing the symptoms associated with ADHD, their involvement is still under investigation. Abnormal levels of these neurotransmitters may be associated with the symptoms of hyperactivity, impulsivity, mood, and aggression often observed in individuals with the disorder.

ANATOMICAL INFLUENCES. Recent studies have implicated alterations in specific areas of the brain in individuals with ADHD. These regions include the frontal lobes, basal ganglia, caudate nucleus and cerebellum (Popper et al., 2003).

PRENATAL, PERINATAL, AND POSTNATAL FACTORS. A recent study is consistent with an earlier finding that links maternal smoking during pregnancy and hyperkinetic-impulsive behavior in offspring (Medscape Health, 2002). Intrauterine exposure to toxic substances, including alcohol, can produce effects on behavior. Fetal alcohol syndrome includes hyperactivity, impulsivity, and inattention as well as physical anomalies (Popper et al., 2003; Sadock & Sadock, 2003).

Perinatal influences that may contribute to ADHD are prematurity, signs of fetal distress, precipitated or prolonged labor, perinatal asphyxia, and low Apgar scores (Clunn, 1991). Postnatal factors that have been implicated include cerebral palsy, epilepsy, and other central nervous system (CNS) abnormalities resulting from trauma, infections, or other neurological disorders (Clunn, 1991; Popper et al., 2003).

Environmental Influences

ENVIRONMENTAL LEAD. Studies continue to provide evidence of the adverse effects on cognitive and behavioral development in children with elevated body levels of lead. Lead is pervasive in our environment, although the government has placed tighter restrictions on the substance in recent years. A possible causal link between elevated lead levels and behavior associated with ADHD is still being investigated.

DIET FACTORS. The possible link between food dyes and additives, such as artificial flavorings and preservatives, was introduced in the mid-1970s. Studies on the effect of food and food-additive allergies remain controversial, largely because of the inconsistencies in the results. Striking improvement in behavior has been reported by some parents and teachers when hyperactive children are placed on a diet free of dyes and additives; however, results are inconclusive.

Another diet factor that has received much attention in its possible link to ADHD is sugar. A number of studies have been conducted in an effort to determine the effect of sugar on hyperactive behavior, and the results strongly suggest that sugar plays no role in hyperactivity. One study reported that ADHD children had fewer problems after a high-carbohydrate breakfast than after a high-protein one (Medscape, 2002).

What has become clear is that the etiological roles of both food additives and sugar have been greatly exaggerated. There are no reliable indications to date that either of these diet components plays a significant role in the development or exacerbation of hyperactivity.

Psychosocial Influences

Disorganized or chaotic environments or a disruption in family equilibrium may predispose some individuals to ADHD. A high degree of psychosocial stress, maternal mental disorder, paternal criminality, low socioeconomic status, and foster care have been implicated (Dopheide & Theesen, 1999).

Other psychosocial influences that have been implicated include family history of alcoholism, hysterical and sociopathic behaviors, and parental history of hyperactivity. Developmental learning disorders may also predispose to ADHD (Clunn, 1991).

Application of the Nursing Process to ADHD

Background Assessment Data (Symptomatology)

A major portion of the problems of a child with ADHD relates to difficulties in performing age-appropriate tasks. These children are highly distractible and have extremely limited attention spans. They often shift from one uncompleted activity to another. Impulsivity, or deficit in inhibitory control, is also common.

Hyperactive children have difficulty forming satisfactory interpersonal relationships. They demonstrate behaviors that inhibit acceptable social interaction. They are disruptive and intrusive in group endeavors. They have difficulty complying with social norms. Some ADHD children are very **aggressive** or oppositional, whereas others exhibit more regressive and immature behaviors. Low frustration tolerance and outbursts of temper are common.

Children with ADHD have boundless energy, exhibiting excessive levels of activity, restlessness, and fidgeting. They have been described as "perpetual motion machines," continuously running, jumping, wiggling, or squirming. They experience a greater than average number of accidents, from minor mishaps to more serious incidents that may lead to physical injury or the destruction of property.

The *DSM-IV-TR* diagnostic criteria for ADHD are presented in Table 21–4.

TABLE 21–4 Diagnostic Criteria for Attention-Deficit/Hyperactivity Disorder

A. Either (1) or (2):
1. Six (or more) of the following symptoms of inattention have persisted for at least 6 months to a degree that is maladaptive and inconsistent with developmental level:
Inattention
a. Often fails to give close attention to details or makes careless mistakes in school work, work, or other activities
b. Often has difficulty sustaining attention in tasks or play activities
c. Often does not seem to listen when spoken to directly
d. Often does not follow through on instructions and fails to finish schoolwork, chores, or duties in the workplace (not because of oppositional behavior or failure to understand instructions)
e. Often has difficulty organizing tasks and activities
f. Often avoids, dislikes, or is reluctant to engage in tasks that require sustained mental effort (such as schoolwork or homework)
g. Often loses things necessary for tasks or activities (e.g., toys, school assignments, pencils, books, or tools)
h. Is often easily distracted by extraneous stimuli
i. Is often forgetful in daily activities
2. Six (or more) of the following symptoms of hyperactivity-impulsivity have persisted for at least 6 months to a degree that is maladaptive and inconsistent with developmental level:
Hyperactivity
a. Often fidgets with hands or feet or squirms in seat
b. Often leaves seat in classroom or in other situations in which remaining seated is expected
c. Often runs about or climbs excessively in situations in which it is inappropriate (in adolescents or adults, may be limited to subjective feelings of restlessness)
d. Often has difficulty playing or engaging in leisure activities quietly
e. Is often "on the go" or often acts as if "driven by a motor"
f. Often talks excessively
Impulsivity
a. Often blurts out answers before questions have been completed
b. Often has difficulty awaiting turn
c. Often interrupts or intrudes on others (e.g., butts into conversations or games)

B. Some hyperactive-impulsive or inattentive symptoms that caused impairment were present before age 7 years.
C. Some impairment from the symptoms is present in two or more settings (e.g., at school or work and at home).
D. There is clear evidence of clinically significant impairment in social, academic, or occupational functioning.
E. The symptoms do not occur exclusively during the course of a pervasive developmental disorder, schizophrenia, or other psychotic disorder and are not better accounted for by another mental disorder (e.g., mood disorder, anxiety disorder, dissociative disorder, or a personality disorder).
Subtypes:
1. **ADHD; combined type:** If both criteria A1 and A2 are met for the past 6 months
2. **ADHD; predominantly inattentive type:** If criterion A1 is met but criterion A2 is not met for the past 6 months
3. **ADHD; predominantly hyperactive-impulsive type:** If criterion A2 is met but criterion A1 is not met for the past 6 months

SOURCE: From APA (2000), with permission.

Diagnosis/Outcome Identification

Based on the data collected during the nursing assessment, possible nursing diagnoses for the child with ADHD include:

Risk for injury related to impulsive and accident-prone behavior and the inability to perceive self-harm

Impaired social interaction related to intrusive and immature behavior

Low self-esteem related to dysfunctional family system and negative feedback

Noncompliance with task expectations related to low frustration tolerance and short attention span

The following criteria may be used for measurement of outcomes in the care of the child with ADHD. The client:

1. Has experienced no physical harm
2. Interacts with others appropriately
3. Verbalizes positive aspects about self
4. Demonstrates fewer demanding behaviors
5. Cooperates with staff in an effort to complete assigned tasks

Planning/Implementation

Table 21–5 provides a plan of care for the child with ADHD, using nursing diagnoses common to the dis-

TABLE 21–5 Care Plan for the Child With Attention-Deficit/Hyperactivity Disorder

Nursing Diagnosis: RISK FOR INJURY

Related to: Impulsive and accident-prone behavior and the inability to perceive self-harm

Outcome Criteria	Nursing Interventions	Rationale
Client will be free of injury.	1. Ensure that client has a safe environment. Remove objects from immediate area on which client could injure self as a result of random, hyperactive movements.	1. Objects that are appropriate to the normal living situation can be hazardous to the child whose motor activities are out of control.
	2. Identify deliberate behaviors that put the child at risk for injury. Institute consequences for repetition of this behavior.	2. Behavior can be modified with aversive reinforcement.
	3. If there is risk of injury associated with specific therapeutic activities, provide adequate supervision and assistance, or limit client's participation if adequate supervision is not possible.	3. Client safety is a nursing priority.

Nursing Diagnosis: IMPAIRED SOCIAL INTERACTION

Related to: Intrusive and immature behavior

Outcome Criteria	Nursing Interventions	Rationale
Client will observe limits set on intrusive behavior and will demonstrate ability to interact appropriately with others.	1. Develop a trusting relationship with the child. Convey acceptance of the child separate from the unacceptable behavior.	1. Unconditional acceptance increases feelings of self-worth.
	2. Discuss with client which behaviors are and are not acceptable. Describe in a matter-of-fact manner the consequences of unacceptable behavior. Follow through.	2. Aversive reinforcement can alter or extinguish undesirable behaviors.
	3. Provide group situations for client.	3. Appropriate social behavior is often learned from the positive and negative feedback of peers.

Nursing Diagnosis: LOW SELF-ESTEEM

Related to: Dysfunctional family system and negative feedback

Outcome Criteria	Nursing Interventions	Rationale
Client will demonstrate increased feelings of self-worth by verbalizing positive statements about self and exhibiting fewer demanding behaviors.	1. Ensure that goals are realistic.	1. Unrealistic goals set client up for failure, which diminishes self-esteem.
	2. Plan activities that provide opportunities for success.	2. Success enhances self-esteem.
	3. Convey unconditional acceptance and positive regard.	3. Affirmation of client as a worthwhile human being may increase self-esteem
	4. Offer recognition of successful endeavors and positive reinforcement for attempts made. Give immediate positive feedback for acceptable behavior.	4. Positive reinforcement enhances self-esteem and may increase the desired behaviors.

Nursing Diagnosis: NONCOMPLIANCE (WITH TASK EXPECTATIONS)

Related to: Low frustration tolerance and short attention span

Outcome Criteria	Nursing Interventions	Rationale
Client will be able to complete assigned tasks independently or with a minimum of assistance.	1. Provide an environment for task efforts that is as free of distractions as possible.	1. Client is highly distractible and is unable to perform in the presence of even minimal stimulation.
	2. Provide assistance on a one-to-one basis, beginning with simple, concrete instructions.	2. Client lacks the ability to assimilate information that is complicated or has abstract meaning.
	3. Ask client to repeat instructions to you.	3. Repetition of the instructions helps to determine client's level of comprehension.
	4. Establish goals that allow client to complete a part of the task, rewarding completion of each step with a break for physical activity.	4. Short-term goals are not as overwhelming to one with such a short attention span. The positive reinforcement (physical activity) increases self-esteem and provides incentive for client to pursue the task to completion.
	5. Gradually decrease the amount of assistance given, while assuring the client that assistance is still available if deemed necessary.	5. This encourages the client to perform independently while providing a feeling of security with the presence of a trusted individual.

order, outcome criteria, and appropriate nursing interventions and rationales.

Evaluation

Evaluation of the care of a client with ADHD involves examining client behaviors following implementation of the nursing actions to determine if the goals of therapy have been achieved. Collecting data by using the following types of questions may provide appropriate information for evaluation.

1. Have the nursing actions directed at client safety been effective in protecting the child from injury?
2. Has the child been able to establish a trusting relationship with the primary caregiver?
3. Is the client responding to limits set on unacceptable behaviors?
4. Is the client able to interact appropriately with others?
5. Is the client able to verbalize positive statements about self?
6. Is the client able to complete tasks independently or with a minimum of assistance? Can he or she follow through after listening to simple instructions?
7. Is the client able to apply self-control to decrease motor activity?

Psychopharmacological Intervention

CNS stimulants are sometimes given to children with ADHD. Those commonly used include dextroamphetamine (Dexedrine), methylphenidate (Ritalin), pemoline (Cylert), and a dextroamphetamine/amphetamine composite (Adderall). The actual mechanism by which these medications improve behavior associated with ADHD is not known. In most individuals, they produce stimulation, excitability, and restlessness. In children with ADHD, the effects include an increased attention span, control of hyperactive behavior, and improvement in learning ability.

Side effects include insomnia, anorexia, weight loss, tachycardia, and temporary decrease in rate of growth and development. Physical tolerance can occur (less with pemoline than with dextroamphetamine or methylphenidate).

In 2002, the U.S. Food and Drug Administration approved atomoxetine (Strattera), a medication specific for treating ADHD. Atomoxetine is a selective norepinephrine reuptake inhibitor. The exact mechanism by which it produces its therapeutic effect in ADHD is unknown. Side effects include headache, nausea and vomiting, upper abdominal pain, dry mouth, decreased appetite, weight loss, constipation, insomnia, increased blood pressure and heart rate, and sexual dysfunction.

Drugs in the antidepressant classification also have been used with some success in the treatment of ADHD. Commonly used medications in this category are bupropion (Wellbutrin), desipramine (Norpramin), nortriptyline (Pamelor), and imipramine (Tofranil).

Bupropion is distributed in a short- and long-lasting form. The side effects are similar to those of the stimulants: tachycardia, dizziness, shakiness, insomnia, nausea, anorexia, and weight loss. Individuals with a history of seizures or eating disorders should not take this medication.

The tricyclic antidepressants are useful for some ADHD symptoms, particularly attention and restlessness. The major side effects include sedation, dry mouth, increased appetite, changes in atrioventricular conduction of the heart, hypertension or hypotension, arrhythmias, and tachycardia. An electrocardiogram should be performed before initiation of therapy.

Route and Dosage Information

Dextroamphetamine (Dexedrine); Dextroamphetamine/Amphetamine Composite (Adderall)

- PO (children age 3 to 5 years old): Initial dosage: 2.5 mg/day. This may be increased in increments of 2.5 mg/day at weekly intervals until the desired response is achieved.
- PO (children age 6 years or older): Initial dosage: 5 mg daily or twice a day. This may be increased in increments of 5 mg/day at weekly intervals until the desired response is achieved. Dosage rarely will exceed 40 mg/day. First dose of tablets or elixir forms may be given on awakening; additional doses at intervals of 4 to 6 hours. Sustained-release forms may be used for once-a-day dosage given in the morning.

Methylphenidate (Ritalin)

- PO (children age 6 and older): Initial dosage: 5 mg before breakfast and lunch. Dosage may be increased gradually in increments of 5 to 10 mg/day at weekly intervals. Maximum daily dosage: 60 mg. Sustained-release form may be used for once-a-day dosage, given in the morning.

Pemoline (Cylert)

- PO (children age 6 and older): Initial dosage: 37.5 mg/day, administered as a single dose each morning. Dosage may be gradually increased at 1-week intervals in increments of 18.75 mg/day until the desired effect is achieved. Effective dosage usually ranges from 56.25 to 75 mg/day. Maximum recommended dose: 112.5 mg/day. Clinical benefit may not be observed for 3 to 4 weeks.

Atomoxetine (Strattera)

- PO (Children and adults weighing more than 70 kg [154 lb]): initial dose: 40 mg/day. Increase after a minimum of 3 days to a target total daily dose of 80 mg, as a single dose in the morning or two evenly divided doses in the morning and late afternoon or early evening. After 2 to 4 weeks, total dosage may be increased to a maximum of 100 mg, if needed.
- PO (Children and adults weighing 70 kg [154 lb] or less): initial dose: 0.5 mg/kg daily. Increase after a minimum of 3 days to a target total daily dose of about 1.2 mg/kg taken as a single dose in the morning or 2 evenly divided doses in the morning and late afternoon or early evening. Maximum daily dose: 1.4 mg/kg or 100 mg daily, whichever is less.

Bupropion (Wellbutrin)

- PO (children age 6 and older): 3 mg/kg/ day.

Imipramine (Tofranil)

- PO (children age 6 and older): initial dose: 1 mg/kg daily in divided doses, with increases every 2 to 3 weeks up to a maximum of 2.5 mg/kg/day.

Nursing Implications

- Assess the client's mental status for changes in mood, level of activity, amount of stimulation, and aggressiveness.
- Ensure that the client is protected from injury. Keep stimuli low and environment as quiet as possible to discourage overstimulation.
- To reduce anorexia, the medication may be administered immediately after meals. The client should be weighed regularly (at least weekly) during hospitalization and at home while on therapy with CNS stimulants because of the potential for anorexia and weight loss and the temporary interruption of growth and development.
- To prevent insomnia, administer last dose at least 6 hours before bedtime. Administer sustained-release forms in the morning.
- In children with behavior disorders, a drug "holiday" should be attempted periodically under direction of the physician to determine effectiveness of the medication and need for continuation.
- Ensure that the parents are aware of the delayed effects of pemoline. Therapeutic response may not be seen for 2 to 4 weeks. The drug should not be discontinued for lack of immediate results.
- Inform parents that over-the-counter (OTC) medications should be avoided while the child is receiving stimulant medication. Some OTC medications, particularly cold and hay fever preparations, contain sympathomimetic agents that could compound the effects of the stimulant and create a drug interaction that may be toxic to the child.
- Ensure that parents are aware that the drug should not be withdrawn abruptly. Withdrawal should be gradual and under the direction of the physician.

CONDUCT DISORDER

With conduct disorder, there is a repetitive and persistent pattern of behavior in which the basic rights of others or major age-appropriate societal norms or rules are violated (APA, 2000). Physical aggression is common. The *DSM-IV-TR* divides this disorder into two subtypes, based on the age at onset:

1. **Childhood-onset type.** This subtype is defined by the onset of at least one criterion characteristic of conduct disorder before age 10 years. Individuals with this subtype are usually boys, frequently display physical aggression, and have disturbed peer relationships. They may have had oppositional defiant disorder during early childhood, usually meet the full criteria for conduct disorder by puberty, and are likely to develop antisocial personality disorder in adulthood.
2. **Adolescent-onset type.** This subtype is defined by the absence of any criteria characteristic of conduct disorder before age 10 years. They are less likely to display aggressive behaviors and tend to have more normal peer relationships than those with childhood-onset type. They are also less likely to have persistent conduct disorder or develop antisocial personality disorder than those with childhood-onset type. The ratio of boys to girls is lower in adolescent-onset type than in childhood-onset type.

Etiological Implications

Biological Influences

GENETICS. Studies with monozygotic and dizygotic twins as well as with non-twin siblings have revealed a significantly higher number of conduct disorders among those who have family members with the disorder (APA, 2000; Fisher, 1997). Although genetic factors appear to be involved in the etiology of conduct disorders, little is yet known about the actual mechanisms involved in genetic transmission. A reasonable assumption is that environmental factors play an important role in the manifestation of the disorder in those who are genetically susceptible.

TEMPERAMENT. The term **temperament** refers to personality traits that become evident very early in life and that may be present at birth. Evidence suggests a genetic component in temperament and an association between temperament and behavioral problems later in life. Studies have shown that, without appropriate intervention, difficult temperament at age 3 has significant links to conduct disorder and movement into care or institutional life at age 17 (Bagley & Mallick, 2000).

BIOCHEMICAL FACTORS. Studies have looked at various chemicals as biological markers. Some studies suggest that children with conduct disorder have lower levels of norepinephrine, are less sensitive to signals of punishment, and less likely to experience anxiety (Fisher, 1997). Studies have also suggested an increase in aggression with decreased serotonin functioning in children. Some investigators have researched the possibility of testosterone association with violence. Fisher (1997) reports, "One study compared children ages 4 to 10 with severe violent behaviors versus non-aggressive peers and showed no difference in the groups with respect to testosterone."

Psychosocial Influences

PEER RELATIONSHIPS. Social groups have a significant impact on a child's development. Peers play an essential role in the socialization of interpersonal competence, and skills acquired in this manner affect the child's long-term adjustment. Studies have shown that poor peer relations during childhood were consistently implicated in the etiology of later deviance (Ladd, 1999). Aggression was found to be the principal cause of peer rejection, thus contributing to a cycle of maladaptive behavior.

Family Influences

The following factors related to family dynamics have been implicated as contributors in the predisposition to conduct disorder (Clunn, 1991; Popper et al., 2003; Sadock & Sadock, 2003):

- Parental rejection
- Inconsistent management with harsh discipline
- Early institutional living
- Frequent shifting of parental figures
- Large family size
- Absent father
- Parents with antisocial personality disorder and/or alcohol dependence
- Association with a delinquent subgroup
- Marital conflict and divorce
- Inadequate communication patterns
- Parental permissiveness

Application of the Nursing Process to Conduct Disorder

Background Assessment Data (Symptomatology)

The classic characteristic of conduct disorder is the use of physical aggression in the violation of the rights of others. The behavior pattern manifests itself in virtually all areas of the child's life (at home and school, with peers, and in the community). Stealing, lying, and truancy are common problems. The child lacks feelings of guilt or remorse.

The use of tobacco, liquor, or nonprescribed drugs and participation in sexual activities occurs earlier than the peer group's expected age. Projection is a common defense mechanism.

Low self-esteem is manifested by a "tough guy" image. Characteristics include poor frustration tolerance, irritability, and frequent temper outbursts. Symptoms of anxiety and depression are common.

Level of academic achievement may be low in relation to age and IQ.

Manifestations associated with ADHD (e.g., attention difficulties, impulsiveness, and hyperactivity) are very common in children with conduct disorder.

The *DSM-IV-TR* diagnostic criteria for conduct disorder are presented in Table 21–6.

Diagnosis/Outcome Identification

Based on the data collected during the nursing assessment, possible nursing diagnoses for the client with conduct disorder include:

Risk for other-directed violence related to characteristics of temperament, peer rejection, negative parental role models, dysfunctional family dynamics

Impaired social interaction related to negative parental role models, impaired peer relations leading to inappropriate social behaviors

TABLE 21–6 Diagnostic Criteria for Conduct Disorder

A. A repetitive and persistent pattern of behavior in which the basic rights of others or major age-appropriate societal norms or rules are violated, as manifested by the presence of three (or more) of the following criteria in the past 12 months, with at least one criterion present in the past 6 months:
   1. **Aggression to people and animals**
      a. Often bullies, threatens, or intimidates others
      b. Often initiates physical fights
      c. Has used a weapon that can cause serious physical harm to others (e.g., a bat, brick, broken bottle, knife, gun)
      d. Has been physically cruel to people
      e. Has been physically cruel to animals
      f. Has stolen when confronting a victim (e.g., mugging, purse snatching, extortion, armed robbery)
      g. Has forced someone into sexual activity
   2. **Destruction of property**
      a. Has deliberately engaged in fire setting with the intention of causing serious damage
      b. Has deliberately destroyed others' property (other than by fire setting)
   3. **Deceitfulness or theft.**
      a. Has broken into someone else's house, building, or car
      b. Often lies to obtain goods or favors or to avoid obligations (i.e., "cons" others)
      c. Has stolen items of nontrivial value without confronting a victim (e.g., shoplifting, but without breaking and entering; forgery)
   4. **Serious violations of rules**
      a. Often stays out at night despite parental prohibitions, beginning before age 13 years
      b. Has run away from home overnight at least twice when living in parental or parental surrogate home (or once without returning for a lengthy period)
      c. Is often truant from school, beginning before age 13 years

B. The disturbance in behavior causes clinically significant impairment in social, academic, or occupational functioning.

C. If the individual is age 18 years or older, criteria are not met for antisocial personality disorder.

Subtypes:
   1. **Childhood-onset type:** Onset of at least one criterion characteristic of conduct disorder prior to age 10
   2. **Adolescent-onset type:** Absence of any criteria characteristic of conduct disorder prior to age 10
   3. **Unspecified onset:** Age at onset is not known

From APA (2000), with permission.

Defensive coping related to low self-esteem and dysfunctional family system

Low self-esteem related to lack of positive feedback and unsatisfactory parent/child relationship

The following criteria may be used for measurement of outcomes in the care of the client with conduct disorder. The client:

1. Has not harmed self or others
2. Interacts with others in a socially appropriate manner
3. Accepts direction without becoming defensive
4. Demonstrates evidence of increased self-esteem by discontinuing exploitative and demanding behaviors toward others

Planning/Implementation

Table 21–7 provides a plan of care for the child with conduct disorder, using nursing diagnoses common to the disorder, outcome criteria, and appropriate nursing interventions and rationales.

Evaluation

Following the planning and implementation of care, evaluation is made of the behavioral changes in the child with conduct disorder. This is accomplished by determining if the goals of therapy have been achieved. Reassessment, the next step in the nursing process, may be initiated by gathering information using the following questions.

1. Have the nursing actions directed toward managing the client's aggressive behavior been effective?
2. Have interventions prevented harm to others or others' property?
3. Is the client able to express anger in an appropriate manner?
4. Has the client developed more adaptive coping strategies to deal with anger and feelings of aggression?
5. Does the client demonstrate the ability to trust others? Is he or she able to interact with staff and peers in an appropriate manner?

TABLE 21–7 Care Plan for Child/Adolescent With Conduct Disorder

Nursing Diagnosis: RISK FOR OTHER-DIRECTED VIOLENCE

Related to: Characteristics of temperament, peer rejection, negative parental role models, dysfunctional family dynamics

Outcome Criteria	Nursing Interventions	Rationale
Client will not harm others or others' property.	1. Observe client's behavior frequently through routine activities and interactions. Become aware of behaviors that indicate a rise in agitation.	1. Recognition of behaviors that precede the onset of aggression may provide the opportunity to intervene before violence occurs.
	2. Redirect violent behavior with physical outlets for suppressed anger and frustration.	2. Excess energy is released through physical activities inducing a feeling of relaxation.
	3. Encourage client to express anger and act as a role model for appropriate expression of anger.	3. Discussion of situations that create anger may lead to more effective ways of dealing with them.
	4. Ensure that a sufficient number of staff is available to indicate a show of strength if necessary.	4. This conveys an evidence of control over the situation and provides physical security for staff.
	5. Administer tranquilizing medication, if ordered, or use mechanical restraints or isolation room only if situation cannot be controlled with less restrictive means.	5. It is the client's right to expect the use of techniques that ensure safety of the client and others by the least restrictive means.

Nursing Diagnosis: IMPAIRED SOCIAL INTERACTION

Related to: Negative parental role models; impaired peer relations leading to inappropriate social behavior

Outcome Criteria	Nursing Interventions	Rationale
Client will be able to interact with staff and peers using age-appropriate, acceptable behaviors.	1. Develop a trusting relationship with the client. Convey acceptance of the person separate from the unacceptable behavior.	1. Unconditional acceptance increases feeling of self-worth.
	2. Discuss with client which behaviors are and are not acceptable. Describe in matter-of-fact manner the consequence of unacceptable behavior. Follow through.	2. Aversive reinforcement can alter or extinguish undesirable behaviors.
	3. Provide group situations for client.	3. Appropriate social behavior is often learned from the positive and negative feedback of peers.

Nursing Diagnosis: DEFENSIVE COPING

Related to: Low self-esteem and dysfunctional family system

Outcome Criteria	Nursing Interventions	Rationale
Client will accept responsibility for own behaviors and interact with others without becoming defensive.	1. Explain to client the correlation between feelings of inadequacy and the need for acceptance from others and how these feelings provoke defensive behaviors, such as blaming others for own behaviors.	1. Recognition of the problem is the first step in the change process toward resolution.
	2. Provide immediate, matter-of-fact, nonthreatening feedback for unacceptable behaviors.	2. Client may not realize how these behaviors are being perceived by others.
	3. Help identify situations that provoke defensiveness and practice through role-play more appropriate responses.	3. Role-playing provides confidence to deal with difficult situations when they actually occur.
	4. Provide immediate positive feedback for acceptable behaviors.	4. Positive feedback encourages repetition, and immediacy is significant for these children who respond to immediate gratification.

Nursing Diagnosis: LOW SELF-ESTEEM

Related to: Lack of positive feedback and unsatisfactory parent/child relationship

Outcome Criteria	Nursing Interventions	Rationale
Client will demonstrate increased feelings of self-worth by verbalizing positive statements about self and exhibiting fewer manipulative behaviors.	1. Ensure that goals are realistic.	1. Unrealistic goals set client up for failure, which diminishes self-esteem.
	2. Plan activities that provide opportunities for success.	2. Success enhances self-esteem.
	3. Convey unconditional acceptance and positive regard.	3. Communicating that client is a worthwhile human being may increase self-esteem.
	4. Set limits on manipulative behavior. Take caution not to reinforce manipulative behaviors by providing desired attention. Identify the consequences of manipulation. Administer consequences matter-of-factly when manipulation occurs.	4. Aversive consequences may work to decrease unacceptable behaviors.
	5. Help client understand that he or she uses this behavior in order to try to increase own self-esteem. Interventions should reflect other actions to accomplish this goal.	5. When the client feels better about self, the need to manipulate others will diminish.

6. Is the client able to accept responsibility for his or her own behavior? Is there less blaming of others?
7. Is the client able to accept feedback from others without becoming defensive?
8. Is the client able to verbalize positive statements about self?
9. Is the client able to interact with others without engaging in manipulation?

OPPOSITIONAL DEFIANT DISORDER

Oppositional defiant disorder is characterized by a pattern of negativistic, defiant, disobedient, and hostile behavior toward authority figures that occurs more frequently than is usually observed in individuals of comparable age and developmental level and interferes with social, academic, or occupational functioning (APA, 2000). The disorder typically begins by 8 years of age and usually not later than early adolescence. It is more prevalent in boys than in girls before puberty, but the rates are more closely equal after puberty. In a significant proportion of cases, oppositional defiant disorder is a developmental antecedent to conduct disorder (APA, 2000).

Etiological Implications

Biological Influences

Because the behaviors associated with oppositional defiant disorder are very similar to those of conduct disorder, with the exception of violation of the rights of others, it is reasonable to speculate that they may share at least *some* of the same biological influences. What role, if any, genetics, temperament, or biochemical alteration plays in the etiology of oppositional defiant disorder has not been determined.

Family Influences

Opposition during various developmental stages is both normal and healthy. Children first exhibit oppositional behaviors at around 10 or 11 months of age, again as a toddler between 18 and 36 months of age, and finally during adolescence. Pathology is only considered when the developmental phase is prolonged or when there is overreaction in the child's environment to his or her behavior.

Some children exhibit these behaviors in a more intense form than others. Sadock and Sadock (2003) report "epidemiological studies of negativistic traits in nonclinical populations found such behavior in between 16 to 22 percent of school-age children."

Some parents interpret average or increased level of developmentally oppositional behavior as hostility and a deliberate effort on the part of the child to be in control. If power and control are issues for parents, or if they exercise authority for their own needs, a power struggle can be established between the parents and the child that sets the stage for the development of oppositional defiant disorder.

Popper and associates (2003) suggest that the following familial influences may play an etiological role in the development of oppositional defiant disorder:

1. Parental problems in disciplining, structuring, and limit setting
2. Identification by the child with an impulse-disor-

dered parent who acts as a role model for oppositional and defiant interactions with other people
3. Parental unavailability (e.g., separation, evening work hours)

Application of the Nursing Process to Oppositional Defiant Disorder

Background Assessment Data (Symptomatology)

Oppositional defiant disorder is characterized by passive-aggressive behaviors such as stubbornness, procrastination, disobedience, carelessness, **negativism**, testing of limits, resistance to directions, deliberately ignoring the communication of others, and unwillingness to compromise. Other symptoms that may be evident are running away, school avoidance, school underachievement, temper tantrums, fighting, and argumentativeness. In severe cases, there may be elective mutism, enuresis, encopresis, or eating and sleeping problems (Harvard Medical School, 2002).

The oppositional attitude is directed toward adults, most particularly the parents. Symptoms of the disorder may or may not be evident in school or elsewhere in the community (APA, 2000).

Usually these children do not see themselves as being oppositional but view the problem as arising from others whom they believe are making unreasonable demands on them. Interpersonal relationships are fraught with difficulty, including those with peers. These children are often friendless, perceiving human relationships as negative and unsatisfactory. School performance is usually poor because of their refusal to participate and their resistance to external demands. The *DSM-IV-TR* (2000) diagnostic criteria for oppositional defiant disorder are presented in Table 21–8.

Diagnosis/Outcome Identification

Based on the data collected during the nursing assessment, possible nursing diagnoses for the client with oppositional defiant disorder include:

Noncompliance with therapy related to negative temperament, denial of problems, underlying hostility
Defensive coping related to retarded ego development, low self-esteem, unsatisfactory parent/child relationship
Low self-esteem related to lack of positive feedback, retarded ego development
Impaired social interaction related to negative temperament, underlying hostility, manipulation of others

The following criteria may be used for measurement of outcomes in the care of the client with oppositional defiant disorder. The client:

1. Complies with treatment by participating in therapies without negativism
2. Accepts responsibility for his or her part in the problem
3. Takes direction from staff without becoming defensive
4. Does not manipulate other people
5. Verbalizes positive aspects about self
6. Interacts with others in an appropriate manner

Planning/Implementation

Table 21–9 provides a plan of care for the child with oppositional defiant disorder, using nursing diagnoses

TABLE 21–8 Diagnostic Criteria for Oppositional Defiant Disorder

A. A pattern of negativistic, hostile, and defiant behavior lasting at least 6 months, during which four (or more) of the following are present:
   1. Often loses temper
   2. Often argues with adults
   3. Often actively defies or refuses to comply with adult requests or rules
   4. Often deliberately annoys people
   5. Often blames others for his or her mistakes or misbehavior
   6. Is often touchy or easily annoyed by others
   7. Is often angry and resentful
   8. Is often spiteful or vindictive
B. The disturbance in behavior causes clinically significant impairment in social, academic, or occupational functioning
C. The behaviors do not occur exclusively during the course of a psychotic or mood disorder.
D. Criteria are not met for conduct disorder, and if the individual is age 18 years or older, criteria are not met for antisocial personality disorder.

From APA (2000), with permission.

TABLE 21–9 Care Plan for the Child/Adolescent With Oppositional Defiant Disorder

Nursing Diagnosis: NONCOMPLIANCE WITH THERAPY

Related to: Negative temperament; denial of problems; underlying hostility

Outcome Criteria	Nursing Interventions	Rationale
Client will participate in and cooperate during therapeutic activities.	1. Set forth a structured plan of therapeutic activities. Start with minimum expectations and increase as client begins to manifest evidence of compliance.	1. Structure provides security, and one or two activities may not seem as overwhelming as the whole schedule of activities presented at one time.
	2. Establish a system of rewards for compliance with therapy and consequences for noncompliance. Ensure that the rewards and consequences are concepts of value to the client.	2. Positive, negative, and aversive reinforcements can contribute to desired changes in behavior.
	3. Convey acceptance of the client separate from the undesirable behaviors being exhibited. ("It is not *you*, but your *behavior*, that is unacceptable")	3. Unconditional acceptance enhances self-worth and may contribute to a decrease in the need for passive-aggression toward others.

Nursing Diagnosis: DEFENSIVE COPING

Related to: Retarded ego development; low self-esteem; unsatisfactory parent/child relationship

Outcome Criteria	Nursing Interventions	Rationale
Client will accept responsibility for own behaviors and interact with others without becoming defensive.	1. Help client recognize that feelings of inadequacy provoke defensive behaviors, such as blaming others for problems, and the need to "get even."	1. Recognition of the problem is the first step toward initiating change.
	2. Provide immediate, nonthreatening feedback for passive-aggressive behavior.	2. Because client denies responsibility for problems, he or she is denying the inappropriateness of behavior.
	3. Help identify situations that provoke defensiveness and practice role-play for more appropriate responses.	3. Role-playing provides confidence to deal with difficult situations when they actually occur.
	4. Provide immediate positive feedback for acceptable behaviors.	4. Positive feedback encourages repetition, and immediacy is significant for these children who respond to immediate gratification.

Nursing Diagnosis: LOW SELF-ESTEEM

Related to: Lack of positive feedback; retarded ego development

Outcome Criteria	Nursing Interventions	Rationale
Client will demonstrate increased feelings of self-worth by verbalizing positive statements about self and exhibiting fewer manipulative behaviors.	1. Ensure that goals are realistic.	1. Unrealistic goals set client up for failure, which diminishes self-esteem.
	2. Plan activities that provide opportunities for success.	2. Success enhances self-esteem.
	3. Convey unconditional acceptance and positive regard.	3. Affirmation of client as worthwhile human being may increase self-esteem.
	4. Set limits on manipulative behavior. Take caution not to reinforce manipulative behaviors by providing desired attention. Identify the consequences of manipulation. Administer consequences matter-of-factly when manipulation occurs.	4. Aversive reinforcement may work to decrease or extinguish unacceptable behaviors.
	5. Help client understand that he or she uses this behavior in order to try to increase own self-esteem. Interventions should reflect other actions to accomplish this goal.	5. When client feels better about self, the need to manipulate others will diminish.

(Continued)

TABLE 21–9 Care Plan for the Child/Adolescent With Oppositional Defiant Disorder *(Continued)*

Nursing Diagnosis: IMPAIRED SOCIAL INTERACTION

Related to: Negative temperament; underlying hostility; manipulation of others

Outcome Criteria	Nursing Interventions	Rationale
Client will be able to interact with staff and peers using age-appropriate, acceptable behaviors.	1. Develop a trusting relationship with the client. Convey acceptance of the person separate from the unacceptable behavior.	1. Unconditional acceptance increases feelings of self-worth and may serve to diminish feelings of rejection that have accumulated over a long period.
	2. Explain to the client about passive-aggressive behavior. Explain how these behaviors are perceived by others. Describe which behaviors are not acceptable and role-play more adaptive responses. Give positive feedback for acceptable behaviors.	2. Role-playing is a way to practice behaviors that do not come readily to the client, making it easier when the situation actually occurs. Positive feedback enhances repetition of desirable behaviors.
	3. Provide peer group situations for the client.	3. Appropriate social behavior is often learned from the positive and negative feedback of peers. Groups also provide an atmosphere for using the behaviors rehearsed in role-play.

common to the disorder, outcome criteria, and appropriate nursing interventions and rationales.

Evaluation

The evaluation step of the nursing process calls for reassessment of the plan of care to determine if the nursing actions have been effective in achieving the goals of therapy. The following questions can be used with the child or adolescent with oppositional defiant disorder to gather information for the evaluation.

1. Is the client cooperating with schedule of therapeutic activities? Is level of participation adequate?
2. Is his or her attitude toward therapy less negative?
3. Is the client accepting responsibility for problem behavior?
4. Is the client verbalizing the unacceptability of his or her passive-aggressive behavior?
5. Is he or she able to identify which behaviors are unacceptable and substitute more adaptive behaviors?
6. Is the client able to interact with staff and peers without defending behavior in an angry manner?
7. Is the client able to verbalize positive statements about self?
8. Is increased self-worth evident with fewer manifestations of manipulation?
9. Is the client able to make compromises with others when issues of control emerge?
10. Are anger and hostility expressed in an appropriate manner? Can the client verbalize ways of releasing anger adaptively?
11. Is he or she able to verbalize true feelings instead of allowing them to emerge through use of passive-aggressive behaviors?

TOURETTE'S DISORDER

The essential feature of this disorder is the presence of multiple motor tics and one or more vocal tics (APA, 2000). They may appear simultaneously or at different periods during the illness. The disturbance causes marked distress or interferes with social, occupational, or other important areas of functioning. The onset of the disorder is before age 18 years and is more common in boys than in girls. The duration of the disorder may extend throughout the lifetime, although there may be periods of remission that last from weeks to years (APA, 2000). The symptoms usually diminish during adolescence and adulthood and, in some cases, disappear altogether by early adulthood.

Etiological Implications

Biological Factors

GENETICS. Tics are noted in two-thirds of relatives of Tourette's disorder clients (Popper, et al., 2003). Twin studies with both monozygotic and dizygotic twins suggest an inheritable component.

Evidence suggests that Tourette's disorder may be transmitted in an autosomal pattern intermediate between dominant and recessive (Sadock & Sadock, 2003).

BIOCHEMICAL FACTORS. Abnormalities in levels of dopamine, serotonin, dynorphin, gamma-aminobutyric acid, acetylcholine, and norepinephrine have been associated with Tourette's disorder (Popper et al., 2003). Neurotransmitter pathways through the basal ganglia, globus pallidus, and subthalamic regions appear to be involved.

STRUCTURAL FACTORS. Neuroimaging brain studies have been consistent in finding dysfunction in the area of the basal ganglia. Enlargement has been found in the caudate nucleus and decreased cerebral blood flow in the left lenticular nucleus (Riddle, Rasmussen, & Woods, 1992; Singer, Reiss, & Brown, 1993).

Environmental Factors

Additional retrospective findings may be implicated in the etiology of Tourette's disorder, such as increased prenatal complications and low birth weight. Greater emotional stress during pregnancy and more nausea and vomiting during the first trimester of pregnancy have been noted in the mothers of children with Tourette's disorder (Leckman, Dolnansky, & Hardin, 1990). It is speculated that these environmental factors may temper the genetic predisposition to Tourette's disorder.

Application of the Nursing Process to Tourette's Disorder

Background Assessment Data (Symptomatology)

The motor tics of Tourette's disorder may involve the head, torso, and upper and lower limbs. Initial symptoms may begin with a single motor tic, most commonly eye blinking, or with multiple symptoms. The *DSM-IV-TR* identifies simple motor tics as eye-blinking, neck-jerking, shoulder-shrugging, facial-grimacing, and coughing. Common complex motor tics include touching, squatting, hopping, skipping, deep knee bends, retracing steps, and twirling when walking.

Vocal tics include various words or sounds such as clicks, grunts, yelps, barks, sniffs, snorts, coughs and, in about 10 percent of cases, a complex vocal tic involving the uttering of obscenities (APA, 2000). Vocal tics may include repeating certain words or phrases out of context, repeating one's own sounds or words **(palilalia),** or repeating what others say **(echolalia).**

The movements and vocalizations are experienced as compulsive and irresistible, but they can be suppressed for varying lengths of time. They are exacerbated by stress and attenuated during periods in which the individual becomes absorbed by an activity. In most cases, tics are diminished during sleep (APA, 2000).

The age at onset of Tourette's disorder can be as early as age 2 years, but the disorder occurs most commonly during childhood (around age 6 to 7 years). Prevalence of the disorder is related to age, affecting many more children (5 to 30 per 10,000) than adults (1 to 2 per 10,000) (APA, 2000).

Diagnosis/Outcome Identification

Based on data collected during the nursing assessment, possible nursing diagnoses for the client with Tourette's disorder include:

Risk for self-directed or other-directed violence related to low tolerance for frustration
Impaired social interaction related to impulsiveness, oppositional and aggressive behavior
Low self-esteem related to shame associated with tic behaviors

The following criteria may be used for measurement of outcomes in the care of the client with Tourette's disorder. The client:

1. Has not harmed self or others
2. Interacts with staff and peers in an appropriate manner
3. Demonstrates self-control by managing tic behavior
4. Follows rules of unit without becoming defensive
5. Verbalizes positive aspects about self

Planning/Implementation

Table 21–10 provides a plan of care for the child or adolescent with Tourette's disorder, using selected nursing diagnoses, outcome criteria, and appropriate nursing interventions and rationales.

Evaluation

Evaluation of care for the child with Tourette's disorder reflects whether the nursing actions have been effective in achieving the established goals. The nursing

TABLE 21–10 Care Plan for the Child or Adolescent With Tourette's Disorder

Nursing Diagnosis: RISK FOR SELF-DIRECTED OR OTHER-DIRECTED VIOLENCE

Related to: Low tolerance for frustration

Outcome Criteria	Nursing Interventions	Rationale
Client will not harm self or others.	1. Observe client's behavior frequently through routine activities and interactions. Become aware of behaviors that indicate a rise in agitation.	1. Stress commonly increases tic behaviors. Recognition of behaviors that precede the onset of aggression may provide the opportunity to intervene before violence occurs.
	2. Monitor for self-destructive behavior and impulses. A staff member may need to stay with the client to prevent self-mutilation.	2. Client safety is a nursing priority.
	3. Provide hand coverings and other restraints that prevent the client from self-mutilative behaviors.	3. Provide immediate external controls against self-aggressive behaviors.
	4. Redirect violent behavior with physical outlets for frustration.	4. Excess energy is released through physical activities and a feeling of relaxation is induced.

Nursing Diagnosis: IMPAIRED SOCIAL INTERACTION

Related to: Impulsiveness; oppositional and aggressive behavior

Outcome Criteria	Nursing Interventions	Rationale
Client will be able to interact with staff and peers using age-appropriate, acceptable behaviors.	1. Develop a trusting relationship with the client. Convey acceptance of the person separate from the unacceptable behavior.	1. Unconditional acceptance increases feelings of self-worth.
	2. Discuss with client which behaviors are and are not acceptable. Describe in matter-of-fact manner the consequences of unacceptable behavior. Follow through.	2. Aversive reinforcement can alter undesirable behaviors.
	3. Provide group situations for client.	3. Appropriate social behavior is often learned from the positive and negative feedback of peers.

Nursing Diagnosis: LOW SELF-ESTEEM

Related to: Shame associated with tic behaviors

Outcome Criteria	Nursing Interventions	Rationale
Client will verbalize positive aspects about self not associated with tic behaviors.	1. Convey unconditional acceptance and positive regard.	1. Communication of client as a worthwhile human being may increase self-esteem.
	2. Set limits on manipulative behavior. Take caution not to reinforce manipulative behaviors by providing desired attention. Identify the consequences of manipulation. Administer consequences matter-of-factly when manipulation occurs.	2. Aversive consequences may work to decrease or extinguish unacceptable behaviors.
	3. Help client understand that he or she uses manipulation to try to increase own self-esteem. Interventions should reflect other actions to accomplish this goal.	3. When client feels better about self, the need to manipulate others will diminish.
	4. If client chooses to suppress tics in the presence of others, provide a specified "tic time," during which he or she "vents" tics, feelings, and behaviors (alone or with staff).	4. Allows for release of tics and assists in sense of control and management of symptoms (Rosner & Pollice, 1991).
	5. Ensure that client has regular one-to-one time with nursing staff.	5. Provides opportunity for educating about illness and teaching management tactics. Assists in exploring feelings around illness and incorporating illness into a healthy sense of self (Rosner & Pollice, 1991).

process calls for reassessment of the plan. Questions for gathering reassessment data may include:

1. Has the client refrained from causing harm to self or others during times of increased tension?
2. Has the client developed adaptive coping strategies for dealing with frustration to prevent resorting to self-destruction or aggression to others?
3. Is the client able to interact appropriately with staff and peers?
4. Is the client able to suppress tic behaviors when he or she chooses to do so?
5. Does the client set a time for "release" of the suppressed tic behaviors?
6. Does the client verbalize positive aspects about self, particularly as they relate to his or her ability to manage the illness?
7. Does the client comply with treatment in a nondefensive manner?

Psychopharmacological Intervention

Medications are used to reduce the severity of the tics in clients with Tourette's disorder. Pharmacotherapy is most effective when it is combined with other forms of therapy, such as education and supportive intervention, individual counseling or psychotherapy, and family therapy (McSwiggan-Hardin, 1995). Some cases of the disorder are mild, and clients choose not to use medication until the symptoms become severe and more intense intervention is warranted. A number of medications have been used to treat Tourette's disorder. The most common ones are discussed here.

HALOPERIDOL (HALDOL). Haloperidol has been the drug of choice for Tourette's disorder. The dosage is 0.05 to 0.075 mg/kg/day in two to three divided doses. Children taking haloperidol can develop the same side effects associated with the neuroleptic as prescribed for psychotic disorders (see Chapter 10). Children should be monitored closely for efficacy and adverse effects of the medication. Because of the potential for adverse effects, haloperidol should be reserved for children with severe symptoms or with symptoms that impede their ability to function in school, socially, or within their family setting (McSwiggan-Hardin, 1995).

PIMOZIDE (ORAP). Pimozide is a neuroleptic with a response rate and side-effect profile similar to that of haloperidol. It is used in the management of severe motor or vocal tics that have failed to respond to more conventional treatment. Pimozide is not recommended for children younger than age 12 years. Dosage is initiated at 1 to 2 mg/day and increased weekly up to 3 to 5 mg/day.

CLONIDINE (CATAPRES). Clonidine is an alpha-adrenergic agonist that is approved for use as an antihypertensive agent. Results of studies on the efficacy of clonidine in the treatment of Tourette's disorder have been mixed. Some physicians use clonidine as a first choice because of the few side effects and relative safety associated with it. Common side effects include dry mouth, sedation, and dizziness or hypotension.

ZIPRASIDONE (GEODON). A recent research study was conducted using ziprasidone for children with Tourette's disorder (Sallee et al., 2000). Ziprasidone was found to safely reduce the severity and frequency of tic symptoms in adolescents and children as young as 7 years old. The benefits of the drug appear to be somewhat less than those achieved with the traditional neuroleptics, but the study participants showed no signs of extrapyramidal symptoms and experienced no appreciable weight gain, both of which are difficult issues with the traditional neuroleptics. However, ziprasidone has a greater capacity to prolong the QT interval compared with several other antipsychotics, which must be taken into consideration. In the study, dosage was initiated at 5 mg/day and titrated up to a maximum of 40 mg/day.

SEPARATION ANXIETY DISORDER

The essential feature of separation anxiety disorder is excessive anxiety concerning separation from the home or from those to whom the person is attached (APA, 2000). The anxiety is beyond that which would be expected for the individual's developmental level and interferes with social, academic, occupational, or others areas of functioning. Onset may occur anytime before age 18 years and is more common in girls than in boys.

Etiological Implications

Biological Influences

GENETICS. Studies have been conducted in which the children of adult clients diagnosed as having separation anxiety disorder were studied. A second method, studying parents and other relatives of children diagnosed as having separation anxiety disorder, also has been used. The results have shown that a greater number of children with relatives who manifest anxiety problems develop anxiety disorders themselves than do children with no such family patterns. The results are significant enough to speculate that there is a hereditary influence in the development of separation anxiety disorder, but the mode of genetic transmission has not been determined.

TEMPERAMENT. It is well established that children differ from birth, or shortly thereafter, on a number of temperamental characteristics. Sadock and Sadock (2003) state:

> The temperamental constellation of behavioral inhibition, excessive shyness, the tendency to withdraw from unfamiliar situations, and separation anxiety are all likely to have a genetic contribution. (p. 1260)

Individual differences in temperaments may be related to the acquisition of fear and anxiety disorders in childhood. This may be referred to as *anxiety proneness* or *vulnerability* and may denote an inherited "disposition" toward developing anxiety disorders.

Environmental Influences

STRESSFUL LIFE EVENTS. Studies have shown a relationship between life events and the development of anxiety disorders (Sadock & Sadock, 2003). It is thought that perhaps children who already are vulnerable or predisposed to developing anxiety disorders may be affected significantly by stressful life events. More research is needed before firm conclusions can be drawn.

Family Influences

Various theories expound on the idea that anxiety disorders in children are related to an overattachment to the mother. Sadock and Sadock (2003) attribute the major determinants of anxiety disorders to transactions relating to separation issues between mother (or mothering figure) and child. The *DSM-IV-TR* (APA, 2000) suggests that children with separation anxiety disorders come from close families.

Some parents may instill anxiety in their children by overprotecting them from expectable dangers or by exaggerating the dangers of the present and the future (Sadock & Sadock, 2003). Some parents may also transfer their fears and anxieties to their children through role modeling. For example, a parent who becomes fearful in the presence of a small, harmless dog and retreats with dread and apprehension teaches the young child by example that this is an appropriate response.

Application of the Nursing Process to Separation Anxiety Disorder

Background Assessment Data (Symptomatology)

Age at onset of this disorder may be as early as preschool age; it rarely begins as late as adolescence. In most cases, the child has difficulty separating from the mother. Occasionally the separation reluctance is directed toward the father, siblings, or other significant individual to whom the child is attached. Anticipation of separation may result in tantrums, crying, screaming, complaints of physical problems, and **clinging** behaviors.

Reluctance or refusal to attend school is especially common in adolescence. Younger children may "shadow," or follow around, the person from whom they are afraid to be separated. During middle childhood or adolescence, they may refuse to sleep away from home (e.g., at a friend's house or at camp). Interpersonal peer relationships are usually not a problem with these children. They are generally well liked by their peers and are reasonably socially skilled.

Worrying is common and relates to the possibility of harm coming to the self or to the attachment figure. Younger children may even have nightmares to this effect.

Specific phobias are common (e.g., fear of the dark, ghosts, animals). Depressed mood is frequently present and often precedes the onset of the anxiety symptoms, which commonly occur following a major stressor. The *DSM-IV-TR* diagnostic criteria for separation anxiety disorder are presented in Table 21–11.

Diagnosis/Outcome Identification

Based on the data collected during the nursing assessment, possible nursing diagnoses for the client with separation anxiety disorder include:

- Anxiety (severe) related to family history, temperament, overattachment to parent, negative role modeling
- Ineffective coping related to unresolved separation conflicts and inadequate coping skills evidenced by numerous somatic complaints
- Impaired social interaction related to reluctance to be away from attachment figure

The following criteria may be used for measurement of outcomes in the care of the client with separation anxiety disorder. The client:

TABLE 21–11 Diagnostic Criteria for Separation Anxiety Disorder

A. Developmentally inappropriate and excessive anxiety concerning separation from home or from those to whom the individual is attached, as evidenced by three (or more) of the following:
   1. Recurrent excessive distress when separation from home or major attachment figures occurs or is anticipated
   2. Persistent and excessive worry about losing, or about possible harm befalling, major attachment figures
   3. Persistent and excessive worry that an untoward event will lead to separation from a major attachment figure (e.g., getting lost or being kidnapped)
   4. Persistent reluctance or refusal to go to school or elsewhere because of fear of separation
   5. Persistently and excessively fearful or reluctant to be alone or without major attachment figures at home or without significant adults in other setting
   6. Persistent reluctance or refusal to go to sleep without being near a major attachment figure or to sleep away from home
   7. Repeated nightmares involving the theme of separation
   8. Repeated complaints of physical symptoms (such as headaches, stomachaches, nausea, or vomiting) when separation from major attachment figures occurs or is anticipated

B. The duration of the disturbance is at least 4 weeks.

C. The onset is before age 18 years.

D. The disturbance causes clinically significant distress or impairment in social, academic (occupational), or other important areas of functioning.

E. The disturbance does not occur exclusively during the course of a pervasive developmental disorder, schizophrenia, or other psychotic disorder and, in adolescents and adults, is not better accounted for by panic disorder with agoraphobia.

From APA (2000), with permission.

1. Is able to maintain anxiety at manageable level
2. Demonstrates adaptive coping strategies for dealing with anxiety when separation from attachment figure is anticipated
3. Interacts appropriately with others and spends time away from attachment figure to do so

Planning/Implementation

Table 21–12 provides a plan of care for the child or adolescent with separation anxiety, using nursing diagnoses common to this disorder, outcome criteria, and appropriate nursing interventions and rationales.

Evaluation

Evaluation of the child or adolescent with separation anxiety disorder requires reassessment of the behaviors for which the family sought treatment. Both the client and the family members have to change their behavior. The following types of questions may provide assistance in gathering data required for evaluating whether the nursing interventions have been effective in achieving the goals of therapy.

1. Is the client able to maintain anxiety at a manageable level—that is, without temper tantrums, "clinging," or screaming?
2. Have complaints of physical symptoms diminished?
3. Has the client demonstrated the ability to cope in more adaptive ways in the face of escalating anxiety?
4. Have the parents identified their role in the separation conflict? Are they able to discuss more adaptive coping strategies?
5. Does the client verbalize an intention to return to school?
6. Have nightmares and fears of the dark subsided?
7. Is the client able to interact with others away from the attachment figure?
8. Has the precipitating stressor been identified? Have strategies for coping with similar stressors in the future been established?

GENERAL THERAPEUTIC APPROACHES

Behavior Therapy

Behavior therapy is based on the concepts of classical conditioning and operant conditioning. Behavior therapy is a common and effective treatment with disruptive behavior disorders. With this approach, rewards are given for appropriate behaviors and withheld when behaviors are disruptive or otherwise inappropriate. The principle behind behavior therapy is that positive reinforcements encourage repetition of desirable behaviors, and aversive reinforcements (punishments) discourage repetition of undesirable behav-

TABLE 21–12 Care Plan for the Client with Separation Anxiety Disorder

Nursing Diagnosis: ANXIETY (SEVERE)

Related to: Family history; temperament; overattachment to parent; negative role modeling

Outcome Criteria	Nursing Interventions	Rationale
Client will maintain anxiety at no higher than moderate level in the face of events that formerly have precipitated panic.	1. Establish an atmosphere of calmness, trust, and genuine positive regard.	1. Trust and unconditional acceptance are necessary for satisfactory nurse/client relationship. Calmness is important because anxiety is easily transmitted from one person to another.
	2. Assure client of his or her safety and security.	2. Symptoms of panic anxiety are very frightening.
	3. Explore the child or adolescent's fears of separating from the parents. Explore with the parents possible fears they may have of separation from the child.	3. Some parents may have an underlying fear of separation from the child, of which they are unaware and which they are unconsciously transferring to the child.
	4. Help parents and child initiate realistic goals (e.g., child to stay with sitter for 2 hr with minimal anxiety; or, child to stay at friend's house without parents until 9 P.M. without experiencing panic anxiety).	4. Parents may be so frustrated with child's clinging and demanding behaviors that assistance with problem solving may be required.
	5. Give, and encourage parents to give, positive reinforcement for desired behaviors.	5. Positive reinforcement encourages repetition of desirable behaviors.

Nursing Diagnosis: INEFFECTIVE COPING

Related to: Unresolved separation conflicts and inadequate coping skills

Evidenced by: Numerous somatic complaints

Outcome Criteria	Nursing Interventions	Rationale
Client will demonstrate use of more adaptive coping strategies (than physical symptoms) in response to stressful situations.	1. Encourage child or adolescent to discuss specific situations in life that produce the most distress and describe his or her response to these situations. Include parents in the discussion.	1. Client and family may be unaware of the correlation between stressful situations and the exacerbation of physical symptoms.
	2. Help the child or adolescent who is perfectionistic to recognize that self-expectations may be unrealistic. Connect times of unmet self-expectations to the exacerbation of physical symptoms.	2. Recognition of maladaptive patterns is the first step in the change process.
	3. Encourage parents and child to identify more adaptive coping strategies that the child could use in the face of anxiety that feels overwhelming. Practice through role-play.	3. Practice facilitates the use of the desired behavior when the individual is actually faced with the stressful situation.

Nursing Diagnosis: IMPAIRED SOCIAL INTERACTION

Related to: Reluctance to be away from attachment figure

Outcome Criteria	Nursing Interventions	Rationale
Client will be able to spend time with staff and peers without excessive anxiety.	1. Develop a trusting relationship with client.	1. This is the first step in helping the client learn to interact with others.
	2. Attend groups with the child and support efforts to interact with others. Give positive feedback.	2. Presence of a trusted individual provides security during times of distress. Positive feedback encourages repetition.
	3. Convey to the child the acceptability of his or her not participating in group in the beginning. Gradually encourage small contributions until client is able to participate more fully.	3. Small successes will gradually increase self-confidence and decrease self-consciousness, so that client will feel less anxious in the group situation.
	4. Help client set small personal goals (e.g., "Today I will speak to one person I don't know").	4. Simple, realistic goals provide opportunities for success that increase self-confidence and may encourage the client to attempt more difficult objectives in the future.

iors. Behavior modification techniques—the system of rewards and consequences—can be taught to parents to be used in the home environment. Consistency is an essential component. In the treatment setting, individualized behavior modification programs are designed for each client.

Family Therapy

Children cannot be separated from their family. Therapy for children and adolescents must involve the entire family if problems are to be resolved. Parents should be involved in designing and implementing the treatment plan for the child and should be involved in all aspects of the treatment process.

The genogram can be used to identify problem areas between family members (see Chapter 8). A genogram provides an overall picture of the life of the family over several generations, including roles that various family members play and emotional distance between specific individuals. Areas for change can be easily identified.

The impact of family dynamics on disruptive behavior disorders has been identified. The impact of disruptive behavior on family dynamics cannot be ignored. Family coping can become severely compromised with the chronic stress of dealing with a behavior-disordered child. It is therefore imperative that the treatment plan for the identified client be instituted within the context of family-centered care. Baggett (1995) states:

> In treating ADHD, the most effective approach is a multimodal program, including the elements of parent involvement, environmental changes, academic or linguistic skill remediation, medication, behavior modification, social skills training, and psychotherapy. (p. 213)

Group Therapy

Group therapy provides children and adolescents with the opportunity to interact in an association of their peers. This can be both gratifying and overwhelming, depending on the child.

Group therapy provides a number of benefits. Appropriate social behavior often is learned from the positive and negative feedback of peers. Opportunity is provided to learn to tolerate and accept differences in others, to learn that it is acceptable to disagree, to learn to offer and receive support from others, and to practice these new skills in a safe environment. It is a way to learn from the experiences of others.

Group therapy with children and adolescents can take several forms. Music therapy groups allow clients to express feelings through music, often when they are unable to express themselves in any other way. Art and activity/craft therapy groups allow individual expression through artistic means.

Group play therapy is the treatment of choice for many children between the ages of 3 and 9 years (Gilbert, 1995). Gilbert (1995) states:

> Play is the most suitable means for children to communicate the content of the unconscious and the distress that the pressures of their environment create. Play also facilitates sublimation; for example, anger and aggression are sublimated and displaced through the use of play equipment. (p. 372)

Psychoeducational groups are very beneficial for adolescents. The only drawback to this type of group is that it works best when the group is closed-ended; that is, once the group has been formed, no one is allowed to join until the group has reached its preestablished closure. Members are allowed to propose topics for discussion. The leader serves as teacher much of the time and facilitates discussion of the proposed topic. Members may, from time to time, be presenters and serve as discussion leaders. Sometimes, psychoeducational groups evolve into traditional therapy discussion groups.

Psychopharmacology

Several of the disorders presented in this chapter are treated with medications. The appropriate pharmacology was presented following the section in which the disorder was discussed. Medication should never be the sole method of treatment. It is undeniable that medication can and does improve quality of life for families of children and adolescents with these disorders. However, research has indicated that medication alone is not as effective as a combination of medication and psychosocial therapy. It is important for families to understand that there is no way to "give him a pill and make him well." The importance of the psychosocial therapies cannot be overstressed. Some clinicians will not prescribe medications for a client unless he or she participates in concomitant psychotherapy sessions. The beneficial effects of the medications promote improved coping ability, which in turn enhances the intent of the psychosocial therapy.

SUMMARY

Child and adolescent psychiatric nursing is a specialty that has been given little attention. Most basic nursing curricula include minimal instruction in child psychiatric nursing. Even though nurses work in many areas that place them in ideal positions to identify emotionally disturbed children, many of them do not have sufficient knowledge of child psychopathology to recognize maladaptive behaviors.

This chapter has presented some of the most prevalent disorders identified by the *DSM-IV-TR* (APA, 2000) as first becoming evident in infancy, childhood, or adolescence. An explanation of various etiological factors was presented for each disorder to assist in the comprehension of underlying dynamics. These included biological, environmental, and family influences.

The nursing process was presented as the vehicle for delivery of care. Symptomatology for each of the disorders provided background assessment data. Nursing diagnoses identified specific behaviors that were targets for change. Both client and family were considered in the planning and implementation. Behavior modification is the focus of nursing intervention with children and adolescents. With families, attention is given to education and referrals to community resources from which they can derive support. Reassessment data provide information for evaluation of nursing interventions in achieving the desired outcomes.

Child psychiatry is an area in which nursing can make a valuable contribution. Nurses who choose this field have an excellent opportunity to serve in the promotion of emotional wellness for children and adolescents. A discussion of psychopharmacological intervention was included for the disorders in which this form of treatment is relevant.

REVIEW QUESTIONS

SELF-EXAMINATION/LEARNING EXERCISE

Select the answer that is most appropriate for each of the following questions:

1. In an effort to help the mild-to-moderately mentally retarded child develop satisfying relationships with others, which of the following nursing interventions is most appropriate?
   a. Interpret the child's behavior for others.
   b. Set limits on behavior that is socially inappropriate.
   c. Allow the child to behave spontaneously, for he or she has no concept of right or wrong.
   d. This child is not capable of forming social relationships.
2. The autistic child has difficulty with trust. With this in mind, which of the following nursing actions would be most appropriate?
   a. Encourage all staff to hold the child as often as possible, conveying trust through touch.
   b. Assign a different staff member each day so child will learn that everyone can be trusted.
   c. Assign the same staff person as often as possible to promote feelings of security and trust.
   d. Avoid eye contact, as it is extremely uncomfortable for the child, and may discourage trust.
3. Which of the following nursing diagnoses would be considered the *priority* in planning care for the autistic child?
   a. Risk for self-mutilation evidenced by banging head against wall
   b. Impaired social interaction evidenced by unresponsiveness to people
   c. Impaired verbal communication evidenced by absence of verbal expression
   d. Disturbed personal identity evidenced by inability to differentiate self from others
4. Which of the following activities would be most appropriate for the child with ADHD?
   a. Monopoly
   b. Volleyball
   c. Pool
   d. Checkers
5. Which of the following groups are most commonly used for drug management of the hyperactive child?
   a. CNS depressants (e.g., diazepam [Valium])
   b. CNS stimulants (e.g., methylphenidate [Ritalin])
   c. Anticonvulsants (e.g., phenytoin [Dilantin])
   d. Major tranquilizers (e.g., haloperidol [Haldol])
6. The child with ADHD has a nursing diagnosis of impaired social interaction. An appropriate nursing intervention for this child is:
   a. To socially isolate the child when interactions with others are inappropriate
   b. To set limits with consequences on inappropriate behaviors
   c. To provide rewards for appropriate behaviors
   d. b and c
   e. All of the above
7. The nursing history and assessment of an adolescent with a conduct disorder might reveal all of the following behaviors *except*:

a. Manipulation of others for fulfillment of own desires
b. Chronic violation of rules
c. Feelings of guilt associated with the exploitation of others
d. Inability to form close peer relationships

8. Certain family dynamics often predispose adolescents to the development of conduct disorder. Which of the following patterns is thought to be a contributing factor?
   a. Parents who are overprotective
   b. Parents who have high expectations for their children
   c. Parents who consistently set limits on their children's behavior
   d. Parents who are alcohol dependent

9. Which of the following is *least* likely to predispose a child to Tourette's disorder?
   a. Absence of parental bonding
   b. Family history of the disorder
   c. Abnormalities of brain neurotransmitters
   d. Structural abnormalities of the brain

10. Which of the following is the drug of choice for Tourette's disorder?
   a. Methylphenidate (Ritalin)
   b. Haloperidol (Haldol)
   c. Imipramine (Tofranil)
   d. Pemoline (Cylert)

Test Your CRITICAL THINKING SKILLS

Jimmy, age 9, has been admitted to the child psychiatric unit with a diagnosis of ADHD. He has been unmanageable at school and at home, and was recently suspended from school for continuous disruption of his class. He refuses to sit in his chair or do his work. He yells out in class, interrupts the teacher and the other students, and lately has become physically aggressive when he cannot have his way. He was suspended after hitting his teacher when she asked him to return to his seat.

Jimmy's mother describes him as a restless and demanding baby who grew into a restless and demanding toddler. He has never gotten along well with his peers. Even as a small child, he would take his friends' toys away from them or bite them if they tried to hold their own with him. His 5-year-old sister is afraid of him and refuses to be alone with him.

During the nurse's intake assessment, Jimmy paced the room or rocked in his chair. He talked incessantly on a superficial level and jumped from topic to topic. He told the nurse that he did not know why he was there. He acknowledged that he had some problems at school but said that was only because the other kids picked on him, and the teacher did not like him. He said he got into trouble at home sometimes but that was because his parents liked his little sister better than they liked him.

The physician has ordered methylphenidate, 5 mg twice a day, for Jimmy. His response to this order is, "I'm not going to take drugs. I'm not sick!"

Answer the following questions related to Jimmy:

1. What are the pertinent assessment data to be noted by the nurse?
2. What is the primary nursing diagnosis for Jimmy?
3. Aside from client safety, to what problems would the nurse want to direct intervention with Jimmy?

IMPLICATIONS OF RESEARCH FOR EVIDENCE BASED PRACTICE

Weissman, M.M., Warner, V., Wickramaratne, P.J., & Kandel, D.B.:

Maternal smoking during pregnancy and psychopathology in offspring followed to adulthood. Journal of the American Academy of Child and Adolescent Psychiatry (1999, July), 38(7), 892–899.

Description of the Study: In this study, 147 offspring and mother pairs were interviewed 3 times over a period of 10 years. All probands and controls were white and group-matched for age. Mothers reported never having smoked during pregnancy (97 offspring) or having smoked more than 10 cigarettes almost daily during pregnancy (50 offspring). Final diagnoses of offspring was made by an experienced clinician who was not involved in the interviewing and was blind to the diagnostic and smoking status of the parent. The clinician independently reviewed all available information, including parent informant, offspring interview, and medical records at each interview and assigned a diagnosis for each offspring.

Results of the Study: It was found that male offspring of mothers who smoked during pregnancy had more than a threefold lifetime risk of conduct disorder, and female offspring had more than a fivefold risk of drug abuse/dependence than those offspring whose mothers did not smoke during pregnancy. Mothers who smoked during pregnancy also had babies with significantly lower birth weight. Nearly 21 percent of the offspring of mothers who smoked during pregnancy, compared with 7 percent of the offspring of mothers who did not smoke, were reported to weigh less than 5.5 pounds at birth.

Implications for Nursing Practice: This study has nursing implications for educating women about the consequences of smoking during pregnancy. Maternal smoking during pregnancy appears to have long-term effects on offspring's behavior and health. The findings suggest the importance of programs aimed at smoking prevention and cessation in women during pregnancy. This is well within the scope of nursing practice.

REFERENCES

American Psychiatric Association (APA). (2000). Diagnostic and statistical manual of mental disorders (4th ed.) Text revision. Washington, DC: American Psychiatric Association.

Baggett, J. (1995). Attention disorders. In B.S. Johnson (Ed.), Child, adolescent & family psychiatric nursing. Philadelphia: J.B. Lippincott.

Bagley, C., & Mallick, K. (2000). Spiraling up and spiraling down: Implications of a long-term study of temperament and conduct disorder for social work with children. Child & Family Social Work 5(4): 291–301.

Clunn, P. (1991). Child psychiatric nursing. St. Louis: Mosby.

Dopheide, J.A. (2001). ADHD Part 1: Current status, diagnosis, etiology/pathophysiology. From the American Pharmaceutical Association 148th Annual Meeting. Retrieved August 11, 2001 from http://www.medscape.com/Medscape/CNO/2001/AphA/AphA-01.html

Dopheide, J.A., & Theesen, K.A. (1999). Disorders of childhood. In J.T. Dipiro, R.L. Talbert, & G.C. Yee (Eds.), Pharmacotherapy: A pathophysiological approach (4th ed.). New York: McGraw-Hill.

Fisher, J.G. (1997). Conduct disorder. Depressive and Manic-Depressive Association of Virginia. Retrieved February 4, 2002 from http://www.dmdav.org/archives/feature4.htm

Gilbert, C. (1995). Group therapy. In B.S. Johnson (Ed.), Child, adolescent & family psychiatric nursing. Philadelphia: J.B. Lippincott.

Harvard Medical School (2002). InteliHealth: Consumer health information. Behavior disorders in children and teens. Retrieved on February 4, 2002 from http://www.intelihealth.com/IH/ihtIH/EMIHC000/20722/8632/187947.html?d=dmtContent

Ladd, G.W. (1999). Peer relationships and social competence during early and middle childhood. Annual Review of Psychology, 50: 333–359.

Leckman, J.F., Dolnansky, E.S., & Hardin, M.T. (1990). Perinatal factors in the expression of Tourette's syndrome: An exploratory study. Journal of the American Academy of Child and Adolescent Psychiatry, 29, 220–226.

McSwiggan-Hardin, M.T. (1995). Tic disorders. In B.S. Johnson (Ed.), Child, adolescent and family psychiatric nursing. Philadelphia: J.B. Lippincott.

Medscape Health (2002). What causes attention-deficit hyperactivity disorder? Retrieved February 3, 2002 from http://health.medscape.com/viewarticle/209223_6

National Institute of Mental Health (NIMH). (2002). Autism. NIH Publication No. 97-Retrieved February 1, 2002 from http://www.nimh.nih.gov/publicat/autism.cfm#aut10

National Institute of Mental Health (NIMH). (2000). Attention Deficit Hyperactivity Disorder (ADHD) – Questions and Answers. Retrieved February 2, 2002 from http://www.nimh.nih.gov/publicat/adhdqa.cfm

Popper, C.W., Gammon, G.D., West, S.A., & Bailey, C.E. (2003). Disorders usually first diagnosed in infancy, childhood, or adolescence. In R.E. Hales, & S.C. Yudofsky (Eds.), Textbook of clinical psychiatry (4th ed.). Washington, DC: The American Psychiatric Publishing.

Riddle, M.A., Rasmussen, A.M., & Woods, S.W. (1992). SPECT imaging of cerebral blood flow in Tourette's syndrome. In T.N. Chase, A.J. Friedhoff, & D.J. Cohen (Eds.), Tourette's syndrome: Genetics, neurobiology, and treatment. New York: Raven.

Rosner, T.A., & Pollice, S.A. (1991). Tourette's syndrome. Journal of Psychosocial Nursing, 29(1), 4–9.

Sadock, B.J., & Sadock, V.A. (2003). Synopsis of psychiatry: Behavioral sciences/clinical psychiatry (9th ed.). Philadelphia: Lippincott Williams & Wilkins.

Sallee, F.T., Kurlan, R., Goetz, C.G., Singer, H., Scahill, L., Law, G., Dittman, V.M., & Chappell, P.B. (2000). Ziprasidone treatment of children and adolescents with Tourette's syndrome: A pilot study. Journal of the American Academy of Child and Adolescent Psychiatry, 39(3): 292–299.

Singer, H.S., Reiss, A.L., & Brown, J.E. (1993). Volumetric MRI changes in the basal ganglia of children with Tourette's syndrome. Neurology, 43, 950–956.

INTERNET REFERENCES

- Additional information about ADHD may be located at the following Web sites:
  - a http://www.chadd.org
  - b http://www.nimh.nih.gov/publicat/adhdmenu.cfm
- Additional information about autism may be located at the following Web sites:
  - a http://www.autism-society.org
  - b http://www.nimh.nih.gov/publicat/autismmenu.cfm
- Additional information about medications to treat ADHD may be located at the following Web sites:
  - a http://www.fadavis.com/townsend
  - b http://www.nimh.nih.gov/publicat/childmedmenu.cfm

22

CHAPTER

Victims of Abuse or Neglect

CHAPTER OUTLINE

KEY TERMS

statutory rape
child sexual abuse
emotional injury
emotional neglect
physical neglect
safe house or shelter
compounded rape reaction
controlled response pattern
expressed response pattern
silent rape reaction
sexual exploitation of a child
cycle of battering
rape
date rape
marital rape
battering
incest

OBJECTIVES

After reading this chapter, the student will be able to:

1. Discuss historical perspectives associated with intimate partner abuse, child abuse, and sexual assault.
2. Describe epidemiological statistics associated with intimate partner abuse, child abuse, and sexual assault.
3. Discuss characteristics of victims and victimizers.
4. Identify etiological implications to abusive behaviors.
5. Describe physical and psychological effects on the victims of intimate partner abuse, child abuse, and sexual assault.
6. Identify nursing diagnoses, goals of care, and appropriate nursing interventions for care of victims of intimate partner abuse, child abuse, and sexual assault.
7. Evaluate nursing care of victims of intimate partner abuse, child abuse, and sexual assault.
8. Discuss various modalities relevant to treatment of victims of abuse.

INTRODUCTION

Abuse—the maltreatment of one person by another—is on the rise in this society. Books, newspapers, movies, and television inundate their readers and viewers with stories of "man's inhumanity to man" (no gender bias intended).

It has been estimated that there are 1.8 million battered wives in the United States, excluding divorced women and women battered on dates (Sadock & Sadock, 2003). More injuries are attributed to **battering** than to all rapes, muggings, and automobile accidents combined. **Rape** is vastly underreported in the United States. Because many of these attacks occurring daily go unreported and unrecognized, sexual assault can be considered a silent, violent epidemic in the United States today.

An increase in the incidence of child abuse and related fatalities has also been documented. Sadock and Sadock (2003) state that "in 1999, about 2.9 million cases of possible child abuse were reported to public social service agencies, and about 826,000 of these cases were substantiated." Child abuse and neglect account for 2,000 to 4,000 deaths each year in the United States.

Abuse affects all populations equally. It occurs among all races, religions, economic classes, ages, and educational backgrounds. The phenomenon is cyclical in that many abusers were themselves victims of abuse as children.

This chapter discusses intimate partner violence, child abuse (including neglect), and sexual assault. Elder abuse is discussed in Chapter 23. Factors that predispose individuals to commit acts of abuse against others, as well as the physical and psychological effects on the victims, are examined.

Nursing of individuals who have experienced abusive behavior from others is presented within the context of the nursing process. Various treatment modalities are described.

HISTORICAL PERSPECTIVES

Family violence is not a new problem; in fact, it is probably as old as humankind and has been documented as far back as Biblical times. In the United States, spouse and child abuse arrived with the Puritans; however, it was not until 1973 that public outrage initiated an active movement against the practice. Child abuse became a mandatory reportable occurrence in the United States in 1968. Responsibility for the protection of elders from abuse rests primarily with the states. In 1987, Congress passed amendments to the Older Americans Act of 1965 that provide for state associations of the Area Agencies on Aging to assess the need for elder abuse prevention services (Frolik & Kaplan, 1995). These events have made it possible for individuals, who once felt powerless to stop the abuse against them, to come forward and seek advice, support, and protection.

Historically, violence against female partners (whether in a married or an unmarried intimate relationship) has not been considered a social problem but rather an unpleasant fact of life. Some individuals have been socialized within their cultural context to accept violence against women in relationships (American Nurses Association [ANA], 1998).

From Roman times until the beginning of the 20th century, women were considered the personal property of men. Very early on in Roman times, women were purchased as brides, and their status, as well as that of their children, was closely akin to that of slaves. Violent beatings and even death occurred if women acted contrary to their husband's wishes or to the social code of the time.

Women historically have been socialized to view themselves as sexual objects. In early Biblical times, women were expected to subjugate themselves to the will of men, and those who refused were often severely punished. Rape is largely a crime against women, although men and children also fall victim to this heinous act. Rape is the extreme manifestation of the domination of one individual over another. Rape is viewed as a ritual of power.

During the Puritan era, "spare the rod and spoil the child" was a theme supported by the Bible. Children were considered the property of their parents and could be treated accordingly. Harsh treatment by parents was justified by the belief that severe physical punishment was necessary to maintain discipline, transmit educational decisions, and expel evil spirits. Change began in the mid-19th and early 20th centuries with the child welfare movement and the passage of laws for the protection of children.

Historical examination reveals an inclination toward violence among human beings from very early in civilization. Little has changed, for violence permeates every aspect of today's society, the victims of which are inundating the healthcare system. Campbell (1992) states "[violence] is costing all of us, in terms of healthcare dollars, human potential squandered, and even in terms of our personal sense of security and well-being."

ETIOLOGICAL IMPLICATIONS

What predisposes individuals to be abusive? Although no one really knows for sure, several theories have been espoused. A brief discussion of ideas associated with biological, psychological, and sociocultural views is presented here.

Biological Theories

Neurophysiological Influences

Various components of the neurological system in both humans and animals have been implicated in both the facilitation and inhibition of aggressive impulses. Areas of the brain that may be involved include the temporal lobe, the limbic system, and the amygdaloid nucleus (Tardiff, 2003).

Biochemical Influences

Studies show that various neurotransmitters—in particular norepinephrine, dopamine, and serotonin—may play a role in the facilitation and inhibition of aggressive impulses (Silver & Yudofsky, 1992). This theory is consistent with the "fight or flight" arousal described by Selye (1956) in his theory of the response to stress (see Chapter 1).

Genetic Influences

Various genetic components related to aggressive behavior have been investigated. Some studies have linked increased aggressiveness with selective inbreeding in mice, suggesting the possibility of a direct genetic link. Another genetic characteristic that was once thought to have some implication for aggressive behavior was the genetic karyotype XYY. The XYY syndrome has been found to contribute to aggressive behavior in a small percentage of cases (Sadock & Sadock, 2003). The evidence linking this chromosomal aberration to aggressive and deviant behavior has not yet been firmly established.

Disorders of the Brain

Organic brain syndromes associated with various cerebral disorders have been implicated in the predisposition to aggressive and violent behavior (Silver & Yudofsky, 1992). Brain tumors, particularly in the areas of the limbic system and the temporal lobes; trauma to the brain, resulting in cerebral changes; and diseases, such as encephalitis (or medications that may effect this syndrome) and epilepsy, particularly temporal lobe epilepsy, have all been implicated.

Psychological Theories

Psychodynamic Theory

The psychodynamic theorists imply that unmet needs for satisfaction and security result in an underdeveloped ego and a weak superego. It is thought that when frustration occurs, aggression and violence supply this individual with a dose of power and prestige that boosts the self-image and validates significance in his or her life that is lacking. The immature ego cannot prevent dominant id behaviors from occurring, and the weak superego is unable to produce feelings of guilt.

Learning Theory

Children learn to behave by imitating their role models, which are usually their parents. Models are more likely to be imitated when they are perceived as prestigious or influential or when the behavior is followed by positive reinforcement (Berndt, 1992). Children may have an idealistic perception of their parents during the very early developmental stages but, as they mature, may begin to imitate the behavior patterns of their teachers, friends, and others. Individuals who were abused as children or whose parents disciplined with physical punishment are more likely to behave in an abusive manner as adults (Tardiff, 2003).

Adults and children alike model many of their behaviors after individuals they observe on television and in movies. Unfortunately, modeling can result in maladaptive as well as adaptive behavior, particularly when children view heroes triumphing over villains by using violence. It is also possible that individuals who have a biological predisposition toward aggressive behavior will be more susceptible to negative role modeling.

Sociocultural Theories

Societal Influences

Although they agree that perhaps some biological and psychological aspects are influential, social scientists believe that aggressive behavior is primarily a product of one's culture and social structure.

American society essentially was founded on a general acceptance of violence as a means of solving problems. The concept of relative deprivation has been shown to have a profound effect on collective violence within a society. Kennedy and associates (1998) have stated:

> Studies have shown that poverty and income are powerful predictors of homicide and violent crime. The effect of the growing gap between the rich and poor is mediated through an undermining of social cohesion, or social capital, and decreased social capital is in turn associated with increased firearm homicide and violent crime.

Indeed, the United States was populated by the violent actions of one group of people over another. Since that time, much has been said and written, and laws have been passed, regarding the civil rights of all people. However, to this day many people would agree that the statement "All men are created equal" is hypocritical in our society.

Societal influences may also contribute to violence when individuals realize that their needs and desires are not being met relative to other people (Tardiff, 2003). When poor and oppressed people find that they have limited access through legitimate channels, they are more likely to resort to delinquent behaviors in an effort to obtain desired ends. This lack of opportunity and subsequent delinquency may even contribute to a subculture of violence within a society.

APPLICATION OF THE NURSING PROCESS

Background Assessment Data

Intimate Partner Abuse

DEFINITION. Several definitions have been set forth for the term *battering*. Marvin (1997) defines the term as:

> A pattern of coercive control founded on and supported by violence or the threat of violence, including punching, choking, biting, hitting, hair-pulling, stabbing, shooting, or threats of this type of violence.

Campbell and Humphreys (1993) define *battering* as "repeated physical and/or sexual assault of an intimate partner within a context of coercive control." Finally, a definition by the National Coalition Against Domestic Violence (2002a) states:

> Battering is a pattern of behavior used to establish power and control over another person through fear and intimidation, often including the threat or use of violence. Battering happens when one person believes they are entitled to control another.

Physical abuse between domestic partners may be known as spouse abuse, domestic or family violence, wife or husband battering, or intimate partner or relationship abuse. United States Bureau of Justice statistics for 1998 (2002) reflected the following: (1) approximately 83 percent of victims of intimate violence were women, (2) women ages 16 to 24 experienced the highest per capita rates of intimate violence, (3) intimate partner violence against men increased significantly. In the same study, approximately 60 percent of women and 50 percent of men reported the victimizations to the police. The most common reason for not reporting among women was "fear of reprisal." Among men, the most common reason for not reporting was that it was a "private or personal matter."

PROFILE OF THE VICTIM. Battered women represent all age, racial, religious, cultural, educational, and socioeconomic groups. They may be married or single, homemakers or business executives. According to Person (1992), many women who are battered have low self-esteem, commonly adhere to feminine sex-role stereotypes, and typically accept the blame for the batterer's actions. Feelings of guilt, anger, fear, and shame are common. They may be isolated from family and support systems.

Many women who are in such relationships grew up in abusive homes and may have left those homes, even married, at a very young age in order to escape the abuse. The battered woman views her relationship as male-dominant, and as the battering continues her ability to see the options available to her and to make decisions concerning her life (and possibly those of her children) decreases. The phenomenon of *learned helplessness* may be applied to the woman's progressing inability to act on her own behalf. Learned helplessness occurs when an individual comes to understand that regardless of his or her behavior, the outcome is unpredictable and usually undesirable.

PROFILE OF THE VICTIMIZER. Men who batter usually are characterized as persons with low self-esteem. Pathologically jealous, they present a "dual personality," exhibit limited coping ability, and have severe stress reactions (Project for Victims of Family Violence, 2000). The typical abuser is very possessive and perceives his spouse as a possession. He becomes threatened when she shows any sign of independence or attempts to share herself and her time with others. Small children are often ignored by the abuser; however, they also become the targets of abuse as they grow older, particularly if they attempt to protect their mother from abuse. The abuser also may use threats of taking the children away as a tactic of emotional abuse.

The abusing man typically wages a continuous campaign of degradation against his female partner. He insults and humiliates her and everything she does at every opportunity. He strives to keep her isolated from others and dependent on him. He demands to know where she is at every moment, and when she tells him, he challenges her honesty. He achieves power and control through intimidation.

THE CYCLE OF BATTERING. In her classic studies of battered women and their relationships, Walker (1979) identified a cycle of predictable behaviors that are repeated over time. The behaviors can be divided into three distinct phases that vary in time and intensity both within the same relationship and among different couples. Figure 22–1 depicts a graphic representation of the **cycle of battering.**

Phase I: The Tension-Building Phase. During this phase, the woman senses that the man's tolerance for frustration is declining. He becomes angry with little provocation but, after lashing out at her, may be quick to apologize. The woman may become very nurturing and compliant, anticipating his every whim in an effort to prevent his anger from escalating. She may just try to stay out of his way.

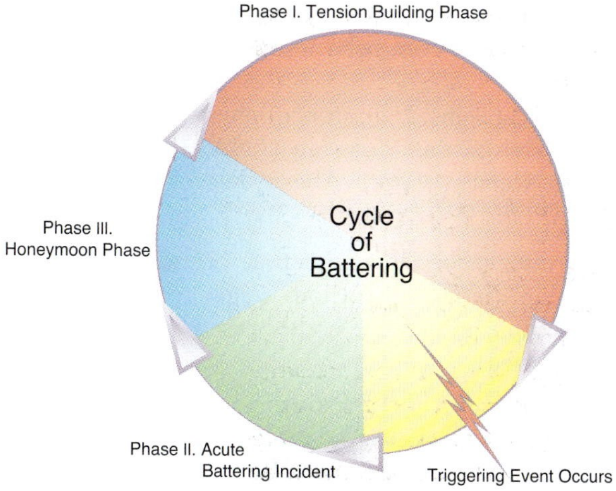

FIGURE 22–1 The cycle of battering. (From Townsend, M.C. (2003), Psychiatric/Mental Health Nursing: Concepts of Care [4th ed.]. Philadelphia: F.A. Davis, p. 776, with permission.)

Minor battering incidents may occur during this phase, and in a desperate effort to avoid dangerous confrontations, the woman accepts the abuse as being legitimate. She denies her anger and rationalizes his behavior (e.g., "I need to do better. He's under so much stress at work. It's the alcohol. If only he didn't drink."). She assumes the guilt for the abuse, even reasoning that perhaps she *did* deserve the abuse, just as her aggressor suggests.

The minor battering incidents continue, and the tension mounts as the woman waits for the impending explosion. The abuser begins to fear that his partner will leave him. His jealousy and possessiveness increase, and he uses threats and brutality to keep her in his captivity. Battering incidents become more intense, after which the woman becomes less and less psychologically capable of restoring equilibrium. She withdraws from him, which he misinterprets as rejection, further escalating his anger toward her. Phase I may last from a few weeks to many months or even years.

Phase II: The Acute Battering Incident. This phase is the most violent and the shortest, usually lasting up to 24 hours. It most often begins with the batterer justifying his behavior to himself. By the end of the incident, however, he cannot understand what has happened, only that in his rage he has lost control over his behavior.

This incident may begin with the batterer wanting to "teach her a lesson." In some instances, the woman may intentionally provoke the behavior. Having come to a point in phase I in which the tension is unbearable, long-term battered women know that once the acute phase is behind them, things will be better.

During phase II, women feel their only option is to find a safe place to hide from the batterer. The beating is severe, and many women can describe the violence in detail, almost as if dissociation from their bodies had occurred. The batterer generally minimizes the severity of the abuse. Help is usually sought only in the event of severe injury or if the woman fears for her life or those of her children.

Phase III: Calm, Loving, Respite ("Honeymoon") Phase. In this phase, the batterer becomes extremely loving, kind, and contrite. He promises that the abuse will never recur and begs her forgiveness. He is afraid she will leave him and uses every bit of charm he can muster to ensure this does not happen. He believes he now can control his behavior, and because now he has "taught her a lesson" he believes she will not "act up" again.

He plays on her feelings of guilt, and she desperately wants to believe him. She wants to believe that he *can* change, and that she will no longer have to suffer abuse. During this phase, the woman relives her original dream of ideal love and chooses to believe that *this* is what her partner is *really* like.

This loving phase becomes the focus of the woman's perception of the relationship. She bases her reason for remaining in the relationship on this "magical" ideal phase and hopes against hope that the previous phases will not be repeated. This hope is evident even in those women who have lived through a number of horrendous cycles.

Although phase III usually lasts somewhere between the lengths of time associated with phases I and II, it can be so short as to almost pass undetected. In most instances, the cycle soon begins again with renewed tensions and minor battering incidents. In an effort to "steal" a few precious moments of the phase III kind of loving, the battered woman becomes a collaborator in her own abusive lifestyle. Victim and batterer become locked together in an intense, symbiotic relationship.

WHY DOES SHE STAY? Probably the most common response that battered women give for staying is that they fear for their life and/or the lives of their children. As the battering progresses, the man gains power and control through intimidation and instilling fear with threats such as, "I'll kill you and the kids if you try to leave." Challenged by these threats and compounded by her low self-esteem and sense of powerlessness, the woman sees no way out. In fact, she may try to leave only to return when confronted by her partner and the psychological power he holds over her. Moss (1991) lists the following other reasons for the woman's staying in the marriage:

1. ***Lack of a support network for leaving.*** Our society glorifies the position of marriage and family, and some women report that family members encourage her to stay in the relationship and "try to work things out."
2. ***Religious beliefs.*** Many religious organizations denounce divorce and encourage the cohesion of the family. Some women have reported that their clergy told them this was "their cross to bear."

The National Coalition Against Domestic Violence (2002b) cites a number of reasons why women stay in an abusive relationship:

1. She realistically fears that the battering will become more violent and maybe even fatal if she attempts to leave.
2. Her friends and family may not support her leaving.
3. She knows the difficulties of single parenting in reduced financial circumstances.
4. There is a mix of good times, love, and hope along with the manipulation, intimidation, and fear.
5. She may not know about or have access to safety and support.

Child Abuse

Erik Erikson (1963) stated, "The worst sin is the mutilation of a child's spirit." Children are vulnerable and relatively powerless, and the effects of maltreatment are infinitely deep and long lasting. Child maltreatment typically includes physical or emotional injury, physical or emotional neglect, or sexual acts inflicted upon a child by a caregiver. The Child Abuse Prevention and Treatment Act (CAPTA), as amended and reauthorized in October 1996, identifies a minimum set of acts or behaviors that characterize maltreatment (National Clearinghouse on Child Abuse and Neglect [NCCAN]) (2002). States may use these as foundations on which to establish state legislation.

PHYSICAL INJURY. Physical injury to a child includes any *nonaccidental physical* injury as a result of punching, beating, kicking, biting, burning, shaking, or otherwise harming a child (NCCAN, 2002). Maltreatment is considered whether or not the caretaker intended to cause harm, or even if the injury resulted from over-discipline or physical punishment. The most obvious way to detect it is by outward physical signs. However, behavioral indicators also may be evident.

Physical Signs. Indicators of physical abuse may include any of the following (ANA, 1998; NCCAN, 2003; Kansas Child Abuse Prevention Council [KCAPC], 1992; Tower, 1992):

1. Bruises, especially numerous bruises of different colors (indicating various stages of healing) over multiple parts of the body; bruises around the head and face
2. Bite marks; skin welts
3. Burns, such as glove-like burns that indicate the hand has been immersed in hot liquid; cigarette burns; burns in the shape of an object such as a poker or iron
4. Fractures, scars, or serious internal injuries
5. Lacerations, abrasions, or unusual bleeding
6. Bald spots indicative of severe hair pulling

Behavioral Signs. Following are common behavioral indicators of physical abuse (KCAPC, 1992;

NCCAN, 2003; Tower, 1992). These behaviors alone do not necessarily indicate physical abuse.

1. Behavioral extremes, including very aggressive or demanding conduct
2. Fear of the parent or caretaker
3. Extreme rage, or passivity and withdrawal
4. Apprehension when other children cry
5. Verbal reporting of abuse
6. Extreme hyperactivity, distractibility, or irritability
7. Disorganized thinking; self-injurious or suicidal behavior
8. Running away from home or engaging in illegal behavior such as drug abuse or stealing
9. Displaying severe depression, flashbacks (including hallucinatory experiences) and dissociative disorders
10. Cheating, lying, or low achievement in school
11. Inability to form satisfactory peer relationships
12. Wearing clothing that covers the body and that may be inappropriate for warm weather
13. Regressiveness; demonstrating age-inappropriate behavior

EMOTIONAL INJURY. **Emotional injury** involves a pattern of behavior on the part of the parent or caretaker that results in serious impairment of the child's social, emotional, or intellectual functioning. Examples of emotional injury include belittling or rejecting the child, ignoring the child, blaming the child for things over which he or she has no control, isolating the child from normal social experiences, and using harsh and inconsistent discipline. Behavioral indicators of emotional injury may include (KCAPC, 1992; NCCAN, 2003; Tower, 1992):

1. Age-inappropriate behaviors
2. Daytime anxiety and unrealistic fears
3. Sleep problems or nightmares
4. Behavioral extremes (e.g., overly happy or affectionate)
5. Social isolation
6. Self-destructive behavior
7. Inappropriate affect (e.g., laughing at something sad)
8. Vandalism, stealing, cheating, substance abuse
9. Rocking, thumb-sucking, enuresis, or other habitual problems
10. Anorexia nervosa (especially in adolescents)

PHYSICAL NEGLECT. **Physical neglect** of a child includes refusal of or delay in seeking healthcare, abandonment, expulsion from the home or refusal to allow a runaway to return home, and inadequate supervision (NCCAN, 2002). The following physical and behavioral characteristics are associated with physical neglect of a child (ANA, 1998; NCCAN, 2003; Tower, 1992):

1. Clothing may be soiled and in need of repair; often fit is too small or too large; may be inappropriate for weather
2. Child always seems hungry; steals and hoards food from others
3. Child often appears listless and tired
4. Child may demonstrate poor hygiene, with bad breath and body odor
5. Medical problems, such as infected sores, and dental problems, such as decayed or abscessed teeth, may be evident
6. Delinquent behavior, such as stealing and vandalism, may be prevalent
7. Poor school performance and attendance record may exist
8. Poor peer relationships may be evident
9. Child may be emaciated or have distended abdomen, indicative of malnutrition

EMOTIONAL NEGLECT. **Emotional neglect** refers to a chronic failure by the parent or caretaker to provide the child with the hope, love, and support necessary for the development of a sound, healthy personality. The following are behavioral indicators of emotional neglect by the parent or caretaker of a child (NCCAN, 2003; KCAPC, 1992):

1. Ignoring the child's presence
2. Rebuffing attempts by the child to establish meaningful interaction
3. Ignoring the child's social, educational, recreational, and developmental needs
4. Denying the child opportunities to receive positive reinforcement

SEXUAL ABUSE OF A CHILD. Various definitions of **child sexual abuse** are available in the literature. CAPTA defines sexual abuse as:

> Employment, use, persuasion, inducement, enticement, or coercion of any child to engage in, or assist any other person to engage in any sexually explicit conduct or any simulation of such conduct for the purpose of producing any visual depiction of such conduct; or the rape, and in cases of caretaker or interfamilial relationships, statutory rape, molestation, prostitution, or other form of sexual exploitation of children, or incest with children. (NCCAN, 2002)

Included in the definition is **sexual exploitation of a child,** in which a child is induced or coerced into engaging in sexually explicit conduct for promoting any performance, and child sexual abuse, in which a child is being used for the sexual pleasure of an adult (parent or caretaker) or any other person.

Incest is the occurrence of sexual contacts or interaction between, or sexual exploitation of, close relatives, or between participants who are related to each other by a kinship bond that is regarded as a prohibition to sexual relations (e.g., caretakers, stepparents, stepsiblings) (Sadock & Sadock, 2003).

INDICATORS OF SEXUAL ABUSE. The following signs and symptoms may be indicators of child sexual abuse (Tower, 1992; KCAPC, 1992; NCCAN, 2003; Sadock & Sadock, 2003).

Physical indicators:

1. Frequent urinary infections
2. Any venereal disease or gonorrhea infection of the throat
3. Difficulty or pain in walking or sitting
4. Foreign matter in the bladder, rectum, urethra, or vagina
5. Sleep problems (e.g., nightmares, insomnia)
6. Rashes or itching in the genital area; scratching the area a great deal or fidgeting when seated
7. Bruises or pain in the genital area
8. Genital or rectal bleeding; vaginal discharge

Behavioral indicators:

1. Seductive behavior, advanced sexual knowledge for the child's age; promiscuity, prostitution
2. Expressing fear of a particular person or place
3. Compulsive masturbation, precocious sex play, excessive curiosity about sex
4. Sexually abusing another child
5. Appearance of an inordinate number of gifts or money from a questionable source
6. Drop in school performance or sudden nonparticipation in school activities
7. Sudden onset of enuresis
8. Excessive anxiety
9. Expression of low self-worth; verbalizations of being "damaged"
10. Excessive bathing
11. Running away from home
12. Suicide attempts

Characteristics of the Abuser

A number of factors have been associated with adults who abuse or neglect their children. Sadock & Sadock (2003) report that 90 percent of parents who abuse their children were severely physically abused by their own mothers or fathers. Murray and Zentner (2001) identify the following as additional characteristics that may be associated with abusive parents:

- Experiencing a stressful life situation (e.g., unemployment; poverty)
- Having few, if any, support systems; commonly isolated from others
- Lacking understanding of child development or care needs
- Lacking adaptive coping strategies; angers easily; has difficulty trusting others
- Expecting the child to be perfect; may exaggerate any mild difference the child manifests from the "usual"

The Incestuous Relationship

A great deal of attention has been given to the study of father-daughter incest. In these cases, there is usually an impaired sexual relationship between the parents. Communication between the parents is ineffective, which prevents them from correcting their problems. Typically, the father is domineering, impulsive, and physically abusing; whereas the mother is passive and submissive and denigrates her role as wife and mother. She is often aware of, or at least strongly suspects, the incestuous behavior between the father and daughter but may believe in or fear her husband's absolute authority over the family. She may deny that her daughter is being harmed and may actually be grateful that her husband's sexual demands are being met by someone other than herself.

Onset of the incestuous relationship typically occurs when the daughter is 8 to 10 years of age and commonly begins with genital touching and fondling. In the beginning, the child may accept the sexual advances from her father as signs of affection. As the incestuous behavior continues and progresses, the daughter usually becomes more bewildered, confused, and frightened, never knowing whether her father will be paternal or sexual in his interactions with her (Sadock & Sadock, 2003).

The relationship may become a love-hate situation on the part of the daughter. She continues to strive for the ideal father-daughter relationship but is fearful and hateful of the sexual demands he places on her. The mother may be alternately caring and competitive as she witnesses her husband's possessiveness and affections directed toward her daughter. Out of fear that his daughter may expose their relationship, the father may attempt to interfere with her normal peer relationships (Sadock & Sadock, 2003).

It has been suggested that some fathers who participate in incestuous relationships may have unconscious homosexual tendencies and have difficulty achieving a stable heterosexual orientation. On the other hand, some men have frequent sex with their wives and several of their own children but are unwilling to seek sexual partners outside the nuclear family because of a need to maintain the public facade of a stable and competent patriarch. Although the oldest daughter in a family is most vulnerable to becoming a participant in father-daughter incest, some fathers form sequential relationships with several daughters. If incest has been reported with one daughter, it should be suspected with all of the other daughters (Murray & Zentner, 2001).

The Adult Survivor of Incest

Several common characteristics have been identified in adults who have experienced incest as children. Basic to these characteristics is a fundamental lack of trust resulting from an unsatisfactory parent-child relationship, which causes low self-esteem and a poor sense of identity. Children of incest often feel trapped because they have been admonished not to talk about the experience and may be afraid, or even fear for their lives, if they are exposed. If they do muster the courage to report the incest, particularly to the mother, they frequently are not believed. This is confusing to the child, who is then left with a sense of self-doubt and the inability to trust his or her own feelings. The child develops feelings of guilt with the realization over the years that the parents are using him or her in an attempt to solve their own problems.

Childhood sexual abuse is likely to distort the development of a normal association of pleasure with sexual activity (Bass & Davis, 1994). Peer relationships are often delayed, altered, inhibited, or perverted. In some instances, individuals who were sexually abused as children completely retreat from sexual activity and avoid all close interpersonal relationships throughout life. Other adult manifestations of childhood sexual abuse in women include diminished libido, vaginismus, nymphomania, and promiscuity. In male survivors of childhood sexual abuse, impotence, premature ejaculation, exhibitionism, and compulsive sexual conquests may occur. Kreidler and Carlson (1991) report the results of various studies that suggest that adult survivors of incest are at risk for being abusers themselves and for experiencing flashbacks, nightmares, drug and alcohol abuse, anxiety attacks, denial, avoidance, emotional numbing, prostitution, depression, suicide, feelings of powerlessness, guilt, victimization, eating and sleeping disorders, sexual dysfunction, and problems with trust and nonsexual intimacy.

The conflicts associated with pain (physical or emotional) and sexual pleasures experienced by children who are sexually abused are commonly manifested symbolically in adult relationships. Women who were abused as children commonly enter into relationships with men who abuse them physically, sexually, or emotionally (Bird, et al., 1992).

Adult survivors of incest who decide to come forward with their stories usually are estranged from nuclear family members. They are blamed by family members for disclosing the "family secret" and often accused of overreacting to the incest. Frequently the estrangement becomes permanent when family members continue to deny the behavior, and the individual is accused of lying. In recent years, a number of celebrities have come forward with stories of their childhood sexual abuse. Some have chosen to make the disclosure only after the death of their parents. Revelation of these past activities can be one way of contributing to the healing process for which incest survivors so desperately strive.

Sexual Assault

DEFINITION. Over the years, a number of definitions have emerged regarding the crime of **rape**, but one theme is common: rape is an act of aggression, not one of passion. Rape has been defined as the expression of power and dominance by means of sexual violence, most commonly by men over women, although men may also be rape victims. Sexual assault is viewed as any type of sexual act in which an individual is threatened or coerced, or forced, to submit against his or her will. Rape, a type of sexual assault, occurs over a broad spectrum of experiences ranging from the surprise attack by a stranger to insistence on sexual intercourse by an acquaintance or spouse.

Date rape is a term applied to situations in which the rapist is known to the victim (Sadock & Sadock, 2003). They may be out on a first date, may have been dating for a number of months, or merely may be acquaintances or schoolmates. College campuses are the location for a staggering number of these types of rapes, a great many of which go unreported. An increasing number of colleges and universities are establishing programs for rape prevention and counseling for victims of rape.

Marital rape, which has been recognized only in recent years as a legal category, is the case in which a spouse may be held liable for sexual abuse directed at a marital partner against that person's will. Historically, with societal acceptance of the concept of women as marital property, the legal definition of rape held an exemption within the marriage relationship. Mahoney (2001) states:

> Today, under at least one section of the sexual offense codes (usually those regarding force), marital rape is a crime in all 50 states. However, since March 1996, only 17 states and the District of Columbia have abolished the marital rape exemption completely.

Statutory rape is defined as unlawful intercourse between a man older than 16 years of age and a woman under the age of consent (Sadock & Sadock, 2003). The age of consent varies from state to state, ranging from age 14 to 21. A man who has intercourse with a woman under the age of consent can be arrested for statutory rape, although the interaction may have occurred between consenting individuals. The charges, when they occur, usually are brought by the young woman's parents.

Profile of the Victimizer

Older profiles of the individual who rapes were described by Abrahamsen (1960) and Macdonald (1971), who identified the rapist's childhood as "mother-dominated" and the mother as "seductive but rejecting" The behavior of the mother toward the son was described as overbearing, with seductive undertones. Mother and son shared little secrets, and she rescued him when his delinquent acts created problems with others. However, she was quick to withdraw her love and attention when he went against her wishes, a rejection that was powerful and unyielding. She was domineering and possessive of the son, a dominance that often continued into his adult life. Macdonald (1971) stated:

> The seductive mother arouses overwhelming anxiety in her son with great anger, which may be expressed directly toward her but more often is displaced onto other women. When this seductive behavior is combined with parental encouragement of assaultive behavior, the setting is provided for personality development in the child which may result in sadistic, homicidal sexual attacks on women in adolescence or adult life.

Many rapists report that they grew up in abusive homes (Scully, 1990). Even when the parental brutality is discharged by the father, the anger may be directed toward the mother who did not protect her child from physical assault. Recent feminist theories suggest that the rapist displaces this anger on the rape victim because he cannot directly express it toward other men (Sadock & Sadock, 2003).

Statistics show that the greatest number of rapists are between the ages of 25 and 44. Of rapists, 51 percent are white, 47 percent are African-American, and the remaining 2 percent come from all other races (Sadock & Sadock, 2003). Many are married or cohabiting at the time of their offenses (Scully, 1990). For those with previous criminal activity, the majority of their convictions are for crimes against property rather than against people. Most rapists do not have histories of mental illness.

The Victim

Rape can occur at any age. Although victims have been reported as young as 15 months old and as old as 82 years, the high-risk age group appears to be 16 to 24 years (Sadock & Sadock, 2003). Of rape victims, 70 to 75 percent are single women, and the attack frequently occurs in or close to the victim's own neighborhood.

Scully (1990), in a study of a prison sample of rapists, found that in "stranger rapes," victims were not chosen for any reason having to do with appearance or behavior but simply because the individual happened to be in a certain place at a certain time. Scully states:

> The most striking and consistent factor in all the stranger rapes, whether committed by a lone assailant or a group, is the unfortunate fact that the victim was "just there" in a location unlikely to draw the attention of a passerby. Almost every one of these men said exactly the same thing, "It could have been any woman," and a few added that because it was dark, they could not even see what their victim looked like very well.

In her study, Scully found that 62 percent of the rapists used a weapon, most frequently a knife. Most suggested that they used the weapon to terrorize and subdue the victim but not to inflict serious injury. The presence of a weapon (real or perceived) appears to be the principal measure of the extent to which a woman resists her attacker.

Rape victims who present themselves for care shortly after the crime has occurred likely may be experiencing an overwhelming sense of violation and helplessness that began with the powerlessness and intimidation experienced during the rape. Burgess (1984) identified two emotional patterns of victim response that may occur within hours after a rape, which healthcare workers may encounter in the emergency department or rape crisis center. In the **expressed response pattern,** the victim expresses feelings of fear, anger, and anxiety through such behaviors as crying, sobbing, smiling, restlessness, and tension. In the **controlled response pattern,** the feelings are masked or hidden, and a calm, composed, or subdued affect is seen.

The following manifestations may be evident in the days and weeks after the attack (Burgess, 1984):

1. Contusions and abrasions about various parts of the body
2. Headaches, fatigue, sleep pattern disturbances
3. Stomach pains, nausea and vomiting
4. Vaginal discharge and itching, burning upon urination, rectal bleeding and pain
5. Rage, humiliation, embarrassment, desire for revenge, and self-blame
6. Fear of physical violence and death

The long-term effects of sexual assault depend largely on the individual's ego strength, social support system, and the way he or she was treated as a victim (Burgess, 1984). Various long-term effects include increased restlessness, dreams and nightmares, and phobias (particularly those having to do with sexual interaction). Some women report that it takes years to get over the experience; they describe a sense of vulnerability and a loss of control over their own lives during this period. They feel defiled and unable to wash themselves clean, and some women are unable to remain living alone in their home or apartment.

Some victims develop a **compounded rape reaction,** in which additional symptoms such as depression and suicide, substance abuse, and even psychotic behaviors may be noted (Burgess, 1984). Another variation has been called the **silent rape reaction,** in which the victim tells no one about the assault. Anxiety is suppressed. and the emotional burden may become overwhelming. The unresolved sexual trauma may not be revealed until the woman is forced to face another sexual crisis in her life that reactivates the previously unresolved feelings.

Diagnosis/Outcome Identification

Nursing diagnoses are formulated from the data gathered during the assessment phase and with background knowledge regarding predisposing factors to the situation. Some common nursing diagnoses for victims of abuse include:

Rape-trauma syndrome related to sexual assault evidenced by verbalizations of the attack; bruises and lacerations over areas of body; severe anxiety.

Powerlessness related to cycle of battering evidenced by verbalizations of abuse; bruises and lacerations over areas of body; fear for her safety and that of her children; verbalizations of no way to get out of relationship.

Delayed growth and development related to abusive family situation evidenced by sudden onset of enuresis, thumb-sucking, nightmares, inability to perform self-care activities appropriate for age.

The following criteria may be used to measure outcomes in the care of abuse victims:

- The client who has been sexually assaulted:
  1. Is no longer experiencing panic anxiety
  2. Demonstrates trust in the primary nurse
  3. Has received immediate attention to physical injuries
  4. Has initiated behaviors consistent with the grief response
- The client who has been physically battered:
  1. Has received immediate attention to physical injuries
  2. Verbalizes assurance of his or her immediate safety
  3. Discusses life situation with primary nurse
  4. Can verbalize choices from which he or she may receive assistance
- The child who has been abused:
  1. Has received immediate attention to physical injuries
  2. Demonstrates trust in primary nurse by discussing abuse through the use of play therapy
  3. Is demonstrating a decrease in regressive behaviors

Planning/Implementation

Table 22–1 provides a plan of care for the client who has been a victim of abuse. Nursing diagnoses are presented along with outcome criteria, appropriate nursing interventions, and rationales for each.

Evaluation

Evaluation of nursing actions to assist victims of abuse must be considered on both a short- and a long-term basis.

Short-term evaluation may be facilitated by gather-

TABLE 22–1 Care Plan for Victims of Abuse

Nursing Diagnosis: RAPE-TRAUMA SYNDROME

Related to: Sexual assault

Evidenced by: Verbalizations of the attack; bruises and lacerations over areas of body; severe anxiety

Outcome Criteria	Nursing Interventions	Rationale
Client will begin a healthy grief resolution, initiating the process of healing (both physically and psychologically).	1. Smith (1987a) relates the importance of communicating the following four phrases to the rape victim: • I am very sorry this happened to you. • You are safe here. • I am very glad you are alive. • You are not to blame. You are a victim. It was not your fault. Whatever decisions you made at the time of the assault were the right ones because you are alive.	1. The woman who has been sexually assaulted fears for her life and must be reassured of her safety. She may also be overwhelmed with self-doubt and self-blame, and these statements instill trust and validate self-worth.
	2. Explain every assessment procedure that will be conducted and why it is being conducted. Ensure that data collection is conducted in a caring, nonjudgmental manner.	2. This may serve to decrease fear/anxiety and increase trust.
	3. Ensure that the client has adequate privacy for all immediate post–crisis interventions. Try to have as few people as possible providing the immediate care or collecting immediate evidence.	3. The post–trauma client is extremely vulnerable. Additional people in the environment increase this feeling of vulnerability and serve to escalate anxiety.
	4. Encourage the client to give an account of the assault. Listen, but do not probe.	4. Nonjudgmental listening provides an avenue for catharsis that the client needs to begin healing. A detailed account may be required for legal follow-up, and a caring nurse, as client advocate, may help to lessen the trauma of evidence collection.
	5. Discuss with the client whom to call for support or assistance. Provide information about referrals for aftercare.	5. Because of severe anxiety and fear, the client may need assistance from others during this immediate post–crisis period. Provide referral information in writing for later reference (e.g., psychotherapist, mental health clinic, community advocacy group).

Nursing Diagnosis: POWERLESSNESS

Related to: Cycle of battering

Evidenced by: Verbalizations of abuse; bruises and lacerations over areas of body; fear for own safety and that of children; verbalizations of no way to get out of relationship

Outcome Criteria	Nursing Interventions	Rationale
Client will recognize and verbalize choices available, thereby perceiving some control over life situation.	1. In collaboration with physician, ensure that all physical wounds, fractures, and burns receive immediate attention. Take photographs if the victim will permit.	1. Client safety is a nursing priority. Photographs may be called in as evidence if charges are filed.
	2. Take the woman to a private area to do the interview.	2. If the client is accompanied by the man who did the battering, she is not likely to be truthful about her injuries.
	3. If she has come alone or with her children, assure her of her safety. Encourage her to discuss the battering incident. Ask questions about whether this has happened before, whether the abuser takes drugs, whether the woman has a safe place to go, and whether she is interested in pressing charges.	3. Some women will attempt to keep secret how their injuries occurred in an effort to protect the partner or because they are fearful that the partner will kill them if they tell.
	4. Ensure that "rescue" efforts are not attempted by the nurse. Offer support, but remember that the final decision must be made by the client.	4. Making her own decision will give the client a sense of control over her life situation. Imposing judgments and giving advice are nontherapeutic.

Outcome Criteria	Nursing Interventions	Rationale
	5. Stress the importance of safety. Smith (1987b) suggests a statement such as, "Yes, it has happened. Now where do you want to go from here?" Burgess (1990) states, "The victim needs to be made aware of the variety of resources that are available to her. These may include crisis hot lines, community groups for women who have been abused, shelters, a variety of counseling opportunities (i.e., couples, individual, or group), and information regarding the victim's rights in the civil and criminal justice system." Following a discussion of these available resources, the woman may choose for herself. If her decision is to return to the marriage and home, this choice also must be respected.	5. Knowledge of available choices decreases the victim's sense of powerlessness, but true empowerment comes only when she chooses to use that knowledge for her own benefit.

Nursing Diagnosis: DELAYED GROWTH AND DEVELOPMENT

Related to: Abusive family situation

Evidenced by: Sudden onset of enuresis, thumb sucking, nightmares, inability to perform self-care activities appropriate for age

Outcome Criteria	Nursing Interventions	Rationale
Client will develop trusting relationship with nurse and report how evident injuries were sustained. Negative regressive behaviors (enuresis, thumb sucking, nightmares) will diminish.	1. Perform complete physical assessment of the child. Take particular note of bruises (in various stages of healing), lacerations, and client complaints of pain in specific areas. Do not overlook or discount the possibility of sexual abuse. Assess for nonverbal signs of abuse: aggressive conduct, excessive fears, extreme hyperactivity, apathy, withdrawal, age-inappropriate behaviors.	1. An accurate and thorough physical assessment is required to provide appropriate care for the client.
	2. Conduct an in-depth interview with the parent or adult who accompanies the child Consider: If the injury is being reported as an accident, is the explanation reasonable? Is the injury consistent with the explanation? Is the injury consistent with the child's developmental capabilities?	2. Fear of imprisonment or loss of child custody may place the abusive parent on the defensive. Discrepancies may be evident in the description of the incident, and lying to cover up involvement is a common defense that may be detectable in an in-depth interview.
	3. Use games or play therapy to gain child's trust. Use these techniques to assist in describing his or her side of the story.	3. Establishing a trusting relationship with an abused child is extremely difficult. He or she may not want to be touched. These types of play activities can provide a nonthreatening environment that may enhance the child's attempt to discuss these painful issues (Celano, 1990).
	4. Determine whether the nature of the injuries warrants reporting to authorities. Specific state statutes must enter into the decision of whether to report suspected child abuse. Individual state statutes regarding what constitutes child abuse and neglect may be found at < http://nccanch.acf.hhs.gov/general/legal/statutes/index.cfm >	4. A report is commonly made if there is reason to suspect that a child has been injured as a result of physical, mental, emotional, or sexual abuse. "Reason to suspect" exists when there is evidence of a discrepancy or inconsistency in explaining a child's injury. Most states require that the following individuals report cases of suspected child abuse: all healthcare workers, all mental health therapists, teachers, child-care providers, firefighters, emergency medical personnel, and law enforcement personnel. Reports are made to the Department of Health and Human Services or a law enforcement agency.

ing information using the following types of questions:

1. Has the individual been reassured of his or her safety?
2. Is this evidenced by a decrease in panic anxiety?
3. Have wounds been properly cared for and provision made for follow-up care?
4. Have emotional needs been attended to?
5. Has trust been established with at least one person to whom the client feels comfortable relating the abusive incident?
6. Have available support systems been identified and notified?
7. Have options for immediate circumstances been presented?

Long-term evaluation may be conducted by health-care workers who have contact with the individual long after the immediate crisis has passed.

1. Is the individual able to conduct activities of daily living satisfactorily?
2. Have physical wounds healed properly?
3. Is the client appropriately progressing through the behaviors of grieving?
4. Is the client free of sleep disturbances (nightmares, insomnia); psychosomatic symptoms (headaches, stomach pains, nausea/vomiting); regressive behaviors (enuresis, thumb-sucking, phobias); and psychosexual disturbances?
5. Is the individual free from problems with interpersonal relationships?
6. Has the individual considered the alternatives for change in his or her personal life?
7. Has a decision been made relative to the choices available?
8. Is he or she satisfied with the decision that has been made?

TREATMENT MODALITIES

Crisis Intervention

The focus of the initial interview and follow-up with the client who has been sexually assaulted is on the rape incident alone. Problems identified but unassociated with the rape are not dealt with at this time. The goal of crisis intervention is to help victims return to their previous lifestyle as quickly as possible (Burgess, 1990).

The client should be involved in the intervention from the beginning. This promotes a sense of competency, control, and decision-making. Because an overwhelming sense of powerlessness accompanies the rape experience, active involvement by the victim is both a validation of personal worth and the beginning of the recovery process. Crisis intervention is time limited—usually 6 to 8 weeks. If problems resurface beyond this time, the victim is referred for assistance from other agencies (e.g., long-term psychotherapy from a psychiatrist or mental health clinic).

During the crisis period, attention is given to coping strategies for dealing with the symptoms common to the post-trauma client. Initially the individual undergoes a period of disorganization during which there is difficulty making decisions, extreme or irrational fears, and general mistrust. Observable manifestations may range from stark hysteria, to expression of anger and rage, to silence and withdrawal. Guilt and feelings of responsibility for the rape, as well as numerous physical manifestations, are common. The crisis counselor will attempt to help the victim draw upon previous successful coping strategies to regain control over his or her life.

If the client is a victim of battering, the counselor ensures that various resources and options are made known to the victim so that she may make a personal decision regarding what she wishes to do with her life. Support groups provide a valuable forum for reducing isolation and learning new strategies for coping with the aftermath of physical or sexual abuse. Particularly for the rape victim, the peer support group provides a therapeutic forum for reducing the sense of isolation she may feel in the aftermath of predictable social and interpersonal responses to her experience.

Sadock and Sadock (2003) state:

> Few women emerge from the assault completely unscathed. The manifestations and the amount of damage depend on the violence of the attack itself, the vulnerability of the woman, and the support system available to her immediately after the attack. A rape victim fares best when she receives immediate support and can ventilate her fear and rage to loving family members, sympathetic physicians, and law enforcement officials. Knowing that she has socially acceptable means of recourse, such as the arrest and conviction of the rapist, can help a rape victim. (p. 892)

The Safe House or Shelter

Most major cities in the United States now have **safe houses or shelters** where women can go to be assured of protection for them and their children. These shelters provide a variety of services, and the women receive emotional support from staff and each other.

Most shelters provide individual and group counseling; help with bureaucratic institutions such as the police, legal representation, and social services; provide child care and children's programming; and aid for the woman in making future plans, such as employment counseling and linkages with housing authorities.

The shelters are usually run by a combination of professional and volunteer staff, including nurses, psychologists, lawyers, and others. Women who have been previously abused are often among the volunteer staff members.

Group work is an important part of the service of shelters. Women in residence range from those in the immediate crisis phase to those who have progressed through a variety of phases of the grief process. Those newer members can learn a great deal from the women who have successfully resolved similar problems. Length of stay varies a great deal from individual to individual, depending on a number of factors, such as outside support network, financial situation, and personal resources.

The shelter provides a haven of physical safety for the battered woman and promotes expression of the intense emotions she may be experiencing regarding her situation. A woman often exhibits depression, extreme fear, or even violent expressions of anger and rage. In the shelter, she learns that these feelings are normal and that others have experienced these same emotions in similar situations. She is allowed to grieve for what has been lost and for what was expected but not achieved. Help is provided in overcoming the tremendous guilt associated with self-blame. This is a difficult step for someone who has accepted responsibility for another's behavior over a long period.

New arrivals at the shelter are given time to experience the relief from the safety and security provided. Making decisions is discouraged during the period of immediate crisis and disorganization. Once the woman's emotions have become more stable, planning begins. Through information from staff and peers, she learns what resources are available to her within the community. Feedback is provided, but the woman makes her own decision about "where she wants to go from here." She is accepted and supported in whatever she chooses to do.

Family Therapy

The focus of therapy with families who use violence is to help them develop democratic ways of solving problems. Studies show that the more a family uses the democratic means of conflict resolution, the less likely they are to engage in physical violence. Families need to learn to deal with problems in ways that can produce mutual benefits for all concerned, rather than engaging in power struggles among family members.

Parents also need to learn effective methods of disciplining children, aside from physical punishment. Methods that emphasize the importance of positive reinforcement for acceptable behavior can be very effective. Family members must be committed to consistent use of this behavior modification technique for it to be successful.

Teaching parents about expectations for various developmental levels may alleviate some of the stress that accompanies these changes. Knowing what to expect from individuals at various stages of development may provide needed anticipatory guidance to deal with the crises commonly associated with these stages.

Therapy sessions with all family members together may focus on problems with family communication. Members are encouraged to express honest feelings in a manner that is nonthreatening to other family members. Active listening, assertiveness techniques, and respecting the rights of others are taught and encouraged. Barriers to effective communication are identified and resolved.

Referrals to agencies that promote effective parenting skills (e.g., parent effectiveness training) may be made. Alternative agencies that may relieve the stress of parenting (e.g., "Mom's day out" programs, sitter-sharing organizations, and day care institutions) also may be considered. Support groups for abusive parents may also be helpful, and assistance in locating or initiating such a group may be provided.

SUMMARY

This chapter provided a discussion of abuse—the maltreatment of one person by another. Intimate partner abuse, child abuse, and sexual assault are all on the rise in this country, and all populations are equally affected.

Abuse of women and children began early in the development of this country when these individuals were considered the property of their husbands and fathers; this physical abuse was considered acceptable. Many women came to believe that they deserved any physical or sexual abuse they encountered.

Various factors have been theorized as influential in the predisposition to violent behavior. Physiological and biochemical influences within the brain have been suggested, as has the possibility of a direct genetic link. Organic brain syndromes associated with various cerebral disorders have been implicated in the predisposition to aggressive and violent behavior.

Psychoanalytical theorists relate the predisposition to violent behavior to underdeveloped ego and a poor self-concept. Learning theorists suggest that children imitate the abusive behavior of their parents. This theory has been substantiated by studies that show that individuals who were abused as children or whose parents disciplined them with physical punishment are more likely to be abusive as adults. Societal influences, such as general acceptance of violence as a means of solving problems, also have been implicated.

Women who are battered usually take blame for their situation. They were reared in abusive families and have come to expect this behavior. Battered women often see no way out of their present situation and may be encouraged by their social support network (family, friends, clergy) to remain in the abusive relationship.

Child abuse includes physical and emotional injury, physical and emotional neglect, and sexual abuse of a child. A child may experience many years of abuse without reporting it because of fear of retaliation by the abuser. Some children report incest experiences to their mothers, only to be rebuffed by her and told to remain secretive about the abuse. Adult survivors of incest often experience a number of physical and emotional manifestations relating back to the incestuous relationship.

Sexual assault is identified as an act of aggression, not passion. Many rapists report growing up in abusive homes, and some theorists relate the predisposition to rape to a "seductive, but rejecting, mother." Rape is a traumatic experience, and many women experience flashbacks, nightmares, rage, physical symptoms, depression, and thoughts of suicide for many years after the occurrence.

Nursing implementation with victims of abuse was discussed in the context of the nursing process. Assessment data, nursing diagnoses, outcome criteria, appropriate nursing interventions with rationale, and standards for evaluation were presented. Additional treatment modalities were described, including crisis intervention with the sexual assault victim, safe shelter for battered women, and therapy for families who use violence.

Problems related to abuse and neglect are becoming a national crisis in the United States. Nurses are in a unique position to intervene at the primary, secondary, and tertiary levels of prevention with the victims of these problematic behaviors.

REVIEW QUESTIONS

SELF-EXAMINATION/LEARNING EXERCISE

Select the answer that is most appropriate for each of the following questions:

Situation: Sharon is a 32-year-old woman who arrives at the emergency department with her three small children. She has multiple bruises around her face and neck. Her right eye is swollen shut.

1. Sharon says to the nurse, "I didn't want to come. I'm really okay. He only does this when he has too much to drink. I just shouldn't have yelled at him." The best response by the nurse is:
   a. "How often does he drink too much?"
   b. "It is not your fault. You did the right thing by coming here."
   c. "How many times has he done this to you?"
   d. "He is not a good husband. You have to leave him before he kills you."

2. In the interview, Sharon tells the nurse, "He's been getting more and more violent lately. He's been under a lot of stress at work the last few weeks, so he drinks a lot when he gets home. He always gets mean when he drinks. I was getting scared. So I just finally told him I was going to take the kids and leave. He got furious when I said that and began beating me with his fists." With knowledge about the cycle of battering, what does this situation represent?
   a. Phase I: Sharon was desperately trying to stay out of his way and keep everything calm.
   b. Phase I: a minor battering incident for which Sharon assumes all the blame.
   c. Phase II: the acute battering incident that Sharon provoked with her threat to leave.
   d. Phase III: the honeymoon phase where the husband believes that he has "taught her a lesson and she won't act up again."

3. The *priority* nursing intervention for Sharon in the emergency department is:
   a. Tending to the immediate care of her wounds
   b. Providing her with information about a safe place to stay
   c. Administering the prn tranquilizer ordered by the physician
   d. Explaining how she may go about bringing charges against her husband.

4. Sharon goes with her children to stay at a women's shelter. She participates in group therapy and receives emotional support from staff and peers. She is made aware of the alternatives open to her. Nevertheless, she decides to return to her home and marriage. The best response by the nurse upon Sharon's departure is:
   a. "I just can't believe you have decided to go back to that horrible man."
   b. "I'm just afraid he will kill you or the children when you go back."
   c. "What makes you think things have changed with him?"
   d. "I hope you have made the right decision. Call this number if you need help."

Situation: Carol is a school nurse. Five-year-old Jana has been sent to her office complaining of nausea. She lies down on the office cot, but eventually vomits and soils her blouse. When Carol removes Jana's blouse to clean it, she notices that Jana has a number of bruises on her arms and torso. Some are bluish in color; others are various shades of green and yellow. She also notices some small scars. Jana's abdomen protrudes on her small, thin frame.

5. From the objective physical assessment, the nurse suspects that:
   a. Jana is experiencing physical and sexual abuse.
   b. Jana is experiencing physical abuse and neglect.
   c. Jana is experiencing emotional neglect.
   d. Jana is experiencing sexual and emotional abuse.

6. Carol tries to talk to Jana about her bruises and scars, but Jana refuses to say how she received them. Another way in which Carol can get information from Jana is to:
   a. Have her evaluated by the school psychologist.
   b. Tell her she may select a "treat" from the treat box (e.g., sucker, balloon, junk jewelry) if she answers the nurse's questions.
   c. Explain to her that if she answers the questions, she may stay in the nurse's office and not have to go back to class.
   d. Use a "family" of dolls to role-play Jana's family with her.

7. Carol strongly suspects that Jana is being abused. What would be the best way for Carol to proceed with this information?
   a. As a healthcare worker, report the suspicion to the Department of Health and Human Services.
   b. Check Jana again in a week and see if there are any new bruises.
   c. Meet with Jana's parents and ask them how Jana got the bruises.
   d. Initiate paperwork to have Jana placed in foster care.

Situation: Lana is an 18-year-old freshman at the state university. She was extremely flattered when Don, a senior star football player, invited her to a party. On the way home, he parked the car in a secluded area by the lake. He became angry when she refused his sexual advances. He began to beat her and finally raped her. She tried to fight him, but his physical strength overpowered her. He dumped her in the dorm parking lot and left. The dorm supervisor rushed Lana to the emergency department.

8. Lana says to the nurse, "It's all my fault. I shouldn't have allowed him to stop at the lake." The nurse's best response is:
   a. "Yes, you're right. You put yourself in a very vulnerable position when you allowed him to stop at the lake."
   b. "You are not to blame for his behavior. You obviously made some right decisions, because you survived the attack."
   c. "There's no sense looking back now. Just look forward, and make sure you don't put yourself in the same situation again."
   d. "You'll just have to see that he is arrested so he won't do this to anyone else."

9. The *priority* nursing intervention with Lana would be:
   a. Help her to bathe and clean herself up.
   b. Provide physical and emotional support during evidence collection.
   c. Provide her with a written list of community resources for rape victims.
   d. Discuss the importance of a follow-up visit to evaluate for sexually transmitted diseases.

10. Lana is referred to a support group for rape victims. She has been attending regularly for 6 months. From this group, she has learned that the most likely reason Don raped her was:
    a. He had had too much to drink at the party and was out of control.
    b. He had not had sexual relations with a girl in many months.
    c. He was predisposed to become a rapist by virtue of the poverty conditions under which he was reared.
    d. He was expressing power and dominance by means of sexual aggression and violence.

INTERNET REFERENCES

- Additional information related to child abuse may be located at the following Web sites:
  - a http://www.childabuse.org/
  - b http://www.fvpf.org
  - c http://www.child-abuse.com
- Additional information related to sexual assault may be located at the following Web sites:
  - a http://www.vaw.umn.edu/Vawnet/mrape.htm
  - b http://www.ncweb.com/org/rapecrisis
- Additional information related to domestic violence may be located at the following Web sites:
  - a http://www.ndvh.org/
  - b http://www.cpsdv.org/
  - c http://home.cybergrrl.com/dv/book/toc.html
  - d http://crisis-support.org/
  - e http://www.ama-assn.org/ama/pub/category/3242.html

Test Your CRITICAL THINKING SKILLS

Sandy is a psychiatric nurse who works at the safe house for battered women. Lisa has just been admitted with her two small children after she was treated in the emergency department. She had been beaten severely by her husband when he was intoxicated last night. She escaped with her children after he passed out in their bedroom.

In her initial assessment, Sandy learns from Lisa that she has been battered by her husband for 5 years, beginning shortly after their marriage. She explained that she "knew he drank quite a lot before we were married, but thought he would stop after we had kids." Instead, the drinking has increased. Sometimes he doesn't even get home from work until 11:00 or midnight, after stopping to drink at the bar with his buddies.

Lately, he has begun to express jealousy and a lack of trust in Lisa, accusing her of numerous infidelities and indiscretions, none of which is true. Lisa says, "If only he wasn't under so much stress on his job, then maybe he wouldn't drink so much. Maybe if I tried harder to make everything perfect for him at home—I don't know. What do you think I should do to keep him from acting this way?"

Answer the following questions related to Lisa:

1. What is an appropriate response to Lisa's question?
2. Identify the priority psychosocial nursing diagnosis for Lisa.
3. What must the nurse ensure that Lisa learns from this experience?

IMPLICATIONS OF RESEARCH FOR EVIDENCE BASED PRACTICE

Sachs, B., Hall, L.A., Lutenbacher, M., and Rayens, M.K.:
Potential for abusive parenting by rural mothers with low-birth-weight children. Image: Journal of Nursing Scholarship (1999); 31(1):21–25.

Description of the Study: The purpose of this study was to describe factors influencing the potential for abusive parenting by rural mothers of low birth weight (LBW) children. The convenience sample in this study included 48 mothers of LBW children, ranging in age from 18 to 39 years, all living in a rural area of the state, and all living with their LBW infant at the time of the study. Average length of the children's hospitalization after birth was 6 weeks, and the average age at time of the study was 9 months. In-home interviews were conducted using structured questionnaires to assess the mothers' everyday stressors, depressive symptoms, functional social support, quality of family relationships, and child abuse potential.

Results of the Study: According to the questionnaires used for measurement, 54 percent of the mothers indicated a high level of depressive symptoms, and 63 percent indicated a high potential for physical child abuse. No significant differences were noted in depressive symptoms and potential for child abuse by birth weight, health status of the child, or time since hospital discharge. Mothers with high child abuse potential reported more everyday stressors and depressive symptoms, less functional social support, and poorer family functioning. Because in this study everyday stressors and the two social support systems (functional social support and quality of family relationships) were examined as predictors of depressive symptoms, it is suggested that everyday stressors exert both a direct and an indirect effect on mothers' potential for child abuse. The strongest predictor of child abuse potential was mothers' depressive symptoms.

Implications for Nursing Practice: The researchers conclude that rural mothers of LBW children are at risk for abusive parenting. This study demonstrated the adverse effects of everyday stressors, minimal social resources, and depressive symptoms on mothers' potential for abusive parenting. Nurses should provide attention to the mental health of mothers living in isolated, rural areas. Information should be made available to these mothers regarding community resources that offer social support and childcare assistance. Nurses could establish and conduct educational programs to improve parenting skills and promote more positive child health outcomes.

REFERENCES

American Nurses Association (ANA). (1998). Culturally competent assessment for family violence. Washington, D.C.: American Nurses Publishing.

Bass, E., & Davis, L. (1994). The courage to heal: A guide for women survivors of child sexual abuse (3rd ed.). New York: HarperCollins Publishers.

Berndt, T.J. (1992). Child development. Ft. Worth, TX: Harcourt Brace Jovanovich, Publishers.

Bird, H.R., Green, A.H., Kranzler, E.M., Rubinstein, B., & Wasserman, G.A. (1992). Stresses and traumas of childhood. In F.I. Kass, J.M. Oldham, & H. Pardes (Eds.), The Columbia University college of physicians and surgeons complete home guide to mental health. New York: Henry Holt and Company.

Burgess, A. (1984). Intrafamilial sexual abuse. In J. Campbell, & J. Humphreys (Eds.), Nursing care of victims of family violence. Reston, VA: Reston Publishing.

Burgess, A. (1990). Victims of family violence: Incest and battering. In A.W. Burgess (Ed.), Psychiatric nursing in the hospital and the community (5th ed.). Norwalk,

Campbell, J. (1992). Violence demands nursing solutions. The American Nurse, 24(4), 4.

Campbell, J., & Humphreys, J. (1993). Nursing care of survivors of family violence. St. Louis: Mosby.

Celano, M.P. (1990). Activities and games for group psychotherapy with sexually abused children. International Journal of Group Psychotherapy, 40(4), 419–428.

Frolik, L.A., & Kaplan, R. L. (1995). Elder law in a nutshell. St. Paul, MN: West Publishing.

Kansas Child Abuse Prevention Council (KCAPC) (1992). A guide about child abuse and neglect. Wichita, KS: National Committee for Prevention of Child Abuse and Parents Anonymous.

Kennedy, B.P., Kawachi, I., Prothrow, S.D., Lochner, K., and Gupta, V. (1998). Social capital, income inequality, and firearm violent crime. Social Science and Medicine,47(1), 7–17.

Kreidler, M.C., & Carlson, R.E. (1991). Breaking the incest cycle: The group as a surrogate family. Journal of Psychosocial Nursing, 29(4), 28–32.

Mahoney, P. (2001). The wife rape information page. Retrieved May 4, 2002 from http://www.wellesley.edu/WCW/projects/mrape.html

Marvin, D.R. (1997). The dynamics of domestic abuse. FBI publications: Law Enforcement Bulletin (July 1997). Retrieved May 3, 2002 from http://www.fbi.gov/publications/leb/1997/july973.htm

Moss, V.A. (1991). Battered women and the myth of masochism. Journal of Psychosocial Nursing, 29(7), 18–23.

Murray, R.B., & Zentner, J.P. (2001). Health promotion strategies through the lifespan (7th ed.). Upper Saddle River, NJ: Prentice Hall.

National Clearinghouse on Child Abuse and Neglect (NCCAN). (2003). Recognizing child abuse and neglect: Signs and symptoms. Retrieved 5-27-04 from http://nccanch.acf.hhs.gov

National Clearinghouse on Child Abuse and Neglect (NCCAN). (2002). What is child maltreatment? Retrieved May 4, 2002 from http://www.calib.com/nccanch/pubs/factsheets/childmal.cfm

National Coalition Against Domestic Violence. (2002a). What is battering? Retrieved May 3, 2002 from http://www.ncadv.org/problem/what.htm

National Coalition Against Domestic Violence. (2002b). Why do women stay? Retrieved May 3, 2002 from http://www.ncadv.org/problem/why2.htm

Person, E.S. (1992). Women's issues at a time of social change. In F.I. Kass, J.M. Oldham, & H. Pardes (Eds.), Columbia University College of physicians and surgeons complete home guide to mental health. New York: Henry Holt and Company.

Project for Victims of Family Violence. (2000). How to help someone you know who is being abused. Retrieved September 7, 2001 from http://www.biz.arkansas.net/lordandedw/warning.htm

Sadock, B.J., & Sadock, V.A. (2003). Synopsis of psychiatry: Behavioral sciences/clinical psychiatry (9th ed.). Philadelphia: Lippincott Williams & Wilkins.

Scully, D. (1990). Understanding sexual violence: A study of convicted rapists. Boston: Unwin Hyman.

Silver, J.M., & Yudofsky, S. (1992). Violence and aggression. In F.I. Kass, J.M. Oldham, & H. Pardes (Eds.), The Columbia University college of physicians and surgeons complete home guide to mental health. New York: Henry Holt and Company.

Smith, L.S. (1987a). Sexual assault: The nurse's role. AD Nurse, 2(2), 24–28.

Smith, L.S. (1987b). Battered women: The nurse's role. AD Nurse, 2(5), 21–24.

Tardiff, K.J. (2003). Violence. In R.E. Hales & S.C. Yudofsky (Eds.), Textbook of clinical psychiatry (4th ed.). Washington, D.C.: The American Psychiatric Publishing.

Tower, C.C. (1992). The role of educators in the prevention and treatment of child abuse and neglect. Retrieved September 7, 2001 from http://www.calib.com/nccanch/pubs/educator/section3.htm

United States Bureau of Justice. (2002). Special Report: Intimate partner violence. Washington, D.C.: U.S. Department of Justice.

CLASSICAL REFERENCES

Abrahamsen D. (1960). The psychology of crime. New York: John Wiley.

Erikson, E.H. (1963). Childhood and society (2nd ed.). New York: W.W. Norton.

Macdonald, J.M. (1971). Rape: Offenders and their victims. Springfield, IL: Charles C. Thomas.

Selye, H. (1956). The stress of life. New York: McGraw-Hill.

Walker, L.E. (1979). The battered woman. New York: Harper & Row.

23

CHAPTER

The Aging Individual

CHAPTER OUTLINE

KEY TERMS

attachment
bereavement overload
disengagement theory
geriatrics
gerontology
geropsychiatry
"granny-bashing"
"granny-dumping"
short-term memory
long-term memory
menopause
osteoporosis
Medicare
Medicaid
reminiscence therapy

OBJECTIVES

After reading this chapter, the student will be able to:

1. Discuss societal perspectives on aging.
2. Describe an epidemiological profile of aging in the United States.
3. Discuss various theories of aging.
4. Describe biological, psychological, sociocultural, and sexual aspects of the normal aging process.
5. Discuss retirement as a special concern to the aging individual.
6. Explain personal and sociological perspectives of long-term care of the aging individual.
7. Describe the problem of elder abuse as it exists in today's society.
8. Discuss the implications of the increasing number of suicides among the elderly population.
9. Apply the steps of the nursing process to the care of aging individuals.

INTRODUCTION

What is it like to grow old? It is not likely that many people in the American culture would state that it is something they want to do. Most would agree, however, that it is "better than the alternative."

Roberts (1991) tells the following often-told tale of Supreme Court Justice Oliver Wendell Holmes, Jr. In the year before he retired at age 91 as the oldest justice ever to sit on the Supreme Court of the United States, Holmes and his close friend Justice Louis Brandeis, then a mere 74 years old, were out for one of their frequent walks on Washington's Capitol Hill. On this particular day, the justices spotted a very attractive young woman approaching them. As she passed, Holmes paused, sighed, and said to Brandeis, "Oh, to be 70 again!" Obviously, being old is relative to the individual experiencing it.

Growing old has not been popular among the youth-oriented American culture. However, with 66 million "baby boomers" reaching their 65th birthdays by the year 2030, greater emphasis is being placed on the needs of an aging population. The disciplines of **gerontology** (the study of the aging process), **geriatrics** (the branch of clinical medicine specializing in problems of the elderly), and **geropsychiatry** (the branch of clinical medicine specializing in psychopathology of the elderly population) are expanding rapidly in response to this predictable demand.

Growing old in a society that has been obsessed with youth may have a critical impact on the mental health of many people. This situation has serious implications for psychiatric nursing.

What is it like to grow old? More and more people will be able to answer this question as the 21st century progresses. Perhaps they will also be asking the question that Roberts (1991) asks: "How did I get here so fast?"

This chapter focuses on physical and psychological changes associated with the aging process, as well as special concerns of the elderly population, such as retirement, long-term care, elder abuse, and rising suicide rates. The nursing process is presented as the vehicle for delivery of nursing care to elderly individuals.

HOW OLD IS *OLD*?

The concept of "old" has changed drastically over the years. Our prehistoric ancestors probably had a life span of 40 years, with an average life span of around 18 years. As civilization developed, mortality rates remained high because of periodic famine and frequent malnutrition. An improvement in the standard of living was not truly evident until about the middle of the 17th century. Since that time, assured food supply, changes in food production, better housing conditions, and more progressive medical and sanitation facilities have contributed to population growth, declining mortality rates, and substantial increases in longevity.

In 1900, the average life expectancy in the United States was 47 years, and only 4 percent of the population was age 65 or older. By 2000, the average life expectancy at birth was 74.1 years for men and 79.5 years for women (National Center for Health Statistics, 2002).

The U.S. Census Bureau has created a system for classification of older Americans:

Older: 55 through 64 years
Elderly: 65 through 74 years
Aged: 75 through 84 years
Very old: 85 years and older

Some gerontologists have elected to use a simpler classification system:

Young old: 60 through 74 years
Middle old: 75 through 84 years
Old old: 85 years and older

So how old is *old*? Obviously, the term cannot be defined by a number. Myths and stereotypes of aging have long obscured our understanding of the aged and the process of aging. Ideas that all elderly individuals are sick, depressed, obsessed with death, senile, and incapable of change affect the way elderly people are treated. They even shape the pattern of aging of the people who believe them. They can become self-fulfilling prophecies—people start to believe they should behave in certain ways and, therefore, act according to those beliefs. Generalized assumptions can be demeaning and interfere with the quality of life for older individuals.

Just as there are many differences in individual adaptation at earlier stages of development, so it is in the elderly person. Erikson (1963) has suggested that the mentally healthy older person possesses a sense of ego integrity and self-acceptance that will help in adapting to the ambiguities of the future with a sense of security and optimism.

Murray and Zentner (2001) state:

> Having accomplished the earlier [developmental] tasks, the person accepts life as his or her own and as the only life for the self. He or she would wish for none other and would defend the meaning and the dignity of the lifestyle. The person has further refined the characteristics of maturity described for the middle-aged adult, achieving both wisdom and an enriched perspective about life and people. (p. 800)

Everyone, particularly healthcare workers, should see aging people as individuals, each with specific needs and abilities, rather than as a stereotypical group. Some individuals may seem "old" at 40, whereas others may not seem "old" at 70. Variables such as attitude, mental health, physical health, and degree of independence strongly influence how an individual perceives himself or herself. Surely, in the final analysis, whether one is considered "old" must be self-determined.

EPIDEMIOLOGICAL STATISTICS

The Population

In 1980, Americans 65 years of age or older numbered 25.5 million. By 2000, these numbers had increased to approximately 35 million, representing 12.4 percent of the population (Administration on Aging [AoA], 2002). This trend is expected to continue, with a projection for 2030 at about 70 million, or 20 percent of the population.

Marital Status

In 2001, of individuals age 65 and older, 73 percent of men and 41 percent of women were married (AoA, 2002). Forty-six percent of all women in this age group were widowed. There were over four times as many widows as widowers because women live longer than men and tend to marry men older than themselves.

Living Arrangements

The majority of individuals age 65 or older live alone, with a spouse, or with relatives (AoA, 2002). At any one time, fewer than 5 percent of people in this age group live in institutions. This percentage increases dramatically with age, ranging from 1.1 percent for persons 65 to 74 years, to 4.7 percent for persons 75 to 84 years, and to 18.2 percent for persons 85 and older. See Figure 23–1 for a distribution of living arrangements.

Economic Status

Approximately 3.4 million persons age 65 or older were below the poverty level in 2001 (AoA, 2002). Older women had a higher poverty rate than older men, and older Hispanic women living alone had the highest poverty rate. Poor people who have worked all their lives can expect to become poorer in old age, and others will become poor only after becoming old. However, there are a substantial number of affluent older persons who enjoy a high quality of life.

Of individuals in this age group, 80 percent owned their own homes in 2001 (AoA, 2002). However, the housing of this population of Americans is usually older and less adequate than that of the younger population; therefore, a higher percentage of income must be spent on maintenance and repairs.

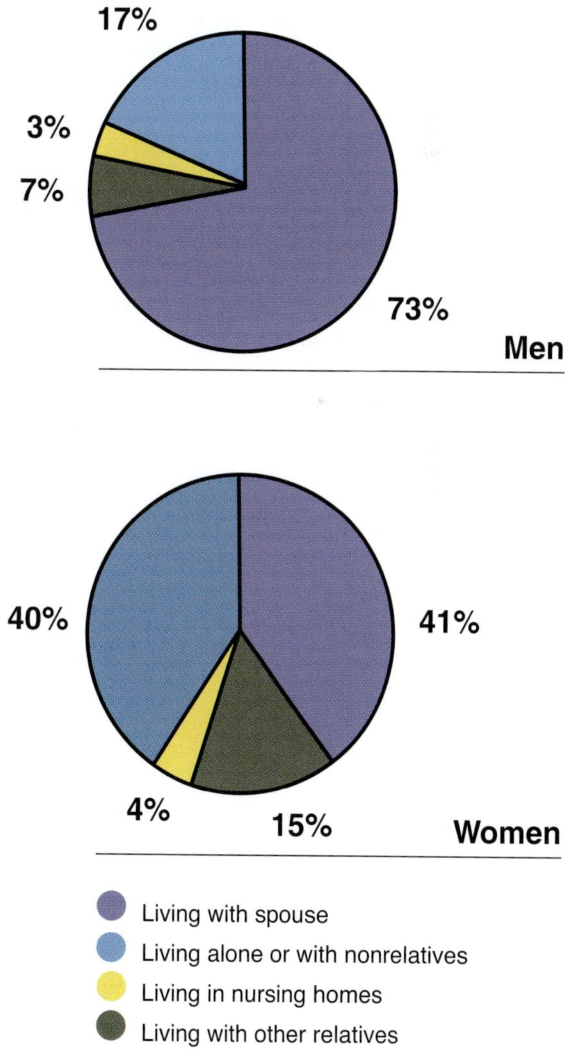

FIGURE 23–1. Living arrangement of persons age 65 and older (2000).

Employment

With the passage of the Age Discrimination in Employment Act in 1967, forced retirement has been virtually eliminated in the workplace. Evidence suggests that involvement in purposeful activity is vital to successful adaptation and perhaps even to survival. Individuals age 65 or older constituted 3 percent of the U.S. labor force in 2001 (AoA, 2002).

Health Status

The number of days in which usual activities are restricted because of illness or injury increases with age. In 2000, 26.1 percent of individuals between 65 and 74 and 45.1 percent of those 75 and older reported that their activities were limited by chronic conditions (AoA, 2002). Most older individuals have at least one chronic medical condition, and many have more than one. The most commonly occurring conditions among the elderly population are arthritis, hypertension, hearing impairments, heart disease, cataracts, orthopedic impairments, sinusitis, and diabetes (AoA, 2002).

Emotional and mental illnesses increase over the life cycle. Depression is particularly prevalent, and suicide is increasing among elderly Americans. Organic mental disease increases dramatically in old age.

THEORIES OF AGING*

Donlon (1999) describes a number of theories related to the aging process. These theories are grouped into two broad categories: biological and psychosocial.

Biological Theories

Biological theories attempt to explain the physical process of aging, including molecular and cellular changes in the major organ systems and the body's ability to function adequately and resist disease. They also attempt to explain why people age differently and what factors affect longevity and the body's ability to resist disease.

*This section was adapted from Donlon, B.C. (1999). In M. Stanley & P.G. Beare (Eds.), Gerontological nursing: A health promotion/protection approach (2nd ed.). Philadelphia: F.A. Davis. With permission.

Genetic Theory

According to genetic theory, aging is an involuntarily inherited process that operates over time to alter cellular or tissue structures (Cristofalo, 1996). This theory suggests that life span and longevity changes are predetermined. Donlon (1999) states:

> Genetic theories posit that the replication process at the cellular level becomes deranged by inappropriate information provided from the cell nucleus. The DNA molecule becomes cross-linked with another substance that alters the genetic information. The cross-linking results in errors at the cellular level that eventually cause the body's organs and systems to fail. (p. 10)

The development of free radicals, collagen, and lipofuscin in the aging body, and of an increased frequency in the occurrence of cancer and autoimmune disorders, provide some evidence for this theory and the proposition that error or mutation occurs at the molecular and cellular level.

Wear-and-Tear Theory

Proponents of this theory believe that the body wears out on a scheduled basis. Free radicals, which are the waste products of metabolism, accumulate and cause damage to important biological structures. Free radicals are molecules with unpaired electrons that exist normally in the body; they also are produced by ionizing radiation, ozone, and chemical toxins. According to this theory, these free radicals cause DNA damage, cross-linkage of collagen, and the accumulation of age pigments.

Environmental Theory

According to this theory, factors in the environment (e.g., industrial carcinogens, sunlight, trauma, and infection) bring about changes in the aging process (Birren & Bengtson, 1998). Although these factors are known to accelerate aging, the impact of the environment is a secondary rather than a primary factor in aging. Science is only beginning to uncover the many environmental factors that affect aging.

Immunity Theory

The immunity theory describes an age-related decline in the immune system. As people age, their ability to defend against foreign organisms decreases and results in susceptibility to diseases such as cancer and infection. Along with the diminished immune function, a rise in the body's autoimmune response occurs, leading to the development of autoimmune diseases such as rheumatoid arthritis and allergies to food and environmental agents.

Neuroendocrine Theory

This theory proposes that aging occurs because of a slowing of the secretion of certain hormones that have an impact on reactions regulated by the nervous system. This is most clearly demonstrated in the pituitary gland, thyroid, adrenals, and the glands of reproduction. Wise, Krajnak, and Kashon (1996) suggest that although credence has been given to a predictable biological clock that controls fertility, there is much more to be learned from the study of the neuroendocrine system in relation to a systemic aging process that is controlled by a "clock."

Psychosocial Theories

Psychosocial theories focus on social and psychological changes that accompany advancing age, as opposed to the biological implications of anatomic deterioration. Several theories have attempted to describe how attitudes and behavior in the early phases of life affect people's reactions during the late phase. This work is called the process of "successful aging."

Personality Theory

Personality theories address aspects of psychological growth without delineating specific tasks or expectations of older adults. These theories suggest that as individuals traverse life experiences, they become increasingly different (Sadavoy, Lazarus, & Jarvik, 1991). In extreme old age, however, people show greater similarity in certain characteristics, probably because of similar declines in biological functioning and societal opportunities.

In a classic study by Reichard, Livson, and Peterson (1962), the personalities of older men were classified into five major categories according to their patterns of adjustment to aging:

1. *Mature men* are considered well-balanced persons who maintain close personal relationships. They accept both the strengths and weaknesses of their age, finding little to regret about retirement and approaching most problems in a relaxed or convivial manner without continually having to assess blame.
2. *"Rocking chair" personalities* are found in passive-dependent individuals who are content to lean on others for support, to disengage, and to let most of life's activities pass them by.
3. *Armored men* have well-integrated defense mechanisms, which serve as adequate protection. Rigid and stable, they present a strong silent front and often rely on activity as an expression of their continuing independence.
4. *Angry men* are bitter about life, themselves, and other people. Aggressiveness is common, as is suspicion of others, especially of minorities or women. With little tolerance for ambiguity or frustration, they have always shown some instability in work and their personal lives, and now feel extremely threatened by old age.
5. *Self-haters* are similar to angry men, except that most of their animosity is turned inward on themselves. Seeing themselves as dismal failures, being old only depresses them more.

The investigators identified the mature, "rocking chair," or armored categories as characteristic of healthy, adjusted individuals and the angry and self-hater categories as those who are less successful in aging. In all cases, the evidence suggested that the personalities of the subjects, although distinguished by age-specific criteria, had not changed appreciably throughout most of adulthood.

Developmental Task Theory

Developmental tasks are the activities and challenges that one must accomplish at specific stages in life to achieve successful aging. Erikson (1963) described the primary task of old age as being able to see one's life as having been lived with integrity. In the absence of achieving that sense of having lived well, the older adult is at risk for becoming preoccupied with feelings of regret or despair.

Disengagement Theory

Disengagement theory describes the process of withdrawal by older adults from societal roles and responsibilities. According to the theory, this withdrawal process is predictable, systematic, inevitable, and necessary for the proper functioning of a growing society.

Older adults were said to be happy when social contacts diminished and responsibilities were assumed by a younger generation. The benefit to the older adult is thought to be in providing time for reflecting on life's accomplishments and for coming to terms with unfulfilled expectations. The benefit to society is thought to be an orderly transfer of power from old to young.

There have been many critics of this theory, and the postulates have been challenged. For many healthy and productive older individuals, the prospect of a slower pace and fewer responsibilities is undesirable.

Activity Theory

In direct opposition to the disengagement theory is the activity theory of aging, which holds that the way to age successfully is to stay active. Multiple studies have validated the positive relationship between maintaining meaningful interaction with others and physical and mental well-being.

Sadock and Sadock (2003) suggest that social integration is the prime factor in determining psychosocial adaptation in later life. Social integration refers to how the aging individual is included and takes part in the life and activities of his or her society. This theory holds that the maintenance of activities is important to most people as a basis for deriving and sustaining satisfaction, self-esteem, and health.

Continuity Theory

This theory emphasizes the individual's previously established coping abilities and personality as a basis for predicting how the person will adjust to the changes of aging. Basic personality traits are said to remain unchanged as a person ages. Furthermore, personality traits typically become more pronounced as a person ages. A person who enjoys the company of others and an active social life will continue to enjoy this lifestyle into old age. One who prefers solitude and a limited number of activities will probably find satisfaction in a continuation of this lifestyle.

Maintenance of internal continuity is motivated by the need for preservation of self-esteem, ego integrity, cognitive function, and social support. As they age, individuals maintain their self-concept by reinterpreting their current experiences so that old values can take on new meanings in keeping with present circumstances. Internal self-concepts and beliefs are not readily vulnerable to environmental change; and external continuity in skills, activities, roles, and relationships can remain remarkably stable into the 70s. Physical illness or death of friends and loved ones may preclude continued social interaction (Sadock & Sadock, 2003).

THE NORMAL AGING PROCESS

Biological Aspects of Aging

Individuals are unique in their physical and psychological aging processes, as influenced by their predisposition or resistance to illness; the effects of their external environment and behaviors; their exposure to trauma, infections, and past diseases; and the health and illness practices they have adopted during their life span (Leventhal, 1991). As the individual ages, there is a quantitative loss of cells and changes in many of the enzymatic activities within cells, resulting in a diminished responsiveness to biological demands made on the body. Age-related changes occur at different rates for different individuals, although in actuality, when growth stops, aging begins. Virtually all growth ceases with puberty (Leventhal, 1991). This section presents a brief overview of the normal biological changes that occur with the aging process.

Skin

One of the most dramatic changes that occur in aging is the loss of elastin in the skin. This effect, as well as changes in collagen, causes aged skin to wrinkle and sag. Excessive exposure to sunlight compounds these changes and increases the risk of developing skin cancer (Williams, 1995).

Fat redistribution results in a loss of the subcutaneous cushion of adipose tissue. Thus, older people lose "insulation" and are more sensitive to extremes of ambient temperature than are younger people (Wiersema & Stanley, 1999). Fewer blood vessels to the skin result in a slower rate of healing.

Cardiovascular System

The age-related decline in the cardiovascular system is thought to be the major determinant of decreased tolerance for exercise and loss of conditioning, and thus the major factor contributing to feelings of agedness and overall decline in energy reserve (Leventhal, 1991). The aging heart is characterized by modest hypertrophy, with reduced ventricular compliance and diminished cardiac output (Sadock & Sadock, 2003; Murray & Zentner, 2001). This results in a decrease in response to work demands and some diminishment of blood flow to the brain, kidneys, liver, and muscles. Heart rate also slows with time. If arteriosclerosis is present, cardiac function is further compromised.

Respiratory System

Thoracic expansion is diminished by an increase in fibrous tissue and loss of elastin. Pulmonary vital capacity decreases, and the amount of residual air increases. Scattered areas of fibrosis in the alveolar septa interfere with exchange of oxygen and carbon dioxide. These changes are accelerated by the use of cigarettes or other inhaled substances. Cough and laryngeal reflexes are reduced, causing decreased ability to defend the airway. Decreased pulmonary blood flow and diffusion ability results in reduced efficiency in responding to sudden respiratory demands.

Musculoskeletal System

Skeletal aging involving the bones, muscles, ligaments, and tendons probably generates the most frequent limitations on activities of daily living experienced by aging individuals. Loss of muscle mass is significant, although this occurs more slowly in men than in women. Demineralization of the bones occurs at a rate of about 1 percent per year throughout the life span in both men and women. However, this increases to approximately 10 percent in women around **menopause**, making them particularly vulnerable to **osteoporosis**.

Individual muscle fibers become thinner and less elastic with age. Muscles become less flexible following disuse. There is diminished storage of muscle glycogen, resulting in loss of energy reserve for increased activity. These changes are accelerated by nutritional deficiencies and inactivity.

Gastrointestinal System

In the oral cavity, the teeth show a reduction in dentine production, shrinkage and fibrosis of root pulp, gingival retraction, and loss of bone density in the alveolar ridges (Leventhal, 1991). There is some loss of peristalsis in the stomach and intestines, and gastric acid production decreases. Levels of intrinsic factor may also decrease, resulting in vitamin B_{12} malabsorption in some aging individuals. A significant decrease in absorptive surface area of the small intestine may be associated with some decline in nutrient absorption. Motility slowdown of the large intestine, combined with poor dietary habits, dehydration, lack of exercise, and some medications, may give rise to problems with constipation.

There is a modest decrease in size and weight of the liver resulting in losses in enzyme activity required to deactivate certain medications by the liver. These age-related changes can influence the metabolism and excretion of these medications. These changes, along with the pharmacokinetics of the drug, must be considered when giving medications to aging individuals.

Endocrine System

A decreased level of thyroid hormones causes a lowered basal metabolic rate. Decreased amounts of adrenocorticotropic hormone may result in less efficient stress response.

Impairments in glucose tolerance are evident in aging individuals (Dellasega, Yonushonis, & Johnson, 1999). Studies of glucose challenges show that insulin levels are equivalent to or slightly higher than those from younger challenged individuals, although peripheral insulin resistance appears to play a significant role in carbohydrate intolerance. The observed glucose clearance abnormalities and insulin resistance in older people may be related to many factors other than biological aging (e.g., obesity, family history of diabetes) and may be influenced substantially by diet or exercise.

Genitourinary System

Age-related declines in renal function occur because of a steady attrition of nephrons and sclerosis within the glomeruli over time (Kee, 1999). The total renal blood flow declines at a steady rate of about 10 percent a year after age 20; therefore, glomerular filtration has decreased approximately 50 percent by age 80 (Pikna, 1994). Elderly people are prone to develop the syndrome of inappropriate antidiuretic hormone secretion, and levels of blood urea nitrogen and creatinine may be elevated slightly. The overall decline in renal functioning has serious implications for physicians in prescribing medications for elderly individuals.

In men, enlargement of the prostate gland is common as aging occurs. Prostatic hypertrophy is associated with an increased risk for urinary retention and may be a cause of urinary incontinence (Williams, 1995). Loss of muscle and sphincter control, as well as the use of some medications, may cause urinary incontinence in women. Not only is this problem a cause of social stigma, but also, if left untreated, it increases the risk of urinary tract infection and local skin irritation. Normal changes in the genitalia are discussed in the section on "Sexual Aspects of Aging."

Immune System

Aging results in changes in both cell-mediated and antibody-mediated immune responses (Larocco, 1994). The size of the thymus gland declines continuously from just beyond puberty to about 15 percent of its original size at age 50. The consequences of these changes include a greater susceptibility to infections and a diminished inflammatory response that results in delayed healing. There is also evidence of an increase in various autoantibodies (e.g., rheumatoid factor) as a person ages, increasing the risk of autoimmune disorders (Pikna, 1994).

Because of the overall decrease in efficiency of the immune system, the proliferation of abnormal cells is facilitated in the elderly individual. Cancer is the best example of aberrant cells allowed to proliferate due to the ineffectiveness of the immune system.

Nervous System

With aging, there is an absolute loss of neurons, which correlates with decreases in brain weight of about 10 percent by age 90 (Murray & Zentner, 2001). Gross morphological examination reveals gyral atrophy in the frontal, temporal, and parietal lobes; widening of the sulci; and ventricular enlargement. However, it must be remembered that these changes have been identified in careful study of adults with normal intellectual function.

The brain has enormous reserve, and little cerebral function is lost over time, although greater functional decline is noted in the periphery (Roussel, 1999). There appears to be a disproportionately greater loss of cells in the cerebellum, the locus ceruleus, the substantia nigra, and olfactory bulbs, accounting for some of the more characteristic aging behaviors such as mild gait disturbances, sleep disruptions, and decreased smell and taste perception (Williams, 1995).

Some of the age-related changes within the nervous system may be a result of alterations in neurotransmitter release, uptake, turnover, catabolism, or receptor functions (Roussel, 1999). A great deal of attention is being given to brain biochemistry and in particular to the neurotransmitters acetylcholine, dopamine, norepinephrine, and epinephrine. These biochemical changes may be responsible for the altered responses of many older persons to stressful events and some biological treatments.

Sensory Systems

VISION. Visual acuity begins to decrease in midlife. Presbyopia (blurred near vision) is the standard marker of aging of the eye. It is caused by a loss of elasticity of the crystalline lens and results in compromised accommodation.

Cataract development is inevitable if the individual lives long enough for the changes to occur. Cataracts are formed when pigment accumulates in the lens fibers and lens proteins become insoluble and rigid (Curtis & Carroll, 1994).

The color in the iris may fade, and the pupil may become irregular in shape. A decrease in production of secretions by the lacrimal glands may cause dryness and result in increased irritation and infection. The pupil may become constricted, requiring an increase in light needed for reading.

HEARING. Hearing changes significantly with the aging process. Gradually over time, the ear loses its sensitivity to discriminate sounds because of damage to the hair cells of the cochlea. The most dramatic decline appears to be in perception of high-frequency sounds.

Although hearing loss is significant in all aging individuals, the decline is more dramatic in men than in women. Men are twice as likely as women are to have hearing loss (Murray & Zentner, 2001).

TASTE AND SMELL. Taste sensitivity decreases over the life span. Taste discrimination decreases, and bitter taste sensations predominate. Sensitivity to sweet and salty tastes is diminished.

The deterioration of the olfactory bulbs is accompanied by loss of smell acuity. The aromatic component of taste perception diminishes.

TOUCH AND PAIN. Organized sensory nerve receptors on the skin continue to decrease throughout the life span; thus, the touch threshold increases with age (Leventhal, 1991). The ability to feel pain also decreases in response to these changes, and the ability to perceive and interpret painful stimuli changes. These changes have critical implications for the elderly in their potential lack of ability to use sensory warnings for escaping serious injury.

Psychological Aspects of Aging

Memory Functioning

Age-related memory deficiencies have been extensively reported in the literature. Although **short-term memory** seems to deteriorate with age, perhaps because of poorer sorting strategies, **long-term memory** does not show similar changes. However, in nearly every instance, well-educated, mentally active people do not exhibit the same decline in memory functioning as their age peers who lack similar opportunities to flex their minds. Nevertheless, with few exceptions, the time required for memory scanning is longer for both recent and remote recall among older people, perhaps more because of social and health factors than any irreversible effects of age (Williams, 1995).

Intellectual Functioning

There appears to be a high degree of regularity in intellectual functioning across the adult age span. Crystallized abilities, or knowledge acquired in the course of the socialization process, tend to remain stable over the adult life span. Fluid abilities, or abilities involved in solving novel problems, tend to decline gradually from young to old adulthood. In other words, intellectual abilities of older people do not decline but do become obsolete. The age of their formal educational experiences is reflected in their intelligence scoring.

Learning Ability

The ability to learn is not diminished by age. Studies, however, have shown that some aspects of learning do change with age. The ordinary slowing of reaction time with age for nearly all tasks or the over-arousal of the central nervous system may account for lower performance levels on tests requiring rapid responses. Under conditions that allow for self-pacing by the participant, differences in accuracy of performance diminish. Ability to learn continues throughout life, although strongly influenced by interests, activity, motivation, health, and income (Williams, 1995). Adjustments do need to be made in teaching methodology and time allowed for learning.

Adaptation to the Tasks of Aging

LOSS AND GRIEF. Individuals experience losses from the very beginning of life. By the time individuals reach their 60s and 70s, they have experienced numerous losses, and mourning has become a lifelong process. Those who are most successful at adapting earlier in life will similarly cope better with the losses and grief inherent in aging (Cath & Sadavoy, 1991). Unfortunately, with the aging process comes a convergence of losses, the timing of which makes it impossible for the aging individual to complete the grief process in response to one loss before another occurs. Because grief is cumulative, this can result in **bereavement overload**, which has been implicated in the predisposition to depression in the elderly.

ATTACHMENT TO OTHERS. Many studies have confirmed the importance of interpersonal relationships at all stages in the life cycle. So important is the need for **attachment** that studies have shown that having a confidant, or the availability of a formal or informal caregiver, is the most critical factor discriminating between elderly who remain in the community and those who are institutionalized (Williams, 1995). These findings are consistent with the activity theory of aging that correlates the importance of social integration with successful adaptation in later life.

MAINTENANCE OF SELF-IDENTITY. Several authors have asserted that self-concept and self-image remain stable and do not become impoverished or negative in old age (Cath & Sadavoy, 1991). A study by Vaillant and Vaillant (1990) found that the factors that favored good psychosocial adjustment in later life were sustained family relationships, maturity of ego defenses, absence of alcoholism, and absence of depressive disorder. Studies show that the elderly have a strong need for and remarkable capability of retaining a persistent self-concept in the face of the many changes that contribute to instability in later life.

DEALING WITH DEATH. Death anxiety among the aging is apparently more of a myth than a reality. Studies have not supported the negative view of death as an overriding psychological factor in the aging process (Cath & Sadavoy, 1991). Various investigators who have worked with dying persons report that it is not death itself, but abandonment, pain, and confusion that are feared. What many desire most is someone to talk with, to show them their life's meaning is not shattered merely because they are about to die (Kübler-Ross, 1969; Murray & Zentner, 2001).

PSYCHIATRIC DISORDERS IN LATER LIFE. The later years constitute a time of especially high risk for emotional distress. Sadock and Sadock, (2003) state:

> Several psychosocial risk factors predispose older people to mental disorders. These risk factors include loss of social roles, loss of autonomy, the deaths of friends and relatives, declining health, increased isolation, financial constraints, and decreased cognitive functioning. (p. 1320)

Dementing disorders are the most common causes of psychopathology in the elderly (Sadock & Sadock, 2003). About half of these disorders are of the Alzheimer's type, which is characterized by an insidious onset and a gradually progressive course of cognitive impairment. No curative treatment is currently available. Symptomatic treatments, including pharmacological interventions, attention to the environment, and family support, can help to maximize the client's level of functioning.

Delirium is one of the most common and important forms of psychopathology in later life. A number of factors have been identified that predispose elderly people to delirium, including structural brain disease, reduced capacity for homeostatic regulation, impaired vision and hearing, a high prevalence of chronic disease, reduced resistance to acute stress, and age-related changes in the pharmacokinetic and pharmacodynamics of drugs. Delirium needs to be recognized and the underlying condition treated as soon as possible. A high mortality is associated with this condition (Williams, 1995).

Depressive disorders are the most common affective illnesses occurring after the middle years. The incidence of increased depression among elderly people is influenced by the variables of physical illness, functional disability, cognitive impairment, and loss of a spouse (Sadock & Sadock, 2003; Williams, 1995). Hypochondriacal symptoms are common in the depressed elderly. Symptomatology often mimics that of dementia, a condition that is referred to as pseudodementia. (See Table 12–3 for a comparison of the symptoms of dementia and pseudodementia.) Suicide is more prevalent in the elderly, with economic status being considered an important influencing factor. Treatment of depression in the elderly individual is with psychotropic medications or electroconvulsive therapy.

Schizophrenia and delusional disorders may continue into old age or may manifest themselves for the first time only during senescence (Blazer, 2003). In many instances, individuals who manifest psychotic disorders early in life show a decline in psychopathology as they age. Late-onset schizophrenia (after age 60) is not common, but when it does occur, it often is characterized by delusions or hallucinations of a persecutory nature. The course is chronic, and treatment is with neuroleptics and supportive psychotherapy.

Most anxiety disorders begin in early to middle adulthood, but some appear for the first time after age 60. Kaplan and Sadock (1998) state:

> The fragility of the autonomic nervous system in older persons may account for the development of anxiety after a major stressor. Because of concurrent physical disability, older persons react more severely to post-traumatic stress disorder than younger persons. (p. 1325)

In older adults, symptoms of anxiety and depression tend to accompany each other, making it difficult to determine which disorder is dominant (Williams, 1995). Personality disorders are uncommon in the elderly population. The incidence of personality disorders among individuals over age 65 is less than 5 percent. Most elderly people with personality disorder have likely manifested the symptomatology for many years.

Sleep disorders are very common in the aging individual. Sleep disturbances affect 50 percent of people age 65 and older who live at home and 66 percent of those who live in long-term care facilities (Bahr, 1999). Some common causes of sleep disturbances among elderly people include age-dependent decreases in the ability to sleep ("sleep decay"); increased prevalence of sleep apnea; depression; dementia; anxiety; pain; impaired mobility; medications; and psychosocial factors such as loneliness, inactivity, and boredom. Benzodiazepines, along with non-pharmacological approaches, are often used as sleep aids with the elderly. Changes in aging associated with metabolism and elimination must be considered when maintenance benzodiazepine therapy is administered for chronic insomnia in the aging client.

Sociocultural Aspects of Aging

Old age brings many important socially induced changes, some of which have the potential for negative effect on both the physical and mental well-being of older people. In American society, old age is defined arbitrarily as being 65 years or older because, historically, that is the age when most people have been able to retire with full Social Security and other pension benefits. (Recent legislation has increased the age beyond 65 years for full Social Security benefits.)

Elderly people in virtually all cultures share some basic needs and interests. There is little doubt that most individuals choose to live the most satisfying life possible until their demise. They want protection from hazards and release from the weariness of everyday tasks. They want to be treated with the respect and dignity that is deserving of individuals who have reached this pinnacle in life; and they want to die with the same respect and dignity.

From the beginning of human culture, the aged have had a special status in society. Even today, in some cultures the aged are the most powerful, the most engaged, and the most respected members of the society. This has not been the case in the modern industrial societies, although trends in the status of the aged differ widely between one industrialized country and another. For example, the status and integration of the aged in Japan have remained relatively high when compared with the other industrialized nations. The aged are awarded a position of honor in cultures that place emphasis on family cohesiveness. In these cultures, the aged are revered for their knowledge and wisdom gained through their years of life experiences (Giger & Davidhizar, 1991).

Many negative stereotypes color the perspective on aging in the United States. Ideas that elderly individuals are always tired or sick, slow and forgetful, isolated and lonely, unproductive, and angry determine the way younger individuals relate to the elderly in this society. Increasing disregard for the elderly has resulted in a type of segregation, as aging individuals voluntarily seek out or are involuntarily placed in special residences for the aged.

Assisted living centers, retirement apartment complexes, and even entire retirement communities intended solely for individuals over age 50, are becoming increasingly common. In 2000, about half (52 percent) of persons age 65 and older lived in nine states, with the majority in California, Florida, and New York (AoA, 2002). It is important for elderly individuals to feel part of an integrated group, and they are migrating to these areas in an effort to achieve this integration. This phenomenon provides additional corroboration for the activity theory of aging and the importance of attachment to others.

Employment is another area in which the elderly experience discrimination. Although compulsory retirement has been virtually eliminated, discrimination still exists in hiring and promotion practices. Many employers are not eager to retain or hire older workers. It is difficult to determine how much of the failure to hire and promote results from discrimination based on age alone and how much of it is related to a realistic and fair appraisal of the aged employee's ability and efficiency. It is true that some elderly individuals are no longer capable of doing as good a job as a younger worker; however, there are many who likely can do a *better* job than their younger counterparts can, given the opportunity. Nevertheless, surveys have shown that some employers accept the negative stereotypes about elderly individuals and believe that older workers are hard to please, set in their ways, less productive, frequently absent, and involved in more accidents.

The status of the elderly may improve with time and as their numbers increase with the aging of the "baby boomers." As older individuals gain political power, the benefits and privileges designed for the elderly will increase. There is power in numbers, and the 21st century promises power for persons age 65 and older.

Sexual Aspects of Aging

Sexuality and the sexual needs of elderly people are frequently misunderstood, condemned, stereotyped, ridiculed, repressed, and ignored. Americans have grown up in a society that has liberated sexual expression for all other age groups, but retains certain Victorian standards regarding sexual expression by the elderly. Negatively stereotyped notions concerning sexual interest and activity of the elderly are common. Some of these include ideas that older people have no sexual interests or desires; that they are sexually undesirable; or that they are all too fragile or too ill to engage in sexual activity. Some people even believe it is disgusting or comical to consider elderly individuals as sexual beings.

These cultural stereotypes undoubtedly play a large part in the misperception many people hold regarding sexuality of the aged, and they may be reinforced by the common tendency of the young to deny the inevitability of aging. With reasonable good health and an interesting and interested partner, there is no inherent reason why individuals should not enjoy an active sexual life well into late adulthood (Masters, Johnson, & Kolodny, 1995).

Physical Changes Associated with Sexuality

Many of the changes in sexuality that occur in later years are related to the physical changes that are taking place at that time of life.

CHANGES IN THE FEMALE. Menopause may begin anytime during the 40s or early 50s. During this time, there is a gradual decline in the functioning of the ovaries and the subsequent production of estrogen, which results in a number of changes. The walls of the vagina become thin and inelastic, the vagina itself shrinks in both width and length, and the amount of vaginal lubrication decreases noticeably. Orgastic uterine contractions may become spastic. All of these changes can result in painful penetration, vaginal burning, pelvic aching, or irritation on urination. In some women, the discomfort may be severe enough to result in an avoidance of intercourse. Paradoxically, these symptoms are more likely to occur with infrequent intercourse of only one time a month or less.

Regular and more frequent sexual activity results in a greater capacity for sexual performance (Masters, Johnson, & Kolodny, 1995). Other symptoms that are associated with menopause in some women include hot flashes, night sweats, sleeplessness, irritability, mood swings, migraine headaches, urinary incontinence, and weight gain.

Some menopausal women elect to take hormone replacement therapy for relief of these changes and symptoms. With estrogen therapy, the symptoms of menopause are minimized or do not occur at all. However, some women choose not to take the hormone because of an increased risk of breast cancer, and when given alone, an increased risk of endometrial cancer. To combat this latter effect, most women also take a second hormone, progesterone. Taken for 7 to 10 days during the month, progesterone decreases the risk of estrogen-induced endometrial cancer. Some physicians are electing to prescribe a low dose of progesterone that is taken, along with estrogen, for the entire month. A combination pill, taken in this manner, is also available.

Results of the Women's Health Initiative, recently reported in the *Journal of the American Medical Association*, indicate that the combination pill is associated with an increased risk of cardiovascular disease and breast cancer (Rossouw et al., 2002). Benefits related to colon cancer and osteoporosis were reported; however, investigators stopped this arm of the study and suggested discontinuation of this type of therapy.

CHANGES IN THE MALE. Testosterone production declines gradually over the years, beginning between ages 40 and 60. A major change resulting from this hormone reduction is that erections occur more slowly and require more direct genital stimulation. There also may be a modest decrease in the firmness of the erection in men older than age 60. The refractory period lengthens with age, increasing the amount of time following orgasm before the man may achieve another erection. The volume of ejaculate gradually decreases, and the force of ejaculation lessens. The testes become somewhat smaller, but most men continue to produce viable sperm well into old age. Prolonged control over ejaculation in middle-aged and elderly men may bring increased sexual satisfaction for both partners.

Sexual Behavior in the Elderly

Coital frequency in early marriage and the overall quantity of sexual activity between age 20 and 40 correlate significantly with frequency patterns of sexual activity during aging (Masters, Johnson, & Kolodny, 1995). Although sexual interest and behavior do appear to decline somewhat with age, studies show that significant numbers of elderly men and women have active and satisfying sex lives well into their 80s. A survey commissioned by the American Association of Retired Persons (AARP) and *Modern Maturity* magazine provided some revealing information regarding the sexual attitudes and behavior of senior citizens. Some statistics from the survey are summarized in Table 23–1. The information from this survey clearly indicates that sexual activity can and does continue well past the 70s for healthy, active individuals who have regular opportunities for sexual expression. Reinisch (1990) states:

> Some sexual patterns established early in life may continue as we age. Those who had lower frequencies of sexual activity in their youth may continue to have sex less frequently, but those who were more active are likely to continue being so in later years. (p. 228)

SPECIAL CONCERNS OF THE ELDERLY

Retirement

Statistics reflect that a larger percentage of Americans of both sexes are living longer and that many of them are retiring earlier. Reasons often given for the increasing pattern of early retirement include health problems, Social Security and other pension benefits, attractive "early out" packages offered by companies, and long-held plans (e.g., turning a hobby into a money-making situation). Even eliminating the mandatory retirement age and the possibility of delaying the age of eligibility for Social Security benefits from 65 to 67 by the year 2027 is not expected to have a significant effect on the trend toward earlier retirement.

Sadock and Sadock (2003) report that of those people who voluntarily retire, most reenter the work force within 2 years. The reasons they give for doing this include negative reactions to being retired, feelings of being unproductive, economic hardship, and loneliness.

About 4.3 million older Americans were in the labor force (working or actively seeking work) in 2001. These included 2.5 million men and 1.8 million women, and constituted 3 percent of the U.S. labor force (AoA, 2002).

TABLE 23–1 AARP/Modern Maturity Survey on Sexual Attitudes and Behavior (A survey of Americans ages 45 and older)

	Ages	Men	Women	Both
Have sex at least once a week	45–59			~ 50%
	60–74	30%	24%	
Have sex at least once a month	45 and older			> 70%
Extremely or very satisfied with their physical relationships	All	67%	61%	
Very satisfied with emotional relationship	All	70%	62%	
Report sexual activity is important to their overall quality of life	All	60%	35%	
Believe non-marital sex is okay	< 60		66%	
	60–74		50%	
	≥ 75		33%	
	All	A majority of men of all ages believe non-marital sex is okay.		
Report having a chronic health problem affecting sex life	All			20%
Report taking hormone replacement therapy	45–59		36%	
	≥ 75		10%	
Report having taken antidepressant therapy	45–59		14%	
	60–74		8%	
Report prostate problems interfere with sex life	All	18%		
Report being treated for prostate problems	All	50%		
Reported being impotent	< 60	2.5%		
	60–74	16%		
	≥ 75	37%		
Report using a medicine, hormone, or other treatment for impotence	All	10%		
Describe their partners as physically attractive	45–59	59%	52%	
	≥ 75	63%	57%	
What would most improve your sex life?	45–59			Less stress/more free time
	≥ 60	Better health		
	60–74		Better health for partner	
	≥ 75		Finding a partner	

Adapted from Jacoby (1999)

Retirement has both social and economical implications for elderly individuals. The role is fraught with a great deal of ambiguity and is one that requires many adaptations on the part of those involved.

Social Implications

Retirement is often anticipated as an achievement in principle, but met with a great deal of ambiguity when it actually occurs. Our society places a great deal of importance on productivity, making as much money as possible, and doing it at as young an age as possible. These types of values contribute to the ambiguity associated with retirement. Although leisure has been acknowledged as a legitimate reward for workers, leisure during retirement historically has lacked the same social value. Adjustment to this life cycle event becomes more difficult in the face of societal values that are in direct conflict with the new lifestyle.

Historically, many women have derived a good deal of their self-esteem from their families—birthing them, rearing them, and being a "good mother." Likewise, many men have achieved self-esteem through work-related activities—creativity, productivity, and earning money. With the termination of these activities may come a loss of self-worth, resulting in depression in some individuals who are unable to adapt satisfactorily. Murray and Zentner (2001) list four developmental tasks related to successful adaptation in retirement:

- Remaining actively involved and having a sense of belonging unrelated to work
- Reevaluating life satisfaction related to family and social relations and spiritual life rather than to work
- Reevaluating the world's outlook, keeping a view of the world that is coherent and meaningful and a view that one's own world is meaningful
- Maintaining a sense of health, integrating mind and body to avoid complaints or illness when work is no longer the focus (p. 811)

American society often identifies an individual by his or her occupation. This is reflected in the conversation of people who are meeting each other for the first time. Undoubtedly, most everyone has asked or been asked at some point in time, "What do you do?" or "Where do you work?" Occupation determines status, and retirement represents a significant change in status. The basic ambiguity of retirement occurs in an individual or society's definition of this change. Is it undertaken voluntarily or involuntarily? Is it desirable or undesirable? Is one's status made better or worse by the change?

In looking at the trend of the past two decades, we may presume that retirement is becoming, and will continue to become, more accepted by societal standards. With more and more individuals retiring earlier and living longer, the growing number of aging people will spend a significantly longer time in retirement. At present, retirement has become more of an institutionalized expectation and there appears to be increasing acceptance of it as a social status.

Economical Implications

Because retirement is generally associated with a 20 to 40 percent reduction in personal income, the standard of living after retirement may be adversely affected (Petras & Petras, 1991). Most older adults derive postretirement income from a combination of Social Security benefits, public and private pensions, and income from savings or investments.

In 2001, the median income in households containing families headed by persons 65 or over was $33,938, and 3.4 million elderly were below the poverty level (AoA, 2002). The rate of those living in poverty was higher among women than among men and higher among African-Americans and Latino Americans than whites.

The Social Security Act of 1935 promised assistance with financial security for elderly Americans. Since then, the original legislation has been modified, yet the basic philosophy remains intact. Its effectiveness, however, is now being questioned. Faced with deficits, the program is forced to pay benefits to those currently retired from both the reserve funds and monies being collected at present. There is genuine concern about future generations, when there may be no reserve funds from which to draw. Because many of the programs that benefit older adults depend on contributions from the younger population, the growing ratio of older Americans to younger people may affect society's ability to supply the goods and services necessary to meet this expanding demand.

Medicare and **Medicaid** were established by the government to provide medical care benefits for elderly and indigent Americans. Medicaid funds are matched by the states, and coverage varies significantly from state to state. Medicare covers only a percentage of healthcare costs; therefore, to reduce risk related to out-of-pocket expenditures, many older adults purchase private "medigap" policies designed to cover charges in excess of those approved by Medicare.

The magnitude of retirement earnings depends almost entirely on preretirement income. The poor will remain poor and the wealthy are unlikely to lower their status during retirement; however, for many in the middle classes, the relatively fixed income sources may be inadequate, possibly forcing them to face financial hardship for the first time in their lives.

Long-Term Care

The concept of long-term care covers a broad spectrum of comprehensive health and wellness and support services to provide the physical, psychological, social, spiritual, and economic needs of people with chronic illness or disabilities (Millsap, 1999). Long-term care facilities are defined by the level of care they provide. They may be skilled nursing facilities, intermediate care facilities, or a combination of the two. Some institutions provide convalescent care for individuals recovering from acute illness or injury, some provide long-term care for individuals with chronic illness or disabilities, and still others provide both types of assistance.

Most elderly individuals prefer to remain in their own homes or in the homes of family members for as long as this can meet their needs without deterioration of family or social patterns. Many elderly individuals are placed in institutions as a last resort only after heroic effects have been made to keep them in their own or a relative's home. The increasing emphasis on home healthcare has extended the period of independence for aging individuals.

In 2000, 4.5 percent of the population age 65 and older lived in nursing homes (AoA, 2002). The percentage increased dramatically with age, ranging from 1.1 percent for persons age 65 to 74, 4.7 percent for persons age 75 to 84, to 18.2 percent for persons age 85 and older. A profile of the "typical" elderly nursing home resident is about 80 years of age, white, female, widowed, with multiple chronic health conditions (Ignatavicius, 1998; Millsap, 1999).

In determining who in our society will need long-term care, several factors have been identified that appear to place people at risk (Ignatavicius, 1998; Williams, 1995). The following risk factors are taken into consideration to predict potential need for services and to estimate future costs.

AGE. Because people grow older in very different ways, and the range of differences becomes greater with the passage of time, age is becoming a less relevant characteristic than it was historically. However, because of the high prevalence of chronic health conditions and disabilities, as well as the greater chance of diminishing social supports associated with advancing age, the 65-and-older population is often viewed as an important long-term care target group.

HEALTH. Level of functioning, as determined by ability to perform various behaviors or activities—such as bathing, eating, mobility, meal preparation, handling finances, judgment, and memory—is a measurable risk factor. The need for ongoing assistance from another person is critical in determining the need for long-term care.

MENTAL HEALTH STATUS. Mental health problems are risk factors in assessing need for long-term care. Many of the symptoms associated with certain mental disorders (especially the dementias) such as memory loss, impaired judgment, impaired intellect, and disorientation would render the individual incapable of meeting the demands of daily living independently.

SOCIOECONOMIC AND DEMOGRAPHIC FACTORS. Low income generally is associated with greater physical and mental health problems among the elderly. Because many elderly individuals have limited finances, they are less able to purchase care resources available outside of institutions (e.g., home healthcare), although Medicare and Medicaid now contribute a limited amount to this type of noninstitutionalized care.

Women are at greater risk of being institutionalized than men are, not because they are less healthy but because they tend to live longer and, thus, are usually older and more likely to be widowed. Whites have a higher rate of institutionalization than nonwhites. This may be related to cultural and financial influences.

MARITAL STATUS, LIVING ARRANGEMENT, AND THE INFORMAL SUPPORT NETWORK. Individuals who are married and living with a spouse are the least likely of all disabled people to be institutionalized. Those who live alone without resources for home care and few or no relatives living nearby to provide informal care are at higher risk for institutionalization.

Attitudinal Factors

Williams (1995) states:

> The diversified highly regulated nursing home of today is a far cry from the nursing home of 30 years ago or the unsupervised, limited service, privately financed home for the poor that was common at the turn of the century. (p. 103)

State and national licensing boards perform periodic inspections to ensure that standards set forth by the federal government are being met. These standards address quality of patient care as well as adequacy of the nursing home facility. Yet, many elderly individuals and their families perceive nursing homes as a place to go to die, and the fact that many of these institutions are poorly equipped, understaffed, and disorganized keeps this societal perception alive. There are, however, many excellent nursing homes that strive to go beyond the minimum federal regulations for Medicaid and Medicare reimbursement. In addition to medical, nursing, rehabilitation, and dental services, social and recreational services are provided to increase the quality of life for elderly people living in nursing homes. These activities include playing cards, bingo, and other games; parties; church activities; books; television; movies; arts and crafts, and other classes. Some nursing homes provide occupational and professional counseling. These facilities strive to enhance opportunities for improving quality of life and for becoming "places to live," rather than "places to die."

Elder Abuse

Abuse of elderly individuals, which at times has been referred to in the media as "**granny-bashing**," is a prevalent and serious form of family violence. Sadock and Sadock (2003) estimate that 10 percent of individuals over age 65 are the victims of abuse or neglect. The abuser is often a relative who lives with the elderly person and may be the assigned caregiver. Typical caregivers who are likely to be abusers of the elderly were described by Murray and Zentner (2001) as being under economic stress, substance abusers, themselves the victims of previous family violence, and exhausted and frustrated by the caregiver role. Identified risk factors for victims of abuse included being a white female age 70 and older, being mentally or physically impaired, being unable to meet daily self-care needs, and having care needs that exceeded the caretaker's ability.

Abuse of elderly individuals may be psychological, physical, or financial. Neglect may be intentional or unintentional. Psychological abuse includes yelling, insulting, harsh commands, threats, silence, and social isolation. Physical abuse is described as striking, shoving, beating, or restraint. Financial abuse refers to misuse or theft of finances, property, or material possessions. Neglect implies failure to do the obviously necessary things that a person cannot perform independently. Unintentional neglect is inadvertent, whereas intentional neglect is deliberate. Additionally, elderly individuals may be the victims of sexual abuse, which is sexual intimacy between two persons that occurs without the consent of one of the persons involved. Another type of abuse, which has been called "**granny-dumping**" by the media, involves abandoning elderly individuals at emergency departments, nursing homes, or other facilities—literally leaving them in the hands of others when the strain of caregiving becomes intolerable. Types of elder abuse are summarized in Table 23–2.

TABLE 23–2 Examples of Elder Abuse

Physical Abuse
Striking, hitting, beating
Shoving
Bruising
Cutting
Restraining
Psychological Abuse
Yelling
Insulting, name-calling
Harsh commands
Threats
Ignoring, silence, social isolation
Withholding of affection
Neglect (intentional or unintentional)
Withholding food and water
Inadequate heating
Unclean clothes and bedding
Lack of needed medication
Lack of eyeglasses, hearing aids, false teeth
Financial Abuse or Exploitation
Misuse of the elderly person's income by the caregiver
Forcing the elderly person to sign over financial affairs to another person against his or her will or without sufficient knowledge about the transaction
Sexual Abuse
Sexual molestation; rape
Any type of sexual intimacy against the elderly person's will

Adapted from Sadock & Sadock (2003) and Murray & Zentner (2001).

Elder victims often minimize the abuse or deny that it has occurred (Sadock & Sadock [2003]). The elderly person may be unwilling to disclose information because of fear of retaliation, embarrassment about the existence of abuse in the family, protectiveness toward a family member, or unwillingness to institute legal action. Adding to this unwillingness to report is the fact that infirm elders are often isolated so their mistreatment is less likely to be noticed by those who might be alert to symptoms of abuse. For these reasons, detection of abuse in the elderly is difficult at best.

Factors Contributing to Abuse

A number of contributing factors have been implicated in the abuse of elderly individuals.

LONGER LIFE. The 65-and-older age group has become the fastest growing segment of the population. Within this segment, the number of elderly older than age 75 has increased most rapidly. This trend is expected to continue well into the 21st century. The 75 and older age group is the one most likely to be physically or mentally impaired, requiring assistance and care from family members. This group also is the most vulnerable to abuse from caregivers.

DEPENDENCY. Dependency appears to be the most common precondition in domestic abuse. Changes associated with normal aging or induced by chronic illness often result in loss of self-sufficiency in the elderly person, requiring that they become dependent on another for assistance with daily functioning. Long life may also consume finances to the point that the elderly individual becomes financially dependent on another as well. This dependence increases the elderly person's vulnerability to abuse.

STRESS. The stress inherent in the caregiver role is a factor in most abuse cases. Some clinicians believe that elder abuse results from individual or family psychopathology. Others suggest that even psychologically healthy family members can become abusive as the result of the exhaustion and acute stress caused by overwhelming caregiving responsibilities. This is compounded in an age group that has been dubbed the "sandwich generation"—those individuals who elected to delay childbearing so that they are now at a point in their lives when they are "sandwiched" between providing care for their children and providing care for their aging parents.

LEARNED VIOLENCE. Children who have been abused or had abusive and violent parents are more likely to evolve into abusive adults. Fulmer (1999) states:

> Violence is a learned behavior that is passed down from generation to generation in some families because violence has been modeled as an acceptable coping behavior, with no substantial penalties for the behavior. This model suggests that a child who grows up in a violent family will also become violent. Some believe that elder mistreatment may be related to retribution on the part of an adult offspring who was abused as a child. (p. 268)

Identifying Elder Abuse

Because so many elderly individuals are reluctant to report personal abuse, healthcare workers need to be able to detect signs of mistreatment when they are in a position to do so. Table 23–2 listed a number of *types* of elder abuse. The following *manifestations* of the various categories of abuse have been identified (Fulmer, 1999; Murray & Zentner, 2001):

- Indicators of psychological abuse include a broad range of behaviors such as the symptoms associated with depression, withdrawal, anxiety, sleep disorders, and increased confusion or agitation.
- Indicators of physical abuse may include bruises, welts, lacerations, burns, punctures, evidence of hair pulling, and skeletal dislocations and fractures.
- Neglect may be manifested as consistent hunger, poor hygiene, inappropriate dress, consistent lack of supervision, consistent fatigue or listlessness, unattended physical problems or medical needs, or abandonment
- Sexual abuse may be suspected when the elderly person is presented with pain or itching in the genital area, bruising or bleeding in external genitalia, vaginal, or anal areas, or unexplained sexually transmitted disease.
- Financial abuse may be occurring when there is an obvious disparity between assets and satisfactory living conditions or when the elderly person complains of a sudden lack of sufficient funds for daily living expenses.

Healthcare workers often feel intimidated when confronted with cases of elder abuse. In these instances, referral to an individual experienced in management of victims of such abuse may be the most effective approach to evaluation and intervention. Healthcare workers are responsible for reporting any suspicions of elder abuse. The investigatory work is then conducted by regulatory agencies, which can determine whether the case is corroborated (Fulmer, 1999). Every effort must be made to ensure the client's safety, but it is important to remember that a competent elderly person has the right to choose his or her healthcare options. As inappropriate as it may seem, some elderly individuals choose to return to the abusive situation. In this instance, he or she should be provided with names and phone numbers to call for assistance if needed. A follow-up visit by an adult protective service representative should be conducted.

Increased efforts need to be made to ensure that healthcare providers have comprehensive training in the detection of and intervention in elder abuse. More research is needed to increase knowledge and understanding of the phenomenon of elder abuse and ultimately to effect more sophisticated strategies for prevention, intervention, and treatment.

Suicide

Although persons older than age 65 comprise only 12.4 percent of the population, they represent a disproportionately high percentage of individuals who commit suicide. Of all suicides, over 20 percent are committed by this age group, and suicide is the 15th leading cause of death among the elderly (Charbonneau, 2003). The group especially at risk appears to be white men. Predisposing factors include loneliness, financial problems, physical illness, loss, and depression (Sadock & Sadock, 2003).

Although the rate of suicide among the elderly remains high, the numbers of suicides among this age group dropped steadily from 1930 to 1980. Investigators who study these trends surmise that this decline was due to increases in services for older people and an understanding of their problems in society. However, from 1980 to 1986 the number of suicides among people age 65 and older increased by 25 percent, which suggests that other factors are contributing to the problem. It has been suggested that increased social isolation may be a contributing factor to suicide among the elderly. The number of elderly individuals who are divorced, widowed, or otherwise living alone has increased. In 1998, among men age 75 years and older the rate for divorced men was 3.4 times and widowed men was 2.6 times that for married men. In the same age group, the suicide rate for divorced women was 2.8 times and widowed women was 1.9 times the rate among married women (Center for Mental Health Services, 2002).

The National Institute of Mental Health [NIMH] (2001) suggests that major depression is a significant predictor of suicide in older adults. Unfortunately, it is widely under-recognized and under-treated by the medical community. The NIMH (2001) states:

> Several studies have found that many older adults who commit suicide have visited a primary care physician very close to the time of the suicide: *20 percent on the same day, 40 percent within 1 week, and 70 percent within 1 month of the suicide.* These findings point to the urgency of enhancing both the detection and the adequate treatment of depression as a means of reducing the risk of suicide among the elderly.

Many elderly individuals express symptoms associated with depression that are never recognized as such. Any sign of helplessness or hopelessness should elicit a supportive intervening response. In assessing suicide intention, direct questions should be asked, but concern and compassion should be used:

- Have you thought life is not worth living?
- Have you considered harming yourself?
- Do you have a plan for hurting yourself?
- Have you ever acted on that plan?
- Have you ever attempted suicide? (Buckwalter, 1999)

Components of intervention with a suicidal elderly person should include demonstrations of genuine concern, interest, and caring; indications of empathy for their fears and concerns; and help in identifying, clarifying, and formulating a plan of action to deal with the unresolved issue. If the elderly person's behavior seems particularly lethal, additional family or staff coverage and contact should be arranged to prevent isolation.

APPLICATION OF THE NURSING PROCESS

Assessment

Assessment of the elderly individual may follow the same framework used for all adults, but with consideration of the possible biological, psychological, sociocultural, and sexual changes that occur in the normal aging process described previously in this chapter. In no other area of nursing is it more important for nurses to practice holistic nursing than with the elderly. Older adults are likely to have multiple physical problems that contribute to problems in other areas of their lives. Obviously, these components cannot be addressed as separate entities. Nursing the elderly is a multifaceted, challenging process because of the multiple changes occurring at this time in the life cycle and the way in which each change affects every aspect of the individual.

Several considerations are unique to assessment of the elderly. Assessment of the older person's thought processes is a primary responsibility. Knowledge about the presence and extent of disorientation or confusion will influence the way in which the nurse approaches elder care.

Information about sensory capabilities is also extremely important. Because hearing loss is common, the nurse should lower the pitch and loudness of his or her voice when addressing the older person. Looking directly into the face of the older person when talking facilitates communication. Questions that require a declarative sentence in response should be asked; in this way, the nurse is able to assess the client's ability to use words correctly. Visual acuity can be determined by assessing adaptation to the dark, color matching, and the perception of color contrast. Knowledge about these aspects of sensory functioning is essential in the development of an effective care plan.

The nurse should be familiar with the normal physical changes associated with the aging process. Examples of some of these changes include:

- Less effective response to changes in environmental temperature, resulting in hypothermia
- Decreases in oxygen use and the amount of blood pumped by the heart, resulting in cerebral anoxia or hypoxia
- Skeletal muscle wasting and weakness, resulting in difficulty in physical mobility
- Limited cough and laryngeal reflexes, resulting in risk of aspiration
- Demineralization of bones, resulting in spontaneous fracturing
- Decrease in gastrointestinal motility, resulting in constipation
- Decrease in the ability to interpret painful stimuli, resulting in risk of injury

Common psychosocial changes associated with aging include:

- Prolonged and exaggerated grief, resulting in depression
- Physical changes, resulting in disturbed body image
- Changes in status, resulting in loss of self-worth

This list is by no means exhaustive. The nurse should consider many other alterations in his or her assessment of the client. Knowledge of the client's functional capabilities is essential for determining the physiological, psychological, and sociological needs of the elderly individual. Age alone does not preclude the occurrence of all these changes. The aging process progresses at a wide range of variance, and each client must be assessed as a unique individual.

Diagnosis/Outcome Identification

Virtually any nursing diagnosis may be applicable to the aging client, depending on individual needs for assistance. Based on normal changes that occur in the elderly, the following nursing diagnoses may be considered.

Physiologically Related Diagnoses

Risk for trauma related to confusion, disorientation, muscular weakness, spontaneous fractures, falls.

Hypothermia related to loss of adipose tissue under the skin, evidenced by increased sensitivity to cold and body temperature below 98.6 degrees.

Decreased cardiac output related to decreased myocardial efficiency secondary to age-related changes, evidenced by decreased tolerance for activity and decline in energy reserve.

Ineffective breathing pattern related to increase in fibrous tissue and loss of elasticity in lung tissue, evidenced by dyspnea and activity intolerance.

Risk for aspiration related to diminished cough and laryngeal reflexes.

Impaired physical mobility related to muscular wasting and weakness, evidenced by need for assistance in ambulation.

Imbalanced nutrition, less than body requirements, related to inefficient absorption from gastrointestinal tract, difficulty chewing and swallowing, anorexia, difficulty in feeding self, evidenced by wasting syndrome, anemia, weight loss.

Constipation related to decreased motility; inadequate diet; insufficient activity or exercise, evidenced by decreased bowel sounds; hard, formed stools; or straining at stool.

Stress incontinence related to degenerative changes in pelvic muscles and structural supports associated with increased age, evidenced by reported or observed dribbling with increased abdominal pressure or urinary frequency.

Urinary retention related to prostatic enlargement, evidenced by bladder distention, frequent voiding of small amounts, dribbling, or overflow incontinence.

Disturbed sensory perception related to age-related alterations in sensory transmission, evidenced by decreased visual acuity, hearing loss, diminished sensitivity to taste and smell, or increased touch threshold.

Disturbed sleep pattern related to age-related decrease in ability to sleep ("sleep decay"), dementia, or medications, evidenced by interrupted sleep, early awakening, or falling asleep during the day.

Pain related to degenerative changes in joints, evidenced by verbalization of pain or hesitation to use weight-bearing joints.

Self-care deficit (specify) related to weakness, confusion, or disorientation, evidenced by inability to feed self, maintain hygiene, dress/groom self, or toilet self without assistance.

Risk for impaired skin integrity related to alterations in nutritional state, circulation, sensation, or mobility.

Psychosocially Related Diagnoses

Disturbed thought processes related to age-related changes that result in cerebral anoxia, evidenced by short-term memory loss, confusion, or disorientation.

Dysfunctional grieving related to bereavement overload, evidenced by symptoms of depression.

Risk for suicide related to depressed mood and feelings of low self-worth.

Powerlessness related to lifestyle of helplessness and dependency on others, evidenced by depressed mood, apathy, or verbal expressions of having no control or influence over life situation.

Low self-esteem related to loss of pre-retirement status, evidenced by verbalization of negative feelings about self and life.

Fear related to nursing home placement, evidenced by symptoms of severe anxiety and statements such as, "Nursing homes are places to go to die."

Disturbed body image related to age-related changes in skin, hair, and fat distribution, evidenced by verbalization of negative feelings about body.

Ineffective sexuality patterns related to dyspareunia, evidenced by reported dissatisfaction with decrease in frequency of sexual intercourse.

Sexual dysfunction related to medications (e.g., antihypertensives) evidenced by inability to achieve an erection.

Social isolation related to total dependence on others, evidenced by expression of inadequacy in or absence of significant purpose in life.

Risk for trauma (elder abuse) related to caregiver role strain.

Caregiver role strain related to severity and duration of the care receiver's illness; lack of respite and recreation for the caregiver, evidenced by feelings of stress in relationship with care receiver; feelings of depression and anger; or family conflict around issues of providing care.

The following criteria may be used for measurement of outcomes in the care of the elderly client.

The Client:

1. Has not experienced injury
2. Maintains reality orientation consistent with cognitive level of functioning
3. Manages own self-care with assistance
4. Expresses positive feelings about self, past accomplishments, and hope for the future
5. Compensates adaptively for diminished sensory perception

Caregivers:

1. Can problem-solve effectively regarding care of elderly client
2. Demonstrate adaptive coping strategies for dealing with stress of caregiver role
3. Openly express feelings
4. Express desire to join support group of other caregivers

Planning/Implementation

In Table 23–3, selected nursing diagnoses are presented for the elderly client. Outcome criteria are included, along with appropriate nursing interventions and rationale for each.

Reminiscence therapy is especially helpful with elderly clients. This therapeutic intervention is highlighted in Table 23–4.

Evaluation

Reassessment is conducted to determine if the nursing actions have been successful in achieving the objectives of care. Evaluation of the nursing actions for the elderly client may be facilitated by gathering information using the following types of questions:

1. Has the client escaped injury from falls, burns, or other means to which he or she is vulnerable because of age?
2. Can caregivers verbalize means of providing a safe environment for the client?
3. Does the client maintain reality orientation at an optimum for his or her cognitive functioning?
4. Can the client distinguish between reality-based and non–reality-based thinking?
5. Can caregivers verbalize ways in which to orient client to reality, as needed?
6. Is the client able to accomplish self-care activities independently to his or her optimum level of functioning?
7. Does the client seek assistance for aspects of self-care that he or she is unable to perform independently?
8. Does the client express positive feelings about himself or herself?

TABLE 23–3 Care Plan for the Elderly Client

Nursing Diagnosis: RISK FOR TRAUMA

Related to: Confusion, disorientation, muscular weakness, spontaneous fractures, falls

Outcome Criteria	Nursing Interventions	Rationale
Client will not experience injury.	1. The following measures may be instituted: a. Arrange furniture and other items in the room to accommodate client's disabilities. b. Store frequently used items within easy access. c. Keep bed in unelevated position. Pad siderails and headboard if client has history of seizures. Keep bedrails up when client is in bed (if permitted by institutional policy). d. Assign room near nurses' station; observe frequently. e. Assist client with ambulation. f. Keep a dim light on at night. g. If client is a smoker, cigarettes and lighter or matches should be kept at the nurses' station and dispensed only when someone is available to stay with client while he or she is smoking. h. Frequently orient client to place, time, and situation. i. Soft restraints may be required if client is very disoriented and hyperactive.	1. To ensure client safety.

Nursing Diagnosis: DISTURBED THOUGHT PROCESSES

Related to: Age-related changes that result in cerebral anoxia

Evidenced by: Short-term memory loss, confusion, or disorientation

Outcome Criteria	Nursing Interventions	Rationale
Client will interpret the environment accurately and maintain reality orientation to the best of his or her cognitive ability.	1. Frequently orient client to reality. Use clocks and calendars with large numbers that are easy to read. Notes and large, bold signs may be useful as reminders. Allow client to have personal belongings.	1. To help maintain orientation and aid in memory and recognition.
	2. Keep explanations simple. Use face-to-face interaction. Speak slowly and do not shout.	2. To facilitate comprehension. Shouting may create discomfort, and in some instances, may provoke anger.
	3. Discourage rumination of delusional thinking. Talk about real events and real people.	3. Rumination promotes disorientation. Reality orientation increases sense of self-worth and personal dignity.
	4. Monitor for medication side effects.	4. Physiological changes in the elderly can alter the body's response to certain medications. Toxic effects may intensify altered thought processes.

Nursing Diagnosis: SELF-CARE DEFICIT (SPECIFY)

Related to: Weakness, disorientation, confusion, or memory deficits

Evidenced by: Inability to fulfill activities of daily living

Outcome Criteria	Nursing Interventions	Rationale
Client will accomplish activities of daily living to the best of his or her ability. Unfulfilled needs will be met by caregivers.	1. Provide a simple, structured environment: a. Identify self-care deficits and provide assistance as required. Promote independent actions as able. b. Allow plenty of time for client to perform tasks. c. Provide guidance and support for independent actions by talking the client through the task one step at a time. d. Provide a structured schedule of activities that do not change from day to day. e. Activities of daily living should follow home routine as closely as possible. f. Allow consistency in assignment of daily caregivers.	1. To minimize confusion.

(Continued)

TABLE 23–3 Care Plan for the Elderly Client *(Continued)*

Nursing Diagnosis: CAREGIVER ROLE STRAIN

Related to: Severity and duration of the care receiver's illness; lack of respite and recreation for the caregiver

Evidenced by: Feelings of stress in relationship with care receiver; feelings of depression and anger; family conflict around issues of providing care

Outcome Criteria	Nursing Interventions	Rationale
Caregivers will achieve effective problem-solving skills and develop adaptive coping mechanisms to regain equilibrium.	1. Assess prospective caregivers' ability to anticipate and fulfill client's unmet needs. Provide information to assist caregivers with this responsibility. Ensure that caregivers are aware of available community support systems from which they can seek assistance when required. Examples include adult day care centers, housekeeping and homemaker services, respite care services, or a local chapter of the Alzheimer's Disease and Related Disorders Association. This organization sponsors a nationwide 24-hour hotline to provide information and link families who need assistance with nearby chapters and affiliates. The hotline number is 800-621-0379.	1. Caregivers require relief from the pressures and strain of providing 24-hour care for their loved one. Studies have shown that elder abuse arises out of caregiving situations that place overwhelming stress on the caregivers.
	2. Encourage caregivers to express feelings, particularly anger.	2. Release of these emotions can serve to prevent psychopathology, such as depression or psychophysiological disorders, from occurring.
	3. Encourage participation in support groups composed of members with similar life situations.	3. Hearing others who are experiencing the same problems discuss ways in which they have coped may help caregiver adopt more adaptive strategies. Individuals who are experiencing similar life situations provide empathy and support for each other.

Nursing Diagnosis: LOW SELF-ESTEEM

Related to: Loss of pre-retirement status

Evidenced by: Verbalization of negative feelings about self and life

Outcome Criteria	Nursing Interventions	Rationale
Client will demonstrate increased feelings of self-worth by expressing positive aspects of self and past accomplishments.	1. Encourage client to express honest feelings in relation to loss of prior status. Acknowledge pain of loss. Support client through process of grieving.	1. Client may be fixed in anger stage of grieving process, which is turned inward on the self, resulting in diminished self-esteem.
	2. If lapses in memory are occurring, devise methods for assisting client with memory deficit. Examples: a. Name sign on door identifying client's room. b. Identifying sign on outside of dining room door. c. Identifying sign on outside of restroom door. d. Large clock, with oversized numbers and hands, appropriately placed. e. Large calendar, indicating one day at a time, with month, day, and year in bold print. f. Printed, structured daily schedule, with one copy for client and one posted on unit wall. g. "News board" on unit wall where current news of national and local interest may be posted.	2. These aids may assist client to function more independently, thereby increasing self-esteem.
	3. Encourage client's attempts to communicate. If verbalizations are not understandable, express to client what you think he or she intended to say. It may be necessary to reorient client frequently.	3. The ability to communicate effectively with others may enhance self-esteem.
	4. Encourage reminiscence and discussion of life review (see Table 23–4). Also discuss present-day events. Sharing picture albums, if possible, is especially good.	4. Reminiscence and life review help client resume progression through the grief process associated with disappointing life events and increase self-esteem as successes are reviewed.

Outcome Criteria	Nursing Interventions	Rationale
	5. Encourage participation in group activities. May need to accompany client at first, until he or she feels secure that the group members will be accepting, regardless of limitations in verbal communication.	5. Positive feedback from group members will increase self-esteem.
	6. Encourage client to be as independent as possible in self-care activities. Provide written schedule of tasks to be performed. Intervene in areas where client requires assistance.	6. The ability to perform independently preserves self-esteem.

Nursing Diagnosis: DISTURBED SENSORY PERCEPTION

Related to: Age-related alterations in sensory transmission

Evidenced by: Decreased visual acuity, hearing loss, diminished sensitivity to taste and smell, and increased touch threshold

Outcome Criteria	Nursing Interventions*	Rationale
Client will attain optimal level of sensory stimulation. Client will not experience injury due to diminished sensory perception.	1. The following nursing strategies are indicated: a. Provide meaningful sensory stimulation to all special senses through conversation, touch, music, or pleasant smells. b. Encourage wearing of glasses, hearing aids, prostheses, and other adaptive devices. c. Use bright, contrasting colors in the environment. d. Provide large-print reading materials, such as books, clocks, calendars, and educational materials. e. Maintain room lighting that distinguishes day from night and that is free of shadows and glare. f. Teach client to scan the environment to locate objects. g. Help client to locate food on plate using "clock" system, and describe food if client is unable to visualize; assist with feeding as needed. h. Arrange physical environment to maximize functional vision. i. Place personal items, call light, within client's field of vision. j. Teach client to watch the person who is speaking. k. Reinforce wearing of hearing aid; if client does not have an aid, use a communication device. l. Communicate clearly, distinctly, and slowly, using a low-pitched voice and facing client; avoid overarticulation. m. Remove as much unnecessary background noise as possible. n. Do not use slang or extraneous words. o. As speaker, position self at eye level and no farther than 6 feet away. p. Get the client's attention before speaking. q. Avoid speaking directly into the client's ear. r. If the client does not understand what is being said, rephrase the statement rather than simply repeating it. s. Help client select foods from the menu that will ensure discrimination between various tastes and smells. t. Ensure that food has been properly cooled so that client with diminished pain threshold is not burned. u. Ensure that bath or shower water is appropriate temperature. v. Use backrubs and massage as therapeutic touch to stimulate sensory receptors.	1. To assist client with diminished sensory perception and because client safety is a nursing priority.

*The interventions for this nursing diagnosis were adapted from Rogers-Seidl (1991).

TABLE 23-4 Reminiscence Therapy and Life Review with the Elderly

Heriot (1999) states: "Stimulation of life memories helps older adults to work through their losses and maintain self-esteem. Life review provides older adults with an opportunity to come to grips with guilt and regrets and to emerge feeling good about themselves." (p. 248)

Studies have indicated that *reminiscence*, or thinking about the past and reflecting on it, may promote better mental health in old age. *Life review* is related to reminiscence, but differs from it in that it is a more guided or directed cognitive process that constructs a history or story in an autobiographical way (Murray & Zentner, 2001).

Elderly individuals who spend time thinking about the past experience an increase in self-esteem and are less likely to suffer depression. Some psychologists believe that life review may help some people adjust to memories of an unhappy past. Others view reminiscence and life review as ways to bolster feelings of well-being, particularly in older people who can no longer remain active.

Reminiscence therapy can take place on a one-to-one basis or in a group setting. In reminiscence groups, elderly individuals share significant past events with peers. The nurse leader facilitates the discussion of topics that deal with specific life transitions, such as childhood, adolescence, marriage, childbearing, grandparenthood, and retirement. Members share both positive and negative aspects, including personal feelings, about these life cycle events.

Reminiscence on a one-to-one basis can provide a way for elderly individuals to work through unresolved issues from the past. Painful issues may be too difficult to discuss in the group setting. As the individual reviews his or her life process, the nurse can validate feelings and help the elderly client come to terms with painful issues that may have been long suppressed. This process is necessary if the elderly individual is to maintain (or attain) a sense of positive identity and self-esteem and ultimately achieve the goal of ego integrity as described by Erikson (1963).

A number of creative measures can be used to facilitate life review with the elderly individual. Having the client keep a journal for sharing may be a way to stimulate discussion (as well as providing a permanent record of past events for significant others). Pets, music, and special foods have a way of provoking memories from the client's past. Photographs of family members and past significant events are an excellent way of guiding the elderly client through his or her autobiographical review.

Care must be taken in the life review to assist clients to work through unresolved issues. Anxiety, guilt, depression, and despair may result if the individual is unable to work through the problems and accept them. Life review can work in a negative way if the individual comes to believe that his or her life was meaningless. However, it can be a very positive experience for the person who can take pride in accomplishments and feel satisfied with his or her life, resulting in a sense of serenity and inner peace in the older adult.

9. Does the client reminisce about accomplishments that have occurred in his or her life?
10. Does the client express some hope for the future?
11. Does the client wear eyeglasses or a hearing aid, if needed, to compensate for sensory deficits?
12. Does the client consistently look at others in the face to facilitate hearing when they are talking to him or her?
13. Does the client use helpful aids, such as signs identifying various rooms, to help maintain orientation?
14. Can the caregivers work through problems and make decisions regarding care of the elderly client?
15. Do the caregivers include the elderly client in the decision-making process, if appropriate?
16. Can the caregivers demonstrate adaptive coping strategies for dealing with the strain of long-term caregiving?
17. Are the caregivers open and honest in expression of feelings?
18. Can the caregivers verbalize community resources to which they can go for assistance with their caregiving responsibilities?
19. Have the caregivers joined a support group?

SUMMARY

Care of the aging individual presents one of the greatest challenges for nursing. The growing population of individuals age 65 and older suggests that the challenge will progress well into the 21st century.

America is a youth-oriented society. It is not desirable to be old; in fact, to some it is repugnant. Most, however, if faced with a choice, would choose growing old to the alternative—death. In some cultures, the elderly are revered and hold a special place of honor within the society, but in highly industrialized countries such as the United States, status declines with the decrease in productivity and participation in the mainstream of society.

Individuals experience many changes as they age. Physical changes occur in virtually every body system. Psychologically, there may be age-related memory deficiencies, particularly for recent events. Intellectual functioning does not decline with age, but length of time required for learning increases.

Aging individuals experience many losses, potentially leading to bereavement overload. They are vulnerable to depression and to feelings of low self-worth. The elderly population represents a disproportionately high percentage of individuals who commit suicide. Dementing disorders are the most frequent causes of psychopathology in the elderly. Sleep disorders are very common.

The need for sexual expression by the elderly is often misunderstood within our society. Although many physical changes occur at this time of life that alter an individual's sexuality, if he or she has reasonably good health and a willing partner, sexual activity can continue well past the 70s for most people.

Retirement has both social and economical implications for elderly individuals. Society often equates an individual's status with occupation, and loss of employment may result in the need for adjustment in the standard of living because retirement income may be reduced by 20 to 40 percent of pre-retirement earnings.

Less than 5 percent of the population age 65 and older live in nursing homes. A profile of the typical elderly nursing home resident is a white woman about 78 years old, widowed, with multiple chronic health conditions. Much stigma is attached to what some still call "rest homes" or "old age homes," and many elderly people still equate them with a place "to go to die."

The strain of the caregiver role has become a major dilemma in our society. Elder abuse is sometimes inflicted by caregivers for whom the role has become overwhelming and intolerable. There is an intense need to find assistance for these people, who must provide care for their loved ones on a 24-hour basis. Home healthcare, respite care, support groups, and financial assistance are needed to ease the burden of this role strain.

Nursing of the elderly individual is accomplished through the six steps of the nursing process. Assessment requires that changes occurring in the normal aging process—biological, psychological, sociocultural, and sexual—be taken into consideration before an accurate plan of care can be formulated.

Nursing of elderly individuals requires a special kind of inner strength and compassion. The following poem, which has become familiar over the years, is excellent in eliciting empathy for what the elderly must feel. I thank the anonymous author for sharing. It conveys a powerful message.

WHAT DO YOU SEE, NURSE?

What do you see, nurse, what do you see?
What are you thinking when you look at me?
A crabbed old woman, not very wise.
Uncertain of habit, with faraway eyes.
Who dribbles her food and makes no reply
When you say in a loud voice, "I do wish you'd try."
Who seems not to notice the things that you do
And forever is losing a stocking or shoe.
Who unresisting or not, lets you do as you will
With bathing and feeding, the long day to fill.
Is that what you're thinking, is that what you see?
Then open your eyes, you're not looking at me.
I'll tell you who I am as I sit there so still.
As I move at your bidding, as I eat at your will.
I'm a small child of ten with a father and mother,
Brothers and sisters who love one another.
A young girl at sixteen with wings on her feet
Dreaming that soon now a lover she'll meet.
A bride soon at twenty—my heart gives a leap
Remembering the vows that I promised to keep.
At twenty-five, now, I have young of my own
Who need me to build a secure happy home.
A woman of thirty, my young now grow fast
Bound to each other with ties that should last.
At forty my young now will soon be gone,
But my man stays beside me to see I don't mourn.
At fifty once more babies play round my knee.
Again we know children, my loved one and me.
Dark days are upon me, my husband is dead.
I look at the future, I shudder with dread.
For my young are all busy rearing young of their own.
And I think of the years and the love I have known.
I'm an old woman now and nature is cruel.
'Tis her jest to make old age look like a fool.
The body it crumbles, grace and vigor depart.
There is now just a stone where I once had a heart.
But inside this old carcass a young girl still dwells.
And now and again my battered heart swells.
I remember the joys, I remember the pain.
And I'm loving and living life all over again.
I think of the years all too few—gone so fast.
And accept the stark fact that nothing can last.
So open your eyes, nurse, open and see.
Not a crabbed old woman—look closer—SEE ME.

Author unknown

REVIEW QUESTIONS

SELF-EXAMINATION/LEARNING EXERCISE

Select the answer that is most appropriate for each of the following questions:

Situation: Stanley, a 72-year-old widower, was brought to the hospital by his son, who reports that Stanley has become increasingly withdrawn. He has periods of confusion and forgetfulness, but most of the time his thought processes are intact. He eats little food and has lost some weight. His wife died 5 years ago and the son reports, "He did very well and didn't even cry." Stanley attended the funeral of his best friend 1 month ago, after which these symptoms began. Stanley has been admitted for testing and evaluation.

1. In her admission assessment, the nurse notices an open sore on Stanley's arm. When she questions him about it he says, "I scraped it on the fence 2 weeks ago. It's smaller than it was." How might the nurse analyze the data?
   a. Stanley was trying to commit suicide.
   b. The delay in healing may indicate that Stanley has developed skin cancer.
   c. A diminished inflammatory response in the elderly increases healing time.
   d. Age-related skin changes and distribution of adipose tissue delay healing in the elderly.

2. Stanley is deaf on his right side. Which is the most appropriate nursing intervention for communicating with Stanley?
   a. Speak loudly into his left ear.
   b. Speak to him from a position on his left side.
   c. Speak face-to-face in a high-pitched voice.
   d. Speak face-to-face in a low-pitched voice

3. Why is it important to have the nurse check the temperature of the water before Stanley takes a shower?
   a. Stanley may catch cold if the water temperature is too low.
   b. Stanley may burn himself because of a higher pain threshold.
   c. Stanley has difficulty discriminating between hot and cold.
   d. The water must be exactly 98.6° F.

4. From the information provided in the situation, which would be the priority nursing diagnosis for Stanley?
   a. Dysfunctional grieving
   b. Imbalanced nutrition: less than body requirements
   c. Social isolation
   d. Risk for injury

5. The physician diagnoses Stanley with major depression. A suicide assessment is conducted. Why is Stanley at high risk for suicide?
   a. All depressed people are at high risk for suicide.
   b. Stanley is in the age group in which the highest percentage of suicides occurs.
   c. Stanley is a white man, recently bereaved, living alone.
   d. His son reports that Stanley owns a gun.

6. Which of the following would be a *priority* nursing intervention with Stanley?
   a. Take blood pressure once each shift.
   b. Ensure that Stanley attends group activities.
   c. Encourage Stanley to eat all of the food on his food tray.
   d. Encourage Stanley to talk about his wife's death.

7. In group exercise, Stanley becomes tired and short-of-breath very quickly. This is most likely caused by:
   a. Age-related changes in the cardiovascular system
   b. Stanley's sedentary lifestyle
   c. The effects of pathological depression
   d. Medication the physician has prescribed for depression
8. Stanley says to the nurse, "I'm all alone now. My wife is gone. My best friend is gone. My son is busy with his work and family. I might as well just go too." Which is the best response by the nurse?
   a. "Are you thinking that you want to die, Stanley?"
   b. "You have lots to live for, Stanley."
   c. "Cheer up, Stanley. It's almost time for activity therapy."
   d. "Tell me about your family, Stanley."
9. Stanley says to the nurse, "I don't want to go to that crafts class. I'm too old to learn anything." Based on knowledge of the aging process, which of the following is a true statement?
   a. Memory functioning in the elderly most likely reflects loss of long-term memories of remote events.
   b. Intellectual functioning declines with advancing age.
   c. Learning ability remains intact, but time required for learning increases with age.
   d. Cognitive functioning is rarely affected in aging individuals.
10. According to the literature, which of the following is most important for Stanley to maintain a healthy, adaptive old age?
   a. To remain socially interactive
   b. To disengage slowly in preparation of the last stage of life
   c. To move in with his son and family
   d. To maintain total independence and accept no help from anyone

Test Your CRITICAL THINKING SKILLS

Mrs. M., age 76, is seeing her primary physician for her regular 6-month physical exam. Mrs. M's husband died 2 years ago, at which time she sold her home in Kansas and came to live in California with her only child, a daughter. The daughter is married and has three children (one in college and two teenagers at home). The daughter reports that her mother is becoming increasingly withdrawn, stays in her room, and eats very little. She has lost 13 pounds since her last 6-month visit. The primary physician refers Mrs. M. to a psychiatrist who hospitalizes her for evaluation. He diagnoses Mrs. M. with major depression.

Mrs. M. tells the nurse, "I didn't want to leave my home, but my daughter insisted. I would have been all right. I miss my friends and my church. Back home, I drove my car everywhere. There's too much traffic out here. They sold my car and I have to depend on my daughter or grandkids to take me places. I hate being so dependent! I miss my husband so much. I just sit and think about him and our past life all the time. I don't have any interest in meeting new people. I want to go home!"

Mrs. M. admits to having some thoughts of dying, although she denies feeling suicidal. She denies having a plan or means for taking her life. "I really don't want to die, but I just can't see much reason for living. My daughter and her family are so busy with their own lives. They don't need me—or even have time for me!"

Answer the following questions about Mrs. M:

1. What would be the *primary* nursing diagnosis for Mrs. M.?
2. Formulate a short-term goal for Mrs. M.
3. From the assessment data, identify the major problem that may be a long-term focus of care for Mrs. M.

IMPLICATIONS OF RESEARCH FOR EVIDENCE BASED PRACTICE

Wright, L.K., Hickey, J.V., Buckwalter, K.C., Kelechi, T., and Hendrix, S.A.:

Spousal interactions in Alzheimer's disease and stroke caregiving: Relationship to care recipients' functional abilities and physical and emotional health. Journal of the American Psychiatric Nurses Association (1998, December) 4(6):169–181.

Description of the study: The objective of this study was to examine spousal interactions along two illness trajectories, Alzheimer's disease (AD) and stroke, and to determine effect of spousal interaction on functional ability and physical and emotional health. The sample in this study included 42 couples equally divided among three groups. One group consisted of 14 persons afflicted with early-phase AD and their spousal caregivers. The second group consisted of 14 persons who had had a stroke and their 14 caregiver spouses. The third group was a control group of 14 healthy couples randomly selected from the community. Demographics were matched among the three groups according to age (mean, 65 years; range 49 to 85 years) and length of marriage (mean, 36 years; range 1 to 57 years). Data was collected in face-to-face interviews at baseline and 6-month follow-up, using various questionnaires to measure cognitive impairment, functional abilities, and physical and emotional health. Spousal interactions were measured by the Dyadic Adjustment Rating (DAR) Scale, with the subscale of "affection" being expanded to include the following items: kissing the spouse, touching the spouse lovingly, caressing, holding hands, putting an arm around the spouse, and sleeping in the same bed. Present interactions were considered during the period of the preceding 2 weeks. Past spousal interactions were referred to as before illness onset for the AD and stroke couples and before retirement for the well couples.

Results of the Study: At baseline assessment, functional ability in both the AD and stroke groups was similar. Quality and quantity of spousal interactions in the AD group was lower than for both the stroke and well group. Little change had occurred in the quality and quantity of spousal interactions after 6 months for all three groups, the one exception being increased quantity of interaction in the AD group. Both AD and stroke groups showed increases in depression at the 6-months follow-up. Spousal interaction was found to be positively correlated to functional ability, physical health, and lower depression in AD care recipients. No significant correlation was found between stroke couples' interactions and stroke care recipients' depression or physical health. Significant correlation was found only with increased functional ability at the 6-month follow-up.

Implications for Nursing Practice: This study revealed that positive spousal interactions are predominantly related to better physical and emotional health in AD care recipients and to increased functional ability in persons who have had a stroke. Implications for nursing include establishing support groups for spouses of individuals who require this type of care. Support from others who are experiencing similar circumstances can be very positive. Working with the care recipients related to their depression is also within the scope of nursing.

REFERENCES

Administration on Aging (AoA). (2002). A profile of older Americans: 2002 Washington, DC: U.S. Department of Health and Human Services.

Bahr, R.T. (1999). Sleep disturbances. In M. Stanley & P.G. Beare (Eds.), Gerontological nursing: A health promotion/protection approach (2nd ed.). Philadelphia: F.A. Davis.

Birren, J.E. & Bengtson, V.L. (1998). Emergent theories of aging. New York: Springer.

Blazer, D.G. (2003). Geriatric psychiatry. In R.E. Hales & S.C. Yudofsky (Eds.), Textbook of clinical psychiatry, (4th ed.). Washington, DC: American Psychiatric Publishing.

Buckwalter, K.C. (1999). Depression and suicide. In M. Stanley & P.G. Beare (Eds.), Gerontological nursing: A health promotion/protection approach (2nd ed.). Philadelphia: F.A. Davis.

Cath, S.H. & Sadavoy, J. (1991). Psychosocial aspects. In J. Sadavoy, L.W. Lazarus, & L.F. Jarvik (Eds.), Comprehensive review of geriatric psychiatry. Washington, DC: American Psychiatric Press.

Center for Mental Health Services. (2002). National Strategy for suicide prevention. Suicide among the elderly. Retrieved April 13, 2002 from http://www.mentalhealth.org/suicideprevention/elderly.asp

Charbonneau, A. (2003). Elderly suicide prevention. Regions VII/VIII Suicide Prevention Planning Meeting. Kansas City, KS: University of Kansas Medical Center, October 29, 2003.

Cristofalo, V.J. (1996). Ten years later: What have we learned about human aging from studies of cell cultures. Gerontologist, 36(6): 737–741.

Curtis, S.M. & Carroll, E.W. (1994). Alterations in vision. In C.M. Porth (Ed.), Pathophysiology: Concepts of altered health states (4th ed.). Philadelphia: Lippincott.

Dellasega, C., Yonushonis, M.E.H., & Johnson, A. (1999). The aging endocrine system. In M. Stanley & P.G. Beare (Eds.), Gerontological nursing: A health promotion/protection approach (2nd ed.). Philadelphia: F.A. Davis.

Donlon, B.C. (1999). Theories of aging. In M. Stanley & P.G. Beare (Eds.), Gerontological nursing: A health promotion/protection approach (2nd ed.). Philadelphia: F.A. Davis.

Fulmer, T. (1999). Elder mistreatment. In M. Stanley & P. G. Beare (Eds.), Gerontological nursing: A health promotion/protection approach (2nd ed.). Philadelphia: F.A. Davis.

Giger, J.N. & Davidhizar, R.E. (1991). Transcultural nursing: Assessment and intervention. St. Louis: Mosby.

Heriot, C.S. (1999). Developmental tasks and development in the later years of life. In M. Stanley & P. G. Beare (Eds.), Gerontological nursing: A health promotion/protection approach (2nd ed.). Philadelphia: F.A. Davis.

Ignatavicius, D.D. (1998). Introduction to long-term care nursing: Principles and practice. Philadelphia: F.A. Davis.

Jacoby, S. (1999). Great sex: What's age got to do with it? Modern Maturity, 42W(5): 40–45.

Kee, C. (1999). The aging renal and urinary system. In M. Stanley & P.G. Beare (Eds.), Gerontological nursing: A health promotion/protection approach (2nd ed.). Philadelphia: F.A. Davis.

Larocco, M. (1994). Inflammation and immunity. In C.M. Porth (Ed.), Pathophysiology: Concepts of altered health states (4th ed). Philadelphia: J.B. Lippincott.

Leventhal, E.A. (1991). Biological aspects. In J. Sadavoy, L.W. Lazarus, & L.F. Jarvik (Eds.), Comprehensive review of geriatric psychiatry. Washington, DC: American Psychiatric Press.

Masters, W.H., Johnson, V.E., & Kolodny, R.C. (1995). Human sexuality (5th ed.). New York: Addison-Wesley Longman.

Millsap, P. (1999). Use of long-term care by older adults. In M. Stanley & P. G. Beare (Eds.), Gerontological nursing: A health promotion/protection approach. (2nd ed.) Philadelphia: F.A. Davis.

Murray, R.B. & Zentner, J.P. (2001). Health promotion strategies

through the life span (7th ed.). Upper Saddle River, NJ: Prentice Hall.
National Center for Health Statistics. (2002). National Vital Statistics Report, Vol. 48, No. 18, March 18, 2002. Retrieved April 9, 2002 from http://www.cdc.gov/nchs/
National Institute of Mental Health [NIMH]. (2001). Older adults: Depression and suicide facts. Retrieved on April 13, 2002 from http://www.nimh.nih.gov/publicat/elderlydepsuicide.cfm
Petras, K. & Petras, R. (1991). The only retirement guide you'll ever need. New York: Poseidon Press.
Pikna, J.K. (1994). Concepts of altered health in older adults. In C.M. Porth (Ed.), Pathophysiology: Concepts of altered health states (4th ed.). Philadelphia: J.B. Lippincott.
Reinisch, J.M. (1990). The Kinsey Institute new report on sex. New York: St. Martin's Press.
Roberts, C.M. (1991). How did I get here so fast? New York: Warner Books.
Rogers-Seidl, F.F. (1991). Geriatric nursing care plans. St. Louis: Mosby.
Rossouw, J.E., Anderson, G.L., et al. (2002, July 17). Risks and benefits of estrogen plus progestin in healthy postmenopausal women: Principal results from the Women's Health Initiative randomized controlled trial. Journal of the American Medical Association, 288(3): 321–333, 366–368.
Roussel, L.A. (1999). The aging neurological system. In M. Stanley & P.G. Beare (Eds.), Gerontological nursing: A health promotion/protection approach (2nd ed.). Philadelphia: F.A. Davis.
Sadavoy, J., Lazarus, L.W. & Jarvik, L.F. (1991). Comprehensive review of geriatric psychiatry. Washington, DC: American Psychiatric Press.
Sadock, B.J. & Sadock, V.A. (2003). Synopsis of psychiatry: Behavioral sciences/clinical psychiatry (9th ed.). Philadelphia: Lippincott Williams & Wilkins.
Vaillant, G. & Vaillant, C.O. (1990). Natural history of male psychosocial health: A 45-year study of predictors of successful aging at age 65. American Journal of Psychiatry, 147, 31–37.
Wiersema, L.A. & Stanley, M. (1999). The aging integumentary system. In M. Stanley & P.G. Beare (Eds.), Gerontological nursing: A health promotion/protection approach (2nd Ed.). Philadelphia: F.A. Davis.
Williams, M.E. (1995). The American Geriatrics Society's complete guide to aging and health. New York: Harmony Books.
Wise, P.M., Krajnak, K.M. & Kashon, M.L. (1996, July 5). Menopause: The aging of multiple pacemakers. Science, 273(5721): 67.

CLASSICAL REFERENCES

Erikson, E.H. (1963). Childhood and society (2nd ed.). New York: WW Norton.
Kübler-Ross, E. (1969). On death and dying. New York: Macmillan.
Reichard, S., Livson, F., & Peterson, P.G. (1962). Aging and personality. New York: John Wiley.

INTERNET REFERENCES

- Additional sources related to aging may be located at the following websites:
  - a http://www.4woman.org/
  - b http://www.aarp.org/
  - c http://www.oaktrees.org/elder/
  - d http://www.acjnet.org/docs/eldabpfv.html
  - e http://www.ssa.gov/
  - f http://www.nfcacares.org/home.html
  - g http://www.nih.gov/nia/
  - h http://www.medicare.gov/
  - i http://www.seniorlaw.com/
  - j http://www.growthhouse.org/cesp.html
  - k http://www.agenet.com/
  - l http://www.aoa.gov/
  - m http://www.senior.com/
  - n http://www.nsclc.org/

24

CHAPTER

Community Mental Health Nursing

CHAPTER OUTLINE

KEY TERMS

deinstitutionalization
prospective payment
diagnostically related groups (DRGs)
primary prevention
secondary prevention
tertiary prevention
case management
community
shelters
storefront clinics
mobile outreach units
case manager

OBJECTIVES

After reading this chapter, the student will be able to:

1. Discuss the changing focus of care in the field of mental health.
2. Define the concepts of care associated with the public health model.
3. Discuss primary prevention of mental illness within the community.
4. Identify populations at risk for mental illness within the community.
5. Discuss nursing intervention in primary prevention of mental illness within the community.
6. Discuss secondary prevention of mental illness within the community.
7. Describe treatment alternatives related to secondary prevention within the community.
8. Discuss tertiary prevention of mental illness within the community as it relates to the chronically and homeless mentally ill.
9. Relate historical and epidemiological factors associated with caring for the chronically and homeless mentally ill within the community.
10. Identify treatment alternatives for care of the chronically and homeless mentally ill within the community.
11. Apply the nursing process to care of the chronically and homeless mentally ill within the community.

INTRODUCTION

This chapter explores the concepts of primary and secondary prevention of mental illness within communities. Additional focus is placed on tertiary prevention of mental illness: treatment with community resources of those who are chronically mentally ill and homeless persons who are mentally ill. Emphasis is given to the role of the psychiatric nurse in the various treatment alternatives within the community setting.

THE CHANGING FOCUS OF CARE

Before 1840, there was no known treatment for individuals who were mentally ill. Because mental illness was perceived as incurable, the only "reasonable" intervention was thought to be removing these ill persons from the community to a place where they would do no harm to themselves or others.

In 1841, Dorothea Dix, a former schoolteacher, began a personal crusade across the land on behalf of clients who were institutionalized with mental illness. The efforts of this self-appointed "inspector" resulted in humane treatment of persons with mental illness and the establishment of a number of hospitals for the mentally ill.

After the movement initiated by Dix, the number of hospitals for persons with mental illness increased, although unfortunately not as rapidly as did the population with mental illness. The demand soon outgrew the supply, and hospitals became overcrowded and understaffed, with conditions that would have sorely distressed Dorothea Dix.

The community mental health movement had its impetus in the 1940s. With establishment of the National Mental Health Act of 1946, the U.S. government awarded grants to the states to develop mental health programs outside of state hospitals. Outpatient clinics and psychiatric units in general hospitals were inaugurated. Then, in 1949, as an outgrowth of the National Mental Health Act, the National Institute of Mental Health (NIMH) was established. The U.S. government has charged this agency with the responsibility for mental health in the United States.

In 1955, the Joint Commission on Mental Health and Illness was established by Congress to identify the nation's mental health needs and to make recommendations for improvement in psychiatric care. In 1961, the Joint Commission published the report, *Action for Mental Health*, in which recommendations were made for treatment of clients with mental illness, training for caregivers, and improvements in education and research of mental illness. With consideration given to these recommendations, Congress passed the Mental Retardation Facilities and Community Mental Health Centers Construction Act (often called the Community Mental Health Centers Act) of 1963. This act called for the construction of comprehensive community health centers, the cost of which would be shared by federal and state governments. The **deinstitutionalization** movement (the closing of state mental hospitals and discharging of individuals with mental illness) had begun.

Unfortunately, many state governments did not have the capability to match the federal funds required for the establishment of these mental health centers. Some communities found it difficult to follow the rigid requirements for services required by the legislation that provided the grant.

In 1980 the Community Mental Health Systems Act, which was to have played a major role in renovation of mental healthcare, was established. Funding was authorized for community mental health centers, services to high-risk populations, ambulatory mental healthcare centers, a prevention unit and associate director for minority concerns at NIMH, and rape research and services (Wilson & Kneisl, 1992). However, before this plan could be enacted, the newly inaugurated administration set forth its intention to diminish federal involvement. Budget cuts reduced the number of mandated services, and federal funding for community mental health centers was terminated in 1984.

Meanwhile, costs of care for hospitalized psychiatric clients continued to rise. The problem of the "revolving door" began to intensify. The chronically mentally ill had no place to go when their illness exacerbated, except back to the hospital. Individuals without support systems remained in the hospital for extended periods because of lack of appropriate community services. Hospital services were paid for by cost-based, retrospective reimbursement: Medicaid, Medicare, and private health insurance. Retrospective reimbursement encouraged hospital expenditure; the more services provided, the more payment received.

This system of delivery of healthcare was interrupted in 1983 with the advent of **prospective payment,** the Reagan administration's proposal of cost containment. It was directed at control of Medicare costs by setting forth preestablished amounts that would be reimbursed for specific diagnoses, or **diagnostically related groups (DRGs)**. Since that time, prospective payment has also been integrated by the states (Medicaid) and by some private insurance companies, drastically affecting the amount of reimbursement for healthcare services.

Mental health services have been influenced by prospective payment. General hospital services to psychiatric clients have been severely restricted. Clients who present with acute symptoms, such as acute psychosis, suicidal ideations or attempts, or manic exacerbations, constitute the largest segment of the psychiatric hospital census. Clients with less serious illnesses (e.g., moderate depression or adjustment disorders) may be hospitalized, but length of stay has been shortened considerably by the reimbursement guidelines. Clients are being discharged from the hospital with a greater need for aftercare than in the past, when hospital stays were longer.

Deinstitutionalization continues to be the changing focus of mental healthcare in the United States. Care for the client in the hospital has become cost prohibitive, whereas care for the client in the community is cost effective. As Shirley Smoyak (1991) has stated:

> How and what healthcare is provided is more of a political and funding issue than one driven by scientific knowledge. That is not to say that science is not important, or that it is not needed, but to emphasize the reality that it is not the number-one factor in how decisions get made to either seek or provide services. (p. 7)

Provision of outpatient mental health services not only is the wave of the future but also has become a necessity today. We must serve the consumer by providing the essential services to assist with health promotion or prevention, to initiate early intervention, and to ensure rehabilitation or prevention of long-term disability.

THE PUBLIC HEALTH MODEL

The premise of the model of public health is based largely on the concepts set forth by Gerald Caplan (1964) during the initial community mental health movement. They include primary prevention, secondary prevention, and tertiary prevention. These concepts no longer have relevance only to mental health nursing but have been widely adapted as guiding principles in many clinical and community settings over a range of nursing specialties.

Primary prevention is defined as reducing the incidence of mental disorders within the population. It targets both individuals and the environment. Emphasis is twofold:

1. Assisting individuals to increase their ability to cope effectively with stress
2. Targeting and diminishing harmful forces (stressors) within the environment

Nursing in primary prevention is focused on the targeting of groups at risk and the provision of educational programs. Examples include:

1. Teaching parenting skills and child development to prospective new parents
2. Teaching physical and psychosocial effects of alcohol and drugs to elementary school students
3. Teaching techniques of stress management to virtually anyone who desires to learn
4. Teaching groups of individuals ways to cope with the changes associated with various maturational stages
5. Teaching concepts of mental health to various groups within the community
6. Providing education and support to unemployed or homeless individuals
7. Providing education and support to other individuals in various transitional periods (e.g., widows and widowers, new retirees, and women entering the work force in middle life)

These are only a few examples of the types of services nurses provide in primary prevention. These services can be offered in a variety of settings that are convenient for the public (e.g., churches, schools, colleges, community centers, YMCAs and YWCAs, workplace of employee organizations, meetings of women's groups, or civic or social organizations such as PTAs, health fairs, and community shelters).

Secondary prevention is reducing the prevalence of psychiatric illness by shortening the duration of the illness (Sadock & Sadock, 2003). This is accomplished through early identification of problems and prompt initiation of effective treatment.

Nursing in secondary prevention focuses on recognition of symptoms and provision of, or referral for, treatment. Examples include:

1. Ongoing assessment of individuals at high risk for illness exacerbation (e.g., during home visits, day care, community health centers, or in any setting where screening of high-risk individuals might occur)
2. Provision of care for individuals in whom illness symptoms have been assessed (e.g., individual or group counseling, medication administration, education and support during period of increased stress [crisis intervention], staffing rape crisis cen-

ters, suicide hotlines, homeless shelters, shelters for abused women, or mobile mental health units)

3. Referral for treatment of individuals in whom illness symptoms have been assessed. Referrals may come from support groups, community mental health centers, emergency services, psychiatrists or psychologists, and day or partial hospitalization. Inpatient therapy on a psychiatric unit of a general hospital or in a private psychiatric hospital may be necessary. Chemotherapy and various adjunct therapies may be initiated as part of the treatment.

Secondary prevention has been addressed extensively in Unit Three of this text. Nursing assessment, diagnosis/outcome identification, plan/implementation, and evaluation were discussed for many of the mental illnesses identified in the *DSM-IV-TR* (APA, 2000). These concepts may be applied in any setting where nursing is practiced.

Tertiary prevention is reducing the residual defects that are associated with severe or chronic mental illness. This is accomplished in two ways:

1. Preventing complications of the illness
2. Promoting rehabilitation that is directed toward achievement of each individual's maximum level of functioning

Sadock and Sadock (2003) suggest that the term *chronic mental illness*, which has historically been associated with long hospitalizations that resulted in loss of social skills and increased dependency, now may also refer to clients from the deinstitutionalized generation. These individuals may never have experienced hospitalization, but they still do not possess adequate skills to live productive lives within the community.

Nursing in tertiary prevention focuses on helping clients learn or relearn socially appropriate behaviors so that they may achieve a satisfying role within the community. Examples include:

1. Consideration of the rehabilitation process at the time of initial diagnosis and treatment planning
2. Teaching the client daily living skills and encouraging independence to his or her maximum ability
3. Referring clients for various aftercare services (e.g., support groups, day treatment programs, partial hospitalization programs, psychosocial rehabilitation programs, group home or other transitional housing)
4. Monitoring effectiveness of aftercare services (e.g., through home health visits or follow-up appointments in community mental health centers)
5. Making referrals for support services when required (e.g., some communities have programs linking individuals with chronic mental disorders to volunteers who serve to develop friendships with the individuals and who may assist with household chores, shopping, and other activities of daily living with which the individual is having difficulty, in addition to participating in social activities with the individual)

Nursing care at the tertiary level of prevention can be administered on an individual or group basis and in a variety of settings, such as inpatient hospitalization, day or partial hospitalization, group home or halfway house, shelters, home healthcare, nursing homes, and community mental health centers.

THE COMMUNITY AS CLIENT

Primary Prevention

Langley (2002) defines community as:

> … a group, population, or cluster of people with at least one common characteristic, such as geographic location, occupation, ethnicity, or health concern. (p. 9)

Primary prevention within communities encompasses the twofold emphasis defined earlier in this chapter. These include:

1. Identifying stressful life events that precipitate crises and targeting the relevant populations at high risk
2. Intervening with these high-risk populations to prevent or minimize harmful consequences

Populations at Risk

One way to view populations at risk is to focus on types of crises that individuals experience in their lives. Two broad categories are maturational crises and situational crises.

Maturational Crises

Maturational crises are crucial experiences that are associated with various stages of growth and development. Erikson (1963) described eight stages of the life cycle during which individuals struggle with developmental "tasks." Crises can occur during any of these stages, although several developmental periods and life-cycle events have been recognized as having increased crisis potential: adolescence, marriage, parenthood, midlife, and retirement.

ADOLESCENCE. The task for adolescence according to Erikson (1963) is *identity versus role confusion.* This is the time in life when individuals ask questions such as "Who am I? Where am I going?" and "What is life all about?"

Adolescence is a transition into young adulthood. It is a very volatile time in most families. Commonly, there is conflict over issues of control. Parents sometimes have difficulty relinquishing even a minimal amount of the control they have had throughout their adolescent's infancy, toddler, and school-age years, when the adolescent seeks to be independent. It may seem that the adolescent is 25 years old one day and 5 years old the next. An often-quoted definition of an adolescent, by an anonymous author, is: "A toddler with hormones and wheels."

At this time, adolescents are "trying out their wings," although they possess an essential need to know that the parents (or surrogate parents) are available if support is required. Mahler, Pine, and Bergman (1975) have termed this vital concept "emotional refueling," and although they were referring to toddlers when they coined the term, it is highly applicable to adolescents as well. In fact, it is believed that the most frequent immediate precipitant to adolescent suicide is loss or threat of loss or abandonment by parents or closest peer relationship.

Adolescents have many issues to deal with and many choices to make. Some of these include issues that relate to self-esteem and body image (in a body that is undergoing rapid changes), peer relationships (with both genders), education and career selection, establishing a set of values and ideals, sexuality and sexual experimentation (including issues of birth control and prevention of sexually transmitted diseases), drug and alcohol abuse, and physical appearance.

Nursing interventions with adolescents, at the primary level of prevention, focuses on providing them with support and accurate information to ease the difficult transition they are undergoing. Educational offerings can be presented in schools, churches, youth centers, or any location in which groups of teenagers gather. Types of programs may include (but are not limited to):

- Alateen groups for adolescents with alcoholic parent(s)
- Other support groups for teenagers who are in need of assistance to cope with stressful situations (e.g., children dealing with divorce of their parents, pregnant teenagers, teenagers coping with abortion, adolescents coping with the death of a parent)
- Educational programs that inform about and validate bodily changes and emotions about which there may be some concerns
- Educational programs that inform about nutritional needs specific for this age group
- Educational programs that inform about sexuality, pregnancy, contraception, and sexually transmitted diseases
- Educational programs that inform about the use and abuse of alcohol and other drugs

MARRIAGE. The "American dream" of the 1950s—especially that of the American woman—was to marry, have two or three children, buy a house in the suburbs, and drive a station wagon. To not be at least betrothed by their mid-20s caused many women to fear becoming an "old maid." Living together without the benefit of marriage was an unacceptable and rarely considered option.

Times have changed considerably in 50 years. Today's young women are choosing to pursue careers before entering into marriage, to continue their careers after marriage, or to not marry at all. Many couples are deciding to live together without being married and, as with most trends, the practice now receives more widespread societal acceptance than it once did.

Why is marriage considered one of the most common maturational crises? Sheehy (1976) writes:

> No two people can possibly coordinate all their developmental crises. The timing of outside opportunities will almost never be the same. But more importantly, each one has an inner life structure with its own idiosyncrasies. Depending on what has gone before, each one will alternate differently between times of feeling full of certainty, hope, and heightened potential and times of feeling vulnerable, unfocused, and scared. (p. 138)

Additional conflicts sometimes also arise when the marriage is influenced by crossovers in religion, ethnicity, social status, or race, although these types of differences have become more individually and societally acceptable than they once were.

Nursing interventions at the primary level of prevention with individuals in this stage of development involve education regarding what to expect at various stages in the marriage. Many high schools now offer courses in marriage and family living in which students role-play through anticipatory marriage and family situations. Nurses could offer these kinds of classes within the community to individuals considering marriage. Too many people enter marriage with the notion that, as sure as the depth of their love, their soon-to-be husband or wife will discontinue "undesirable" traits and change into the perceived ideal spouse. Primary prevention with these individuals involves:

- Encouraging honest communication
- Determining what each person expects from the relationship
- Ascertaining whether or not each individual can accept compromise

This type of intervention can be effective in individual or couple's therapy or in support and educational groups of couples experiencing similar circumstances.

PARENTHOOD. Murray and Zentner (2001) state:

> The coming of the child is a crisis, a turning point in the couple's life in which old patterns of living must be changed for new ways of living and new values. With the advent of parenthood, a couple is embarking on a journey from which there is no return. To put it simply, parents cannot quit. The child's birth brings finality to many highly valued privileges and a permanence of responsibilities. (p. 326)

There is perhaps no developmental stage that creates upheaval equal to the arrival of a child. Even when the child is desperately wanted and pleasurably anticipated, his or her arrival usually results in some amount of chaos within the family system.

Because the family operates as a system, the addition of a new member influences all parts of the system as a whole. If it is a first child, the relationship between the spouses is likely to be affected by the demands of caring for the infant on a 24-hour basis. If there are older children, they may resent the attention showered on the new arrival and show their resentment in a variety of creative ways.

The concept of having a child (particularly the first one) is often romanticized, with little or no consideration given to the realities and responsibilities that accompany this "bundle of joy." Many young parents are shocked to realize that such a tiny human can create so many changes in so many lives. It is unfortunate that parenting is one of the most important positions an individual will hold in life and one for which he or she is often least prepared.

Nursing intervention at the primary level of prevention with the developmental stage of parenthood must begin long before the child is even born. How do we prepare individuals for parenthood? *Anticipatory guidance* is the term used to describe the interventions used to help new parents know what they might expect. Volumes have been written on the subject, but it is also important for expectant parents to have a support person or network with whom they can talk, express feelings, excitement, and fears. Nurses can provide the following type of information to help ease the transition into parenthood (Mercer, 2000; Murray & Zentner, 2001; Spock & Parker, 1998):

1. Prepared childbirth classes: what most likely will happen but with additional information about possible variations from what is expected.
2. Information about what to expect after the baby arrives: **Parent-infant bonding:** expectant parents should know that it is common for parent-infant bonding not to occur immediately. The strong attachment will occur as parent and infant get to know each other. **Changing husband-wife relationships:** the couple should be encouraged to engage in open honest communication and role-playing of typical situations that are likely to arise after the baby becomes a part of the family. **Clothing and equipment:** expectant parents need to know what is required to care for a newborn child. Family economics, space available, and lifestyle should be considered. **Feeding:** advantages and disadvantages of both breast-feeding and formula feeding should be presented. The couple should be supported in whatever method is chosen. Anticipatory guidance related to technique should be provided for one or both methods, as the expectant parents request. **Other expectations:** it is important for expectant parents to receive anticipatory guidance about the infant's sleeping and crying patterns, bathing the infant, care of the circumcision and cord, toys that provide stimulation of the newborn's senses, aspects of providing a safe environment, and when to call the physician.
3. Stages of growth and development: it is very important for parents to understand what behaviors should be expected at what stage of development. It is also important to know that their child may not necessarily follow the age guidelines associated with these stages. However, a substantial deviation from these guidelines should be reported to their physician.

MIDLIFE. What is middle age? A colleague once remarked that upon turning 50 years of age she stated, "Now I can say I am officially middle-aged … until I began thinking about how few individuals I really knew who were 100!"

Midlife crises are not defined by a specific number. Various sources in the literature identify these conflicts as occurring anytime between age 35 and 65 years.

What is a midlife crisis? This, too, is very individual, but a number of patterns have been identified within three broad categories:

1. **An alteration in perception of the self.** One's perception of self may occur slowly. One may suddenly become aware of being "old" or "middle-aged." Murray and Zentner (2001) state:

> The individual looks in the mirror and sees changes that others may have noticed for some time. Gray thinning hair and wrinkles, coarsening features, decreased muscular tone, weight gain, varicosities, and capillary breakage may be the first signs of impending age and may suddenly become frighteningly apparent to the individual. (p. 699)

Other biological changes that occur naturally with the aging process may also affect the crises that occur at this time. In women, a gradual decrease in the production of estrogen initiates menopause, which results in a variety of physical and emotional symptoms. Some physical symptoms include "hot flashes," vaginal dryness, cessation of menstruation, loss of reproductive ability, night sweats, insomnia, headaches, and minor memory disturbances. Emotional symptoms include anxiety, depression, crying for no reason, and temper outbursts.

Although the menopausal period in men is not as evident as it is in women, most clinicians subscribe to the belief that men undergo a climacteric experience related to the gradual decrease in production of testosterone. Although sperm production diminishes with advancing age, there is usually no complete cessation, as there is of ovum production in women at menopause (Scanlon & Sanders, 1999). Some men experience hot flashes, sweating, chills, dizziness, and heart palpitations (Murray & Zentner, 2001), whereas others may experience severe depression and an overall decline in physical vigor (Sadock & Sadock, 2003). An alteration in sexual functioning is common (see Chapter 23).

2. **An alteration in perception of others.** A change in relationship with adult children requires a sensitive shift in caring. Wright and Leahey (1994) state:

> The family of origin must relinquish the primary roles of parent and child. They must adapt to the new roles of parent and separate adult. This involves renegotiation of emotional and financial commitments. There is decreased investment in caretaking activities by the parents and increased investment in physical separation and independent living by the young adult. (p. 69)

These experiences are particularly difficult when parents' values conflict with the relationships and types of lifestyles their children choose. An alteration in perception of one's parents also begins to occur during this time. Having always looked to parents for support and comfort, the middle-aged individual may suddenly find that the roles are beginning to reverse. Aging parents may look to their children for assistance with making decisions regarding their everyday lives and for assistance with chores that they have previously accomplished independently. When parents die, middle-aged individuals must come to terms with their own mortality. The process of recognition and resolution of one's own finitude begins in earnest at this time.

3. **An alteration in perception of time.** Middle age has been defined as the end of youth and the beginning of old age. Individuals often experience a sense that time is running out: "I haven't done all I want to do or accomplished all I intended to accomplish!" Depression and a sense of loss may occur as individuals realize that some of the goals established in their youth may indeed go unmet.

"The empty nest" syndrome has been identified as the adjustment period parents experience when the last child leaves home to establish an independent residence. The crisis is often more profound for the mother who has devoted her life to nurturing her family. As the last child leaves, she may perceive her future as uncertain and meaningless. Some women who have devoted their lives to rearing their children decide to develop personal interests and pursue personal goals once the children are grown. This occurs at a time when many husbands have begun to decrease what may have been a compulsive drive for occupational security during the earlier years of their lives. This disparity in common goals may create conflict between husband and wife. At a time when she is experiencing more value in herself and her own life, he may begin to feel less valued. This may also relate to a decrease in the amount of time and support from the wife to which the husband has become accustomed. This type of role change will require numerous adaptations on the part of both spouses.

Finally, an alteration in one's perception of time may be related to the societal striving for eternal youth. Murray and Zentner (2001) state:

> Whether a man or a woman, the person who lacks self-confidence and who cannot accept the changing body, has a compulsion to try cosmetics, clothes, hair styles, and the other trappings of youth in the hope that the physical attributes of youth will be attained. The person tries to regain a youthful figure and face, perhaps through surgery; tints the hair to cover signs of gray; and turns to hormone creams to restore the skin. (pp. 731–732)

This yearning for youth may take the form of sexual promiscuity or extramarital affairs with much younger individuals, in an effort to prove that one "still has what it takes." Some individuals reach for the trappings of youth with regressive-type behaviors, such as the middle-aged man who buys a motorcycle and joins a motorcycle gang and the 50-year-old woman who wears miniskirts and flirts with her daughter's boyfriends. These individuals may be denying their own past and experience. With a negative view of self, they strongly desire to relive their youth.

Nursing intervention at the primary level of prevention with the developmental stage of midlife involves providing accurate information regarding changes that occur during this time of life and support for adapting to these changes effectively. These interventions might include:

1. Nutrition classes to inform individuals in this age group about the essentials of diet and exercise. Educational materials on how to avoid obesity or reduce weight can be included, along with the importance of good nutrition.
2. Assistance with ways to improve health (e.g., quit smoking, cease or reduce alcohol consumption, reduce fat intake).
3. Discussions of the importance of having regular physical examinations, including Pap and breast examinations for women and prostate examinations for men. Monthly breast self-examinations should be taught and yearly mammograms encouraged.
4. Classes on menopause should be given. Provide information about what to expect. Myths that abound regarding this topic should be expelled. Support groups for women (and men) undergoing the menopausal experience should be formed.
5. Support and information related to physical changes occurring in the body during this time of life. Assist with the grief response that some individuals will experience in relation to loss of youth, "empty nest," and sense of identity.
6. Support and information related to care of aging parents should be given. Individuals should be referred to community resources for respite and assistance before strain of the caregiver role threatens to disrupt the family system.

RETIREMENT. Retirement, which is often anticipated as an achievement in principle, may be met with a great deal of ambivalence when it actually occurs. Our society places a great deal of importance on productivity and on earning as much money at as young an age as possible. These types of values contribute to the ambivalence associated with retirement. Although leisure has been acknowledged as a legitimate reward for workers, leisure during retirement has never been accorded the same social value. Adjustment to this life-cycle event becomes more difficult in the face of societal values that are in direct conflict with the new lifestyle.

Historically, many women have derived much of their self-esteem from having children, rearing children, and being a "good mother." Likewise, many men have achieved self-esteem through work-related activities—creativity, productivity, and earning money. With the termination of these activities comes a loss of self-worth. Depression may be the result for some individuals who are unable to adapt satisfactorily.

It would appear that retirement is becoming, and will continue to become, more accepted by societal standards. With more and more individuals retiring earlier and living longer, the growing number of aging persons will spend a significantly longer time in retirement. At present, retirement has become more of an institutionalized expectation, and there appears to be increasing acceptance of it as a social status.

Nursing intervention at the primary level of prevention with the developmental task of retirement involves providing information and support to individuals who have retired or are considering retirement. Support can be on a one-to-one basis to assist these individuals to sort out their feelings regarding retirement. Murray and Zentner (2001) state:

> The retiree may be faced with these questions: Can I face loss of job satisfaction? Will I feel the separation from people close to me at work? If I need continued employment on a part-time basis to supplement Social Security payments, will the old organization provide it, or must I adjust to a new job? Shall I remain in my present home or seek a different one because of easier maintenance or reduced cost of upkeep? Might a different climate be better, and if so, will I miss my relatives and neighbors? (p. 812)

Support can also be provided in a group environment. Support groups of individuals undergoing the same types of experiences can be extremely helpful.

Nurses can form and lead these types of groups to assist retiring individuals through this critical period. These groups can also serve to provide information about available resources that offer assistance to individuals in or nearing retirement, such as information concerning Medicare, Social Security, and Medicaid; information related to organizations that specialize in hiring retirees; and information regarding ways to use newly acquired free time constructively.

Situational Crises

Situational crises are acute responses that occur because of an external circumstantial stressor. The number and types of situational stressors are limitless and may be real or exist only in the perception of the individual. Some types of situational crises that put individuals at risk for mental illness include the following.

POVERTY. A number of studies have identified poverty as a direct correlation to emotional illness. This may have to do with the direct consequences of poverty, such as inadequate and crowded living conditions, nutritional deficiencies, medical neglect, unemployment, or being homeless.

HIGH RATE OF LIFE CHANGE EVENTS. Miller and Rahe (1997) found that frequent changes in life patterns due to a large number of significant events occurring in close proximity tend to decrease a person's ability to deal with stress, and physical or emotional illness may be the result. These include life change events such as death of a loved one, divorce, being fired from job, a change in living conditions, a change in place of employment or residence, physical illness, or a change in body image because of loss of a body part or function.

ENVIRONMENTAL CONDITIONS. Environmental conditions can create situational crises. Tornados, floods, hurricanes, and earthquakes have wreaked devastation on thousands of individuals and families in recent years.

TRAUMA. Individuals who have encountered traumatic experiences must be considered at risk for emotional illness. These include traumatic experiences usually considered outside the range of usual human experience, such as military combat, being a victim of violent personal assault, undergoing torture, being taken hostage or kidnapped, or being the victim of a natural or manmade disaster (APA, 2000).

Nursing intervention at the primary level of prevention with individuals experiencing situational crises is aimed at maintaining the highest possible level of functioning and offering support and assistance with problem solving during the crisis period. Interventions for nursing of clients in crisis include the following:

1. Use a reality-oriented approach. The focus of the problem is on the here and now.
2. Remain with the individual who is experiencing panic anxiety.
3. Establish a rapid working relationship by showing unconditional acceptance, by active listening, and by attending to immediate needs.
4. Discourage lengthy explanations or rationalizations of the situation; promote an atmosphere for verbalization of true feelings.
5. Set firm limits on aggressive, destructive behaviors. At high levels of anxiety, behavior is likely to be impulsive and regressive. Establish at the outset what is acceptable and what is not, and maintain consistency.
6. Clarify the problem that the individual is facing. The nurse does this by describing his or her perception of the problem and comparing it with the individual's perception of the problem.
7. Help the individual determine what he or she believes precipitated the crisis.
8. Acknowledge feelings of anger, guilt, helplessness, and powerlessness, taking care not to provide positive feedback for these feelings.
9. Guide the individual through a problem-solving process by which he or she may move in the direction of positive life change:
   a. Help the individual confront the source of the problem that is creating the crisis response;
   b. Encourage the individual to discuss changes he or she would like to make; jointly determine whether desired changes are realistic;
   c. Encourage exploration of feelings about aspects that cannot be changed, and explore alternative ways of coping in these situations;
   d. Discuss alternative strategies for creating changes that are realistic;
   e. Weigh benefits and consequences of each alternative;
   f. Assist the individual to select alternative coping strategies that will help alleviate future crisis.
10. Identify external support systems and new social networks from which the individual may seek assistance in times of stress.

Nursing, at the level of primary prevention, focuses largely on education of the consumer to prevent initiation or exacerbation of mental illness. An example of just one type of teaching plan for use in primary prevention situations is presented in Table 24–1.

TABLE 24–1 Client Education for Primary Prevention: Drugs of Abuse

Class of Drugs	Effects	Symptoms of Overdose	Trade Names	Common Names	Effects on the Body (Chronic or High-Dose Use)
CNS Depressants					
Alcohol	Relaxation, loss of inhibitions, lack of concentration, drowsiness, slurred speech, sleep	Nausea, vomiting; shallow respirations; cold, clammy skin; weak, rapid pulse; coma; possible death.	Ethyl alcohol, beer, gin, rum, vodka, bourbon, whiskey, liqueurs, wine, brandy, sherry, champagne.	Booze, alcohol, liquor, drinks, cocktails, high balls, nightcaps, moonshine, white lightning, firewater.	Peripheral nerve damage, skeletal muscle wasting, encephalopathy, psychosis, cardiomyopathy, gastritis, esophagitis, pancreatitis, hepatitis, cirrhosis of the liver, leukopenia, thrombocytopenia, sexual dysfunction.
Other (barbiturates and nonbarbiturates)	Same as alcohol.	Anxiety, fever, agitation, hallucinations, disorientation, tremors, delirium, convulsions, possible death.	Seconal Nembutal Amytal Valium Librium Chloral hydrate Equanil, Miltown	Red birds Yellow birds Blue birds Blues/yellows Green & whites Mickies Downers	Decreased REM sleep, respiratory depression, hypotension, possible kidney or liver damage, sexual dysfunction.
CNS Stimulants					
Amphetamines and related drugs	Hyperactivity, agitation, euphoria, insomnia, loss of appetite.	Cardiac arrhythmias, headache, convulsions, hypertension, rapid heart rate, coma, possible death.	Dexedrine, Didrex, Tenuate, Preludin, Ritalin, Plegine, Cylert, Ionamin, Sanorex	Uppers, pep pills, wakeups, bennies, eye-openers, speed, black beauties, sweet A's	Aggressive, compulsive behavior; paranoia; hallucinations; hypertension.
Cocaine	Euphoria, hyperactivity, restlessness, talkativeness, increased pulse, dilated pupils.	Hallucinations, convulsions, pulmonary edema, respiratory failure, coma, cardiac arrest, possible death.	Cocaine hydrochloride	Coke, flake, snow, dust, happy dust, gold dust, girl, cecil, C, toot, blow, crack	Pulmonary hemorrhage; myocardial infarction; ventricular fibrillation.
Opioids	Euphoria, lethargy, drowsiness, lack of motivation.	Shallow breathing, slowed pulse, clammy skin, pulmonary edema, respiratory arrest, convulsions, coma, possible death.	Heroin Morphine Codeine Dilaudid Demerol Methadone Percodan Talwin Opium	Snow, stuff, H, Harry, horse M, morph, Miss Emma Schoolboy Lords Doctors Dollies Perkies T's Big O, black stuff	Respiratory depression, constipation, fecal impaction, hypotension, decreased libido, retarded ejaculation, impotence, orgasm failure.
Hallucinogens	Visual hallucinations, disorientation, confusion, paranoid delusions, euphoria, anxiety, panic, increased pulse.	Agitation, extreme hyperactivity, violence, hallucinations, psychosis, convulsions, possible death.	LSD PCP Mescaline DMT STP	Acid, cube, big D Angel dust, Hog crystal Mesc Businessman's trip Serenity and peace	Panic reaction, acute psychosis, flashbacks.
Cannabinols	Relaxation, talkativeness, lowered inhibitions, euphoria, mood swings.	Fatigue, paranoia, delusions, hallucinations, possible psychosis.	Cannabis Hashish	Marijuana, pot, grass, joint, Mary Jane, MJ Hash, rope, Sweet Lucy	Tachycardia, orthostatic hypotension, chronic bronchitis, problems with infertility, amotivational syndrome.

Secondary Prevention

Populations at Risk

Secondary prevention within communities relates to using early detection and prompt intervention with individuals experiencing mental illness symptoms. The same maturational and situational crises that were presented in the previous section on primary prevention are used to discuss intervention at the secondary level of prevention.

Maturational Crises

ADOLESCENCE. The need for intervention at the secondary level of prevention in adolescence occurs when disruptive and age-inappropriate behaviors become the norm, and the family can no longer cope adaptively with the situation. All levels of dysfunction are considered, from dysfunctional family coping to the need for hospitalization of the adolescent.

Nursing intervention with the adolescent at the secondary level of prevention may occur in the community setting at community mental health centers, physician's offices, schools, public health departments, and crisis intervention centers. They may work with families to problem solve and improve coping and communication skills, or they may work on a one-to-one basis with the adolescent in an attempt to modify behavior patterns.

Adolescents may be hospitalized for a variety of reasons. The *DSM-IV-TR* (APA, 2000) identifies a number of problems, the severity of which would determine whether the adolescent required inpatient care. Conduct disorders, adjustment disorders, eating disorders, substance-related disorders, depression, and anxiety disorders are the most common diagnoses for which adolescents are hospitalized. Nursing care of adolescents in the hospital setting focuses on problem identification and stabilization of the crisis situation. Once stability has been achieved, clients are commonly discharged to outpatient care. If an adolescent's home situation has been deemed unsatisfactory, the state may take custody and the child is then discharged to a group or foster home. Care plans for intervention with the adolescent at the secondary level of prevention can be found in Chapter 21.

MARRIAGE. Problems in a marriage are as far-reaching as the individuals who experience them. Problems that are common to the disruption of a marriage relationship include substance abuse on the part of one or both partners and disagreements on issues of sex, money, children, gender roles, and infidelity, among others. Murray and Zentner (2001) state:

> Staying married to one person and living with the frustrations, conflicts, and boredom that any close and lengthy relationship imposes requires constant work by both parties. (p. 613)

Nursing intervention at the secondary level of prevention with individuals encountering marriage problems may include one or more of the following:

1. Counseling with the couple or with one of the spouses on a one-to-one basis
2. Referral to a couples' support group
3. Identification of the problem and possible solutions; support and guidance as changes are undertaken
4. Referral to a sex therapist
5. Referral to a financial advisor
6. Referral to parent effectiveness training

Murray and Zentner (2001) state:

> When marriage fails and bonds are broken, aloneness, anger, mistrust, hostility, guilt, shame, a sense of betrayal, fear, disappointment, loss of identity, anxiety, and depression, alone or in combination, can appear in both the divorcee and the one initiating the divorce. (p. 677)

In Miller and Rahe's (1997) life change questionnaire, only death of a spouse or other family member scored higher than divorce in severity of stress experienced. This is an area in which nurses can intervene to help ease the transition and prevent emotional breakdown. In community health settings, nurses can lead support groups for newly divorced individuals. They can also provide one-to-one counseling for individuals experiencing the emotional chaos engendered by the dissolution of a marriage relationship.

Divorce also has an impact on the children involved. Nurses can intervene with the children of divorce in an effort to prevent dysfunctional behaviors associated with the breakup of a marriage.

PARENTHOOD. Intervention at the secondary level of prevention with parents can be required for a number of reasons. A few of these include:

1. Physical, emotional, or sexual abuse of a child
2. Physical or emotional neglect of a child
3. Birth of a child with special needs
4. Diagnosis of a terminal illness in a child
5. Death of a child

Nursing intervention at the secondary level of prevention includes being able to recognize the physical and behavioral signs that indicate possible abuse of a child. The child may be cared for in the emergency room or as an inpatient on the pediatric unit or child psychiatric unit of a general hospital.

Nursing intervention with parents may include teaching effective methods of disciplining children, aside from physical punishment. Methods that emphasize the importance of positive reinforcement for acceptable behavior can be very effective. Family members must be committed to consistent use of this behavior modification technique for it to be successful.

Parents should also be informed about behavioral expectations at the various levels of development. Knowledge of what to expect from children at various stages of development may provide needed anticipatory guidance to deal with the crises commonly associated with these various stages.

Therapy sessions with all family members together may focus on problems with family communications. Members are encouraged to express honest feelings in a manner that is nonthreatening to other family members. Active listening, assertiveness techniques, and respect for the rights of others are taught and encouraged. Barriers to effective communication are identified and resolved.

Referrals to agencies that promote effective parenting skills may be made (e.g., parent effectiveness training). Alternative agencies that may provide relief from the stress of parenting may also be considered (e.g., "Mom's day out" programs, sitter-sharing organizations, and day care institutions). Support groups for abusive parents may also be helpful and assistance in locating or initiating such a group may be provided.

The nurse can assist parents who are grieving the loss of a child or the birth of a child with special needs by helping them to express their true feelings associated with the loss. Feelings such as shock, denial, anger, guilt, powerlessness, and hopelessness need to be expressed in order for the parents to progress through the grief response.

Home healthcare assistance can be provided for the family of a child with special needs. This can be done by making referrals to other professionals, such as speech, physical, and occupational therapists, medical social workers, psychologists, and nutritionists. If the child with special needs is hospitalized, the home health nurse can provide specific information to hospital staff that may be helpful in providing continuity of care for the client and help in the transition for the family.

Nursing intervention also includes providing assistance in the location of and referral to support groups that deal with loss of a child or birth of a child with special needs. Some nurses may serve as leaders of these types of groups in the community.

MIDLIFE. Nursing care at the secondary level of prevention during midlife becomes necessary when the individual is unable to integrate all of the changes that are occurring during this period. An inability to accept the physical and biological changes, the changes in relationships between themselves and their adult children and aging parents, and the loss of the perception of youth may result in depression for which the individual may require help to resolve.

RETIREMENT. Retirement can also result in depression for individuals who are unable to satisfactorily grieve for the loss of this aspect of their lives. This is more likely to occur if the individuals have not planned for retirement and if they have derived most of their self-esteem from their employment.

Nursing intervention at the secondary level of prevention with depressed individuals takes place in both inpatient and outpatient settings. Severely depressed clients with suicidal ideations will need close observation in the hospital setting, whereas those with mild to moderate depression may be treated in the community. A nursing care plan for the client with depression is found in Chapter 15. These concepts apply to the secondary level of prevention and may be used in all nursing care settings.

The physician may elect to use pharmacotherapy with antidepressants. Nurses may intervene by providing information to the client about what to expect from the medication, possible side effects, adverse effects, and how to self-administer the medication.

Situational Crises

Nursing care at the secondary level of prevention with clients undergoing situational crises occurs only if crisis intervention at the primary level failed and the individual is unable to function socially or occupationally. Exacerbation of mental illness symptoms requires intervention at the secondary level of prevention. These disorders were addressed extensively in Unit 3. Nursing assessment, diagnosis and outcome identification, plan and implementation, and evaluation were discussed for many of the mental illnesses identified in the *DSM-IV-TR* (APA, 2000). These skills may be applied in any setting where nursing is practiced.

A case study situation of nursing care at the secondary level of prevention in a community setting is presented in Table 24–2.

Tertiary Prevention

Individuals with Chronic Mental Illness

Historical and Epidemiological Aspects

In 1955, more than half a million individuals resided in public mental hospitals. Recent statistics indicate that approximately 100,000 persons with mental illness inhabit these institutions on a long-term basis (Sadock & Sadock, 2003).

Deinstitutionalization of persons with chronic mental illness began in the 1960s as national policy change and with a strong belief in the individual's right to freedom. Other considerations included the deplorable conditions of some of the state asylums, the introduction of neuroleptic medications, and the cost-effectiveness of caring for these individuals in the community setting.

Deinstitutionalization began to occur rapidly and without sufficient planning for the needs of these individuals as they reentered the community. Those who were fortunate enough to have support systems to provide assistance with living arrangements and sheltered employment experiences most often received the outpatient treatment they required. However, those without adequate support managed to survive on

TABLE 24–2 Secondary Prevention Case Study: Parenthood

The identified patient was a petite, doll-like 4-year-old girl named Tanya. She was the older of two children in a Latino family. The other child was a boy named Joseph, age 2. The mother was 5 months pregnant with their third child. The family had been referred to the nurse after Tanya was placed in foster care following a report to Department of Human Services (DHS) by her nursery school teacher that the child had marks on her body suspicious of child abuse.

The parents, Paulo and Annette, were in their mid-20s. Paulo had lost his job at an aircraft plant 3 months ago and had since been unable to find work. Annette brought in a few dollars from cleaning houses for other people, but the family was struggling to survive.

Paulo and Annette were angry at having to see the nurse. After all, "Parents have the right to discipline their children." The nurse did not focus on the *intent* of the behavior, but instead looked at factors in the family's life that could be viewed as stressors. This family had multiple stressors: poverty, the father's unemployment, the age and spacing of the children, the mother's chronic fatigue from work at home, as well as in other people's homes, and finally, having a child removed from the home against the parents' wishes.

During therapy with this family, the nurse discussed the behaviors associated with various developmental levels. She also discussed possible deviations from these norms and when they should be reported to the physician. The nurse and the family discussed Tanya's behavior, and how it compared with the norms.

The parents also discussed their own childhoods. They were able to relate some of the same types of behaviors that they observed in Tanya. However, they both admitted that they came from families whose main method of discipline was physical punishment. Annette had been the oldest child in her large family, and had been expected to "keep the younger ones in line." When she had not done so, she was punished with her father's belt. She expressed anger toward her father, although she had never been allowed to express it at the time.

Paulo's father had died when he was a small boy, and Paulo had been expected to be the "man of the family." He worked at odd jobs from the time he was very young to bring money into the home. Because of this, he had little time for the usual activities of childhood and adolescence. He held much resentment toward the young men who "had everything and never had to work for it."

Paulo and Annette had high expectations for Tanya. In effect, they expected her to behave in a manner well beyond her developmental level. These expectations were based on the reflections of their own childhoods. They were uncomfortable with the spontaneity and playfulness of childhood, for they had had little personal experience with these behaviors. When Tanya balked and expressed the verbal assertions common to early childhood, Paulo and Annette interpreted these behaviors as defiance toward them, and retaliated with anger in the manner in which they had been parented.

With the parents, the nurse explored feelings and behaviors from their past so that they were able to understand the correlation to their current behaviors. They learned to negotiate ways to deal with Tanya's age-appropriate behaviors. In combined therapy with Tanya, they learned how to relate to her childishness, and even how to enjoy playing with both of their children.

The parents ceased blaming each other for the family's problems. Annette had spent a good deal of her time deprecating Paulo for his lack of support of his family, and Paulo blamed Annette for being "unable to control her daughter." Communication patterns were clarified, and life in the family became more peaceful.

Without a need to "prove himself" to his wife, Paulo's efforts to find employment met with success, as he no longer felt the need to turn down jobs that he knew his wife would perceive to be beneath his capabilities. Annette no longer works outside the home, and both she and Paulo participate in the parenting chores. Tanya and her siblings continue to demonstrate age-appropriate developmental progression.

a meager existence or were forced to join the ranks of the homeless. Some ended up in nursing homes meant to provide care for individuals with physical disabilities.

Large segments of our population with chronic mental illness problems are left untreated: the elderly, the "working poor," the homeless, and those individuals previously covered by funds that have been cut by various social reforms (Talley & Coleman, 1992). These circumstances have promoted in individuals with chronic mental illness a greater number of crisis-oriented emergency department visits and hospital admissions, and repeated confrontations with law enforcement officials.

The community-based mental health system is not working for the chronically mentally ill. The Coalition of Psychiatric Nursing Organizations has developed a position paper in which barriers to care are described and essential services delineated (Krauss, 1993). The Coalition identified the following five barriers:

1. **Public attitudes.** A social stigma still exists regarding attitudes toward mental illness, even in light of the fact that in 1998, 44.3 million adults had some form of mental disorder. In fact, a study by the NIMH reports that one in five adults in the United States suffers from a diagnosable mental disorder in a given year (NIMH, 2002). The unfortunate fact is that having cancer is considered more "socially appropriate" than having a mental disorder.
2. **Fragmented systems.** Our nation's health policy ignores the biopsychosocial aspects of illness. Body and mind cannot be separated, yet our system is not properly prepared to meet the general healthcare needs on a holistic level. Because of fragmented and diminished services, many consumers cannot achieve the level of care required to maintain a satisfactory community existence.
3. **Poverty and race.** Poor people have limited access to mental health services because of economics and cultural implications, yet studies show that poverty increases one's risk of psychiatric illness by twofold. Children born into poverty are two to three times more likely to develop emotional or behavioral problems (Krauss, 1993).
4. **Private insurance.** Coverage for mental health services by private insurance companies is and always has been far less comprehensive than for physical illness. Benefits and reimbursements are lower, and deductibles and copayments are higher. Some individuals who have insurance coverage will not file claims for mental healthcare for fear that they may suffer repercussions from disclosure of such information.
5. **Public funding.** Public funding of mental health services comes from various state and federal sources. Most is apportioned to pay for costly inpatient treatment of individuals who require acute care because of decompensation of their illness (which may have been prevented if less costly outpatient care had been available).

The Coalition outlined the following essential services for mental health reform:

1. **Primary care mental health services.** Krauss (1993) states:

> Community-based primary care settings should serve as an essential consumer pathway to mental health services. Such settings must be prepared to provide mental health promotion and education programs, case finding, diagnostic assessments, routine treatment, and referral.

2. **Universal access to a basic mental health package.** The Coalition advocates a universal minimum-benefit package that ensures access to mental health services (both inpatient and outpatient) to all individuals across the life span.
3. **Long-term care.** The Coalition recommends assurance of long-term or rehabilitative services for clients with mental impairment. The Coalition proposes, "Such care should be financed by public funds and sliding-scale service fees, and authorized by a care coordinator or case manager."
4. **Managed care.** The Coalition views the concept of managed care as a "cost-effective monitoring system for the delivery of mental health services," and a way to "ensure that maximum value is received from the resources used in the production and delivery of healthcare services."

If these proposals became reality, it would surely mean improvement in the care of individuals who are chronically mentally ill. Many nurse leaders see this period of healthcare reform as an opportunity for nurses to expand their roles and assume key positions in education, prevention, assessment, and referral. Nurses are, and will continue to be, in key positions to assist chronically mentally ill clients to remain as independent as possible, to manage their illness within the community setting, and to strive to minimize the number of hospitalizations required.

Treatment Alternatives

COMMUNITY MENTAL HEALTH CENTERS. The goal of community mental health centers in caring for the chronically mentally ill is to improve coping ability and prevent exacerbation of acute symptoms. A major obstacle in meeting this goal has been the lack of advocacy or sponsorship for clients who require services from a variety of sources. This has placed responsibility for healthcare on an individual with mental illness who is often barely able to cope with everyday life (Pittman, 1989). **Case management** is becoming a recommended method of treatment for individuals with a chronic mental illness.

The ANA (1992a) has endorsed case management as an effective method of providing care for clients in the community who require long-term assistance, and nurses as uniquely qualified case managers:

> Nurses bring broad-based and unique skills and knowledge to case management. The role of the nurse as a coordinator of care has been integral to defining nursing practice for decades. The coordination of services and care is the primary function of case managers. This role is a logical extension of the nursing role. (p. 14)

Bower (1992) has identified five core components and nursing role functions that blend with the steps of the nursing process to form a framework for nursing case management. The core components include:

- **Interaction.** The nurse must develop a trusting relationship with the client, family members, and other service providers. During an initial screening, the nurse determines if the client is eligible for case management according to preestablished guidelines and, if not, refers the client for appropriate assistance elsewhere.
- **Assessment: establishment of a database.** The nurse conducts a comprehensive assessment of the client's physical health status, functional capability, mental status, personal and community support systems, financial resources, and environmental conditions. The data are then analyzed and appropriate nursing diagnoses formulated.
- **Planning.** A service care plan is devised with client participation. The plan should include mutually agreed-on goals, specific actions directed toward goal achievement, and selection of essential resources and services through collaboration among healthcare professionals, the client, and the family or significant others.
- **Implementation.** In this phase, the client receives the needed services from appropriate providers. In some instances, the nursing case manager is also a provider of care, whereas in others, he or she is only the coordinator of care.
- **Evaluation.** The case manager continuously monitors and evaluates the client's responses to interventions and progress toward preestablished goals. Regular contact is maintained with client, family or significant others, and direct service providers. Ongoing care coordination continues until outcomes have been achieved. The client may then be discharged or assigned to inactive status, as appropriate.

A case study of nursing case management within a community mental health center is presented in Table 24–3.

DAY-EVENING TREATMENT/PARTIAL HOSPITALIZATION PROGRAMS. Day or evening treatment programs (also called partial hospitalization) are designed to prevent institutionalization or to ease the transition from inpatient hospitalization to community living. Various types of treatment are offered. Many include therapeutic community (milieu) activities; individual, group, and family therapies; psychoeducation; alcohol and drug education; crisis intervention; therapeutic recreational activities; and occupational therapy. Many programs offer medication administration and monitoring as part of their care.

Partial hospitalization programs generally offer a comprehensive treatment plan formulated by an interdisciplinary team of psychiatrists, psychologists, nurses, occupational and recreational therapists, and social workers.

Wilkinson (1991) describes a specialty program within the framework of a day-treatment program. Because individuals with chronic mental illness are frequently noncompliant with psychotropic medications, Wilkinson and colleagues established a medication clinic and medication group, each of which met on a weekly basis to provide education and support of individuals on long-term psychopharmacological therapy. During medication clinic appointments, clients are evaluated in relation to effectiveness of and side effects or adverse reactions associated with their medication. Medication groups are assembled according to type of drug being used (e.g., individuals taking antipsychotics compose one group, and those taking antidepressants are in another). The groups are time limited and led by the psychiatric clinical nurse specialist, who provides education and support as needed. As a result of these efforts, Wilkinson reports a 96 per-

TABLE 24–3 Nursing Case Management in the Community Mental Health Center: A Case Study

Michael, 73 years old with a history of multiple psychiatric admissions, has lived in various adult foster homes and boarding houses for the past 10 years. He was originally diagnosed as having schizophrenia, but he was recently rediagnosed as having bipolar disorder, mania. His symptoms are well controlled with lithium 300 mg three times a day, which is prescribed by the outpatient psychiatrist.

The nurse practitioner/case manager in the outpatient clinic coordinates Michael's care, advocates for his needs, and counsels him regarding his health problems. She orders routine blood tests to assess his lithium levels. When Michael experienced visual disturbances, she referred him for an emergency eye evaluation. He was found to have a retinal detachment and was sent to a local VA hospital for emergency surgery. After his eye surgery, the nurse practitioner arranged transportation to his follow-up visits with the eye doctor and instructed him about his eye care and instillation of his eye drops. Michael did not like putting eye drops in his eye and tended to neglect doing it. Because he also had glaucoma and required ongoing treatment with pilocarpine and timolol maleate eye drops twice daily, he needed a great deal of education and reassurance to continue using the eye drops.

In addition to routine quarterly visits for ongoing case management, the nurse practitioner also performs his annual health assessment consisting of history, review of systems, mental status exam, and physical assessment. During Michael's last physical examination, the nurse practitioner detected a thyroid mass and referred him for a complete evaluation including thyroid function tests, a thyroid scan, and evaluation by a surgeon and an endocrinologist. She discussed his thyroid problem with the surgeon and the endocrinologist, and they determined that Michael would best benefit from thyroid replacement therapy (i.e., levothyroxine sodium 0.1 mg daily).

Because Michael eats all of his meals in restaurants, the nurse was concerned about his diet. A brief diet review revealed that his diet was low in vitamin C. He was then instructed in which foods and juices he should include in his daily menu. The nurse practitioner discussed ways that Michael could get the best nutrition for the least cost.

Michael is currently living in a boarding house and is totally responsible for taking his own medication, attending to his activities of daily living, and managing his own money. He has very limited income and depends on donations for many of his clothing needs.

Despite his age, he is quite active and alert. He attends many VA-sponsored social activities and does daily volunteer work at the VA, such as pushing wheelchairs, running errands, and escorting other veterans to clinic appointments. His nurse case manager arranged for him to receive free lunches as a reward for some of his volunteer activities.

Nursing case management has helped this elderly man with chronic psychiatric illness and many years of hospitalization to live independently within the community setting.

From Pittman (1989), with permission.

cent success rate with medication compliance and subsequent client adjustment to community living.

Nurses take a leading role in the administration of partial hospitalization programs. They lead groups, provide crisis intervention, conduct individual counseling, act as role models, and make necessary referrals for specialized treatment. Use of the nursing process provides continual evaluation of the program, and modifications can be made as necessary. Pittman, Parsons, and Peterson (1990) state:

> Day programs for the chronically mentally ill have been shown to be effective in preventing hospitalization. They help to facilitate the transition from the hospital back into the mainstream of the community. They can improve the quality of life of the deinstitutionalized person by providing social skills training, adding structure and support to the person's daily life, and providing opportunities for socialization. (p. 11)

COMMUNITY RESIDENTIAL FACILITIES. Community residential facilities for persons with chronic mental illness are known by many names: group homes, halfway houses, foster homes, boarding homes, sheltered care facilities, transitional housing, independent living programs, social-rehabilitation residences, and others. These facilities differ by the purpose for which they exist and the activities that they offer.

Some of these facilities provide food, shelter, housekeeping, and minimal supervision and assistance with activities of daily living. Others offer a variety of therapies and serve as a transition between hospital and independent living. In addition to the basics, services might include individual and group counseling, medical care, job training or employment assistance, and leisure-time activities.

A wide variety of personnel staffs these facilities. Some facilities have live-in professionals who are available at all times, some have professional staff who are on call for intervention during crisis situations, and some are staffed by volunteers and individuals with little knowledge or background for understanding and treating persons who are chronically mentally ill.

The concept of transitional housing for the chronically mentally ill is sound and has proved, in many instances, to be a successful means of therapeutic support and intervention for maintaining them within the community. However, without guidance and planning, transition to the community can be futile. These individuals may be ridiculed and rejected by the community. They may be targets of unscrupulous individuals who take advantage of their inability to care for themselves satisfactorily. These behaviors may increase maladaptive responses to the demands of community living and exacerbate the mental illness. A period of structured reorientation to the community in a living situation that is supervised and monitored by professionals is more likely to result in a successful transition for the individual with chronic mental illness.

PSYCHIATRIC HOME HEALTHCARE. For the chronically mentally ill who no longer live in a structured, supervised setting, home healthcare may be the element that helps to keep the individual living independently. To receive home healthcare, individuals must validate their homebound status for the prospective payer (Medicare, Medicaid, most insurance companies, and Veteran's Administration [VA] benefits). An acute psychiatric diagnosis is not enough to qualify for the service. The plan of treatment and subsequent charting must explain why the client's psychiatric disorder keeps him or her at home and justify the need for home services.

Homebound clients most often have diagnoses of depression, dementia, anxiety disorders, bipolar affective disorder, and schizophrenia (Duffey & Miller, 1996). Many elderly clients are homebound because of medical conditions that impair mobility and necessitate home care.

Nurses who provide psychiatric home care must have an in-depth knowledge of psychopathology, psychopharmacology, and how medical and physical problems can be influenced by psychiatric impairments (Finkelman, 1997). These nurses must be highly adept at performing biopsychosocial assessments. They must be sensitive to changes in behavior that signal that the client is decompensating psychiatrically or medically so that early intervention may be implemented.

Another important job of the psychiatric home health nurse is monitoring compliance with the regimen of psychotropic medications. Some clients who are receiving injectable medications remain on home healthcare only until they can be placed on oral medications. Those clients receiving oral medications require close monitoring for compliance and assistance with the uncomfortable side effects of some of these drugs. Medication noncompliance is responsible for approximately two-thirds of psychiatric hospital readmissions. Home health nurses can assist clients with this problem by helping them to see the relationship between control of their psychiatric symptoms and compliance with their medication regimen.

Client populations that benefit from psychiatric home health nursing include:

1. **Elderly clients.** These individuals may not have a psychiatric diagnosis, but they may be experiencing emotional difficulties that have arisen from medical, sociocultural, or developmental factors. Depressed mood and social isolation are common.
2. **Persons with chronic mental illness.** These individuals have a history of psychiatric illness and hospitalization. They require long-term medications and continual supportive care. Common diagnoses include recurrent major depression, schizophrenia, and borderline personality disorder.
3. **Individuals in acute crisis.** These individuals are in need of crisis intervention and and/or short-term psychotherapy.

The American Nurses Association (ANA) (1992b) defines home health nursing as:

> The practice of nursing applied to a patient with a health deficit in the patient's place of residence. Patients and their designated caregivers are the focus of home health nursing practice. The goal of care is to initiate, manage, and evaluate the resources needed to promote the patient's optimal level of well-being. (p. 5)

Medicare requires that psychiatric home nursing care be provided by "psychiatrically trained nurses" whom they define as "…nurses who have special training and/or experience beyond the standard curriculum required for a registered nurse" (Health Care Financing Administration [HCFA], 2002).

The guidelines that cover psychiatric nursing services are not well defined by HCFA. This has presented some reimbursement problems for psychiatric nurses in the past. The HCFA statement regarding psychiatric nursing services is presented in Table 24–4.

Finkelman (1997) suggests that the ideal candidate for a psychiatric home health nurse has a minimum of 1 year of medical-surgical nursing experience, as well as several years of psychiatric inpatient treatment experience. Further training and experience in psychotherapy is viewed as an asset. However, psychotherapy is not the primary focus of psychiatric home nursing care. In fact, most reimbursement sources say they will not pay for exclusively insight-oriented "therapy" (Duffey & Miller, 1996). Peplau (1995) states, "Hands-on care, health teaching, coordination of care, and supervision of home health aides are all nursing functions in psychiatric home care." Crisis intervention is common in psychiatric home nursing care.

TABLE 24–4 HCFA Guidelines for Psychiatric Home Nursing Care

Psychiatric Evaluation, Therapy, and Teaching

The evaluation, psychotherapy, and teaching activities needed by a patient suffering from a diagnosed psychiatric disorder that requires active treatment by a psychiatrically trained nurse and the costs of the psychiatric nurse's services may be covered as a skilled nursing service. Psychiatrically trained nurses are nurses who have special training and/or experience beyond the standard curriculum required for a registered nurse. The services of the psychiatric nurse are to be provided under a plan of care established and reviewed by a physician.

Health Care Financing Administration, 2002.

The psychiatric home health nurse provides comprehensive nursing care, incorporating interventions for physical and psychosocial problems into the treatment plan. The interventions are based on the client's mental and physical health status, cultural influences, and available resources. The nurse is accountable to the client at all times during the therapeutic relationship. Nursing interventions are carried out with appropriate knowledge and skill, and referrals are made when the need is outside the scope of nursing practice. Continued collaboration with other members of the healthcare team (e.g., psychiatrist, social worker, psychologist, occupational therapist, and/or physical therapist) is essential for maintaining continuity of care.

A case study of psychiatric home healthcare and the nursing process is presented in Table 24–5. A plan of care for Mrs. C (the client in the case study) is presented in Table 24–6. Nursing diagnoses are presented, along with outcome criteria, appropriate nursing interventions, and rationale for each.

TABLE 24–5 Psychiatric Home Healthcare and the Nursing Process: A Case Study

Assessment

Mrs. C, age 76, has been living alone in her small apartment for 6 months since the death of her husband, to whom she had been married for 51 years. Mrs. C had been an elementary school teacher for 40 years, retiring at age 65 with an adequate pension. She and her husband had no children. A niece looks in on Mrs. C regularly. It was she who contacted Mrs. C's physician when she observed that Mrs. C was not eating properly, was losing weight, and seemed to be increasingly isolating herself. She had not left her apartment in weeks. Her physician referred her to psychiatric home healthcare.

On her initial visit, Carol, the psychiatric home health nurse, conducted a preliminary assessment revealing the following information about Mrs. C:

1. Blood pressure 90/60 mm Hg
2. Height 5 ft 5 in; weight 102 lb
3. Poor skin turgor; dehydration
4. Subjective report of occasional dizziness
5. Subjective report of loss of 20 lb since death of husband
6. Oriented to time, place, person, and situation.
7. Memory (remote and recent) intact
8. Flat affect
9. Mood is dysphoric and tearful at times, but client is cooperative.
10. Denies thoughts to harm self, but states, "I feel so alone; so useless."
11. Subjective report of difficulty sleeping
12. Subjective report of constipation

Diagnosis/Outcome Identification

The following nursing diagnoses were formulated for Mrs. C:

1. Dysfunctional grieving related to death of husband evidenced by symptoms of depression such as withdrawal, anorexia, weight loss, difficulty sleeping, dysphoric/tearful mood.
2. Risk for injury related to dizziness and weakness from lack of activity, low blood pressure, and poor nutritional status.
3. Social isolation related to depressed mood and feelings of worthlessness, evidenced by staying home alone, refusing to leave her apartment.

Outcome Criteria. The following criteria were selected as measurement of outcomes in the care of Mrs. C:

1. Experiences no physical harm/injury
2. Is able to discuss feelings about husband's death with nurse
3. Sets realistic goals for self
4. Is able to participate in problem solving regarding her future
5. Eats a well-balanced diet with snacks to restore nutritional status and gain weight
6. Drinks adequate fluid daily
7. Sleeps at least 6 hours per night and verbalizes feeling well rested

(Continued)

TABLE 24–5 Psychiatric Home Healthcare and the Nursing Process: A Case Study *(Continued)*

8. Shows interest in personal appearance and hygiene, and is able to accomplish self-care independently
9. Seeks to renew contact with previous friends and acquaintances
10. Verbalizes interest in participating in social activities

Plan/Implementation

A plan of care for Mrs. C is presented in Table 24–6.

Evaluation

Mrs. C was started the second week taking trazodone (Desyrel) 150 mg at bedtime. Her sleep was enhanced, and within 2 weeks she showed a noticeable improvement in mood. She began to discuss how angry she felt about being alone in the world. She admitted that she had felt anger toward her husband but experienced guilt and tried to suppress that anger. As she was assured that these feelings were normal, they became easier for her to express.

The nurse arranged for a local teenager to do some weekly grocery shopping for Mrs. C and contacted the local Meals on Wheels program, which delivered her noon meal to her every day. Mrs. C began to eat more and slowly to gain a few pounds. She still has an occasional problem with constipation but verbalizes improvement with the addition of vegetables, fruit, and a daily stool softener prescribed by her physician.

Mrs. C used her walker until she felt she was able to ambulate without assistance. She reports that she no longer experiences dizziness, and her blood pressure has stabilized at around 100/70 mm Hg.

Mrs. C has joined a senior citizens group and attends activities weekly. She has renewed previous friendships and formed new acquaintances. She sees her physician monthly for medication management and visits a local adult day health center for regular blood pressure and weight checks. Her niece still visits regularly, but her favorite relationship is the one she has formed with her constant canine companion, Molly, whom Mrs. C rescued from the local animal shelter and who continually demonstrates her unconditional love and gratitude.

TABLE 24–6 Care Plan for Psychiatric Home Health Care of Depressed Elderly Person (Mrs. C)

Nursing Diagnosis: DYSFUNCTIONAL GRIEVING

Related to: Death of husband

Evidenced by: Symptoms of depression such as withdrawal, anorexia, weight loss, difficulty sleeping, and dysphoric/tearful mood

Outcome Criteria	Nursing Interventions	Rationale
Mrs. C will demonstrate adaptive grieving behaviors and evidence of progression toward resolution.	1. Assess Mrs. C's position in the grief process.	1. Accurate baseline data are required to plan accurate care for Mrs. C.
	2. Develop a trusting relationship by showing empathy and caring. Be honest and keep all promises. Show genuine positive regard.	2. These interventions provide the basis for a therapeutic relationship.
	3. Explore feelings of anger and help Mrs. C direct them toward the source. Help her understand it is appropriate and acceptable to have feelings of anger and guilt about her husband's death.	3. Knowledge of acceptability of the feelings associated with normal grieving may help to relieve some of the guilt that these responses generate.
	4. Encourage Mrs. C to review honestly the relationship she had with her husband. With support and sensitivity, point out reality of the situation in areas where misrepresentations may be expressed.	4. Mrs. C must give up an idealized perception of her husband. Only when she is able to see both positive and negative aspects about the relationship will the grieving process be complete.
	5. Determine if Mrs. C has spiritual needs that are going unfulfilled. If so, contact spiritual leader for intervention with Mrs. C.	5. Recovery may be blocked if spiritual distress is present and care is not provided.
	6. Refer Mrs. C to physician for medication evaluation.	6. Antidepressant therapy may help Mrs. C to function while confronting the dynamics of her depression.

Nursing Diagnosis: RISK FOR INJURY

Related to: Dizziness and weakness from lack of activity, low blood pressure, and poor nutritional status

Outcome Criteria	Nursing Interventions	Rationale
Mrs. C will not experience physical harm or injury.	1. Assess vital signs at every visit. Report to physician should they fall below baseline.	1. Client safety is a nursing priority.
	2. Encourage Mrs. C to use walker until strength has returned.	2. The walker will help to prevent Mrs. C from falling.
	3. Visit Mrs. C during mealtimes and sit with her while she eats. Encourage her niece to do the same. Ensure that easy to prepare, nutritious foods for meals and snacks are available in the house and that they are items that Mrs. C likes.	3. She is more likely to eat what is convenient and what she enjoys.
	4. Contact local meal delivery service (e.g., Meals on Wheels) to deliver some of Mrs. C's meals.	4. This would ensure that she receives at least one complete and nutritious meal each day.
	5. Weigh Mrs. C each week.	5. Weight gain is a measurable, objective means of assessing whether Mrs. C is eating.
	6. Ensure that diet contains sufficient fluid and fiber.	6. Adequate dietary fluid and fiber will help to alleviate constipation. She may also benefit from a daily stool softener.

Nursing Diagnosis: SOCIAL ISOLATION

Related to: Depressed mood and feelings of worthlessness

Evidenced by: Staying home alone, refusing to leave apartment

Outcome Criteria	Nursing Interventions	Rationale
Mrs. C will renew contact with friends and participate in social activities.	1. As nutritional status is improving and strength is gained, encourage Mrs. C to become more active. Take walks with her; help her perform simple tasks around her house.	1. Increased activity enhances both physical and mental status.
	2. Assess lifelong patterns of relationships.	2. Basic personality characteristics will not change. Mrs. C will very likely keep the same style of relationship development that she had in the past.
	3. Help her identify present relationships that are satisfying and activities that she considers interesting.	3. She is the person who truly knows what she likes, and these personal preferences will facilitate success in reversing social isolation.
	4. Consider the feasibility of a pet.	4. There are many documented studies of the benefits to elderly individuals of companion pets.
	5. Suggest possible alternatives that Mrs. C may consider as she seeks to participate in social activities. These may include foster grandparent programs, senior citizens centers, church activities, craft groups, and volunteer activities. Help her to locate individuals with whom she may attend some of these activities.	5. She is more likely to attend and participate if she does not have to do so alone.

CARE FOR THE CAREGIVERS. Another aspect of psychiatric home healthcare is to provide support and assistance to primary caregivers. When family is the provider of care on a 7-day-a-week, 24-hour-a-day schedule for a loved one with a chronic mental disorder, it can be very exhausting and very frustrating. A care plan for primary caregivers is presented in Table 24–7.

TABLE 24–7 Care Plan for Primary Caregiver of Client with Chronic Mental Illness

Nursing Diagnosis: CAREGIVER ROLE STRAIN

Related to: Severity and duration of the care receiver's illness and lack of respite and recreation for the caregiver

Evidenced by: Feelings of stress in relationship with care receiver, feelings of depression and anger, family conflict around issues of providing care

Outcome Criteria	Nursing Interventions	Rationale
Caregivers will achieve effective problem-solving skills and develop adaptive coping mechanisms to regain equilibrium.	1. Assess prospective caregivers' abilities to anticipate and fulfill client's unmet needs. Provide information to assist caregivers with this responsibility. Ensure that caregivers encourage client to be as independent as possible.	1. Caregivers may be unaware of what the client can realistically accomplish. They may be unaware of the nature of the illness.
	2. Ensure that caregivers are aware of available community support systems from whom they can seek assistance when required. Examples include respite care services, day treatment centers, and adult day care centers.	2. Caregivers require relief from the pressures and strain of providing 24-hour care for their loved one. Studies have shown that abuse arises out of caregiving situations that place overwhelming stress on the caregivers.
	3. Encourage caregivers to express feelings, particularly anger.	3. Release of these emotions can serve to prevent psychopathology, such as depression or psychophysiological disorders, from occurring.
	4. Encourage participation in support groups comprised of members with similar life situations. Provide information about support groups that may be helpful: a. National Alliance for the Mentally Ill (800) 950-NAMI b. Association on Mental Retardation (800) 424-3688 c. Association for Retarded Citizens (301) 565-3842 d. Alzheimer's Disease and Related Disorders Association (800) 272-3900	4. Hearing others who are experiencing the same problems discuss ways in which they have coped may help the caregiver adopt more adaptive strategies. Individuals who are experiencing similar life situations provide empathy and support for each other.

THE HOMELESS POPULATION

Historical and Epidemiological Aspects

Dr. Richard Lamb (1992) has stated:

> Alec Guinness, in his memorable role as a British Army colonel in *Bridge on the River Kwai*, exclaims at the end of the film when he finally realizes he has been working to help the enemy, "What have I done?" As a vocal advocate and spokesperson for deinstitutionalization and community treatment of severely mentally ill patients for well over two decades, I often find myself asking that same question.

The number of homeless in the United States has been estimated at somewhere between 250,000 and 4 million. It is difficult to determine the true scope of the problem because even the statisticians who collect the data have difficulty defining homeless persons. Criteria have included: "those people who sleep in shelters or public spaces" (Susser, Conover, & Struening, 1990). This approach results in underestimates because available shelter services are insufficient to meet the numbers of homeless people (U.S. Conference of Mayors, 2001).

According to the Stewart B. McKinney Act, a person is considered homeless who:

> lacks a fixed, regular, and adequate night-time residence; and...has a primary night-time residency that is : (A) a supervised publicly or privately operated shelter designed to provide temporary living accommodations, (B) an institution that provides a temporary residence for individuals intended to be institutionalized, or (C) a public or private place not designed for, or ordinarily used as, a regular sleeping accommodation for human beings. (National Coalition for the Homeless [NCH], 1999b)

Two methods of counting the homeless are commonly used (NCH, 1999a). The point-in-time method attempts to count all the people who are literally homeless on a given day or during a given week. The second method (called *period prevalence counts*) examines the number of people who are homeless over a given period. This second method may result in a more accurate count because the extended time period would allow for including the people who are homeless 1 day (or week) but find employment and affordable housing later, removing them from the count of homeless persons. At the same time during this extended period, others would lose housing and become homeless.

Who are the Homeless?

The U.S. Conference of Mayors (2001) reports that during the past year requests for emergency shelter increased in the survey cities by an average of 13 percent. Homeless persons are increasingly a heterogeneous group. The NCH (1999b) provides the following demographics:

AGE. Studies have produced a variety of statistics related to age of the homeless: 25 percent are younger than 18 years of age; individuals between the ages of 31 and 50 comprise 51 percent; and persons age 55 through 60 have been estimated at 2.5 to 19.4 percent.

GENDER. More men than women are homeless. The U.S. Conference of Mayors (2001) study found that single men comprise 40 percent of the urban homeless population and single women 14 percent.

FAMILIES. Families with children are among the fastest growing segments of the homeless population. Families comprise 40 percent of the urban homeless population, but research indicates that this number is likely higher in rural areas, where families, single mothers, and children make up the largest group of homeless people.

ETHNICITY. The study by the U.S. Conference of Mayors (2001) found that the homeless population was 50 percent African-American, 35 percent Caucasian, 12 percent Hispanic, 2 percent Native American, and 1 percent Asian. The ethnic makeup of homeless populations varies according to geographic location.

Mental Illness and Homelessness

It is thought that approximately 22 percent of the homeless population suffers from some form of mental illness (U.S. Conference of Mayors, 2001). Who are these individuals, and why are they homeless? Some blame the deinstitutionalization movement. Persons with mental illness who were released from state and county mental hospitals and who did not have families with whom they could reside sought residence in board and care homes of varying quality. Halfway houses and supportive group living arrangements were helpful but scarce. Many of those with families returned to their homes, but because families received little if any instruction or support, the consequences of their mentally ill loved one returning to live at home were often turbulent, resulting in the individual frequently leaving home.

Types of Mental Illness Among the Homeless

A number of studies have been conducted, primarily in large, urban areas, which have addressed the most common types of mental illness identified among homeless individuals. Schizophrenia is frequently described as the most common diagnosis. Other prevalent disorders include bipolar affective disorder, substance abuse and dependence, depression, personality disorders, and organic mental disorders. Many exhibit psychotic symptoms, many are former residents of long-term care institutions for the mentally ill, and many have such a strong desire for independence that they isolate themselves in an effort to avoid being identified as a part of the mental health system. Many of them are clearly a danger to themselves or others, yet they do not see themselves as ill (Torrey, 1997).

Contributing Factors to Homelessness Among the Mentally Ill

DEINSTITUTIONALIZATION. As previously stated, deinstitutionalization is frequently implicated as a contributing factor to homelessness among the mentally ill. Deinstitutionalization began out of expressed concern by mental health professionals and others who described the "deplorable conditions" under which mentally ill individuals were housed.

The advent of psychotropic medications and the community mental health movement began a growing philosophical view that mentally ill individuals receive better and more humanitarian treatment in the community than in state hospitals far removed from their homes. It was believed that commitment and institutionalization in many ways deprived these individuals of their civil rights (Lamb, 1992). Not the least of the motivating factors for deinstitutionalization was the financial burden these clients placed on state governments.

In fact, deinstitutionalization has not failed completely. About 50 percent of the mentally ill population—those who have insight into their illness and need for medication—have done reasonably well since leaving the hospital (Torrey, 1997). It is the other 50 percent who lack such insight and often stop taking their medication that end up on the streets.

However, because the vast increases in homelessness did not occur until the 1980s, the release of severely mentally ill people from institutions cannot be solely to blame. A number of other factors have been implicated.

POVERTY. Cuts in various government entitlement programs have depleted the allotments available for chronically mentally ill individuals living in the community. The job market is prohibitive for individuals whose behavior is incomprehensible or even frightening to many. The stigma and discrimination associated with mental illness may be diminishing slowly, but it is highly visible to those who suffer from its effects.

A SCARCITY OF AFFORDABLE HOUSING. Wallsten (1992) states:

> Economic policies and issues have contributed to the growing numbers and different profiles of the homeless. Urban redevelopment projects eliminated a considerable amount of low-cost housing options for poor people. A growing number of impoverished families have been doubling and tripling up in single housing units as affordable housing becomes more scarce. A sizable proportion of residents in these renewal areas were poor elderly renting rooms in houses, residential hotels, and missions. (p. 21)

In addition, the number of single-room-occupancy (SRO) hotels has diminished drastically. These SRO hotels provided a means of relatively inexpensive housing for chronic psychiatric clients. Although some people believe that these facilities nurtured isolation, they provided adequate shelter from the elements for their occupants. So many individuals currently frequent the shelters of our cities that there is concern that the shelters are becoming mini-institutions for the chronically mentally ill.

OTHER FACTORS. The U.S. Conference of Mayors (2001) identified several other factors that may contribute to homelessness. They include:

- **Lack of affordable healthcare.** For families barely able to scrape together enough money to pay for day-to-day living, a catastrophic illness can create the level of poverty that starts the downward spiral to homelessness.
- **Domestic violence.** The study by the U.S. Conference of Mayors (1998) revealed that 46 percent identified domestic violence as a primary cause of homelessness. Battered women are often forced to choose between an abusive relationship and homelessness.
- **Addiction disorders.** For individuals with alcohol or drug addictions, in the absence of appropriate treatment, the chances increase for being forced into life on the street. The following have been cited as obstacles to addiction treatment for homeless persons: lack of health insurance; lack of documentation; waiting lists; scheduling difficulties; daily contact requirements; lack of transportation; ineffective treatment methods; lack of supportive services; and cultural insensitivity.

Community Resources for the Homeless

INTERFERING FACTORS. Among the many issues that complicate service planning for the homeless mentally ill is this population's penchant for mobility. Frequent relocation confounds service delivery and interferes with providers' efforts to ensure appropriate care. Some chronically mentally ill individuals may be affected by homelessness only temporarily or intermittently. These individuals are sometimes called the "episodically homeless." Others move around within neighborhoods or cities as needs change and based on whether or not they can obtain needed services. A large number of the homeless mentally ill population exhibits continuous unbounded movement over wide geographical areas.

Not all of the homeless mentally ill population is mobile. Some studies have indicated that a large percentage remains in the same location over a number of years. Healthcare workers must identify movement patterns of the homeless in their area in order at least to try to bring the best care possible to this unique population. This may indeed mean delivering services to those individuals who do not seek out services on their own.

HEALTH ISSUES. Life as a homeless person can have severe consequences in terms of health. Exposure to the elements, poor diet, sleep deprivation, risk of violence, injuries, and little or no healthcare lead to a precarious state of health and exacerbate any preexisting illnesses (Glasser, 1994). One of the major afflictions is alcoholism. Currently, alcohol abuse affects an estimated two-fifths of the U.S. homeless population, with the majority being men. Compared to other homeless individuals, those who abuse alcohol are at greater risk for neurological impairment, heart disease and hypertension, chronic lung disease, gastrointestinal (GI) disorders, hepatic dysfunction, and trauma.

Thermoregulation is a health problem for all homeless individuals because of their exposure to all kinds of weather. It is a compounded problem for the homeless alcoholic who spends much time in an altered level of consciousness.

It is difficult to determine whether mental illness is a cause or an effect of homelessness. Some behaviors that may seem deviant to some people in actuality may be adaptations to life on the street. It has been suggested that some homeless individuals seek hospitalization in psychiatric institutions in an attempt to get off the streets for a while.

A recent increase in the incidence of tuberculosis, especially the drug-resistant form, has been noted. A number of factors have been implicated in the increase of this disease, including the growth of the number of people living in congregate living situations and an increase of poverty and homelessness.

Dietary deficiencies are a continuing problem for homeless individuals. Not only is the homeless person commonly in a poor nutritional state, but also the condition itself exacerbates a number of other health problems. Homeless people suffer from higher mortality rates and a greater number of serious disorders than their counterparts in the general population.

Sexually transmitted diseases, such as gonorrhea and syphilis, are a serious problem for homeless persons. One of the most serious sexually transmitted diseases prevalent among homeless individuals is human immunodeficiency virus (HIV) infection. Street life is precarious for individuals whose systems are immunosuppressed by the HIV. Rummaged food scraps are often spoiled, and exposure to the elements is a continuous threat. HIV-infected individuals who stay in **shelters** are often exposed to the infectious diseases of others, which can be life-threatening in their vulnerable condition.

HIV disease is increasing among the homeless population. The NCH (1999c) reports that one study revealed a seropositive rate of 2.3 percent for homeless persons under the age of 25. Another suggested that up to 50 percent of persons living with HIV/AIDS are expected to need housing assistance of some kind during their lifetimes.

Homeless children have special health needs. Studies have indicated an increased rate of respiratory infections, minor skin ailments, ear disorders, GI disorders, infestational ailments, developmental delays, and psychological problems among homeless children, when compared with control samples (Sherman, 1998; Rafferty & Shinn, 1991).

Types of Resources Available

HOMELESS SHELTERS. The system of shelters for the homeless in the United States varies widely, from converted warehouses that provide cots or floor space on which to sleep overnight to significant operations that provide a multitude of social and healthcare services. They are run by volunteers and paid professionals and are sponsored by churches, community governments, and a variety of social agencies.

It is impossible, then, to describe a "typical" shelter. One profile may be described as the provision of lodging, food, and clothing to individuals who are in need of these services. Some shelters also provide medical and psychiatric evaluations, first aid and other healthcare services, and even referral for case management services by nurses or social workers.

Individuals who seek services from the shelter are generally assigned a bed or cot, issued a set of clean linen, provided a place to shower, shown laundry facilities, and offered a meal in the shelter kitchen or dining hall. Most shelters attempt to separate dormitory areas for men and women, with various consequences for those who violate the rules.

Shelters cover expenses through private and corporate donations, church sponsorships, and government grants. From the outset, shelters were conceptualized as "temporary" accommodations for individuals who needed a place to spend the night. Realistically, they have become permanent lodging for homeless individuals with little hope for improving their situation. Some individuals use shelters for their mailing address.

In the early 1980s, New York City instituted the Work Experience Program (WEP), which required all employable residents to work 20 hours a week for a $12.50 stipend. Evaluation of the program suggested that WEP kept the residents busy and enhanced their self-esteem, preventing idleness and depression. Since 1995, under a comprehensive program of welfare reform, more than 250,000 people have moved through the WEP (Human Resources Administration [HRA], 2002).

Shelters provide a safe and supportive environment for homeless individuals who have no other place to go. Some homeless people who inhabit shelters use the resources offered to improve their lot in life, whereas others become hopelessly dependent on the shelter's provisions. To a few, the availability of a shelter may even mean the difference between life and death.

HEALTHCARE CENTERS AND STOREFRONT CLINICS. Some communities have established "street clinics" to serve the homeless population. Many of these clinics are operated by nurse practitioners who work in consultation with physicians in the area. In recent years, some of these clinics have provided clinical rotation sites for nursing students in their community health rotation. Some have been staffed by faculties of nursing schools that have established group practices in the community setting.

A wide variety of services are offered at these clinics, including administering medications, assessing vital signs, screening for tuberculosis and other communicable diseases, giving immunizations and flu shots, changing dressings, and administering first aid (Brunner & Suddarth, 1992). Physical and psychosocial assessments, health education, and supportive counseling are also frequent interventions.

Mayo (1992), reporting on the Nurse Clinic for the Homeless at Charleston's Interfaith Crisis Ministry, related that the most frequent health problems for which the homeless presented themselves at the clinic were foot injuries and infections; ingrown toenails; respiratory infections; problems with eyes, ears, nose, and throat; skin conditions such as rashes and lice infestation; GI problems including ulcers, flu, vomiting, and diarrhea; and accidental injuries involving musculoskeletal damage from trauma or work-related injuries. Referrals are made to local hospitals and physicians who provide pro bono services when necessary.

Nursing in **storefront clinics** for the homeless provides many special challenges, not the least of which is poor working conditions. These clinics often operate under severe budgetary constraints with inadequate staffing, supplies, and equipment, in high-crime neighborhoods in rundown facilities that provide inadequate heat in the winter, poor to no air-conditioning in the summer, broken plumbing, vermin infestation, and a scarcity of secure parking facilities.

Frustration is often high among nurses who work in these clinics, as they are seldom able to see measurable progress in their homeless clients. Maintenance of health management is virtually impossible for many individuals who have no resources outside the healthcare setting. When return appointments for preventive care are made, the lack of follow-through is high.

MOBILE OUTREACH UNITS. Outreach programs literally reach out to the homeless in their own environment in an effort to provide healthcare. Volunteers and paid professionals form teams to drive or walk around and seek out homeless individuals who are in need of assistance. They offer coffee, sandwiches, and blankets in an effort to show concern and establish trust. If assistance can be provided at the site, it is done so. If not, every effort is made to ensure that the individual is linked with a source that can provide the necessary services.

Mobile outreach units assist homeless individuals who are in need of physical or psychological care. Blau (1992) presents the following report about the Center City Project, established in 1984 by the Philadelphia Office of Mental Health and Mental Retardation to address the special needs of homeless persons with mental illness:

> The project consisted of a network of twenty-one service sites that provided aggressive outreach to the homeless. Careful planning linked services, so that an outreach team could bring someone they engaged on the street to an intake center. From there, the homeless could be referred to a "low-demand" facility to ease their way into the system, and then, as their capacity to tolerate rules increased, to a facility offering specialized care. (p. 129)

The emphasis of outreach programs is to accommodate the homeless who refuse to seek treatment elsewhere. Most target the mentally ill segment of the population. When trust has been established, and the individual agrees to come to the team's office, medical and psychiatric treatment is initiated. Involuntary hospitalization is initiated when an individual is deemed harmful to self or others, or otherwise meets the criteria for being considered "gravely disabled."

The Homeless Client and the Nursing Process

Nursing process with the homeless client is demonstrated by the following case study:

CASE STUDY

ASSESSMENT

Joe, age 66, is brought to the community health clinic by two of his peers, who report: "He just had a fit. He needs a drink bad!" Joe is dirty, unkempt, has visible tremors of the upper extremities, and is weak enough to require assistance when ambulating. He is cooperative as the nurse completes the intake assessment. He is coherent, although thought processes are slow. He is disoriented to time and place. He appears somewhat frightened as he scans the unfamiliar surroundings. He is unable to tell the nurse when he had his last drink. He reports no physical injury, and none is observable.

Joe carries a small bag with a few personal items inside, including a Department of Veteran's Affairs (VA) benefit card, identifying him as a veteran of the Vietnam War. The nurse finds a cot for Joe to lie down, ensures that his vital signs are stable, and telephones the number on the VA card.

The clinic nurse discovers that Joe is well known to the admissions personnel at the VA. He has a 35-year history of schizophrenia, with numerous hospitalizations. At the time of his last discharge, he was taking fluphenazine (Prolixin) 10 mg twice a day. He told the clinic nurse that he took the medication for a few months after he got out of the hospital but then did not have the prescription refilled. He could not remember when he had last taken fluphenazine.

Joe also has a long history of alcohol-related disorders and has participated in the VA substance rehabilitation program three times. He has no home address and receives his VA disability benefit checks at a shelter address. He reports that he has no family. The nurse arranges for VA personnel to drive Joe from the clinic to the VA hospital, where he is admitted for detoxification. She sets up a case management file for Joe and arranges with the hospital to have Joe return to the clinic after discharge.

DIAGNOSIS/OUTCOME IDENTIFICATION

The following nursing diagnosis was formulated for Joe:

Ineffective health maintenance related to ineffective coping skills evidenced by abuse of alcohol, lack of follow-through with neuroleptic medication, and lack of personal hygiene.

Ongoing criteria were selected as outcomes for Joe. They include:

1. Follows the rules of the group home and maintains his residency status
2. Attends weekly sessions of group therapy at the VA day treatment program
3. Attends weekly sessions of Alcoholics Anonymous and maintains sobriety
4. Reports regularly to the health clinic for injections of fluphenazine
5. Volunteers at the VA hospital 3 days a week
6. Secures and retains permanent employment.

PLAN/IMPLEMENTATION

During Joe's hospitalization, the clinic nurse remained in contact with his case. Joe received complete physical and dental examinations and treatment during his hospital stay. The clinic nurse attended the treatment team meeting for Joe as his outpatient case manager. It was decided at the meeting to try giving Joe injections of fluphenazine decanoate because of his history of noncompliance with his daily oral medications. The clinic nurse would administer the injection every 4 weeks.

At Joe's follow-up clinic visit the nurse explains to Joe that she has found a group home where he may live with others who have personal circumstances similar to his. At the group home, meals will be provided and the group home manager will ensure that Joe's basic needs are fulfilled. A criterion for remaining at the residence is for Joe to remain alcohol free. Joe is agreeable to these living arrangements.

With Joe's concurrence, the clinic nurse also performs the following interventions:

1. Goes shopping with Joe to purchase some new clothing, allowing Joe to make decisions as independently as possible
2. Helps Joe move into the group home and introduces him to the manager and residents
3. Helps Joe change his address from the shelter to the group home so that he may continue to receive his VA benefits
4. Enrolls Joe in the weekly group therapy sessions of the day treatment facility connected with the VA hospital
5. Helps Joe locate the nearest Alcoholics Anonymous group and identifies a sponsor who will ensure that Joe gets to the meetings
6. Sets up a clinic appointment for Joe to return in 4 weeks for his fluphenazine injection; telephones Joe 1 day in advance to remind him of his appointment
7. Instructs Joe to return to or call the clinic if any of the following symptoms occur: sore throat, fever, nausea and vomiting, severe headache, difficulty urinating, tremors, skin rash, or yellow skin or eyes
8. Assists Joe in securing transportation to and from appointments
9. Encourages Joe to set realistic goals for his life and offers recognition for follow-through
10. When Joe is ready, discusses employment alternatives with him; suggests the possibility of starting with a volunteer job (perhaps as a VA hospital volunteer)

EVALUATION

Evaluation of the nursing process with homeless clients who are mentally ill must be highly individualized. Statistics show that chances for relapse with this population are high. Therefore, it is extremely important that outcome criteria be realistic so as not to set the client up for failure.

SUMMARY

The trend in psychiatric care is shifting from that of inpatient hospitalization to a focus of outpatient care within the community. This trend is largely due to the need for greater cost-effectiveness in the provision of medical care to the masses. The community mental health movement began in the 1960s with the closing of state hospitals and the deinstitutionalization of many chronically mentally ill individuals.

Mental healthcare within the community targets primary prevention (reducing the incidence of mental disorders within the population), secondary prevention (reducing the prevalence of psychiatric illness by shortening the course of the illness), and tertiary prevention (reducing the residual defects that are associated with severe or chronic mental illness). Primary prevention focuses on identification of populations at risk for mental illness, increasing their ability to cope with stress, and targeting and diminishing harmful forces within the environment. The focus of secondary prevention is accomplished through early identification of problems and prompt initiation of effective treatment. Tertiary prevention focuses on preventing complications of the illness and promoting rehabilitation that is directed toward achievement of the individual's maximum level of functioning.

Registered nurses serve as providers of psychiatric/mental healthcare in the community setting. Nurses provide outpatient care for chronically mentally ill individuals in community mental health centers, in day and evening treatment programs, in partial hospitalization programs, in community residential facilities, and with psychiatric home healthcare.

The homeless mentally ill provide a special challenge for the community mental health nurse. Care is provided within homeless shelters, at healthcare centers or storefront clinics, and through mobile outreach programs.

REVIEW QUESTIONS

SELF-EXAMINATION/LEARNING EXERCISE

Select the answer that is most appropriate for each of the following questions:

1. Which of the following represents a nursing intervention at the primary level of prevention?
   a. Teaching a class in parent effectiveness training
   b. Leading a group of adolescents in drug rehabilitation
   c. Referring a married couple for sex therapy
   d. Leading a support group for battered women
2. Which of the following represents a nursing intervention at the secondary level of prevention?
   a. Teaching a class about menopause to middle-aged women
   b. Providing support in the emergency room to a rape victim
   c. Leading a support group for women in transition
   d. Making monthly visits to the home of a client with schizophrenia to ensure medication compliance
3. Which of the following represents a nursing intervention at the tertiary level of prevention?
   a. Serving as case manager for a mentally ill homeless client
   b. Leading a support group for newly retired men
   c. Teaching prepared childbirth classes
   d. Caring for a depressed widow in the hospital
4. John, a homeless person, has just come to live in the shelter. The shelter nurse is assigned to his care. Which of the following is a priority intervention on the part of the nurse?
   a. Referring John to a social worker
   b. Developing a plan of care for John
   c. Conducting a behavioral and needs assessment on John
   d. Helping John apply for Social Security benefits
5. John has a history of paranoid schizophrenia and noncompliance with medications. Which of the following medications might be the best choice of neuroleptic for John?
   a. Haldol
   b. Navane
   c. Lithium carbonate
   d. Prolixin decanoate
6. Ann is a psychiatric home health nurse. She has just received an order to begin regular visits to Mrs. W, a 78-year-old widow who lives alone. Mrs. W's primary care physician has diagnosed her as depressed. Which of the following criteria would qualify Mrs. W for home health visits?
   a. Mrs. W never learned to drive and has to depend on others for her transportation.
   b. Mrs. W is physically too weak to travel without risk of injury.
   c. Mrs. W refuses to seek assistance as suggested by her physician, "because I don't have a psychiatric problem."
   d. Mrs. W says she would prefer to have home visits than go to the physician's office.

7. Based on a needs assessment, which of the following problems would Ann address during her first visit?
   a. Dysfunctional grieving
   b. Social isolation
   c. Risk for injury
   d. Sleep pattern disturbance
8. Mrs. W says to Ann, "What's the use? I don't have anything to live for anymore." Which is the best response on the part of the nurse?
   a. "Of course you do, Mrs. W. Why would you say such a thing?"
   b. "You seem so sad. I'm going to do my best to cheer you up."
   c. "Let's talk about why you are feeling this way."
   d. "Have you been thinking about harming yourself in any way?
9. The physician orders trazodone (Desyrel) for Mrs. W, 150 mg to take at bedtime. Which of the following statements about this medication would be appropriate for Ann to make in teaching Mrs. W about trazodone?
   a. "You may feel dizzy when you stand up, so go slowly when you get up from sitting or lying down."
   b. "You must be sure and not eat any chocolate when you are taking this medicine."
   c. "We will need to draw a sample of blood to send to the lab every month when you are on this medication."
   d. "If you don't feel better right away with this medicine, the doctor can order a different kind for you."
10. Three predominant client populations have been identified as benefiting most from psychiatric home healthcare. Which of the following is not included among this group?
   a. Elderly individuals
   b. Individuals living in poverty
   c. Chronically mentally ill individuals
   d. Individuals with acute mental health problems

IMPLICATIONS OF RESEARCH FOR EVIDENCE BASED PRACTICE

Hatton, D.C.:

Managing health problems among homeless women with children in a transitional shelter. Image: Journal of Nursing Scholarship, 29(1):33–37.

Description of the Study: This study was conducted to examine the health concerns of homeless women with children, to analyze how they managed various ailments and when and how they sought assistance from healthcare providers. The study was conducted at a shelter for homeless women that serves 600 to 700 women a year. The convenience sample included 13 Hispanic, 11 white, and 6 African-American women ranging in age from 20 to 30 years. All but two of the women had children, and the two without children were pregnant. Data was gathered through in-depth, semi-structured interviews. Subjects were asked to evaluate their health, express any concerns they had about particular diseases, discuss the last time they saw a healthcare provider, describe various symptoms they experienced and how they managed them, and report how they decided on various treatments.

Results of the Study: Typically, the respondents reported that they dealt with health problems before entering the shelter by "overcoming it alone." They ignored signs and symptoms of illness and hoped they would go away. As for lack of management of healthcare problems, four patterns of consequence emerged: shame (too embarrassed to seek help for a specific problem); fear (afraid that if they admit to having some kind of problem they may lose their children); lack of information (limited information about their children's and their own health needs, and where to seek it); and lack of eligibility (unable to seek care or medication because they could not afford it and were ineligible for government assistance). Most of the women, when asked to describe their health, tended to describe their mental health concerns and minimize physical concerns. They reported alcohol/drug abuse, bipolar disorders, depression, suicidal behaviors, self-mutilation, and anxiety, giving little consideration to conditions such as cystitis, otitis media, and sexually transmitted disease.

Implications for Nursing Practice: The author concluded that, even when the homeless women with children received supportive services from their transitional living situation, they continued to have difficulty knowing when health problems needed professional attention, and generally attempted to deal with the problems by overcoming them alone. Clinical nursing interventions that address shame, fear, lack of information, and eligibility for services could improve health outcomes among women and children living in transitional shelters.

REFERENCES

American Nurses Association (ANA). (1992a). Case management by nurses. Washington, DC: American Nurses Publishing.

American Nurses Association (ANA). (1992b). A statement on the scope of home health nursing practice. Washington, DC: American Nurses Publishing.

American Psychiatric Association (APA). (2000). Diagnostic and statistical manual of mental disorders (4th ed.). Text revision. Washington, DC: American Psychiatric Association.

Blau, J. (1992). The visible poor: Homelessness in the United States. New York: Oxford University Press.

Bower, K.A. (1992). Designing case management programs. Case management by nurses. Washington, DC: American Nurses Publishing.

Brunner, L.S. & Suddarth, D.S. (1992). Textbook of medical-surgical nursing (7th ed.). Philadelphia: J.B. Lippincott.

Duffey, J.M. & Miller, M.P. (1996, June). Toward resolving the issue: In-home psychiatric nursing. Journal of the American Psychiatric Nurses Association, 2(3), 104–106.

Finkelman, A.W. (1997). Psychiatric home care. Gaithersburg, MD: Aspen Publications.

Glasser, I. (1994). Homelessness in global perspective. New York: G.K. Hall.

Healthcare Financing Administration (HCFA). (2002). Home health agency manual: Chapter II: Coverage of Services. Retrieved May 27, 2002 http://www.hcfa.gov/pubforms/11_hha/hh00.htm

Human Resources Administration (HRA). (2002). New York City welfare reform program. Retrieved May 26, 2002 from http://www.ci.nyc.ny.us/html/serv_welfarework.html

Krauss, J.B. (1993). Healthcare reform: Essential mental health services. Waldorf, MD: American Nurses Publishing.

Lamb, H.R. (1992). Perspectives on effective advocacy for homeless mentally ill persons. Hospital and Community Psychiatry, 43(12), 1209–1212.

Langley, C. (2002). Community-based nursing practice: An overview in the United States. In J.M. Sorrell & G.M. Redmond (Eds.), Community-based nursing practice: Learning through students' stories. Philadelphia: F.A. Davis.

Mayo, K. (1992 Nov-Dec). Homelessness in the south: Excerpts from student journals. Imprint, 64–67.

Mercer, R.T. (2000). Transitions to parenthood. Nurse Week. Retrieved May 24, 2002 from http://nurse.cyberchalk.com/nurse/courses/nurseweek/nw1850/menu.html

Miller, M.A. & Rahe, R.H. (1997). Life changes scaling for the 1990s. Journal of Psychosomatic Research, 43(3), 279–292.

Murray, R. & Zentner, J. (2001). Health promotion strategies through the life span (7th ed.). Upper Saddle River, NJ: Prentice Hall.

National Coalition for the Homeless (NCH). (1999a). How many people experience homelessness? Retrieved May 26, 2002 from http://nch.ari.net/numbers.html

National Coalition for the Homeless (NCH). (1999b). Who is homeless? Retrieved May 26, 2002 from http://www.national-homeless.org/who.html

National Coalition for the Homeless (NCH). (1999c). HIV/AIDS and homelessness. Retrieved December 31, 2003 from http://www.nationalhomeless.org/hivaids.html

National Institute of Mental Health (NIMH). (2002). Mental disorders in America: The numbers count. Retrieved May 25, 2002 from http://www.nimh.nih.gov/publicat/numbers.cfm

Peplau, H. E. (1995). Some unresolved issues in the era of biopsychosocial nursing. Journal of the American Psychiatric Nurses Association,1(3), 92–96.

Pittman, D.C. (1989). Nursing case management: Holistic care for the deinstitutionalized chronically mentally ill. Journal of Psychosocial Nursing, 27(11), 23–27.

Pittman, D.C., Parsons, R. & Peterson, R.W. (1990). Easing the way: A multifaceted approach to day treatment. Journal of Psychosocial Nursing, 28(11), 6–11.
Rafferty, Y. & Shinn, M. (1991). The impact of homelessness on children. American Psychologist, 46(11), 1170–1179.
Sadock, B.J. & Sadock, V.A. (2003). Synopsis of psychiatry: Behavioral sciences/ clinical psychiatry (9th ed.). Philadelphia: Lippincott Williams & Wilkins.
Scanlon, V.C. & Sanders, T. (1999). Essentials of anatomy and physiology (3rd ed.). Philadelphia: F.A. Davis.
Sherman, P. (1998, October). Healthcare for homeless children: A clinician's perspective. Healing Hands, 2(6). Retrieved May 26, 2002 from http://www.nhchc.org/hands/1998/oct/octhands.html
Smoyak, S.A. (1991). Psychosocial nursing in public versus private sectors: An introduction. Journal of Psychosocial Nursing, 29(8), 6–12.
Spock, B. & Parker, S.J. (1998). Baby and child care (7th ed.). New York: Pocket Books.
Susser, E., Conover, S., & Struening, E.L. (1990). Mental illness in the homeless: Problems of epidemiologic method in surveys of the 1980s. Community Mental Health Journal, 26(5), 391–414.
Talley, B.S. & Coleman, M.A. (1992). The chronically mentally ill: Issues of individual freedom versus societal neglect. Journal of Community Health Nursing, 9(1), 33–41.
Torrey, E.F. (1997). Madness in the streets. Retrieved September 10, 2001, from http://www.nami-nyc-metro.org/Torrey/deinst.html
U.S. Conference of Mayors. (2001). A status report on hunger and homelessness in America's cities: 2001. Washington, DC: U.S. Conference of Mayors.
U.S. Conference of Mayors. (1998). A status report on hunger and homelessness in America's cities: 1998. Washington, DC: U.S. Conference of Mayors.
Wallsten, S.M. (1992). Geriatric mental health: A portrait of homelessness. Journal of Psychosocial Nursing, 30(9), 20–24.
Wilkinson, L. (1991). A collaborative model: Ambulatory pharmacotherapy for chronic psychiatric patients. Journal of Psychosocial Nursing, 29(12), 26–29.
Wilson, H.S. & Kneisl, C.R. (1992). Psychiatric nursing (4th ed.). Menlo Park, CA: Addison-Wesley Health Sciences Division.
Wright, L.M. & Leahey, M. (1994). Nurses and families: A guide to family assessment and intervention (2nd ed.).Philadelphia: F.A. Davis.

CLASSICAL REFERENCES

Caplan, G. (1964). Principles of preventive psychiatry. New York: Basic Books.
Erikson, E. (1963). Childhood and society (2nd ed.). New York: W.W. Norton.
Mahler, M., Pine, F., & Bergman, A. (1975). The psychological birth of the human infant. New York: Basic Books.
Sheehy, G. (1976). Passages: Predictable crises of adult life. New York: Bantam Books.

25
CHAPTER

The Bereaved Individual

CHAPTER OUTLINE

KEY TERMS

loss
grief
anticipatory grieving
delayed grief
bereavement overload
shiva
velorio
luto
hospice
advance directives

OBJECTIVES

After reading this chapter, the student will be able to:

1. Describe various types of loss that trigger the grief response in individuals.
2. Discuss theoretical perspectives of grieving as proposed by Elisabeth Kübler-Ross, John Bowlby, George Engel, and J. William Worden.
3. Differentiate between normal and maladaptive responses to loss.
4. Discuss grieving behaviors common to individuals at various stages across the life span.
5. Describe customs associated with grief in individuals of various cultures.
6. Formulate nursing diagnoses and goals of care for individuals experiencing the grief response.
7. Describe appropriate nursing interventions for individuals experiencing the grief response.
8. Identify relevant criteria for evaluating nursing care of individuals experiencing the grief response.
9. Describe the concept of hospice care for people who are dying and their families.
10. Discuss the use of advance directives for individuals to provide directions about their future medical care.

INTRODUCTION

Loss is the experience of separation from something of personal importance. Loss is anything that is perceived as such by the individual. The separation from loved ones or the giving up of treasured possessions, for whatever reason; the experience of failure, real or perceived; or life events that create change in a familiar pattern of existence—all can be experienced as loss, and all can trigger behaviors associated with the grieving process. Loss and bereavement are universal events encountered by all beings that experience emotions. Following are examples of some notable forms of loss:

1. A significant other (person or pet), through death, divorce, or separation for any reason.
2. Illness or debilitating conditions. Examples include (but are not limited to) diabetes, stroke, cancer, rheumatoid arthritis, multiple sclerosis, Alzheimer's disease, hearing or vision loss, and spinal cord or head injuries. Some of these conditions not only incur a loss of physical and/or emotional wellness, but may also result in the loss of personal independence.
3. Developmental/maturational changes or situations, such as menopause, andropause, infertility, "empty nest," aging, impotence, or hysterectomy.
4. A decrease in self-esteem, if one is unable to meet self-expectations or the expectations of others (even if these expectations are only perceived by the individual as unfulfilled). This includes a loss of potential hopes and dreams.
5. Personal possessions that symbolize familiarity and security in a person's life. Separation from these familiar and personally valued external objects represents a loss of material extensions of the self.

Some texts differentiate the terms **mourning** and **grief** by describing mourning as the psychological process (or stages) through which the individual passes on the way to successful adaptation to the loss of a valued object. Grief may be viewed as the subjective states that accompany mourning, or the emotional work involved in the mourning process. For purposes of this text, grief work and the process of mourning are collectively referred to as the *grief response.*

This chapter examines human responses to the experience of loss. Care of bereaved individuals is presented in the context of the nursing process.

THEORETICAL PERSPECTIVES ON LOSS AND BEREAVEMENT

Stages of Grief

Behavior patterns associated with the grief response include many individual variations. However, sufficient similarities have been observed to warrant characterization of grief as a syndrome that has a predictable course with an expected resolution. Early theorists, including Kübler-Ross (1969), Bowlby (1961), and Engel (1964), described behavioral stages through which individuals advance in their progression toward resolution. A number of variables influence one's progression through the grief process. Some individuals may reach acceptance, only to revert back to an earlier stage; some may never complete the sequence; and some may never progress beyond the initial stage. A comparison of the similarities among these three models is presented in Table 25–1.

A more contemporary grief specialist, J. William Worden (2002), offers a set of tasks that must be processed in order to complete the grief response. He suggests that it is possible for a person to accomplish some of these tasks and not others, resulting in an incomplete bereavement, and thus impairing further growth and development.

Elisabeth Kübler-Ross

These well-known stages of the grief process were identified by Kübler-Ross in her extensive work with dying patients. Behaviors associated with each of these stages can be observed in individuals experiencing the loss of any concept of personal value.

Stage I: Denial. In this stage, the individual does not acknowledge that the loss has occurred. He or she may say, "No, it can't be true!" or "It's just not possible." This stage may protect the individual against the psychological pain of reality.

Stage II: Anger. This is the stage when reality sets in. Feelings associated with this stage include sadness, guilt, shame, helplessness, and hopelessness. Self-blame or blaming of others may lead to feelings of anger toward the self and others. The anxiety level may be elevated, and the individual may experience confusion and a decreased ability to function independently. He or she may be preoccupied with an idealized image of what has been lost. Numerous somatic complaints are common.

Stage III: Bargaining. At this stage in the grief re-

TABLE 25 – 1 Stages of the Normal Grief Response

A Comparison of Models by Elisabeth Kubler-Ross, John Bowlby, and George Engel

STAGES				
Kubler-Ross	**Bowlby**	**Engel**	**Possible Time Dimension**	**Behaviors**
I. Denial	I. Numbness/Protest	I. Shock/Disbelief	Occurs immediately upon experiencing the loss. Usually lasts no more than 2 weeks.	Individual refuses to acknowledge that the loss has occurred.
II. Anger	II. Disequilibrium	II. Developing Awareness	In most cases begins within hours of the loss. Peaks within 2 to 4 weeks.	Anger is directed toward self or others. Ambivalence and guilt may be felt toward the lost object.
III. Bargaining				The individual fervently seeks alternatives to improve current situation.
		III. Restitution		Attends to various rituals associated with the culture in which the loss has occurred.
IV. Depression	III. Disorganization and despair	IV. Resolution of the loss	A year or more.	The actual work of grieving. Preoccupation with the lost object. Feelings of helplessness and loneliness occur in response to realization of the loss. Feelings associated with the loss are confronted.
V. Acceptance	IV. Reorganization	V. Recovery		Resolution is complete. The bereaved person experiences a reinvestment in new relationships and new goals. Terminally ill persons express a readiness to die.

sponse, the individual attempts to strike a bargain with God for a second chance, or for more time. The person acknowledges the loss, or impending loss, but holds out hope for additional alternatives, as evidenced by statements such as, "If only I could ..." or "If only I had ...".

Stage IV: Depression. In this stage, the individual mourns for that which has been or will be lost. This is a very painful stage, during which the individual must confront feelings associated with having lost someone or something of value (called *reactive* depression). An example might be the individual who is mourning a change in body image. Feelings associated with an impending loss (called *preparatory* depression) are also confronted. Examples include permanent lifestyle changes related to the altered body image or even an impending loss of life itself. Regression, withdrawal, and social isolation may be observed behaviors with this stage. Therapeutic intervention should be available, but not imposed, and with guidelines for implementation based on client readiness.

Stage V: Acceptance. At this time, the individual has worked through the behaviors associated with the other stages and accepts or is resigned to the loss. Anxiety decreases, and methods for coping with the loss have been established. The client is less preoccupied with what has been lost and increasingly interested in other aspects of the environment. If this is an impending death of self, the individual is ready to die. The person may become very quiet and withdrawn, seemingly devoid of feelings. These behaviors are an attempt to facilitate the passage by slowly disengaging from the environment.

John Bowlby

John Bowlby hypothesized four stages in the grief process. He implies that these behaviors can be observed in all individuals who have experienced the loss of something or someone of value, even in babies as young as 6 months of age.

Stage I: Numbness or Protest. This stage is characterized by a feeling of shock and disbelief that the loss has occurred. Reality of the loss is not acknowledged.

Stage II: Disequilibrium. During this stage, the individual has a profound urge to recover what has been lost. Behaviors associated with this stage include a preoccupation with the loss, intense weeping and expressions of anger toward the self and others, and feelings of ambivalence and guilt associated with the loss.

Stage III: Disorganization and Despair. Feelings of despair occur in response to realization that the loss has occurred. Activities of daily living become increasingly disorganized, and behavior is characterized by restlessness and aimlessness. Efforts to regain productive patterns of behavior are ineffective, and the individual experiences fear, helplessness, and hopelessness. Somatic complaints are common. Perceptions of visualizing or being in the presence of that which has been lost may occur. Social isolation is common, and the individual may feel a great deal of loneliness.

Stage IV: Reorganization. The individual accepts or becomes resigned to the loss. New goals and patterns of organization are established. The individual begins a reinvestment in new relationships and indicates a readiness to move forward within the environment. Grief subsides and recedes into valued remembrances.

George Engel

Stage I: Shock and Disbelief. The initial reaction to a loss is a stunned, numb feeling and refusal by the individual to acknowledge the reality of the loss. Engel states that this stage is an attempt by the individual to protect the self "against the effects of the overwhelming stress by raising the threshold against its recognition or against the painful feelings evoked thereby."

Stage II: Developing Awareness. This stage begins within minutes to hours of the loss. Behaviors associated with this stage include excessive crying and regression to a state of helplessness and a childlike manner. Awareness of the loss creates feelings of emptiness, frustration, anguish, and despair. Anger may be directed toward the self or toward others in the environment who are held accountable for the loss.

Stage III: Restitution. In this stage, the various rituals associated with loss within a culture are performed. Examples include funerals, wakes, special attire, a gathering of friends and family, and religious practices customary to the spiritual beliefs of the bereaved. Participation in these rituals is thought to assist the individual to accept the reality of the loss and to facilitate the recovery process.

Stage IV: Resolution of the Loss. This stage is characterized by a preoccupation with the loss. The concept of the loss is idealized, and the individual may even imitate admired qualities of that which has been lost. Preoccupation with the loss gradually decreases over a year or more, and the individual eventually begins to reinvest feelings in others.

Stage V: Recovery. Obsession with the loss has ended, and the individual is able to go on with his or her life.

J. William Worden

Worden views the bereaved as active and self-determining rather than passive participants in the grief process. He proposes that bereavement includes a set of tasks that must be reconciled in order to complete the grief process. Worden's four tasks of mourning include the following.

Task I. Accepting the Reality of the Loss. When something of value is lost, it is common for individuals to refuse to believe that the loss has occurred. Behaviors include misidentifying individuals in the environment for their lost loved one, retaining possessions of the lost loved one as though he or she has not died, and removing all reminders of the lost loved one so as not to have to face the reality of the loss. Worden (2002) states:

> Coming to an acceptance of the reality of the loss takes time since it involves not only an intellectual acceptance but also an emotional one. The bereaved person may be intellectually aware of the finality of the loss long before the emotions allow full acceptance of the information as true. (p. 29)

Belief and denial are intermittent when grappling with this task. It is thought that traditional rituals such as the funeral help some individuals move toward acceptance of the loss.

Task II. Working Through the Pain of Grief. Pain associated with a loss includes both physical pain and emotional pain. This pain must be acknowledged and worked through. To avoid or suppress it serves only to delay or prolong the grieving process. People accomplish this by refusing to allow themselves to think painful thoughts, by idealizing or avoiding reminders of that which has been lost, and by using alcohol or drugs. The intensity of the pain and the manner in which it is experienced are different for all individuals. However, the commonality is that it *must* be experienced. Failure to do so generally results in some form of depression that commonly requires therapy, which then focuses on working through the pain of grief that the individual failed to work through at the time of the loss. In this very difficult task II, individuals must "indulge the pain of loss—to feel it and to know that one day it will pass" (Worden, 2002).

Task III. Adjusting to an Environment that has Changed Because of the Loss. It usually takes a number of months for a bereaved person to realize what his or her world will be like without that which has been lost. In the case of a lost loved one, how the environment changes will depend on the types of roles that person fulfilled in life. In the case of a changed lifestyle, the individual will be required to make adaptations to his or her environment in terms of the change as they are presented in daily life. In addition, those individuals who had defined their identity through that which has been lost will require an adjustment to their own sense of self. Worden (2002) states:

> The coping strategy of redefining the loss in such a way that it can redound to the benefit of the survivor is often part of the successful completion of Task III. (p. 33)

If the bereaved person experiences failures in his or her attempt to adjust in an environment without their valued concept, feelings of low self-esteem may result. Regressed behaviors and feelings of helplessness and inadequacy are common. Worden (2002) states:

> [Another] area of adjustment may be to one's sense of the world. Loss through death can challenge one's fundamental life values and philosophical beliefs—beliefs that are influenced by our families, peers, education, and religion as well as life experiences. The bereaved person searches for meaning in the loss and its attendant life changes in order to make sense of it and to regain some control of his or her life. (p. 34)

To be successful in task III, bereaved individuals must develop new skills to cope and adapt to their new environment without the lost concept. Successful achievement of this task determines the outcome of the mourning process—that of continued growth or a state of arrested development.

Task IV. Emotionally Relocating That Which Has Been Lost and Moving on With Life. This task allows the bereaved person to identify a special place for what has been lost. Individuals need not purge from their history or find a replacement for that which has been lost. Instead, there is a kind of continued presence of the lost concept in the life of the bereaved. The lost concept is *relocated* in the life of the bereaved. Successful completion of task IV involves letting go of past attachments and forming new ones. However, there is also the recognition that although the relationship between the bereaved and what has been lost is changed, it is nonetheless still a relationship. Worden (2002) suggests that one never loses memories of a significant relationship. He states:

> For many people, Task IV is the most difficult one to accomplish. They get stuck at this point in their grieving and later realize that their life in some way stopped at the point the loss occurred. (p. 37)

Worden (2002) relates the story of a teenaged girl who had a difficult time adjusting to the death of her father. After 2 years, when she began to finally fulfill some of the tasks associated with successful grieving, she wrote these words that express rather clearly what bereaved people in task IV are struggling with: "There are other people to be loved, and it doesn't mean that I love Dad any less."

LENGTH OF THE GRIEF PROCESS

Stages of grief allow bereaved persons an orderly approach to the resolution of mourning. Each stage presents tasks that must be overcome through a painful experiential process. Engel (1964) has stated that successful resolution of the grief response is thought to have occurred when a bereaved individual is able "to remember comfortably and realistically both the pleasures and disappointments of [that which is lost]." Length of the grief process depends on the individual and can last for a number of years without being maladaptive. The acute phase of normal grieving usually lasts 6 to 8 weeks—longer in older adults—but complete resolution of the grief response may take much longer. Sadock and Sadock (2003) state:

> Traditionally, grief lasts about 6 months to 1 year, as the grieving person experiences the calendar year at least once without the lost person. Some signs and symptoms of grief may persist much longer than 1 or 2 years, and a

> survivor may have various grief-related feelings, symptoms, and behavior throughout life. In general, the acute grief symptoms gradually lessen, and within 1 or 2 months, the grieving person is able to eat, sleep, and return to functioning. (pp. 62–63)

A number of factors influence the eventual outcome of the grief response. The grief response can be more difficult if:

- The bereaved person was strongly dependent on or perceived that which was lost as an important means of physical and/or emotional support.
- The relationship with that which was lost was highly ambivalent. A love-hate relationship may instill feelings of guilt that can interfere with the grief work.
- The individual has experienced a number of recent losses. Grief tends to be cumulative, and if previous losses have not been resolved, each succeeding grief response becomes more difficult.
- The loss is that of a young person. Grief over loss of a child is often more intense than it is over the loss of an elderly person.
- The state of the person's physical or psychological health is unstable at the time of the loss.
- The bereaved person perceives (whether real or imagined) some responsibility for the loss.

The grief response may be facilitated if:

- The individual has the support of significant others to assist him or her through the mourning process.
- The individual has the opportunity to prepare for the loss. Grief work is more intense when the loss is sudden and unexpected. The experience of *anticipatory grieving* is thought to facilitate the grief response that occurs at the time of the actual loss.

Worden (2002) states:

> There is a sense in which mourning can be finished, when people regain an interest in life, feel more hopeful, experience gratification again, and adapt to new roles. There is also a sense in which mourning is never finished. [People must understand] that mourning is a long-term process, and the culmination [very likely] will not be to a pre-grief state. (pp. 46–47)

ANTICIPATORY GRIEF

Anticipatory grieving is the experiencing of the feelings and emotions associated with the normal grief response before the loss actually occurs. One dissimilar aspect relates to the fact that conventional grief tends to diminish in intensity with the passage of time. Conversely, anticipatory grief may increase in intensity as the expected loss becomes imminent.

Although anticipatory grief is thought to facilitate the actual mourning process following the loss, there may be some problems. In the case of a dying person, difficulties can arise when the family members complete the process of anticipatory grief, and detachment from the dying person occurs prematurely. The person who is dying experiences feelings of loneliness and isolation as the psychological pain of imminent death is faced without family support. Sadock and Sadock (2003) describe another example of difficulty associated with premature completion of the grief response:

> Once anticipatory grief has been expended, the bereaved person may find it difficult to reestablish a previous relationship; this phenomenon is experienced with the return of persons long gone (for example, to war or confined to concentration camps) and of persons thought to have been dead. (p. 63)

Anticipatory grieving may serve as a defense for some individuals to ease the burden of loss when it actually occurs. It may prove to be less functional for others who, because of interpersonal, psychological, or sociocultural variables, are unable in advance of the actual loss to express the intense feelings that accompany the grief response.

MALADAPTIVE RESPONSES TO LOSS

When, then, is the grieving response considered to be maladaptive. Three types of pathological grief reactions have been described. These include delayed or inhibited grief, an exaggerated or distorted grief response, and chronic or prolonged grief.

Delayed or Inhibited Grief

Delayed or inhibited grief refers to the absence of evidence of grief when it ordinarily would be expected. Many times, cultural influences, such as the expectation to keep a "stiff upper lip," cause the delayed response.

Delayed or inhibited grief is potentially pathological because the person is simply not dealing with the reality of the loss. He or she remains fixed in the denial stage of the grief process, sometimes for many years. When this occurs, the grief response may be triggered, sometimes many years later, when the individual experiences a subsequent loss. Sometimes the grief process is triggered spontaneously or in response to a seemingly insignificant event. Overreaction to another person's loss may be one manifestation of **delayed grief.**

The recognition of delayed grief is critical because, depending on the profoundness of the loss, the failure of the mourning process may prevent assimilation of the loss and thereby delay a return to satisfying living. Delayed grieving most commonly occurs because of ambivalent feelings toward that which has been lost, outside pressure to resume normal function, or perceived lack of internal and external resources to cope with a profound loss.

Distorted (Exaggerated) Grief Response

In the distorted grief reaction, all of the symptoms associated with normal grieving are exaggerated. Feelings of sadness, helplessness, hopelessness, powerlessness, anger, and guilt, as well as numerous somatic complaints, render the individual dysfunctional in terms of management of daily living. Murray and Zentner (2001) describe an exaggerated grief reaction in the following way:

> An intensification of grief to the point that the person is overwhelmed, demonstrates prolonged maladaptive behavior, manifests excessive symptoms and extensive interruptions in healing, and does not progress to integration of the loss, finding meaning in the loss, and resolution of the mourning process. (p. 858)

When the exaggerated grief reaction occurs, the individual remains fixed in the anger stage of the grief response. This anger may be directed toward others in the environment to whom the individual may be attributing the loss. However, many times the anger is turned inward on the self. When this occurs, depression is the result. Depressive mood disorder is a type of exaggerated grief reaction.

Chronic or Prolonged Grieving

Some authors have discussed a chronic or prolonged grief response as a type of maladaptive grief response. Care must be taken in making this determination because, as was stated previously, length of the grief response depends on the individual. An adaptive response may take years for some people. A prolonged process may be considered maladaptive when certain behaviors are exhibited. Prolonged grief may be a problem when behaviors such as maintaining personal possessions aimed at keeping a lost loved one alive (as though he or she will eventually reenter the life of the bereaved) or disabling behaviors that prevent the bereaved from adaptively performing activities of daily living are in evidence. Another example is of a widow who refused to participate in family gatherings following the death of her husband. For many years until her own death, she took a sandwich to the cemetery on holidays, sat on the tombstone, and ate her "holiday meal" with her husband. Other bereaved individuals have been known to set a place at the table for the deceased loved one long after the completed mourning process would have been expected.

Normal versus Maladaptive Grieving

Several authors have identified one crucial difference between normal and maladaptive grieving: the loss of self-esteem. Kaplan, Sadock, and Grebb (1994) assert that "marked feelings of worthlessness" are indicative of depression rather than uncomplicated bereavement. Eisendrath (1996) affirms:

> Grief is usually accompanied by intact self-esteem, whereas depression is marked by a sense of guilt and worthlessness. (p. 939)

It is thought that this major difference between normal grieving and a maladaptive grieving response (the feeling of worthlessness or low self-esteem) ultimately precipitates depression.

APPLICATION OF THE NURSING PROCESS

Background Assessment Data: Concepts of Death—Developmental Issues

Children

BIRTH TO AGE 2. Infants are unable to recognize and understand death, but they can experience the feelings of loss and separation. Infants who are separated from their mother may become quiet, lose weight, and sleep less. Children at this age will likely sense changes in the atmosphere of the home where a death has occurred. They often react to the emotions of adults by becoming more irritable and crying more.

AGES 3 TO 5. Preschoolers and kindergartners have some understanding about death but often have difficulty distinguishing between fantasy and reality. They believe death is reversible, and their thoughts about death may include magical thinking. For example, they may believe that their thoughts or behaviors caused a person to become sick or to die.

Children of this age are capable of understanding at least some of what they see and hear from adult conversations or media reports. They become frightened if they feel a threat to themselves or their loved ones. They are concerned with safety issues and require a great deal of personal reassurance that they will be protected. Regressive behaviors, such as loss of bladder or bowel control, thumb sucking, and temper tantrums are common. Changes in eating and sleeping patterns may also occur.

AGES 6 TO 9. Children at this age are beginning to understand the finality of death. They are able to understand a more detailed explanation of why or how the person died, although death is often associated with old age or with accidents. They may believe that death is contagious and avoid association with individuals who have experienced a loss by death. Death is often personified in the form of a "bogey man" or a monster—someone who takes people away or someone whom they can avoid if they try hard enough. It is difficult for them to perceive their own death. Normal grief reactions at this age include regressive and aggressive behaviors, withdrawal, school phobias, somatic symptoms, and clinging behaviors.

AGES 10 TO 12. Preadolescent children are able to understand that death is final and eventually affects everyone, including themselves. They are interested in the physical aspects of dying and the final disposition of the body. They may ask questions about how the death will affect them personally. Feelings of anger, guilt, and depression are common. Peer relationships and school performance may be disrupted. There may be a preoccupation with the loss and a withdrawal into the self. They will require reassurance of their own safety and self-worth.

Adolescents

Adolescents are usually able to view death on an adult level. They understand death to be universal and inevitable; however, they have difficulty tolerating the intense feelings associated with the death of a loved one. They may or may not cry. They may withdraw into themselves or attempt to go about usual activities in an effort to avoid dealing with the pain of the loss. Some teens exhibit acting-out behaviors, such as aggression and defiance. It is often easier for adolescents to discuss their feelings with peers than with their parents or other adults. Some adolescents may show regressive behaviors, whereas others react by trying to take care of their loved ones who are also grieving. In general, individuals of this age group have an attitude of immortality. Although they understand that their own death is inevitable, the concept is so far-reaching as to be imperceptible.

Adults

The adult's concept of death is influenced by cultural and religious backgrounds (Murray & Zentner, 2001). Behaviors associated with grieving in the adult were discussed in the section on "Theoretical Perspectives on Loss and Bereavement."

Elderly Adults

Bateman (1999) states,

> For the older adult, the later years have been described by philosophers and poets as the "season of loss." Loss of one's occupational role upon retirement, loss of control and competence, loss in some life experiences, loss of material possessions, and loss of dreams, loved ones, and friends must be understood and accepted if the older adult is to adapt effectively. (p. 144)

By the time individuals reach their 60s and 70s, they have experienced numerous losses, and mourning has become a lifelong process. Those who are most successful at adapting earlier in life will similarly cope better with the losses and grief inherent in aging (Cath & Sadavoy, 1991). Unfortunately, with the aging process comes a convergence of losses, the timing of which makes it impossible for the aging individual to complete the grief process in response to one loss before another occurs. Because grief is cumulative, this can result in **bereavement overload,** the person is less able to adapt and reintegrate, and mental and physical health is jeopardized (Halstead, 1999). Bereavement overload has been implicated as a predisposing factor in the development of depressive disorder in the elderly person.

Depression is a common symptom in the grief response to significant losses. It is important to understand the difference between the depression of normal grieving and the disorder of clinical depression. Some of these differences are presented in Table 25–2.

TABLE 25–2 Normal Grief Reactions versus Symptoms of Clinical Depression

Normal Grief	Clinical Depression
Self-esteem intact	Self-esteem is disturbed
May openly express anger	Usually does not directly express anger
Experiences a mixture of "good and bad days"	Persistent state of dysphoria
Able to experience moments of pleasure	Anhedonia is prevalent
Accepts comfort and support from others	Does not respond to social interaction and support from others
Maintains feeling of hope	Feelings of hopelessness prevail
May express guilt feelings over some aspect of the loss	Has generalized feelings of guilt
Relates feelings of depression to specific loss experienced	Does not relate feelings to an experience
May experience transient physical symptoms	Expresses chronic physical complaints

Adapted from Periyakoil (2001) and Sadock & Sadock (2003).

Background Assessment Data: Concepts of Death—Cultural Issues

As previously stated, bereavement practices are greatly influenced by cultural and religious backgrounds. It is important for healthcare professionals to have an understanding of these individual differences in order to provide culturally sensitive care to their clients. Clinicians must be able to identify and appreciate what is culturally expected or required, because failure to carry out expected rituals may hinder the grief process and result in unresolved grief for some bereaved individuals. Table 25–3 provides a set of guidelines for assessing culturally specific death rituals. Following is a discussion of selected culturally specific death rituals.

African-Americans

Customs of bereaved African-Americans are similar to those of the American culture of the same religion and social class, with a blending of cultural practices from the African heritage. The majority of African-Americans are Protestant, largely Baptist and Methodist (Campinha-Bacote, 1998). Campinha-Bacote (1998) states:

> One response to hearing about a death of a family member or close member in the African-American culture is *falling-out*, which is manifested by sudden collapse and paralysis and the inability to see or speak. However, the individual's hearing and understanding are still intact. Healthcare providers must be knowledgeable about the African-American culture to recognize this condition as a cultural response to the death of a family member and not a medical condition requiring emergency intervention. (p. 65)

Funeral services may differ from the traditional European-American service with ceremonies and rituals modified by the musical rhythms and patterns of speech and worship that are unique to African-Americans. Feelings are expressed openly and publicly at the funeral, and eulogies are extremely important. Services usually conclude with a viewing of the body and burial at a cemetery. Burial rather than cremation is usually chosen (American Association of Retired Persons [AARP], 2002).

Many African-Americans attempt to maintain a strong connection with their loved ones who have died. This connection may take the form of communication with the deceased's spirit through mediums who are believed to possess this special capability.

TABLE 25–3 Guidelines for Assessing Culturally Specific Death Rituals

Death Rituals and Expectations

1. Identify culturally specific death rituals and expectations.
2. Explain the purpose of death rituals and mourning practices.
3. What are specific burial practices, such as cremation?

Responses to Death and Grief

1. Identify cultural expectations of responses to death and grief.
2. Explore the meaning of death, dying, and the afterlife.

Purnell & Paulanka (1998). With permission.

Asian-Americans

CHINESE-AMERICANS. Death and bereavement in the Chinese tradition are centered on ancestor worship. Chinese people have an intuitive fear of death and avoid references to it. Matocha (1998) states:

> The purchase of insurance may be avoided because of a fear that it is inviting death. The color white is associated with death and is considered bad luck. Black is also a bad luck color. Red is the ultimate good luck color. (p. 178)

The Chinese often do not express their emotions openly. Mourners are recognized by black armbands and white strips of cloth tied around their heads (Matocha, 1998). Traditionally, for a year following a death, a place for the deceased is set at table with a bowl of rice, meat and vegetables, and chopsticks (AARP, 2002).

JAPANESE-AMERICANS. The dominant religion among the Japanese is Buddhism. On death of a loved one, the body is prepared by close family members. This is followed by a 2-day period of visitation by family and friends, during which there is prayer, burning of incense, and presentation of gifts (AARP, 2002). Funeral ceremonies are held at the Buddhist temple, and cremation is common.

VIETNAMESE-AMERICANS. Buddhism is the predominant religion among the Vietnamese. Attitudes toward death are influenced by the Buddhist emphasis on cyclic continuity and reincarnation (Nowak, 1998). Many Vietnamese believe that birth and death are predestined (AARP, 2002).

Most Vietnamese people prefer to die at home, and most do not approve of autopsy. Cremation is common. The final moments before the funeral procession is a time of prayer for the immediate family. Individuals in mourning wear white clothing for 14 days. During the following year, men wear black armbands and women wear white headbands (Nowak, 1998). The 1-year anniversary of an individual's death is celebrated. Nowak (1998) states:

> Priests and monks should only be called at the request of the client or family. Clergy visitation is usually associated with last rites by the Vietnamese, especially those influenced by Catholicism, and can actually be upsetting to hospitalized clients. Sending flowers may be startling, as flowers usually are reserved for the rites of the dead. (p. 467)

Filipino-Americans

Following a death in the Filipino community, a wake is held with family and friends. This wake usually takes place in the home of the deceased and lasts up to a week before the funeral. A large proportion of Filipinos are Catholic (AARP, 2002). Miranda, McBride, and Spangler (1998) state:

> When resources are available among Catholic families, nine days of *pabasa* (novenas) are held in the home or in the church. These special prayers ask God's blessing for the deceased. Food and refreshments are served after each prayer day. Sometimes the last day of the novena takes on the atmosphere of a *fiesta* or a celebration. Filipino families in the United States follow variations of this ritual according to their social and economic circumstances. (p. 261)

Most follow the traditional custom of wearing dark clothing—black armbands for men and black dresses for women—for 1 year after the death, at which time ritualistic mourning officially ends. Emotional outbursts of uncontrolled crying are common expressions of grief. Fainting as a bereavement response is common (Miranda, McBride, & Spangler, 1998). Burial of the body is most common, but cremation is acceptable.

Jewish-Americans

Traditional Judaism believes in an afterlife, where the soul continues to flourish, where what is not understood in this life becomes clear, and where people are judged and rewarded on the goodness of their actions during their life (Selekman, 1998). Taking one's own life is forbidden and the person who commits suicide may be denied full burial honors by ultraconservative Jews; however, the more liberal view is to emphasize the needs of the survivors.

A dying person is never left alone. At death, the face is covered with a cloth, and the body is treated with respect. Autopsy is only allowed if it is required by law, the deceased person has requested it, or it may save the life of another (Selekman, 1998).

For the funeral, the body is wrapped in a shroud and placed in a wooden, unadorned casket. No wake and no viewing are part of a Jewish funeral. Cremation is prohibited. Selekman (1998) states:

> After the funeral, mourners are welcomed to the home of the closest relative. Outside the front door is water to wash one's hands before entering, which is symbolic of cleansing the impurities associated with contact with the dead. The water is not passed from person to person, just as it is hoped that the tragedy is not passed. At the home, a meal is served to all the guests. This "meal of condolence" is traditionally provided by the neighbors. (p. 386)

The 7-day period beginning with the burial is called ***shiva***. During this time, mourners do not work, and no activity is permitted that diverts attention from thinking about the deceased. Mourning lasts 30 days for a relative and 1 year for a parent, at which time a tombstone is erected and a graveside service is held (Selekman, 1998).

Mexican-Americans

Most Mexican-Americans view death as a natural part of life. The predominant religion is Catholic, and many of the death rituals are a reflection of these religious beliefs. A vigil by family members is kept over the sick or dying person. Following the death, large numbers of family and friends gather for a ***velorio***, a festive watch over the body of the deceased person before burial (Purnell, 1998), and a novena of prayers is offered for the soul of the deceased (AARP, 2002).

Mourning is called ***luto*** and is symbolized by wearing black, black and white, or dark clothing and by subdued behavior (AARP, 2002). Often the bereaved refrain from attending movies or social events and from listening to radio or watching television. For middle-aged or elderly Mexican-Americans, the period of bereavement may last for 2 years or more. These mourning behaviors do not indicate a sign of respect for the dead; instead, they demonstrate evidence that the individual is grieving for a loved one. Purnell (1998) states:

> More traditional Mexican-Americans may continue their native practice of erecting altars in their homes to honor deceased relatives on the anniversary of their death. The dead are honored, sometimes annually, with candles, decorations, and bringing the deceased's favorite meal to a picnic at the grave site. (p. 411)

Native Americans

More than 500 Native American tribes are now recognized by the U.S. government. Although many of the tribal traditions have been modified throughout the years, some of the traditional Native American values have been preserved.

The Navajo of the Southwest, the largest Native American tribe in the United States, do not bury the body of a deceased person for 4 days after death. Beliefs require that a cleansing ceremony take place before burial to prevent the spirit of the dead person from trying to assume control of someone else's spirit (Still & Hodgins, 1998). The dead are buried with their shoes on the wrong feet and rings on their index fingers. The Navajo generally do not express their grief openly and are reluctant to touch the body of a dead person. Still and Hodgins (1998) state:

> One death taboo involves talking with clients concerning a fatal disease or illness. Effective discussions require that the issue be presented in the third person. The health-care provider must never suggest that the client is dying. To do so would imply that the provider wishes the client dead. If the client does die, it would imply that the provider might have evil powers. (p. 440)

Nursing Diagnosis/Outcome Identification

From analysis of the assessment data, appropriate nursing diagnoses are formulated for the client and family experiencing grief and loss. From these identified diagnoses, accurate planning of nursing care is executed. Possible nursing diagnoses for grieving persons include:

- Risk for dysfunctional grieving related to loss of a valued concept/object; loss of a loved one
- Risk for spiritual distress related to complicated grief process

The following criteria may be used for measurement of outcomes in the care of the grieving client. The client:

1. Acknowledges awareness of the loss
2. Is able to express feelings about the loss
3. Verbalizes stages of the grief process and behaviors associated with each
4. Expresses personal satisfaction and support from spiritual practices

Planning/Implementation

Table 25–4 provides a plan of care for the grieving person. Selected nursing diagnoses are presented, along with outcome criteria, appropriate nursing interventions, and rationales for each.

Evaluation

In the final step of the nursing process, a reassessment is conducted to determine if the nursing actions have been successful in achieving the objectives of care. Evaluation of the nursing actions for the grieving client may be facilitated by gathering information using the following types of questions:

1. Has the client discussed the recent loss with staff and family members?
2. Is the client able to verbalize feelings and behaviors associated with each stage of the grieving process and recognize his or her own position in the process?

TABLE 25–4 Care Plan for the Grieving Person

Nursing Diagnosis: RISK FOR DYSFUNCTIONAL GRIEVING

Related to: Loss of a valued concept/object; loss of a loved one

Evidenced by: Feelings of sadness, anger, guilt, self-reproach, anxiety, loneliness, fatigue, helplessness, shock, yearning, and numbness

Outcome Criteria	Nursing Interventions	Rationale
Client will progress through the grief process in a healthful manner toward resolution.	1. Assess client's stage in the grief process.	1. Accurate baseline data are required to provide appropriate assistance.
	2. Develop trust. Show empathy, concern, and unconditional positive regard.	2. Developing trust provides the basis for a therapeutic relationship.
	3. Help the client actualize the loss by talking about it. "When did it happen? How did it happen?" and so forth.	3. Reviewing the events of the loss can help the client come to full awareness of the loss.
	4. Help the client identify and express feelings. Some of the more problematic feelings include:	4. Until client can recognize and accept personal feelings regarding the loss, grief work cannot progress.
	a. Anger. The anger may be directed at the deceased, at God, displaced onto others, or retroflected inward on the self. Encourage the client to examine this anger and validate the appropriateness of this feeling.	a. Many people will not admit to angry feelings, believing it is inappropriate and unjustified. Expression of this emotion is necessary to prevent fixation in this stage of grief.
	b. Guilt. The client may feel that he or she did not do enough to prevent the loss. Help the client by reviewing the circumstances of the loss and the reality that it could not be prevented.	b. Feelings of guilt prolong resolution of the grief process.
	c. Anxiety and helplessness. Help the client to recognize the way that life was managed before the loss. Help the client to put the feelings of helplessness into perspective by pointing out ways that he or she managed situations effectively without help from others. Role-play life events and assist with decision-making situations.	c. The client may have fears that he or she may not be able to carry on alone.
	5. Interpret normal behaviors associated with grieving and provide client with adequate time to grieve.	5. Understanding of the grief process will help prevent feelings of guilt generated by these responses. Individuals need adequate time to accommodate to the loss and all its ramifications. This involves getting past birthdays and anniversaries of which the deceased was a part.
	6. Provide continuing support. If this is not possible by the nurse, then offer referrals to support groups. Support groups of individuals going through the same experiences can be very helpful for the grieving individual.	6. The availability of emotional support systems facilitates the grief process.
	7. Identify pathological defenses that the client may be using (e.g., drug/alcohol use, somatic complaints, social isolation). Assist the client in understanding why these are not healthy defenses and how they delay the process of grieving.	7. The bereavement process is impaired by behaviors that mask the pain of the loss.
	8. Encourage the client to make an honest review of the relationship with that which has been lost. Journal keeping is a facilitative tool with this intervention.	8. Only when the client is able to see both positive and negative aspects related to the loss will the grieving process be complete.

Nursing Diagnosis: RISK FOR SPIRITUAL DISTRESS

Related to: Dysfunctional grieving over loss of valued object

Evidenced by: Anger toward God, questioning meaning of own existence, inability to participate in usual religious practices

Outcome Criteria	Nursing Interventions	Rationale
Client will express achievement of support and personal satisfaction from spiritual practices.	1. Be accepting and nonjudgmental when client expresses anger and bitterness toward God. Stay with the client.	1. The nurse's presence and nonjudgmental attitude increase the client's feelings of self-worth and promote trust in the relationship.
	2. Encourage the client to ventilate feelings related to meaning of own existence in the face of current loss.	2. Client may believe he or she cannot go on living without lost object. Catharsis can provide relief and put life back into realistic perspective.
	3. Encourage the client as part of grief work to reach out to previously used religious practices for support. Encourage client to discuss these practices and how they provided support in the past.	3. Client may find comfort in religious rituals with which he or she is familiar.
	4. Ensure client that he or she is not alone when feeling inadequate in the search for life's answers.	4. Validation of client's feelings and assurance that they are shared by others offer reassurance and an affirmation of acceptability.
	5. Contact spiritual leader of client's choice, if he or she requests.	5. These individuals serve to provide relief from spiritual distress and often can do so when other support persons cannot.

3. Has obsession with and idealization of the loss subsided?
4. Is anger toward that which has been lost expressed appropriately?
5. Is the client able to participate in usual religious practices and feel satisfaction and support from them?
6. Is the client seeking out interaction with others in an appropriate manner?
7. Is the client able to verbalize positive aspects about his or her life, past relationships, and prospects for the future?

ADDITIONAL ASSISTANCE

Hospice

Hospice is a program that provides palliative and supportive care to meet the special needs of people who are dying and their families. Hospice care provides physical, psychological, spiritual, and social care for the person for whom aggressive treatment is no longer appropriate. Various models of hospice exist, including freestanding institutions that provide both inpatient and home care; those affiliated with hospitals in which hospice services are provided within the hospital setting; and hospice organizations that provide home care only. Historically, the hospice movement in the United States has evolved mainly as a system of home-based care.

Hospice helps clients achieve physical and emotional comfort so that they can concentrate on living life as fully as possible. Clients are urged to stay active for as long as they are able—to take part in activities they enjoy, and to focus on the quality of life.

The National Hospice and Palliative Care Organization (2000) has published standards of care based on principles that are directed at the hospice program concept. These principles of care are presented in Table 25–5.

Hospice follows an interdisciplinary team approach to provide care for the terminally ill individual in the familiar surroundings of the home environment. The interdisciplinary team consists of nurses, attendants (homemakers, home health aides), physicians, social workers, volunteers, and other healthcare workers from other disciplines as required for individual clients.

TABLE 25–5 Principles of Care – National Hospice and Palliative Care Organization

Access, Rights and Ethics

Access: The hospice offers palliative care to terminally ill patients and their families regardless of age, gender, nationality, race, creed, sexual orientation, disability, diagnoses, availability of primary caregiver, or ability to pay.

Rights: The hospice respects and honors the rights of each patient and family it serves.

Ethics: The hospice assumes responsibility for ethical decision making and behavior related to the provision of hospice care.

Bereavement Care and Services

Addressing issues related to loss, grief, and bereavement begins at the time of admission to the hospice with the initial assessment and continues throughout the course of care. Bereavement services are provided to help patients, families, and caregivers cope with the multitude of losses that occur during the illness and eventual death of the patient. Bereavement services are offered based on a number of factors including the individual assessment, intensity of grief, coping ability of the survivors, and their needs as perceived by each patient, family, and caregiver.

Clinical Care and Services

The desired outcomes of hospice intervention are safe and comfortable dying, self-determined life closure, and effective grieving, all as determined by the patient and family/caregivers. The interdisciplinary team identifies, assists, and respects the desires of the patient and family/caregivers in the facilitation of these outcomes through treatment, prevention, and promotion of strategies based on continuous assessment.

Coordination and Continuity of Care

The hospice provides coordinated and uninterrupted service and assures continuity of care across settings, from admission through discharge and subsequent bereavement care.

Human Resources

Hospice organizational leaders ensure that the number and qualifications of staff and volunteers are appropriate to the scope of care and services provided by the hospice program.

Interdisciplinary Team

The hospice interdisciplinary team, in collaboration with the patient, family, and caregiver, develops and maintains a patient, family, and caregiver-directed, individualized, safe and coordinated plan of palliative care.

Leadership and Governance

Hospice has an organizational leadership structure that permits and facilitates action and decision making by those individuals closest to any issue or process.

Management of Information

The hospice identifies and collects information needed to operate in an efficient manner. Such information is handled in a manner that respects the patient, family, and hospice's confidentiality.

Performance Improvement and Outcomes Measurement

The hospice defines a systematic, planned approach to improving performance. This approach is authorized and supported by the governing body and leaders.

Safety and Infection Control

The hospice provides for the safety of all staff and promotes the development and maintenance of a safe environment for patients and families served.

Adapted From: National Hospice and Palliative Care Organization, *Standards of Practice for Hospice Programs* (2000). Alexandria VA: Author. Item #711077 available from NHPCO 1-800-646-6460.

The hospice approach is based on seven components: the interdisciplinary team, pain and symptom management, emotional support to client and family, pastoral and spiritual care, bereavement counseling, 24-hour on-call nurse/counselor, and staff support. These are the ideal, and not all hospice programs may include all of these services.

Interdisciplinary Team

NURSES. A registered nurse usually acts as case manager for care of hospice clients. The nurse assesses the client's and family's needs, establishes the goals of care, supervises and assists caregivers, evaluates care, serves as client advocate, and provides educational information as needed to client, family, and caregivers. He or she also provides physical care when needed, including IV therapy.

ATTENDANTS. These individuals are usually the members of the team who spend the most time with the client. They assist with personal care and all activities of daily living. Without these daily attendants, many individuals would be unable to spend their remaining days in their home. Attendants may be noncertified and provide basic housekeeping services; they may be certified nursing assistants who assist with personal care; or they may be licensed vocational or practical nurses that provide specialized care, such as dressing changes or tube feedings.

PHYSICIANS. The client's primary physician and the hospice medical consultant have input into the care of the hospice client. Orders may continue to come from the primary physician, whereas pain and symptom management may come from the hospice consultant. Ideally, these physicians attend weekly client care conferences and provide in-service education for hospice staff as well as others in the medical community.

SOCIAL WORKERS. The social worker assists the client and family members with psychosocial issues, including those associated with the client's condition, financial issues, legal needs, and bereavement concerns. The social worker provides information on community resources from which client and family may receive support and assistance. Some of the functions of the nurse and social worker may overlap at times.

TRAINED VOLUNTEERS. Volunteers are vital to the hospice concept. They provide services that may otherwise be financially impossible. They are specially selected and extensively trained, and they provide services such as transportation, companionship, respite care, recreational activities, light housekeeping, and in general are sensitive to the needs of families in stressful situations.

REHABILITATION THERAPISTS. Physical therapists may assist hospice clients in an effort to minimize physical disability. They may assist with strengthening exercises and provide assistance with special equipment needs. Occupational therapists may help the debilitated client learn to accomplish activities of daily living as independently as possible. Other consultants, such as speech therapists, may be called upon for the client with special needs.

DIETITIAN. A nutritional consultant may be helpful to the hospice client who is experiencing nausea and vomiting, diarrhea, anorexia, and weight loss. A nutritionist can ensure that the client is receiving the proper balance of calories and nutrients.

COUNSELING SERVICES. The hospice client may require the services of a psychiatrist or psychologist if there is a history of mental illness, or if dementia or depression has become a problem. Other types of counseling services are available to provide assistance in dealing with the special needs of each client.

Pain and Symptom Management

Improved quality of life at all times is a primary goal of hospice care. Thus, a major intervention for all caregivers is to ensure that the client is as comfortable as possible, whether experiencing pain or other types of symptoms common in the terminal stages of an illness.

Emotional Support

Members of the hospice team encourage clients and families to discuss the eventual outcome of the disease process. Some individuals find discussing issues associated with death and dying uncomfortable, and if so, their decision is respected. However, honest discussion of these issues provides a sense of relief for some people, and they are more realistically prepared for the future. It may even draw some clients and families closer together during this stressful time.

Pastoral and Spiritual Care

Hospice philosophy supports the individual's right to seek guidance or comfort in the spiritual practices most suited to that person. The hospice team members help the client obtain the spiritual support and guidance for which he or she expresses a preference.

Bereavement Counseling

Hospice provides a service to surviving family members or significant others after the death of their loved one. This is usually provided by a bereavement counselor, but when one is not available, volunteers with special training in bereavement care may be of service. A grief support group may be helpful for the bereaved and provide a safe place for them to discuss their own fears and concerns about the death of a loved one.

Twenty-Four-Hour On-Call

The standards of care set forth by the National Hospice and Palliative Care Organization state that care shall be available 24 hours a day, 7 days a week. A nurse or counselor is usually available by phone or for home visits around the clock. The knowledge that emotional or physical support is available at any time, should it be required, provides considerable support and comfort to significant others or family caregivers.

Staff Support

Team members (all who work closely and frequently with the client) often experience emotions similar to those of the client or their family and/or significant others. They may experience anger, frustration, or fears of death and dying—all of which must be addressed through staff support groups, team conferences, time off, and adequate and effective supervision. Burnout is a common problem among hospice staff. Stress can be reduced, trust enhanced, and team functioning more effective if lines of communication are kept open among all members (medical director through volunteer), if information is readily accessible through staff conferences and inservice education, and if staff know they are appreciated and feel good about what they are doing.

Advance Directives

The term **advance directives** refers to a living will or a durable power of attorney for healthcare (also called a healthcare proxy). Either document allows an individual to provide directions about his or her future medical care.

A living will is a written document made by a competent individual that provides instructions that should be used when that individual is no longer able to express his or her wishes for healthcare treatment. The durable power of attorney for healthcare is a written form that gives another person legal power to make decisions regarding healthcare when an individual is no longer capable of making such decisions. Some states have adopted forms that combine the intent of the durable power of attorney for healthcare (i.e., to have a proxy) and the intent of the living will (i.e., to state choices for end-of-life medical treatment).

Doctors usually follow clearly stated directives. It is important that the physician be informed that an advanced directive exists and what the specific wishes of the client are. In most states, healthcare professionals are legally bound to honor the client's wishes (Norlander, 2001). However, there is often no legal enforcement of a living will. Guido (1997) states:

> There is no protection for the practitioner against criminal or civil liability, and many physicians have been afraid to proceed under a living will's direction for fear that family members or the state will file charges of wrongful death. (p. 136)

Norlander (2001) suggests the following reasons why advance directives sometimes are not honored:

- The advance directive is not available at the time treatment decisions need to be made. This is especially true in emergencies.
- The advance directive is not clear. Statements such as "no heroic measures" can be interpreted in many different ways.
- The healthcare proxy is unsure of the client's wishes.

Advance directives allow the client to be in control of decisions at the end of life. It is also a way to spare family and loved ones the burden of making choices without knowing what is most important to the person who is dying.

SUMMARY

Loss is the experience of separation from something of personal importance. Loss is anything that is perceived as such by the individual. Loss of any concept of value to an individual triggers the grief response.

Elisabeth Kübler-Ross identified five stages that individuals pass through on their way to resolution of a loss. These include denial, anger, bargaining, depression, and acceptance. John Bowlby described similar stages that he identified in the following manner: stage I, numbness or protest; stage II, disequilibrium; stage III, disorganization and despair; and stage IV, reorganization. George Engel's stages include shock and disbelief, developing awareness, restitution, resolution of the loss, and recovery. J. William Worden, a more contemporary clinician, has proposed that bereaved individuals must accomplish a set of tasks in order to complete the grief process. These four tasks include accepting the reality of the loss, working through the pain of grief, adjusting to an environment that has changed because of the loss, and emotionally relocating that which has been lost and moving on with life.

The length of the grief process is highly individual, and it can last for a number of years without being maladaptive. The acute stage usually lasts a couple of months, but resolution lasts much longer. Kübler-Ross suggests that a calendar year of experiencing significant events and anniversaries without the lost concept may be required.

Anticipatory grieving is the experiencing of the feelings and emotions associated with the normal grief process in response to anticipation of the loss. Anticipatory grieving is thought to facilitate the grief process when the actual loss occurs.

Three types of pathological grief reactions have been described. These include the following:

- Delayed or inhibited grief in which there is absence of evidence of grief when it ordinarily would be expected.
- Distorted or exaggerated grief response in which the individual remains fixed in the anger stage of the grief process and all of the symptoms associated with normal grieving are exaggerated.
- Chronic or prolonged grieving in which the individual is unable to let go of grieving behaviors after a extended period of time and in which behaviors are evident that indicate the bereaved individual is not accepting that the loss has occurred.

Several authors have identified one crucial difference between normal and maladaptive grieving: the loss of self-esteem. Feelings of worthlessness are indicative of depression rather than uncomplicated bereavement.

Grieving behaviors characteristic of children, adolescents, adults, and elderly individuals were described. A discussion of cultural grieving behaviors associated with African-Americans, Asian-Americans, Filipino-Americans, Jewish-Americans, Mexican-Americans, and Native Americans was included. Care of individuals experiencing uncomplicated bereavement was presented in the context of the nursing process. A discussion of hospice care and the use of advance directives was presented.

REVIEW QUESTIONS

SELF-EXAMINATION/LEARNING EXERCISE

Select the answer that is most appropriate for each of the following questions:

1. Which of the following is most likely to initiate a grief response in an individual?
   a. Death of the pet dog
   b. Being told by her doctor that she has begun menopause
   c. Failing an exam
   d. "a" only
   e. All of the above
2. Nancy, who is dying of cancer, says to the nurse, "I just want to see my new grandbaby. If only God will let me live until she is born. Then I'll be ready to go." This is an example of which of Kübler-Ross' stages of grief?
   a. Denial
   b. Anger
   c. Bargaining
   d. Acceptance
3. Gloria, a recent widow, states, "I'm going to have to learn to pay all the bills. Hank always did that. I don't know if I know if I can handle all of that." This is an example of which of the tasks described by Worden?
   a. Task I: accepting the reality of the loss
   b. Task II: working through the pain of grief
   c. Task III: adjusting to an environment that has changed because of the loss
   d. Task IV: emotionally relocating that which has been lost and moving on with life
4. Engel identifies which of the following as successful resolution of the grief process?
   a. When the bereaved person can talk about the loss without crying
   b. When the bereaved person no longer talks about that which has been lost
   c. When the bereaved person puts all remembrances of the loss out of sight
   d. When the bereaved person can discuss both positive and negative aspects about what has been lost
5. Which of the following is thought to facilitate the grief process?
   a. The ability to grieve in anticipation of the loss
   b. The ability to grieve alone without interference from others
   c. Having recently grieved for another loss
   d. Taking personal responsibility for the loss
6. When Frank's wife of 34 years dies, he is very stoic, handles all the funeral arrangements, doesn't cry or appear sad, and comforts all of the other family members in their grief. Two years later, when Frank's best friend dies, Frank has sleep disturbances, difficulty concentrating, loss of weight, and difficulty performing on his job. This is an example of which of the following maladaptive responses to loss?
   a. Delayed grieving
   b. Distorted grieving
   c. Prolonged grieving
   d. Exaggerated grieving

7. A major difference between normal and maladaptive grieving has been identified by which of the following?
   a. There are no feelings of depression in normal grieving.
   b. There is no loss of self-esteem in normal grieving.
   c. Normal grieving lasts no longer than 1 year.
   d. In normal grief, the person does not show anger toward the loss.
8. Which grief reaction can the nurse anticipate in a 10-year-old child?
   a. Statements that the deceased person will soon return
   b. Regressive behaviors, such as loss of bladder control
   c. A preoccupation with that which has been lost
   d. Thinking that they may have done something to cause the death
9. Which of the following is a correct statement when attempting to distinguish normal grief from clinical depression?
   a. In clinical depression, anhedonia is prevalent.
   b. In normal grieving, the person has generalized feelings of guilt.
   c. The person who is clinically depressed relates feelings of depression to a specific loss.
   d. In normal grieving, there is a persistent state of dysphoria.
10. Which of the following is ***not*** true regarding grieving by an adolescent?
    a. Adolescents may not show their true feelings about the death.
    b. Adolescents tend to have an immortal attitude.
    c. Adolescents do not perceive death as inevitable.
    d. Adolescents may exhibit acting-out behaviors as part of their grief.

IMPLICATIONS OF RESEARCH FOR EVIDENCED-BASED PRACTICE

Douglas, R. & Brown, H.N.:

Patients' Attitudes toward Advance Directives.
Journal of Nursing Scholarship (2002), 34(1), 61–65.

Description of the Study: This study was conducted to investigate hospitalized patients' attitudes toward advanced directives. It explored patients' reasons for completing or not completing advance directive forms, and examined demographic differences between patients who did and did not complete advance directive forms. Subjects consisted of a convenience sample of 30 hospitalized patients. Criteria required that the patients (1) speak English, (2) be at least 18 years of age, (3) be oriented to time and place, and (4) have been approached by an RN regarding advance directives, as documented in the patient chart. Data were collected over a 3-week period in the oncology and medical-telemetry units of a teaching hospital in central North Carolina. Interviews were conducted using an adapted advance directive attitude survey (ADAS) in which subjects were asked 5 general questions regarding perceptions of personal health, whether they had ever received information on advance directives, whether they had ever completed an advance directive, and whether they had ever had a discussion with their primary physician or family members about end-of-life care. Demographic data were also obtained. The tool was based on a 4-point Likert scale from 1 (strongly disagree) to 4 (strongly agree). Higher scores indicate favorable attitudes toward advance directives.

Results of the Study: Subjects ranged in age from 24 to 85 years, with a mean age of 57 years. Nineteen were Caucasian, ten were African-American, and one was Hispanic. Ten had completed grade school or junior high, 13 completed high school, 4 completed college, and 3 had master's degrees or beyond. Twelve subjects had been diagnosed with cancer, five with respiratory disorders, four with sickle cell disease, three with cardiac disorders, two with vascular disorders, and one each with gastrointestinal, musculoskeletal, neurological, and dermatological disorders. Twenty-three subjects had received information on advance directives and seven said they had received no information. Thirteen of the subjects had completed advance directives and seventeen had not.

Participants with the highest mean scores were African-American, female, age 35 to 49 years, with a high school education. No subject in the-20-to-30 age group had completed an advanced directive, whereas 62 percent of subjects over age 65 had done so. The two people with the lowest scores both disagreed with the statement that an advance directive would make sure that their family knew what treatment they desired and they would receive the treatment they desired. The 13 participants who had completed advance directives cited the following reasons for doing so: (a) desire not to be placed on life support, (b) desire to name someone to make decisions in event of incapacitation, (c) desire to make decisions easier for spouse or family, (d) failing health, and (e) advancing age. The 17 who had not completed advance directives cited the following reasons: (a) keep putting it off, (b) not necessary at this point in my life, (c) uncomfortable making decisions about life support, (d) never heard of advance directives before, (e) form was too long, (f) trust husband to make those decisions, and (g) advance directives are unnecessary.

Implications for Nursing Practice: The authors suggest that nurses need to explain what advance directives are when asking patients if they have an advance directive. They state: "[Nurses] can explore alternative ways to educate patients about advance directives (e.g., videotape), and follow up with patients who have requested information to see if they have additional questions or need assistance completing an advance directive." They also suggest that nurses need to inform physicians when patients have advance directives. As patient advocates, nurses have the responsibility for making sure that patients understand the purpose of advance directives and what is involved in completing an advance directive, and for ensuring that patients' end-of-life care is executed according to their wishes.

INTERNET REFERENCES

- Additional references related to bereavement may be located at the following Web sites:
  - a http://www.journeyofhearts.org
  - b http://www.nhpco.org
  - c http://www.aarp.org/griefandloss/
  - d http://www.hospicefoundation.org
  - e http://www.bereavement.org
  - f http://www.partnershipforcaring.org/
  - g http://www.aahpm.org
  - h http://www.hpna.org

REFERENCES

American Association of Retired Persons (AARP). (2002). Grief and loss: People of African heritage in America. Retrieved September 3, 2002, from www.aarp.org/griefandloss/articles/46_b.html

Bateman, A.L. (1999). Understanding the process of grieving and loss: A critical social thinking perspective. Journal of the American Psychiatric Nurses Association, 5(5), 139–147.

Campinha-Bacote, J. (1998). African-Americans. In L.D. Purnell & B.J. Paulanka (Eds.), Transcultural healthcare: A culturally competent approach. Philadelphia: F.A. Davis.

Cath, S.H. & Sadavoy, J. (1991). Psychosocial aspects. In J. Sadavoy, L.W. Lazarus, & L.F. Jarvik (Eds.), Comprehensive review of geriatric psychiatry. Washington, DC: American Psychiatric Press.

Eisendrath, S.J. (1996). Psychiatric disorders. In L.M. Tierney, S.J. McPhee, & M.A. Papadakis (Eds.), Current medical diagnosis and treatment (35th ed.). Norwalk, CT: Appleton & Lange.

Guido, G.W. (1997). Legal issues in nursing (2nd ed.). Stamford, CT: Appleton & Lange.

Halstead, H.L. (1999). Spirituality in older adults. In M. Stanley and P.G. Beare (Eds.), Gerontological nursing: A health promotion/protection approach (2nd ed.). Philadelphia: F. A. Davis.

Kaplan, H.I., Sadock, B.J. & Grebb, J.A. (1994). Synopsis of psychiatry: Behavioral sciences, clinical psychiatry (7th ed.). Baltimore: Williams & Wilkins.

Matocha, L. K. (1998). Chinese Americans. Transcultural healthcare: A culturally competent approach. Philadelphia: F.A. Davis.

Miranda, B.F., McBride, M.R., & Spangler, Z. (1998). Filipino-Americans. Transcultural healthcare: A culturally competent approach. Philadelphia: F.A. Davis.

Murray, R.B. & Zentner, J.P. (2001). Health promotion strategies through the life span (7th ed.). Upper Saddle River, NJ: Prentice Hall.

National Hospice and Palliative Care Organization (NHPCO). (2000). Standards of Practice for hospice programs. Alexandria, VA: NHPCO.

Norlander, L. (2001). To comfort always: A nurse's guide to end of life care. Washington, DC: American Nurses Publishing.

Nowak, T.T. (1998). Vietnamese-Americans. Transcultural healthcare: A culturally competent approach. Philadelphia: F.A. Davis.

Periyakoil, V.J. (2001). Is it grief or depression? End-of-Life Physician Education Resource Center. Retrieved October 27, 2002, from www.eperc.mcw.edu/educate/flash/fastfact/226.htm

Purnell, L.D. (1998). Mexican-Americans. Transcultural healthcare: A culturally Competent approach. Philadelphia: F.A. Davis.

Purnell, L.D. & Paulanka, B.J. (1998). Transcultural healthcare: A culturally competent approach. Philadelphia: F.A. Davis.

Sadock, B.J. & Sadock, V.A. (2003). Synopsis of psychiatry: Behavioral sciences/clinical psychiatry (9th ed.). Philadelphia: Lippincott Williams & Wilkins

Selekman, J. (1998). Jewish-Americans. Transcultural healthcare: A culturally competent approach. Philadelphia: F.A. Davis.

Still, O. & Hodgins, D. (1998). Navajo Indians. Transcultural healthcare: A culturally competent approach. Philadelphia: F.A. Davis.

Worden, J. W. (2002). Grief counseling and grief therapy: A handbook for the mental health practitioner (3rd ed.). New York: Springer.

CLASSICAL REFERENCES

Bowlby, J. (1961). Processes of mourning. International Journal of Psychoanalysis, 42, 22.

Engel, G. (1964). Grief and grieving. American Journal of Nursing, 64, 93.

Kübler-Ross, E. (1969). On death and dying. New York: Macmillan.

APPENDICES

APPENDIX A

DSM-IV-TR Classification: Axes I and II Categories and Codes*

DISORDERS USUALLY FIRST DIAGNOSED IN INFANCY, CHILDHOOD, OR ADOLESCENCE

Mental Retardation

NOTE: *These are coded on Axis II.*

317 Mild Mental Retardation
318.0 Moderate Retardation
318.1 Severe Retardation
318.2 Profound Mental Retardation
319 Mental Retardation, Severity Unspecified

Learning Disorders

315.00 Reading Disorder
315.1 Mathematics Disorder
315.2 Disorder of Written Expression
315.9 Learning Disorder Not Otherwise Specified (NOS)

Motor Skills Disorder

315.4 Developmental Coordination Disorder

Communication Disorders

315.31 Expressive Language Disorder
315.32 Mixed Receptive-Expressive Language Disorder
315.39 Phonological Disorder
307.0 Stuttering
307.9 Communication Disorder NOS

Pervasive Developmental Disorders

299.00 Autistic Disorder
299.80 Rett Disorder
299.10 Childhood Disintegrative Disorder
299.80 Asperger's Disorder
299.80 Pervasive Developmental Disorder NOS

Attention-Deficit and Disruptive Behavior Disorders

314.xx Attention-Deficit/Hyperactivity Disorder
314.01 Combined Type
314.00 Predominantly Inattentive Type
314.01 Predominantly Hyperactive-Impulsive Type
314.9 Attention-Deficit/Hyperactivity Disorder NOS
312.xx Conduct Disorder
.81 Childhood-Onset Type
.82 Adolescent-Onset Type
.89 Unspecified Onset
313.81 Oppositional Defiant Disorder
312.9 Disruptive Behavior Disorder NOS

Feeding and Eating Disorders of Infancy or Early Childhood

307.52 Pica
307.53 Rumination Disorder
307.59 Feeding Disorder of Infancy or Early Childhood

*Reprinted with permission from the Diagnostic and Statistical Manual of Mental Disorders, (4th Edition) Text Revision. Copyright 2000, American Psychiatric Association.

Tic Disorders

307.23 Tourette's Disorder

307.22 Chronic Motor or Vocal Tic Disorder

307.21 Transient Tic Disorder

307.20 Tic Disorder NOS

Elimination Disorders

— Encopresis

787.6 With Constipation and Overflow Incontinence

307.7 Without Constipation and Overflow Incontinence

307.6 Enuresis (Not Due to a General Medical Condition)

Other Disorders of Infancy, Childhood, or Adolescence

309.21 Separation Anxiety Disorder

313.23 Selective Mutism

313.89 Reactive Attachment Disorder of Infancy or Early Childhood

307.3 Stereotypic Movement Disorder

313.9 Disorder of Infancy, Childhood, or Adolescence NOS

DELIRIUM, DEMENTIA, AND AMNESTIC AND OTHER COGNITIVE DISORDERS

Delirium

293.0 Delirium Due to… *(indicate the general medical condition)*

—Substance Intoxication Delirium *(refer to Substance-Related Disorders for substance-specific codes)*

—Substance Withdrawal Delirium *(refer to Substance-Related Disorders for substance-specific codes)*

— Delirium Due to Multiple Etiologies *(code each of the specific etiologies)*

780.09 Delirium NOS

Dementia

294.xx Dementia of the Alzheimer's Type, With Early Onset

.10 Without Behavioral Disturbance

.11 With Behavioral Disturbance

294.xx Dementia of the Alzheimer's Type, With Late Onset

.10 Without Behavioral Disturbance

.11 With Behavioral Disturbance

290.xx Vascular Dementia

.40 Uncomplicated

.41 With Delirium

.42 With Delusions

.43 With Depressed Mood

294.1x Dementia Due to HIV Disease

294.1x Dementia Due to Head Trauma

294.1x Dementia Due to Parkinson's Disease

294.1x Dementia Due to Huntington's Disease

294.1x Dementia Due to Pick's Disease

294.1x Dementia Due to Creutzfeldt-Jakob Disease

294.1x Dementia Due to *(indicate the general medical condition not listed above)*

— Substance-Induced Persisting Dementia *(refer to Substance-Related Disorders for substance-specific codes)*

— Dementia Due to Multiple Etiologies *(code each of the specific etiologies)*

294. 8 Dementia NOS

Amnestic Disorders

294.0 Amnestic Disorder Due to *(indicate the general medical condition)*

—Substance-Induced Persisting Amnestic Disorder *(refer to Substance-Related Disorders for substance-specific codes)*

294.8 Amnestic Disorder NOS

Other Cognitive Disorders

294.9 Cognitive Disorder NOS

MENTAL DISORDERS DUE TO A GENERAL MEDICAL CONDITION NOT ELSEWHERE CLASSIFIED

293.89 Catatonic Disorder Due to *(indicate the general medical condition)*

310.1 Personality Change Due to *(indicate the general medical condition)*

293.9 Mental Disorder NOS Due to *(Indicate the general medical condition)*

SUBSTANCE-RELATED DISORDERS

Alcohol-related disorders

Alcohol Use Disorders

303.90 Alcohol Dependence
305.00 Alcohol Abuse

Alcohol-Induced Disorders

303.00 Alcohol Intoxication
291.81 Alcohol Withdrawal
291.0 Alcohol Intoxication Delirium
291.0 Alcohol Withdrawal Delirium
291.2 Alcohol-Induced Persisting Dementia
291.1 Alcohol-Induced Persisting Amnestic Disorder
291.x Alcohol-Induced Psychotic Disorder
  .5 With Delusions
  .3 With Hallucinations
291.89 Alcohol-Induced Mood Disorder
291.89 Alcohol-Induced Anxiety Disorder
291.89 Alcohol-Induced Sexual Dysfunction
291.89 Alcohol-Induced Sleep Disorder
291.9 Alcohol Related Disorder NOS

Amphetamine (or Amphetamine-Like)-Related Disorders

Amphetamine Use Disorders

304.40 Amphetamine Dependence
305.70 Amphetamine Abuse

Amphetamine-Induced Disorders

292.89 Amphetamine Intoxication
292.0 Amphetamine Withdrawal
292.81 Amphetamine Intoxication Delirium
292.xx Amphetamine-Induced Psychotic Disorder
  .11 With Delusions
  .12 With Hallucinations
292.84 Amphetamine-Induced Mood Disorder
292.89 Amphetamine-Induced Anxiety Disorder
292.89 Amphetamine-Induced Sexual Dysfunction
292.89 Amphetamine-Induced Sleep Disorder
292.9 Amphetamine-Related Disorder NOS

Caffeine-Related Disorders

Caffeine-Induced Disorders

305.90 Caffeine Intoxication
292.89 Caffeine-Induced Anxiety Disorder
292.89 Caffeine-Induced Sleep Disorder
292.9 Caffeine-Related Disorder NOS

Cannabis-Related Disorders

Cannabis Use Disorders

304.30 Cannabis Dependence
305.20 Cannabis Abuse

Cannabis-Induced Disorders

292.89 Cannabis Intoxication
292.81 Cannabis Intoxication Delirium
292.xx Cannabis-Induced Psychotic Disorder
  .11 With Delusions
  .12 With Hallucinations
292.89 Cannabis-Induced Anxiety Disorder
292.9 Cannabis-Related Disorder NOS

Cocaine-Related Disorders

Cocaine Use Disorders

304.20 Cocaine Dependence
305.60 Cocaine Abuse

Cocaine-Induced Disorders

292.89 Cocaine Intoxication
292.0 Cocaine Withdrawal
292.81 Cocaine Intoxication Delirium
292.xx Cocaine-Induced Psychotic Disorder
  .11 With Delusions
  .12 With Hallucinations
292.84 Cocaine-Induced Mood Disorder
292.89 Cocaine-Induced Anxiety Disorder
292.89 Cocaine-Induced Sexual Dysfunction
292.89 Cocaine-Induced Sleep Disorder
292.9 Cocaine-Related Disorder NOS

Hallucinogen-Related Disorders

Hallucinogen Use Disorders

304.50 Hallucinogen Dependence
305.30 Hallucinogen Abuse

Hallucinogen-Induced Disorders

292.89 Hallucinogen Intoxication
292.89 Hallucinogen Persisting Perception Disorder (Flashbacks)
292.81 Hallucinogen Intoxication Delirium
292.xx Hallucinogen-Induced Psychotic Disorder
.11 With Delusions
.12 With Hallucinations
292.84 Hallucinogen-Induced Mood Disorder
292.89 Hallucinogen-Induced Anxiety Disorder
292.9 Hallucinogen-Related Disorder NOS

Inhalant-Related Disorders

Inhalant Use Disorders

304.60 Inhalant Dependence
305.90 Inhalant Abuse

Inhalant-Induced Disorders

292.89 Inhalant Intoxication
292.81 Inhalant Intoxication Delirium
292.82 Inhalant-Induced Persisting Dementia
292.xx Inhalant-Induced Psychotic Disorder
.11 With Delusions
.12 With Hallucinations
292.84 Inhalant-Induced Mood Disorder
292.89 Inhalant-Induced Anxiety Disorder
292.9 Inhalant-Related Disorder NOS

Nicotine-Related Disorders

Nicotine Use Disorders

305.1 Nicotine Dependence

Nicotine-Induced Disorders

292.0 Nicotine Withdrawal
292.9 Nicotine-Related Disorder NOS

Opioid-Related Disorders

Opioid Use Disorders

304.00 Opioid Dependence
305.50 Opioid Abuse

Opioid-Induced Disorders

292.89 Opioid Intoxication
292.0 Opioid Withdrawal
292.81 Opioid Intoxication Delirium
292.xx Opioid-Induced Psychotic Disorder
.11 With Delusions
.12 With Hallucinations
292.84 Opioid-Induced Mood Disorder
292.89 Opioid-Induced Sexual Dysfunction
292.89 Opioid-Induced Sleep Disorder
292.9 Opioid-Related Disorder NOS

Phencyclidine (or Phencyclidine-Like)-Related Disorders

Phencyclidine Use Disorders

304.60 Phencyclidine Dependence
305.90 Phencyclidine Abuse

Phencyclidine-Induced Disorders

292.89 Phencyclidine Intoxication
292.81 Phencyclidine Intoxication Delirium
292.xx Phencyclidine-Induced Psychotic Disorder
.11 With Delusions
.12 With Hallucinations
292.84 Phencyclidine-Induced Mood Disorder
292.89 Phencyclidine-Induced Anxiety Disorder
292.9 Phencyclidine-Related Disorder NOS

Sedative-, Hypnotic-, or Anxiolytic-Related Disorders

Sedative, Hypnotic, or Anxiolytic Use Disorders

304.10 Sedative, Hypnotic, or Anxiolytic Dependence
305.40 Sedative, Hypnotic, or Anxiolytic Abuse

Sedative-, Hypnotic-, or Anxiolytic-Induced Disorders

292.89 Sedative, Hypnotic, or Anxiolytic Intoxication

292.0 Sedative, Hypnotic, or Anxiolytic Withdrawal

292.81 Sedative, Hypnotic, or Anxiolytic Intoxication Delirium

292.81 Sedative, Hypnotic, or Anxiolytic Withdrawal Delirium

292.82 Sedative-, Hypnotic-, or Anxiolytic-Induced Persisting Dementia

292.83 Sedative-, Hypnotic-, or Anxiolytic-Induced Persisting Amnestic Disorder

292.xx Sedative-, Hypnotic-, or Anxiolytic-Induced Psychotic Disorder

.11 With Delusions

.12 With Hallucinations

292.84 Sedative-, Hypnotic-, or Anxiolytic-Induced Mood Disorder

292.89 Sedative-, Hypnotic-, or Anxiolytic-Induced Anxiety Disorder

292.89 Sedative-, Hypnotic-, or Anxiolytic-Induced Sexual Dysfunction

292.89 Sedative-, Hypnotic-, or Anxiolytic-Induced Sleep Disorder

292.9 Sedative-, Hypnotic-, or Anxiolytic-Related Disorder NOS

Polysubstance-Related Disorder

304.80 Polysubstance Dependence

Other (or Unknown) Substance-Related Disorders

Other (or Unknown) Substance Use Disorders

304.90 Other (or Unknown) Substance Dependence

305.90 Other (or Unknown) Substance Abuse

Other (or Unknown) Substance-Induced Disorders

292.89 Other (or Unknown) Substance Intoxication

292.0 Other (or Unknown) Substance Withdrawal

292.81 Other (or Unknown) Substance-Induced Delirium

292.82 Other (or Unknown) Substance-Induced Persisting Dementia

292.83 Other (or Unknown) Substance-Induced Persisting Amnestic Disorder

292.xx Other (or Unknown) Substance-Induced Psychotic Disorder

.11 With Delusions

.12 With Hallucinations

292.84 Other (or Unknown) Substance-Induced Mood Disorder

292.89 Other (or Unknown) Substance-Induced Anxiety Disorder

292.89 Other (or Unknown) Substance-Induced Sexual Dysfunction

292.89 Other (or Unknown) Substance-Induced Sleep Disorder

292.9 Other (or Unknown) Substance-Related Disorder NOS

SCHIZOPHRENIA AND OTHER PSYCHOTIC DISORDERS

295.xx Schizophrenia

.30 Paranoid type

.10 Disorganized type

.20 Catatonic type

.90 Undifferentiated type

.60 Residual type

295.40 Schizophreniform Disorder

295.70 Schizoaffective Disorder

297.1 Delusional Disorder

298.8 Brief Psychotic Disorder

297.3 Shared Psychotic Disorder

293.xx Psychotic Disorder Due to *(indicate the general medical condition)*

.81 With Delusions

.82 With Hallucinations

— Substance-Induced Psychotic Disorder *(refer to Substance-Related Disorders for substance-specific codes)*

298.9 Psychotic Disorder NOS

MOOD DISORDERS

(Code current state of Major Depressive Disorder or Bipolar I Disorder in fifth digit: 0 = unspecified; 1 = mild; 2 = moderate; 3 = severe, without psychotic features; 4 = severe, with psychotic features; 5 = in partial remission; 6 = in full remission.)

Depressive Disorders

296.xx Major Depressive Disorder
- .2x Single episode
- .3x Recurrent

300.4 Dysthymic Disorder

311 Depressive Disorder NOS

Bipolar Disorders

296.xx Bipolar I Disorder
- .0x Single Manic Episode
- .40 Most Recent Episode Hypomanic
- .4x Most Recent Episode Manic
- .6x Most Recent Episode Mixed
- .5x Most Recent Episode Depressed
- .7 Most Recent Episode Unspecified

296.89 Bipolar II Disorder *(specify current or most recent episode: Hypomanic or Depressed)*

301.13 Cyclothymic Disorder

296.80 Bipolar Disorder NOS

293.83 Mood Disorder Due to *(indicate the general medical condition*

—Substance-Induced Mood Disorder *(refer to Substance-Related Disorders for substance-specific codes)*

296.90 Mood Disorder NOS

ANXIETY DISORDERS

300.01 Panic Disorder Without Agoraphobia

300.21 Panic Disorder With Agoraphobia

300.22 Agoraphobia Without History of Panic Disorder

300.29 Specific Phobia

300.23 Social Phobia

300.3 Obsessive-Compulsive Disorder

309.81 Posttraumatic Stress Disorder

308.3 Acute Stress Disorder

300.02 Generalized Anxiety Disorder

293.89 Anxiety Disorder Due to *(indicate the general medical condition)*

—Substance-Induced Anxiety Disorder *(refer to Substance-Related Disorders for substance-specific codes)*

300.00 Anxiety Disorder NOS

SOMATOFORM DISORDERS

300.81 Somatization Disorder

300.82 Undifferentiated Somatoform Disorder

300.11 Conversion Disorder

307.xx Pain Disorder
- .80 Associated with Psychological Factors
- .89 Associated with Both Psychological Factors and a General Medical Condition

300.7 Hypochondriasis

300.7 Body Dysmorphic Disorder

300.82 Somatoform Disorder NOS

FACTITIOUS DISORDERS

300.xx Factitious Disorder
- .16 With Predominantly Psychological Signs and Symptoms
- .19 With Predominantly Physical Signs and Symptoms
- .19 With Combined Psychological and Physical Signs and Symptoms

300.19 Factitious Disorder NOS

DISSOCIATIVE DISORDERS

300.12 Dissociative Amnesia

300.13 Dissociative Fugue

300.14 Dissociative Identity Disorder

300.6 Depersonalization Disorder

300.15 Dissociative Disorder NOS

SEXUAL AND GENDER IDENTITY DISORDERS

Sexual Dysfunctions

Sexual Desire Disorders

302.71 Hypoactive Sexual Desire Disorder

302.79 Sexual Aversion Disorder

Sexual Arousal Disorders

302.72 Female Sexual Arousal Disorder
302.72 Male Erectile Disorder

Orgasmic Disorders

302.73 Female Orgasmic Disorder
302.74 Male Orgasmic Disorder
302.75 Premature Ejaculation

Sexual Pain Disorders

302.76 Dyspareunia (Not Due to a general medical condition)

306.51 Vaginismus (Not Due to a general medical condition)

Sexual Dysfunction Due to a General Medical Condition

625.8 Female Hypoactive Sexual Desire Disorder Due to *(indicate the general medical condition)*

608.89 Male Hypoactive Sexual Desire Disorder Due to *(indicate the general medical condition)*

607.84 Male Erectile Disorder Due to *(indicate the general medical condition)*

625.0 Female Dyspareunia Due to *(indicate the general medical condition)*

608.89 Male Dyspareunia Due to *(indicate the general medical condition)*

625.8 Other Female Sexual Dysfunction Due to *(indicate the general medical condition)*

608.89 Other Male Sexual Dysfunction Due to *(indicate the general medical condition)*

—Substance-Induced Sexual Dysfunction *(refer to Substance-Related Disorders for substance-specific codes)*

302.70 Sexual Dysfunction NOS

Paraphilias

302.4 Exhibitionism
302.81 Fetishism
302.89 Frotteurism
302.2 Pedophilia
302.83 Sexual Masochism
302.84 Sexual Sadism
302.3 Transvestic Fetishism
302.82 Voyeurism
302.9 Paraphilia NOS

Gender Identity Disorders

302.xx Gender Identity Disorder
.6 In Children
.85 In Adolescents or Adults
302.6 Gender Identity Disorder NOS
302.9 Sexual Disorder NOS

EATING DISORDERS

307.1 Anorexia Nervosa
307.51 Bulimia Nervosa
307.50 Eating Disorder NOS

SLEEP DISORDERS

Primary Sleep Disorders

Dyssomnias

307.42 Primary Insomnia
307.44 Primary Hypersomnia
347 Narcolepsy
780.59 Breathing-Related Sleep Disorder
307.45 Circadian Rhythm Sleep Disorder
307.47 Dyssomnia NOS

Parasomnias

307.47 Nightmare Disorder
307.46 Sleep Terror Disorder
307.46 Sleepwalking Disorder
307.47 Parasomnia NOS

Sleep Disorders Related to Another Mental Disorder

307.42 Insomnia Related to *(indicate the Axis I or Axis II Disorder)*

307.44 Hypersomnia Related to *(indicate the Axis I or Axis II Disorder)*

Other Sleep Disorders

780.xx Sleep Disorder Due to *(indicate the general medical condition)*
.52 Insomnia type
.54 Hypersomnia type

.59 Parasomnia type

.59 Mixed type

—Substance-Induced Sleep Disorder *(refer to Substance-Related Disorders for substance-specific codes)*

IMPULSE CONTROL DISORDERS NOT ELSEWHERE CLASSIFIED

312.34 Intermittent Explosive Disorder

312.32 Kleptomania

312.33 Pyromania

312.31 Pathological Gambling

312.39 Trichotillomania

312.30 Impulse Control Disorder NOS

ADJUSTMENT DISORDERS

309.xx Adjustment Disorder

.0 With Depressed Mood

.24 With Anxiety

.28 With Mixed Anxiety and Depressed Mood

.3 With Disturbance of Conduct

.4 With Mixed Disturbance of Emotions and Conduct

.9 Unspecified

PERSONALITY DISORDERS

NOTE: *These are coded on Axis II.*

301.0 Paranoid Personality Disorder

301.20 Schizoid Personality Disorder

301.22 Schizotypal Personality Disorder

301.7 Antisocial Personality Disorder

301.83 Borderline Personality Disorder

301.50 Histrionic Personality Disorder

301.81 Narcissistic Personality Disorder

301.82 Avoidant Personality Disorder

301.6 Dependent Personality Disorder

301.4 Obsessive-Compulsive Personality Disorder

301.9 Personality Disorder NOS

OTHER CONDITIONS THAT MAY BE A FOCUS OF CLINICAL ATTENTION

Psychological Factors Affecting Medical Condition

316 *Choose name based on nature of factors:*

Mental Disorder Affecting Medical Condition

Psychological Symptoms Affecting Medical Condition

Personality Traits or Coping Style Affecting Medical Condition

Maladaptive Health Behaviors Affecting Medical Condition

Stress-Related Physiological Response Affecting Medical Condition

Other or Unspecified Psychological Factors Affecting Medical Condition

Medication-Induced Movement Disorders

332.1 Neuroleptic-Induced Parkinsonism

333.92 Neuroleptic Malignant Syndrome

333.7 Neuroleptic-Induced Acute Dystonia

333.99 Neuroleptic-Induced Acute Akathisia

333.82 Neuroleptic-Induced Tardive Dyskinesia

333.1 Medication-Induced Postural Tremor

333.90 Medication-Induced Movement Disorder NOS

Other Medication-Induced Disorder

995.2 Adverse Effects of Medication NOS

Relational Problems

V61.9 Relational Problem Related to a Mental Disorder or General Medical Condition

V61.20 Parent-Child Relational Problem

V61.10 Partner Relational Problem

V61.8 Sibling Relational Problem

V62.81 Relational Problem NOS

Problems Related to Abuse or Neglect

V61.21 Physical Abuse of Child
V61.21 Sexual Abuse of Child
V61.21 Neglect of Child
— Physical Abuse of Adult
V61.12 (if by partner)
V62.83 (if by person other than partner)
— Sexual Abuse of Adult
V61.12 (if by partner)
V62.83 (if by person other than partner)

Additional Conditions That May Be a Focus of Clinical Attention

V15.81 Noncompliance with Treatment
V65.2 Malingering
V71.01 Adult Antisocial Behavior
V71.02 Childhood or Adolescent Antisocial Behavior
V62.89 Borderline Intellectual Functioning (coded on Axis II)
780.9 Age-Related Cognitive Decline
V62.82 Bereavement
V62.3 Academic Problem
V62.2 Occupational Problem
313.82 Identity Problem
V62.89 Religious or Spiritual Problem
V62.4 Acculturation Problem
V62.89 Phase of Life Problem

ADDITIONAL CODES

300.9 Unspecified Mental Disorder (nonpsychotic)
V71.09 No Diagnosis or Condition on Axis I
799.9 Diagnosis or Condition Deferred on Axis I
V71.09 No Diagnosis on Axis II
799.9 Diagnosis Deferred on Axis II

Appendix B

NANDA Nursing Diagnoses: Taxonomy II*

EXCHANGING

- Imbalanced nutrition: More than body requirements
- Imbalanced nutrition: Less than body requirements
- Risk for imbalanced nutrition: More than body requirements
- Risk for infection
- Risk for imbalanced body temperature
- Hypothermia
- Hyperthermia
- Ineffective thermoregulation
- Autonomic dysreflexia
- Risk for autonomic dysreflexia
- Constipation
- Perceived constipation
- Diarrhea
- Bowel incontinence
- Risk for constipation
- Impaired urinary elimination
- Stress urinary incontinence
- Reflex urinary incontinence
- Urge urinary incontinence
- Functional urinary incontinence
- Total urinary incontinence
- Risk for urge urinary incontinence
- Urinary retention
- Ineffective tissue perfusion (specify type: renal, cerebral, cardiopulmonary, gastrointestinal, peripheral)
- Risk for imbalanced fluid volume
- Excess fluid volume
- Deficient fluid volume
- Risk for deficient fluid volume
- Decreased cardiac output
- Impaired gas exchange
- Ineffective airway clearance
- Ineffective breathing pattern
- Impaired spontaneous ventilation
- Dysfunctional ventilatory weaning response
- Risk for injury
- Risk for suffocation
- Risk for poisoning
- Risk for trauma
- Risk for aspiration
- Risk for disuse syndrome
- Latex allergy response
- Risk for latex allergy response
- Ineffective protection
- Impaired tissue integrity
- Impaired oral mucous membrane
- Impaired skin integrity
- Risk for impaired skin integrity
- Impaired dentition
- Decreased intracranial adaptive capacity
- Disturbed energy field

COMMUNICATING

- Impaired verbal communication

RELATING

- Impaired social interaction
- Social isolation
- Risk for loneliness
- Ineffective role performance
- Impaired parenting
- Risk for impaired parenting
- Risk for impaired parent/infant/child attachment
- Sexual dysfunction
- Interrupted family processes

*NANDA Nursing Diagnoses: Definitions & Classification 2003–2004. (2003). Philadelphia: NANDA International. With permission.

- Caregiver role strain
- Risk for caregiver role strain
- Dysfunctional family processes: Alcoholism
- Parental role conflict
- Ineffective sexuality patterns

VALUING

- Spiritual distress
- Risk for spiritual distress
- Readiness for enhanced spiritual well-being
- Ineffective coping
- Impaired adjustment
- Defensive coping
- Ineffective denial
- Disabled family coping
- Compromised family coping
- Readiness for enhanced family coping
- Readiness for enhanced community coping
- Ineffective community coping
- Ineffective therapeutic regimen management
- Noncompliance (specify)
- Ineffective family therapeutic regimen management
- Ineffective community therapeutic regimen management
- Effective therapeutic regimen management
- Decisional conflict (specify)
- Health-seeking behaviors (specify)

MOVING

- Impaired physical mobility
- Risk for peripheral neurovascular dysfunction
- Risk for perioperative-positioning injury
- Impaired walking
- Risk for falls
- Wandering
- Impaired wheelchair mobility
- Impaired transfer ability
- Impaired bed mobility
- Activity intolerance
- Fatigue
- Risk for activity intolerance
- Disturbed sleep pattern
- Sleep deprivation
- Deficient diversional activity
- Impaired home maintenance
- Ineffective health maintenance
- Delayed surgical recovery
- Adult failure to thrive
- Feeding self-care deficit
- Impaired swallowing
- Ineffective breast-feeding
- Interrupted breast-feeding
- Effective breast-feeding
- Ineffective infant feeding pattern
- Bathing/hygiene self-care deficit
- Dressing/grooming self-care deficit
- Toileting self-care deficit
- Delayed growth and development
- Risk for delayed development
- Risk for disproportionate growth
- Relocation stress syndrome
- Risk for relocation stress syndrome
- Risk for disorganized infant behavior
- Disorganized infant behavior
- Readiness for enhanced organized infant behavior

PERCEIVING

- Disturbed body image
- Chronic low-self-esteem
- Situational low self-esteem
- Risk for situational low self-esteem
- Disturbed personal identity
- Disturbed sensory perception (specify: visual, auditory, kinesthetic, gustatory, tactile, olfactory)
- Unilateral neglect
- Hopelessness
- Powerlessness
- Risk for powerlessness

KNOWING

- Deficient knowledge (specify)
- Impaired environmental interpretation syndrome
- Acute confusion
- Chronic confusion
- Disturbed thought processes
- Impaired memory

FEELING

- Acute pain
- Chronic pain
- Nausea
- Dysfunctional grieving
- Anticipatory grieving

- Chronic sorrow
- Risk for other-directed violence
- Self-mutilation
- Risk for self-mutilation
- Risk for self-directed violence
- Risk for suicide
- Post-trauma syndrome
- Rape-trauma syndrome
- Rape-trauma syndrome: Compound reaction
- Rape-trauma syndrome: Silent reaction
- Risk for post-trauma syndrome
- Anxiety
- Death anxiety
- Fear

APPENDIX C

Assigning Nursing Diagnoses to Client Behaviors

Following is a list of client behaviors and the NANDA nursing diagnoses that correspond to the behaviors and that may be used in planning care for the client exhibiting the specific behavioral symptoms.

Behaviors	**NANDA Nursing Diagnoses**
Aggression; hostility	Risk for injury; Risk for other-directed violence
Anorexia or refusal to eat	Imbalanced nutrition: Less than body requirements
Anxious behavior	Anxiety (Specify level)
Confusion; memory loss	Confusion, acute/chronic; Disturbed thought processes
Delusions	Disturbed thought processes
Denial of problems	Ineffective denial
Depressed mood or anger turned inward	Dysfunctional grieving
Detoxification; withdrawal from substances	Risk for injury
Difficulty making important life decision	Decisional conflict (specify)
Difficulty with interpersonal relationships	Impaired social interaction
Disruption in capability to perform usual responsibilities	Ineffective role performance
Dissociative behaviors (depersonalization; derealization)	Disturbed sensory perception (kinesthetic)
Expresses feelings of disgust about body or body part	Disturbed body image
Expresses lack of control over personal situation	Powerlessness
Flashbacks, nightmares, obsession with traumatic experience	Post-trauma syndrome
Hallucinations	Disturbed sensory perception (auditory; visual)
Highly critical of self or others	Low self-esteem (chronic; situational)
HIV positive; altered immunity	Ineffective protection
Inability to meet basic needs	Self-care deficit (feeding; bathing/hygiene; dressing/grooming; toileting)
Insomnia or hypersomnia	Disturbed sleep pattern
Loose associations or flight of ideas	Impaired verbal communication
Manic hyperactivity	Risk for injury
Manipulative behavior	Ineffective coping
Multiple personalities; gender identity disturbance	Disturbed personal identity
Orgasm, problems with; lack of sexual desire	Sexual dysfunction
Overeating, compulsive	Risk for imbalanced nutrition: More than body requirements
Phobias	Fear
Physical symptoms as coping behavior	Ineffective coping
Projection of blame; rationalization of failures; denial of personal responsibility	Defensive coping

Behaviors	NANDA Nursing Diagnoses
Ritualistic behaviors	Anxiety (severe); Ineffective coping
Seductive remarks; inappropriate sexual behaviors	Impaired social interaction
Self-mutilative behaviors	Self-mutilation; Risk for self-mutilation
Sexual behaviors (difficulty, limitations, or changes in; reported dissatisfaction)	Ineffective sexuality patterns
Stress from caring for chronically ill person	Caregiver role strain
Stress from locating to new environment	Relocation stress syndrome
Substance use as a coping-behavior	Ineffective coping
Substance use (denies use is a problem)	Ineffective denial
Suicidal	Risk for suicide; Risk for self-directed violence
Suspiciousness	Disturbed thought processes; Ineffective coping
Vomiting, excessive, self-induced	Risk for deficient fluid volume
Withdrawn behavior	Social isolation

MENTAL STATUS ASSESSMENT

Gathering the correct information about the client's mental status is essential to the development of an appropriate plan of care. The mental status examination is a description of all the areas of the client's mental functioning. The following are the components that are considered critical in the assessment of a client's mental status.

IDENTIFYING DATA

1. Name
2. Sex
3. Age
4. Race/culture
5. Occupational/financial status
6. Educational level
7. Significant other
8. Living arrangements
9. Religious preference
10. Allergies
11. Special diet considerations
12. Chief complaint
13. Medical diagnosis

GENERAL DESCRIPTION

Appearance

1. Grooming and dress
2. Hygiene
3. Posture
4. Height and weight
5. Level of eye contact
6. Hair color and texture
7. Evidence of scars, tattoos, or other distinguishing skin marks
8. Evaluation of client's appearance compared with chronological age

Motor Activity

1. Tremors
2. Tics or other stereotypical movements
3. Mannerisms and gestures
4. Hyperactivity
5. Restlessness or agitation
6. Aggressiveness
7. Rigidity
8. Gait patterns
9. Echopraxia
10. Psychomotor retardation
11. Freedom of movement (range of motion)

Speech Patterns

1. Slowness or rapidity of speech
2. Pressure of speech
3. Intonation
4. Volume
5. Stuttering or other speech impairments
6. Aphasia

General Attitude

1. Cooperative/uncooperative
2. Friendly/hostile/defensive
3. Uninterested/apathetic
4. Attentive/interested
5. Guarded/suspicious

EMOTIONS

Mood

1. Sad
2. Depressed
3. Despairing

4. Irritable
5. Anxious
6. Elated
7. Euphoric
8. Fearful
9. Guilty
10. Labile

Affect

1. Congruence with mood
2. Constricted or blunted (diminished amount/range and intensity of emotional expression)
3. Flat (absence of emotional expression)
4. Appropriate or inappropriate (defines congruence of affect with the situation or with the client's behavior)

THOUGHT PROCESSES

Form of Thought

1. Flight of ideas
2. Associative looseness
3. Circumstantiality
4. Tangentiality
5. Neologisms
6. Concrete thinking
7. Clang associations
8. Word salad
9. Perseveration
10. Echolalia
11. Mutism
12. Poverty of speech (restriction in the amount of speech)
13. Ability to concentrate
14. Attention span

Content of Thought

1. Delusions: a. Persecutory; b. Grandiose; c. Reference; d. Control or influence; e. Somatic; f. Nihilistic
2. Suicidal or homicidal ideas
3. Obsessions
4. Paranoia/suspiciousness
5. Magical thinking
6. Religiosity
7. Phobias
8. Poverty of content (vague, meaningless responses)

PERCEPTUAL DISTURBANCES

1. Hallucinations: a. Auditory; b. Visual; c. Tactile; d. Olfactory; e. Gustatory
2. Illusions
3. Depersonalization (altered perception of the self)
4. Derealization (altered perception of the environment)

SENSORIUM AND COGNITIVE ABILITY

1. Level of alertness/consciousness
2. Orientation: a. Time; b. Place; c. Person; d. Circumstances
3. Memory: a. Recent; b. Remote; c. Confabulation
4. Capacity for abstract thought

IMPULSE CONTROL

1. Ability to control impulses related to the following: a. Aggression; b. Hostility; c. Fear; d. Guilt; e. Affection; f. Sexual feelings

JUDGMENT AND INSIGHT

1. Ability to solve problems
2. Ability to make decisions
3. Knowledge about self: a. Awareness of limitations; b. Awareness of consequences of actions; c. Awareness of illness
4. Adaptive/maladaptive use of coping strategies and ego defense mechanisms

APPENDIX E

CRITICAL PATHWAYS OF CARE*

I. Critical Pathway of Care for Client in Alcohol Withdrawal

Estimated Length of Stay: 7 Days—Variations from Designated Pathway Should be Documented in Progress Notes

Nursing Diagnoses and Categories of Care	Time Dimension	Goals and/or Actions	Time Dimension	Goals and/or Actions	Time Dimension	Discharge Outcome
Risk for injury related to CNS agitation					Day 7	Client shows no evidence of injury obtained during ETOH withdrawal
Referrals	Day 1	Psychiatrist Assess need for: Neurologist Cardiologist Internist			Day 7	Discharge with follow-up appointments as required
Diagnostic studies	Day 1	Blood alcohol level Drug screen (urine and blood) Chemistry profile Urinalysis Chest X-ray ECG	Day 4	Repeat of selected diagnostic studies as necessary.		
Additional assessments	Day 1 Day 1–5 Ongoing Ongoing	VS q4h I&O Restraints p.r.n. Assess withdrawal symptoms: tremors, nausea/vomiting, tachycardia, sweating, high blood pressure, seizures, insomnia, hallucinations	Day 2–3 Day 6 Day 4	VS q8h if stable DC I&O Marked decrease in objective withdrawal symptoms	Day 4–7 Day 7	VS b.i.d.; remain stable Discharge; absence of objective withdrawal symptoms
Medications	Day 1 Day 2 Day 1–6 Day 1–7	*Librium 200 mg in divided doses Librium 160 mg in divided doses Librium p.r.n. Maalox ac & hs **Note:* Some physicians may elect to use Serax or Tegretol in the detoxification process	Day 3 Day 4	Librium 120 mg in divided doses Librium 80 mg in divided doses	Day 5 Day 6 Day 7	Librium 40 mg DC Librium Discharge; no withdrawal symptoms

(Continued)

*NOTE: With the advent of shorter hospital says, adjustments may need to be made in the time dimensions on these critical pathways of care (CPCs). These CPCs are intended to provide guidelines from which the student or practitioner can base client care.

I. Critical Pathway of Care for Client in Alcohol Withdrawal *(Continued)*

Nursing Diagnoses and Categories of Care	Time Dimension	Goals and/ or Actions	Time Dimension	Goals and/ or Actions	Time Dimension	Discharge Outcome
Client education			Day 5	Discuss goals of AA and need for outpatient therapy	Day 7	Discharge with information regarding AA attendance or outpatient treatment
Imbalanced nutrition: Less than body requirements					Day 7	Nutritional condition has stabilized.
Referrals	Day 1	Consult dietitian	Day 1–7	Fulfill nutritional needs		
Diet	Day 1	Bland as tolerated; fluids as tolerated	Day 2–3	Frequent, small, meals; easily digested foods; advance as tolerated	Day 4–7	High-protein, high-carbohydrate diet
Additional assessments	Day 1–7	Weight I&O Skin turgor Color of mucous membranes				
Medications	Day 1–7	Thiamine 100 mg po (or injection, depending on condition of pt.) Multiple vitamin tablet Folate 1 mg po				
Client education			Day 4 Day 5	Principles of nutrition; foods for maintenance of wellness Reinforce teaching	Day 6–7	Client demonstrates ability to select appropriate foods for healthy diet

II. Critical Pathway of Care for Client with Schizophrenic Psychosis

Estimated Length of Stay: 14 Days—Variations from Designated Pathway Should be Documented in Progress Notes

Nursing Diagnosis and Categories of Care	Time Dimension	Goals and/or Actions	Time Dimension	Goals and/or Actions	Time Dimension	Discharge Outcome
Disturbed thought processes/Disturbed sensory perception			Day 7	Client is able to differentiate between what is real and what is not real	Day 14	Client experiences no delusional thinking or hallucinations.
Referrals	Day 1	Psychiatrist Psychologist Social worker Clinical nurse specialist Music therapist Occupational therapist Recreational therapist			Day 14	Discharge with follow-up appointments as required.
Diagnostic studies	Day 1 Day 3–5	Drug screen Chemistry profile CT scan, MRI, PET, EEG. (These may be ordered to examine structure and function of the brain.)				
Additional assessments	Day 1 Day 1	VS every shift. Assess for: delusions, hallucinations, loose associations, inappropriate affect, excitement/stupor, panic anxiety, suspiciousness.	Day 2–14 Day 2–5	Ongoing assessments Establish trust with at least one person.	Day 2–14 Day 14	VS daily if stable. No evidence of delusions, hallucinations, loose associations, inappropriate affect, excitement/stupor, panic anxiety, suspiciousness.
Medications	Day 1	Antipsychotic medication (scheduled and p.r.n.). May need order for concentrate and injectable form. Antiparkinsonian medication (p.r.n.)	Day 1–14	Assess for effectiveness and side effects of medications.	Day 14	Client is discharged with medications.
Client education			Day 7	Discuss correlation between increased anxiety and psychotic symptoms. Discuss ways to deescalate anxiety.	Day 12–13	Reinforce teaching.
			Day 10	Discuss importance of taking medications regularly, even when feeling well. Discuss possible side effects of medications and when to see the doctor.	Day 14	Client verbalizes understanding of information presented prior to discharge.

(Continued)

II. Critical Pathway of Care for Client with Schizophrenic Psychosis *(Continued)*

Nursing Diagnosis and Categories of Care	Time Dimension	Goals and/ or Actions	Time Dimension	Goals and/ or Actions	Time Dimension	Discharge Outcome
Risk for violence: Self-directed or other-directed	Day 1	Environment is made safe for client and others.	Ongoing	Client does not harm self or others.	Day 14	Client is discharged without harm to self or others.
Referrals	Day 1	Alert hostility management team of the admission of a potentially violent client. For relaxation therapy: Music therapist Clinical nurse specialist Stress management specialist Psychiatrist: May give order for mechanical restraints to be used if needed.			Day 14	Discharge with follow-up appointments as required.
Additional assessments	Day 1	Assess for signs of impending violent behavior: increase in psychomotor activity; angry affect; verbalized persecutory delusions or frightening hallucinations.	Day 2–14	Assessments are ongoing.		
Medications	Day 1	Use antipsychotic medications (p.r.n.) when signs of agitation begin.	Day 1–14	Use medications, isolation/seclusion, or mechanical restraints. If client refuses medications, administer following application of restraints.	Day 14	Client is discharged with medications.
Client education			Day 3–12	Teach relaxation techniques; discuss activities in which client could participate to relieve pent-up tension; discuss signs and symptoms of escalating anxiety.	Day 12–13 Day 14	Reinforce teaching. Client verbalizes understanding of information presented prior to discharge.

CT = computed tomography; MRI = magnetic resonance imaging; PET = positron-emission tomography; EEG = electroencephalogram.

III. Critical Pathway of Care for the Depressed Client

Estimated Length of Stay: 7 Days—Variations from Designated Pathway Should be Documented in Progress Notes

Nursing Diagnoses and Categories of Care	Time Dimension	Goals and/ or Actions	Time Dimension	Goals and/ or Actions	Time Dimension	Discharge Outcome
Risk for suicide	Day 1	Environment is made safe for client.	Ongoing	Client does not harm self.	Day 7	Client is discharged without harm to self.
Referrals	Day 1	Psychiatrist: May give order to isolate if risk is great or may do ECT For relaxation therapy: Music therapist Clinical nurse specialist Stress management specialist			Day 7	Discharge with follow-up appointments as required.
Additional assessments	Day 1	Suicidal assessment: • ideation • gestures • threats • plan • means • anxiety level • thought disorder	Day 2–7	Ongoing assessments.	Day 7	Client discharged. Denies suicidal ideations.
	Day 1	Secure no-suicide contract.				
Medications	Day 1	Antidepressant medication, as ordered. Antianxiety agents p.r.n.	Day 1–7	Assess for effectiveness and side effects of medications. Be alert for sudden lifts in mood.	Day 7	Discharged with antidepressant medications.
Client education	Day 3–6	Teach relaxation techniques. Discuss resources outside the hospital from whom client may seek assistance when feeling suicidal.	Day 6–7	Reinforce teaching.	Day 7	Discharge with understanding of instruction given.
Dysfunctional grieving	Day 1	Assess stage of fixation in grief process.			Day 7	Discharge with evidence of progression toward resolution of grief.
Referrals	Day 1	Psychiatrist Psychologist Social worker Clinical nurse specialist Music therapist Occupational therapist Recreational therapist Chaplain			Day 7	Discharge with follow-up appointments as required.

(Continued)

III. Critical Pathway of Care for the Depressed Client *(Continued)*

Nursing Diagnoses and Categories of Care	Time Dimension	Goals and/ or Actions	Time Dimension	Goals and/ or Actions	Time Dimension	Discharge Outcome
Diagnostic studies		Any of the following tests *may* be ordered:				
	Day 1	Drug screen Chemistry profile				
	Day 2–3	Urine test for norepinephrine and serotonin Dexamethasone-suppression test A measure of TSH response to administered TRH Serum and urine studies for nutritional deficiencies.				
Medications	Day 1	Antidepressant medication, as ordered. Antianxiety agent p.r.n.	Day 1–7	Assess for effectiveness and side effects of medications.	Day 7	Client is discharged with medications.
Diet	Day 1	If antidepressant medication is MAO inhibitor: low tyramine			Day 7	Client has experienced no symptoms of hypertensive crisis.
Additional assessments	Day 1	VS every shift	Day 2–7	VS daily if stable.	Day 7	Mood and affect appropriate. No evidence of thought disorder. Participates willingly and appropriately in activities.
	Day 1	Assess: • Mental status • Mood, affect • Thought disorder • Communication patterns • Level of interest in environment • Participation in activities • Weight	Day 2–7	Ongoing assessments.		
Client education	Day 1	Orient to unit	Day 4	Discuss importance of taking medications regularly, even when feeling well or if feeling medication is not helping. Discuss possible side effects of medication and when to see the physician. Teach which foods to eliminate from diet if taking MAO inhibitor.	Day 7	Client is discharged. Verbalizes understanding of information presented prior to discharge.
			Day 5–6	Reinforce teaching.		

IV. Critical Pathway of Care for the Client Experiencing a Manic Episode

Estimated Length of Stay: 7 Days—Variations from Designated Pathway Should be Documented in Progress Notes

Nursing Diagnoses and Categories of Care	Time Dimension	Goals and/ or Actions	Time Dimension	Goals and/ or Actions	Time Dimension	Discharge Outcome
Risk for injury/ violence	Day 1	Environment is made safe for client and others.	Ongoing	Client does not harm self or others.	Day 7	Client has not harmed self or others.
Referrals	Day 1	Psychiatrist Clinical nurse specialist Internist (may need to determine if symptoms are caused by other illness or medication side effects) Neurologist (may want to check for brain lesion) Alert hostility management team			Day 7	Discharge with follow-up appointments as required.
Diagnostic studies	Day 1	Drug screen Electrolytes Lithium level Chemistry profile	Day 5	Lithium level	Day 7	Lithium level and discharge with instructions to return monthly to have level drawn.
Additional assessments	Day 1 Ongoing Ongoing	VS q4h Restraints p.r.n. Assess for signs of impending violent behavior: increase in psychomotor activity, angry affect, verbalized persecutory delusions or frightening hallucinations.	Day 2–7	Ongoing assessments		
Medications	Day 1	Antipsychotic medications, scheduled and p.r.n. *Lithium carbonate 600 mg t.i.d. or q.i.d. **Note:* Physician may elect to use an anticonvulsant (e.g., valproic acid; carbamazepine)	Day 2–7	Administer medications as ordered and observe for effectiveness and side effects.	Day 7	Client is discharged on maintenance dose lithium carbonate (or other mood-stabilizing agent).
Client education			Day 4 Day 6	Teach about lithium: Continue to take medication even when feeling okay. Teach symptoms of toxicity. Emphasize importance of monthly blood levels. Teach about other medications client may be taking. Reinforce teaching.	Day 7	Client is discharged with written instructions and verbalizes understanding of material presented.

(Continued)

IV. Critical Pathway of Care for the Client Experiencing a Manic Episode (*Continued*)

Nursing Diagnoses and Categories of Care	Time Dimension	Goals and/ or Actions	Time Dimension	Goals and/ or Actions	Time Dimension	Discharge Outcome
Imbalanced nutrition: Less than body requirements					Day 7	Nutritional condition and weight have stabilized.
Referrals	Day 1	Consult dietitian	Day 1–7	Fulfill nutritional needs.		
Diet	Day 1	High-protein, high-calorie nutritious finger foods. Juice and snacks as tolerated.	As mania subsides	Regular diet with foods of client's choice.		
Diagnostic studies	Day 1	Chemistry profile Urinalysis	Day 2–7	Repeat of selected diagnostic studies as required.		
Additional assessments	Day 1–7	Weight I&O Skin turgor Color of mucous membranes				
Medications	Day 1–7	Multiple vitamin/mineral tab				
Client education			Day 4 Day 6	Principles of nutrition; foods for maintenance of wellness; adequate sodium; 6–8 glasses of water/day. Contact dietitian if weight gain becomes a problem. Reinforce teaching	Day 5–7	Client demonstrates ability to select appropriate foods for healthy diet and verbalizes understanding of material presented.

V. Critical Pathway of Care for the Posttrauma Client

Estimated Length of Stay: 7 Days—Variations from Designated Pathway should be Documented in Progress Notes

Nursing Diagnoses and Categories of Care	Time Dimension	Goals and/ or Actions	Time Dimension	Goals and/ or Actions	Time Dimension	Discharge Outcome
Posttrauma Syndrome	Day 1	Reassurance of client safety.	Ongoing	Environment is made safe for client.	Day 7	Client is able to carry out activities of daily living. Fewer flashbacks, nightmares.
Referrals	Day 1	Psychiatrist Psychologist Social worker Clinical nurse specialist Music therapist Occupational therapist Recreational therapist Chaplain			Day 7	Discharge with follow-up appointments as required.
Diagnostic studies	Day 1	Drug screen; EKG; EEG; Chemistry profile				
	Day 2–5	MMPI Impact of event scale (IES)				
Medications	Day 1	Antidepressant medication, as ordered (SSRIs, tricyclics or MAO inhibitors). Antianxiety medication, as ordered (benzodiazepines); may be given p.r.n. because of addictive quality. Clonidine or propranolol (for intrusive thoughts and hyperarousal). Sedative/hypnotics for sleep disturbances; may be given p.r.n.	Day 1–7	Assess for effectiveness and side effects of medications. Administer addictive medications judiciously and taper dosage.	Day 7	Discharged with scripts as ordered by physician (e.g., antidepressants; clonidine; propranolol).

(Continued)

V. Critical Pathway of Care for the Posttrauma Client *(Continued)*

Nursing Diagnoses and Categories of Care	Time Dimension	Goals and/ or Actions	Time Dimension	Goals and/ or Actions	Time Dimension	Discharge Outcome
Additional assessments	Day 1	VS every shift Assess: • Mental status • Mood swings • Anxiety level • Social interaction • Ability to carry out activities of daily living • Suicide ideation • Sleep disturbances • "Flashbacks" • Presence of guilt feelings	Day 2–7	VS daily if stable Ongoing assessments	Day 7	Anxiety is maintained at manageable level. Mood is appropriate. Interacts with others. Carries out activities of daily living independently. Denies suicide ideation. Sleeps without medication. Is able to interrupt flashbacks with adaptive, coping strategies. Has worked through feelings of guilt.
Diet	Day 1	Client's choice or low-tyramine if taking MAO inhibitor	Day 2–7	Same	Day 7	Client eats well-balanced diet.
Client education	Day 1	Orient to unit	Day 3–4	Stages of grief Side effects of medications Coping strategies Low-tyramine diet Community resources Support group Importance of not mixing drugs and alcohol.	Day 7	Client is discharged. Verbalizes understanding of information presented before discharge.
			Day 6	Reinforce teaching.		

VI. Critical Pathway of Care for Client with Anorexia Nervosa

Estimated Length of Stay: 28 Days—Variations from Designated Pathway should be Documented in Progress Notes

Nursing Diagnoses and Categories of Care	Time Dimension	Goals and/ or Actions	Time Dimension	Goals and/ or Actions	Time Dimension	Discharge Outcome
Imbalanced nutrition: Less than body requirements. Risk for deficient fluid volume.	Ongoing	Client will gain 3 lb/wk and maintain adequate state of hydration			Day 28	Client will exhibit no signs or symptoms of malnutrition or dehydration.
Referrals	Day 1 and ongoing	Consult dietitian	Day 2–28	Fulfill nutritional needs. Client consumes 75% of food provided and at least 1000 ml fluid/day.		
Diagnostic studies	Day 1	Electrolytes Electrocardiogram Blood urea nitrogen/creatinine Urinalysis Complete blood count Thyroid function	Day 14	Repeat of selected diagnostic studies.	Day 28	All laboratory values are within normal limits.
Additional assessments	Daily; q shift	Vital signs	Day 7–28	Vital signs within normal limits.	Day 22–28	Client is able to refrain from self-induced vomiting.
	Daily; q shift	Input & output	Day 7–28	Appropriate balance is achieved.		
	Day 1	Weight	Day 2–28	Client gains approximately $^1/_2$ lb/day.		
	Day 1	Monitor for purging following meals.	Day 1–21	Client bathroom is locked for 1 hr following meals.		
Client education	Day 1	Unit orientation; behavior modification plan	Day 7–14	Principles of nutrition; foods for maintenance of wellness.	Day 15–18	Client demonstrates ability to select appropriate foods for healthy diet.
Ineffective denial	Day 1	Client will cooperate with orientation to unit and explanation of behavior modification plan	Day 2–28	Client cooperates with therapy to restore nutritional status.	Day 18–28	Client accepts that eating behaviors are maladaptive and demonstrates ability to cope more adaptively.
Referrals	Day 7 (or when physical condition is stable)	Psychologist; social worker; psychodramatist	Day 8–28	Client attends group psychotherapies daily.	Day 28	Client verbalizes ways to gain control in life situation.
Additional assessments	Day 1–17	Assess client's ability to trust; use of manipulation to achieve control	Day 14	Client has developed trusting relationship with at least one staff member on each shift.	Day 28	Client no longer manipulates others to achieve control.

(Continued)

VI. Critical Pathway of Care for Client with Anorexia Nervosa *(Continued)*

Nursing Diagnoses and Categories of Care	Time Dimension	Goals and/ or Actions	Time Dimension	Goals and/ or Actions	Time Dimension	Discharge Outcome
Client education	Day 1 and ongoing as required	Describe privileges and responsibilities of behavior modification program. Explain consequences of noncompliance.	Day 21	Discuss role of support groups for individuals with eating disorders.	Day 28	Client and family verbalize intention to attend community support group.
Disturbed body image; Low self-esteem	Day 7	Client acknowledges that attention will not be given to the discussion of body image and food	Day 21	Client acknowledges misperception of body image as fat and verbalizes positive self-attributes.	Day 28	Client perceives body image correctly, is not obsessed with food, and has given up the need for perfection.
Referrals	Day 1 (or when condition is stable)	Occupational therapy; recreational therapy; music therapy; art therapy	Day 2–28	Client attends therapy sessions on a daily basis.	Day 28	Through self-expression, client has gained self-awareness and verbalizes positive attributes of self.
Additional assessments	Day 7	Compare specific measurements of client's body with client's perceived calculations. Clarify discrepancies.	Day 8–28	Discuss strengths and weaknesses. Client should strive to achieve self-acceptance.	Day 28	Client verbalizes acceptance of self, including "imperfections"
Medications	At physician's discretion	For associated symptoms: Antidepressant (e.g., SSRI) and/or Antianxiety (e.g., benzodiazepine)			Day 28	Discharge with medications as required.
Client education	Day 14–28	Discuss alternative coping strategies for dealing with feelings. Have client keep diary of feelings, particularly when thinking about food. Discuss action and side effects of medications.			Day 28	Client demonstrates adaptive coping strategies unrelated to eating behaviors for dealing with feelings. Client verbalizes understanding of need for and side effects of medications.

GLOSSARY

A

abreaction. "Remembering with feeling;" bringing into conscious awareness painful events that have been repressed, and reexperiencing the emotions that were associated with the events.

acquired immunodeficiency syndrome (**AIDS**). A condition in which the immune system becomes deficient in its efforts to prevent opportunistic infections, malignancies, and neurological disease. It is caused by the human immunodeficiency virus (HIV), which is passed from one individual to another through body fluids.

acupoints. In Chinese medicine, acupoints represent areas along the body that link pathways of healing energy.

acupressure. A technique in which the fingers, thumbs, palms, or elbows are used to apply pressure to certain points along the body. This pressure is thought to dissolve any obstructions in the flow of healing energy and to restore the body to a healthier functioning.

acupuncture. A technique in which hair-thin, sterile, disposable, stainless-steel needles are inserted into points along the body to dissolve obstructions in the flow of healing energy and restore the body to a healthier functioning.

adaptation. Restoration of the body to homeostasis following a physiological and/or psychological response to stress.

ADC. See AIDS dementia complex.

adjustment disorder. A maladaptive reaction to an identifiable psychosocial stressor that occurs within 3 months after onset of the stressor. The individual shows impairment in social and occupational functioning, or exhibits symptoms that are in excess of a normal and expectable reaction to the stressor.

advance directives. A document, usually a living will or durable power of attorney for healthcare, which allows an individual to provide directions about his or her future medical care.

affect. The behavioral expression of emotion; may be appropriate (congruent with the situation); inappropriate (incongruent with the situation); constricted or blunted (diminished range and intensity); or flat (absence of emotional expression).

aggression. Harsh physical or verbal actions intended (consciously or unconsciously) to harm or injure another.

aggressiveness. Behavior that defends an individual's own basic rights by violating the basic rights of others (as contrasted with assertiveness).

agoraphobia. The fear of being in places or situations from which escape might be difficult (or embarrassing) or in which help might not be available in the event of a panic attack.

agranulocytosis. Extremely low levels of white blood cells. Symptoms include sore throat, fever, and malaise. This may be a side effect of long-term therapy with some antipsychotic medications.

AIDS. See acquired immunodeficiency syndrome (AIDS).

AIDS dementia complex (**ADC**). A neuropathological syndrome, possibly caused by chronic HIV encephalitis and myelitis, and manifested by cognitive, behavioral, and motor symptoms that become more severe with progression of the disease.

akathesia. Restlessness; an urgent need for movement. A type of extrapyramidal side effect associated with some antipsychotic medications.

akinesia. Muscular weakness; or a loss or partial loss of muscle movement; a type of extrapyramidal side effect associated with some antipsychotic medications.

Alcoholics Anonymous (**AA**). A major self-help organization for the treatment of alcoholism. It is based on a 12-step program to help members attain and maintain sobriety. Once individuals have achieved sobriety, they in turn are expected to help other alcoholic persons.

allopathic medicine. Traditional medicine. The type traditionally, and currently, practiced in the United States and taught in U.S. medical schools.

alternative medicine. Practices that differ from usual traditional (allopathic) medicine.

altruism. One curative factor of group therapy (identified by Yalom) in which individuals gain self-esteem through mutual sharing and concern. Providing assistance and support to others creates a positive self-image and promotes self-growth.

altruistic suicide. Suicide based on behavior of a group to which an individual is excessively integrated.

amenorrhea. Cessation of the menses; may be a side effect of some antipsychotic medications.

amnesia. An inability to recall important personal information that is too extensive to be explained by ordinary forgetfulness.

amnesia, continuous. The inability to recall events occurring after a specific time up to and including the present.

amnesia, generalized. The inability to recall anything that has happened during the individual's entire lifetime.

amnesia, localized. The inability to recall all incidents associated with a traumatic event for a specific time following the event (usually a few hours to a few days).

amnesia, selective. The inability to recall only certain incidents associated with a traumatic event for a specific time following the event.

amnesia, systematized. The inability to remember events that relate to a specific category of information, such as one's family, a particular person, or an event.

anger. An emotional response to one's perception of a situation. Anger has both positive and negative functions.

anhedonia. The inability to experience or even imagine any pleasant emotion.

anomic suicide. Suicide that occurs in response to changes that occur in an individual's life that disrupt cohesiveness from a group and cause that person to feel without support from the formerly cohesive group.

anorexia. Loss of appetite.

anorexigenics. Drugs that suppress appetite.

anorgasmia. Inability to achieve orgasm.

anosmia. Inability to smell.

anticipatory grief. A subjective state of emotional, physical, and social responses to an anticipated loss of a valued entity. The grief response is repeated once the loss actually occurs, but it may not be as intense as it might have been if anticipatory grieving has not occurred.

antisocial personality disorder. A pattern of socially irresponsible, exploitative, and guiltless behavior, evident in the tendency to fail to conform to the law, develop stable relationships, or sustain consistent employment; exploitation and manipulation of others for personal gain is common.

anxiety. Vague diffuse apprehension that is associated with feelings of uncertainty and helplessness.

aphasia. Inability to communicate through speech, writing, or signs, caused by dysfunction of brain centers.

aphonia. Inability to speak.

apraxia. Inability to carry out motor activities despite intact motor function.

ascites. Excessive accumulation of serous fluid in the abdominal cavity, occurring in response to portal hypertension caused by cirrhosis of the liver.

assault. An act that results in a person's genuine fear and apprehension that he or she will be touched without consent. Nurses may be guilty of assault for threatening to place an individual in restraints against his or her will.

assertiveness. Behavior that enables individuals to act in their own best interests, to stand up for themselves without undue anxiety, to express their honest feelings comfortably, or to exercise their own rights without denying those of others.

associative looseness. Sometimes called loose associations, a thinking process characterized by speech in which ideas shift from one unrelated subject to another. The indivdual is unaware that the topics are unconnected.

ataxia. Muscular incoordination.

attachment theory. The hypothesis that individuals who maintain close relationships with others into old age are more likely to remain independent and less likely to be institutionalized than those who do not.

attitude. A frame of reference around which an individual organizes knowledge about his or her world. It includes an emotional element and can have a positive or negative connotation.

autism. A focus inward on a fantasy world and distorting or excluding the external environment; common in schizophrenia.

autistic disorder. The withdrawal of an infant or child into the self and into a fantasy world of his or her own creation. There is marked impairment in interpersonal functioning and communication and in imaginative play. Activities and interests are restricted and may be considered somewhat bizarre.

autocratic. A leadership style in which the leader makes all decisions for the group. Productivity is very high with this type of leadership, but morale is often low because of the lack of member input and creativity.

autoimmunity. A condition in which the body produces a disordered immunological response against itself. In this situation, the body fails to differentiate between what is normal and what is a foreign substance. When this occurs, the body produces antibodies against normal parts of the body to such an extent as to cause tissue injury.

autonomy. Independence; self-governance. An ethical principle that emphasizes the status of persons as autonomous moral agents whose right to determine their destinies should always be respected.

aversive stimulus. A stimulus that follows a behavioral response and decreases the probability that the behavior will recur; also called punishment.

axon. The cellular process of a neuron that carries impulses away from the cell body.

azidothymidine (**AZT**). An antiviral agent used to treat individuals with AIDS.

B

battering. A pattern of repeated physical assault, usually of a woman by her spouse or intimate partner. Men are also battered, although this occurs much less frequently.

battery. The unconsented touching of another person. Nurses may be charged with battery should they participate in the treatment of a client without his or her consent and outside of an emergency.

behavior modification. A treatment modality aimed at changing undesirable behaviors, using a system of reinforcement to bring about the modifications desired.

belief. A belief is an idea that one holds to be true. It can be rational, irrational, taken on faith, or a stereotypical idea.

beneficence. An ethical principle that refers to one's duty to benefit or promote the good of others.

bereavement overload. An accumulation of grief that occurs when an individual experiences many losses over a short period and is unable to resolve one before another is experienced. This phenomenon is common among the elderly.

binge and purge. A syndrome associated with eating disorders, especially bulimia, in which an individual consumes thousands of calories of food at one sitting, and then purges using laxatives or self-induced vomiting.

bioethics. The term used with ethical principles that refer to concepts within the scope of medicine, nursing, and allied health.

biofeedback. The use of instrumentation to become aware of processes in the body that usually go unnoticed and to bring them under voluntary control (e.g., the blood pressure or pulse); used as a method of stress reduction.

bipolar disorder. Characterized by mood swings from profound depression to extreme euphoria (mania), with intervening periods of normalcy. Psychotic symptoms may or may not be present.

body image. One's perception of his or her own body. It may also be how one believes others perceive his or her body. (See also physical self.)

borderline personality disorder. A disorder characterized by a pattern of intense and chaotic relationships, with affective instability, fluctuating and extreme attitudes regarding other people, impulsivity, direct and indirect self-destructive behavior, and lack of a clear or certain sense of identity, life plan, or values.

boundaries. The level of participation and interaction between individuals and between subsystems. Boundaries denote physical and psychological space individuals identify as their own. They are sometimes referred to as limits. Boundaries are appropriate when they permit appropriate contact with others and prevent excessive interference. Boundaries may be clearly defined (healthy) or rigid or diffuse (unhealthy).

C

cachexia. A state of ill health, malnutrition, and wasting; extreme emaciation.

cannabis. The dried flowering tops of the hemp plant. It produces euphoric effects when ingested or smoked and is commonly used in the form of marijuana or hashish.

carcinogen. Any substance or agent that produces or

increases the risk of developing cancer in humans or lower animals.

case management. A healthcare delivery process, the goals of which are to provide quality healthcare, decrease fragmentation, enhance the client's quality of life, and contain costs. A case manager coordinates the client's care from admission to discharge and sometimes following discharge. Critical pathways of care are the tools used for the provision of care in a case management system.

case manager. The individual responsible for negotiating with multiple healthcare providers to obtain a variety of services for a client.

catatonia. A type of schizophrenia that is typified by stupor or excitement; stupor characterized by extreme psychomotor retardation, mutism, negativism, and posturing, excitement by psychomotor agitation, in which the movements are frenzied and purposeless.

catharsis. One curative factor of group therapy (identified by Yalom), in which members in a group can express both positive and negative feelings in a nonthreatening atmosphere.

cell body. The part of the neuron that contains the nucleus and is essential for the continued life of the neuron.

chi. In Chinese medicine, the healing energy that flows through pathways in the body called meridians.

chiropractic medicine. A system of alternative medicine based on the premise that the relationship between structure and function in the human body is a significant health factor and that such relationships between the spinal column and the nervous system are important because the normal transmission and expression of nerve energy are essential to the restoration and maintenance of health.

child sexual abuse. Any sexual act, such as indecent exposure or improper touching to penetration (sexual intercourse) that is carried out with a child.

Christian ethics. The ethical philosophy that states one should treat others as moral equals, and recognize the equality of other persons by permitting them to act as we do when they occupy a position similar to ours; sometimes referred to as "the ethic of the golden rule."

circadian rhythm. A 24-hour biological rhythm controlled by a "pacemaker" in the brain that sends messages to other systems in the body. Circadian rhythm influences various regulatory functions, including the sleep-wake cycle, body temperature regulation, patterns of activity such as eating and drinking, and hormonal and neurotransmitter secretion.

circumstantiality. In speaking, the delay of an individual to reach the point of a communication, owing to unnecessary and tedious details.

civil law. Law that protects the private and property rights of individuals and businesses.

clang associations. A pattern of speech in which the choice of words is governed by sounds. Clang associations often take the form of rhyming.

classical conditioning. A type of learning that occurs when an unconditioned stimulus (UCS) that produces an unconditioned response (UCR) is paired with a conditioned stimulus (CS), until the CS alone produces the same response, which is then called a conditioned response (CR). Pavlov's example: food (i.e., UCS) causes salivation (i.e., UCR); ringing bell (i.e., CS) with food (i.e., UCS) causes salivation (i.e., UCR), ringing bell alone (i.e., CS) causes salivation (i.e., CR).

codependency. An exaggerated dependent pattern of learned behaviors, beliefs, and feelings that make life painful. It is a dependence on people and things outside the self, along with neglect of the self to the point of having little self-identity.

cognition. Mental operations that relate to logic, awareness, intellect, memory, language, and reasoning powers.

cognitive development. A series of stages described by Piaget through which individuals progress, demonstrating at each successive stage a higher level of logical organization than at each previous stage.

cognitive maturity. The capability to perform all mental operations needed for adulthood.

cognitive therapy. A type of therapy in which the individual is taught to control thought distortions that are considered to be a factor in the development and maintenance of emotional disorders.

common law. Laws that are derived from decisions made in previous cases.

community. A group of people living close to and depending to some extent on each other.

compensation. Covering up a real or perceived weakness by emphasizing a trait one considers more desirable.

complementary medicine. Practices that differ from usual traditional (allopathic) medicine, but may in fact supplement it in a positive way.

compounded rape reaction. Symptoms that are in addition to the typical rape response of physical complaints, rage, humiliation, fear, and sleep disturbances. They include depression and suicide, substance abuse, and even psychotic behaviors.

concrete thinking. Thought processes that are focused on specifics rather than on generalities and immediate issues rather than eventual outcomes. Individuals who are experiencing concrete thinking are unable to comprehend abstract terminology.

confidentiality. The right of an individual to the assurance that his or her case will not be discussed outside the boundaries of the healthcare team.

contextual stimulus. Conditions present in the environment that support a focal stimulus and influence a threat to self-esteem.

contingency contracting. A written contract between individuals used to modify behavior. Benefits and consequences for fulfilling the terms of the contract are delineated.

controlled response pattern. The response to rape in which feelings are masked or hidden, and a calm, composed, or subdued affect is seen.

counselor. One who listens as the client reviews feelings related to difficulties he or she is experiencing in any aspect of life; one of the nursing roles identified by H. Peplau.

covert sensitization. An aversion technique used to modify behavior that relies on the individual's imagination to produce unpleasant symptoms. When the individual is about to succumb to undesirable behavior, he or she visualizes something that is offensive or even nauseating in an effort to block the behavior.

criminal law. Law that provides protection from conduct deemed injurious to the public welfare. It provides for punishment of those found to have engaged in such conduct.

crisis. Psychological disequilibrium in a person who confronts a hazardous circumstance that constitutes an important problem, which for the time he or she can neither escape nor solve with usual problem-solving resources.

crisis intervention. An emergency type of assistance in which the intervener becomes a part of the individual's life situation. The focus is to provide guidance and support to help mobilize the resources needed to resolve the crisis and restore or generate an improvement in previous level of functioning. Usually lasts no longer than 6 to 8 weeks.

critical pathways of care. An abbreviated plan of care that provides outcome-based guidelines for goal achievement within a designated length of time.

culture. A particular society's entire way of living, encompassing shared patterns of belief, feeling, and knowledge that guide people's conduct and are passed down from generation to generation.

curandera. A female folk healer in the Latino culture.

curandero. A male folk healer in the Latino culture.

cycle of battering. Three phases of predictable behaviors that are repeated over time in a relationship between a batterer and a victim: tension-building phase; the acute battering incident; and the calm, loving, respite (honeymoon) phase.

cyclothymia. A chronic mood disturbance involving numerous episodes of hypomania and depressed mood, of insufficient severity or duration to meet the criteria for bipolar disorder.

D

date rape. A situation in which the rapist is known to the victim. This may occur during dating or with acquaintances or schoolmates.

defamation of character. An individual may be liable for defamation of character by sharing with others information about a person that is detrimental to his or her reputation.

deinstitutionalization. The removal of mentally ill individuals from institutions and the subsequent plan to provide care for these individuals in the community setting.

delayed grief. Also called *inhibited grief.* The absence of evidence of grief when it ordinarily would be expected.

delirium. A state of mental confusion and excitement characterized by disorientation for time and place, often with hallucinations, incoherent speech, and a continual state of aimless physical activity.

delusions. False personal beliefs, not consistent with a person's intelligence or cultural background. The individual continues to have the belief in spite of obvious proof that it is false and/or irrational.

dementia. Global impairment of cognitive functioning that is progressive and interferes with social and occupational abilities.

dendrites. The cellular processes of a neuron that carries impulses toward the cell body.

denial. Refusal to acknowledge the existence of a real situation and/or the feelings associated with it.

density. The number of people in a given environmental space, influencing interpersonal interaction.

depersonalization. An alteration in the perception or experience of the self so that the feeling of one's own reality is temporarily lost.

derealization. An alteration in the perception or

experience of the external world so that it seems strange or unreal.

detoxification. The process of withdrawal from a substance to which one has become dependent.

diagnostically related groups (DRGs). A system used to determine prospective payment rates for reimbursement of hospital care based on the client's diagnosis.

Diagnostic and Statistical Manual of Mental Disorders, 4th edition, Text Revision (DSM-IV-TR). Standard nomenclature of emotional illness published by the American Psychiatric Association (APA) and used by all healthcare practitioners. It classifies mental illness and presents guidelines and diagnostic criteria for various mental disorders.

directed association. A technique used to help clients bring into consciousness events that have been repressed. Specific thoughts are guided and directed by the psychoanalyst.

discriminative stimulus. A stimulus that precedes a behavioral response and predicts that a particular reinforcement will occur. Individuals learn to discriminate between various stimuli that will produce the responses they desire.

disengagement. In family theory, disengagement refers to extreme separateness among family members. It is promoted by rigid boundaries or lack of communication among family members.

disengagement theory. The hypothesis that there is a process of mutual withdrawal of aging persons and society from each other that is correlated with successful aging. This theory has been challenged by many investigators.

displacement. Feelings are transferred from one target to another that is considered less threatening or neutral.

disulfiram. A drug that is administered to individuals who abuse alcohol as a deterrent to drinking. Ingestion of alcohol when disulfiram is in the body results in a syndrome of symptoms that can produce a great deal of discomfort, and can even result in death if the blood alcohol level is high.

double-bind communication. Communication described as contradictory that places an individual in a "double bind." It occurs when a statement is made and succeeded by a contradictory statement or when a statement is made accompanied by nonverbal expression that is inconsistent with the verbal communication.

dyspareunia. Pain during sexual intercourse.

dysthymia. A depressive neurosis. The symptoms are similar to, if somewhat milder than, those ascribed to major depression. There is no loss of contact with reality.

dystonia. Involuntary muscular movements (spasms) of the face, arms, legs, and neck; may occur as an extrapyramidal side effect of some antipsychotic medications.

E

echolalia. The parrot-like repetition, by an individual with loose ego boundaries, of the words spoken by another.

echopraxia. An individual with loose ego boundaries attempting to identify with another person by imitating movements that the other person makes.

ego. One of the three elements of the personality identified by Freud as the rational self or "reality principle." The ego seeks to maintain harmony between the external world, the id, and the superego.

ego defense mechanisms. Strategies employed by the ego for protection in the face of threat to biological or psychological integrity. (See individual defense mechanisms.)

egoistic suicide. The response of an individual who feels separate and apart from the mainstream of society.

electroconvulsive therapy (ECT). A type of somatic treatment in which electric current is applied to the brain through electrodes placed on the temples. A grand mal seizure produces the desired effect. This is used with severely depressed patients refractory to antidepressant medications.

emaciated. The state of being excessively thin or physically wasted.

emotional injury of a child. A pattern of behavior on the part of the parent or caretaker that results in serious impairment of the child's social, emotional, or intellectual functioning.

emotional neglect of a child. A chronic failure by the parent or caretaker to provide the child with the hope, love, and support necessary for the development of a sound, healthy personality.

empathy. The ability to see beyond outward behavior and sense accurately another's inner experiencing. With empathy, one can accurately perceive and understand the meaning and relevance in the thoughts and feelings of another.

enmeshment. Exaggerated connectedness among family members. It occurs in response to diffuse boundaries in which there is overinvestment, overinvolvement, and lack of differentiation between individuals or subsystems.

esophageal varices. Veins in the esophagus become distended because of excessive pressure from defective blood flow through a cirrhotic liver.

essential hypertension. Persistent elevation of blood pressure for which there is no apparent cause or associated underlying disease.

ethical dilemma. A situation that arises when, based on moral considerations, an appeal can be made for taking each of two opposing courses of action.

ethical egoism. An ethical theory espousing that what is "right" and "good" is what is best for the individual making the decision.

ethics. A branch of philosophy dealing with values related to human conduct, to the rightness and wrongness of certain actions, and to the goodness and badness of the motives and ends of such actions.

ethnicity. The concept of people identifying with each other because of a shared heritage.

exhibitionism. A paraphilic disorder characterized by a recurrent urge to expose one's genitals to a stranger.

expressed response pattern. Pattern of behavior in which the victim of rape expresses feelings of fear, anger, and anxiety through such behavior as crying, sobbing, smiling, restlessness, and tenseness; in contrast to the rape victim who withholds feelings in the controlled response pattern.

extinction. The gradual decrease in frequency or disappearance of a response when the positive reinforcement is withheld.

extrapyramidal symptoms (EPS). A variety of responses that originate outside the pyramidal tracts and in the basal ganglion of the brain. Symptoms may include tremors, chorea, dystonia, akinesia, akathisia, and others. May occur as a side effect of some antipsychotic medications.

F

false imprisonment. The deliberate and unauthorized confinement of a person within fixed limits by the use of threat or force. A nurse may be charged with false imprisonment by placing a patient in restraints against his or her will in a non-emergency situation.

family structure. A family system in which the structure is founded on a set of invisible principles that influence the interaction among family members. These principles are established over time and become the "laws" that govern the conduct of various family members.

family system. A system in which the parts of the whole may be the marital dyad, parent-child dyad, or sibling groups. Each of these subsystems is further divided into subsystems of individuals.

family therapy. A type of therapy in which the focus is on relationships within the family. The family is viewed as a system in which the members are interdependent, and a change in one creates change in all.

fetishism. A paraphilic disorder characterized by recurrent sexual urges and sexually arousing fantasies involving the use of non-living objects.

fight or flight. A syndrome of physical symptoms that result from an individual's real or perceived perception that harm or danger is imminent.

flexible boundary. A personal boundary is flexible when, because of unusual circumstances, individuals can alter limits that they have set for themselves. Flexible boundaries are healthy boundaries.

flooding. Sometimes called implosive therapy, this technique is used to desensitize individuals to phobic stimuli. The individual is "flooded" with a continuous presentation (usually through mental imagery) of the phobic stimulus until it no longer elicits anxiety.

focus charting.® A type of documentation that follows a data, action, and response (DAR) format. The main perspective is a client "focus," which can be a nursing diagnosis, a client's concern, change in status, or significant event in the client's therapy. The focus cannot be a medical diagnosis.

folk medicine. A system of healthcare within various cultures that is provided by a local practitioner, not professionally trained, but who uses techniques specific to that culture in the art of healing.

free association. A technique used to help individuals bring to consciousness material that has been repressed. The individual is encouraged to verbalize whatever comes into his or her mind, drifting naturally from one thought to another.

frotteurism. A paraphilic disorder characterized by the recurrent preoccupation with intense sexual urges or fantasies involving touching or rubbing against a nonconsenting person.

fugue. A sudden unexpected travel away from home or customary work locale with the assumption of a new identity and an inability to recall one's previous identity; usually occurring in response to severe psychosocial stress.

G

gains. The reinforcements an individual receives for somaticizing.

gains, primary. The receipt of positive reinforcement

for somaticizing by being able to avoid difficult situations because of physical complaint.

gains, secondary. The receipt of positive reinforcement for somaticizing through added attention, sympathy, and nurturing.

gains, tertiary. The receipt of positive reinforcement for somaticizing by causing the focus of the family to switch to him or her and away from conflict that may be occurring within the family.

Gamblers Anonymous (GA). An organization of inspirational group therapy, modeled after Alcoholics Anonymous (AA), for individuals who desire to, but cannot, stop gambling.

gender identity disorder. A sense of discomfort associated with an incongruence between biologically assigned gender and subjectively experienced gender.

generalized anxiety disorder. A disorder characterized by chronic (at least 6 months), unrealistic, and excessive anxiety and worry.

genogram. A graphic representation of a family system. It may cover several generations. Emphasis is on family roles and emotional relatedness among members. Genograms facilitate recognition of areas requiring change.

genotype. The total set of genes present in an individual at the time of conception, and coded in the DNA.

genuineness. The ability to be open, honest, and "real" in interactions with others; the awareness of what one is experiencing internally and the ability to project the quality of this inner experiencing in a relationship.

geriatrics. The branch of clinical medicine specializing in the care of the elderly and concerned with the problems of aging.

gerontology. The study of normal aging.

geropsychiatry. The branch of clinical medicine specializing in psychopathology of the elderly.

gonorrhea. A sexually transmitted disease caused by the bacterium *N. gonorrhoeae* and resulting in inflammation of the genital mucosa. Treatment is with antibiotics, particularly penicillin. Serious complications occur if the disease is left untreated.

"granny-bashing." Media-generated term for abuse of the elderly.

"granny-dumping." Media-generated term for abandoning elderly individuals at emergency departments, nursing homes, or other facilities—literally, leaving them in the hands of others when the strain of caregiving becomes intolerable.

grief. A subjective state of emotional, physical, and social responses to the real or perceived loss of a valued entity. Change and failure can also be perceived as losses. The grief response consists of a set of relatively predictable behaviors that describe the subjective state that accompanies mourning.

grief, exaggerated. A reaction in which all of the symptoms associated with normal grieving are exaggerated out of proportion. Pathological depression is a type of exaggerated grief.

grief, inhibited. The absence of evidence of grief when it ordinarily would be expected.

grief, prolonged. Grief characterized by lack of resumption of normal activities of daily living within 4 to 8 weeks of a loss.

group therapy. A therapy group, founded in a specific theoretical framework, led by a person with an advanced degree in psychology, social work, nursing, or medicine. The goal is to encourage improvement in interpersonal functioning.

gynecomastia. Enlargement of the breasts in men; may be a side effect of some antipsychotic medications.

H

hallucinations. False sensory perceptions not associated with real external stimuli. Hallucinations may involve any of the five senses.

hepatic encephalopathy. A brain disorder resulting from the inability of the cirrhotic liver to convert ammonia to urea for excretion. The continued rise in serum ammonia results in progressively impaired mental functioning, apathy, euphoria or depression, sleep disturbances, increasing confusion, and progression to coma and eventual death.

histrionic personality disorder. Conscious or unconscious overly dramatic behavior used for drawing attention to oneself.

HIV wasting syndrome. An absence of concurrent illness other than HIV infection, and presence of the following: fever, weakness, weight loss, and chronic diarrhea.

homosexuality. A sexual preference for persons of the same gender.

hospice. A program that provides palliative and supportive care to meet the special needs arising out of the physical, psychosocial, spiritual, social, and economic stresses that are experienced during the final stages of illness and during bereavement.

human immunodeficiency virus (HIV). The virus that is the etiological agent that produces the immunosuppression resulting in AIDS.

humors. The four body fluids described by Hippocrates: blood, black bile, yellow bile, and phlegm. Hippocrates associated insanity and mental illness with these four fluids.

hypersomnia. Excessive sleepiness or seeking excessive amounts of sleep.

hypertensive crisis. A potentially life-threatening syndrome that results when an individual taking MAOIs eats a product high in tyramine. Symptoms include severe occipital headache, palpitations, nausea and vomiting, nuchal rigidity, fever, sweating, marked increase in blood pressure, chest pain, and coma. Foods with tyramine include aged cheeses or other aged, overripe, and fermented foods; broad beans; pickled herring; beef or chicken liver; preserved meats; beer and wine; yeast products; chocolate; caffeinated drinks; canned figs; sour cream; yogurt; soy sauce; and some over-the-counter cold medications and diet pills.

hypnosis. A treatment for disorders brought on by repressed anxiety. The individual is directed into a state of subconsciousness and assisted, through suggestions, to recall certain events that he or she cannot recall when conscious.

hypochondriasis. The unrealistic preoccupation with fear of having a serious illness.

hypomania. A mind form of mania. Symptoms are excessive hyperactivity, but not severe enough to cause marked impairment in social or occupational functioning or to require hospitalization.

hysteria. A polysymptomatic disorder characterized by recurrent, multiple somatic complaints often described dramatically.

I

id. One of the three components of the personality identified by Freud as the "pleasure principle." The id is the locus of instinctual drives; is present at birth; and compels the infant to satisfy needs and seek immediate gratification.

identification. An attempt to increase self-worth by acquiring certain attributes and characteristics of an individual one admires.

illusion. A misperception of a real external stimulus.

implosion therapy. See flooding.

incest. Sexual exploitation of a child under 18 years of age by a relative or non-relative who holds a position of trust in the family.

informed consent. Permission granted to a physician by a client to perform a therapeutic procedure, before which information about the procedure has been presented to the client with adequate time given for consideration about the pros and cons.

insomnia. Difficulty initiating or maintaining sleep.

insulin coma therapy. The induction of a hypoglycemic coma aimed at alleviating psychotic symptoms; a dangerous procedure, questionably effective, no longer used in psychiatry.

integration. The process used with individuals with dissociative identity disorder in an effort to bring all the personalities together into one; usually achieved through hypnosis.

intellectualization. An attempt to avoid expressing actual emotions associated with a stressful situation by using the intellectual processes of logic, reasoning, and analysis.

interdisciplinary care. A concept of providing care for a client in which members of various disciplines work together with common goals and shared responsibilities for meeting those goals.

intimate distance. The closest distance individuals will allow between themselves and others. In the United States, this distance is 0 to 18 inches.

introjection. The beliefs and values of another individual are internalized and symbolically become a part of the self to the extent that the feeling of separateness or distinctness is lost.

isolation. The separation of a thought or a memory from the feeling tone or emotions associated with it (sometimes called emotional isolation).

J

justice. An ethical principle reflecting that all individuals should be treated equally and fairly.

K

Kantianism. The ethical principle espousing that decisions should be made and actions taken out of a sense of duty.

Kaposi's sarcoma. Malignant areas of cell proliferation initially in the skin and eventually in other body sites; thought to be related to the immunocompromised state that accompanies AIDS.

kleptomania. A recurrent failure to resist impulses to steal objects not needed for personal use or monetary value.

Korsakoff's psychosis. A syndrome of confusion, loss of recent memory, and confabulation in alcoholics, caused by a deficiency of thiamine. It often occurs together with Wernicke's encephalopathy and may be termed Wernicke-Korsakoff's syndrome.

L

la belle indifference. A symptom of conversion disorder in which there is a relative lack of concern that is out of keeping with the severity of the impairment.

laissez-faire. A leadership type in which the leader lets group members do as they please. There is no direction from the leader. Member productivity and morale may be low, owing to frustration from lack of direction.

lesbian. A female homosexual.

libel. An action with which an individual may be charged for sharing with another individual, in writing, information that is detrimental to someone's reputation.

libido. Freud's term for the psychic energy used to fulfill basic physiological needs or instinctual drives such as hunger, thirst, and sexuality.

limbic system. The part of the brain that is sometimes called the "emotional brain." It is associated with feelings of fear and anxiety; anger and aggression; love, joy, and hope; and with sexuality and social behavior.

long-term memory. Memory for remote events, or those that occurred many years ago. The type of memory that is preserved in the elderly individual.

loss. The experience of separation from something of personal importance.

luto. The word for mourning in the Mexican-American culture that is symbolized by wearing black, black and white, or dark clothing and by subdued behavior.

M

magical thinking. A primitive form of thinking in which an individual believes that thinking about a possible occurrence can make it happen.

maladaptation. A failure of the body to return to homeostasis following a physiological and/or psychological response to stress, disrupting the individual's integrity.

malpractice. The failure of one rendering professional services to exercise that amount of skill and learning commonly applied, under all the circumstances, in the community by the average, prudent, reputable member of the profession with the result of injury, loss, or damage to the recipient of those services or to those entitled to rely upon them.

managed care. A concept purposefully designed to control the balance between cost and quality of care. Examples of managed care are health maintenance organizations (HMOs) and preferred provider organizations (PPOs). The amount and type of healthcare that the individual receives is determined by the organization providing the managed care.

mania. A type of bipolar disorder in which the predominant mood is elevated, expansive, or irritable. Motor activity is frenzied and excessive. Psychotic features may or may not be present.

mania, delirious. A grave form of mania characterized by severe clouding of consciousness and representing an intensification of the symptoms associated with mania. The symptoms of delirious mania have become relatively rare since the availability of antipsychotic medications.

marital rape. Sexual violence directed at a marital partner against that person's will.

marital schism. A state of severe, chronic disequilibrium and discord within the marital dyad, with recurrent threats of separation.

marital skew. A marital relationship in which there is lack of equal partnership. One partner dominates the relationship and the other partner.

masochism. Sexual stimulation derived from being humiliated, beaten, bound, or otherwise made to suffer.

Medicaid. A system established by the federal government to provide medical care benefits for indigent Americans. Medicaid funds are matched by the states, and coverage varies significantly from state to state.

Medicare. A system established by the federal government to provide medical care benefits for elderly Americans.

meditation. A method of relaxation in which an individual sits in a quiet place and focuses total concentration on an object, word, or thought.

melancholia. A severe form of major depressive episode. Symptoms are exaggerated, and interest or pleasure in virtually all activities is lost.

menopause. The period marking the permanent cessation of menstrual activity; usually occurs at approximately 48 to 51 years of age.

mental health. The successful adaptation to stressors from the internal or external environment, evidenced by thoughts, feelings, and behaviors that are age-appropriate and congruent with local and cultural norms.

mental illness. Maladaptive responses to stressors from the internal or external environment, evidenced by thoughts, feelings, and behaviors that are incongruent with the local and cultural norms, and interfere with the individual's social, occupational, and/or physical functioning.

mental imagery. A method of stress reduction that employs the imagination. The individual focuses imagination on a scenario that is particularly relaxing to him or her (e.g., a scene on a quiet seashore, a mountain atmosphere, or floating through the air on a fluffy white cloud).

meridians. In Chinese medicine, pathways along the body in which the healing energy (chi) flows, and which are links between acupoints.

migraine personality. Personality characteristics that have been attributed to the migraine-prone person. The characteristics include perfectionistic, overly conscientious, somewhat inflexible, neat and tidy, compulsive, hard worker, intelligent, exacting, and places a very high premium on success, setting high (sometimes unrealistic) expectations on self and others.

milieu. French for "middle;" the English translation connotes "surroundings, or environment."

milieu therapy. Also called therapeutic community, or therapeutic environment, this type of therapy consists of a scientific structuring of the environment in order to effect behavioral changes and to improve the individual's psychological health and functioning.

mobile outreach units. Programs in which volunteers and paid professionals drive or walk around and seek out homeless individuals who need assistance with physical or psychological care.

modeling. Learning new behaviors by imitating the behaviors of others.

mood. An individual's sustained emotional tone, which significantly influences behavior, personality, and perception.

moral behavior. Conduct that results from serious critical thinking about how individuals ought to treat others; reflects respect for human life, freedom, justice, or confidentiality.

moral-ethical self. That aspect of the personal identity that functions as observer, standard setter, dreamer, comparer, and most of all evaluator of who the individual says he or she is. This component of the personal identity makes judgments that influence an individual's self-evaluation.

mourning. The psychological process (or stages) through which the individual passes on the way to successful adaptation to the loss of a valued object.

multidisciplinary care. A concept of providing care for a client in which individual disciplines provide specific services for the client without formal arrangement for interaction between the disciplines.

N

narcissistic personality disorder. A disorder characterized by an exaggerated sense of self-worth. These individuals lack empathy and are hypersensitive to the evaluation of others.

narcolepsy. A disorder in which the characteristic manifestation is sleep attacks. The individual cannot prevent falling asleep, even in the middle of a sentence or performing a task.

natural law theory. The ethical theory that has as its moral precept to "do good and avoid evil" at all costs. Natural law ethics are grounded in a concern for the human good, which is based on man's ability to live according to the dictates of reason.

negative reinforcement. Increasing the probability that a behavior will recur by removal of an undesirable reinforcing stimulus.

negativism. Strong resistance to suggestions or directions; exhibiting behaviors contrary to what is expected.

negligence. The failure to do something that a reasonable person, guided by those considerations, which ordinarily regulate human affairs, would do, or doing something that a prudent and reasonable person would not do.

neologism. New words that an individual invents that are meaningless to others but have symbolic meaning to the psychotic person.

neuroendocrinology. The study of hormones functioning within the neurological system.

neuroleptic. Antipsychotic medication used to prevent or control psychotic symptoms.

neuroleptic malignant syndrome (NMS). A rare but potentially fatal complication of treatment with neuroleptic drugs. Symptoms include severe muscle rigidity, high fever, tachycardia, fluctuations in blood pressure, diaphoresis, and rapid deterioration of mental status to stupor and coma.

neuron. A nerve cell; consists of a cell body, an axon, and dendrites.

neurotic disorder. A psychiatric disturbance, characterized by excessive anxiety and/or depression, disrupted bodily functions, unsatisfying interpersonal relationships, and behaviors that interfere with routine functioning. There is no loss of contact with reality.

neurotransmitter. A chemical that is stored in the axon terminals of the presynaptic neuron. An electrical impulse through the neuron stimulates the release of the neurotransmitter into the synaptic cleft, which in turn determines whether another electrical impulse is generated.

nonassertiveness. Individuals who are nonassertive (sometimes called passive) seek to please others at the expense of denying their own basic human rights.

nonmaleficence. The ethical principle that espouses abstaining from negative acts toward another, including acting carefully to avoid harm.

nursing diagnosis. A clinical judgment about individual, family, or community responses to actual and potential health problems/life processes. Nursing diagnoses provide the basis for selection of nursing interventions to achieve outcomes for which the nurse is accountable.

nursing process. A dynamic, systematic process by which nurses assess, diagnose, identify outcomes, plan, implement, and evaluate nursing care. It has been called "nursing's scientific methodology." Nursing process gives order and consistency to nursing intervention.

O

obesity. The state of having a body mass index of 30 or above.

object constancy. The phase in the separation/individuation process when the child learns to relate to objects in an effective, constant manner. A sense of separateness is established, and the child is able to internalize a sustained image of the loved object or person when out of sight.

obsessive-compulsive disorder. Recurrent thoughts or ideas (obsessions) that an individual is unable to put out of his or her mind, and actions that an individual is unable to refrain from performing (compulsions). The obsessions and compulsions are severe enough to interfere with social and occupational functioning.

oculogyric crisis. An attack of involuntary deviation and fixation of the eyeballs, usually in the upward position. It may last for several minutes or hours and may occur as an extrapyramidal side effect of some antipsychotic medications.

operant conditioning. The learning of a particular action or type of behavior that is followed by reinforcement.

opportunistic infection. Infections with any organism, but especially fungi and bacteria, that occur due to the opportunity afforded by the altered physiological state of the host. Opportunistic infections have long been a defining characteristic of AIDS.

orgasm. A peaking of sexual pleasure, with release of sexual tension and rhythmic contraction of the perineal muscles and pelvic reproductive organs.

osteoporosis. A reduction in the mass of bone per unit of volume, which interferes with the mechanical support function of bone. This process occurs because of demineralization of the bones, and is escalated in women about the time of menopause.

overt sensitization. A type of aversion therapy that produces unpleasant consequences for undesirable behavior. An example is the use of disulfiram therapy with alcoholics, which induces an undesirable physical response if the individual has consumed any alcohol.

P

palilalia. Repeating one's own sounds or words (a type of vocal tic associated with Tourette's disorder).

panic disorder. A disorder characterized by recurrent panic attacks, the onset of which are unpredictable, and manifested by intense apprehension, fear, or terror, often associated with feelings of impending doom, and accompanied by intense physical discomfort.

paradoxical intervention. In family therapy, "prescribing the symptom." The therapist requests that the family continue to engage in the behavior that they are trying to change. Tension is relieved, and the family is able to view more clearly the possible solutions to their problem.

paralanguage. The gestural component of the spoken word. It consists of pitch, tone, and loudness of spoken messages, the rate of speaking, expressively placed pauses, and emphasis assigned to certain words.

paranoia. A term that implies extreme suspiciousness. Paranoid schizophrenia is characterized by persecutory delusions and hallucinations of a threatening nature.

paraphilias. Repetitive behaviors or fantasies that involve non-human objects, real or simulated suffering or humiliation, or nonconsenting partners.

parasomnia. Unusual or undesirable behaviors that occur during sleep (e.g., nightmares, sleep terrors, and sleepwalking).

passive-aggressive behavior. Behavior that defends an individual's own basic rights by expressing resistance to social and occupational demands. Sometimes called indirect aggression, this behavior takes the form of sly, devious, and undermining actions that express the opposite of what they are really feeling.

pathological gambling. A failure to resist impulses to gamble and gambling behavior that compromises, disrupts, or damages personal, family, or vocational pursuits.

pedophilia. Recurrent urges and sexually arousing fantasies involving sexual activity with a prepubescent child.

peer assistance programs. A program established by the American Nurses Association to assist impaired nurses. The individuals who administer these efforts are nurse members of the state associations, as well as nurses who are in recovery themselves.

perseveration. Persistent repetition of the same word or idea in response to different questions.

persistent generalized lymphadenopathy (PGL). A condition common in HIV-infected individuals in whom there are lymph nodes greater than 1 cm in diameter at two extrainguinal sites persisting for 3 months or longer, not attributed to other causes, and not associated with other substantial constitutional symptoms.

personal distance. The distance between individuals who are having interactions of a personal nature, such as a close conversation. In the U.S. culture, personal distance is approximately 18 to 40 inches.

personal identity. An individual's self-perception that defines one's functions as observer, standard setter, and self-evaluator. It strives to maintain a stable self-image and relates to what the individual strives to become.

personal self. See personal identity.

personality. Deeply ingrained patterns of behavior, which include the way one relates to, perceives, and thinks about the environment and oneself.

pharmacoconvulsive therapy. The chemical induction of a convulsion used in the past for the reduction of psychotic symptoms, a type of therapy no longer used in psychiatry.

phencyclidine HCl. An anesthetic used in veterinary medicine; used illegally as a hallucinogen, referred to as PCP or angel dust.

phenotype. Characteristics of physical manifestations that identify a particular genotype. Examples of phenotypes include eye color, height, blood type, language, and hairstyle. Phenotypes may be genetic or acquired.

phobia. An irrational fear.

phobia, social. The fear of being humiliated in social situations.

phobia, specific. A persistent fear of a specific object or situation, other than the fear of being unable to escape from a situation (agoraphobia) or the fear of being humiliated in social situations (social phobia).

physical neglect of a child. The failure on the part of the parent or caregiver to provide for a child's basic needs, such as food, clothing, shelter, medical-dental care, and supervision.

physical self. A personal appraisal by an individual of his or her physical being and includes physical attributes, functioning, sexuality, wellness-illness state, and appearance.

PIE charting. More specifically called "APIE," this method of documentation has an assessment, problem, intervention, and evaluation (APIE) format and is a problem-oriented system used to document nursing process.

***Pneumocystis carinii* pneumonia (PCP)**. The most common life-threatening opportunistic infection seen in patients with AIDS. Symptoms include fever, exertional dyspnea, and nonproductive cough.

positive reinforcement. A reinforcement stimulus that increases the probability that the behavior will recur.

postpartum depression. Depression that occurs during the postpartum period. It may be related to hormonal changes, tryptophan metabolism, or alterations in membrane transport during the early postpartum period. Other predisposing factors may also be influential.

post-traumatic stress disorder (PTSD). A syndrome of symptoms that develop following a psychologically distressing event that is outside the range of usual human experience (e.g., rape, war). The individual is unable to put the experience out of his or her mind, has nightmares, flashbacks, and panic attacks.

posturing. The voluntary assumption of inappropriate or bizarre postures.

preassaultive tension state. Behaviors predictive of potential violence. They include excessive motor activity, tense posture, defiant affect, clenched teeth and fists, and other arguing, demanding, and threatening behaviors.

precipitating event. A stimulus arising from the internal or external environment that is perceived by an individual as taxing or exceeding his or her resources and endangering his or her well-being.

predisposing factors. A variety of elements that influence how an individual perceives and responds to a stressful event. Types of predisposing factors include genetic influences, past experiences, and existing conditions.

Premack principle. This principle states that a frequently occurring response (R1) can serve as a positive reinforcement for a response (R2) that occurs less frequently. For example, a girl may talk to friends on the phone (R2) only if she does her homework (R1).

premature ejaculation. Ejaculation that occurs with minimal sexual stimulation or before, upon, or shortly after penetration and before the person wishes it.

premenstrual dysphoric disorder. A disorder that is characterized by depressed mood, anxiety, mood swings, and decreased interest in activities during the week before menses and subsiding shortly after the onset of menstruation (*DSM-IV*, APA, 1994).

presenile. Pertaining to premature old age as judged by mental or physical condition. In presenile onset dementia, initial symptoms appear at age 65 or younger.

priapism. Prolonged painful penile erection; may occur as an adverse effect of some antidepressant medications, particularly trazodone.

primary prevention. Reduction of the incidence of mental disorders within the population by helping individuals to cope more effectively with stress and by trying to diminish stressors within the environment.

privileged communication. A doctrine, common to most states, that grants certain privileges under which they may refuse to reveal information about and communications with clients.

problem-oriented recording (POR). A system of documentation that follows a subjective, objective, assessment, plan, implementation, and evaluation (SOAPIE) format. It is based on a list of identified patient problems to which each entry is directed.

progressive relaxation. A method of deep muscle relaxation in which each muscle group is alternately tensed and relaxed in a systematic order with the person concentrating on the contrast of sensations experienced from tensing and relaxing.

projection. Attributing to another person feelings or impulses unacceptable to oneself.

prospective payment. The program of cost containment within the healthcare profession directed at setting forth preestablished amounts that would be reimbursed for specific diagnoses.

pseudocyesis. A condition in which an individual has nearly all the signs and symptoms of pregnancy but is not pregnant; a conversion reaction.

pseudodementia. Symptoms of depression that mimic those of dementia.

pseudohostility. A family interaction pattern characterized by a state of chronic conflict and alienation among family members. This relationship pattern allows family members to deny underlying fears of tenderness and intimacy.

pseudomutuality. A family interaction pattern characterized by a facade of mutual regard with the purpose of denying underlying fears of separation and hostility.

psychodrama. A specialized type of group therapy that employs a dramatic approach in which patients become "actors" in life situation scenarios. The goal is to resolve interpersonal conflicts in a less-threatening atmosphere than the real-life situation would present.

psychodynamic nursing. Being able to understand one's own behavior, to help others identify felt difficulties, and to apply principles of human relations to the problems that arise at all levels of experience.

psychoimmunology. The study of the implications of the immune system in psychiatry.

psychomotor retardation. Extreme slowdown of physical movements. Posture slumps; speech is slowed; digestion becomes sluggish. Common in severe depression.

psychophysiological. Referring to psychological factors contributing to the initiation or exacerbation of a physical condition. Either a demonstrable organic pathology or a known pathophysiological process is involved.

psychosomatic. See psychophysiological.

psychotic disorder. A serious psychiatric disorder in which there is a gross disorganization of the personality, a marked disturbance in reality testing, and the impairment of interpersonal functioning and relationship to the external world.

public distance. Appropriate interactional distance for speaking in public or yelling to someone some distance away. U.S. culture defines this distance as 12 feet or more.

pyromania. An inability to resist the impulse to set fires.

R

rape. The expression of power and dominance by means of sexual violence, most commonly by men over women, although men may also be rape victims. Rape is considered an act of aggression, not of passion.

rapport. The development between two people in a relationship of special feelings based on mutual acceptance, warmth, friendliness, common interest, a sense of trust, and a nonjudgmental attitude.

rationalization. Attempting to make excuses or formulate logical reasons to justify unacceptable feelings or behaviors.

reaction formation. Preventing unacceptable or undesirable thoughts or behaviors from being expressed by exaggerating opposite thoughts or types of behaviors.

receptor sites. Molecules that are situated on the cell membrane of the postsynaptic neuron that will accept only molecules with a complementary shape. These complementary molecules are specific to certain neurotransmitters that determine whether an electrical impulse will be excited or inhibited.

reciprocal inhibition. Also called counterconditioning, this technique serves to decrease or eliminate a behavior by introducing a more adaptive behavior, but one that is incompatible with the unacceptable behavior (e.g., introducing relaxation techniques to an anxious person; relaxation and anxiety are incompatible behaviors).

reframing. Changing the conceptual or emotional setting or viewpoint in relation to which a situation is experienced and placing it in another frame that fits the "facts" of the same concrete situation equally well or even better, and thereby changing its entire meaning. The behavior may not actually change, but the consequences of the behavior may change because of a change in the meaning attached to the behavior.

regression. A retreat to an earlier level of development and the comfort measures associated with that level of functioning.

religiosity. Excessive demonstration of or obsession with religious ideas and behavior; common in schizophrenia.

reminiscence therapy. A process of life review by elderly individuals that promotes self-esteem and provides assistance in working through unresolved conflicts from the past.

repression. The involuntary blocking of unpleasant feelings and experiences from one's awareness.

residual stimuli. Certain beliefs, attitudes, experiences, or traits that may contribute to an individual's low self-esteem.

retarded ejaculation. Delayed or absent ejaculation, even though the man has a firm erection and has had more than adequate stimulation.

retrograde ejaculation. Ejaculation of the seminal fluid backwards into the bladder; may occur as a side effect of antipsychotic medications.

right. That which an individual is entitled (by ethical or moral standards) to have, or to do, or to receive from others within the limits of the law.

rigid boundaries. A person with rigid boundaries is "closed" and difficult to bond with. Such a person has a narrow perspective on life, sees things one way, and cannot discuss matters that lie outside his or her perspective.

ritualistic behavior. Purposeless activities that an individual performs repeatedly in an effort to decrease anxiety (e.g., hand washing); common in obsessive-compulsive disorder.

S

sadism. Recurrent urges and sexually arousing fantasies involving acts (real, not simulated) in which the psychological or physical suffering (including humiliation) of the victim is sexually exciting.

safe house or shelter. An establishment set up by many cities to provide protection for battered women and their children.

scapegoating. Occurs when hostility exists in a marriage dyad and an innocent third person (usually a child) becomes the target of blame for the problem.

schizoid personality disorder. A profound defect in the ability to form personal relationships or to respond to others in any meaningful, emotional way.

schizotypal personality disorder. A disorder characterized by odd and eccentric behavior, not decompensating to the level of schizophrenia.

secondary prevention. Healthcare that is directed at reduction of the prevalence of psychiatric illness by shortening the course (duration) of the illness. This is accomplished through early identification of problems and prompt initiation of treatment.

self-concept. The composite of beliefs and feelings that one holds about oneself at a given time, formed from perceptions of others' reactions. The self-concept consists of the physical self, or body image; the personal self or identity; and the self-esteem.

self-consistency. The component of the personal identity that strives to maintain a stable self-image.

self-esteem. The amount of regard or respect that individuals have for themselves. It is a measure of worth that they place on their abilities and judgments.

self-expectancy. The component of the personal identity that is the individual's perception of what he or she wants to be, to do, or to become.

self-ideal. See self-expectancy.

senile. Pertaining to old age and the mental or physical weakness with which it is sometimes associated. In senile-onset dementia, the first symptoms appear after age 65.

sensate focus. A therapeutic technique used to treat individuals and couples with sexual dysfunction. The technique involves touching and being touched by another and focusing attention on the physical sensations encountered thereby. Clients gradually move through various levels of sensate focus that progress from nongenital touching to touching that includes the breasts and genitals; touching done in a simultaneous, mutual format rather than by one person at a time; and touching that extends to and allows eventually for the possibility of intercourse.

seroconversion. The development of evidence of antibody response to a disease or vaccine. The time at which antibodies may be detected in the blood.

sexual exploitation of a child. The inducement or coercion of a child into engaging in sexually explicit conduct for promoting any performance (e.g., child pornography).

shaman. The Native American "medicine man" or folk healer.

shaping. In learning, one shapes the behavior of another by giving reinforcements for increasingly closer approximations to the desired behavior.

shelters. A variety of places designed to help the homeless, ranging from converted warehouses that provide cots or floor space on which to sleep overnight to significant operations that provide a multitude of social and healthcare services.

"ship of fools." The term given during the Middle Ages to sailing boats filled with severely mentally ill people that were sent out to sea with little guidance and in search of their lost rationality.

shiva. In the Jewish culture, following a death, the 7-day period beginning with the burial is called *shiva.*

short-term memory. The ability to remember events that occurred very recently. This ability deteriorates with age.

silent rape reaction. The response of a rape victim in which he or she tells no one about the assault.

slander. An action with which an individual may be charged for orally sharing information that is detrimental to a person's reputation.

social distance. The distance considered acceptable in interactions with strangers or acquaintances, such as at a cocktail party or in a public building. U.S. culture defines this distance as 4 to 12 feet.

social skills training. Educational opportunities through role-play for the person with schizophrenia to learn appropriate social interaction skills and functional skills that are relevant to daily living.

somatization. A method of coping with psychosocial stress by developing physical symptoms.

splitting. A primitive ego defense mechanism in which the person is unable to integrate and accept both positive and negative feelings. In their view, people—including themselves—and life situations are all good or all bad. This trait is common in borderline personality disorder.

statutory law. A law that has been enacted by legislative bodies, such as a county or city council, state legislature, or the U.S. Congress.

statutory rape. Unlawful intercourse between a man over age 16 and a female under the age of consent. The man can be arrested for statutory rape even when the interaction has occurred between consenting individuals.

stereotyping. The process of classifying all individuals from the same culture or ethnic group as identical.

stimulus generalization. The process by which a conditioned response is elicited from all stimuli similar to the one from which the response was learned.

storefront clinic. Establishments that have been converted into clinics that serve the homeless population.

stress. A state of disequilibrium that occurs when there is a disharmony between demands occurring within an individual's internal or external environment and his or her ability to cope with those demands.

stress management. Various methods used by individuals to reduce tension and other maladaptive responses to stress in their lives; includes relaxation exercises, physical exercise, music, mental imagery, or any other technique that is successful for a person.

stressor. A demand from within an individual's internal or external environment that elicits a physiological and/or psychological response.

sublimation. The rechanneling of personally and/or socially unacceptable drives or impulses into activities that are tolerable and constructive.

subluxation. The term used in chiropractic medicine to describe vertebrae in the spinal column that have become displaced, possibly pressing on nerves and interfering with normal nerve transmission.

substance abuse. Use of psychoactive drugs that poses significant hazards to health and interferes with social, occupational, psychological, or physical functioning.

substance dependence. Physical dependence is identified by the inability to stop using a substance despite attempts to do so; a continual use of the substance despite adverse consequences; a developing tolerance; and the development of withdrawal symptoms upon cessation or decreased intake. Psychological dependence is said to exist when a substance is perceived by the user to be necessary to maintain an optimal state of personal well-being, interpersonal relations, or skill performance.

substitution therapy. The use of various medications to decrease the intensity of symptoms in an individual who is withdrawing from, or experiencing the effects of excessive use of, substances.

subsystems. The smaller units of which a system is composed. In family systems theory, the subsystems are composed of husband-wife, parent-child(ren), or sibling-sibling.

superego. One of the three elements of the personality identified by Freud that represents the conscience and the culturally determined restrictions that are placed on an individual.

suppression. The voluntary blocking from one's awareness of unpleasant feelings and experiences.

surrogate. One who serves as a substitute figure for another.

symbiotic relationship. A type of "psychic fusion" that occurs between two people; it is unhealthy in that severe anxiety is generated in one or both if separation is indicated. A symbiotic relationship is normal between infant and mother.

sympathy. The actual sharing of another's thoughts and behaviors. Differs from empathy, in that with empathy one experiences an objective understanding of what another is feeling, rather than actually sharing those feelings.

synapse. The junction between two neurons. The small space between the axon terminals of one neuron and the cell body or dendrites of another is called the synaptic cleft.

syphilis. A sexually transmitted disorder caused by the spirochete *Treponema pallidum* and resulting in a chancre on the skin or mucous membranes of the sexual organs. If left untreated, may go systemic. End-stage disease can have profound effects, such as blindness or insanity.

systematic desensitization. A treatment for phobias in which the individual is taught to relax and then asked to imagine various components of the phobic stimulus on a graded hierarchy, moving from that which produces the least fear to that which produces the most.

T

tangentiality. The inability to get to the point of a story. The speaker introduces many unrelated topics, until the original topic of discussion is lost.

tardive dyskinesia. Syndrome of symptoms characterized by bizarre facial and tongue movements, a stiff neck, and difficulty swallowing. It may occur as an adverse effect of long-term therapy with some antipsychotic medications.

technical expert. Peplau's term for one who understands various professional devices and possesses the clinical skills necessary to perform the interventions that are in the best interest of the client.

temperament. A set of inborn personality characteristics that influence an individual's manner of reacting to the environment, and ultimately influences his or her developmental progression.

territoriality. The innate tendency of individuals to own space. Individuals lay claim to areas around them as their own. This phenomenon can have an influence on interpersonal communication.

tertiary prevention. Healthcare that is directed toward reduction of the residual effects associated with severe or chronic physical or mental illness.

therapeutic group. Differs from group therapy in that there is a lesser amount of theoretical foundation. Focus is on group relations, interactions between group members, and the consideration of a selected issue. Leaders of therapeutic groups do not require the extent of educational preparation required of group therapy leaders.

thought-stopping technique. A self-taught technique that an individual uses each time he or she wishes to eliminate intrusive or negative, unwanted thoughts from awareness.

time out. An aversive stimulus or punishment during which the individual is removed from the environment where the unacceptable behavior is being exhibited.

token economy. In behavior modification, a type of contracting in which the reinforcers for desired behaviors are presented in the form of tokens, which may then be exchanged for designated privileges.

tort. The violation of a civil law in which an individual has been wronged. In a tort action, one party asserts that wrongful conduct on the part of the other has caused harm, and compensation for harm suffered is sought.

transsexualism. A disorder of gender identity or gender dysphoria (unhappiness or dissatisfaction with one's gender) of the most extreme variety. The individual, despite having the anatomical characteristics of a given gender, has the self-perception of being of the opposite gender, and may seek to have gender changed through surgical intervention.

transvestic fetishism. Recurrent urges and sexually arousing fantasies involving dressing in the clothes of the opposite gender.

triangles. A three-person emotional configuration, which is considered the basic building block of the family system. When anxiety becomes too great between two family members, a third person is brought in to form a triangle. Triangles are dysfunctional in that they offer relief from anxiety through diversion rather than through resolution of the issue.

trichotillomania. The recurrent failure to resist impulses to pull out one's own hair.

type A personality. The personality characteristics attributed to individuals prone to coronary heart disease, including excessive competitive drive, chronic sense of time urgency, easy anger, aggressiveness, excessive ambition, and inability to enjoy leisure time.

type B personality. The personality characteristics attributed to individuals who are not prone to coronary heart disease; includes characteristics such as ability to perform even under pressure but without the competitive drive and constant sense of time urgency experienced by the type A personality. Type Bs can enjoy their leisure time without feeling guilty, and they are much less impulsive than type A individuals; that is, they think things through before making decisions.

type C personality. The personality characteristics attributed to the cancer-prone individual. Includes characteristics such as suppression of anger, calm, passive, puts the needs of others before their own, but holds resentment toward others for perceived "wrongs."

tyramine. An amino acid found in aged cheeses or other aged, overripe, and fermented foods; broad beans; pickled herring; beef or chicken liver; preserved meats; beer and wine; yeast products; chocolate; caffeinated drinks; canned figs; sour cream; yogurt; soy sauce; and some over-the-counter cold medications and diet pills. If foods high in tyramine content are consumed when an individual is taking MAOIs, a potentially life-threatening syndrome called hypertensive crisis can result.

U

unconditional positive regard. Carl Rogers' term for the respect and dignity of an individual regardless of his or her unacceptable behavior.

undoing. A mechanism used to symbolically negate or cancel out a previous action or experience that one finds intolerable.

universality. One curative factor of groups (identified by Yalom) in which individuals realize that they are not alone in a problem and in the thoughts and feelings they are experiencing. Anxiety is relieved by the support and understanding of others in the group who share similar experiences.

utilitarianism. The ethical theory that espouses "the greatest happiness for the greatest number." Under this theory, action would be taken based on the results that will produce the most good (happiness) for the most people.

V

vaginismus. Involuntary constriction of the outer one-third of the vagina that prevents penile insertion and intercourse.

values. Personal beliefs about the truth, beauty, or worth of a thought, object, or behavior that influences an individual's actions.

values clarification. A process of self-discovery by which people identify their personal values and their value rankings. This process increases awareness about why individuals behave in certain ways.

velorio. In the Mexican-American culture, following a death, large numbers of family and friends gather for a *velorio*, a festive watch over the body of the deceased person before burial.

voyeurism. Recurrent urges and sexually arousing fantasies involving the act of observing unsuspecting people, usually strangers, who are naked, in the process of disrobing, or engaging in sexual activity.

W

waxy flexibility. A condition by which the individual with schizophrenia passively yields all movable parts of the body to any efforts made at placing them in certain positions.

Wernicke's encephalopathy. A brain disorder caused by thiamine deficiency and characterized by visual disturbances, ataxia, somnolence, stupor, and, without thiamine replacement, death.

word salad. A group of words that are put together in a random fashion without any logical connection.

Y

yin and yang. The fundamental concept of Asian health practices. Yin and yang are opposite forces of energy such as negative/positive, dark/light, cold/hot, hard/soft, and feminine/masculine. Food, medicines, and herbs are classified according to their yin and yang properties and are used to restore a balance, thereby restoring health.

yoga. A system of beliefs and practices, the ultimate goal of which is to unite the human soul with the universal spirit. In Western countries, yoga uses body postures, along with meditation and breathing exercises, to achieve a balanced, disciplined workout that releases muscle tension, tones the internal organs, and energizes the mind, body, and spirit, so that natural healing can occur.

APPENDIX G

ANSWERS TO REVIEW QUESTIONS

CHAPTER 1. MENTAL HEALTH AND MENTAL ILLNESS

1. c	2. d	3. b	4. a	5. b
6. d	7. c	8. d	9. c	10. b

CHAPTER 2. CONCEPTS OF PERSONALITY DEVELOPMENT

1. b	2. c	3. d	4. b	5. b
6. b	7. a	8. c	9. a	10. b

CHAPTER 3. BIOLOGICAL IMPLICATIONS

1. c	2. e	3. f	4. b	5. d
6. g	7. a	8. c	9. b	10. a

CHAPTER 4. ETHICAL AND LEGAL ISSUES

1. c	2. a	3. e	4. d	5. b
6. d	7. b	8. e	9. a	10. c

CHAPTER 5. RELATIONSHIP DEVELOPMENT AND THERAPEUTIC COMMUNICATION

1. c 2. a 3. d 4. b
5. a. Nontherapeutic technique: Disagreeing
   b. The correct answer. Therapeutic technique: Voicing doubt
6. a. The correct answer. Therapeutic technique: Giving recognition
   b. Nontherapeutic technique: Complimenting—a judgment on the part of the nurse.
7. a. Nontherapeutic: Giving reassurance
   b. Nontherapeutic: Disapproving
   c. Nontherapeutic: Introducing an unrelated topic
   d. Nontherapeutic: Indicating an external source of power
   e. The correct answer. Therapeutic technique: Exploring
8. a. Nontherapeutic: Requesting an explanation
   b. Nontherapeutic: Belittling feelings expressed
   c. Nontherapeutic: Rejecting
   d. The correct answer. Therapeutic technique: Formulating a plan of action
9. Therapeutic response: "Do you think you should tell him?" Technique: Reflecting.
   Nontherapeutic response: "Yes, you must tell your husband about your affair with your boss." Technique: Giving advice.
10. a. The correct answer. Therapeutic technique: Reflecting.
    b. Nontherapeutic: Requesting an explanation.
    c. Nontherapeutic: Indicating an external source of power.
    d. Nontherapeutic: Giving advice.
    e. Nontherapeutic: Defending.
    f. Nontherapeutic: Making stereotyped comments.

CHAPTER 6. THE NURSING PROCESS IN PSYCHIATRIC/MENTAL HEALTH NURSING

1. a	2. c	3. b	4. b	5. c
6. b	7. e	8. d	9. a	10. c

CHAPTER 7. MILIEU—THE THERAPEUTIC ENVIRONMENT

1. A scientific structuring of the environment in order to effect behavioral changes and to improve the psychological health and functioning of the individual.
2. The goal of milieu therapy/therapeutic community is for the client to learn adaptive coping, interaction, and relationship skills that can be generalized to other aspects of his or her life.

3. c	4. b	5. a	6. d	7. f
8. h	9. b	10. i	11. g	12. j
13. a	14. e	15. c	16. k	17. m
18. l	19. d			

CHAPTER 8. INTERVENTION IN GROUPS

1. A group is defined as "a collection of individuals whose association is founded upon shared commonalities of interest, values, norms, or purpose."
2. a. Teaching; Laissez-faire
   b. Supportive/therapeutic; Democratic
   c. Task; Autocratic

3. b	4. i	5. k	6. h	7. e
8. j	9. a	10. d	11. f	12. g
13. c	14. e	15. h	16. f	17. d
18. a	19. c	20. g	21. b	

CHAPTER 9. INTERVENING IN CRISES

1. c	2. d	3. a	4. b	5. c
6. a	7. d	8. b	9. b	10. d
11. c	12. a	13. b	14. c	15. e

CHAPTER 10. PSYCHOPHARMACOLOGY

1. a	2. c	3. d	4. b	5. c
6. b	7. a	8. b	9. d	10. b

CHAPTER 11. COMPLEMENTARY AND PSYCHOSOCIAL THERAPIES

1. c	2. e	3. f	4. b	5. g
6. a	7. d	8. c	9. d	10. a
11. a	12. b	13. d		

CHAPTER 12. DELIRIUM, DEMENTIA, AND AMNESTIC DISORDERS

1. c	2. d	3. b	4. a	5. b
6. c	7. d	8. a	9. b	10. d

CHAPTER 13. SUBSTANCE-RELATED DISORDERS

1. a	2. c	3. b	4. b	5. a
6. c	7. a	8. b	9. d	10. a

CHAPTER 14. SCHIZOPHRENIA AND OTHER PSYCHOTIC DISORDERS

1. b	2. b	3. c	4. d	5. d
6. a	7. c	8. b	9. c	10. d

CHAPTER 15. MOOD DISORDERS

1. c	2. b	3. a	4. d	5. c
6. b	7. c	8. a	9. c	10. b

CHAPTER 16. ANXIETY DISORDERS

1. d	2. c	3. d	4. a	5. b
6. c	7. b	8. c	9. a	10. d

CHAPTER 17. ANXIETY-RELATED DISORDERS

1. c	2. f	3. a	4. d	5. g
6. e	7. h	8. b	9. a	10. d
11. c	12. d	13. b	14. a	15. d

CHAPTER 18. DISORDERS OF HUMAN SEXUALITY

1. b	2. c	3. d	4. a	5. b
6. b	7. d	8. a	9. e	10. c

CHAPTER 19. EATING DISORDERS

1. c	2. a	3. b	4. b	5. c
6. b	7. c	8. b	9. c	10. a

CHAPTER 20. PERSONALITY DISORDERS

1. d	2. a	3. b	4. d	5. a
6. b	7. c	8. c	9. d	10. b

CHAPTER 21. CHILDREN AND ADOLESCENTS

1. b	2. c	3. a	4. b	5. b
6. d	7. c	8. d	9. a	10. b

CHAPTER 22. VICTIMS OF ABUSE OR NEGLECT

1. b	2. c	3. a	4. d	5. b
6. d	7. a	8. b	9. b	10. d

CHAPTER 23. THE AGING INDIVIDUAL

1. c	2. d	3. b	4. a	5. c
6. d	7. a	8. a	9. c	10. a

CHAPTER 24. COMMUNITY MENTAL HEALTH NURSING

1. a	2. b	3. a	4. c	5. d
6. b	7. c	8. d	9. a	10. b

CHAPTER 25. THE BEREAVED INDIVIDUAL

1. e	2. c	3. c	4. d	5. a
6. a	7. b	8. c	9. a	10. c

APPENDIX H

SAMPLE CLIENT TEACHING GUIDES

BENZODIAZEPINES

Patient Medication Instruction Sheet

Patient Name ______________________ **Drug Prescribed** ______________________

Directions for Use ______________________

Examples and Uses of this Medicine:

Benzodiazepines are used to treat moderate to severe anxiety: alprazolam [Xanax], chlordiazepoxide [Librium], clonazepam [Klonopin], clorazepate [Tranxene], diazepam [Valium], lorazepam [Ativan], and oxazepam [Serax]. Some are used to treat insomnia (sleeplessness): flurazepam [Dalmane], temazepam [Restoril], and triazolam [Halcion]. Some are used for muscle spasms and to treat seizure disorders.

Before Using this Medicine, Be Sure to tell your Doctor if you:

- Are allergic to any medicine
- Have glaucoma
- Are pregnant, plan to be, or are breast-feeding
- Are taking any other medications

Side Effects of this Medicine:

REPORT THE FOLLOWING SIDE EFFECTS TO YOUR DOCTOR IMMEDIATELY:

- Mental confusion or depression
- Hallucinations (seeing, hearing, or feeling things not there)
- Skin rash or itching
- Sore throat and fever
- Unusual excitement, nervousness, irritability, or trouble sleeping

SIDE EFFECTS THAT MAY OCCUR BUT NOT REQUIRE A DOCTOR'S ATTENTION UNLESS THEY PERSIST LONGER THAN A FEW DAYS:

- Blurred vision, or other changes in vision
- Clumsiness, dizziness, lightheadedness, or slurred speech
- Constipation, diarrhea, nausea, vomiting, or stomach pain
- Difficulty in urination
- Drowsiness, headache, or unusual tiredness or weakness

Other Instructions While Taking This Medication:

- Take this medicine only as your doctor has directed. Do not take more of it or do not take it more often than prescribed. If large doses are taken for a prolonged period, it may become habit-forming.
- If you are taking this medicine several times a day and you forget a dose, if it is within an hour or so of the missed dose, go ahead and take it. Otherwise, wait and take the next dose at regular time. Do not double up on a dose if you forget one. Just keep taking the prescribed dosage.
- Do not stop taking the drug abruptly. Can produce serious withdrawal symptoms, such as depression, insomnia, anxiety, abdominal and muscle cramps, tremors, vomiting, sweating, convulsions, delirium. Discuss with the doctor before stopping this medication.
- Do not consume other CNS depressants (including alcohol) when taking this medication.
- Do not take nonprescription medication without approval from physician.
- Rise slowly from the sitting or lying position to prevent a sudden drop in blood pressure.

BUSPIRONE (BuSpar)

Patient Medication Instruction Sheet

Patient Name________________________
Directions for Use________________________

Uses of this Medicine:

BuSpar is used in the treatment of anxiety disorders. It is also sometimes used to treat the symptoms of premenstrual syndrome.

Before Using this Medicine, Be Sure to tell your Doctor if you:

- Are allergic to any medicine
- Are pregnant, plan to be, or are breast-feeding
- Are taking any other medications

Side Effects of this Medicine:

REPORT THE FOLLOWING SIDE EFFECTS TO YOUR DOCTOR IMMEDIATELY:

- Mental confusion or depression
- Hallucinations (seeing, hearing, or feeling things not there)
- Skin rash or itching
- Unusual excitement, nervousness, irritability, or trouble sleeping
- Persistent headache
- Involuntary movements of the head or neck muscles

SIDE EFFECTS THAT MAY OCCUR BUT NOT REQUIRE A DOCTOR'S ATTENTION UNLESS THEY PERSIST LONGER THAN A FEW DAYS:

- Dizziness; lightheadedness
- Drowsiness
- Nausea
- Fatigue
- Headache that subsides

Other Instructions While Taking This Medication:

- Take this medicine only as your doctor has directed. Do not take more of it or do not take it more often than prescribed.
- If you are taking this medicine several times a day and you forget a dose, if it is within an hour or so of the missed dose, go ahead and take it. Otherwise, wait and take the next dose at regular time. Do not double up on a dose if you forget one. Just keep taking the prescribed dosage.
- Do not consume other CNS depressants (including alcohol) when taking this medication.
- Do not take nonprescription medication without approval from physician.
- Rise slowly from the sitting or lying position to prevent a sudden drop in blood pressure.

TRICYCLIC ANTIDEPRESSANTS

Patient Medication Instruction Sheet

Patient Name ______________________ **Drug Prescribed** ______________________
Directions for Use ______________________

Examples and Uses of this Medicine:
Tricyclic antidepressants are used to treat symptoms of depression: amitriptyline [Elavil], amoxapine [Asendin], desipramine [Norpramin], doxepin [Sinequan], imipramine [Tofranil], nortriptyline [Aventyl], protriptyline [Vivactil], and trimipramine [Surmontil]. Doxepin is used to treat depression with anxiety. Clomipramine [Anafranil] is used to treat obsessive-compulsive disorder. Imipramine is used to treat enuresis (bedwetting) in children.

Before Using this Medicine, Be Sure to tell your Doctor if you:

- Are allergic to any medicine
- Have glaucoma
- Have a history of heart problems
- Are pregnant, plan to be, or are breast-feeding
- Are taking any other medications
- Have a history of seizures or high blood pressure

Side Effects of this Medicine:

REPORT THE FOLLOWING SIDE EFFECTS TO YOUR DOCTOR IMMEDIATELY:

- Seizures
- Difficulty urinating
- Irregular heartbeat or chest pain
- Hallucinations
- Skin rash
- Sore throat and fever
- Unusual amount of restlessness and excitement
- Confusion; disorientation

SIDE EFFECTS THAT MAY OCCUR BUT MAY NOT REQUIRE A DOCTOR'S ATTENTION:

- Drowsiness
- Dry mouth
- Nausea
- Sensitivity to the sun (may burn easily)
- Headache
- Constipation

Other Instructions While Taking This Medication:

- Continue to take the medication even though you still have symptoms. It may take as long as 4 weeks before you start feeling better.
- Use caution when driving or operating dangerous machinery. Drowsiness and dizziness can occur. If these side effects don't go away or get worse, report them to the doctor.
- Do not stop taking the drug abruptly. To do so might produce withdrawal symptoms, such as nausea, vertigo, insomnia, headache, malaise, and nightmares. Tell the doctor when you want to stop taking it.
- Use sunscreens and wear protective clothing when spending time outdoors.
- Rise slowly from a sitting or lying position to prevent a sudden drop in blood pressure.
- Take frequent sips of water, chew sugarless gum, or suck on hard candy if dry mouth is a problem.
- You may take this medication with food if nausea is a problem.
- Do not drink alcohol when taking this medication.
- Do not consume other medications (including over-the-counter medications) without the physician's approval when taking this medication. Many medications contain substances that, in combination with tricyclic antidepressants, could be dangerous.

SELECTIVE SEROTONIN REUPTAKE INHIBITORS (SSRIs)

Patient Medication Instruction Sheet

Patient Name ______________________ **Drug Prescribed** ______________________
Directions for Use ____

Examples and Uses of this Medicine:
SSRIs are used to treat symptoms of depression: citalopram [Celexa], fluoxetine [Prozac], paroxetine [Paxil], and sertraline [Zoloft]. Some are used to treat obsessive-compulsive disorder: fluvoxamine [Luvox], fluoxetine, [Prozac], paroxetine [Paxil], and sertraline [Zoloft]. Also bulimia nervosa: fluoxetine [Prozac], and panic disorder: sertraline [Zoloft] and paroxetine [Paxil].

Before Using this Medicine, Be Sure to tell your Doctor if you:

- Are allergic to any medicine
- Are pregnant, plan to be, or are breast-feeding
- Are taking any other medications
- Have diabetes

Side Effects of this Medicine:

REPORT THE FOLLOWING SIDE EFFECTS TO YOUR DOCTOR IMMEDIATELY:
- Skin rash
- Fever
- Unusual excitement, nervousness, irritability, or trouble sleeping
- Loss of appetite and weight loss
- Seizures
- Difficulty breathing
- Increased sensitivity to sunburn

SIDE EFFECTS THAT MAY OCCUR BUT MAY NOT REQUIRE A DOCTOR'S ATTENTION:
- Drowsiness
- Dizziness
- Nausea
- Headache
- Impotence or loss of sexual desire (this should be reported to physician if it is troubling to the patient)

Other Instructions While Taking This Medication:
- Continue to take the medication even though you still have symptoms. It may take as long as 4 weeks before you start feeling better.
- Use caution when driving or operating dangerous machinery. Drowsiness and dizziness can occur. If these side effects don't go away or get worse, report them to the doctor.
- Use sunscreens and wear protective clothing when spending time outdoors.
- Rise slowly from a sitting or lying position to prevent a sudden drop in blood pressure.
- Take frequent sips of water, chew sugarless gum, or suck on hard candy if dry mouth is a problem.
- You may take this medication with food if nausea is a problem.
- Avoid drinking alcohol when taking this medication.
- Do not consume other medications (including over-the-counter medications) without the physician's approval when taking this medication. Many medications contain substances that, in combination with SSRI antidepressants, could be dangerous.

MONOAMINE OXIDASE INHIBITORS (MAOIs)

Patient Medication Instruction Sheet

Patient Name ______________________________ **Drug Prescribed** ___________________________
Directions for Use ____

Examples and Uses of this Medicine:
MAOIs are used to treat the symptoms of depression: isocarboxazid [Marplan], phenelzine [Nardil], tranylcypromine [Parnate].

Before Using this Medicine, Be Sure to tell your Doctor if you:
- Are allergic to any medicine
- Have a history of liver or kidney disease
- Have been diagnosed with pheochromocytoma
- Have a history of severe or frequent headaches
- Are pregnant, plan to be, or are breast-feeding
- Have a history of hypertension
- Have a history of heart disease
- Are taking (or have taken in the last 2 weeks) **any** other medication

Side Effects of this Medicine:
REPORT THE FOLLOWING SIDE EFFECTS TO YOUR DOCTOR IMMEDIATELY:
- Severe, pounding headache
- Rapid or pounding heartbeat
- Stiff or sore neck
- Chest pain
- Nausea and vomiting
- Seizures

THE FOLLOWING SIDE EFFECTS SHOULD ALSO BE REPORTED TO THE DOCTOR:
- Dark urine
- Yellowing of eyes or skin
- Hallucinations
- Fainting
- Hyperexcitable
- Confusion
- Fever
- Skin rash
- Disorientation

SIDE EFFECTS THAT MAY OCCUR BUT MAY NOT REQUIRE A DOCTOR'S ATTENTION:
- Constipation
- Diarrhea (unless severe and persistent)
- Dizziness
- Dry Mouth
- Fatigue
- Drowsiness
- Nausea
- Decreased sexual ability

Other Instructions While Taking This Medication:
- Continue to take the medication even though you still have symptoms. It may take as long as 4 weeks before you start feeling better.
- Use caution when driving or operating dangerous machinery. Drowsiness and dizziness can occur.
- Do not stop taking the drug abruptly. To do so might produce withdrawal symptoms, such as nausea, vertigo, insomnia, headache, malaise, and nightmares. Tell the doctor when you want to stop taking it.
- Rise slowly from a sitting or lying position to prevent a sudden drop in blood pressure.
- Take frequent sips of water, chew sugarless gum, or suck on hard candy if dry mouth is a problem.
- You may take this medication with food if nausea is a problem. Do not drink alcohol.
- Do not consume other medications (including over-the-counter medications) without the physician's approval when taking this medication. Many medications contain substances that, in combination with MAOI antidepressants, could be dangerous.
- Do not consume the following foods or medication when taking MAOIs (or for 2 weeks after you stop taking them): aged cheese, raisins, red wine (especially Chianti), beer, chocolate, colas, coffee, tea, sour cream, beef/chicken livers, game meat, canned figs, soy sauce, meat tenderizer (MSG), pickled herring, smoked/processed meats (lunch meats, sausage, pepperoni), yogurt, yeast products, broad beans, sauerkraut, cold remedies, diet pills, or nasal decongestants. To do so could cause a life-threatening condition.
- Be sure to tell any doctor or dentist that you see that you are taking this medication.

LITHIUM

Patient Medication Instruction Sheet

Patient Name ______________________ **Drug Prescribed** ______________________
Directions for Use ____

Uses of this Medicine:
Lithium is used for treatment of manic episodes associated with bipolar disorder. Taking lithium regularly also prevents manic episodes or causes fewer, less serious manic episodes in a person with bipolar disorder.

Before Using this Medicine, Be Sure to tell your Doctor if you:

- Are allergic to any medicine
- Have heart, kidney, or thyroid disease
- Are pregnant, plan to be, or are breast-feeding
- Are taking any other medication, particularly diuretics, haloperidol, NSAIDs, fluoxetine, or carbamazepine

Side Effects of this Medicine:

REPORT THE FOLLOWING SIDE EFFECTS TO YOUR DOCTOR IMMEDIATELY:

- Lack of coordination
- Persistent nausea and vomiting
- Slurred speech
- Blurred vision
- Ringing in the ears
- Jerking of arms and legs
- Severe diarrhea
- Confusion

SIDE EFFECTS THAT MAY OCCUR BUT MAY NOT REQUIRE A DOCTOR'S ATTENTION UNLESS THEY PERSIST:

- Mild hand tremors
- GI upset; nausea
- Diarrhea
- Dizziness
- Dry mouth

Other Instructions While Taking This Medication:

- Take this medicine exactly as it is prescribed. Do not take more of it or more often than it is prescribed. Sometimes it takes several weeks of taking this medication before you begin to feel better. At some point, you doctor may make an adjustment in the dosage.
- Do not drive or operate dangerous machinery until your response to the medication is adjusted. Drowsiness or dizziness can occur.
- Do not stop taking the medication even if you are feeling fine and don't think you need it. Symptoms of mania can occur.
- Take this medication with food or milk to lessen stomach upset, unless otherwise directed by your doctor.
- Use a normal amount of salt in your food. Drink 8–10 glasses of water each day. Avoid drinks that contain caffeine (that have a diuretic effect). Have blood tests taken to check lithium level every month, or as advised by physician.
- Avoid consuming alcoholic beverages and nonprescription medications without approval from physician.
- Use extra care in hot weather and during activities that cause you to sweat heavily, such as hot baths, saunas, or exercising. The loss of too much water and salt from your body can lead to serious side effects from this medicine.
- Be sure to get enough salt and water in the diet during times of sickness that can deplete the body of water, such as high fever, nausea and vomiting, and diarrhea.
- Carry card at all times identifying the name of medications being taken.

ANTIPSYCHOTICS (Conventional)

Patient Medication Instruction Sheet

Patient Name ______________________ **Drug Prescribed** ______________________
Directions for Use ____

Examples: Chlorpromazine (Thorazine), Perphenazine (Trilafon), Thioridazine (Mellaril), Triflupromazine (Vesprin), Molindone (Moban), Fluphenazine (Prolixin), Prochlorperazine (Compazine), Trifluoperazine (Stelazine), Loxapine (Loxitane), Pimozide (Orap), Mesoridazine (Serentil), Promazine (Sparine), Thiothixene (Navane), Haloperidol (Haldol)

Uses of this Medicine: Used in the management of psychotic symptoms, acute agitated states, and some are used to treat nausea and vomiting.

Before Using this Medicine, Be Sure to tell your Doctor if you:

- Are allergic to any medicine
- Have history of seizures
- Have liver or heart disease
- Have any other medical problem
- Are pregnant, plan to be, or are breast-feeding
- Are taking any other medications (prescription or over-the-counter)
- Have any blood disorders

Side Effects of this Medicine:

REPORT THE FOLLOWING SIDE EFFECTS TO YOUR DOCTOR IMMEDIATELY:

- Difficulty urinating
- Shuffling walk
- Yellow eyes and skin
- Wormlike movements of the tongue
- Fainting
- Skin rash
- Sore throat
- Seizures
- Fever
- Muscle spasms or stiffness
- Excitement or restlessness
- Jerky movements of head, face, or neck
- Unusual bleeding; easy bruising
- Unusually fast heartbeat

SIDE EFFECTS THAT MAY OCCUR BUT MAY NOT REQUIRE A DOCTOR'S ATTENTION:

- Dry mouth
- Nausea
- Weight gain
- Blurred vision
- Decreased sweating
- Dizziness
- Constipation
- Increased sensitivity to sunburn
- Drowsiness

Other Instructions While Taking This Medication:

- Use caution when driving or operating dangerous machinery. Drowsiness and dizziness can occur.
- Do not stop taking the drug abruptly after long-term use. To do so might produce withdrawal symptoms, such as nausea, vomiting, gastritis, headache, tachycardia, insomnia, tremulousness.
- Use sunscreens and wear protective clothing when spending time outdoors. Skin is more susceptible to sunburn, which can occur in as little as 30 minutes.
- Rise slowly from a sitting or lying position to prevent a sudden drop in blood pressure.
- Take frequent sips of water, chew sugarless gum, or suck on hard candy, if experiencing a problem with dry mouth.
- Dress warmly in cold weather and avoid extended exposure to very high or low temperatures. Body temperature is harder to maintain with this medication.
- Do not drink alcohol when on antipsychotic therapy. These drugs potentiate each other's effects.
- Do not consume other medications (including over-the-counter products) without physician's approval. Many medications contain substances that interact with antipsychotics in a way that may be harmful.
- Continue to take medication, even if feeling well and as though it is not needed. Symptoms may return if medication is discontinued.
- Some of these medications may turn the urine pink to red or reddish brown. This is harmless.

ANTIPSYCHOTICS (Atypical)

Patient Medication Instruction Sheet

Patient Name ______________________ **Drug Prescribed** ______________________
Directions for Use ______________________

Examples:
- Risperidone (Risperdal)
- Clozapine (Clozaril)
- Olanzapine (Zyprexa)
- Quetiapine (Seroquel)
- Ziprasidone (Geodon)

Uses of this Medicine: Used in the management of schizophrenia, bipolar mania, and dementia-related psychotic symptoms.

Before Using this Medicine, Be Sure to tell your Doctor if you:
- Are allergic to any medicine
- Have history of seizures
- Have liver or heart disease
- Have any blood disorders
- Are pregnant, plan to be, or are breast-feeding
- Are taking any other medications (prescription or over-the-counter)
- Have any other medical problem

Side Effects of this Medicine:

REPORT THE FOLLOWING SIDE EFFECTS TO YOUR DOCTOR IMMEDIATELY:
- Difficulty urinating
- Shuffling walk
- Yellow eyes and skin
- Wormlike movements of the tongue
- Fainting
- Skin rash
- Sore throat
- Seizures
- Fever
- Muscle spasms or stiffness
- Excitement or restlessness
- Jerky movements of head, face, or neck
- Unusual bleeding; easy bruising
- Unusually fast heartbeat

SIDE EFFECTS THAT MAY OCCUR BUT MAY NOT REQUIRE A DOCTOR'S ATTENTION:
- Dry mouth
- Nausea
- Weight gain
- Blurred vision
- Decreased sweating
- Dizziness
- Constipation
- Increased sensitivity to sunburn
- Drowsiness

Other Instructions While Taking This Medication:
- Use caution when driving or operating dangerous machinery. Drowsiness and dizziness can occur.
- Do not stop taking the drug abruptly after long-term use. To do so might produce withdrawal symptoms, such as nausea, vomiting, gastritis, headache, tachycardia, insomnia, tremulousness.
- Use sunscreens and wear protective clothing when spending time outdoors. Skin is more susceptible to sunburn, which can occur in as little as 30 minutes.
- Rise slowly from a sitting or lying position to prevent a sudden drop in blood pressure.
- Take frequent sips of water, chew sugarless gum, or suck on hard candy, if you have dry mouth.
- Dress warmly in cold weather and avoid extended exposure to very high or low temperatures. Body temperature is harder to maintain with this medication.
- Do not drink alcohol when on antipsychotic therapy. These drugs potentiate each other's effects.
- Do not consume other medications (including over-the-counter products) without physician's approval. Many medications contain substances that interact with antipsychotics in a way that may be harmful.
- Continue to take medication, even if feeling well and as though it is not needed. Symptoms may return if medication is discontinued.
- Report weekly (if receiving clozapine therapy) to have blood levels drawn and to obtain a weekly supply of the drug.

CNS STIMULANTS (Amphetamines, Methylphenidate, & Pemoline)

Patient Medication Instruction Sheet

Patient Name ______________________ **Drug Prescribed** ______________________
Directions for Use ____

Examples and Uses of this Medicine:

These medications are used in the treatment of narcolepsy and in Attention Deficit Hyperactivity Disorder (ADHD) in children and adults. Examples include: amphetamine sulfate, dextroamphetamine sulfate [Dexedrine], methamphetamine [Desoxyn], methylphenidate [Ritalin], pemoline [Cylert], and dextroamphetamine/amphetamine mixture [Adderall].

Before Using this Medicine, Be Sure to tell your Doctor if you:

- Are allergic to any medicine
- Have glaucoma
- Have a history of tics or Tourette's disorder
- Have a history of heart disease
- Have a history of hyperthyroidism
- Have any other medical problem
- Are pregnant, plan to be, or are breast-feeding
- Are taking any other medications
- Have arteriosclerosis
- Have high blood pressure
- Have taken an MAOI within 14 days

Side Effects of this Medicine:

REPORT THE FOLLOWING SIDE EFFECTS TO YOUR DOCTOR IMMEDIATELY:

- Insomnia
- Rapid, pounding heartbeat
- Restlessness or agitation
- Severe, persistent headache
- Skin rash

SIDE EFFECTS THAT MAY OCCUR BUT MAY NOT REQUIRE A DOCTOR'S ATTENTION:

- Dry mouth
- Dizziness
- Constipation
- Anorexia
- Nausea

Other Instructions While Taking This Medication:

- Use caution in driving or operating dangerous machinery. Dizziness can occur.
- Do not stop taking the drug abruptly. To do so can cause fatigue and mental depression. Tell the physician if you wish to discontinue this medication.
- Take medication no later than 6 hours before bedtime to prevent insomnia.
- Do not take other medications (including over-the-counter drugs) without physician's approval. Many medications contain substances that, in combination with CNS stimulants, can be harmful.
- Diabetic clients should monitor blood sugar two or three times a day or as instructed by the physician. Be aware of need for possible alteration in insulin requirements because of changes in food intake, weight, and activity.
- Avoid consumption of large amounts of caffeinated products (coffee, tea, colas, chocolate). They may increase restlessness and stimulation.
- Carry a card or other identification at all times describing medications being taken.

CNS STIMULANTS (Anorexigenics)

Patient Medication Instruction Sheet

Patient Name ______________________ **Drug Prescribed** ______________________
Directions for Use ____

Examples and Uses of this Medicine:

These medications are used in the management of exogenous obesity, in conjunction with a reduced-calorie diet. Examples include: benzphetamine [Didrex], diethylpropion [Tenuate], phendimetrazine [Prelu-2; Plegine], phentermine [Fastin; Ionamin; Adipex-P], and sibutramine [Meridia].

Before Using this Medicine, Be Sure to tell your Doctor if you:

- Are allergic to any medicine
- Have glaucoma
- Have a history of tics or Tourette's disorder
- Have a history of heart disease
- Have a history of hyperthyroidism
- Have any other medical problem
- Are pregnant, plan to be, or are breast-feeding
- Are taking any other medications
- Have arteriosclerosis
- Have high blood pressure
- Have taken an MAOI within 14 days
- Have a history of seizures

Side Effects of this Medicine:

REPORT THE FOLLOWING SIDE EFFECTS TO YOUR DOCTOR IMMEDIATELY:

- Insomnia
- Rapid, pounding heartbeat
- Restlessness or agitation
- Severe, persistent headache
- Skin rash
- Sore throat or fever
- Fainting

SIDE EFFECTS THAT MAY OCCUR BUT MAY NOT REQUIRE A DOCTOR'S ATTENTION:

- Dry mouth
- Dizziness
- Constipation
- Anorexia
- Nausea
- Blurred vision

Other Instructions While Taking This Medication:

- Use caution in driving or operating dangerous machinery. Dizziness can occur.
- Do not stop taking the drug abruptly. To do so can cause fatigue and mental depression. Tell the physician if you wish to discontinue this medicine.
- Take medication no later than 6 hours before bedtime to prevent insomnia.
- Do not take other medications (including over-the-counter drugs) without physician's approval. Many medications contain substances that, in combination with CNS stimulants, can be harmful.
- Diabetic clients should monitor blood sugar two or three times a day or as instructed by the physician. Be aware of need for possible alteration in insulin requirements because of changes in food intake, weight, and activity.
- Avoid consumption of large amounts of caffeinated products (coffee, tea, colas, chocolate). They may increase restlessness and stimulation.
- Take medication as prescribed by physician. Do not take larger dose or more frequently than prescribed. This medication can become habit-forming.
- Follow reduced-calorie diet and program of regular exercise. Do not exceed the recommended dose if the appetite suppressant effect diminishes. Contact the doctor.

DEPRESSION

What is Depression?

It is normal to feel "blue" sometimes. In fact, feelings of sadness or disappointment are quite common, particularly in response to a loss, a failure, or even a change. Depression is different from just feeling "blue" or unhappy. The severity of the feelings, how long they last, and the presence of other symptoms are some of the factors that separate normal sadness from depression. Depression is more common in women that it is in men, and the probability increases with age.

What are the Symptoms of Depression? (From the National Institute of Mental Health)

- Persistent sad, anxious or "empty" feeling
- Loss of interest or pleasure in ordinary activities, including sex
- Decreased energy, fatigue, feeling "slowed down"
- Sleep problems (insomnia, oversleeping, early-morning waking)
- Eating problems (loss of appetite or weight, weight gain)
- Difficulty concentrating, remembering, or making decisions or helplessness
- Recurring aches and pains that don't respond to treatment
- Irritability
- Excessive crying
- Feelings of hopelessness or pessimism
- Feelings of guilt, worthlessness,
- Recurring aches and pains that don't respond to treatment
- Thoughts of death or suicide; a suicide attempt

What Causes Depression?

The causes of depression are not fully known. It is most likely caused by a combination of factors.

Genetic. A lot of research has been done to determine if depression is hereditary. Although no direct mode of hereditary transmission has been discovered, it has been found that depression does run in families. You are more likely to get depressed if a close biological relative has or has had the illness.

Biological. Depression is thought to be caused by a chemical imbalance in the brain. Neurotransmitters called serotonin, norepinephrine, and dopamine have been found to be deficient in people with depressive symptoms.

Hormonal. In women, the female hormones estrogen and progesterone most likely pay a role in depression. These hormones contribute to premenstrual depression, postpartum depression, and depression associated with menopause.

Medication side effects. Some medications, such as steroids, hormones, cancer chemotherapy, and antiparkinsonian agents, cause depression as a side effect.

Nutrition deficiencies. Deficiencies in Vitamins B_1, B_6, B_{12}, and C, and niacin, iron, folic acid, zinc, and protein may produce symptoms of depression.

How is Depression Diagnosed?

A mental health specialist, such as a psychiatrist, social worker, or psychologist, is the best source for a diagnosis of depression. A pencil and paper screening test may be administered, but generally, depression is diagnosed based on symptoms and other criteria.

What is the Treatment for Depression?

Patients with depression have a number of treatment options, including psychotherapy and antidepressant medication. It has been found that either one of these options may be effective, however a combination of the two has been shown to be more effective than either treatment alone. For those who fail to improve with medications and/or psychotherapy, other techniques, such as electroconvulsive therapy (ECT), has proven to be safe and effective for treating depressive symptoms.

Other Contacts:

National Foundation for Depressive Illness, Box 225720, NY, NY 10116, 1-800-239-1265, http://www.depression.org

Nat'l Depressive & Manic-Depressive Assn., 730 Franklin St., Ste. 501, Chicago, IL 60610, 1-800-826-3632, http://www.ndmda.org/

National Alliance for the Mentally Ill, 2107 Wilson Blvd, Ste. 300, Arlington, VA 22201, 1-800-950-6264, http://www.nami.org

BIPOLAR DISORDER

What is Bipolar Disorder?
Bipolar is sometimes called manic-depressive illness. It is indicated by moods that swing between two opposite extremes:

- Periods of mania (when the mood is elevated and the person is very excited or irritable)
- Periods of depression (when the person is sad and withdrawn)

What are the Symptoms of Bipolar Disorder?
The symptoms of bipolar disorder, depression are the same as those experienced by a person who gets depressed (but does not have bipolar disorder). They are sadness, fatigue, sleep problems, weight changes, inability to concentrate, loss of interest or pleasure in life, and thoughts or attempts of suicide.

Symptoms of bipolar disorder, mania include being very excited, irritable, distracted, and unable to sleep. They have thoughts that race through their head and sometimes they believe things that are not true. They talk excessively and move about constantly. They may be angry and suspicious, and can become violent. Some manic people spend a lot of money and abuse substances. Some manic patients may have thoughts of suicide.

Some people have mixed symptoms in which they experience symptoms of depression part of the day and symptoms of mania part of the day.

Bipolar disorder affects men and women equally. It can occur in childhood, adolescence, adulthood, or late in life.

What Causes Bipolar Disorder?
Genetic. Bipolar disorder has a strong hereditary factor. It occurs more often within families, and individuals who have close biological relatives with the illness are more likely to get the disease themselves.

Biological. Bipolar disorder is thought to be caused by a chemical imbalance in the brain. Neurotransmitters called dopamine and norepinephrine have been found to be elevated in people with manic symptoms.

Medication side effects. Certain medications, such as steroids, amphetamines, and tricyclic antidepressants, have the potential for initiating a manic episode.

How is Bipolar Disorder Diagnosed?
Bipolar disorder is often difficult to diagnose, and an individual with symptoms should be seen by a mental health professional. A careful history, taken with the help of family if possible, of all episodes of depression, mania, or both, must be completed. Patients often deny problems with mania. Other illnesses, such as attention deficit hyperactive disorder, schizophrenia, substance abuse, thyroid disorders, adrenal disorders, and certain neurological disorders, which can all cause mood swings, must be ruled out.

What is the Treatment for Bipolar Disorder?
The goals of treating bipolar disorder are to:

1. Treat the episodes of mania and depression when they occur.
2. Decrease the number of episodes that occur
3. Help the patient function as effectively as possible between episodes

Treatment is with mood-stabilizing drugs, such as lithium, valproic acid, carbamazepine, or lamotrigine. Antipsychotic medications, such as risperidone, olanzapine, or quetiapine, are sometimes given.

Psychotherapy has shown to be helpful in patients with bipolar disorder to assist in the management of everyday stressors and to help prevent relapse.

Other Contacts:
Nat'l Depressive & Manic-Depressive Assn., 730 Franklin St., Ste. 501, Chicago, IL 60610, 1-800-826-3632, http://www.ndmda.org/

National Alliance for the Mentally Ill, 2107 Wilson Blvd, Ste. 300, Arlington, VA 22201, 1-800-950-6264, http://www.nami.org

POST-TRAUMATIC STRESS DISORDER (PTSD)

What is PTSD?

PTSD is an anxiety disorder, the symptoms of which occur following exposure to an extreme traumatic stressor. The stressor that triggers these symptoms is outside the norm of human experience, and includes events such as military combat, violent personal assault, being kidnapped or taken hostage, terrorist attack, being tortured, being a prisoner of war, natural or manmade disasters, severe automobile accidents, or being diagnosed with a life-threatening illness (*DSM-IV-TR*, 2000).

What are the Symptoms of PTSD?

- Recurrent and distressing thoughts about the event
- Nightmares about the event and sleeping problem
- Flashbacks and reliving the event
- Inability to remember parts of the event
- Avoids people or activities that remind of the event
- Emotional withdrawal
- Difficulty concentrating
- Irritability or outbursts of anger
- Exaggerated startle response
- Decreased interest or participation in activities
- Guilt for surviving when other died

What Causes PTSD?

No one really knows why some people develop PTSD and others do not. Some theories include:

- Conditioned learning (people learn throughout their life to respond to stress in certain ways.)
- Ineffective coping strategies (some people naturally have stronger ability to cope than others.)
- Extreme severity and long duration of the stressor (it is thought that the more severe the stressor is and the longer it lasts, the more likely the person is to develop PTSD.)
- Absence of support systems (whether a person has significant others in his or her life to offer support in time of extreme stress affects the outcome of the response.)
- Presence of preexisting psychopathology (some individuals who already have an emotional problem may be more likely to develop PTSD in response to an extreme stressor.)
- People with a family history of anxiety disorders, who have a history of childhood abuse or neglect, or who experienced early separation from parents seem more highly predisposed to develop PTSD.

How is PTSD Diagnosed?

A physical examination to rule out physical illness is conducted. The patient must tell the physician about any anxiety disorders or depression within the family, and mention any other contributing factors, such as a history of having experienced a traumatic event. PTSD is best diagnosed by a mental health professional.

What is the Treatment for PTSD?

Group therapy and family therapy are effective treatments for PTSD in association with prescribed medications. Cognitive/behavioral therapy is also recommended. The following medications have been useful in individuals with PTSD:

- Sertraline (Zoloft) and paroxetine (Paxil) are the only two medications approved by the FDA specifically for PTSD. Other SSRIs (fluoxetine [Prozac], citalopram [Celexa], and fluvoxamine [Luvox] have also been effective.
- Other antidepressants have also been effective: bupropion (Wellbutrin), mirtazapine (Remeron), nefazodone (Serzone), and venlafaxine (Effexor).
- Tricyclic and MAOI antidepressants have been successful with some individuals.
- Benzodiazepines may relieve anxiety, but are not recommended because they are addictive.
- The antihypertensives propranolol (Inderal) and clonidine (Catapres), as well as lithium and carbamazepine (Tegretol) have been successful in alleviating nightmares, intrusive recollections, insomnia, startle responses, and angry outburst associated with PTSD.

Other Contacts:

Int'l Society for Traumatic Stress Studies, 60 Revere Dr., Ste 500, Northbrook, IL 60062, 847-480-9028, http://wwwistss.org

National Alliance for the Mentally Ill, 2107 Wilson Blvd, Ste. 300, Arlington, VA 22201, 1-800-950-6264, http://www.nami.org

OBSESSIVE-COMPULSIVE DISORDER (OCD)

What is OCD?
OCD is an anxiety disorder in which a person has recurring thoughts or images (called **obsessions**) and/or repetitive, ritualistic-type behaviors that the individual is unable to keep from doing (called **compulsions**). An individual with OCD may try to suppress these thoughts or behaviors, but is unable to do so. The individual knows that the thoughts or behaviors are irrational, but feels powerless to stop.

What are the Symptoms of OCD?
The most common obsessions include:

- Repeated thoughts about contamination (e.g., may lead to fear of shaking hands or touching objects)
- Repeated doubts (e.g., repeatedly wondering if they locked the door or turned off an appliance)
- A need to have things in a certain order (e.g., feels intense anxiety when things are out of place)
- Thoughts of aggression (e.g., to hurt a loved one)
- Sexual imagery (e.g., recurring pornographic image)

The most common compulsions include:

- Washing and cleaning (e.g., excessive handwashing or housecleaning)
- Counting (e.g., counting the number of times that something is done)
- Checking (e.g., checking something that one has done, over and over)
- Requesting or demanding assurances from others
- Repeating actions (e.g., going in and out of a door, or up and down from a chair)
- Ordering (e.g., arranging and rearranging clothes or other items)
- The obsessions and compulsions seem to be worse in the face of emotional stress.

What Causes OCD?
The exact causes of OCD are unclear. There appear to be certain contributing factors to the disorder. These include:

- **Biochemical.** OCD may be caused by a disturbance in the chemistry of the brain involving the neurotransmitter serotonin.
- **Genetics.** OCD seems to run in families. Researchers are still looking for specific genetic factors that may contribute to an inherited risk.
- **Learning Theory.** Some clinicians believe that OCD may be the result of certain patterns of learned behavior in one's early family development.

How is OCD Diagnosed?
OCD has differing amounts of severity. Some people are able to hide their illness or learn to live with it. In other instances, individuals may not be able to do anything but carry out their rituals, thereby causing a great deal of interference in their lives. Most individuals wait until the illness is severe enough that it is interfering with their social or occupational functioning before they seek treatment. A diagnosis should be made by a mental health professional.

What is the Treatment for OCD?
Antidepressants have been used with success in the treatment of OCD. Clomipramine (Anafranil) was first to be approved by the FDA for this purpose. Because of their effectiveness and low side-effect profile, the SSRIs have become the first line of treatment for OCD. Other antidepressants that have also shown to be effective include nefazodone (Serzone), venlafaxine (Effexor), and mirtazapine (Remeron).

In addition to medication, psychosocial techniques, such as cognitive-behavioral therapy, individual psychotherapy, and relaxation training have been helpful for some individuals with OCD.

Other Contacts:
The Obsessive Compulsive Foundation, 337 Notch Hill Rd., North Branford, CT 06471, 203-315-2190, http://www.ocfoundation.org

National Alliance for the Mentally Ill, 2107 Wilson Blvd, Ste. 300, Arlington, VA 22201, 1-800-950-6264, http://www.nami.org

PANIC DISORDER

What is Panic Disorder?

Panic disorder is characterized by periodic attacks of anxiety, feelings of terror, and intense physical discomfort. They usually last about 15 to 30 minutes. The individual feels nervous and fearful between attacks. The attacks can occur spontaneously or in response to a particular situation. They may occur daily, then remit for months, or they may occur weekly for months at a time.

What are the Symptoms of Panic Disorder?

- Fast, pounding heartbeat
- Shortness of breath
- Nausea
- Fear of going insane
- Chills or hot flashes
- Sweating
- A choking feeling
- Dizziness
- Fear of dying
- Trembling or shaking
- Chest pain
- Feelings of unreality
- Numbness

What Causes Panic Disorder?

The exact cause of panic disorder is unclear. There appear to be certain contributing factors to the disorder:

- **Biochemical.** OCD may be caused by a disturbance in the chemistry of the brain involving the neurotransmitter norepinephrine.
- **Genetics.** Panic disorder seems to run in families. Many people with panic disorder have close relatives with the disorder.
- **Psychodynamics.** This theory suggests that panic disorder may be caused by the inability to solve the early childhood conflict of dependence vs. independence.

How is Panic Disorder Diagnosed?

A physical examination to rule out physical illness is conducted. The patient should report any anxiety disorders or depression in other family members and other contributing factors, such as excessive caffeine use, recent life changes, or stressful events. Panic disorder is best diagnosed by a mental health professional.

What is the Treatment for Panic Disorder?

A combination of psychosocial therapy and medication is the treatment of choice for panic disorder. Medications include: Benzodiazepines (alprazolam [Xanax], lorazepam [Ativan], and clonazepam [Klonopin]). Care must be used in taking these medications, because they are addictive. Antidepressants such as the SSRIs are particularly effective and are often first-line treatment for panic disorder. The tricyclics clomipramine [Anafranil] and imipramine [Tofranil] have also been successful in treating this disorder. Individual psychotherapy, cognitive-behavioral therapy, and relaxation training are helpful.

Other Contacts:

Anxiety Disorders Association of America, 11900 Parklawn Dr., Ste 100, Rockville, MD 20852, 301-231-9350, http://www.adaa.org

National Anxiety Foundation, 3135 Custer Dr., Lexington, KY 40517. 606-272-7166, http://lexington-on-line.com/nafmasthead.html

National Alliance for the Mentally Ill, 2107 Wilson Blvd, Ste. 300, Arlington, VA 22201, 1-800-950-6264, http://www.nami.org

EATING DISORDERS

What are Eating Disorders?
The categories of eating disorders include anorexia nervosa, bulimia nervosa, and binge eating. These disorders deal with food obsessions, distorted body images, and obsessional thinness. In reality, they have little to do with food and more to do with psychological and emotional factors. Ninety percent of eating disorders are in women.

What are the Symptoms of Eating Disorders?
In **anorexia nervosa,** the individual has an intense fear of gaining weight. She sees herself as fat, even though she may only weigh 85 percent or less of expected weight. She may eat very little, and sometimes self-induces vomiting after eating. She exercises excessively. She generally stops having periods. Her blood pressure and temperature are low and her heartbeat is slow. In **bulimia nervosa,** the individual eats huge amounts of food and follows with self-induced vomiting (purging). They often abuse laxatives and diuretics. Their weight is usually within normal range. In **binge eating disorder**, the individual eats huge amounts of food, but does not purge. Weight gain can progress to obesity.

What Causes Eating Disorders?
- **Genetics.** Eating disorders appear to run in families. There is thought to be a hereditary link
- **Biological.** Eating disorders may be associated with a disturbance in the chemistry of the brain involving the neurotransmitters serotonin and norepinephrine.
- **Family dynamics.** Some clinicians believe that eating behaviors become maladaptive when there are issues of power and control within the family. Perfectionism is expected by the parents in order to achieve love and affection. Distorted eating patterns may be viewed by the adolescent as a way to gain and remain in control.

How are Eating Disorders Diagnosed?
Denial (on the part of both the parent and the child) is common in eating disorders. The disorder may progress to a serious condition before treatment is sought. In anorexia nervosa, the individual may be emaciated, not having periods, and a distorted self-image. In bulimia, the diagnosis is made if there are at least two bulimic episodes per week for 3 months. Lab work is completed: blood count, electrolytes, protein levels, EKG, and chest x-ray. A bone-density test may be administered.

What is the Treatment for Eating Disorders?
Hospitalization is common for nutritional stabilization is common for anorexia and sometimes for bulimia. For the anorexic person, behavior modification with weight gain is the goal. Cognitive-behavioral therapy, interpersonal psychotherapy, and family therapy are used, along with medication. Medications for eating disorders include antidepressants (the SSRIs) for anorexia, bulimia, and binge eating; appetite stimulants for anorexia; and anorexigenics for obesity.

Other Contacts:
National Association of Anorexia Nervosa and Associated Disorders, P.O. Box 7, Highland Park, IL 60035 847-831-3438, http://www.anad.org

Anorexia Nervosa and Related Eating Disorders, Box 5102, Eugene, OR 97405. 541-344-1144, http://www.anred.com

Eating Disorders Awareness and Prevention, 603 Stewart Street, Suite 803, Seattle, WA 98101 1-800-931-2237, http://www.edap.org

SCHIZOPHRENIA

What is Schizophrenia?

Schizophrenia is a severe, chronic, and often disabling brain disease. It causes severe mental disturbances that disrupt normal thought, speech, and behavior. It can affect anyone at any age, but most cases develop between adolescence and age 30. Schizophrenia impairs a person's ability to think clearly, make decisions, and relate to others.

What are the Symptoms of Schizophrenia?

- Delusions (false ideas)
- Hallucinations (hearing, seeing, or feeling things that are not there)
- Confused thinking
- Speech that does not make sense
- Lack of feeling or emotional expression
- Lack of pleasure or interest in life
- Lack of ability to complete activities
- Suspiciousness
- Difficulty socializing with others

What causes Schizophrenia?

The cause of schizophrenia is unknown. Several theories exist:

- **Genetics.** Genetics appears to play a role, as schizophrenia seems to run in families.
- **Biochemical.** An excess of the neurotransmitter dopamine is thought to play a role in the cause of the disorder. Abnormalities in other neurotransmitters have also been suggested.
- **Brain abnormalities.** Structural and cellular changes in the brain have been noted in people with schizophrenia.
- **Other.** Scientists are currently investigating viral infections that occur early in life and mild brain damage from complications during birth as contributing to the development of schizophrenia.

How is Schizophrenia Diagnosed?

To be diagnosed with schizophrenia, a person must have psychotic, "loss-of-reality" symptoms for at least 6 months and show increasing difficulty in normal functioning. The doctor will rule out other problems that cause psychotic symptoms, such as drugs, mania, major depression, autistic disorder, or personality disorders. Diagnosis should be made by a mental health professional.

What is the Treatment for Schizophrenia?

Hospitalization is necessary to treat severe delusions, hallucinations, or inability for self-care. A combination of psychosocial therapy and medication has been effective in treating schizophrenia. Individual psychotherapy, behavioral therapy, social skills training, and family therapy are appropriate, along with antipsychotic medication. Conventional antipsychotics include chlorpromazine [Thorazine], fluphenazine [Prolixin], haloperidol [Haldol], thiothixene [Navane], trifluoperazine [Stelazine], perphenazine [Trilafon], thioridazine [Mellaril], and molindone [Moban]. Newer atypical antipsychotics have fewer side effects and include risperidone [Risperdal], clozapine [Clozaril], olanzapine [Zyprexa], quetiapine [Seroquel], and ziprasidone [Geodon]. Medications must be taken daily for maintenance of symptoms. Certain ones may be taken by injection at 1-to-4-week intervals.

Other Contacts:

National Alliance for the Mentally Ill, 2107 Wilson Blvd, Ste. 300, Arlington, VA 22201, 1-800-950-6264, http://www.nami.org

World Fellowship for Schizophrenia and Allied Disorders, 869 Yonge St., Suite 104, Toronto, Ontario, M4W 2H2, Canada, http://www.world-schizophrenia.org

ALZHEIMER'S DISEASE

What is Alzheimer's Disease?

Alzheimer's disease is a type of dementia characterized by a loss of intellectual abilities involving impairment of memory, judgment, and abstract thinking, coordination of movement, and changes in personality. An estimated 4 million people in the United States have Alzheimer's disease.

What are the symptoms of Alzheimer's Disease?

Early Stages

Forgetfulness (loses things; forgets names) self
Confusion with performing simple tasks
Confusion about month or season
Difficulty making decisions
Increasing loss of interest in activities
Depression; anger
Difficulty completing sentences or finding the right words
Reduced and/or irrelevant conversation
Visibly impaired movement or coordination, including slowing of movements, halting gait, and reduced sense of balance

Later Stages

Unable to dress, groom, and toilet
Forgets names of close relatives
Withdrawal; apathy
Disorientation to surroundings
Urinary and fecal incontinence
Wandering
Loss of language skills

What causes Alzheimer's Disease?

- **Genetics.** Hereditary factors appear to play a role in the development of Alzheimer's disease.
- **Biological.** Imbalance in the neurotransmitter acetylcholine. Levels of serotonin and norepinephrine may also be affected.
- **Brain changes.** Twisted nerve cell fibers, called neurofibrillary tangles, and a high concentration of plaques of a protein known as beta amyloid are found in the brains of people with Alzheimer's disease.
- **Head injury.** Injury to the head can accelerate the development of Alzheimer's in people who are susceptible to it.
- **Down syndrome.** People with Down syndrome are especially susceptible to Alzheimer's disease.

How is Alzheimer's Disease Diagnosed?

Family members report difficulties with memory, language, behavior, reasoning, and orientation. The physician then conducts a history and physical examination. Diagnostic laboratory tests are performed. CT scans or MRI may be used to rule out tumors or stroke. The neurologist will perform a mental status exam and possibly other cognitive and functional-ability tests.

What is the treatment for Alzheimer's Disease?

Treatment for Alzheimer's disease involves assistance with hygiene, dressing, grooming, toileting, and food preparation. Safety is an important issue, particularly as the individual begins to have difficulty with balance and coordination, and if he or she tends to wander. Individuals with Alzheimer's disease require help with all activities of daily living, and as the disease progresses, usually requires institutionalization. Some medications have been approved for treating the symptoms of Alzheimer's disease. These include: tacrine (Cognex), donepezil (Aricept), rivastigmine (Exelon), and galantamine (Reminyl). These medications have been shown to slow the progression of cognitive, functional, and behavioral symptoms in some individuals with Alzheimer's disease.

Other Contacts:

Alzheimer's Association, 919 N. Michigan Ave, Ste. 1000, Chicago, IL 60611, 1-800-272-3900, http://www.alz.org

Alzheimer's Disease Education and Referral Center, PO Box 8250, Silver Spring, MD 20907, 1-800-438-4380, http://www.alzheimers.org

ALCOHOLISM

What is Alcoholism?

Alcoholism is a disease in which an individual is dependent upon alcohol. About 9 million persons in the United States have this disease. It is a lifelong illness, is incurable, and the only cure is total abstinence from alcohol.

What are the Symptoms of Alcoholism?

Alcoholism may begin with social drinking or drinking to relieve stress and tension. As the individual continues to drink, tolerance develops, and the amount required to achieve the desired effect increases steadily. This progresses to blackouts—periods of drinking time that the individual is unable to remember. The disease has now progressed to the point that the individual requires alcohol to prevent withdrawal symptoms, yet denial of problems is common. Binges occur leading to physical illness and/or loss of consciousness. Abstaining from alcohol at this point can lead to tremors, hallucinations, convulsions, and severe agitation. Chronic alcoholism leads to many serious physical problems involving the heart, brain, and gastrointestinal system.

What Causes Alcoholism?

- **Genetic.** Alcoholism is thought to have a strong hereditary component.
- **Biological.** There may be a connection between alcoholism and certain neurotransmitters that form addictive substances in the brain when they combine with the products of alcohol metabolism.
- **Social learning.** Drinking alcohol may be learned early in the family of origin, thereby leading to a problem with drinking.
- **Cultural.** The incidence of alcohol abuse and dependence is higher in some cultures than others.

How is Alcoholism Diagnosed?

Alcoholism is diagnosed when the use of alcohol interferes with any aspect of the individual's life. The individual continues to drink even though he or she understands the negative consequences. When dependence occurs, the individual develops a tolerance and requires more and more of the substance. A syndrome of withdrawal symptoms occurs when the individual stops drinking or drastically cuts down on the amount consumed.

What is the treatment for Alcoholism?

- **Rehabilitation programs.** Help the individual get dry and, through therapy, to work toward achieving and maintaining sobriety.
- **Alcoholics Anonymous.** Self-help support groups made up of alcoholics who work to help each other achieve and maintain sobriety.
- **Medications.** Disulfiram (Antabuse) is a deterrent therapy. Individuals who drink alcohol when taking this drug become very ill. Naltrexone (ReVia) and nalmefene (Revex) have been used with some success in the treatment of alcoholism.

Other Contacts:

Alcoholics Anonymous, PO Box 459, Grand Central Station, New York, NY 10163, 212-870-3400, http://www.alcoholics-anonymous.org

National Institutes of Health, National Institute on Alcohol Abuse and Alcoholism, 6000 Executive Blvd.—Willco Building, Bethesda, MD 20892, http://www.niaaa.nih.gov

HIV DISEASE

What is HIV Disease?

HIV disease is a condition in which the individual suffers from severe suppression of the immune system related to infection with the human immunodeficiency virus (HIV). Because of this immunosuppression, the individual is highly susceptible to many diseases.

What are the symptoms of HIV Disease?

- Rapid weight loss
- Dry cough
- Memory loss, depression, and other neurological disorders
- Red, brown, pink, or purplish blotches, on or under the skin, or inside the mouth, nose, or eyelids
- White spots on the tongue, in the mouth, or in the throat
- Recurring fever or profuse night sweats
- Profound and unexplained fatigue
- Swollen lymph glands in the armpits, groin, or neck
- Diarrhea that lasts for more than a week
- Pneumonia

What causes HIV Disease?

The HIV virus is passed from one person to another through homosexual and heterosexual contact, through transfusion with infected blood products, and by being stuck with a needle infected with HIV. In addition, pregnant women can pass HIV to their baby during pregnancy or delivery, as well as through breast-feeding.

To prevent transmission: Use latex-rubber condoms against sexual transmission, do not share needles or syringes, do not share toothbrushes, razors, or other implements that may be contaminated with blood or body fluids, and avoid becoming pregnant if at risk for HIV infection. Individuals with HIV should ensure that all food is well cooked, avoid crowds, avoid traveling in countries with poor sanitation, avoid vaccines that contain live organisms, and consult physician before obtaining a pet.

How is HIV Disease Diagnosed?

There are two types of blood tests used to diagnose HIV infection: one that detects the presence of HIV-specific antibodies that the body produces in response to the virus and another type that detects the presence of the virus itself.

What is the Treatment for HIV Disease?

- **Medication.** Antiretroviral agents are used to interfere with the replication of the HIV virus. Other medications such as antibiotics, antifungal agents, antiviral agents, and antineoplastic agents are used to treat other conditions associated with HIV disease. Antianxiety agents, antidepressants, mood-stabilizing drugs, and antipsychotics may be prescribed for relief from associated symptoms that may accompany HIV disease.
- **Nutrition.** Some individuals with HIV have a wasting syndrome that includes major weight loss, chronic diarrhea, weakness, and fever. Loss of appetite, malnutrition, and wasting may be treated with dronabinol (Marinol), megestrol (Megace), somatropin (Serostim).

Other Contacts:

Centers for Disease Control and Prevention, 1600 Clifton Rd., Atlanta, GA 30333, 1-800-311-3435, AIDS Hotline: 1-800-342-2437, http://www.cdc.gov/hiv/pubs/facts.htm

AVERT, 4 Brighton Rd., Horsham, West Sussex, RH13 5BA, England, http://www.avert.org

ATTENTION-DEFICIT/HYPERACTIVITY DISORDER (ADHD)

What is ADHD?

ADHD is a behavior disorder that is characterized by hyperactivity, impulsiveness, inattention, or a combination of these behaviors that are more frequent and severe than would be expected for the age. It is usually not diagnosed before age 4, and is more common in boys than it is in girls. ADHD can also be a disorder in adults.

What are the Symptoms of ADHD?

There are three subtypes of the disorder:

1. **ADHD, Inattentive type:** has difficulty paying attention; does not listen when spoken to; is easily distracted; does not follow through on instructions; has difficulty organizing tasks and activities.
2. **ADHD, Hyperactive-Impulsive type:** has trouble sitting still; gets up out of seat at times when expected to remain seated; cannot play quietly; talks excessively; blurts out answers before questions are completed; has difficulty waiting turn; often interrupts or intrudes on others.
3. **ADHD, Combined type:** displays a combination of behaviors associated with the above two types.

What Causes ADHD?

- **Genetics.** Hereditary factors appear to be a factor in the development of ADHD.
- **Biochemical.** Low levels of dopamine and norepinephrine have been implicated as a cause of ADHD.
- **Perinatal factors.** Perinatal factors implicated: problem pregnancies and difficult deliveries; maternal smoking and use of alcohol or other drugs during pregnancy; exposure during pregnancy to environmental toxins.
- **Environmental factors.** Exposure to environmental lead may be an influential factor.
- **Early family life.** A chaotic family environment, a disruption in boding during the first 3 years of life, and infant malnutrition may be a contributing factor to ADHD.

How is ADHD Diagnosed?

ADHD is difficult to diagnose. A mother's description of her child's behavior can be the most accurate and reliable guide for diagnosing ADHD. A detailed history of the child's behavior will be matched against a standardized checklist used to define the disorder. The physician will inquire about problem behaviors at home and school, about sibling relationships, recent life changes, family history of ADHD, eating and sleeping patterns, and speech and language development. A medical history will be taken of the child and of the mother's pregnancy and delivery. A physical examination will be conducted. Screening tests may be used to test neurological, intellectual, and emotional development.

What is the treatment for ADHD?

Behavior modification and family therapy, in combination with medication, is used to treat ADHD. Medications include: CNS stimulants, including methylphenidate (Ritalin); dextroamphetamine (Dexedrine); pemoline (Cylert); and dextroamphetamine/amphetamine composite (Adderall). Other medications used for ADHD include the antidepressant bupropion (Wellbutrin) and most recently, the selective serotonin reuptake inhibitors (SSRIs).

Other Contacts:

National Institute of Mental Health, 6001 Executive Blvd, Rm. 8184, MSC 9663, Bethesda, MD 20892, 301-443-4513, http://www.nimh.nih.gov/publicat/adhdmenu.cfm

National Attention Deficit Disorder Association, 1788 Second Street, Suite 200, Highland Park, IL 60035, 847-432-ADDA, http://www.add.org

INDEX

Note: Page numbers followed by f indicate figures; page numbers followed by t indicate tables; and page numbers followed by g refer to glossary entries.

A

D

E

F

O

P

Q

R

S

T